A guide to evidence-based integrative and complementary medicine

A guide to evidence-based integrative and complementary medicine

Vicki Kotsirilos
MBBS, FACNEM
Chair, Royal Australian College of General Practitioners (RACGP) – AIMA Working Party
Adjunct Senior Lecturer, Department of Epidemiology and Preventive Medicine, School of Public Health and Preventive Medicine, Monash University, Melbourne, Victoria

Luis Vitetta
PhD, GradDipNutrEnvironMed, GradDipIntegrMed
Director, Centre for Integrative Clinical and Molecular Medicine, School of Medicine, University of Queensland, Brisbane, Queensland

Avni Sali
MBBS, PhD, FRACS, FACS, FACNEM
Founding Director, National Institute of Integrative Medicine
Honorary Professor, Centre for Integrative Clinical and Molecular Medicine, School of Medicine, University of Queensland, Brisbane, Queensland

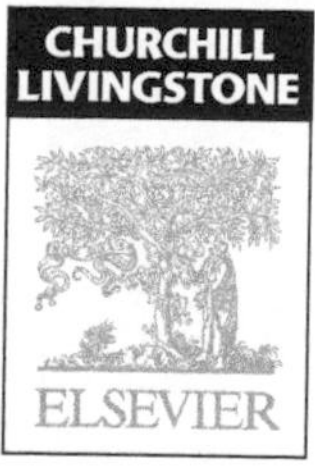

Sydney Edinburgh London New York Philadelphia St Louis Toronto

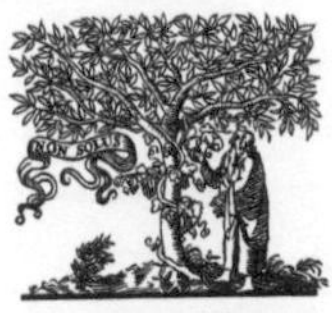

Churchill Livingstone
is an imprint of Elsevier

Elsevier Australia. ACN 001 002 357
(a division of Reed International Books Australia Pty Ltd)
Tower 1, 475 Victoria Avenue, Chatswood, NSW 2067

Complementary medicine and pharmacology are ever-changing fields. Standard safety precautions must be followed but, as new research and clinical experience broaden our knowledge, changes in treatment become necessary or appropriate. The authors and publisher have, in so far as it is possible, taken every care to ensure that the information contained within the text is as accurate and as up-to-date as possible. Readers are, however, advised always to check available product information with the herb, supplement or drug manufacturer to verify the recommended dose, the method and duration of administration, and contraindications. It is the responsibility of the treating person to determine dosages and the best treatment for the patient. Neither the publisher nor the editors assume any responsibility for any injury and/or damage to persons or property.

National Library of Australia Cataloguing-in-Publication Data

---

A guide to evidence-based integrative and complementary medicine / editors Vicki Kotsirilos, Luis Vitetta, Avni Sali

9780729539081 (pbk.)

Alternative medicine – Textbooks.

Integrative medicine – Textbooks.

Kotsirilos, Vicki.

Vitetta, Luis.

Sali, Avni.

615.5

Publisher: Sophie Kaliniecki
Developmental Editor: Neli Bryant
Publishing Services Manager: Helena Klijn
Project Coordinator: Karen Griffiths
Edited by Forsyth Publishing Services
Editorial coordination by Sarah Newton-John
Proofread by Forsyth Publishing Services
Cover and internal design by Russell Jeffery
Index by Michael Ferreira
Typeset by TNQ Books and Journals Pvt. Ltd.
Moved to Digital Printing 2016

Contents

Foreword

A Guide to Evidence-based Complementary and Integrative Medicine is a long-awaited book written by three very experienced Australian practitioners and educators in this discipline. The authors, Vicki Kotsirilos, Luis Vitetta, and Avni Sali, who are graduates of Monash University and the University of Melbourne, have injected more than 100 years of collective experience into this ambitious and erudite book. Dr Vicki Kotsirilos has practised as a general practitioner for many years and over time has developed special expertise in evidence-based complementary medicine, which she integrates into her orthodox practice. This book represents a collaboration between Vicki, Associate Professor Luis Vitetta and Professor Avni Sali. The result is an interesting blend of complementary clinical and scientific information and practice. Avni Sali, a distinguished surgeon, has been a great advocate of holistic health care from his medical student days. His passion for the integration of mainstream medicine and complementary medicine culminated in his development of the Graduate School of Integrative Medicine at Swinburne University of Technology and subsequently the National Institute of Integrative Medicine, of which he is foundation director. For these visionary projects, he was joined by Associate Professor Luis Vitetta who is now Director of the Centre for Integrative Clinical and Molecular Medicine at the University of Queensland.

The book commences with an overview of integrative and complementary medicine, including nutritional assessment and therapies. This makes the reader aware of the reality that this medical practice, with the emphasis on whole person care and healthy lifestyle, is now accepted with and integrated into mainstream medical practice.

However, this book provides another dimension, with its broad overview of complementary practice. An important feature of the text is the enormous amount of material on evidence-based medicine, and this means long lists of references. It makes sense that the authors have to justify their discipline with meticulously researched evidence. I do know for a fact that the authors are obsessive and prolific surveyors of the medical literature, including the latest scientific journals, papers and review articles. This attention to detail is evident in the text. At the end of each chapter, there is a table that uses NHMRC guidelines to summarise the level of evidence for each of the proposed therapies. There is also a section entitled 'Clinical tips handout', which permits the practitioner to print this patient-friendly information to give to patients.

The book, which is intended for postgraduate medical and health practitioners, gives the readers a fascinating insight into this often misunderstood area. The authors are to be congratulated on achieving such a detailed and scientific reference work in this popular and emerging field of health practice.

Professor John Murtagh AM
BSc, BEd (Melb), MBBS, MD, DipObst(RCOG), FRACGP

Preface

We are pleased to present *A Guide to Evidence-based Integrative and Complementary Medicine,* a comprehensive textbook on the non-pharmacological treatments for common medical practice problems, with the support of current scientific evidence. Non-pharmacological approaches include advice on lifestyle and behavioural factors, prevention strategies, mind–body medicine, stress management, dietary changes, exercise and sleep advice, encouraging appropriate exposure to sunshine, living in an environment free of chemicals and using evidence-based complementary medicines, such as acupuncture, hypnosis and herbal and nutritional supplements, that positively impact on people's lives and the treatment of their disease(s). Only proven therapies from current research are included, particularly from Cochrane reviews and research from systematic reviews, randomised control trials and published cohort studies. It is hoped that publication of this book will help to drive prevention and treatment strategies that will improve community health and promote wellness.

This book is designed help educate health practitioners on the latest science and evidence for lifestyle and non-drug approaches to health care. The growing body of research in this area will help to play an increasingly important role in shaping the future of medicine. We have made great efforts to collate this evidence up to 2009-2010, although the evidence for integrative medicine (IM) and complementary medicine (CM) is growing rapidly on a daily basis.

Worldwide studies indicate that lifestyle factors play a key role in contributing to diseases, particularly chronic diseases. For example, a report released by the Australian Institute of Health and Welfare found that more than three-quarters of Australians suffer from at least one chronic condition, such as heart disease, asthma, diabetes or arthritis. The report highlights that Australians are not doing enough about the lifestyle risk factors associated with chronic diseases. They found that more than 85% of adults are not consuming enough vegetables, almost 50% of adults are not consuming enough fruit, about 54% of adult Australians are either overweight or obese and about 21% of adults smoke tobacco. It is essential that lifestyle advice is included as a first-line approach in the management of many conditions, particularly chronic diseases.

The term 'complementary medicine' (CM) broadly describes a number of different therapies that may or may not have much in common, ranging from mind–body therapies, such as hypnosis, spiritual healing and meditation, to herbal medicine, nutritional supplements and bioenergetic healing. This can be a problem when defining this area, so it is always best to focus on these therapies individually, not collectively as a group, and to determine from the science which of the therapies have evidence, which are safe and can play a valid role in clinical care, and for which specific condition each is suited.

It is for this reason that the term 'integrative medicine' is preferable. It describes a style of practice in which the practitioner and patient choose the appropriate therapy or medicine for the treatment of the condition. Acupuncture may be suitable for some patients but not for others; surgery may be suitable for some patients but not for others; herbs may be suitable for some conditions but not for others, and so on.

The scientific evidence for many CMs is growing, with positive systematic reviews and meta-analyses, including Cochrane reviews. Some worthy of mention that may play a role as first-line treatments include: cranberry herb for the prevention of recurrent urinary tract infections in young women; music therapy for depression; St John's wort herb for mild, moderate and severe depression; various herbs for irritable bowel syndrome; yoga, relaxation and exercise for menopausal symptoms; *Pygeum africanum* herb extract for benign prostate hypertrophy; fish oils for hypertryglyceridaemia; acupuncture for migraine and tension headaches; and garlic supplement for hypertension.

However, there are both negative and positive trials for many CMs, which we have also addressed and included in the various chapters to provide a balanced picture. This may not mean that the therapy or supplement does not work. One needs to ask why are there differences in the results? There are many explanations for this, such as differences in the quality and methodology of the trial(s) used for the CM, variations in the dosage or quality of a herb or nutritional supplement used in the trial(s), or the actual method used for some therapies such as yoga, meditation and massage. All these factors need to be taken into account when carefully exploring the evidence for CMs. When the evidence for CMs is consistently negative, and particularly when it is associated with potential risks, it is time to consider abandoning that treatment, especially if the risks outweigh any clinical benefit.

Publication bias is not uncommon for CM trials, but is also seen for all trials in general medicine. The absence of evidence for CMs does not mean a therapy does not work, but rather indicates that further testing is needed. So while the integration of CM poses many challenges to the health profession, CMs should be viewed in some cases as positive, as they may provide valid and safer options for health care. This is particularly relevant to the patient who has suffered side-effects from pharmaceutical medication or where surgery is contraindicated and alternative, safer approaches are needed.

This book also extensively covers risks and common adverse events associated with CMs, both in the main text and in all the clinical tips for patients. There is a common misconception that CMs are harmless and pose no risks. All herbs have pharmacological activity and so can potentially cause a reaction in a sensitive individual or an interaction with medication. It is worth noting that, overall, CMs are relatively safe compared with pharmaceutical medicines, with significantly fewer reports of adverse effects considering their widespread community use, although under-reporting may be contributing to this finding.

We have tried to make this book as user-friendly as possible for the busy health practitioner by summarising the scientific evidence. We have used the NHMRC guidelines grading system and summarised the evidence by formatting it into a table at the end of each chapter. This will help practitioners to view the evidence at a glance, which is particularly useful during a busy consultation when they are often time-limited. Furthermore, we have provided a one- to two-page patient summary sheet at the end of each chapter. The clinical tips are guided by our own years of clinical experience in successfully treating many patients with various conditions and chronic diseases. Both the clinical tips and the patient summaries can easily be copied to guide the practitioner during a consultation without having to read the entire text and to give to patients to take home. The clinical tips also cover risk factors so that patients can be well informed about any potential harm.

We hope that you will find this textbook valuable for your own learning and that it will enhance your clinical experience by providing safer options for health care through practising a more integrative approach. Referral to and working closely with qualified, respected health practitioners may be necessary. We also hope it assists you to successfully treat your own patients so as to improve their overall wellbeing, their quality of health and, of course, their quality of life.

Dr Vicki Kotsirilos
Associate Professor Luis Vitetta
Professor Avni Sali
November 2010
Melbourne, Australia

Acknowledgments

Special thanks are due to our family members for all their support and patience during the busy time of writing this textbook: Fred, Christopher and Cassandra Karalis; Susan and Gemma Vitetta; Hana, Radek, Lenka and Filip Sali. We also take this opportunity to thank one another as co-authors for working continuously as a dedicated and committed team to complete the vision of this textbook. We sincerely thank Elsevier, our publishers, for supporting and trusting our vision.

We are fortunate to have had the help of medical and health practitioners who are experts in their field to write some of the chapters in this textbook and would like to thank them sincerely for their contribution. In alphabetical order, they are: Dr Jenny Altermatt, Professor Manohar Garg, Mr Greg de Jong, Dr Antigone Kouris-Blazos, Dr Andrew Pipingas, Ms Danielle Sestito, Dr Katherine Sevar, Dr Gillian Singleton and Dr Lily Tomas.

The publications *Australian Doctor* and *Medical Observer* played a role in the development of this book by providing the opportunity for collaboration and contributing articles. Vicki Kotsirilos would like to express special gratitude to *Australian Doctor*, which gave her the opportunity to write regular articles for Australian doctors based on the scientific evidence for IM, something that had never been done before, and inspired her to write this textbook. She would also like to thank *Medical Observer* for the continued opportunity to contribute her thoughts on the subject through opinion columns and through other means.

Thank you to our teachers in life

Vicki Kotsirilos: I would like to express my thanks to: my parents and siblings for their respect, trust and support throughout my life and for teaching me valuable life skills; Mr Steven Cotham, my year 7 science/biology teacher, who inspired my interest in school; Professor John Murtagh and Professor Fritz Guldner, as my early teachers and mentors in medicine at Monash University; Professor Avni Sali, Professor Ian Brighthope, Dr Richard Hetzel and Dr Ian Gawler, Australian pioneers in integrative medicine who inspired my interest in this field; Dr Craig Hassed and Dr Steven Sommer for their kind-heartedness, wisdom and guidance; Professor Michael Kidd, Professor Kerryn Phelps and Professor Morton Rawlin for their passion and ongoing support; and Ms Anne Kantor, a special, humble lady, who has touched the hearts of many, including mine, with her kindness and generosity.

Luis Vitetta: I would like to acknowledge Professor Avni Sali and Emeritus Professor of Medicine Gabriel Kune, lifelong mentors and friends who, with their visionary guidance in science and medicine, provided the impetus for lateral thinking; otherwise very little would have been possible. I also thank Emeritus Professor of Biochemistry Anthony W Linnane, Fellow of the Royal Society: through his accomplishments in cellular biology and many discussions, I have come to understand the philosophy that is 'excellence in science and medical research'.

Avni Sali: I would like to acknowledge Jean Osborne, my year 3 teacher, who had confidence in me becoming a doctor; Professor Rod Andrew, who gave me the opportunity to do medicine at Monash University; Professor Hugh Dudley, who encouraged me to do a PhD in his department; Professor Phillip Hunt, Dr Roy Bean and Dr Ainsle Meares for inspiring me to look at other ways; Professor Sir Andrew Kay and Professor Gabriel Kune for their valuable support and Professor Iain Wallace for his vision and courage in allowing me to establish the first postgraduate medical school in integrative medicine.

About the authors

Dr Vicki Kotsirilos MBBS, FACNEM

Dr Vicki Kotsirilos is a medical practitioner who combines orthodox medicine with evidence-based complementary medicine such as acupuncture, hypnosis, counselling, herbal and nutritional medicine. In 1992 she founded the Australasian Integrative Medicine Association (AIMA) to represent medical practitioners in Australia and New Zealand who integrate various forms of evidence-based complementary medicine and therapies in their clinical practices. In 1994 the AIMA affiliated with the Australian Medical Association in Victoria, and since 1997 it has been recognised as a special interest group by the Royal Australian College of General Practitioners (RACGP). In 2004 the AIMA developed a joint working party with the RACGP, which Dr Kotsirilos chairs, to address the appropriate and ethical use of complementary medicine by the medical profession.

Dr Kotsirilos has served on a number of government committees, including the Professional Services Review, the Australian Drug Reaction Advisory Committee and the Complementary Medicines Evaluation Committee of the Therapeutics Goods Administration. She is passionate about the value of integrative medicine and is committed to assisting health practitioners to learn more about this valuable area of health care. She has published articles in a wide range of medical journals and popular magazines, lectures regularly to doctors and has spoken at numerous medical and public conferences.

Associate Professor Luis Vitetta PhD, GradDipNutrEnvironMed, GradDipIntegrMed

Luis Vitetta is Associate Professor and Director of the Centre for Integrative Clinical and Molecular Medicine, University of Queensland School of Medicine. Previously he was Senior Research Fellow and Associate Professor at the Centre for Molecular Biology and Medicine at the Epworth Medical Centre in Melbourne, and from 2000 to 2005 he was the Deputy Head and Director of Research of the Graduate School of Integrative Medicine at Swinburne University. His research interests include mind–body medicine, nutrition/functional foods/pro-oxidant cellular signalling systems, herbal medicines and the function of the immune system. He is an invited speaker at numerous local and international conferences.

Professor Avni Sali MBBS, PhD, FRACS, FACS, FACNEM

Professor Avni Sali is the founding Director of National Institute of Integrative Medicine in Melbourne and an honorary professor of the Faculty of Health Sciences, University of Queensland. His research interests lie mainly in integrative medicine and include clinical aspects, behaviour, nutrition, herbal medicine and exercise. His clinical expertise in integrative medicine includes cause of disease, cancer, difficult clinical problems and health advice. Professor Sali has helped to pioneer health promotion and integrative medicine in Australia, with particular emphasis on the importance of nutrition, exercise and the mind. He has been teaching in this area since 1978 and is a frequent speaker at local, state, national and international meetings. He has written and contributed to a number of books and has published more than 300 articles in medical journals. Professor Sali was instrumental in the establishment of the Graduate School of Integrative Medicine, Swinburne University of Technology in Melbourne, and was its first head. He is President of the Australasian Integrative Medicine Association (AIMA) and the International Council of Integrative Medicine (ICIM).

Contributors

Jennifer Altermatt MBBS, FRACGP
Medical general practitioner, Warranwood, Victoria, Australia
Skin cancer practitioner, Blackburn and Mitcham, Victoria, Australia

Manohar Garg PhD, MND, MSc (Biochem), BSc (Hons), RNutr 2
Professor and Director, Nutraceuticals Research Group, School of Biomedical Sciences and Pharmacy, Faculty of Health, University of Newcastle, Callaghan, New South Wales, Australia
President, Nutrition Society of Australia

Greg de Jong BAppSc(Physio), GradDipClinNutr
Physiotherapist and nutritionist, Pambula, New South Wales, Australia
Medical journalist
Stress management/life balance program creator and facilitator

Antigone Kouris-Blazos PhD, BSc, GradDipDietetics, DipBotanicMed
Accredited practising dietitian, Melbourne, Victoria, Australia
Managing editor of www.healthyeatingclub.org

Andrew Pipingas PhD, BAppSci(Dist)
Senior Lecturer and Unit Leader, Ageing Research, Brain Sciences Institute, Swinburne University of Technology, Hawthorn, Victoria, Australia
Chief Investigator, National Institute of Complementary Medicine (NICM), Collaborative Centre for Neurocognition

Miss Danielle Sestito BSci (Psychology/Psychophisiology)
Student Swinburne University of Technology, Hawthorn, Victoria

Katherine Sevar MBChB, DCH
Psychiatry Registrar, Austin Health, Melbourne, Victoria, Australia

Gillian Singleton MBBS(Hons), FRACGP, FARGP
General practitioner, Monash University, Clayton, Victoria, Australia
Member, Royal Australian College of General Practitioners – AIMA Joint Working Party
Member, Detention Health Advisory Group (DeHAG)

Lily Tomas MBBS, BSc(Med), MACNEM
General practitioner, Pambula, New South Wales, Australia
Vice President, Australasian Integrative Medical Association (AIMA)
Member, Royal Australian College of General Practitioners – AIMA Joint Working Party
Editor, *Journal of Integrative Medicine*

Reviewers

Dr Elen ApThomas MBBS, DRANZCOG
Integrative medicine GP, Gold Coast, Queensland, Australia

David Colquhoun MBBS, FRACP
Cardiologist, Brisbane, Queensland
Associate Professor of Medicine, University of Queensland, Australia

Josephine M Hallinan MBBS, BSc

Judy Humphries PhD, ND
Lecturer in complementary medicine, School of Rural Medicine, University of New England, Armidale, New South Wales, Australia

Lisa Macdonald MBBS (Sydney), FRACGP, Dip Bowen Therapy, ACNEM, AIMA
Holistic doctor, Mt Tamborine, Queensland, Australia

David Mitchell MBBS, FAMAC
Acupuncture physician, integrative medicine GP, Adelaide, South Australia, Australia

Alison Moffatt BMedSc, MBBS (Hons)
Psychiatry Registrar, Hunter New England Mental Health, Newcastle, New South Wales, Australia

Azita Moradi MBBS, MPM, FRANZCP
Consultant psychiatrist
Lecturer, Monash University, Faculty of Medicine, Nursing and Health Sciences, Melbourne, Victoria, Australia

Phil Rasmussen MPharm, MNIMH, MPS, Dip Herb Med, MNHAA, MNZAMH
Medical herbalist and pharmacist, Auckland, New Zealand
Honorary lecturer, Faculty of Health Sciences, University of Auckland, Auckland, New Zealand

Kathryn J Steadman BPharm(Hons), PhD, MRPharmS, MPS
Senior Lecturer, School of Pharmacy, University of Queensland, Brisbane, Queensland, Australia

Suzi Wigge MBBS, FRACGP, Dip TCM, Dip RM
Integrative medical practitioner, traditional Chinese medicine, acupuncturist, herbalist, Sydney, New South Wales, Australia

Abbreviations

AI	adequate intake
BMI	body mass index
CAM	complementary and alternative medicine
CBT	cognitive behaviour therapy
CI	confidence interval
CM	complementary medicine
EAR	estimated average requirements
FVC	forced vital capacity
GI	glycaemic index
HR	hazard ratio
IM	integrative medicine
MA	meta-analysis
OR	odds ratio
RCT	randomised control trial
RDI	recommended dietary intake
RR	relative risk
SR	systematic review
TCM	traditional Chinese medicine

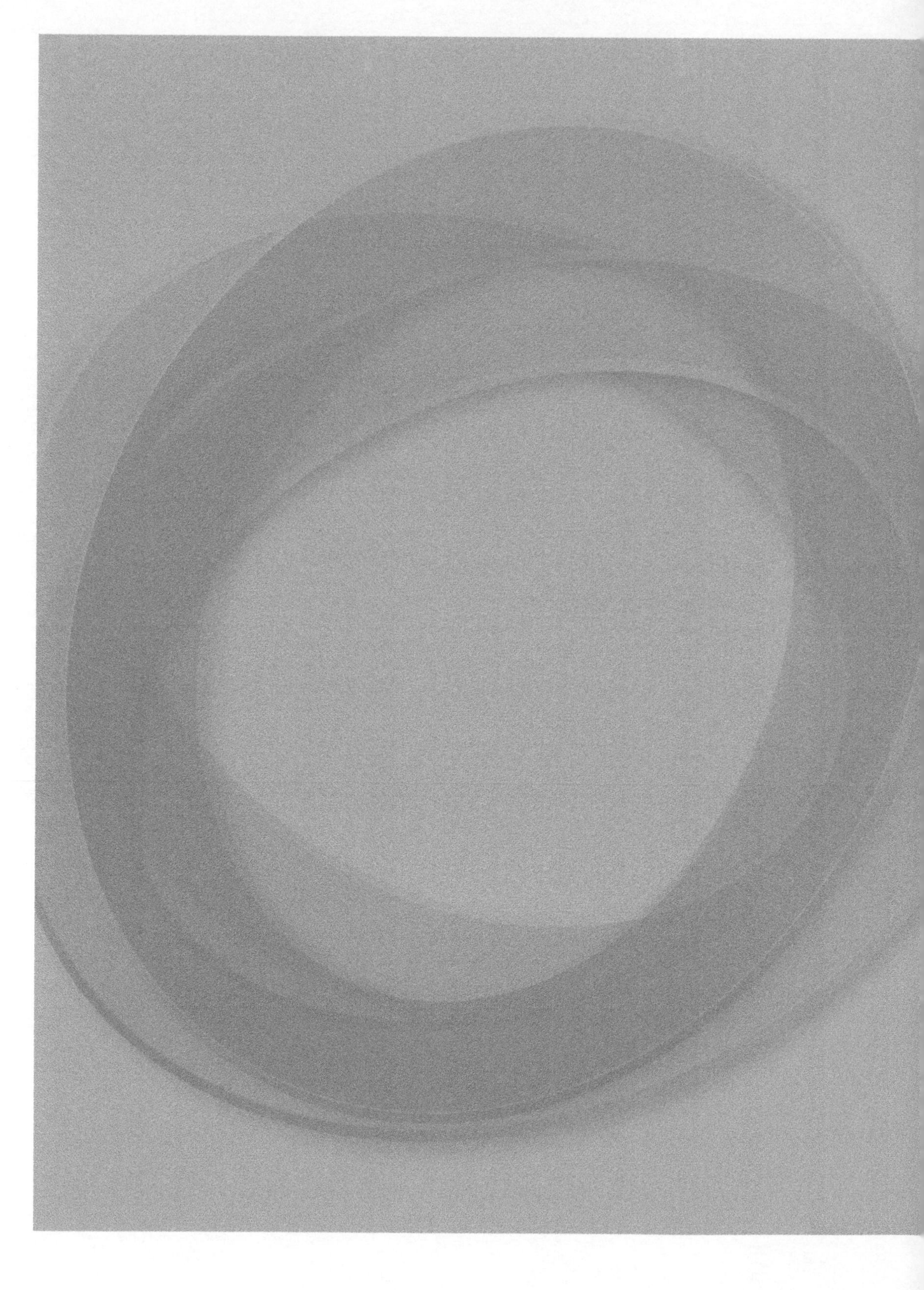

Part 1

Integrative and complementary medicine

Chapter 1

Introduction

Clinicians have always performed the role of health care providers, where the family doctor has always been viewed as the logical interface with the community's health needs. Integrative medicine (IM) is an established paradigm shift in medicine in areas such as the North American continent, India and China. Whereas in other areas of the world it is a developing movement, such as in continental Europe, especially Scandinavia, the Middle East and Australia. [1,2]

Integrative medicine is recognised as the practice of medicine in a way that relates to complete patient care. IM includes practices currently beyond the scope of conventional medical teachings. However, it neither rejects conventional therapies nor uncritically accepts alternative/complementary ones. It implicitly emphasises principles that may or may not be associated with complementary and alternative medicine (CAM) modalities such as:

- *Whole person medicine*. IM views patients beyond simply the physical picture of their symptoms. They are managed as mental/emotional beings who are members of communities and societies. These other dimensions of human life are relevant to health since antiquity and essential for the accurate diagnosis and effective treatment of disease.[3]
- *The natural healing power of the organism*. IM assumes that the body has an innate capacity for healing. The primary goal of treatment should be to support, facilitate, and augment that innate capacity to improve the wellbeing of the sick patient, not necessarily a cure.
- *The importance of lifestyle to improve the wellbeing of the sick patient, not necessarily a cure*. Health or disease results from interactions between genes and all aspects of lifestyle and environment, including diet, physical activity, rest, sunshine exposure, fresh air and sleep, life stressors (the balance between pleasure events and distressful events),[4] the quality of relationships and work. A plethora of studies demonstrate that positive lifestyle changes significantly reduce the risk and progression of a number of major chronic diseases such as cardiovascular disease (e.g. myocardial infarction and stroke), diabetes, and cancer.
  In a study of 23 153 German participants, aged 35 to 65 years, from the European Prospective Investigation Into Cancer and Nutrition–Potsdam study, found that adhering to just 4 lifestyle factors — namely, never smoking, having a body mass index less than 30, performing 3.5 hours/week or more of physical activity, and adhering to healthy dietary principles (high intake of fruits, vegetables, and whole-grain bread and low meat consumption) — significantly reduces the risk of developing a chronic disease by up to 78%.[5]
- *The critical role of the doctor–patient relationship*. Throughout history people have accorded the doctor–patient relationship special, even sacred, status. When a medically trained person sits with a patient and listens with full attention to his or her story, that alone can initiate healing before any treatment is offered. This latter pattern of care constitutes the basic essence of IM.[3]

Western medicine and science has created some wonderfully useful ways of treating diseases and developing skills in surgery. Our goal should be not to replace conventional medicine, but to expand its boundaries and build a scientific foundation for integrating less well understood approaches to improve the functional status of patients and to provide a range of validated treatment options.

The medical profession is confronted by changing community attitudes, so a growing awareness of such therapies by the medical profession would seem to be in harmony with the growing public awareness for a more holistic form of health care.

Holistic health — caring for the whole person

The holistic model is traced back to the Hippocratic school of medicine (*circa* 400 BC) and the oath of Maimoides (*circa* the 12th century AD) which have fashioned and defined the unique obligations that clinicians have toward their patients and their medical practices. Disease and illness was viewed as an 'effect' from imbalance and explored causes of disease from the environment and natural phenomena such as air, water, and food. Early health practitioners used the term *vis medicatrix naturae*, meaning the healing power of nature, to describe the body's ability to heal itself. Furthermore, the Hippocratic oath states: 'first, do no harm'. It is important despite which style of medicine we use, whether it is a pharmaceutical agent, surgical approach or a natural therapy, that we do no harm to patients.

The World Health Organization (WHO) definition for optimal health suggests this should be inclusive of physical, social, psychological, emotional and spiritual wellbeing. The holistic or health model looks at maximising or supporting all aspects of a person's health, which will then lead to the disease being healed by the body.

The health practitioner's aim is to help empower patients to be active participants in their own healing process and to encourage personal responsibility for their health to improve quality of care and quality of life. The goal is not just to treat the illness, but to focus on promoting health and wellness.

Establishing and maintaining optimal health and balance is vital to prevention and treatment. Wellness is a state of being healthy characterised by positive emotions, thoughts and actions. Wellness is inherent in everyone, no matter what 'disease' is present. If wellness is truly recognised, focused upon and experienced, the individual will heal more quickly, not just through direct treatment of the 'disease' alone.

Holistic medicine also includes the integration of various safe, evidence-based complementary therapies and medicines that may provide a gentler, safer and, in some cases, more empowering approach to health care. Many medical and health practitioners worldwide are integrating various ethical non-pharmaceutical modalities into their clinical practice as part of the holistic approach. These forms of therapies aim to enhance a healthy lifestyle, work with the natural healing process, empower patients to be active participants in their own healing process and nurture the whole person. Where such therapies can be safely used, they include counselling, meditation and relaxation therapies, hypnosis, primary preventative medicine and lifestyle management, acupuncture, nutritional medicine, herbal medicine, environmental medicine, and physical and manipulative medicine. These therapies work in harmony with the natural healing processes of the body. Natural medicines, when used properly, generally are well tolerated and rarely cause side-effects. They generally support the body's healing mechanisms, rather than take over the body's processes.[6]

It is important to remain open-minded and flexible, both philosophically and in research methodology, with such an approach to treating individuals. We must recognise that healing primarily comes from the individual and mostly depends on their motivation level.

Integrative medicine

Integrative medicine (IM) refers to the blending of conventional and complementary medicines and therapies with the aim of using the most appropriate of either or both modalities to care for the patient as a whole.[7]

This closely reflects both the Hippocratic oath and the WHO definition discussed above. However, although some may view IM as synonymous with CAM, this was never so, nor was it ever the case. CAM comprises many therapeutic modalities that are not taught in a conventional medical syllabus, based on the ideas that range from those that are sensible and worth including in mainstream medicine to those that are extremely imprudent and a few that are very perilous. Neither the word *alternative* nor *complementary* captures the essence of IM.[8] The former suggests a replacement of conventional therapies by others whereas the latter suggests therapies of varying value that may be used as adjuncts.

IM embraces a holistic approach to clinical practice encouraging patient involvement in self-health care, prevention and interventions that focus on health maintenance by paying attention to all relative components of lifestyle, including diet, exercise, stress management, and the emotional wellbeing of the patient. IM also integrates evidence-based complementary medicines that are safe and may positively impact on the healing process and quality of life for the patient.

IM does not reject or compete with conventional health care but rather seeks to broaden conventional health care by providing the health practitioner, doctor and patient with options to improve health that can work alongside conventional health care.

IM emphasises a number of issues including:[9]

- a focus on wellness and illness prevention
- being holistic in nature by focusing on physical, psychological, spiritual, social and lifestyle issues

- incorporating evidence-based, safe and ethical complementary therapies and medicines
- individualising the approach to any particular patient or clinical situation using the best of all available modalities in conjunction with informed patient choice
- integrating all of the above into conventional medical care
- acknowledging that advances in health care will be dependent on scientific advances, improvements in health care delivery systems, and cultural change as well as practitioner and patient education.

When considering any therapy it is important to balance the risks, the benefits, the evidence, the costs, and the alternatives, such as other therapies or doing nothing.

Complementary and alternative medicine (CAM)

Complementary and alternative medicine, as defined by the National Centre for Complementary and Alternative Medicine (NCCAM), is a group of diverse medical and health care systems, practices, and products that are not presently considered to be part of conventional medicine (see Table 1.1).[10]

As the evidence-base for some CAM increases, medical practitioners have a legal obligation to inform patients of the efficacy of relevant complementary therapies as treatment options, and to simultaneously be aware of the potential for adverse events and interactions that CAMs, such as nutritional and herbal supplements, may have when co-administered with pharmaceutical drugs or when a patient denies good orthodox care for any unproven CAM.[11] Knowledge in the efficacy of a complementary medicine or therapy is essential when making clinical decisions for patient care to help weigh against potential risks, such as adverse reactions or delays in useful conventional treatment. This highlights the importance of medical practitioners having at least basic education in the area of CAM to enable them to communicate and inform patients about what therapies are appropriate to the individual. Education on potential risks such as nutrient toxicity, especially with single nutrient use, and any potential interactions with pharmaceuticals is also essential.

Popularity of IM and CAM

Worldwide reports demonstrate that a large proportion of the public are using CAM and its popularity is increasing. For example, in

Table 1.1 NCCAM classifications [10]

NCCAM classifies natural, complementary and alternative medicines into 5 categories, or domains	
1 Alternative medical systems	Alternative medical systems are built upon complete systems of theory and practice such as homeopathic and naturopathic medicine, Traditional Chinese medicine and Ayurveda.
2 Mind–body interventions	These interventions include counselling, patient support groups, meditation, prayer, spiritual healing, and therapies that use creative outlets such as art, music, or dance.
3 Biologically based therapies	These therapies include the use of herbs, foods, vitamins, minerals, dietary supplements.
4 Manipulative and body-based methods	These methods include chiropractic or osteopathic manipulation, and massage.
5 Energy therapies	Energy therapies involve the use of energy fields. They are of 2 types: 1 biofield therapies such as qigong, reiki, therapeutic touch 2 bioenergetic therapies involving the use of pulsed electromagnetic fields, such as pulsed fields, magnetic fields, or alternating-current fields and/or alternating- and direct-current fields.

Australia up to 70% of the population are using CAM.[12] In the United States, up to 62% of adults use CAM.[13] It is therefore vital that health and medical practitioners are well informed about the evidence in these areas.

In many respects, the enthusiasm to use CAM is largely driven by the public. The community has greater access to information and various complementary medicine practitioners and therapies. There are often various reasons why a patient will want to trial CAM. These include philosophical and cultural reasons — wanting a more holistic approach to health care, when there are no longer any other orthodox approaches to assist in their health care, especially if they have suffered any adverse events from orthodox treatments. Generally, patients who use CAM are not rejecting orthodox medicine but are looking for options to improve wellbeing. Unfortunately, medical practitioners underestimate the extent of use of CAM by patients.[14, 15] This is of great concern, considering the potential for adverse events such as herb–drug interactions and coordinating the overall management of the patient.

Cultural aspects in determining type of CAM use

The WHO estimates that approximately 60% of medicine that is practiced worldwide is traditional medicine.[16] Traditional Chinese medicine (TCM) is practised in many Asian countries, Ayurveda medicine in India, Unani medicine in the Middle-East, Pakistan and India, while Kampo medicine is used in Japan. Biomedicine or conventional medicine is the predominant medicine practised in developed countries and its formation has also been influenced by cultural factors.[17]

Many of these therapies have been used for centuries, and some for thousands of years, and have a long traditional use in some societies and cultures, being highly entrenched in their health care system. There may be little scientific evidence for these therapies, but some inherent safety considering long-term use, in some cases up to 2000 years.

Although it is correct to offer patients conventional medical treatment for acute illnesses, for a chronic illness though for which there is no 'right' answer it is likely that the best treatment is that which best matches the patient's belief systems and cultural understanding. For example, a patient of Asian background may be very keen to use either herbal medicine or acupuncture. Under these circumstances it is mandatory that the practitioner is aware of possible toxicity, interactions with conventional medicines and the cost of such therapy.

IM strategies and healing

A holistic approach to health care involves giving comprehensive lifestyle advice that is inclusive of physical, social, psychological, emotional and spiritual wellbeing. In this way, we are encouraging and promoting our patients to take personal responsibility and be active participants for their own health. The focus needs to be on wellness, and not specifically on the disease. Positive lifestyle changes and a typical integrative approach to assist healing that can work alongside conventional medicine to improve health outcome or quality of life are listed in Table 1.2.

Health practitioner/doctor and patient satisfaction

Holistic health care offers an enormous amount of satisfaction and joy to the health practitioner, working with patients to help restore good health. The patients are often satisfied with this style of medicine and this, in turn, equally satisfies the doctors practising holistic health care. It empowers patients by providing them individually prescribed options for treating their health condition. Failure to treat or cure patients may occur due to a number of factors, such as lack of motivation, not changing lifestyle, choosing the wrong therapy, lack of commitment to the therapy for various reasons (e.g. financial, lack of support, peer pressure, non-believers etc). It is important to be aware and sensitive to these factors by being intuitive and listening to patients' needs carefully, and with clinical experience fine tune treatment modalities accordingly.

Furthermore, patients and doctors need to have access to quality information about complementary medicine to make well-informed decisions.

The health practitioner(HP)/doctor–patient relationship is precious, patient–centred and can result in a positive therapeutic outcome. It positively affects medical care and patient satisfaction. The HP/doctor–patient relationship is based on:

- kindness, compassion, and respect
- genuine caring, honesty, and trust
- the intention to heal
- empowering the patient (and the HP/doctor)
- good communication
- active listening and empathy.

Most studies actually indicate that over 80% of patients are satisfied with their general practitioner especially if they see the same doctor frequently.[18] A questionnaire

Table 1.2 Summary of lifestyle and IM strategies

Lifestyle suggestions	Diet/exercise/stress management/sleep Behavioural changes (avoidance of smoking, alcohol) Fun, laughter, joy; being in touch with nature; forgiveness Religion; spiritual belief Creative activities
Mind–body approaches	Stress management, meditation, relaxation therapies; breathing techniques Counselling — attitudinal healing, cognitive behavioural therapy Social support and/or support groups Group therapy Hypnosis; self-hypnosis Imagery and creative visualising techniques; positive thinking; mind training Communication; self-expression Personal development Biofeedback Spiritual healing; religion; prayer; exploring meaning and purpose in life
Environmental advice	Clean Air Fresh filtered water Organic foods Sun exposure (more or less) Soothing, relaxing sounds Chemical exposure (work and home) Avoiding household and work surroundings
Exercise	Swimming, walking, cycling, yoga, tai chi, qigong
Dietary suggestions	Low glycaemic index diet Mediterranean diet Asian diet Low-fat diet
Nutrient supplementation	Vitamins Minerals Fish oils Amino acids
Herbal therapies	Herbs Aromatherapy
Physical therapies	Acupuncture Manipulation Massage TENS machine Hydrotherapy
Energetic	Reiki Reflexology Homeopathy

Table 1.3 Encourage patient responsibility

The holistic health care practitioner encourages patient responsibility by:
Empowering patients to be active participants in their health care
Promoting self-care
Helping patients to make informed decisions and choices
Respecting choices
Being honest about limitations

Table 1.4 The well-informed patient

The well-informed patient:
Chooses not to be passive
Actively sources material and information about their disease
Works together with their health care practitioner to achieve common goals based on mutual respect
Participates in their own health care
Is motivated to get better
Needs close monitoring and discussion if they refuse orthodox treatment — this requires careful documentation in clinical notes

of 869 patients demonstrated that trust and commitment was positively associated with adherence to treatment. Positive relationships were also associated with adherence to treatment and commitment, and between trust and commitment, that led to positive lifestyle choices, such as healthy eating habits.[19] The researchers concluded:

> Patients' trust in their physician and commitment to the relationship offer a more complete understanding of the patient–physician relationship. In addition, trust and commitment favourably influence patients' health behaviours.[18]

It is also vital that patients are encouraged to take responsibility for their health and be well informed about all treatments (conventional or complementary) that are safe and suitable for their health care (see Tables 1.3 and 1.4).

Respect for the patient and their choice of treatment, compassion, trust and empathetic understanding all positively influence the HP/doctor–patient relationship, and help adherence to therapeutic regimens (see Table 1.5).[20, 21, 22]

Other factors that influence the HP/doctor–patient relationship:

- the tone of the clinician's voice
- the clinician's stress levels
- the amount of talking by the clinician; is it excessive or not enough?
- clinician self-awareness of: voice, body posture and any non-verbal cues
- do clinicians hold on to patients when care is limited……?

Respect and care of the patient

Care of any patient needs to be flexible and respectful of their individual needs and choices. It does require that the practitioner has a basic understanding of CAM and is willing to be honest with the patient and consider referral to a trusted, appropriately trained health practitioner (medically or non-medically trained) if their knowledge is limited. Hence, there is a great need to further educate the medical profession on the efficacy and safety of CAM.

The other area of concern is if the patient is led into particular CAM that is non-evidence based and leads to delay of potentially useful orthodox treatments. This situation is often seen in vulnerable groups, such as patients with cancer looking for cures.

HP/doctor–patient relationship and the 'doctor' as the teacher

The doctor–patient relationship also refers here to the health practitioner–patient relationship as the basic principles of care are similar. Interestingly, the original meaning of the word '*doctore*' is teacher. Thus as doctor's we are also educator's for lifestyle and health. Patient needs vary from one patient to another. Therefore, it is mandatory to remain flexible and vary approaches using treatment according to an individual's needs at the time. Many studies demonstrate that active listening, spending time with a patient, displaying a sympathetic, understanding, caring and warm attitude not only helps to develop patient trust, but also enhances the healing response (also known as placebo). To achieve all of this requires longer consultations.

The value of long clinical consultations

Longer patient-centred consultations are of benefit for those patients with chronic disease or mental health problems. The Australasian Integrative Medicine Association (AIMA) evaluated the evidence of long clinical consultations and

Table 1.5 Hallmarks essential to the HP/doctor–patient relationship

Respect	Compassion	Trust	Empathy	Appropriate touch
Philosophical beliefs Cultural background Personal experiences Choices	Deep awareness of the suffering of another coupled with the wish to relieve suffering	Integral to HP/doctor–patient relationship and influences healthy behaviour patterns	Empathy is the capacity to imagine what another person is feeling without feeling it yourself; the patient feels understood	Can convey • sympathy • empathy • reassurance Felt to be seen, heard, understood Be sensitive to the patient — use touch thoughtfully, not automatically Varies person to person Varies consultation to consultation

the impact on quality of health. The results demonstrated that long consultations:[23]

- improved the therapeutic relationship, trust, rapport, and answers to questions
- enhanced health outcomes
- enhanced handling of psychosocial problems
- decreased medication prescriptions
- increased lifestyle advice
- reduced litigation
- enhanced both patient and doctor satisfaction.

The thorough documentation of patient notes was essential with all medical notes but more so in particular with longer clinical consultations. Furthermore, it was reported that it is essential to write accurate notes to record informed choices made with patients, including refusal of treatment and why; known as 'informed refusal'.

The IM consultation is extensive in order to allow the following essential components to be included by the clinician.

Mind–body medicine

- **Evaluation of lifestyle stressors.** A key aspect of the extended consultation is to ascertain the patient's life stressors, which can be important cumulative risk factors for the pathogenesis of various chronic diseases.
- **Providing advice on relaxation techniques and stress reduction/management.** Numerous recent studies have demonstrated a significant and efficacious effect afforded to patients by relaxation and meditation techniques in managing lifestyle stressors. It should also be noted that there are many other stress-reduction modalities that can be employed, such as exercise in a natural environment, massage therapy, music therapy, aromatherapy and art therapy, for stress reduction/management.
- **Providing advice on lifestyle factors,** such as sleep restoration. There are various studies that demonstrate that sleep deprivation can significantly contribute to the pathogenesis of fatigue, depression, type II diabetes mellitus (T2DM) and cardiac disease.
- **Providing advice on behavioural factors** that may impact on disease outcomes e.g. drug, smoking and alcohol consumption.
- **Exercise and appropriate sunshine exposure.** There are numerous studies that have reported on the important value of exercise, not only in the prevention of illness but in the treatment of illness. Combined with prudent sunlight exposure, this assists to provide increased levels of serotonin, melatonin and vitamin D, all of which are essential for good health and enhanced immune function.
- **Nutritional history**. It is a well established fact that nutrition plays a critical role in the prevention of almost all illnesses.
- **Nutritional and herbal supplements.** Evidence-based medicine supports the use of nutrition and herbal supplements. Supplements such as folic acid during pregnancy have been demonstrated to prevent congenital abnormalities and reduce the risk of cognitive deficits. Vitamin D deficiency is common and widespread.
- **Referral to other health professionals** who can assist the patient with the necessary specific expertise can be essential in certain disease states (e.g. meditation, yoga, acupuncture).[24]

The plant analogy

If given the 'right conditions', the body has an innate capacity to heal. The body is equipped with natural healing mechanisms. A good analogy of this is the sick plant. Most gardeners know that plants can thrive well by providing the 'right conditions', such as: the right amount of sunlight; fresh air; nutrient-dense soil (occasionally supplementing with nutrients through fertilising); a stable, nurturing environment free of chemicals; and adequate water. Even if a plant appears unwell, changing any of these conditions can aid the recovery of the plant. If we apply this concept to the unwell person, their needs are very similar. Human needs for maintaining and restoring good health include: plenty of fresh air; exercise; adequate water; sunlight; good nutritious unprocessed foods; a peaceful environment free of chemicals, excessive noise and light; good quality sleep; contact with nature and people; meaning and joy in our lives; and minimising psychological stress.

Dis–ease

The term *dis–ease* literally means the person is *not at ease* and illness is the body's expression of imbalance that requires the necessary fundamental changes to bring about balance, ease and wellness. It is important for the patient to recognise that their current circumstances and lifestyle have contributed to their current health situation. Therefore, if patients are expected to gain maximum benefit from treatment, they need to fully commit themselves to a number of positive lifestyle changes. The illness, therefore, should be viewed as positive, as it is the body's expression that changes are necessary and this is the opportunity to change one's life and adopt healthier behaviour patterns to allow this to occur.

Stress

Most illnesses have a psychological component as a precipitator and/or as a consequence of the illness. Stress plays a major role in most diseases and stress management should be regularly prescribed to our patients. A common question one should ask patients is:

What was happening in your life at the onset of your illness?

This question often gives us a good clue as to what major stressors may have contributed to the onset or aggravation of the illness. Providing the time to listen to patients and 'hearing their stories' can have profound healing effects on them.

It is important to emphasise to patients to listen to their bodies, follow their own intuition and learn to love oneself. If people are stressed and don't care for themselves, they won't follow our advice to exercise, eat right, to not smoke or drink alcohol. As health practitioners, we can play a vital role in helping to guide our patients towards better health, positive lifestyle changes and behaviour patterns through guidance, appropriate counselling and being suitable role models.

Communication with allied and CAM practitioners

It is well established that patients are not communicating with medical practitioners about the use of CAM.[25, 26] What is not so well established is to what degree the CAM practitioners and regular doctors are communicating. Medical practitioners (MPs) have an established tradition of communicating with each other e.g. specialists (consultants) with general practitioners (GPs). A specialist knows that in general the GP will have some idea about the content of what they are communicating, as medical graduates would have had at least some exposure to do with the various medical specialties during their medical courses and postgraduate training. If a homeopath was to communicate with a GP there are major difficulties as most GPs would either have no or little knowledge or understanding of homeopathy and the language behind it. Many patients do not communicate with their regular doctor about CAM use for fear of being misunderstood or jeopardising their doctor–patient relationship. However, studies indicate that patients prefer that GPs were more educated about the CAMs they use, so that they can then better communicate with their doctors about their use of CAMs.[12]

There is a greater need to have more interaction between CAM and doctors when the patient chooses to see a CAM practitioner. An increasing number of medical practices include MPs plus various non-medical CAM practitioners and they are proving to be very popular with patients. Many of these medical practices have routine meetings to discuss the management of the patient. Other means of improving communication include letter writing, emails or phone discussions, especially with CAM practitioners at other clinics.

Referrals to regulated CAM practitioners such as osteopaths, chiropractors (in most states and territories of Australia) and TCM practitioners (Australia), reduces the risk of incompetent management. If the CAM practitioner is a member of a professional body this can provide evidence of at least some training, standards and guidelines for safe practise.

It is also reassuring to the MP if it is known that the CAM practitioner has adequate experience and in particular is aware of their limitations and knows when to refer back to a MP. The MP should initially be involved if a diagnosis has to be made but this would not be necessary if a patient wanted, for example, dietary advice or wanted to learn relaxation techniques which could be obtained from a CAM practitioner. As a ground rule, MPs differentiate between medical and CAM practitioners and have expressed greater confidence in medical colleagues who practice complementary medicine.[27, 28]

There are unresolved issues to do with referrals by MPs to CAM practitioners and these include:[29]

- Should a doctor refer a patient so the patient can be assessed regarding suitability for a complementary therapy?
- What information should the patient be given about the benefits and risks to do with the therapy?
- Should the doctor forward personal information to the therapist and vice versa?
- When should a CAM practitioner refer to a MP?
- What are the circumstances under which a patient is referred by one CAM practitioner to another?

Ethical and legal Issues

A report on ethical and legal issues at the interface of CAM and conventional medicine suggests that when MPs are faced with patients wanting to trial CAM they should:[30]

- be honest with patient's direct questioning about CAM
- establish the patient's understanding of CAM and why they use it
- take into account the burden of the patient's illness and provide material of their expressed preferences
- discuss the risks and benefits of both CAM and orthodox treatment
- adequately inform the patient about available CAMs that have been shown to be safe and effective, and those that are shown to be ineffective
- become familiar with qualified and competent CAM practitioners (both medical and non-medical) to whom referrals are made
- continue their relationship with the patient, and continue to monitor their health
- keep communication with the patient open and respectful.

The abovementioned points serve as useful guidelines for MPs in consultations involving CAM.

Evidence-based medicine (EBM)

The definition of evidence-based medicine (EBM) is 'the conscientious, explicit and judicious use of current best evidence in making decisions about the care of individual patients'.[31] EBM integrates the best external evidence with individual clinical expertise and patients' choice. Furthermore it is noted that absence of evidence does not mean a therapy does not work.[32]

EBM is a common term described as:

> the conscientious, explicit, and judicious use of current best evidence in making decisions about the care of individual patients. The practice of evidence-based medicine means integrating individual clinical expertise with the best available external clinical evidence from systematic research. By individual clinical expertise we mean the proficiency and judgment that individual clinicians acquire through clinical experience and clinical practice.[31]

This definition emphasises that whilst scientific evidence is important in clinical judgment, clinical experience and expertise also play a major role in the care and choice of treatment for a patient.

EBM encourages doctors to look for well-structured, randomised placebo-controlled prospective studies (Level II evidence) and systematic reviews of such studies (Level I evidence) to support clinical practice, but as yet there are few of these for the majority of CAMs.

'Outcome studies' may be more appropriate for holistic models of health, such as TCM and traditional Ayurveda medicine, where a more individualised and holistic approach to treatment occurs. Randomised control trials (RCTs) may be suitable for the holistic approaches but need to be creative but still technically possible. Very little good quality research exists for these therapies. Lack of evidence is not necessarily associated with lack of patient benefit.

Biomedical focus on evidence-based medicine and evidence-based research affecting IM and CAM

Scientific evidence is the basis and is pivotal to biomedicine. Evidence on efficacy and safety should be the basis of defining which CAMs are useful and which are not. To date, research in CAM has been limited due to a number of factors such as funding, the type of CAM used, the quality of the studies, the ability to patent a product and so forth, to make any firm conclusions about their potential role in health care. In saying this, there is also a large body of scientific evidence emerging for

CAM worldwide. This evidence should be made accessible to the health profession and public, and also integrated into recommended national guidelines of treatment for specific health conditions. Once a therapy or medicine, be it orthodox or complementary, has scientific evidence to prove its efficacy and safety, then the medical practitioner has a legal and ethical obligation to use the best treatment possible for the individual patient.

There are many CAMs that are not evidence-based to date. This may not mean that they are ineffective as funding may have not been allocated to research these therapies/medicines. However, until they are tested they need to be used cautiously.

National and Health Medical Research Council (NHMRC) guidelines to research

Since 1999, the National and Health Medical Research Council (NHMRC)[33] has created useful guidelines to identify the varying levels of scientific evidence using a scale from I–IV. These guidelines help to identify which medicines or therapies carry greater weight in research, with Level I considered as superior research and Level IV considered the least superior: Refer to Table 1.6

To date, there is a growing body of clinical studies ranging from Level I–IV scientific evidence (NHMRC guidelines) for complementary medicines. Throughout this textbook reference is made using the NHMRC guidelines.

Table 1.6 NHMRC levels of evidence

Level I	From a systematic review of all relevant randomised controlled trials, meta-analyses.
Level II	From at least 1 properly designed randomised controlled clinical trial.
Level IIIa	From well-designed pseudo-randomised controlled trials (alternate allocation or some other method).
Level IIIb	From comparative studies (including systematic reviews of such studies) with concurrent controls and allocation not randomised, cohort studies, case-control studies, or interrupted time series with a parallel control group.
Level IIIc	From comparative studies with historical control, 2 or more single-arm studies or interrupted time series without a parallel control group.
Level IV	Opinions of respected authorities based on clinical experience, descriptive studies or reports of expert committees.
Level V	Represents minimal evidence from testimonials.

Cochrane collaboration

A worldwide network of researchers called the Cochrane collaboration prepare, disseminate and continuously update systematic reviews of randomised clinical trials in all areas of health care. A CAM field is set up and is bringing together evidence for CAM. This involves a conjoint effort of many scientific researchers and centres throughout the world.

A list of CAM Cochrane reviews and protocols can be accessed via:

http://www.compmed.umm.edu/cochrane/Reviews2002.pdf

Conclusion

The use of CAM should have certain boundaries. Its use should not be to the exclusion of a clearly indicated, safe, effective and superior orthodox therapy. In making choices patients need to be informed about the range of reasonable options of orthodox and complementary therapies. Based on clear information patients should then be allowed to make their choices as to what treatment they wish to pursue if they are low risk and have some proven efficacy. It is easier to recommend CAMs when they have evidence for safety and efficacy. There is now a growing body of scientific evidence to support CAMs such as some herbal medicines, acupuncture, nutritional medicine, and stress management techniques which work with the natural healing process of the body.

The basic principles of holistic health care include:

- the patient must be motivated and have an intention to heal, therefore the patient must be a willing participant in their own health care
- the health practitioner and/or doctor should have an intention to help the patient with compassion, understanding and kindness
- developing a good health practitioner/doctor–patient therapeutic relationship in a safe atmosphere is essential and listening carefully and intently to what they are saying

- all healing is self-healing; the CAM practitioner role is to empower patients to help heal themselves, to take charge and have personal responsibility of their health
- recognising that illness can be seen as positive and is an opportunity for positive change and growth, such as developing positive behaviour patterns
- the health practitioner and/or doctor should be a role model for good health and always endeavour to educate and encourage the patient to adopt healthy behaviour patterns and a healthy lifestyle.

This book summarises the key scientific and management strategies using an IM approach to treat common health problems faced by medical and health practitioners in everyday medical practices.

References

1 Kotsirilos V. Complementary and alternative medicine. Part 2-evidence and implications for GPs. Australian Family Physician 2005;34(8):689–91.

2 See websites for the Royal Australian College of General Practitioners (RACGP — http://www.racgp.org.au) and the Australasian Integrative Medicine Association (AIMA — http://www.aima.net.au/).

3 Snyderman R, Weil AT. Integrative medicine: bringing medicine back to its roots. Arch Intern Med 2002;162(4):395–7.

4 Vitetta L, Anton B, Cortizo F, et. al. Mind-body medicine: stress and its impact on overall health and longevity. Ann N Y Acad Sci 2005;1057:492–505.

5 Ford ES, Bergmann MM, Kröger J, et. al. Healthy living is the best revenge: findings from the European Prospective Investigation Into Cancer and Nutrition–Potsdam study. Arch Intern Med. 2009;169(15):1355–62.

6 Kotsirilos V. Complementary and alternative medicine. Part 1-what does it all mean? Australian Family Physician 2005;34(7):595–7.

7 RACGP-AIMA Joint Position Statement of the RACGP and AIMA, Complementary Medicine, 2004. Online. Available: http://www.racgp.org.au/Content/NavigationMenu/Advocacy/RACGPpositionstatements/2006compmedstatement.pdf (accessed 14-04-09)

8 Vitetta L. Integration is here to stay. Editorial. J Compl Med 2008;7(6):7.

9 Integrative Medicine Statement. See Statement Chapters in RACGP Curriculum for Australian General Practice. Online. Available: http://www.racgp.org.au/curriculum (accessed 14-04-09)

10 National Center for Complementary and Alternative Medicine (NCCAM). What is Complementary and Alternative Medicine (CAM)?May 2002, USA. Last modified: 21 October 2002. Online. Available: http://nccam.nih.gov/health/whatiscam/ (accessed 14-08-09)

11 Brophy E. Informed consent and complementary medicine. J Comp Med 2003:223–8.

12 Easton K. Complementary medicines: attitudes and information needs of consumers and health care professionals. Prepared for the National Prescribing Service Limited (NPS). July 2007.

13 Patricia M, Barnes MA, Eve Powell-Griner, et. al. Complementary and alternative medicine use among adults: United States. Seminars in Integrative Medicine, June 2004;2(2):54–71.

14 Kristoffersen SS, cited in Drew AK, Myers SP. Safety issues in herbal medicine: implications for the health professions. MJA 1997;166:538–41.

15 Nahin RL, Straus SE. Research into complementary and alternative medicine: problems and potential. BMJ 322 (7279):161.

16 World Health Organization. Media Centre fact sheets. Online. Available: http://www.who.int/mediacentre/factsheets/fs134/en/ (accessed Jan 2010)

17 Cassidy CM et. al. Commentary on terminology and therapeutic principles: challenges in classifying complementary and alternative medicine practices. J Altern Comp Med 2002;8:893–5.

18 Potiriadis M, Chondros P, Gilchrist G, et. al. How do Australian patients rate their general practitioner? A descriptive study using the General Practice Assessment Questionnaire. MJA 2008;189(4):215–19.

19 Berry LL, Parish JT, Janakiraman R, et. al. Patients' commitment to their primary physician and why it matters. Ann Fam Med 2008;6(1):6–13.

20 Marie-Thérèse Lussier, Claude Richard. Feeling understood. Expression of empathy during medical consultations. Canadian Family Physician 2007;53:640–1.

21 Squier RW. A model of empathic understanding and adherence to treatment regimens in practitioner–patient relationships. Soc Sci Med 1990;30(3):325–39.

22 Branch WT, Malik TK. Using 'windows of opportunities' in brief interviews to understand patients' concerns. JAIMA 1993;269(13):1667–8.

23 Cohen M, Kotsirilos V, Hassed C, et. al. Long Consultations and Quality of Care: AIMA Position Statement. Journal of the Australasian Integrative Medicine Association (JAIMA) Oct 2002;19:19–22.

24 Sali A, Vitetta L. Integrative medicine. In: the Mix. Australian Doctor 2007; 20 April: 39–40.

25 MacLennan AH, Wilson DH, Taylor AW. The escalating cost and prevalence of alternative medicine. Prev Med. 2002;35:166–73.

26 Tillem J. Utilisation of complementary and alternative medicine among rheumatology patients. Integrative Medicine. 2000;2:143–4.

27 Marshall R, Gee R, Israel N, et. al. The use of alternative therapies by Auckland general practitioners. NZ Med J 1990;103:213–15.

28 Pirotta Marie, Cohen Marc, Kotsirilos Vicki, et. al. Complementary therapies: have they become accepted in General Practice? MJA 2000;172:105–9.

29 Brophy E. Referral to CM practitioners — legal and ethical issues. J Comp Med 2003;2:42–8.

30 Kerridge I, McPhee J. Ethical and legal issues at the interface of complementary medicine and conventional medicine. Medical Journal of Australia 2004;181:164–6.

31 Sackett DL, Rosenberg WMC, Muir Gray JA, et. al. Editorial: Evidence based medicine: what it is and what it isn't. BMJ 1996;312:71–2. Online. Available: http://www.bmj.com/cgi/content/full/312/7023/71?eaf (accessed 13-01-09)

32 Douglas G Altman, J Martin Bland. Absence of evidence is not evidence of absence. BMJ 1995; 311: 19 August: 485.

33 National Health and Medical Research Council (NHMRC). A guide to the development, implementation and evaluation of clinical practice guidelines. Commonwealth of Australia, Canberra, 1999.

Chapter 2

Nutritional assessment and therapies

With contribution from Dr Antigone Kouris-Blazos

Introduction

The importance of nutrition in general medical practice has paralleled the increasing prevalence of lifestyle related disorders such as obesity, diabetes, and heart disease. In fact, alongside dermatology and psychological disorders, nutritional disorders are among the most common problems encountered by doctors and there is pressure for the general practitioner to provide competent nutritional assessment, diagnosis and therapy.[1] It has been estimated that over 70% of patients seen in general practice are at high risk of having or developing a nutritional deficiency and many patients will exhibit symptoms suggestive of nutritional inadequacy or imbalance which is contributing to their illness.[2, 3]

The Australian National Health Survey in 2004–5 reported that 86% of Australians between 18–64 years do not consume the recommended 5 serves of vegetables each day and 46% do not consume the recommended 2 serves of fruit each day.[4] In 2008 rising petrol and food prices (especially for fresh produce but not for processed/take away foods) were reported to potentially affect shopping trends with less fresh produce being purchased.[5] Furthermore, the costs of healthy foods such as bread and milk is rising far greater than the cost of nutrient poor energy dense foods (such as cakes, soft drinks and biscuits), which will impact on food choices and the diet in lower socioeconomic groups.[6]

This may be further compounded by emerging evidence from the UK and US (Australian data lacking) that there has been declining levels of minerals in our fruit and vegetables over the last 50 years, especially for magnesium dropping by about 45% (see page 23 'Dietary history and assessing food and nutrient intake'). Markovic and Natoli report paradoxical nutrient deficiencies such as zinc, iron, vitamin C and D and folate in the obese and overweight due to eating high-energy foods that are also high in saturated fats, salt and sugar, with poor nutrient content.[7] The authors note that this condition is under-recognised and therefore not treated. The Public Health Association of Australia released a report in 2009 'A Future for our Food: addressing public health, sustainability and equity from paddock to plate' outlining the urgent need for Australian food policy to encourage food choices that are environmentally sustainable and address the re-emergence of nutrient-deficiency related diseases.[8]

The Australian dietary guidelines and core food groups are currently undergoing revision. The Public Health Association of Australia would like to see the new guidelines address the re-emergence of nutrient-deficiency related disease and food sustainability. Specific recommendations include: reduced total intake of animal products; reduced reliance on ruminant meat; promotion of sustainable proteins, especially legumes, nuts, eggs and chicken; promotion of seasonal fruit and vegetables, legumes and grains that are grown using production methods appropriate to the region. The report highlights that shifting less than 1 day per week's worth of calories from red meat and dairy products to chicken, fish, eggs, or legume-based diet achieves more green house gas reduction than buying all locally sourced food. In addition, consuming less meat and more plant-based foods may be 1 type of measure that will lead to increased sustainability and reduced environmental costs of food production systems.[8]

The Australian National Children's Nutrition and Physical Activity Survey also highlights the growing epidemic of obesity in children — estimated at 17% of children considered overweight and 6% obese in Australia — with poor quality diets with significant nutritional shortfalls, particularly vitamin D, E, iodine and iron.[9]

Suboptimal intake of vitamins from diet is common in the general population, particularly children and the elderly, and a risk factor for chronic diseases such as cardiovascular disease, neural tube defects, colon and breast cancer, osteopenia and fractures.[10]

Other risk groups identified include vegans, drug and alcohol-dependent individuals, hospitalised patients and patients with malabsorption.

If these trends continue nutritional deficiencies may become more commonplace in the community. Doctors, dietitians, nurses and other allied health professionals may need to become more active and skilled at detecting signs and symptoms of nutritional deficiencies/insufficiencies. Improving the nutritional status of patients will help improve clinical outcomes/wellness and reduce morbidity and mortality and is thus of increasing importance to comprehensive medical care. In order to determine whether a patient's nutritional status needs improving, a nutritional assessment is required.

Nutritional assessment will identify the high-risk patient (see Table 2.1) for nutrient inadequacies or excesses which in turn will contribute to a nutritional diagnosis. Once the diagnosis is made it is then possible to put in place the nutritional therapy of the patient.

Table 2.1 Identifying patients at high risk of nutrient deficiency or insufficiency

- Patients with chronic illnesses (especially bowel problems, other functional disorders, such as chronic fatigue, psychiatric illness).
- Patients on certain and many medications (poly-pharmacy).
- Senior patients, recent surgery, injured/severe trauma, burns, sepsis, protracted fever, recent discharge from hospital.
- Crash dieters or patients on chronic low calorie diets (<1300kcal/day).
- Poor/altered food intake (e.g. due to restricted food budget, food supply, rising food prices, food storage, poor cooking skills).
- Some vegetarians, some athletes and those with food allergies or sensitivities to particular foods.
- Sedentary patients, especially those who are office/housebound (with little sun exposure or opportunity for incidental activity); the elderly.
- Pregnant/breastfeeding women and those who excessively bleed during menstruation.
- Women with young children.
- Excess alcohol (more than 1 drink per day for women and 2 drinks per day for men), smoking or illegal drug users.
- Disabled patients, dental/chewing problems, widowers, socially isolated/living alone.

(Source: adapted from Wahlqvist M, Kouris-Blazos A. Nutrition — is diet enough? J Comp Med 2002: 46)[11]

Nutritional assessment is based on information gathered from:

1. medical history and genetic predisposition (see Table 2.3)
2. examination for nutrition-related signs and symptoms (see Table 2.2)
3. anthropometry (weight history, BMI, waist circumference, body composition using electrical impedance or skinfold measurements)
4. socioeconomic history (living arrangements, financial problems) and lifestyle history (physical activity, alcohol, smoking, stress, gambling, sleep)
5. medication (potential adverse or beneficial effects on nutritional status (see also Chapter 37, Herb–nutrient–drug interactions)
6. vitamin and herbal supplement use — potential adverse effects (especially if far exceeding the recommended dietary intakes) or beneficial effects on nutritional status and interaction with medications (see also Chapter 37, Herb–nutrient–drug interactions)
7. dietary history (food pattern, cuisine/culture, food variety, intake and frequency of specific foods like fish, nuts, legumes)
8. laboratory tests (see Table 2.5).

Medical history

The medical history may reveal a disease that interferes with the patient's ability to eat (e.g. Cerebrovascular accident and Parkinson's disease) or the body's use of nutrients (increased excretion of magnesium and chromium in diabetes or reduced absorption of several nutrients in Crohn's disease). The genetic predisposition may also provide clues e.g. reported weight loss or diarrhoea could be due to coeliac disease which runs in the family.

Signs and symptoms of nutritional deficiencies

Clinical symptoms and anthropometric measurements will provide further clues to the nutritional puzzle. However, symptoms (manifestations reported by the patient) and signs (observations made by a clinician) can occur late in the development of the nutritional problem. Thus diagnosis of a nutritional deficiency cannot usually be made solely on the basis of a clinical examination. This is mainly because many nutrition-related signs and symptoms are non-specific and can occur for non-nutritional reasons. Usually the presence of a group of related clinical signs and symptoms is a better indication than a single sign or symptom.[12] For example, the finding of follicular hyperkeratosis isolated to the back of a patient's arms is a fairly common, normal finding. On the other hand if it is widespread on a person who consumes little fruit and vegetables and smokes regularly (increasing vitamin C requirements) vitamin C deficiency is a possible cause. Not surprisingly, the tissues with the fastest turnover rates are the most likely to show signs of nutrient deficiencies or excesses e.g. hair, skin and lingual papillae (an indirect reflection of the status of the villae of the gut)[13] (see Tables 2.2 and 2.3 for clinical signs and symptoms of possible nutritional deficiencies).

Table 2.2 Presentations and signs (can include) to consider with specific vitamin deficiencies (rare or sub-clinical deficiency in Western populations)

Micronutrient	Signs
Vitamin A	Conjuctival xerosis Bitot spot Perifollicular hyperkeratosis
Vitamin B1	Peripheral neuropathy Cardiac arrythmias Cardiac failure
Vitamin B2	Magenta tongue (Glossitis) Angular stomatitis 'Shark skin'
Vitamin B3	Strawberry tipped tongue (Glossitis) Swollen gums Dermatitis Peripheral neuropathy Hyperpigmentation
Vitamin B6	Glossitis, seborrhoea Peripheral neuropathy Symmetrical sensory and motor deficits
Vitamin B12	Glossitis Angular stomatitis Hyperpigmentation Peripheral neuropathy and sub–acute combined degeneration
Vitamin B complex/folate	Glossitis Angular stomatitis and hyperpigmentation
Vitamin C	Bleeding and swollen gums Swollen eyelids Perifollicular petechiae Follicular hyperkeratosis Scorbutic rosary and joint pain
Vitamin D	Rickets–bowing of long bone and rachitic rosary Osteoporosis
Calcium (Ca) and/or magnesium (Mg)	Positive Chvostek sign
Iron (Fe)	Koilonychia, leucoplakia, Plummer–Vinson syndrome
Zinc (Zn)	Acne, stretch marks, white spots on nail
Iodine (I)	Weight gain

Table 2.3 Clinical symptoms and signs of nutrient deficiencies/insufficiencies

Clinical symptoms and signs	Consider low intake/deficiency (may warrant blood/urine/faeces testing)
HEAD	
appetite poor	Zn[i, v], Mg[iii], Fe[iii], B1[vi], B3[vi], folate[vi], excess vit A[i]
nausea (esp with fatty foods)	B3[vi]
fatigue/tiredness/irritable	B6[vi], B12[vi], folate[vi], Zn[i, v, vi], vit C[vi], Fe[iii, vi], chromium (Cr)[vi], thyroid, excess vit A[v], protein[vi]
sugar cravings/hyperglycaemia	insulin resistance, Mg, Cr[iii, v, vi], Zn, vit E
moody/depressed	protein[vi], B1[vi], B3[iii], B6[iii, vi], B12[vi], vit C[vi], Mg[vi], Zn[iii], iodine, thyroid, vit D
anxiety/agitation	Cr[vi], Mg[vi], vit D[vi]
migraine	B2[vi], coenzyme Q_{10} (CoQ_{10})
headache	B3[iii], B12[vi], folate[vi], Fe[iii], Mg if cervicocranial, excess vit A[i, iii]
sleep disturbance	B6[vi], Mg[vi], vit C[vi]
sleep onset delay	vit D[vi]
poor dream recall	B6[vi]
insomnia/restless sleep	vit D[vi], Ca[vi], B3[iii]
non-refreshing sleep	Mg[vi]
night sweats-back of head/scalp	vit D[vi]
low libido	Fe (women) [iii], Zn (men), low testosterone, thyroid
impaired memory/cognition/dementia	B1[iv, vi], B12[iii, iv, vi], B3[iii, iv, v], folate[iv, vi], Fe[vi], Zn[vi], iodine
HAIR/SCALP	
hair thinning/loss/alopecia	protein[iv], B2[vi], EFA[vi], Zn[iii, vi], Fe[vi], Biotin[i, iii, v, vi], excess vit A[iii], excess selenium (Se[iii]) thyroid[i], iodine
dry dull hair	essential fatty acid (EFA)[vi], vit A[vi]
easily plucked hair	protein[iv]
dry coarse/brittle hair	protein[iv], biotin[iv], Fe[vi], Zn[i, vi], Iodine, hypothyroid, EFA[vi], excess vit A[i, iii]
depigmentation/dyschromotrichia	copper (Cu)[i], Se[i]
hair growth arrest	Zn[i]
diaphoresis of scalp (night)	vit D[vi]
dry flaking hair and scalp	vit A, Zn, Se
dandruff	Zn[vi], Mg[vi], biotin[vi], Se
prematurely graying hair	Cu[vi], Biotin[vi], vit B12[iii, vi]
coiled/cork screw hairs	vit C[iii] (hair shaft flat instead of round in cross section)

EYES	
tearing/burning/itching	vit B2[v]
dark/crimson under eye circles	Fe, allergy[vi], liver problems
dry thickened conjunctiva xerophthalmia/xerosis	vit A[i, vi], Zn[i], Biotin[iii] (conjunctivitis)
pale conjunctiva	Fe[iii]
muddy sclera	vit C[vi]
yellow sclera	liver function[i, vi]
photosensitivity	vit B2[iii, vi], Zn[iii]
bitot spots/white thick patches	vit A[i], Zn[i]
impaired night vision	vit A[iii, vi], Zn[iii]
long sightedness	vit D[vi]
impaired visual acuity/blurred	EFA[vi], xs vit A[i]
pterygium (thickness)	vit C[vi], B3[vi], EFA[vi]
twitching eye/spasms facial muscles	Mg[i, iii, vi], Ca[i, iii], K[i]
macular/retinal degeneration	age, lutein, zeaxanthin, excess blood sugar
NOSE	
scaling/red folds nasolabial seborrhea	vit B2[iii, vi] (red greasy folds), B6[iii], omega-6[iii] (dry folds)
poor smell/anosmia	Zn[v, vi], vit A[v]
EARS	
noise intolerance	Mg[vi]
post aural flush	Zn[vi], EFA[vi]
tinnitus	Fe[iii]
TONGUE/MOUTH	
dark red raw/swollen/glossitis painful 'raw beef' appearance	vit B3[i, iii, iv, v], B12[i, iii, iv, v], folate[i, iv, v], Fe[i, iv, v, vi]
bright red smooth/glossitis	vit B2[i, iv], B6[i, iii, iv, v], B12[i, iv], folate[i, iv, v], Fe[i, iv, v, vi], biotin[i, v]
large beefy tongue	hypothyroid[i], iodine[i]
magenta/blue tongue	vit B2[i, iii, v], Biotin[i]
white/pale smooth	Fe[i]
yellow/brown tongue	bowel dysfunction/dysbiosis[vi], low HCL[vi]
berry like red tongue	vit B complex[i]
fissured/creviced tongue	vit B3[iv, v]
scalloped tongue	Mg[vi], vit B3[vi]

strawberry tip/cherry tip tongue	vit B3[vi], B6[vi]
burning sensation of mouth/throat	D[vi]
lips cheilosis (burning/soreness)	vit B2[iii, iv, v], B3[iii, iv], B6[iv, v]
angular stomatitis	vit B1[i], B2[i, iii, iv, v], B3[i, iii, iv], B6[iii, iv], folate[v], B12[i, v], Fe[i]
halitosis	vit B3[vi], low HCL, dysbiotic bacteria, hypothyroid; liver problems
periodontal disease/loose teeth	vit C[vi], CoQ_{10}[vi], Ca[vi]
bleeding gums/gingivitis	vit C[i, iii, iv], B2[iv], vitK[vi], xs vit A (red gingiva around teeth)[i, iii]
gum recession	protein[vi], CoQ_{10}[vi]
mouth ulcers	vit B12[vi], vit A[vi], folate[vi]
crimson crescents back of mouth	food sensitivies[vi]
intense thirst	xs vit D[vi], B1/wet beri beri[iii]
impaired taste	Zn[i, v], vit A[iii]
loss of tooth enamel	Ca[iv]
HANDS/NAILS	
finger pulp atrophy	protein[vi]
cold hands	Fe[iii], Mg[vi], vit E[vi], EFA[vi], thyroid
vertical corrugations — pronounced (beaded nails)	vit B[ii], protein[vi], Zn[vi], diabetes[ii], thyroid[ii], Addisons[ii]
vertical corrugations — unpronounced	Age[i], RA[i], PVD[i], Lichen planus[i]
pronounced central ridge	Fe[i], folate[i], protein[i]
horizontal grooves/Beau's lines	protein[vi], past severe illness/surgery[ii], MI[ii], Zn[i], Se[i], Ca[ii]
leukonychia (white spots)	Zn[vi]
half moons base of nails	vit B6[vi]
dry thin brittle nails	protein[vi], malnutrition[ii] EFA[vi], Fe[vi], Ca/osteopenia[ii], thyroid[ii]
peeling/splitting nails	Ca[vi] protein[vi]
spoon shaped/brittle nails	Fe[i, iii, vi], low cysteine/methionine[i], diabetes[i]
soft/papery/bitten nails	Zn[vi], protein[vi]
growth arrest/thickened nails	protein[vi], Zn[i]
yellow nails	vit E[vi]
black/red thickened nails	xs Se[i]
egg shell nails	vit A[vi]
clubbed nails	lung problems[ii], IBD[ii], coeliac[ii], hyperthyroid[ii]
brown nail beds or skin creases	vit B12[iii]

white nail beds	Se[iii]
paronychia	excess Se[iii], Zn[iii]
MUSCLE	
generalised muscle pain/ache tender muscles	B1[iv], vit E[v], Ca[i], [v], Mg[i, vi], potasium (K)[i, v], Se[i, iii], vit D[v, vi], coma, iodine CoQ_{10} (if on statins), vit C[iii]
cramps	Ca[iii], [v], Mg[vi], vit B5[vi], Fe[iii], K, Na, vit C[iii], vit D[vi]
muscle twitching/spasms (hyper-reflexia)	B6[v], Mg[i, iii, v, vi], Ca[i, iii], K[i], vit D[vi]
muscle atrophy face, hands, chest, loss of tissue recoil back of hand	protein[vi], B1[vi]
calf/muscle tenderness	vit E[v] (intermittent claudication), B complex[iv], [vi]
muscle weakness/wasting (difficulty up/down stairs)[iii]	protein[iv], vit D[v], K[v], Ca, thiamin
decreased muscle reflexes	B complex[vi], vit E[vi]
SKIN	
excessive ageing of skin/wrinkles	vit E[vi]
perifollicular hyperkeratosis (toad skin) commonly seen on upper arms/thighs	vit A[i, iv, vi,] Zn[i], B complex[iii], vit C[iii, v], EFA[iii]
perifollicular petechiae/ haemorrhages	vit C[i, iii, v], vit K[i, iii] (causes petechiae unrelated to hair; sometimes seen with prolonged antibiotic treatment)
shark skin/dyssebacea (sebum plugs in follicles/face/body)	vit B2[iii]
oily scaly seborrheic dermatitis esp nasolabial folds/eyebrows/ forehead	vit B2[iii, v](nasolabial/scrotum), vit B3[iii], vit B6[i, iii, v], Biotin[vi,] Cu[i], EFA[vi]
dry scaly/coarse dermatitis	Zn[iii, v], Iodine[i], vit B3[iii], omega-6[i, iii], omega-3[vi], vit C[v], vit E, biotin[i, v], vitA[v], vit A excess[i], [iii], [v]
dry 'fish scale', 'flaky paint'	vit A[iv], Zn[iv, v] especially on the legs
hyperpigmentation non scaly macules/patches	insulin resistance[vi], vit A, Zn[iii, v], vit C, vit B12[iii], vit B6[vi], folate[iii], EFA, evening primrose oil (EPO), vit B3[iv] (see also dermatitis)
hyperpigmented scaly dermal patches on face/limbs (pellagra)	vit B1, vit B3[i], biotin[i, v], Zn[iii, v], EFA
unusual skin rash	vit B6 or excess supplement use
spider veins	vit C[vi]
liver spots (ceroid accumulation)	vit E[vi]
eczema	biotin[vi], Zn[iii], omega-3[vi], omega-6/EPO[i], [iii], gluten[i]
rosacea	vit B2, hypochlorhydria/gastric dysfunction[vi], dysbiotic bacteria/H pylori infection[vi]

psoriasis	vit D[vi], EFA[vi], vit A[iv], Zn[iii]
acne	EFA[vi], Zn[vi], vit A[vi], vit C[iii], dysbiotic bacteria, bowel dysbiosis[vi], high GI diet/insulin resistance[vi]
stretchmarks	Zn[vi], vit E[vi], Bvi[vi]
wound healing/lesions on pressure areas	vit A, B6[vi], vit C[v, vi], Zn[i, iii, v], EFA[vi], protein[vi], biotin[vi]
easy bruising	vit K[iv], [vi], dysbiotic bacteria[vi], protein, vit C[iv], [vi], blood thinning medication
blood mottling arms/legs	vit B6[vi]
itchy skin/rashes	liver problems
NERVES/PAIN/BONES	
impaired coordination/balance, disorientation/ataxic gait	vit B1[i], [vi], B12[iii], [v] (neurological changes can occur without haematologic changes), B3[iv], vit E[iv], [vi]
neuropathy (weakness, ataxia, pins/needles, parasthesia, foot/wrist drop, reduced tendon reflexes, numbness of fingers/feet/lips/tongue fine tactile sense, vibratory sense, position sense)	vit B1[i, iv, vi], B2[iii, vi], B6[iii, iv], B12[iv, v], carnitine, EPO, vit B6 toxicity[iii], folate[iii], Mg[i], Ca[i], K[i], omega-3[iii], Cr[iii], [v]Fe[vi], vit E[iv, v], lipoic acid
neuralgia/paralysis/paresthesia	vit B1[iv], B3[iii], B12[iii, iv, v] Mg[iv, v]
tetany	Ca[iv, v], Mg[iv], K[v]
diminished reflexes	Iodine[iv]
postural hypotension	vit B6/B complex[vi], Fe[vi] (general hypotension)
bone/joint pain	vit C[iv, v, vi], xs vit A[iv, v], vit D[iv, v], Ca[v], omega-3[vi], Zn[vi], Boron[vi]
low bone density	excess vit A[v] Ca[v], Mg[v], vit D[v], Ca[v], Zn, vit K
DIGESTION	
constipation/bloating	Fe[iii], B3[vi], low HCL/enzymes, gluten, food intolerances, dysbiosis, candida management, vit D excess
diarrhoea	Fe[iii], excess Mg/vit C[i], Zn[i], B3[iii, vi], B12[iii] folate[v], biotin[v], fructose, fructans
belching/flatulence/reflux	vit B12[iii], low hydrochloric acid (HCL), H Pylori, allergen, lactose, fructose
poor digestion	vit B3[vi], low stomach acid (HCl)[vi]
MENSTRUAL	
delayed/<flow periods/irregular oligomenorrhoea/sub-fertility	Fe[iii], vit E[vi], EFAs[vi], insulin resistance[vi], Zn[vi]
mastalgia	vit E[vi], vit A[vi], omega-3[vi]/EFA imbalance[vi]
PMS	vit B6[vi], Ca[vi], Mg[vi], EFA[vi]
dysmennorrhoea/menorrhagea	Ca[vi]

LEGS/FEET	
heels — hyperkeratosis/dry/cracked	vit E[vi], EFA[vi]
soles — hyperkeratosis	vit A[vi]
cold feet/<peripheral perfusion	vit E[vi], EFA[vi], Mg[vi], vit B6, thyroid (vit A, Zn, I, Fe)
burning paresthesias in feet	vit B5[iii], B1[iii]
arch collapse	protein[vi]
calf muscle tenderness	vit E[vi], B1[iii]
oedema	K, Mg, vit B1[i, iii], Fe[iii], protein[iv], quercetin
GROWTH	
poor	Fe[i], Zn[i, vi], Iodine[i, iii], protein[i], energy[i], vit D[i], Ca, omega-6[iii], vitA[v]
IMMUNITY/INFECTIONS/CANCER	
immuno-dysfunction	Zn[iii] Se[vi], vit C[vi], vit E[vi], vit D

i McLaren DS. A Colour Atlas and Text of Diet-Related Disorders. 2nd edn. London England: Wolfe & Mosby — Year book Europe Ltd, 1992.
ii Medscape. Examining the Fingernails When Evaluating Presenting Symptoms in Elderly Patients. Online. Available: www.medscape.com (accessed 7 Aug 2008).
iii McLaren DS. Clinical manifestations of human vitamin and mineral disorders: a resume. In: Shils M, Olson JA, Shike M, Ross C. Modern Nutrition in Health and Disease. 9th edn. Williams & Wilkins, 1999;485–503.
iv Newton MJ, Halsted CH. Clinical and functional assessment of adults. In: Shils M, Olson JA, Shike M, Ross C. Modern Nutrition in Health and Disease. 9th edn. Williams & Wilkins, 1999;895–902.
v Heimburger DC, Ard JD. Handbook of Clinical Nutrition. 4th edn. Mosby Elsevier 2006.
vi Sydney-Smith M. Nutritional Assessment. J Comp Medicine 2006; Jan-Feb 28–40; and Nutritional Assessment Workshop Seminar slides, March 2008.

Important note: The list in Table 2.3 is not definitive and is based on combined clinical experience and scientific evidence. Assessment and treatment should be based on your own clinical judgment (i.e. dietary history and physical examination) and confirmed with pathology testing. Symptoms may also occur from other non-nutritional related diseases.

A thorough medical and nutritional history, together with a thorough physical examination is necessary to detect nutrient deficiencies (occasionally this may be subtle i.e. nutritional insufficiency). When taking a nutritional history, if limited by time, ask patients to recall what they ate and drank in the last 24–48 hours and/or ask them to bring a 1-week food diary at their next consultation. If time permits, then a more extensive dietary assessment would be helpful as discussed under *Dietary history and assessing food and nutrient intake* in this chapter. Examples of symptoms suggestive of nutrient deficiencies include gum bleeding (vitamin C), numbness of feet (folic acid and B1 deficiency), night blindness (vitamin A), poor immunity and recurrent infections (vitamins A, C, D and zinc), poor appetite (B group vitamins and zinc), muscle cramps (calcium, magnesium), tremor (magnesium), poor memory (B group vitamins, folic acid and various minerals e.g. magnesium), loss of libido (B group vitamins, folic acid), tiredness (any nutrient), mood disorders (B group vitamins, vitamin C and zinc), poor wound healing (protein, zinc, vitamin C), sore tongue (several B group vitamins) and loss of taste (zinc). Physical examination of the patient may identify a number of signs suggestive of nutrient deficiency (see Tables 2.2 and 2.3).

Anthropometry

Anthropometry is a measurement and study of the human body and its parts and capacities and can provide information on body muscle mass, fat reserves and fat distribution. Unintentional weight loss during illness often reflects loss of lean body mass, especially if rapid and not caused by diuresis. Body mass index (BMI) alone is not ideal in determining health risk because it does not reflect the amount of muscle or distribution of fat mass. The waist circumference is a good indicator of abdominal obesity but it does not differentiate between visceral/internal fat (the one linked to chronic diseases) and the more inert subcutaneous abdominal fat. Convenient and inexpensive electrical impedance devices are increasingly being used by clinicians to determine muscle mass, fat mass, visceral fat and body water. When assessing health risks associated with a patient's weight, it may be useful to remember that higher weight in the elderly has been associated with lower mortality risk — staying in the 'normal' BMI range during young adulthood is recommended but slowly gaining weight during the elderly years does not seem to pose a health risk. On the other hand, obesity during young adulthood and being underweight during the elderly years leads to higher mortality rates.[14] Furthermore, if a patient does a lot of exercise but is still overweight this poses a lower mortality risk than being slim and unfit.[15] There is also emerging evidence of a subgroup of *healthy obese* that could be genetically determined or could relate to the dietary pathway in becoming overweight. For example, becoming overweight on a Mediterranean diet may not pose the same health risk as becoming overweight on a Western diet. This possibility has been identified in elderly Greek migrants in Australia that despite being overweight had lower mortality rates than their leaner Anglo-Celtic counterparts.[16]

Socioeconomic/lifestyle circumstances

Socioeconomic circumstances, in particular education, may highlight a financial inability to buy foods; for example, in situations such as gambling addiction or where there are poor kitchen facilities in which to prepare food.

Medications

A medication history may reveal possible drug nutrient interactions that lead to nutrient deficiencies or excesses. (See Chapter 37, Herb–nutrient–drug interactions.)

Some of the top nutrient-depleting drugs include: proton pump inhibitors and histamine receptor antagonists; loop and thiazide diuretics; corticosteroids; bile acid sequestrants; some antibiotics; oestrogens; anticonvulsants; benzodiazepines; aspirin; colchicine; laxatives; antacids.

Dietary history and assessing food and nutrient intake

A dietary history can be used to indicate whether the diet: may be under or oversupplying nutrients or energy; is made up primarily by easily digested, low nutrient, high-GI snacks; is low in plant food; or if meals are being skipped. A dietary history can be provided by the patient as a food diary in which the patient writes down everything consumed during a 7-day period. Alternatively, a dietary history can be taken from the patient by the clinician by asking the patient a few key questions about usual food intake over the last few days or months — this takes around 5–10 minutes. A food diary can provide a lot of useful data for the clinician but patients may change their food intake as a result of this process and the clinician may not get a true picture of the patient's food intake. Also, it is quite tedious going through pages of handwritten notes kept by the patient. For this reason many dietitians prefer the dietary history method, which gathers data on:

1. **Food distribution** across the day and if patients have a high protein food at every meal. A study in 867 of free-living individuals[17] reported that food intake in the morning created better satiety and was linked to a reduced total amount of food ingested for the day; on the other hand intake in the late night appeared to lack satiating value and resulted in greater overall daily intake. Consuming low energy dense high protein foods throughout the day can reduce overall intake by increasing satiety. In other words, this study suggests that it is not wise to under eat during the first part of the day and appears to be linked to circadian and diurnal rhythms.
2. **Food intake frequency and food portions**; for example, how many times a week do you consume red meat (Figure 2.1) and how large are the food portions — for example, is the meat serve the size of a deck of cards (= 100g) or is the cheese serve the size of a matchbox (= 30g) (Figure 2.2)? Another way to look at portion sizes is to use your hand. One serving of protein should be about the size of the palm of your hand or about ¼ plate. The recommended serving of green vegetables and salad greens could be the size of 2 fists (½ plate), while starchy items like potatoes or pasta should be served in a portion about the size of 1 tightly clenched fist (¼ plate). Finally, how closely do the patient's food servings resemble the recommended 'plate' servings (Figure 2.3).

A general dietary history from a patient can be obtained within 5–10 minutes. A more detailed dietary history using the information as in Figure 2.1.

1) FOOD DISTRIBUTION - describe basic foods eaten for main meals and snacks and identify how food is distributed across the day and whether patient has a tendency to skip meals e.g Breakfast: cereal + milk; Lunch: sandwich; Dinner: main meal; Snacks: fruit; ascertain food portions by comparing patient food serves to recommended "plate" *(Fig 2.3)*

2) FOOD FREQUENCY - How often does patient eat following foods on a daily or weekly basis? (this can be filled in by clinician or by patient)

TICK ONE box when ONE serving is consumed in a typical DAY or WEEK (for half serves draw a diagonal line through the box). **Shaded boxes indicate minimum recommended serves; unshaded boxes either indicates less is best or recommended serving has not yet been established or recommended serving may depend on medical condition e.g. eggs or energy requirements.**

DAILY INTAKE

Vegetables (except potatoes)									

1 serve= ½ cup cooked or 1 cup salad/raw (a minimum of 5 serves is required for an adequate diet, but more is good)
PS: a variety of different coloured vegetables recommended across week, especially dark green leafy vegetables

Cereal group (wholegrain only)									

1 serve = 1 thin (30-40g) slice bread, ½ thick/large (60g) slice bread, ½ medium bread roll, ¼ large pita bread, 3 wholegrain crispbreads, 1/3 cup cooked brown rice, ½ cup cooked wholemeal pasta or quinoa, ½ cup flake type breakfast cereal or ¼ cup oats/muesli or 2 wheat/oat breakfast biscuits PS: prefer wholegrain bread or crispbread to dry biscuits

Dairy/Ca fortified Soy/rice milk									

1 serve = 250ml cow's milk or goat/sheep's milk or calcium fortified soy/rice milk, ½ cup evaporated milk, 200g yoghurt (prefer reduced fat natural), 2 slices (40g) cheese (prefer reduced fat/salt), ½ cup (130g) ricotta, 150g tofu (calcium set) PS: cottage cheese is high in protein but low in calcium; rice milk is low in protein; custard/icecream have less calcium and more calories

Fruit (whole)									

1 serve = one average sized fruit, 2 small fruits, ½ mango, handful of grapes/berries/strawberries, 1 large wedge rockmelon/ watermelon, 1 cup honeydew or pineapple, ¾ cup canned fruit drained, 10 dried apricots, 1-2 tbs sultanas, 4 dried apple rings
PS: a minimum of 2 serves is required for an adequate diet, but more is acceptable

Added good fats									

1 serve = one tsp oil or oil spread = 5g fat (PS 1 tbs = 4 tsp or 20g fat), 25g avocado (⅛), 2tsp peanut butter/tahini.
PS: variety of different oils recommended, including extra virgin olive oil; a total of 40-80g fat can be eaten daily from added and hidden good fats

Sugar/Jam/honey									

1 serve = one tsp (PS 1 tbs = 4 tsp) (limited intake recommended)

Coffee									
Tea English									
Tea Green									

Water									

Treats									

1 serve = 3 plain sweet biscuits, 4 savoury dry biscuits, medium piece cake, 25g packet crisps, 30g milk chocolate, 1 scoop ice cream, 2 glasses soft drink, 5 lollies (limited intake recommended no more than 2 serves per day).

Figure 2.1 Taking a dietary history from your patient[18]

Copyright: Kouris-Blazos A 2010; adapted from Kouris-Blazos A & Wahlquist ML, HEC Healthy Eating Pyramid 2001, www.healthyeatingclub.org, 2001

WEEKLY INTAKE

Nuts/seeds/spread									

1 serve (or meat alternative) = handful (1/3 cup) nuts (prefer unsalted), 2 tbs (¼ cup) seeds, 2tbs peanut butter/nut or seed paste. PS: vegetarians need to eat nuts and seeds daily; one serving replaces a serving of meat.

Potatoes									

1 serve = 1 medium, ½ cup mashed

Pasta/Rice white									

1 serve = ½ cup cooked pasta, 1/3 cup cooked rice (limited intake recommended – prefer wholegrain, see cereal group)

Eggs									

1 serve (or meat alternative) = one large egg PS: up to 6 eggs a week recommended ; vegetarians need to eat eggs regularly; one serving replaces a serving of meat.

Fish									

1 serve = 150g cooked or canned (drained) PS: for adequate marine omega 3 intake fatty fish needs to be consumed 3 times a week (but may not be sustainble) or a fish oil supplement may be needed at 500mg EPA + DHA/day for all adults and children (or 1000mg for those with heart disease). If unable to eat fish then foods with high plant omega 3 recommended (linseed, chia seeds, walnuts, canola oil, eggs)

Red meat/Turkey									

1 serve = 100g cooked (size of palm of hand), ½ cup mince, 2 small lamb chops, 2 thin slices roast meat (no more than 455g red meat per week); PS: for adequate iron intake by premenopausal women red meat may need to be consumed 3 times a week or other high iron foods needed; for adequate zinc intake by male adults red meat/turkey may need to be consumed 3 times a week or other high zinc foods needed

Chicken									
Pork (fresh)									

1 serve = 100g cooked (e.g half chicken breast), medium pork chop

Processed meat									

1 serve = 50g (limited intake recommended)

Legume/tofu meal									

1 serve (meat alternative) = 1 cup cooked white beans/lentils/chickpeas/peas, 100g tofu/tempeh/TVP/nut meat etc.
PS: Try to include a vegetarian style meal with legumes at least once-twice a week; vegetarians need to eat legumes and/or nuts daily; one serving replaces a serving of meat

Fruit juice									

1 serve = 150 ml juice (no more than one serve recommended/day)

Dark chocolate									

1 serving = 15g or 3 small squares

Alcohol										

1 serving = 100ml wine, 300ml beer, 30ml spirit, 60ml sherry; no more than 1 standard drink for women or 2 for men recommended and must include 2 alcohol free days per week

Treats										

1 serving = see daily intake (limited intake recommended)

Fast food										

e.g fried food, hamburgers (limited intake recommended)

Figure 2.1, cont'd

Size Up Your Portions!

It's a good idea to measure foods so you know exactly how much you're eating. But if measuring cups or a food scale isn't available, you can estimate your portion size.

One fist is approximately 240 ml of cold and hot beverages, or 1 cup of broccoli or mashed potatoes.

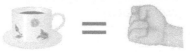

One hand cupped is about 1/2 cup of pasta, rice, polenta, hot cereal, grits, fruit salad, beans, okra, tofu, or cottage cheese, or 30 grams of nuts.

30 g =

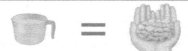

Two hands cupped is about 1 cup of cold cereal, soup, salad, and mixed dishes like casseroles.

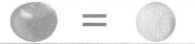

A deck of cards (or the palm of your hand) is about 90g of cooked meat, such as a hamburger patty, chicken breast, or fish fillet.

90 g =

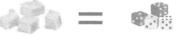

A medium apple or other fruit is about the size of a tennis ball.

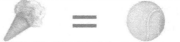

30g of cheese is about the size of 4 dice.

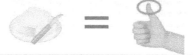

1/2 cup of ice cream or frozen yogurt is about the size of a tennis ball.

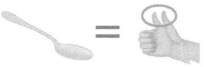

1 teaspoon of butter or peanut butter is about the size of the tip of your thumb.

Two thumbs together is about 1 tablespoon of peanut butter, salad dressing, sour cream, mayonnaise, or dip.

Figure 2.2 Estimating portion sizes[19]

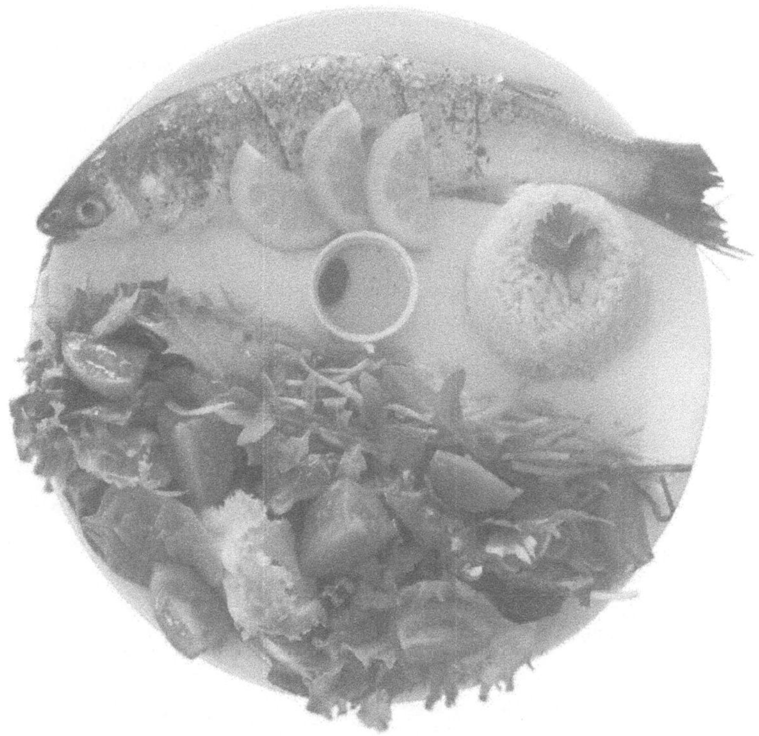

Figure 2.3 Recommended 'plate' servings
Photo: Antigone Kouris-Blazos

Servings: ***½ plate of vegetables*** **(1 cup cooked or 2 cups raw);** ***¼ plate starchy food*** **(1/2 cup pasta or 1/3 cup rice or 1 slice bread or 2 small potatoes);** ***¼ plate high protein food*** **(100g cooked red meat/chicken/pork or 150g cooked fish fillet or 250g whole fish or 1 cup legumes or 1 large egg);** ***1–2 tablespoons unsaturated oil; season food*** **with vinegar or lemon juice as this helps to lower the glycaemic index of the meal and flavour with herbs/spices (if using salt prefer iodised salt).**

Note: Serving food from a smaller plate (e.g. from a 30cm plate to a 25cm plate) can result in about 22% fewer calories being served as long as vegetable intake is not reduced (www.smallplatemovement.org).

Assessing food intake and nutrient intake

Various models and guides have been developed over the years to assess adequacy of food intake — not only with respect to obtaining an adequate intake of nutrients but also for health protection and promotion. Models and guides have been developed by:

- the Australian Government Department of Health (5 food groups in 1940s, food plate 1998)
- Nutrition Australia (formerly known as Australian Nutrition Foundation — Healthy Eating Pyramid 1980s)
- The National Health and Medical Research Council (NHMRC) core food groups (1995) currently being revised for a new food guidance system for Australia, (to be released in 2011)
- nutrition scientists developing their own tools, such as:
  - *the food variety checklist by Australian Professor Mark Wahlqvist (1989)*
  - *the Mediterranean diet pyramid developed in 1995 by American Professor Walter Willet*[20]
  - *the Healthy Eating Pyramid developed by the Department of Nutrition, Harvard School of Public Health, Harvard College (Figure 2.4) which*

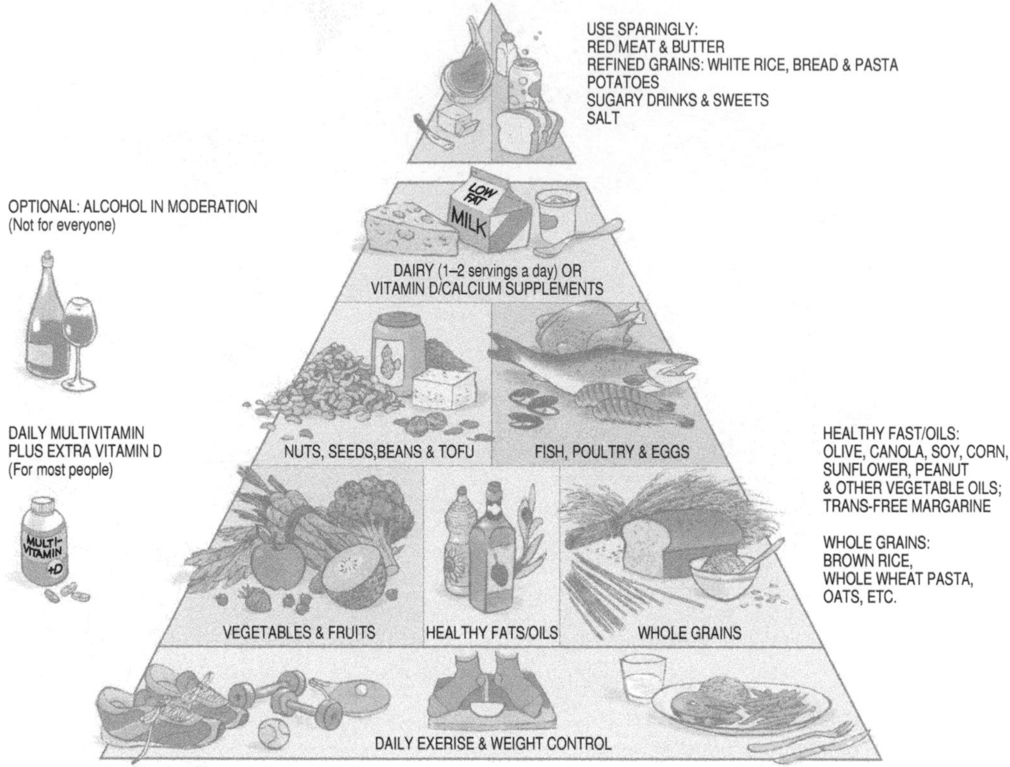

Figure 2.4 The Healthy Eating Pyramid[29]

Copyright © 2008. For more information about The Healthy Eating Pyramid, please see The Nutrition Source, Department of Nutrition, Harvard School of Public Health, http://www.thenutritionsource.org, and Eat, Drink, and Be Healthy, by Walter C Willett, MD and Patrick J Skerrett (2005), Free Press/Simon & Schuster Inc.

is similar to the Mediterranean food pyramid but emphasises foods known to have healing benefits, plant-based choices, variety and balance, support of a healthful environment and mindful eating.

The interest in the Mediterranean diet was reignited in the 1990s when a Greek-Australian team of researchers showed that adhering to the principals of a Mediterranean food pattern conferred longevity in people aged over 70,[21] especially when legumes were consumed.[22] The Mediterranean diet represents the dietary pattern that has been widely reported to be a model of healthy eating[23] that contributes significantly to a favourable health status[24], including prevention of diabetes,[25] cancer,[26] cardiovascular and heart disease[27] and even obesity/weight loss.[28]

The food serves calculated from the dietary history can be compared to the recommended food serves (shaded boxes in Fig 2.1). The closer the patient's intake is to the recommended daily servings for meat and alternatives, fruit, dairy, cereals, and vegetables the more nutritionally adequate it will be. To investigate the intake of particular nutrients, food composition tables or lists of good food sources of nutrients can be used (see Appendix 1). The adequacy of energy and nutrient intakes can then be compared to the recommended dietary intake (see Table 2.4 and Figure 2.5).

When the food and nutrient data is combined with other sources of information (e.g. clinical signs, laboratory tests) it can help confirm or rule out the possibility of suspected nutritional problems. A sufficient intake of a nutrient does not guarantee adequate nutrition status for an individual (e.g. medication or chronic diarrhoea may be increasing excretion of minerals) and an insufficient intake does not always indicate a deficiency, but such findings warn of possible problems. A variety of computer programs and patient questionnaires are available that permit rapid estimation of nutrient intake. These can be completed before or after the consultation, with the aid of practice staff. However, many of these nutrient analysis programs are based on food composition tables that have been periodically

Energy requirements = BMR (basal metabolic rate) x Activity factor

Basal Metabolic Requirements (Schofield Equation)

Answer is in kilojoules (divide by 4.18 to convert to kcal)

W = weight kg (use current weight or ideal/preferred weight)

	Men	Women
10–17 yrs	74W+2754	56W+2898
18-29	63W+2896	62W+2036
30-59	48W+3653	34W+3538
>60	49W+2459	38W+2755
60-74	49.9W+2930	38.6W+2875
Over 75	35W+3434	41W+2610

Activity Factor (AF)

Answer is in kilojoules (divide by 4.18 to convert to kcal)

BMR x 1.1 no exercise
BMR x 1.2 low exercise (less than twice/week)
BMR x 1.3 low-medium exercise (low intensity 3–6 times/week) e.g. walking 30 min
BMR x 1.4 medium exercise (medium intensity 3–6 times a week) e.g. walking 60 min or 30 min jog
BMR x 1.5 high (high intensity 3–6 times a week) e.g. gym

Calculating Protein Requirements
= ideal weight (kg) x 0.9 x Activity factor

ideal weight = 23 x (height in m^2) (ideal weight based on BMI of 23)

Figure 2.5 Calculating energy and protein requirements

updated for some foods but not all foods. For instance, the nutrient composition data for Australian fruits and vegetables is over 20 years old in the Australian food composition tables, therefore calculated nutrient intakes using these programs may not reflect actual intake.

There is emerging evidence from the UK and USA that there have been declining levels of many nutrients in fruit and vegetables over the last 50 years with magnesium levels dropping by 45%, calcium and iron levels dropping by 20%, copper by 80%, vitamin C by 20% and riboflavin by 40%. These changes have been linked to changes in soil quality and plant cultivars having a higher water content (referred to as the *dilution effect*) suggesting that crop yield may have been favoured over nutrient content.[30, 31, 32] Many Australians are not eating the recommended amount of fruit and vegetables and these data suggest we may need to eat even larger serves of fruit and vegetables!

Laboratory tests

The laboratory test will, to some extent, help the clinician confirm their suspicions and assist them in reaching a nutritional diagnosis. Sample nutritional testing may include those tests detailed in Table 2.5.[3, 34]

There are limitations in using plasma, serum or cellular conentrations of nutrients as these are subject to homeostatic control, tend to reflect very recent uptake or supplementation and not

Table 2.4 Recommended dietary intakes per day for men and women aged >19 years, 2006

	Men	Women	Upper level[1]	Undesirable or toxic level
Protein	70g	50g	15–25% energy	
Fat [2]	50–80g	50–80g	20–35% energy	
Saturated+Trans[2]	<30g	<30g	<10% energy	
Linoleic omega-6	13g	8g	5–10% energy	
Linolenic omega-3	1.3g	0.8g	0.4–0.5% energy	
DHA/EPA omega-3	160mg (610mg [3])	90mg (430mg[3])	3000mg	
Fibre	30g (38g[3])	25g (28g[3])		
Carbohydrate [2]	150–250g	150–250g	45–50% energy	
Water	3.4 L (2.6L[3])	2.8L (2.1L[3])		
Thiamin B1	1.2mg	1.1mg	20–25mg	Non toxic >25mg
Riboflavin B2	1.4mg	1.2mg	20–25mg	Non toxic >25mg
Nicotinic acid B3	16mg	14mg	35mg	>50mg
Nicotinamide			900mg	>1000mg
Pyridoxine B6	1.5mg	1.4mg	50mg	>200mg[4]
Cobalamin B12	2.4ug	2.4ug	1000ug	Non toxic >1000ug[4]
Folate	400ug (300–600ug[3])	400ug (300–600ug[3])	1000ug (from food & supplements)	Non toxic >1000ug[5]
Pantothenic acid	6mg	4mg	10–25mg	Non toxic >10 000ug
Biotin	30ug	25ug	30–70ug	Non toxic >2mg
Vit A retinol equivalents	900ug/3000IU (1500ug/5000IU[3])	700ug/2300IU (1220ug/4000IU[3])	3000ug/10000IU	>10 000ug >30 000IU
Carotenes	(5800ug[3])	(5000ug[3])		
Vit C ascorbic acid	45mg (220mg[3])	45mg (190mg[3])	2000mg	>2000mg

	Men	Women	Upper level	Undesirable or toxic level
Vit D D2/D3 cholecalciferol	5–15ug/200–600IU (19ug/800IU) if sun deprived need ≥25ug/1000IU	5–15ug/200–600IU (14ug/600IU) if sun deprived need ≥25ug/1000IU	80ug/3200IU	>250ug/> 10 000IU
Vit E a-tocopherol#	10mg/15IU (19mg[3])	7mg/10IU (19mg[3])	300mg/400IU	1000mg/1500IU
Vit K phylloquinone	70ug	60ug	?	?
Choline (lecithin contains Phosphatidyl Choline)	550mg	425mg	3500mg	>9000mg
Potassium#	3800mg (4700mg[3])	2800mg (4700mg[3])	?	?
Calcium	1100mg	1100mg	2500mg	>2500mg[6]
Phosphorus	1000mg	1000mg	4000mg	>4000mg
Zinc	14mg	8mg	40mg (take with 2mg copper)	>300mg
Iron	8mg	<50 yrs 18mg >50 yrs 8mg	45mg 100–200mg/ day to correct deficiency	>200mg
Magnesium	420mg	320mg	350mg (from supps only)	>1000mg
Iodine	150ug	150ug	1100ug	
Selenium	70ug	60ug	400ug	>900ug
Molybdenum	45ug	45ug	2000ug	
Copper#	1.7mg	1.2mg	10mg	
Chromium#	35ug	25ug	300ug	>600ug
Manganese#	5.5mg	5mg	?	
Fluoride#	4mg	3mg	10mg	
Sodium#	460–920mg	460–920mg	2300mg/ 100mmol 1600mg for HPT	

1 intake above the Upper Level (UL) may place individual at risk of adverse effects from excessive nutrient intake
2 based on 1500–2000 kilocalories
3 values in brackets are recommended for chronic disease prevention
4 some evidence that high intakes reduce kidney function and increase vascular event[36]
5 some evidence that high intakes are linked to cancer and reduced kidney function and vascular events[37]
6 some evidence that calcium supplements increase the risk of coronary heart disease in older women [33]

(Source: adapted from 2006 Revised Tables for Australia, National Health and Medical Research Council)[38]

All values are Recommended Dietary intakes or RDIs (except those marked with # =AI adequate intake) — intake at or above the RDI has a low probability of inadequacy

Table 2.5 Sample nutritional tests [3, 34]

Protein	serum albumin, TIBC, transferrin, urinary excretion 3–methylhistidine; Urea mmol/l: Creatinine umol/l ratio (the average urea/creat ratio is around 0.08 and the majority of results tend to be less than 0.15; values lower than 0.08 suggest low protein intake and values higher than 0.15 are associated with dehydration, high protein meals, excessive protein tissue catabolism, upper gastrointestinal tract (GIT) bleeds etc.)
Fatty acids	plasma and erythrocyte essential fatty acids
Carbohydrate	fasting insulin/hyperinsulinaemia, glucose tolerance test (GTT) (with insulin and C-peptide), HbA1c, fructosamine
Vitamins	
Vitamin A	plasma retinol/carotene
Thiamin (B1)	whole blood thiamin (preferred), plasma thiamin, erythrocyte transketolase activity before or after stimulation with thiamine pyrophosphate, erythrocyte thiamin diphosphate, urinary thiamin
Riboflavin (B2)	whole blood riboflavin, urinary riboflavin, percentage activation of erythrocyte glutathione reducatse by flavinadenine dinucleotide (FAD)
Niacin (B3)	urinary N1–methyl-nicotinamide or erythrocyte NAD:NADP ratio
Pyridoxine (B6)	erythrocyte pyridoxal and pyridoxine
Folate	erythrocyte folate
Cobalamin (B12)	serum B12 (does not pick up all cases of deficiency), urinary methylmalonic acid or holotrans-cobalamine or active B_{12} (more accurate)
Biotin	whole blood biotin, urinary biotin (more accurate)
Homocysteine	serum homocysteine
Vitamin C	plasma vitamin C, urinary vitamin C
Vitamin D	serum 25–OH vitamin D (preferred), serum 1,25 OH vitamin D
Vitamin E	serum tocopherol
Vitamin K	prothrombin time
CoQ_{10}	serum coenzyme Q_{10}
Antioxidants	serum or plasma total antioxidant status
Minerals	
Calcium	24–hour urinary calcium excretion, plasma ionised calcium, serum PTH, 25-OH vit D, bone mineral densitometry (DEXA)
Chromium	serum and urine chromium used clinically only to detect toxic levels
Copper	erythrocyte copper, serum copper, urine copper
Iodine	urine iodine/creatinine ratio (consistent hydration required to compare iodine in different urine samples); repeated urine samples (at least 2–3 samples) are needed to diagnose iodine status preferably taken at the same time e.g. morning urine, first void; iodine supplements need to be stopped at least 24 hrs before urine collection
Iron	serum iron, TIBC, ferritin, transferrin saturation

Continued

Table 2.5 Sample nutritional tests [3, 34]—cont'd

Zinc	24–hour urinary zinc excretion which allows some assessment of turnover, erythrocyte/leucocyte zinc, serum zinc (unreliable measure), plasma zinc (more reliable than serum zinc) together with serum albumin (an important zinc-binding protein which may affect values)
Magnesium	low serum Mg usually indicates a true magnesium deficiency but a normal serum Mg does not rule out a deficiency — up to 20% depletion without change in serum Mg (unreliable measure); erythrocyte/leucocyte Mg and 24–hour urinary magnesium excretion possibly better than serum Mg as it reflects intracellular Mg but normal or even elevated levels may occur in frank deficiency states; 24-hour urinary magnesium excretion after intravenous loading is the most accurate with an excretion level 80% of the infused amount being indicative of deficiency
Selenium	serum or whole blood selenium
Food intolerances*	no reliable blood test currently available to identify food intolerances — elimination diet currently best tool to identify foods/chemicals causing symptoms
Food allergy*	blood IgG levels for 40–93 foods — this is not a reliable test

*Skin prick for allergies and elimination diet and oral re-challenging test for food intolerances are considered gold standard.

longer term nutritional status. Supplements should be ceased a few days before blood testing.[34]

Nutritional therapy and micronutrients

Recommended daily intake

Micronutrients are nutrients, such as vitamins, minerals and essential fatty acids that are required by the body in small quantities (usually less than 1g/day),[35] as opposed to macronutrients that include proteins, carbohydrates and fats. This topic has been a controversial and highly debated area amongst leading nutritionists, but there is an increasing body of scientific evidence to support the use of micronutrients as therapeutic agents. There is no doubt in anybody's mind that our natural source of micronutrients should be from food. A diet of fresh fruit, vegetables, whole-grains, meats, legumes, raw nuts and seeds, and dairy foods (if tolerant to cow's, goat's or sheep's milk) should provide all of the necessary nutrients. However, as discussed, it is not always possible for individuals to obtain their required daily allowance of nutrients from food.

The National Health and Medical Research Council (NHMRC) updated its recommended daily intake of nutrients in 2006; the first time in 15 years.[39, 33] The update brings with it a new set of definitions. The recommended intakes are now referred as 'Nutrient Reference Values' (NRV). 'Estimated Average Requirements' (EAR) was established for all nutrients, which is the level estimated to meet the requirements of half of the healthy individuals in a particular life stage and gender group. If the data were normally distributed and sufficiently robust to calculate an EAR then a Recommended Dietary Intake (RDI) was defined as the EAR plus 2 standard deviations; that is, most EAR values are 20% less than the RDIs. When there were insufficient or inconsistent data to calculate an EAR, an Adequate Intake (AI) was set. The AI is defined as the median intake of a given nutrient as obtained from the National Nutrition Surveys of Australia and New Zealand. Furthermore, an Upper Limit (UL) was set for the first time for all nutrients that included intake from all sources and was based on the possibility of adverse effects. The NRVs also include a recommendation for an Acceptable Macronutrient Distribution Range or AMDR expressed in terms of total energy consumed. The AMDR for protein has increased allowing for a higher intake than previously recommended (up to 25% energy intake). There is also the Suggested Dietary Target (SDT) for chronic disease prevention for many micronutrients, fibre and omega-3 fatty acids for which there is evidence that intakes higher than EAR, RDI or AI may confer a health advantage. In the revised NRVs, the RDIs for the following nutrients increased: iron (for women only); calcium, zinc (for men only); magnesium; and B group vitamins. The RDI for vitamin E was changed to AI (and an SDT was set) because the key evidence, published in the early 1960s, does not allow for a valid analysis of the vitamin E dose-response curve.

A number of population studies and surveys have shown that the majority of people in the community fail to meet RDI levels for many common nutrients.[43, 41] For instance, the Commonwealth Department of Health, [43, 41] following a national dietary survey in 1983 on adults and in 1985 on children, concluded that there were problems of excess in the average Australian diet, particularly of sugar and fat intake, and a high prevalence of obesity. The studies indicated that a significant proportion of the population did not reach RDI levels. This was seen mostly in females, and in the Asian and Southern European population. Micronutrients that these populations were mostly deficient in included vitamins A, calcium, zinc and iron.

A survey of children and teenagers in 2007 continues to highlight the nutritional shortfalls of the diets of Australian children and teenagers, with less than 5% meeting the guideline for recommended vegetable intake and only 1% of teenagers consuming 3 serves of fruit daily when fruit juice was excluded (24% met the recommendation when juice was included) and egg intake was low at less than 2 eggs per week.[42] The study also reported the following average percentages of children aged 9–16 years not achieving the minimal EARs for key nutrients: calcium (60%); folate (15%); vitamin A (12%); magnesium (30%); zinc (10%); iodine (10%); and iron (3%). However, when intakes were compared to RDIs (or optimal intake) the percentage of children not achieving RDIs was much higher than those for EARs (since RDIs are about 20% higher than EARs).

Nutrient deficiency

There are various reasons for nutrient deficiencies occurring. One factor is over-consumption of processed and packaged foods, causing:[40]

1. destruction of the nutrient balance often inherent from the 'whole' food
2. loss of essential nutrients and bulk, especially complex carbohydrates and fibre
3. excess intake of total calories in the form of fats and refined sugars.

Nutritional deficiencies are becoming more common because of emerging food insecurity and the changing quality of the food supply, especially iodine, selenium, magnesium, zinc, and vitamin D. Special cultivars of plants that can absorb and bind organically greater amounts of these nutrients might be the answer in addressing nutrient deficiencies in plants rather than food fortification with micronutrients. Apart from food processing, risk factors for micronutrient deficiency also includes the following:[43]

- Decreased nutrient intake — stress, psychiatric disorders (e.g. anorexia, depression), crash dieters or people on chronic low energy diets for weight loss, poor appetite, food processing and lack of nutritious food, diseases of the mouth and chewing, chronic illness, sedentary lifestyle, alcohol and drug abuse. Decreased nutrient intake is found particularly in population groups such as: teenagers; vegetarians; those with allergies or sensitivities to particular foods; indigenous peoples; and the homeless and elderly, especially if institutionalised or in those that are house bound.
- Decreased absorption — chronic illness, thyroid disorders, gastrointestinal tract illness (virtually all, including irritable bowel syndrome), medication, alcohol and drug abuse.
- Decreased storage — liver disease, alcohol and fat storage disorder, chronic illness.
- Increased utilisation — a number of illnesses (e.g. recurrent infections), catabolic stress (trauma, major infection, surgery), chronic illness (cancer, HIV etc.), pregnancy and lactation, very heavy exercise, a number of medications (eg. anti-neoplastic drugs, colchicine, oral contraceptive pill, anticonvulsants, tetracyclines — see Chapter 37, Herb–nutrient–drug interactions), smoking, alcohol and drug abuse.
- Increased excretion — medication such as laxatives, anticonvulsants, diuretics (see Chapter 37, Herb–nutrient–drug interactions). Dietary fibre can bind minerals and increase their excretion.[5]

The problem with RDI levels is that it is based on the 'healthy' population. It does not take into consideration the 'unwell or sick' individual who requires significantly higher levels of micronutrients than the suggested RDI figures, and it is not designed to apply to individual needs (e.g. at times of stress, ill health, lifestyle factors etc.) that may vary with changing lifecycle patterns.

When there is disturbance of more than 1 of the above mechanisms together with a processed diet, there is an even greater risk of deficiency of nutrients in individuals.

Megadoses versus multivitamins

A Cochrane review based on a meta-analysis of 68 randomised primary and secondary prevention trials (n = 232 606) that tested antioxidant supplements concluded that high doses of vitamins A, E and b-carotene (but not vitamin C or selenium) can significantly increase all-cause mortality when given singly or with other antioxidant supplements.[44] This review, however, focused on antioxidant vitamins used at high doses rather than lower dose multivitamins. Furthermore, the review looked at 815 antioxidant trials but included only 68 of them in its analysis. Two excluded from this review (published in the Journal of the National Cancer Institute and the Lancet) found substantial benefits and reduced mortality from intake of antioxidant supplements. If these 2 large studies had been included, none of the reported effects on increased mortality would have been significant, with the exception of the effects of beta-carotene.

The research on multivitamin supplement usage is more positive and has prompted many nutrition experts to rethink their stance on this issue (see below). Several studies have shown taking low dose multivitamins can reduce health risks such as all-cause mortality, ischaemic heart disease and cancer in men but not in women (RR 0.63 in men versus RR 1.03 in women, in 13 000 French adults taking a single capsule daily multivitamin over a 7.5 year period), especially where the diet is of poor quality and lacking in nutrient-dense foods.[45] A study on people (n = 1056) using (1) multiple supplements (2) a single multivitamin supplement and (3) non-users of multivitamins produced some interesting findings. More than 50% of the multiple supplement users took a multivitamin, B complex, vitamin C, carotenoids, vitamin E, calcium/vitamin D, fish oil, flavonoids, lecithin, alfalfa, CoQ_{10} with resveratrol, glucosamine, and a herbal immune supplement. The majority of women also took evening primrose oil and probiotic and men took zinc, garlic, saw palmetto and a protein soy supplement. A greater degree of supplement use was associated with more favourable concentrations of serum homocysteine, C-reactive protein, high density lipoprotein cholesterol, triglycerides as well as lower risk of prevalent elevated blood pressure and diabetes even when confounders were controlled, such as education, income, BMI.[46] Another study on 8555 women from the US Nurses Health study showed that regular use of multivitamin supplements may decrease the risk of ovulatory infertility.[47]

Farvid et. al.[48] randomised 69 people with type 2 diabetes to 4 groups to receive 1 of the following daily supplements for 3 months: Group 1 200mg Mg, 30mg Zn; Group 2 200mg vitamin C and 100IU vitamin E; Group 3 minerals plus vitamins; Group 4: placebo. After 3 months Group 2 (vitamins) and Group 3 (vitamins and minerals) had improved glomerular (but not tubular) kidney function with reduced excretion of urinary albumin. Group 3 experienced additional benefits: reductions in systolic and diastolic blood pressure, fasting serum glucose and malondialdehyde concentration, increases in HDL cholesterol and apolipoprotein A1 levels. This study not only supports the use of multivitamins in diabetes but suggests a synergistic action of vitamin and mineral therapy with the combination achieving better results than vitamins or minerals alone.

Harvard University Healthy Eating Pyramid

Nutrition scientists at Harvard University School of Public Health developed their own version of a *Healthy Eating Pyramid* in 2006[49] based upon the best available scientific evidence linking diet and health independent of businesses and organisations with vested interests (see Figure 2.4). The Harvard University experts agreed that there was enough evidence to recommend a multivitamin daily (which appears alongside their pyramid). However, some scientists believe there is not enough scientific evidence to recommend either for or against taking a daily multivitamin.[50] The Harvard scientists argue this is a short-sighted point of view[49] since it may never be possible to conduct randomised trials that are long enough to test the effects of multiple vitamins on risks of cancers, Alzheimer's disease, and other degenerative conditions. They conclude that, balancing the weight of all of the evidence — from epidemiological studies on diet and health, to biochemical studies on the minute mechanisms of disease — the potential health benefits of taking a standard daily multivitamin far outweigh the potential risks.[51]

Prescribing micronutrient supplements

How can micronutrients be of help?

1. Micronutrients may be used to correct deficiencies in the unwell for relief of symptoms (Table 2.6).
2. Micronutrients have a therapeutic action as evidenced by increasing studies and are effective in the treatment of a number of diseases (Table 2.7).

When a plant is looking unwell, amongst other ways, we improve the quality of the soil by changing the soil (analogous to improving the food source) and adding fertiliser rich in micronutrients. We can use this concept as an analogy for improving human health.

Table 2.6 Circumstances that place patients at risk of nutrient deficiency and suggested supplementation

Food habits	Consider short-term (or long-term if food habits cannot be altered) low-dose supplementation with:*
At risk individuals (see Table 2.1), especially patients following reduced energy diets (<1500kcal/day) for several months, elderly, polypharmacy, GI disorders	Multivitamin, Ca, Mg, Fe, Zn, B complex, fibre
Not eating recommended number of food serves (but if eating vegemite will not need B complex) (see Table 2.4)	Multivitamin, Ca, Mg, Fe, Zn, B complex, fibre
High intake of sugar, refined carbohydrates/white flour, processed foods, pre-cooked meals, take away food	Multivitamin, Mg, Chromium, Zn, fibre
Excess alcohol	Multivitamin, Ca, Mg, K, Fe, Zn, Se, folate, thiamin and other B vitamins, vit C/D/E
Eating out more than twice a week for dinner, especially at fast food restaurants	Multivitamin, fibre
Fatty fish consumed less than 3 times a week	Omega-3 EPA/DHA
Low intake of animal foods (if 2 brazil nuts consumed daily Se intake adequate; if vegemite or bananas/walnuts/pecans/ potatoes consumed daily then B6 may be adequate)	Fe, Zn, Se, B12, B6
Total avoidance of animal foods and fish (vegan diet)	B12, Iodine, Fe, Zn, Ca, omega-3, vit D, vitamin A (some medical conditions affect conversion of beta carotene from plant foods to vitamin A)
Low intake of dairy or calcium fortified soy foods (<3 serves/ day) For food cultures that do not habitually consume milk products, a low intake of certain soup broths (soups made form bones can be high in calcium, especially if acid ingredients such as vinegar or lemon are used, which facilitate dissolution of bones), prawns, fish with soft bones, tofu Chinese cabbage, broccoli, and bok choy may suggest inadequate calcium intake)	Ca, B2
Low intake of dairy, eggs, carrots, sweet potato, dark green leafy vegetables and avoidance of organ meats (e.g. liver)	Vitamin A
Reduced carbohydrate diets or low intake of wholegrain cereals/ breakfast cereals (<3 serves/day), not compensated by adequate meat, fish, legumes, nuts	B1, Mg, Zn, Cr
Low intake of fish/seaweed (less than once a week), iodised bread, or use of un-iodised salt or un-iodised milo or multivitamin not containing iodine (especially important for pregnant/lactating women and children)	Iodine
Low intake of dark green leafy vegetables (<3 times a week) e.g. spinach, endives, kale, chickory, Chinese greens, nuts (<3 times a week), wholegrain cereals/breakfast cereals (<3 serves/day), legumes (<once a week)	Mg, Zn, folate, fibre

Low intake of fruit and vegetables	Vit C, folate, b carotene, Mg, fibre
Low intake of flax seeds, chia seeds, canola/soybean oil or spreads, walnuts, pumpkin seeds, tofu	Omega-3 linolenic
Low intake of unsaturated oils/spreads (<1 tbs/day) and nuts/ seeds (whole/spread) or fatty fruit (avocado) or sweet potato	Vit E, omega-6 linoleic Omega-3 linolenic
Low intake of eggs, fatty fish, sun exposed mushrooms, vitamin D fortified foods (milk, oil spreads), inadequate sun exposure (more important)	Vit D (deficiency can lead to reduced absorption of Mg, Ca, and Zn)

*Ideally, it is best to do blood/urine tests to check levels before supplementation is commenced but this may not be possible for some nutrients (because they may not be covered by public medical system or tests may not accurately measure nutrient levels in body). In this situation supplementation (with fortified drinks or capsules) should be low dose, around the RDI levels or below the upper tolerable level (Table 2.4). However, if blood/urine tests show deficiency, a much higher dose above the RDI will be needed.
Note: use this table in conjunction with Appendix 1 'Food sources of macronutrients, micronutrients, phytonutrients and chemicals'.
(source: www.healthyeatingclub.com)

Table 2.7 Some conditions(s) that may be prevented or improved with nutrient administration

Conditions	Supplementation
Prevention of neural tube defects in ongoing pregnancies[53, 54, 55]	B12, folate
Mood disturbance/insomnia,[56] depression, affective disorder[57, 58] Psychiatric disorders[58]	Vitamin C, E, folic acid B group vitamins (B1,B2, B6, B12) Biotin, nicotinamide Tryptophan, magnesium, vitamin D
Atherosclerosis, coronary artery disease, cardiovascular disease, stroke[59–68]	Omega-3 fatty acids (fish oils) Vitamins A, C, E Folate, vitamin D
HIV, AIDS[69, 70] (Improving T cell levels)	Vitamin A, Zinc micronutrients
Cervical cancer[71, 72]	Carotenoids, vitamins C and possibly E and D Folate and vitamin B12
Oral cavity and pharyngeal cancers[72]	Carotenoids, vitamins C and possibly E
Gastric cancer[73] Gastrointestinal cancer[74, 75]	Vitamins A, C, E Selenium, B6, vitamin D
Prevention of bronchial squamous metaplasia in smokers[76]	Folate Vitamin B12
Common cold[77–80]	Vitamin C, zinc
Respiratory infections in hospitalised elderly[79]	Vitamin C
Diabetes[81–85] Diabetic neuropathy[85, 87]	Vitamin C, E, magnesium Chromium, evening primrose oil, omega-3 fatty acids Gestational vitamin B6 Lipoic acid Vitamin B12, vitamin D
Infantile atopic dermatitis[88, 89]	Evening primrose oil (omega-6–GLA)

Hypercholesterolaemia[90, 91, 92]	Vitamin C, garlic
Acute measles[93, 94]	Vitamin A
Thyroid (low T3/4 ratio)[95]	Selenium, iodine, Zn, Fe
Miscarriage[96]	Selenium Zinc
Myocardial infarction[97–102]	Vitamins A, C, E magnesium, coenzyme Q10
Angina[101, 103, 104]	Beta–carotene, magnesium, vitamin E
Arrhythmia[105, 109, 110]	Selenium, magnesium, vitamin C Coenzyme Q_{10} Fish oils
Autism[106, 107]	Vitamin B6 Magnesium Vitamin C
Tardive Dyskinesia[108]	Vitamin E
Nausea/vomiting and vertigo during pregnancy[111, 112]	Vitamin B6 Multivitamin Multimineral
Chemotherapy-induced neuropathy[113]	Vitamin E
Parkinson's disease[114, 115]	Coenzyme Q_{10}
Bladder cancer[116]	Vitamins A, C, E Vitamin B6 Zinc, selenium
Poor sperm quality (esp. in smokers)[117]	Vitamin C, zinc, selenium
The elderly[117, 118]	Multivitamin Beta–carotene Vitamins C, E
Age–related macular degeneration[121]	Beta–carotene, vitamins C, E
Atopic eczema[122]	Evening primrose oil
Preterm delivery[123, 124]	Zinc
Short stature in infants, children and adolescents[124–126]	Zinc
Smoking[127]	Vitamin C
Iron deficiency[128]	Vitamin C
↓ risk of basal cell carcinoma[129]	Vitamin A, E
Fibromyalgia[130]	Magnesium, malic acid
Hypertension[131–136]	Fish oil (omega–3 fatty acids), coenzyme Q_{10}, magnesium, garlic Vitamin D

Preeclampsia/pregnancy induced hypertension[137–138]	Magnesium, calcium
Mastalgia[139]	Evening primrose oil, vitamin E
Hip fracture prevention[140, 141]	Calcium Vitamin D3
Osteoporosis[142]	Magnesium, calcium, vitamin D3 (>400IU/day)
Muscle soreness[143]	Vitamin C, vitamin D, magnesium, thiamin
Immune function[144–146]	Garlic, vitamin D, Zn Vitamin A Multivitamin/multimineral
Asthma[147, 148]	Vitamin C, antioxidants
Status Asthmaticus[149]	Magnesium (iv)
Hearing loss[150] (noise induced)	Magnesium, vitamin B12
Tinnitus[151]	Vitamin B12
Multiple sclerosis[152]	Vitamin D
Pulmonary function[153] (asthma, COAD, ARF)	Magnesium
Pulmonary hypertension in newborn[154]	Magnesium
Convulsions in preeclampsia[155]	Magnesium
Cataract[156]	Vitamin C
Acute pancreatitis[157, 158]	Sodium Selenite
Rheumatoid arthritis[159]	Omega-3 fatty acid (fish oils)
Coronary artery bypass graft[160, 161]	Vitamin E, A
Favourable lipoprotein profiles[162]	Vitamin C
Growth of infants small for gestational age[163]	Zinc
Tardive Dyskinesia[164]	Vitamin E
Lipoprotein profile (favourable)[165]	Vitamin c, fish oils
Recurrent herpes labialis[166]	Vitamin C, bioflavanoids
Mortality reduction[167]	Vitamin D

Note: For more detail see chapters in this book regarding specific conditions.

What if a patient presents with vague symptoms such as ‘tiredness’ and their dietary history reveals that their diet could be improved although a specific vitamin deficiency cannot be identified? What if the clinician feels they do not have time to provide dietary counselling and the patient can’t afford a dietitian? Is it acceptable to use a multivitamin supplement or fortified protein drink instead of, or in addition to, dietary counselling? The answer is yes but the clinician ought to solve the problem with food as often as possible. Some patients may need long-term supplementation if they are unable to improve their diet or if they have certain conditions or take certain medications.[11]

Cautions when prescribing supplements

One must be cautious when prescribing nutrients, especially in the presence of kidney and/or liver disease. In most cases, there are minimal side-effects. Table 2.4 provides upper safe levels for each nutrient.

In general, *avoid mega-dose vitamins and mega-fortified foods* (e.g. folate — see below) as these may have adverse effects. Vitamin D, vitamin B12 and iron are an exception, as many people need more than the RDA due to deficiencies identified in blood tests. Also *avoid 'super' supplements* which tend to have wild health claims — if they sound too good to be true, they probably are. Many vitamins and minerals operate in a synergistic fashion so it is best they are taken together rather than individually. Unless the diet is very poor, a low dose multivitamin can be taken intermittantly (a few times a week as a top-up) and it is probably prudent to take a break from a daily mutivitamin for a while. Long-term high-dose individual supplementation is not advised and it is preferable to increase patient's consumption of nutrient-dense foods before instituting long-term supplement therapy.

Vitamin E

The adult safe upper intake level (UL) for vitamin E is set at 400IU/300mg daily. Vitamin E has a blood thinning effect. In 1 study of 28 519 men, vitamin E supplementation at the low dose of about 50IU *synthetic* vitamin E per day caused an increase in fatal hemorrhagic strokes.[52] Based on its blood thinning effects, there are concerns that vitamin E could cause problems if it is combined with blood thinning medications, such as warfarin (Coumadin), heparin, clopidogrel (Plavix), ticlopidine (Ticlid), pentoxifylline (Trental), and aspirin. However, a study has shown that Vitamin E does not interfere with the anticoagulation response of warfarin.[166]

A study that evaluated vitamin E plus aspirin did in fact find an additive effect.[167] There is also at least a remote possibility that vitamin E could also interact with supplements that possess a mild blood thinning effect, such as garlic, policosanol, and ginkgo. Individuals with bleeding disorders, such as haemophilia, and those about to undergo surgery or labour and delivery should also approach vitamin E with caution. In addition, vitamin E might temporarily enhance the body's sensitivity to its own insulin in individuals with type 2 diabetes[168] but may raise blood pressure in people with diabetes.[169] Some evidence suggests that long-term usage of vitamin E at high doses (>400IU/day) might increase overall death rate, for reasons that are unclear.[170] Vitamin E may help to prevent heart disease in people with diabetes.[171] A number of these studies have used *synthetic* vitamin E and this may explain differences in safety between the studies. Also, ideally vitamin E should be given with vitamin C in order to allow vitamin E to function most effectively.[172]

Folate

A standard multivitamin usually has the RDI for folic acid, so one may need to avoid foods that have high amounts of folic acid added to them.

The US Institute of Medicine[173] recommends against obtaining more than 1000mg per day of folic acid from supplements or fortified food; folate intake from food is not a concern.[174] Excess folic acid supplementation can mask the signs of a vitamin B12 deficiency (up to 1 in 6 older people either don't get enough vitamin B12 or don't absorb it efficiently). Too much folic acid can hide the signs of anaemia, an early warning of a vitamin B12 deficiency. This could allow the problem to progress to the point of causing confusion, dementia, and/or severe and irreversible damage to the nervous system. There is some concern that too much folic acid can accelerate the growth of existing tumours and may increase the risk for colorectal, breast[175] and prostate cancer.[176] It is thought that folate can protect against colorectal cancer if commenced earlier in life.[177] Although these studies are limited, and other, similar studies have shown no association between folic acid and increased cancer risk, they sound a warning about consuming too much folic acid supplementation that deserves further investigation.

Vitamin C

The safe tolerable upper intake level for vitamin C from supplements and diet is 2000mg. Even within the safe intake range for vitamin C, some individuals may develop diarrhoea and abdominal discomfort which resolves on dose reduction. Long-term high dose vitamin C intake has not been linked with kidney stone formation but there may be certain individuals who are particularly at risk for vitamin C-induced kidney stones.[178] People with a history of kidney stones and those with kidney failure and who have a defect in vitamin C or oxalate metabolism should probably restrict vitamin C intake to approximately 100mg daily. High-dose vitamin C should also be avoided in glucose-6–phosphate dehydrogenase deficiency, iron overload, or a history of intestinal surgery.

Weak evidence suggests that vitamin C, when taken in high doses, might reduce the blood thinning effects of warfarin (Coumadin) and heparin. Heated disagreement exists regarding whether it is safe or appropriate to combine antioxidants such as vitamin C with standard chemotherapy drugs. The reasoning behind the concern is that some chemotherapy drugs may work in part by creating free radicals that destroy cancer cells, and antioxidants might interfere with this beneficial effect. However, there is no good evidence that antioxidants actually interfere with chemotherapy drugs, but there is growing evidence that they do not.[179]

However, new research on stem cells suggests that high (but not low) doses of antioxidants such as vitamins C and E can increase DNA damage, increasing potentially the risk of developing cancer.[180]

The maximum safe dosages of vitamin C for people with severe liver or kidney disease have not been determined. Large doses of oral or intravenous vitamin C in patients with renal impairment should be avoided.

Vitamin A, β carotene

Nutrient toxicity, especially with prolonged use, is a concern. Most supplements in Australia have warnings of this on their labels. For instance, signs of vitamin A toxicity include skin dryness. Vitamin A supplementation in excess of 2500IU per day in pregnant women is associated with fetal teratogenicity.[181] Beta–carotene is a safer form of vitamin A. However, beta–carotene in high doses should be avoided in smokers and asbestos-related lung disease as it may increase the risk of lung cancer in these situations.[182] This study has been criticised because *synthetic* β-carotene rather than the natural form was used.

Vitamin B6

High prolonged doses of vitamin B6 (>50mg/day) can cause headache, epistaxis and peripheral neuropathy (usually reversible, upon withdrawal of vitamin B6 although in some cases can cause permanent damage).

Zinc

The safe tolerable upper intake level for zinc from supplements and diet is 40mg. Long-term use of oral zinc at dosages of 100mg or more daily can cause a number of toxic effects, including severe copper deficiency and reduced iron absorption leading to anaemia, impaired immunity and heart problems. Zinc at a dose of more than 50mg daily might reduce levels of HDL cholesterol. In addition, very weak evidence hints that use of zinc supplements might increase risk of prostate cancer in men.[183]

Magnesium

The safe tolerable upper intake level for magnesium from supplements is 350mg. This level of daily supplemental magnesium intake is not likely to pose a risk of diarrhoea or gastrointestinal disturbance in almost all individuals. The initial symptom of excess magnesium supplementation is diarrhoea — a well-known side-effect of magnesium that is used therapeutically as a laxative. Individuals with impaired kidney function are at higher risk for adverse effects of magnesium supplementation, and symptoms of magnesium toxicity have occurred in people with impaired kidney function taking moderate doses of magnesium-containing laxatives or antacids. Elevated serum levels of magnesium (hypermagnesemia) may result in a fall in blood pressure (hypotension). Some of the later effects of magnesium toxicity, such as lethargy, confusion, disturbances in normal cardiac rhythm, and deterioration of kidney function, are related to severe hypotension. As hypermagnesemia progresses, muscle weakness and difficulty breathing may occur. Severe hypermagnesemia may result in cardiac arrest. However, there are some conditions that may warrant higher doses of magnesium under medical supervision.[184]

Selenium

The tolerable upper intake level for selenium is 400mcg/day based on the prevention of hair and nail brittleness and early signs of chronic selenium toxicity. Highly excessive selenium intake, beginning at about 900mcg daily, can cause selenium toxicity. Signs include skin rashes, a garlic breath odour, fatigue, depression, nervousness, emotional instability, nausea, vomiting, gastrointestinal disturbances and in some cases loss of hair and fingernails. Maximum safe doses of selenium for individuals with severe liver or kidney disease have not been established. There is some evidence that supplementing selenium over the long-term in areas where selenium is already adequate in the diet may increase the risk of diabetes and perhaps hypercholesterolemia.

Chromium

The tolerable upper intake level for chromium is 300µg/day. There is some evidence that if chromium is taken in high enough amounts, it may be converted from its original safe form (chromium 3) into a known carcinogen, chromium 6.[185] The risk of chromium toxicity (kidney, liver, bone marrow damage) is believed to be higher in individuals who already have liver or kidney disease. There are also several concerns about the picolinate form of chromium in particular. Picolinate can alter levels of neurotransmitters. This has led to concern among some experts that chromium picolinate might be harmful for individuals with depression, bipolar disease, or schizophrenia. Finally, there are also concerns, still fairly theoretical and uncertain, that chromium picolinate could cause adverse effects on DNA.[186]

Iodine

The tolerable upper intake level for iodine is 1100mcg/day. The World Health Organization warns iodine deficiency is widespread and contributing to worldwide health problems. Iodine deficiency is commonly found in Western countries and populations regarded as iodine sufficient. This emerging deficiency is due to a number of factors including depletion in soils, farmed fish and low intake of iodised salt. For instance, recent studies demonstrate almost half of all Australian primary school children are mild to moderately iodine deficient.[187]

Consequently, the Foods Standard Australia New Zealand now recommend Australians use iodised salt. Iodine is necessary for the synthesis of thyroid hormones. Consequently, severe iodine deficiency can result in hypothyroidism, goitre and cretinism. Borderline iodine deficiency may give rise to clinical symptoms of hypothyroidism without deranged thyroid hormone values, and give rise to sub-clinical thyroid dysfunction leading to health problems resembling hypothyroidism or diseases that have been associated with the occurrence of hypothyroidism such as obesity in adults and children, attention deficit hyperactivity disorder (ADHD), psychiatric disorders, fibromyalgia, neuropsychological consequences such as mental and growth retardation, learning difficulties, and possibly malignancies.[188]

Most food sources of iodine include seafood, iodised bread, iodised milo and iodised salt. The Japanese diet is high in kelp and seaweed which may also be an important factor contributing to low body weight in the Japanese population. Iodine deficiency (or borderline deficiency) may be a factor contributing to weight gain of some populations. According to US researchers, many prenatal multivitamins did not contain the recommended daily dose of iodine crucial for normal fetal neurocognitive development.[189]

Conclusion

So with the careful use of micronutrients, health practitioners are in an excellent position to prescribe supplements to some of our patients as an adjunct to aid healing where needed. It is encouraging to see a growing body of scientific evidence supporting this area of medicine although further studies are required before we can conclude their usefulness. In all circumstances, we must encourage a proper, varied, unprocessed diet as a natural source of nutrients. A multivitamin provides some insurance against deficiencies but is far less important for health than a balanced healthy diet.

Nutrition depends not only on food consumption but on energy expenditures associated with basal metabolic rate, the amount of physical activity performed, body composition, and metabolic conditions. Also there exists significant nutritional differences between individuals, age groups, lifestyles, lifecycles (pregnancy and lactation) and under different food consumption conditions. The nutrition–health relationship is primarily dependant on the capacity a human being has to adapt to and maintain metabolic balance throughout life. This adjustment is easier the more that the food consumed agrees with the functional capacity of the genetic profile and the interaction between nutrients–genes and the environment.[190] The greater the efficiency of the system the better the health achieved over longer periods of time.

Nutrigenomics is an emerging area of research where diet and nutritional therapy will one day be matched to a patient's genetic profile. Micronutrients which play a central part in metabolism and in the maintenance of tissue function may also require supplementation in other Western settings.

Nutritional assessments have an important role to play in lifestyle interventions for preventing disease and in chronic disease management. This is especially so in the elderly population, for example, where nutritional options that include micronutrient supplementations provide additional beneficial options, especially as the aged are particularly prone to inadequate nutritional status because of factors such as age-related physiological and social changes, occurrence of chronic diseases, use of medications, and decreased mobility.

References

1 Wahlqvist ML, Strauss B. Clinical Nutrition in primary health care. Australian Family Physician 1992;21:1485–92.

2 Kyle UG, Unger P, Dupertuis YM, et. al. Body composition in 995 acutely ill or chronically ill patients at hospital admission: a controlled population study. J Am Diet Assoc 2002;102(7):944–55.

3 Sydney-Smith J. Nutritional Assessment. J Comp Med 2006;28–40.

4 Australian Bureau of Statistics 2004–2005 National Health Survey: Summary of results. Report No. 4364.0. Canberra. ABS 2006. Online. Available: http://www.ausstats.abs.gov.au/ausstats/subscriber.nsf/0/3B1917236618A042CA25711F00185526/$File/43640_2004–05.pdf (accessed January 2009).

5 Larsen K, Ryan C, Abraham AB. The Secure and Sustainable Food Systems for Victoria, Victorian Eco-Innovation Lab (VEIL), Research Report no 1, University of Melbourne, April 2008. Online. Available: http://www.scribd.com/doc/6539650/Sustainable-and-Secure-Food-Systems-for-Victoria (accessed January 2009).

6 Burns K, Sacks G, Gold L. Longitudinal study of Consumer Price Index (CPI) trends in core and non-core foods in Australia. ANZ J Pub Health 2008;32(5):450–3.
7 Markovic T, Natoli S. Paradoxical nutrient deficiency in overweight and obesity: the importance of nutrient density. Medical Journal of Australia 2009;190:149–51.
8 Public Health Association Australia. A Future for Food: Addressing public health, sustainability and equity from paddock to plate. Online. Available: http://www.phaa.net.au/futureforfood.php (accessed Feb 2009).
9 CSIRO and The University of South Australia. 2007 Australian National Children's Nutrition and Physical Activity Survey. Department of Health and Ageing. 2008.
10 Fletcher RH, Fairfield, KM. Journal of the American Medical Association. 2002;287(23):3116–26, 3127–9.
11 Wahlqvist M, Kouris-Blazos A. Nutrition — is diet enough. J Comp Med 2002;1(3) Nov-Dec; 46–8.
12 Rutishauser I. Nutritional Assessment and Monitoring. In: Food and Nutrition. Allen & Unwin, Sydney, 2002.
13 Heimburger DC, Ard JD. Handbook of Clinical Nutrition (4th edn). Elsevier, Philadelphia, 2006.
14 Corrada MM, Kawas CH, Mozaffar F, et. al. Association of body mass index and weight change with all-cause mortality in the elderly. Am J Epidemiol 2006;163(10):938–49.
15 Lee CD, Blair SN, Jackson AS. Cardiorespiratory fitness, body composition, and all-cause and cardiovascular disease mortality in men. AJCN 1999;69(3):373–80.
16 Kouris-Blazos A. Morbidity Mortality paradox of 1st generation Greek Australians. Asia Pac J Clin Nutr 2002;11:S569–S575.
17 de Castro JM. The time of day of food intake influences overall intake in humans. J Nutr 2004;134:104–11.
18 Adapted from Kouris-Blazos A & Wahlqvist ML. HEC Healthy Eating Pyramid. 2001. Online. Available: www.healthyeatingclub.com (accessed Sept 2009)
19 Abbott Glucerna. Online. Available: http://glucerna.com./smart_nutrition/npwd.aspx (accessed Sept 2009).
20 Kouris-Blazos A. Dietary advice and food guidance systems. In: Food and Nutrition. Allen & Unwin, Sydney, 2002;532–57.
21 Trichopoulou A, Kouris-Blazos A, Wahlqvist ML, et. al. Diet and overall survival in elderly people. BMJ 1995;311:1457–60.
22 Darmadi-Blackberry I, Wahlqvist ML, Kouris-Blazos A, et. al. Legumes: the most important dietary predictor of survival in older people of different ethnicities. Asia Pac J Clin Nutr 2004;13(2):217–20.
23 Sofi F, Cesari F, Abbate R, et. al. Adherence to Mediterranean diet and health status: meta-analysis. BMJ 2008;337:a1344. doi: 10.1136/bmj.a1344.
24 Hu FB. Dietary pattern analysis: a new direction in nutritional epidemiology. Curr Opin Lipidol 2002;13:3–9.
25 Martínez-González MA, de la Fuente-Arrillaga C, Nunez-Cordoba JM, et. al. Adherence to Mediterranean diet and risk of developing diabetes: prospective cohort study. BMJ 2008;336:1348–51.
26 Benetou V, Trichopoulou A, Orfanos P, et. al. Greek EPIC cohort. Conformity to traditional Mediterranean diet and cancer incidence: the Greek EPIC cohort. Br J Cancer 2008;99(1):191–5.
27 Harriss LR, English DR, Powles J, et. al. Dietary patterns and cardiovascular mortality in the Melbourne Collaborative Cohort Study. AJCN 2007;86(1):221–9.
28 Shai I, Schwarzfuchs D, Henkin Y, et. al. Weight loss with a low-carbohydrate, Mediterranean, or low-fat diet. NEJM 2008;359:229–41.
29 For an online version of this pyramid go to www.thenutritionsource.org or http://www.hsph.harvard.edu/nutritionsource/.
30 Mayer AM. Historical changes in the mineral content of fruits and vegetables. Br Food J 1997;99(6):207–11.
31 White PJ, Broadley MR. Historical variation in the mineral composition of edible horticultural products. J Hort Sci and Biotech 2005;80:660–7.
32 Davis DR, Epp MD, Riordan HD. Changes in USDA food composition data for 43 garden crops 1950 to 1999. J Am Coll Nutr 2004;23:669–82.
33 Australian Government Department of Health and Ageing, National Health and Medical Research Council and Ministry of Health New Zealand. Nutrient Reference Values for Australia and New Zealand, Including Recommended Dietary Intakes. Commonwealth of Australia 2006. Online. Available: www.nhmrc.gov.au/publications (accessed Sept 2007).
34 Heimburger DC, Ard JD. Handbook of Clinical Nutrition (4th edn). Mosby Elsevier, 2006.
35 Helman AD. Vitamins, Mineral and Other Nutrients in Clinical Practice: a GP Guide Arbor Communications P/L Vic, 1991.
36 Andrew A et. al. Effect of B-vitamin therapy on progression of diabetic nephropathy: a randomised control trial. JAMA 2010;303(16):1603–9.
37 Ebbing M et. al. Cancer incidence and mortality after treatment with folic acid and B12. JAMA 2009;302:2119–26.
38 Pentti et. al. Use of calcium supplements and risk of coronary heart disease. Maturitas 2009;63(1):73–8.
39 National Health and Medical Research Council. Recommended dietary intakes. Australian Government Publishing Service (AGPS), Canberra, 1989.
40 Dept Community Services and Health. National dietary survey of adults: 1983. No. 2: dietary intakes. AGPS, Canberra 1987.
41 Dept Community Services and Health. National dietary survey of schoolchildren (aged 10–15 years): 1985. No. 2: dietary intakes. AGPS, Canberra 1989.
42 Martinez JA, Parra MD, Santos JL, et. al. Genotype-dependent response to energy-restricted diets in obese subjects: towards personalized nutrition. Asia Pac J Clin Nutr 2008;17:(Suppl 1):119–22.
43 Helman AD. Vitamins, Minerals and other Nutrients in Clinical Practice, a GP guide. Arbor Communications Pty Ltd, ISBN:0 646 07837.
44 Bjelakovic G, Nikolova D, Gluud LL, et. al. Antioxidant supplements for prevention of mortality in healthy participants and patients with various diseases. Cochrane Database Sys Rev 2008;April 16,(2):7176.
45 Herchberg S, Galan P, Preziosi P, et. al. The SU.VI.MAX Study: a randomized, placebo-controlled trial of the health effects of antioxidant vitamins and minerals. Arch Intern Med 2004;164(21):2335–42.
46 Block G, Jensen CD, Norkus EP, et. al. Usage patterns, health and nutritional status of long-term multiple dietary supplement users: a cross-sectional study. Nutrition Journal 2007;6:30.
47 Chavarro JE, Rich-Edwards JW, Rosner BA, et. al. Use of multivitamins, intake of B vitamins and risk of ovulatory infertility. Fertil Steril 2008;89:668–76.
48 Farvid MS, Jalali M, Siassi F, et. al. Comparison of the effects of vitamins and/or mineral supplementation on glomerular and tubular dysfunction in type 2 diabetes. Diabetes Care 2005;28:2458–64.

49 Online. Available: http://www.hsph.harvard.edu/nutritionsource/what-should-you-eat/multivitamin/index.html. Updated in 2008 (accessed Jan 2009).
50 National Institutes of Health State-of-the-Science Conference Statement: multivitamin/mineral supplements and chronic disease prevention. AJCN 2007;85:257S-264S.
51 Ames BN, McCann JC, Stampfer MJ, et. al. Evidence-based decision making on micronutrients and chronic disease: long-term randomized controlled trials are not enough. Am J Clin Nutr. 2007;86:522–3 (author reply 523–4).
52 Leppala JM, Virtamo J, Fogelholm R, et. al. Controlled trial of alpha-tocopherol and beta-carotene supplements on stroke incidence and mortality in male smokers. Arterioscler Thromb Vasc Biol 2000;20:230–5.
53 Kirke PN, Molloy AM, Daly LE, et. al. Materal plasma folate and vitamin B12 are independent risk factors for NTDs. Quar J Med 1993;86:703–8.
54 Wolff T, Witkop CT, Miller T, et. al. U.S. Preventive Services Task Force. Folic acid supplementation for the prevention of neural tube defects: an update of the evidence for the U.S. Preventive Services Task Force. Ann Internal Medicine 2009 May 5;150(9):632–9.
55 Molloy AM, Kirke PN, Troendle JF, et. al. Maternal vitamin B12 status and risk of neural tube defects in a population with high neural tube defect prevalence and no folic Acid fortification. Pediatrics 2009 Mar;123(3):917–23.
56 Benton D, Haller J, Fordy J. Vitamin supplementation for 1 year improves mood. Neuropsychobiology 1995;32:98–105.
57 Benkelfat C, Ellenbogen MA, Dean P, et. al. Mood-lowering effects of Trytophan depletion: enhanced susceptibility in young men at genetic risk for major affective disorder. Arch Gen Psych 1994;687–97.
58 Hofle KH. Magnesium in psychotherapy. Magn Res 1988;1:99.
59 Keli SO, Hertog MGL, Feskens EJM, et. al. Dietary flavinoids, antioxidants vitamins and the incidence of stroke. The Zulphen Study. Arch Intern Med 1996;156:637–42.
60 Hopkins PN, Wu LL, Wu J, et. al. Higher plasma homocysteine and increased susceptibility to adverse effects of low folate in early familial coronary artery disease. Arteriosc Throm Vas Biol 1995;15:1314–20.
61 Abbey M. The importance of vitamin E in reducing cardiovascular risk. Nutrition Reviews 1995;53(9):S28–S32.
62 Verlarigieri AJ, Bush MJ. Effects of d-a-Tocopherol Supplementation on experimentally induced primate atherosclerosis. J Am Coll Nutr 1992;11:131–8.
63 Cordova C, Musca A, Viola F, et. al. Influence of ascorbic acid on platelet aggregation in vitro and in vivo. Atherosclerosis 1981;41.15–19.
64 Bordia A, Paliwol DK, Jain K, et. al. Acute effect of ascorbic acid on fibronylitic activity. Atherosclerosis 1978;30:351–354.
65 Stampfer MJ, Hennekens CH, Manson JE, et. al. Vitamin E consumption and the risk of coronary disease in women. NEJM 1993;328:1444–9.
66 Rimm EB, Stampfer MJ, Ascherio A, et. al. Vitamin E consumption and the risk of coronary disease in men. NEJM 1993;328:1450–6.
67 Kritchevsky SB, Shimakawa T, Tell GS, et. al. Dietary antioxidants and carotid artery wall thickness. Circulation 1995;92:2142–50.
68 Stephens NG, Parsons A, Schofield PM, et. al. Randomised trial of vitamin E in patients with coronary disease: Cambridge Heart Antioxidant Study (CHAOS). Lancet 1996;347:781–6.
69 Baum MK, Shor-Posner G, Lu Y, et. al. Micronutrients and HIV-1 disease progression. AIDS 1995;9:1051–6.
70 Odeh M. The role of zinc in Acquired Immunodeficiency Syndrome. J Int Med 1992;231:463–9.
71 Flagg EW, Coates RJ, Greenberg RS. Epidemiologic studies of antioxidants and cancer in humans. J Am Coll Nutr 1995;14(5):419–27.
72 Alberg AJ, Selhub J, Shah KV, et. al. The risk of cervical cancer in relation to serum concentrations of folate, vitamin B12, and Homocysteine. Can Epidem Biomark Prevent 2000;9:761–4.
73 Hansson LE, Nyren O, Bergstrom R, et. al. Nutrients and gastric cancer risk. A population-based case-control study in Sweden Int J Cancer 1994;57:638–644.
74 Bjelakovic G, Nikolova D, Simonetti RG, et. al. Antioxidant supplements for prevention of gastrointestinal cancers: a systematic review and meta-analysis. Lancet 2004 Oct 2–8; 364(9441):1219–28.
75 Theodoratou E, Farrington SM, Tenesa A, et. al. Dietary vitamin B6 intake and the risk of colorectal cancer. Can Epidem Biomark Prevent 2008;17(1):171–82.
76 Saito M, Kato H, Tsuchida T, et. al. Chemoprevention effects on bronchial squamous metaplasia by folate and vitamin B12 in heavy smokers. Chest 1994;102(2):496–9.
77 Hemila H. Does Vitamin C alleviate the symptoms of the common cold? Scand J Infect Dis 1994;26:1–6.
78 Mossad SB, Macknin ML, Medendorp SV, et. al. Zinc gluconate lozenges for treating the common cold. A randomised double-blind, placebo-controlled study. Ann Int Med 1996;125(2):81–8.
79 Hunt C. The clinical effects of vitamin C supplementation in elderly hospitalised patients with acute respiratory infection. Int J Vit Nut Res 1994;64:212–19.
80 Prasad AS, Beck FWJ, Bao B, et. al. Duration and severity of symptoms and levels of Plasma Interleukin-1 Receptor Antagonist, Soluble Tumor Necrosis Factor Receptor, and Adhesion Molecules in patients with common cold treated with zinc acetate. J Infect Dis 2008;197(6):795–802.
81 Keen H. Treatment of diabetic neuropathy with gamma-linolenic acid. Diabetes Care 1993;16(1): 8–15.
82 Paolisso G, Balbi V, Volpe C, et. al. Metabolic benefits deriving from chronic vitamin C supplementation in aged non-insulin dependent diabetics. J Am Coll Nut 1995;14(4):387–92.
83 Thompson KH, Godin DV. Micronutrients and antioxidants in the progression of diabetes (Review). Nutr Res 1995;15(9):1377–1410.
84 Wilson BE, Gondy A. Effects of chromium supplementation on fasting insulin levels and lipid parameters in healthy, non-obese young subjects. Diabet Res Clin Pract 1995;28:179–84.
85 Jamal GA. The use of gamma-linolenic acid in the prevention and treatment of diabetic neuropathy. Diabet Med 1994;11(2):145–9.
86 Norris JM, Yin X, Lamb MM, et. al. Omega-3 polyunsaturated fatty acid intake and islet autoimmunity in children at increased risk for type 1 diabetes. JAMA 2007;298(12):1420–8.

87 Yaqub BA, Siddique A, Sulimani R. Effects of Methylcobalamin on Diabetic Neuropathy. Clin Neurol Neurosurg 1992;94:105–11.

88 Biagi PL, Bordoni A, Hrelia S, et. al. The effect of gamma-linolenic acid on clinical status, red cell fatty acid composition and membrane microviscosity in infants with atopic dermatitis. Drugs Exp Clin Res 1994;20(2):77–84.

89 Fiocchi A, Sala M, Signoroni P, et. al. The efficacy and safety of gamma-linolenic acid in the treatment of infantile atopic dermatitis. J Int Med Res 1994;22(1):24–32.

90 Ginter E. Pretreatment serum-cholesterol and response to ascorbic acid. Lancet 1979;2(8149):958–9.

91 Jain AK, Vargas R, Gotzkowsky S, et. al. Can Garlic Reduce Levels of Serum Lipids? A Controlled Clinical Study. Amer J Med 1993;94:632–4.

92 Warshafsky S, Kamer RS, Sivak SL. Effect of garlic on total serum cholesterol-A meta-analysis. Ann Inter Med 1993;119:599–605.

93 Rosales FJ. Vitamin A supplementation of vitamin A deficient measles patients lowers the risk of measles-related pneumonia in zambian children. J Nutr 2002;132(12):3700–3.

94 Frieden TR, Sowell AL, Henning KJ, et. al. Vitamin A levels and severity of measles: New York City. Am J Dis Child 1992;(146):182–6.

95 Olivieri O, Girelli D, Stanzial AM, et. al. Selenium, zinc and thyroid hormones in healthy subjects: low T3/T4 ratio in the elderly is related to impaired selenium status. Bio Trac Ele Res 1996;51:31–42.

96 Barrington JW, Lindsay P, James D, et. al. Selenium deficiency and miscarriage: a possible link. Br.J Obst Gyn 1996;103:130–2.

97 Singh RB, Niaz MA, Rastogi SS, et. al. Usefulness of antioxidant vitamins in suspected acute myocardial infarction (the Indian experiment of infarct survival-3). Amer J Cardiol 1996;77:232–6.

98 Brodsky MA. Magnesium, Myocardial Infarction and Arrhythmias. J Am Coll Nut 1992;11(5):607.

99 Millane TA, Camm AJ. Magnesium and the Myocardium. Br Heart J 1992;68:441–2.

100 Thogerson A, Johnson O, Wester PO. Effects of intravenous magnesium sulfate in suspected acute myocardial infarction on acute arrythmias and long-term outcome. Int J Cardiol 1995;49:143–51.

101 Hampton EM, Whang DD, Whang R. Intravenous magnesium therapy in acute myocardial infarction. Ann Pharmocoth 1994;28:212–19.

102 Gaziano JM, Manson JE, Ridker PM, et. al. Beta-carotene therapy for chronic stable angina. Circulation 1990;82:(Suppl. 111):111–201 abstract.

103 Rapola JM, Virtamo J, Haukka JK, et. al. Effect of vitamin E and betacarotene on the incidence of angina pectoris. A randomised, double blind, controlled trial. JAMA 1996;275:693–698.

104 Lehr D. The Possible beneficial effect of selenium administration in antiarrhythmic therapy. J Am Coll Nutri 1994;13(5):496–8.

105 Crestanello JA, Doliba NM, Doliba NM, et. al. Effect of coenzyme Q_{10} supplementation on mitochondrial function after myocardial ischemia reperfusion. J Surg Res 2002;102(2):221–8.

106 Dolske MC, Spollen J, McKay S. A preliminary trial of ascorbic acid as supplemental therapy for autism. Prog Neuropsychopharmacol Biol Psychiatry. 1993;17(5):765–74.

107 Martineau J, Barthelemy C, Roux S, et. al. Electrophysiological effects of fenfluramine or combined vitamin b6 and magnesium on children with autistic behaviour. Develop Med Child Neurol 1989;31:721–7.

108 Adler LA, Peselow E, Rotrosen J, et. al Vitamin E Treatment of Tardive Dyskinesia. Am J Psych 1993;150(9):1405–7.

109 England MR, Gordon G, Salem M, et. al. Magnesium Administration and Dysrhythmias After Cardiac Surgery: A Placebo-controlled, Double-Blind, Radomized Trial. JAMA 1992;268;2395–402.

110 Shepherd J, Jones J, Frampton GK, et. al. Intravenous magnesium sulphate and sotalol for prevention of atrial fibrillation after coronary artery bypass surgery: a systematic review and economic evaluation. Health Technol Assess 2008;12(28):1–118.

111 Vutyavanich T, Wongtrangan S, Ruangsri R. Pyridoxine for nausea and vomiting of pregnancy: a randomised, double-blind, placebo-controlled trial. Am J Obstet Gynecol 1995;173:881–4.

112 Czeizel AE, Dudas FG, et. al. The effect of periconceptional multivitamin-mineral supplementation on vertigo, nausea and vomitting in the first trimester of pregnancy. Arch Gynecol Obstet 1992;251:181–5.

113 Argyriou AA, Chroni E, Koutras A, et. al. Vitamin E for prophylaxis against chemotherapy-induced neuropathy: a randomized controlled trial. Neurology 2005;64:26–31.

114 Shults CW, Oakes D, Kieburtz K, et. al. Effects of coenzyme Q_{10} in early Parkinson disease: evidence of slowing of the functional decline. Archives of Neurology 2002;59:1541–50.

115 Shults CW, et. al. Effects of coenzyme Q_{10} in early Parkinson disease: evidence of slowing of the functional decline. Arch Neurol 2002, 59:1541–50.

116 Lamm D, Riggs DR, Shriver JS, et. al. Megadose vitamins in bladder cancer: a double-blind clinical trial. J Urol 1994;141:21–6.

117 Dawson EB, Harris WA, Teter MC, et. al. Effect of ascorbic acid supplementation on the sperm quality of smokers. Fertility and Sterility 1992;58:1034–9.

118 Heseker H, Schneider R. Requirement and supply of Vitamin C, E and betacarotene for elderly men and women. Eur J Cli Nut 1994;13:57–61.

119 Roebothan BV, Chandra RK. Relationship between nutritional status and immune function of elderly people. Age and Ageing 1994;23:49–53.

120 Woo J, Ho Sc, et. al. Nutritional status of elderly patients during recovery from chest infection and the role of nutritional supplementation assessed by a prospective randomised single blind trial. Age and Ageing 1994;23:40–8.

121 West S, Vitale S, Hallfrisch J, et. al. Are antioxidants or supplements protective for age related macular degeneration? Arch Opthalmol 1994;112:222–7.

122 Schanlin-Karrila M, Mattila L, Jansen CT, et. al. Evening primrose oil in the treatment of atopic eczema: effect on clinical status, plasma phospholipid fatty acids and circulating blood prostaglandins. B J Dermatol 1987;117:11–19.

123 Scholl TO, Hediger ML, Schall JL, et. al. Low zinc intake during pregnancy: its association with preterm and very preterm delivery. Am J Epid 1993;137:1115–23.

124 Simmer K, Lort-Phillips L, James C, et. al. A double-blind trial of zinc supplementation in pregnancy. Eur J Clin Nutr 1991, 45:139–144.

125 Apgar J. Zinc and reproduction: an update. J Nutr Biochem 1992;3: 266–77.

126 Castilloduran C, Garcia H, Venegas P, et. al. Zinc supplementation increases growth velocity of male children and adolescents with short stature. Acta Paediatrica 1994;83:833–7.

127 Schectman G, Byrd JC, Hoffmann R. Ascorbic acid requirements for smokers: analysis of a population survey. Am J Clin Nutr 1991;53:1466–70.
128 Hunt JR, Gallagher SK, Johnson LK. Effect of ascorbic acid on apparent iron absorption by women with low iron stores. Am J Clin Nutr 1994;59:1381–5.
129 Wei Q, Matanoski G, et. al. Vitamin supplementation and reduced risk of basal cell carcinoma. J Clin Epidem 1994;47:829–36.
130 Abraham GE, Glechas JD. Management of fibromyalgia: rationale for the use of magnesium and malic acid. J Nut Med 1992;3:49–59.
131 Digiesi V, Cantini F, Oradei A, et. al. coenzyme Q_{10} in essential hypertension. Mol Aspects Med 1994;15:s257–63.
132 Shibutani Y, Sakamoto K, Katsuno S, et. al. Relation of serum and erythrocyte magnesium levels to blood pressure and a family history of hypertension. ACTA Paeditr Scand 1990;79:316–21.
133 Champagne CM. Magnesium in hypertension, cardiovascular disease, metabolic syndrome, and other conditions: a review. Nutr Clin Pract 2008;23(2):142–51.
134 Appel LJ, Miller ER III, Seidler AJ, et. al. Does supplementation of diet with 'fish oil' reduce blood pressure? A meta-analysis of controlled clinical trials. Arch Intern Med 1993;153:1429–38.
135 Silagy C, Neil A. A meta-analysis of the effect of garlic on blood pressure. J Hypertension 1994; 463–8.
136 Witteman JCM, Grobbee DE, Derk FHM, et. al. Reduction of blood pressure with oral magnesium supplementation in women with mild to moderate hypertension. Am Clin Nutr 1994;60:129–35.
137 Bucher HC, Guyatt GH, Cook RJ. Effect of calcium supplementation on pregnancy-induced hypertension and preeclampsia. A meta-analysis of randomized controlled trials. JAMA 1996;275:1113–17.
138 Gateley CA, Miers M, Mansel RE, et. al. Drug treatments for mastalgia: 17 years experience in the Cardiff Mastalgia Clinic. J R Soc Med 1992;85(1):12–15.
139 Jackson C, Gaugris S, Sen SS, Hosking D. The effect of cholecalciferol (vitamin D3) on the risk of fall and fracture: a meta-analysis. QJM 2007;100(4):185–92.
140 Chapuy MC, Arlot ME, Duboeuf F, et. al. Vitamin D and calcium to prevent hip fractures in elderley women. NEJM 1992;327(23):1637–42.
141 Sojka JE. Magnesium supplementation and osteoporosis. Nutr Rev 1995;53:71–4.
142 Kaminski M, Boal R. An effect of ascorbic acid on delayed-onset muscle soreness. Pain 1992;50:317–21.
143 Semba, Richard D, et. al. Abnormal T-Cell subset proportions in vitamin-a deficient children. Lancet 1993 Jan 2;341:5–8.
144 Chandra RK. Effect of vitamin and trace element supplementation on immune responses and infection in elderly subjects. Lancet 1992;340:1124–7.
145 Brosche T, Platt D. On the Immunomodulatory action of garlic (Allium sativum L.). Medizinische Welt 1993;44:309–13.
146 Hatch GE. Asthma, inhaled oxidants and dietary antioxidants. Amer J Clin Nutr 1995;61:625S-30S.
147 Bielory L, Rinki G. Asthma and vitamin C. Ann Aller 1994;73:89–96.
148 Sydow M, Crozier TA, Zielmann S, et. al. High-dose intravenous magnesium sulfate in the management of life-threatening Status Asthmaticus. Intens Care Med 1993;19:467–71.
149 Attias J, Weisz G, Almog S, et. al. Oral magnesium intake reduces permanent hearing loss by noise exposure. Amer J Otolaryng 1994;15:26–32.
150 Shemesh Z, Attias J, Ornan M, et. al. Vitamin B12 deficiency in patients with chronic tinnitus and noise-induced hearing loss. Amer J Otolaryng 1993;14(2):94–9.
151 Munger KL, Zhang SM, O'Reilly E, et. al. Vitamin D intake and incidence of multiple sclerosis. Neurology 2004;62(1):60–5.
152 Landon RA, Young EA. Role of magnesium in regulation of lung function. J Amer Diet Assoc 1993;93(6):674–7.
153 Abu-Osba YK, Galal O, Manasra K, et. al. Treatment of severe persistent pulmonary hypertension in the newborn with magnesium sulfate. Arch of Dis in Child 1992;67:31–5.
154 Sibai BM. Magnesium sulfate is the ideal anticonvulsant in preeclampsia. Am J Obst Gyn 1990;162:1141–5.
155 Hankinson SE, et. al. Nutrient intake and cataract extraction in women: a prospective study. BMJ 1992;305:335–9.
156 Kuklinski, B, Zimmermann T, Schweder R. Reducing the lethality in acute pancreatitis with sodium selenite. Med Klin 1995;90:36–41.
157 Kuklinski, B, Buchner M, Schweder R, et. al. Acute pancreatitis. A free radical disease. decrease of lethality by sodium selenite therapy. Z Gesamte Inn Med 1991;46:S145–S149.
158 Geusens P, Wouters C, et. al. Long-term effect of omega-3–fatty acid supplementation in active rheumatoid arthritis. Arthr Rheum 1994;37:824–9.
159 Yau TM, Weisel RD, Mickle DAG, et. al. Vitamin E for coronary bypass operations. A prospective, double-blind, radomized trial. J Thorac Cardiovasc Surg 1994;108:302–10.
160 Ferreira RF, Milei J, Llesuy S, et. al. Antioxidant action of vitamins A and E in patients submitted to coronary artery bypass surgery. Vascular Surgery 1991;25:191–5.
161 Knekt P, Reunanen A, et. al. Antioxidant vitamin intake and coronary mortality in a longitudinal population study. Am J Epidemiol 1994;139: 1180–9.
162 Castilloduran C, Rodriguez A, Venegas G, et. al. Zinc supplementation and growth of infants born small for gestational age. J. Paediatrics 1995;127:206–11.
163 Lohr JB, Caligiuri MP. A double-blind placebo-controlled study of vitamin E treatment of tardive dyskinesia. J of Clin Psych 1996;57:4:167–73.
164 Gatto LM, Hallen GK, Brown AJ, et. al. Ascorbic acid induces a favourable lipoprotein profile in women. J Amer Coll Nutr 1996;15(2):154–8.
165 Terezhalmy GT. The use of water-soluble bioflavinoid-ascorbic acid complex in the treatment of recurrent Herpes Labialis. Oral Surgery 1978;45(1)56–62.
166 Autier P, Gandini S. Vitamin D supplementation and total mortality: a meta-analysis of randomized controlled trials. Arch Intern Med 2007;167(16):1730–7.
167 Kim JM, White RH. Effect of vitamin E on the anticoagulant response to warfarin. Am J Cardiol 1996;77(7):545–6.
168 Liede KE, Haukka JK, Saxen LM, et. al. Increased tendency towards gingival bleeding caused by joint effect of alpha-tocopherol supplementation and acetylsalicylic acid. Ann Med 1998;30:542–6.

169 Paolisso G, D'Amore A, Giugliano D, et. al. Pharmacologic doses of vitamin E improve insulin action in healthy subjects and non-insulin-dependent diabetic patients. AJCN 1993;57:650–6.
170 Ward NC, Hodgson JM, Puddey IB, et. al. Vitamin E increases blood pressure in type 2 diabetic subjects, independent of vascular function and oxidative stress. Asia Pac J Clin Nutr 2005;14(suppl):S41.
171 Bjelakovic G, Nikolova D, Gluud LL, et. al. Mortality in randomized trials of antioxidant supplements for primary and secondary prevention: systematic review and meta-analysis. JAMA 2007;297:842–57.
172 Milman U, Blum S, Shapira C, et. al. Vitamin E supplementation reduces cardiovascular events in a subgroup of middle-aged individuals with both type 2 diabetes mellitus and the haptoglobin 2–2 genotype. A prospective double-blinded clinical trial. Arterioscler Thromb Vasc Biol 2007:ATVBAHA.107.153965.
173 Burke KE. Interaction of vitamins C and E as better cosmeceuticals. Dermatol Ther 2007;20(5):314–21.
174 Institute of Medicine. Dietary Reference Intakes for Thiamin, Riboflavin, Niacin, Vitamin B6, Folate, Vitamin B12, Pantothenic Acid, Biotin, and Choline. National Academy Press, Washington, DC, 1999.
175 Cole BF, Baron JA, Sandler RS, et. al. Folic acid for the prevention of colorectal adenomas: a randomized clinical trial. JAMA 2007;297:2351–9.
176 Mason JB, Dickstein A, Jacques PF, et. al. A temporal association between folic acid fortification and an increase in colorectal cancer rates may be illuminating important biological principles: a hypothesis. Cancer Epidem Biom Prevent 2007;16:1325–9.
177 Stevens VL, Rodriguez C, Pavluck AL, et. al. Folate nutrition and prostate cancer incidence in a large cohort of US men. Amer J Epidemiol 2006; 163:989–96.
178 Hubner RA, Houlston RS. Folate and colorectal cancer prevention. Br J Cancer 2009;100(2):233–9.
179 Wandzilak, T, D'Andre S, Davis P, et. al. Effect of High Dose Vitamin C on Urinary Oxalate Levels. J Urol 1994;151: 834–7.
180 Drisko JA, Chapman J, Hunter VJ. The use of antioxidant therapies during chemotherapy. Gynecol Oncol 2003;88:434–9.
181 Li TS, Marban E. Physiological levels of reactive oxygen species are required to maintain genomic stability in stem cells. Stem Cells 2010; 4 May.
182 Underwood B. Maternal Vitamin A status and its importance in infancy and early childhood. Am J Clin Nutr 1994;59:517S–24S.
183 Bardia A, Imad M, Tleyjey IM, et. al. Mayo Foundation for Medical Education and Research efficacy of antioxidant supplementation in reducing primary cancer incidence and mortality: systematic review and meta-analysis. Mayo Clin Proc 2008;83:23–34.
184 Leitzmann MF, Stampfer MJ, Wu K, et. al. Zinc supplement use and risk of prostate cancer. JNCI 2003;95:1004–7.
185 Food and Nutrition Board, Institute of Medicine. Magnesium. Dietary Reference Intakes: Calcium, Phosphorus, Magnesium, Vitamin D, and Fluoride. National Academy Press, Washington DC, 1997:190–249. [National Academy Press].
186 Food and Nutrition Board, Institute of Medicine. Chromium. Dietary Reference Intakes for Vitamin A, Vitamin K, Boron, Chromium, Copper, Iodine, Iron, Manganese, Molybdenum, Nickel, Silicon, Vanadium, and Zinc. National Academy Press, Washington DC, 2001:197–223.
187 Mulyani I, Levina A, Lay PA. Biomimetic oxidation of chromium (III): Does the antidiabetic activity of chromium (iii) involve carcinogenic chromium(vi). Angew Chem Int Ed Engl. 2004;43:4504–7.
188 The prevalence and severity of iodine deficiency in Australia. Prepared for the Australian Population Health Development Principal Committee of the Australian Health Ministers Advisory Committee December, 2007. Online. Available: http://www.foodstandards.gov.au/_srcfiles/Item%2002%2005%20–%20Attachment%201%20–%20%20Prevalence%20and%20severity%20of%20iodine%20deficiency%20in%20Australia.pdf#search=%22iodine%22 (accessed 02-02-09).
189 Verheesen RH, Schweitzer CM. Iodine deficiency, more than cretinism and goiter. Med Hypotheses 2008 November;5(71):645–8.
190 New England J of Med 2009;360:939–40.
191 Gorduza EV, Indrei LL, Gorduza VM. Nutrigenomics in postgenomic era. Rev Med Chir Soc Med Nat Iasi 2008;112(1):152–64.

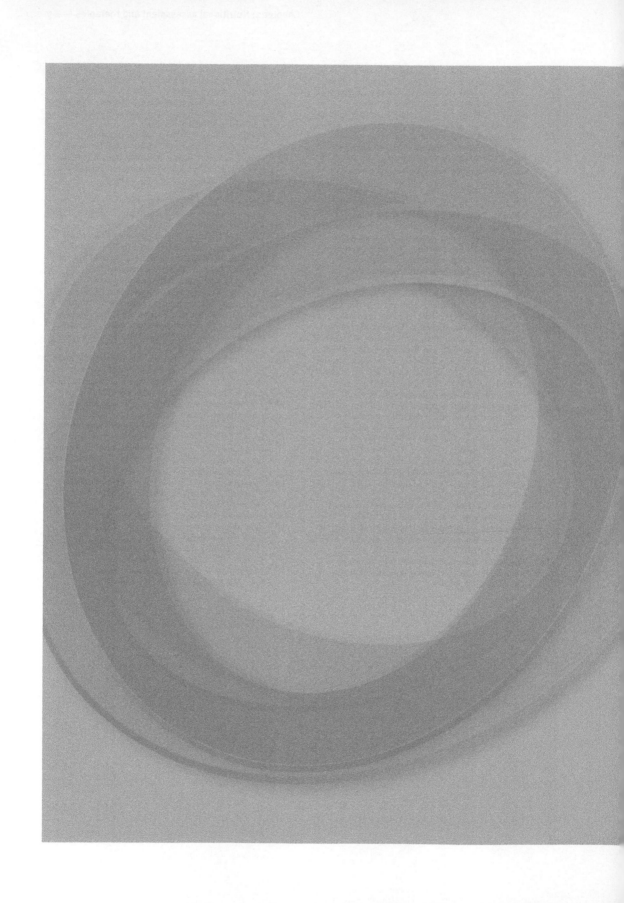

Part 2

Integrative and complementary approaches to common clinical problems

Chapter 3

Age-related macular degeneration (AMD) and cataracts

Introduction

AMD

Age-related macular degeneration (AMD) and cataracts are the 2 leading eye diseases of advanced age. AMD is the leading cause of blindness in the elderly worldwide, affecting 30–50 million people. The World Health Organization (WHO) statistics from the most recent WHO global eye disease surveys conducted in 2002 reported that 8.7% of worldwide blindness was due to AMD, the third leading cause of worldwide blindness after cataract and glaucoma.[1] Conservatively, the WHO has estimated that 14 million persons worldwide could be blind or severely visually impaired because of AMD.[2, 3] The majority of these impaired individuals and the millions more who are visually impaired from this condition live in developed countries.

The large population-based Beaver Dam Eye Study discovered that the prevalence of large extracellular ocular deposits known as drusen, a hallmark sign of AMD, was 2% in persons 43–54 years of age and 24% in persons over 75 years of age in the US.[4] It has also been reported that late AMD is the most common cause of untreatable blindness in the Western world, with a prevalence that is 0.05% before the age of 50 years and that rises to 11.8% after 80 years of age.[5]

Numerous large population studies have identified important factors as to the epidemiology of AMD. The Age-Related Eye Disease Study (AREDS) found that 20.2% of individuals with an early stage diagnosis of AMD progressed to advanced disease over a 5-year period, a rate of 4.0% per year. Similar annual rates of progression, between 2.5% and 4.8%, were reported in the Rotterdam Study and Blue Mountains Eye Study (BMES) respectively.[6, 7] Recently a report by Taylor and colleagues estimated that the progression rate for mild to moderate visual impairment was approximately 32%, and that the rate from moderate to severe visual impairment was 46%.[8] The basis for this estimate was derived from the 2–3 year progression data that originated from the Macular Photocoagulation Study (MPS), the Treatment of AMD with Photodynamic Therapy (TAP) study and the Vertiporfin in Photodynamic (VIP) Therapy study. These reported rates are slightly higher than the rates of 16% and 17% per year reported by the Melbourne Visual Impairment Project (MVIP) study. Taylor and colleagues also showed that the incidence of mild visual impairment in individuals who were 40 years or older was 0.10% per year and, for moderate and severe visual impairment in this same group, it was 0.04% and 0.11% per year, respectively.[9]

However, as life expectancies are observed to increase in all parts of the world the prevalence of AMD is also expected to increase. It is likely that in the following decades, many millions of people worldwide will suffer blindness or severe visual impairment from AMD.[10–17]

Cataracts

A recent review has reported that *cataract*, (opacification of the lens) is one of the commonest causes of loss of useful vision, with an estimated prevalence of 16 million people affected worldwide.[18] Prevalence studies for cataract are made difficult by a lack of uniform grading scores for the clinically observed opacities of the lens. Several population studies have been reported though, that demonstrate an increasing risk for cataract development with increasing age.[19, 20, 21,]

The Framingham Eye Study from the US, reported in 1977,[19] that the proportion of people with age-related cataracts causing loss of vision of 20/30 (6/9) or worse was 15·5% for all ages and 45·9% for those 75 years or older. In the 1992 Beaver Dam Eye Study,[20, 21] which used a similar definition of loss of vision, the reported proportions were 38·8% of men and 45·9% of women older than 74 years.

Data from other studied populations demonstrate a wide range of rates, such as 82% of 75–85 year olds in India and 53% of 75–85 year olds in Tibet.[22, 23]

Lifestyle and lifetime risk factors

A recent report by the US Preventive Services Task Force has identified a number of risk factors for the prevention of AMD and cataracts (Table 3.1).[24]

The reviewed epidemiological literature conclusively reports that the older ages are causal for the development of AMD and cataracts.[22, 25]

Genetic predispositions

Family history, white race, black race

Family history is a consistent risk factor identified in most epidemiological studies of AMD that have been conducted. Familial aggregation studies have shown that there is a genetic contribution that has been readily identified in up to 25% of AMD cases.[26] Moreover, studies with twins also support a genetic basis for the disease, with the concordance of clinical features (i.e. drusen and pigmentary changes) for both early and late onset of the disease being approximately twice as high in identical (monozygotic) twins compared to non-identical (dizygotic) twins.[27, 28]

Numerous population studies have investigated the racial differences observed in the prevalence of AMD.[29, 30, 31] Recently, in an eye disease prevalence investigation Bressler et. al.[32] have described the differences in frequency of early fundus lesions associated with AMD by racial group in an extended study of the Salisbury Eye Evaluation population cohort. The study confirmed that white persons are generally more likely than black persons to have medium or large drusen, focal pigment abnormalities, and advanced AMD. Also racial differences were prominent for non-neovascular AMD features only when present in the central zone.

The Salisbury Eye Evaluation study has also reported racial differences in lens opacities, confirming that cataract was a highly significant problem in the African-American population more so than in the white population.[33, 34]

Table 3.1 Scientifically proven robust risk factors for AMD and cataracts

AMD	Cataracts
Older age groups	Older age groups
Family history	Female gender
White race	Black race
Smoking	Smoking
Alcohol use (heavy)	Alcohol use
	Exposure to ultraviolet light B
	Diabetes (+associated pathologies)
	Corticosteroid use

Smoking

There is robust evidence that causally associates AMD and cataract to smoking.[22, 35, 36, 37]

Alcohol

A recent systematic review and meta-analysis has concluded that heavy alcohol consumption that consists of more than 3 standard drinks per day is associated with an increased risk of early AMD.[38] The link between alcohol and cataract is less robust — a relationship between alcohol consumption and an increased risk of cataract has been reported from cross-sectional studies, but with several prospective cohort studies failing to confirm this association.[39, 40]

Exposure to UVB

Over-exposure to ultraviolet B has also been concluded to be causally associated to lens opacifications as reported by numerous studies.[41, 42, 43]

Diabetes

The prevalence and causes of visual impairment in an epidemiologic study of aged, urban individuals in Denmark reported that diabetic retinopathy in that country has a prevalence of 5.6%.[44] A recent study from the US has reported that the prevalence of diabetic retinopathy among persons with diagnosed diabetes was 9.9% and in that survey of self-reported age-related eye diseases there were approximately 1.3 million people in the US with diabetic retinopathy.[45]

Steroid and/or corticosteroid medications

The association of cataract with systemic corticosteroid therapy was first postulated in 1960.[46] Later reviews of the scientific literature concluded that steroids remained a risk for the development of cataract.[47, 48] Recently a report on steroid-induced posterior subcapsular cataracts concluded that it remains a serious concern even though some reports indicated that the evidence for glucocorticoid-protein adduct formation in the lens was inconclusive.[49]

Obesity

A prospective cohort study in a hospital-based retinal practice investigated and followed up patients that were 60 years or older, with some sign of non-advanced AMD and visual acuity of 20/200 or better in at least 1 eye.[50] This study documented that overall and abdominal obesity increased the risk for progression to advanced AMD, and more physical activity tended to decrease risk.

Recently the association between changes in waist-hip ratio, a measure of abdominal obesity, and AMD in a total of 12 515 persons aged 45–64 years, from a population-based cohort study from 1987 to 1989, was followed up over 6 years.[51]

The study concluded that middle-aged persons who had a 3% or greater reduction in waist-hip ratio over time were less likely to have AMD, particularly among those who were initially obese.

High glycaemic index foods (versus low glycaemic index foods)

The eye experiences numerous biological and histological changes as it ages. The ageing process together with a lifetime of exposure to light induces redox signalling imbalances, which then can lead to damage to the retinal pigment epithelium, drusen formation and retinal pigment epithelium dysfunction. Drusen, a marker of AMD, which accumulate between Bruch's membrane and the retinal pigment epithelium, may become targets for activated dendritic cells and can activate complement cascades.

As has been previously demonstrated in this section and within the framework of cellular metabolic dysfunction, dietary factors are known risk factors for AMD. The National Health and Nutrition Examination Survey (NHANES III) demonstrated that, in the population over 65 years of age, 18–20% have diabetes, with 40% having either diabetes or its precursor form of impaired glucose tolerance. Hyperglycaemia itself can promote the formation of advanced glycation end products. Hyperglycaemia damages blood vessels leading to various micro- and macro-vascular diseases such as diabetic retinopathy, which is the main microvascular complication of diabetes and the most common cause of blindness in working populations.[52]

The Blue Mountain Eye Study reported on the risk associated with high glycaemic index foods in its study population.[53] The study concluded that a high glycaemic index diet was a risk factor for early AMD; the recognised precursor of sight-threatening late AMD. It was also noted that low glycaemic index foods, such as oatmeal, could protect against early AMD. This was consistent with an earlier study that advised that persons at risk of AMD progression, especially those at high risk of advanced AMD, could benefit from consuming smaller amounts of refined carbohydrates.[54]

A recent dietary/food composition and consumption study investigated a number of nutritional factors and the risk of AMD.[55] It was reported that consuming diets that provided low glycaemic index foods and higher intakes of nutrients were associated with the greatest reduction in risk for prevalent drusen and advanced AMD.

Environmental

Sunlight/UVB exposure

There is no total accord on the role of light exposure in the development of AMD. A 10-year prospective study has demonstrated that prolonged exposure to sunlight may be associated with increased risk of earlier development of AMD but not AMD progression.[56, 57] Furthermore, this study also found a protective effect from the use of a hat and sunglasses in reducing the incidence of early AMD. An earlier Australian case control study, however, had failed to find a link between sunlight exposure and AMD.[58]

Pesticide exposure

It has been reported that exposure to pesticides may increase the risk of macular degeneration. Studies from Japan have linked organophosphate exposure to Saku disease, which involves retinal degeneration and other adverse ocular effects.[59] Moreover, in an early study from India the prevalence of macular degeneration was higher among pesticide workers exposed to the organophosphate fenthion than among unexposed controls.[60]

Physical activity

AMD

As part of the Beaver Dam Eye population-based study, a 15-year cumulative incidence of AMD was determined through 4 examination phases at 5-year intervals.[61] The study showed that there was a protective effect of physical activity for incident exudative AMD, independent of body mass index and other confounders. Moreover the study also suggested a possible modifiable behaviour that might be protective against developing AMD.

A recent study tested whether the risk of AMD could be decreased with vigorous physical activity.[62] This was a prospective study of self-reported clinically diagnosed macular degeneration in male (n = 29 532) and female (n = 12 176) runners followed prospectively for 7.7 years. The study reported that higher doses of vigorous exercise (running — risk for AMD decreased 10% per km per day increment in running distance) was associated with a lower incident AMD risk independent of weight, cardiorespiratory fitness, and cigarette use. Hence, compared to men and women running < 2 km per day, those averaging 2 to 4 km per day had 19% lower adjusted risk, and those averaging ≥ 4 km per day had 42% to 54% lower adjusted AMD risk.

Cataracts

Similarly, a prospective study investigated physical activity and incident cataract.[63] The risk for incident cataract increased with BMI, such that the risk in men > 27.5 kg/m^2 was 88% larger than in men < 20 kg/m^2. Men's cataract risk declined significantly in relation to running distance, even when adjusted for BMI. Men who ran ≥64 km/week had 35% lower risk for cataract than those reporting < 16 km/week (28% lower risk when adjusted for BMI). Furthermore, men with greater cardiorespiratory fitness were at significantly less risk for development of cataract than were the least fit men.

Nutrition

Diets

Vegetables

Early descriptive reports[64] hypothesised that there was an inverse relationship between increased consumption of foods rich in certain carotenoids (an important constituent of the retinal pigments), in particular dark green, leafy vegetables, and a decreased risk of developing advanced or exudative AMD.

A recent descriptive study that measured the regular dietary intake of antioxidants and the associated lowered risk of incident AMD reported that an above-median intake of all 4 nutrients — beta-carotene, vitamin C, vitamin E, and zinc — from foods was associated with a 35% reduced risk for incident AMD in elderly persons.[65]

In a further prospective observational study of plant food consumption from a large cohort of female health professionals, higher dietary intakes of lutein and/or zeaxanthin (refer also to later sections this chapter) and vitamin E from food and supplements were associated with significantly decreased risks of cataract.[66]

Meats

A recent epidemiological study has shown that higher consumption of fresh and processed red meat intake was positively associated with early AMD.[67] Specifically the study reported that consumption of chicken ≥ 3.5 times/week versus <1.5 times/week was inversely associated with late AMD. Moreover that the data suggested that different meats may differently affect AMD risk and that hence this may be a target for lifestyle modification.

Fats (animal fats versus fish fats)

A cross-sectional study that assessed whether dietary intake of fat or fish is associated with AMD showed that the amount and type of dietary fat intake may be associated with AMD.[37, 68] That this could be the situation was apparent from a recent study that evaluated the associations between past dietary fat intake and the prevalence of AMD and found that a diet low in trans-unsaturated fat and rich in omega-3 fatty acids and olive oil may reduce the risk of AMD.[69]

A prospective cohort study was undertaken to advise patients with a high risk for advanced forms of AMD about preventive measures through an evaluation program of the relationships between dietary fat intake and the progression of early or intermediate AMD to the advanced stages of the disease associated with visual loss. This study showed that:[70]

- higher total fat intake increased the risk of progression to the advanced forms of AMD, with a relative risk of 2.90 for the highest fat-intake quartile relative to the lowest fat-intake quartile
- animal fat intake was associated with a twofold increased risk of progression, although the trend for increasing risk with higher animal fat intake was not significant
- higher vegetable fat intake (not including olive oil) had a stronger relationship with increased risk of AMD progression with a relative risk of 3.82 for the highest quartile compared with the lowest quartile

- saturated, and trans-unsaturated fats increased the likelihood of progression
- olive oil was protective
- processed baked goods, which are higher in some of these fats, increased the rate of AMD progression approximately twofold; higher fish intake was associated with a lower risk of AMD progression among participants with lower linoleic acid intake
- nuts were protective.

Among individuals with the early or intermediate stages of AMD, total and specific types of fat intake, as well as some fat-containing food groups, modified the risk of progression to advanced AMD.

An AREDS study that examined the association of dietary omega-3 long-chain polyunsaturated fatty acid and fish intake with incident neovascular AMD and central geographic atrophy (CGA) reported that the data strongly suggested that dietary omega-3 long-chain polyunsaturated fatty acid intake was associated with a decreased risk of progression from bilateral drusen to CGA.[71]

A systematic review and meta-analysis from the same year confirmed that consumption of fish and foods rich in omega-3 fatty acids may be associated with a lower risk of AMD. However, it also reported that there was insufficient evidence from the current literature, with few prospective studies and no randomised clinical trials, to support their routine consumption for AMD prevention.[72]

In an elderly Australian cohort from 2009, 3654 participants that were examined at baseline and 2454 participants who were examined 5 and/or 10 years later were assessed for AMD.[73] The study provided significant evidence for protection against early AMD from regular consumption of fish. Greater consumption of omega-3 polyunsaturated fatty acids and low intakes of foods rich in linoleic acid afforded a similar protection. It was also noted that regular consumption of nuts may also reduce AMD risk.

Salt consumption

A large Australian population-based cross-sectional study[74] of 2873 patients (mean age 65 years), from the Blue Mountains area, reported that low intakes of salt in the diet reduced the risk of cataracts. Of these participants, 620 already had cortical cataracts, 350 had nuclear cataracts and 160 had posterior subcapsular cataracts. After controlling for additional risk factors for cataract formation, people with the highest quintile of sodium intake had twice the risk of developing posterior subcapsular cataracts than those in the lowest quintile of sodium intake.

Supplements

Vitamins and minerals

The incidence of eye diseases, most notably AMD and cataracts, is expected to increase sharply in the next few decades with the increasing number of people surviving to old age. Population studies have tracked the use of antioxidant vitamins for the prevention or the delay in the progression of eye diseases.

AMD

Antioxidants (Beta-carotene, vitamin C, vitamin E, Zinc)

The Beaver Dam Eye Study pointed to the importance of micronutrients in the prevention of progression of eye diseases. Significant, but modest, inverse associations were observed between intakes of pro–vitamin A carotenoids and dietary vitamin E and the incidence of large drusen and between zinc and the incidence of pigmentary abnormalities. No significant inverse associations though were found between antioxidants or zinc intake and the incidence of overall early AMD.[75]

Randomised placebo-controlled trials (by the AREDS study group) investigating high levels of antioxidant consumption of vitamins and minerals such as C and E, beta-carotene, and zinc have reported that people without contraindications, such as smoking, should consider taking a supplement of antioxidants plus zinc that could be of benefit in preventing progression of AMD.[76]

Systematic reviews provide additional recommendations that include that people with AMD, or early signs of the disease, could experience some benefit from taking supplements as used in the AREDS trial.[77] The author also alluded to the potential harms of high-dose antioxidant supplementation which included an increased risk of lung cancer in smokers with beta-carotene, heart failure in people with vascular disease or diabetes using high dose vitamin E, and hospitalisation for genitourinary conditions for those people using high dose zinc.[77, 78]

Recent randomised trials with single vitamins, namely beta–carotene, has demonstrated no beneficial or harmful effects on the incidence of AMD.[79] These randomised data relative to 12 years of treatment among a large population of apparently healthy men indicated that long-term supplementation with beta-carotene neither decreased nor increased the risk of AMD.

The evidence is somewhat contentious though given that systematic reviews have reported that there is insufficient evidence to support the role of dietary antioxidants, including the use of dietary antioxidant supplements, for the primary prevention of early AMD or to delay its progression.[78, 80]

However, while there is no definitive treatment presently available for AMD, the most recent evidence recommends that vitamin supplements with high doses of antioxidants used for primary prevention may reduce the incidence of AMD.[81] This together with previous research by the National Eye Institute (AREDS) and others suggest benefit in the secondary prevention of dry AMD for some patients and some improvement in visual acuity.

B Group Vitamins

Observational epidemiologic and clinical studies indicate a direct association between homocysteine concentration in the blood and the risk of AMD.[78, 82, 83, 84]

A recent US study conducted a randomised double-blind placebo-controlled trial including 5442 female health care professionals 40 years or older with pre-existing cardiovascular disease or 3 or more cardiovascular disease risk factors. They examined the effect of combined folic acid (2.5mg/day), pyridoxine hydrochloride (vitamin B6 50mg/day), and cyanocobalamin (vitamin B_{12}, 1mg/day) therapy to lower homocysteine levels versus placebo. A total of 5205 of these women did not have a diagnosis of AMD at baseline.[81] At the end of the study they reported that after an average of 7.3 years of treatment and follow-up, there were 55 cases of AMD in the combination treatment group and 82 in the placebo group. For visually significant AMD, there were 26 cases in the combination treatment group and 44 in the placebo group These randomised trial data from a large cohort of women at high risk of cardiovascular disease indicates that daily supplementation with a combination of folic acid, pyridoxine, and cyanocobalamin may significantly reduce the risk of AMD.

Vitamin D

A cross-sectional association study of serum vitamin D and early and advanced AMD, assessed from non-mydriatic fundus photographs, were evaluated in the third National Health and Nutrition Examination Survey.[85] This was a multistage nationally representative probability sample of non-institutionalised individuals (n = 7752; 11% with AMD). This study showed that consistent use versus non-use of vitamin D from supplements was inversely associated with early AMD only in individuals who did not consume milk daily. Moreover, even though additional studies are required to confirm these results, it was concluded that this study provided evidence that vitamin D may protect against AMD.

Cataract

Antioxidants (Vitamins C, E)

Population studies investigating the use of antioxidant vitamins and cataract incidents reported that the results provided significant evidence that there was a lower risk for cataract among users of multivitamin supplements and a stronger relationship for long-term use.[86, 87] A nutritional assessment study of long-term intake of vitamins and carotenoids reported that the data support a role for vitamin C in diminishing the risk of cortical cataracts in women aged < 60 years and for carotenoids in diminishing the risk of posterior subcapsular cataracts in women who had never smoked.[88]

Randomised clinical trials with antioxidants have also been conducted for the prevention of cataract. The AREDS group has also reported that the use of a high-dose formulation of vitamin C, vitamin E, and beta-carotene in a relatively well-nourished older adult cohort had no apparent effect on the 7-year risk of development or progression of age-related lens opacities or visual acuity loss.[89]

Furthermore, an additional large randomised trial of apparently healthy female health professionals with 9.7 years of treatment and follow-up indicated that 600IU natural-source vitamin E taken every other day provided no benefit for age-related cataract or subtypes.[90]

Other nutritional supplements

Omega-3 Essential Fatty Acids (EFAs)

EFAs that humans require for healthy metabolic functions include alpha-linolenic acid, (short-chain omega-3 fatty acid), docosahexaenoic acid (DHA), and eicosapentaenoic acid (EPA) (both long-chain omega-3 fatty acids). Alpha-linolenic acid is the dietary precursor to both DHA and EPA and can be converted to a long-chain omega-3 fatty acid.[91, 92, 93] Importantly and related to eye physiological structure and function, DHA is present in high concentrations in the retinal outer segments, and its deficiency has been reported to be associated with the initiation of the onset of AMD.[94] Moreover, long-chain omega-3 fatty acids may also protect against unbalanced oxygenic,[95] inflammatory and age-related retinal damage,[93] which have been reported to be key pathogenic processes in AMD development.[96]

To date there have been few prospective studies[37, 97–101] and no randomised clinical trials investigating the efficacy of EFAs in preventing AMD. However a recent systematic review and meta-analysis does suggest that consumption of fish and foods rich in omega-3 fatty acids may be associated with a lower risk of AMD.[102]

Recently it was reported that dietary lipid intake in the form of EFAs is a lifestyle and/or nutritional modifiable factor that could significantly influence the likelihood of developing sight-threatening forms of AMD.[103]

Phytochemicals

Lutein and zeaxanthin xanthophyll

Lutein and zeaxanthin give the macula lutea its characteristic yellow appearance.

There is cumulative evidence on the consumption of lutein, carotenoid and zeaxanthin xanthophyll (in whole food or supplemental form), the resulting concentrations in the serum, and tissue distribution throughout the body, particularly in the retina, play a role in the development of AMD.[104]

The observational study, Carotenoids in Age-Related Eye Disease (CAREDS), concluded that diets rich in lutein plus zeaxanthin may protect against intermediate AMD in healthy women.[105, 106] In addition, the population-based Pathologies Oculaires Liees-a l'Age (POLA) study also was strongly suggestive of a protective role of the xanthophylls, in particular zeaxanthin, for the protection against AMD as well as cataract.[107]

Other epidemiological studies have shown that elevated serum levels and/or intake of several antioxidants, such as carotenoids, vitamin E and ascorbic acid, are associated with a diminished risk for cataracts.[108, 109] A case control study though failed to show that the serum status of carotenoids and tocopherols in patients with age-related cataracts was significantly different between cases and controls.[110]

Studies have found that lutein and xeanthins can be increased in the serum following an oral dose.[111] A more recent study that investigated the effect of the carotenoid, lutein, supplemented at doses of 2.5, 5.0, and 10mg/day for 6 months on distribution of these carotenoids and their metabolites in the serum of elderly human participants, with and without AMD reported similar findings.[112] The increase in the serum levels of lutein and/or zeaxanthin correlated with increases in the serum levels of their metabolites that have previously been identified in the ocular tissues. Hence it was concluded that elderly human participants with and without AMD can safely take supplements of lutein up to 10mg/day for 6 months with no apparent toxicity or side-effects.

A small study that investigated 17 patients clinically diagnosed with age-related cataracts were randomised in a double-blind study involving dietary supplementation with lutein (15mg; n = 5), alpha-tocopherol (100mg; n = 6), or placebo (n = 6), 3 times a week for up to 2 years demonstrated that visual function in patients who received the lutein supplements improved, suggesting that a higher intake of lutein, through lutein-rich fruit and vegetables or supplements, may have significantly beneficial effects on the visual performance of people with age-related cataracts.[113]

A further small study that investigated the long-term supplementation of lutein (mean 13 months range 4–20 months for participants diagnosed with AMD; mean 26 months range 16–36 months for participants diagnosed with cataract) found that serum lutein levels were maintained and that it was associated with improved visual function of the participants.[114]

Notwithstanding this evidence the US Food and Drug Administration (FDA) reviewed intervention and observational studies that evaluated the role of lutein and zeaxanthin in reducing the risk of AMD and cataracts and concluded that no credible evidence exists for a health claim about the intake of lutein or zeaxanthin and the risk of AMD or cataracts.[115]

A recent report post the FDA's review, the 6–12 month Lutein Xanthophyll Eye Accumulation study involving 102 healthy caucasian males who received daily supplementation of either lutein (11mg), zeaxanthin (13mg), or a combination (10mg lutein, 12mg zeaxanthin), or placebo, a significant improvement was reported in macular pigment optical density responses were observed compared to placebo. This clinical trial did not report any adverse event due to the supplemental phytonutrient doses and it reported increased bioavailability, showing a 27-fold increase in plasma xanthophyll concentrations.[116] In previous clinical trials, lutein and zeaxanthin were also reported to be safe at higher doses and to improve macular pigment optical density, visual acuity, and glare sensitivity.

Furthermore, it should be noted that currently evaluation of nutritional factors, specifically lutein and/or zeaxanthin and omega-3 fatty acids, is being tested in a multi-centre controlled, randomised trial — the Age-Related Eye Disease Study 2 (AREDS2).[106] This is a randomised controlled clinical trial which started enrolling participants in the northern hemisphere in the autumn of 2006. The primary outcome of this trial is to determine whether oral supplementation with macular xanthophylls (lutein at 10mg/day and zeaxanthin at 2mg/day) or omega-3 long-chain polyunsaturated fatty acids (LCPUFAs; DHA eicosapentaenoic acid at a total of 1g/day) will decrease the risk of progression to advanced AMD, as compared with placebo. This study should further clarify the role, especially of these carotenoids in preventing AMD and or cataract.

A recent review has recommended[108] that for persons with intermediate risk of AMD (such as bilateral large drusen) or advanced AMD (such as unilateral neovascular AMD or geographic atrophy involving the centre of fovea), the AREDS-type supplements are recommended because they are proven to reduce the risk of developing advanced AMD by 25% according to the following formulation.[108]

AREDS-type supplement intermediate AMD (extensive intermediate drusen, large drusen, and no advanced AMD) advanced AMD (neovascular AMD or central geographic atrophy) in one eye:
AREDS formulation
Vitamin C 500mg
Vitamin E 400IU
Beta-carotene 15mg
Zinc oxide 80mg
Cupric oxide 2mg

There are a number of additional emerging phytochemicals that have been reported to be promising in ocular physiology health.[117]

Anthocyanins

Blackcurrant anthocyanins have been found to be widely distributed in their intact forms in the plasma, ocular tissues, and whole eye after oral and intraperitoneal administration in animal models. Four anthocyanins were identified after intravenous administration in the aqueous humor, cornea, choroid, and retina, as well as small amounts in the vitreous and lens areas demonstrating the potential ocular protective benefits from oral intakes of anthocyanins.[118]

Anthocyanins are water-soluble flavonoid pigments that have been reported to have potent antioxidants and are known to reduce inflammatory processes and regulate redox signalling.[119]

Participants in a parallel-designed, placebo-controlled, clinical trial who were given 300mg/day of capsules containing purified anthocyanins isolated from bilberry (*Vaccinium myrtillus*) and blackcurrant (*Ribes nigrum)* for 3 weeks displayed 15–45% reductions of NFkB inflammatory markers.[120]

Resveratrol

Resveratrol, a polyphenolic compound isolated from red wine, has been shown to have protective benefits against inflammation and also involved in the regulation of redox signalling both *in vitro* and *in vivo*.[121, 122]

Studies have demonstrated that treatment with 50 and 100 μmol/L resveratrol significantly reduced proliferation of retinal pigment epithelium cells by 10% and 25%, respectively.[123] Further, in an animal model, rats supplemented with 40mg/kg body weight of resveratrol for 4 days were reported to have a reduced frequency of cataract development.[124]

Herbal medicines

Ginkgo biloba

Small early studies, such as phase I placebo-controlled cross-over, have demonstrated benefit in ocular functions. A trial with 11 patients investigated the effects of 40mg of *Ginkgo biloba* extract administered 3 times per day for 2 days on ocular blood flow. *Ginkgo biloba* extract increased blood flow to the ophthalmic artery, while no change was observed in the placebo group.[125] In a further prospective, randomised, placebo-controlled, cross-over trial that investigated the effects of 40mg of *Ginkgo biloba* extract administered for 4 weeks demonstrated improvements in pre-existing visual field damage in patients, but no improvements in intraocular pressure.[126]

Epigallocatechin gallate (EGCG)

EGCG is the principal flavonoid present in green tea. EGCG has been reported to confer neuroprotection of retinas injured by ischemia/reperfusion.[127]

Moreover, a recent investigation was conducted to deduce as to whether inclusion of EGCG in the drinking water of albino rats attenuated the effect of a light insult to the retina.[128] This study showed that orally administered EGCG blunted the detrimental effect of light to the retina of albino rats where the photoreceptors were primarily affected.

A recent human study with 18 ocular hypertension patients and 18 patients with open-angle glaucoma were randomly assigned to an oral placebo or EGCG over a 3-month period in a randomised, placebo-controlled, double-blind, cross-over design clinical trial.[129] The study concluded that although it could not provide evidence for long-term benefit of EGCG supplementation in open angle glaucoma, and the observed effect was small, the results suggest that EGCG might favourably influence inner retinal function in eyes with early to moderately advanced glaucomatous damage.

Physical therapies

Acupuncture

Experimental studies with laboratory animals have reported the usefulness of electro-acupuncture in preventing selenite-induced cataract formation.[130] The study showed that electro-acupuncture effectively decreased selenite-induced cataract formation rate in pup rats when needles were applied at specific acu-points.

A recent study assessed the effectiveness of acupuncture in reducing anxiety in patients having cataract surgery under topical anaesthesia.[131] The study design was a prospective randomised double-blind controlled trial. Anxiety levels before and after cataract surgery in 3 groups (A = no acupuncture, B = true acupuncture starting 20 minutes before surgery, C = sham acupuncture starting 20 minutes before surgery) were compared using the visual analogue scale. Twenty-five patients scheduled for inpatient phacoemulsification surgery were enrolled in each group. All surgeries were performed using topical anaesthesia. The study concluded that acupuncture was effective in reducing anxiety related to cataract surgery under topical anaesthesia.

Conclusion

The most common form of retinal degeneration, macular degeneration, is the leading cause of decreased visual acuity and loss of central vision among older adults in industrialised countries, followed by cataract.

While there is no curative treatment at present, various interventions can reduce the risk of developing AMD or cataract and limit disease progression if it occurs.

Clearly there are non-modifiable factors that may predispose an individual to the development of AMD or cataract, such as a family history and racial differences. However, numerous lifestyle intervention changes that people could adopt can significantly decrease the risk of developing AMD or cataract and even reduce the progression of the disease. Lifestyle interventions such as reducing alcohol intake and smoking cessation can significantly assist to reduce risk.

Evaluating environmental insults is also important in minimising risks. Patients should be advised to minimise exposure to UV B without eye protection.

Adopting prudent nutritional and physical activity practices can further enhance overall health and reduce risks not just for eye diseases but for all the major chronic diseases.

The use of a good multivitamin and/or mineral supplement has numerous advantages in reducing the risk of developing eye diseases by assisting to maintain metabolic health. Within this framework of scientific evidence there is an emerging literature that suggests that phytochemicals such as lutein and zeaxanthins, and to a lesser extent anthocyanins, resveratrol and some herbal medicines such as *Ginko biloba* and tea catechins, may provide protection and significantly delay the progression of eye diseases — extended clinical trials are however necessary. Table 3.2 summarises the best evidence for lifestyle, CM and therapies for AMD and cataracts.

Table 3.2 Levels of evidence for lifestyle and complementary medicines/therapies in the management of AMD and cataracts

Modality	Level I	Level II	Level IIIa	Level IIIb	Level IIIc	Level IV	Level V
Lifestyle modifications (see also Table 3.1)							
Smoking (AMD and cataract)	x						
Alcohol (AMD and cataract)	x						
Diabetes (cataract)	x						
Corticosteroid use (cataract)	x						
Obesity	x						
High glycaemic index food Consumption	x						
Non-modifiable factors (see also Table 3.1)							
Older age groups (AMD and cataract)	x						

Continued

Table 3.2 Levels of evidence for lifestyle and complementary medicines/therapies in the management of AMD and cataracts—cont'd

Modality	Level I	Level II	Level IIIa	Level IIIb	Level IIIc	Level IV	Level V
Family history (AMD)	x						
Female race (AMD)	x						
Black race (cataract)	x						
Environmental							
UV B exposure (cataract)	x						
Pesticide exposure					x		
Physical activity				x			
Nutrition — diets							
Vegetable consumption				x			
Meat consumption				x			
Fats — saturated consumption				x			
Salt consumption				x			
Supplements and/or nutraceuticals (vitamins and minerals)							
Multivitamin and/or mineral complex	x						
Beta-carotene				x			
Vitamin C				x			
Vitamin E					x		
Vitamin D				x			
B Group vitamins					x		
Zinc				x			
Supplements other							
EFAs (fish fats)			x				
Phytochemicals							
Lutein and/or zeaxanthin			x				
Anthocyanins					x		
Resveratrol					x		
Herbal medicines							
Ginkgo biloba				x			
EGCG				x			
Physical therapies							
Acupuncture					x		

Level I — from a systematic review of all relevant randomised controlled trials — meta-analyses.
Level II — from at least 1 properly designed randomised controlled clinical trial.
Level IIIa — from well-designed pseudo-randomised controlled trials (alternate allocation or some other method).
Level IIIb — from comparative studies (including systematic reviews of such studies) with concurrent controls and allocation not randomised, cohort studies, case-control studies, or interrupted time series with a parallel control group.
Level IIIc — from comparative studies with historical control, 2 or more single-arm studies, or interrupted time series without a parallel control group.
Level IV — opinions of respected authorities based on clinical experience, descriptive studies or reports of expert committees.
Level V — represents minimal evidence that represents testimonials.

Clinical tips handout for patients — AMD and cataracts

1 Lifestyle advice

Sleep

- Restore normal sleep patterns. Most adults require about 7 hours sleep. (See Chapter 22 for more advice.)

Sunshine

- Eye protection should be worn in the form of sunglasses at all times when exposed to the sun for prolonged periods of time.
- Amount of exposure varies with local climate.
- At least 15 minutes of sunshine needed daily for vitamin D and melatonin production — especially before 10 a.m. and after 3 p.m. when the sun exposure is safest during summer. Much more exposure is required in winter, when supplementation needs to be considered.
- Ensure gradual adequate skin exposure to sun; avoid sunscreen and excess clothing to maximise levels of vitamin D.
- More time in the sun is required for dark skinned people.
- Direct exposure to about 10% of body (hands, arms, face), without sunscreen and not through glass.
- Vitamin D is obtained in the diet from fatty fish, eggs, liver and fortified foods (some milks and margarines); however, it is unlikely that adequate vitamin D concentrations can be obtained from diet alone.

2 Physical activity/exercise

- Exercise for 30 minutes or more daily. If exercise is not regular, commence with 5 minutes daily and slowly build up to at least 30 minutes. Outdoor exercise with nature, fresh air and sunshine is ideal (e.g. brisk walking, light jogging, cycling, swimming, stretching). Weight-bearing exercises or resistance exercise are beneficial. The more time you spend outdoors the better.
- Yoga may be of help; other examples: qiqong, tai chi.

3 Mind–body medicine

- Stress management programs are important for life-stressor management; for example, six 40 minute sessions for patients to understand the nature of their symptoms, the symptoms' relationship to stress and the practice of regular relaxation exercises.
- Regular meditation practice at least 10-20 minutes daily.

Breathing

- Be aware of breathing from time to time. Notice if tendency to hold breath or over-breathe. Always aim to relax the breath and the muscles around the chest wall.

Rest and stress management

- Recurrent stress may cause a return of symptoms. Relaxation is important for a healthy lifestyle.
- Reduce workload and resolve conflicts. Contact family, friends, church, social or other groups for support.
- Listening to relaxation music and daily baths help.
- Massage therapy reduces stress.
- Exercise can reduce stress.
- Hypnotherapy and biofeedback may be of help.
- Cognitive behavioural therapy and psychotherapy are extremely helpful.
- Fun —it is important to have fun in life. Joy can be found even in the simplest tasks, such as being with friends with a sense of humour, funny movies/videos, comedy, hobbies, dancing, playing with pets and children.

4 Environment

- Avoid smoking, environmental pollutants, chemicals — at work and in the home.

5 Dietary changes

- Eat more fruit and vegetables — a variety of colours and those in season.
- Eat regular healthy low GI meals.
- Consume more dietary fibre — nuts (e.g. walnuts, peanuts); seeds; beans (e.g. lentils, soybeans) sprouts (e.g. alfalfa, mung bean).
- Eat more fish (daily if possible), especially deep sea fish; canned fish is okay (mackerel, salmon, sardines, cod, tuna, salmon).
- Use cold pressed olive oil and avocado oil.
- Eat dark chocolate — preferably 85% or more of cocoa.
- Eat low GI wholegrains/cereals (variety) — rice (brown, basmati, Mahatmi, Doongara), traditional rolled oats,

buckwheat flour, wholegrain organic breads (rye bread, Essene, spelt, Kamut), brown pasta, millet, amaranth etc.

- Increase intake of foods that are high in lutein and/or zeaxanthin levels, such as:
  - egg yolk (high source)
  - corn (a vegetable with high lutein concentration)
  - orange and red capsicum (a vegetable with high zeaxanthin concentration)
  - dark, leafy, green vegetables (high in lutein but not zeaxanthin).
- To a lesser degree also consume:
  - *kiwi fruit, oranges, grapes.*
- Reduce red meat intake — preferably use red lean meat (e.g. lamb, kangaroo) and white meat (e.g. free range organic chicken)
- Reduce dairy intake — low fat dairy products such as yoghurt and occasionally cheeses are okay, unless there is a dairy intolerance.
- Drink more water: 1–2 litres a day.
- Drink teas (e.g. especially organic green tea, black tea) and vegetable juices.
- Moderate alcohol intake — restrict intake to no more than 1–2 glasses daily (non-sweet) as it is a brain depressant and can disturb sleep.
- Avoid artificial sweeteners — replace with honey (e.g. Yellow Box and Stringy Bark have lowest GI)
- Avoid hydrogenated fats, salt, fast foods, added sugar (e.g. as in soft drinks, lollies, biscuits, cakes and processed foods such as white bread, white pasta, pastries)
- Avoid chemical additives — preservatives, colourings and flavours

6 Physical therapies

Various forms of acupuncture and other physical therapies may be very useful for the treatment of various of eye conditions.

7 Supplements

Fish oils

- Indication: fish oils 2–4g (1g fish oil containing EPA 180mg/DHA 120mg) daily depending on fish consumption.
- Dosage: take with meals. Adult: 1g 1–2 capsules twice daily. Child 500mg 1 to 2 x daily (500mg — 1g daily EPA and DHA); can be used in pregnancy or lactation as tolerated.
- Side-effects: often well tolerated especially if taken with meals. Very mild and rare side-effects — for example, gastrointestinal upset; allergic reactions (e.g. rash); breathing problems if allergic to seafood; blood thinning effects in very high doses > 10g daily (may need to stop fish oil supplements 2 weeks prior to surgery).
- Contraindications: sensitivity reaction to seafood; drug interactions; caution when taking high doses of fish oils >4g per day together with warfarin (your doctor should check your INR test).

Vitamins B group

Folate

- Indication: elevated homocysteine.
- Dosage: 0.25–0.5–1mg daily as in a multivitamin and mineral supplement.
- Side-effects: very mild and rare.
- Contraindications: avoid in anaemia until assessed by a doctor.

Vitamins B6 and B12

- Indication: elevated homocysteine can reduce vitamin B12.
- Dosage: upper level of intake of vitamin B6 should not exceed 50mg/day.
- Results: uncertain.
- Side-effects: avoid overuse of single vitamin products (e.g. oral and injectable forms of vitamin B6) or concomitant use of multivitamin products could result in some patients routinely exceeding the upper limit for vitamins associated with severe toxicity. Toxicity in high doses of vitamin B6 includes peripheral neuropathy, such as tingling, burning and numbness of limbs.
- Contraindications: avoid in anaemia until assessed by a doctor.

Vitamin D3 (cholecalciferol 1000IU)

Doctors should check blood levels and suggest supplementation if levels are low.

Vitamin C and Vitamin E (best given together)

Vitamin C

- Indication: can reactivate vitamin E. May help prevent progression of AMD.
- Dosage: 500–1000mg daily or as tolerated.
- Side-effects: with high doses can cause nausea, heartburn, abdominal cramps and diarrhoea.
- Contraindications: can increase iron absorption. Use with caution if glucose-6 phosphate dehydrogenase deficiency.

Vitamin E (natural form)

- Indication: may prevent progression of AMD.
- Dosage: 200–500–1000IU daily (D-alpha-tocopherol or mixed isomers).
- Side-effects: doses below 1500IU daily are very unlikely to result in haemorrhage, diarrhoea, flatulence, nausea, heart palpitations.
- Contraindications: use with caution if bleeding disorder or if taking with blood thinning medication. If using very high dose, reduce dose before surgery.

Zinc

- Indication: may prevent progression of AMD.
- Dosage: usual dosage in adult no more than 5–10mgs zinc sulfate daily. Zinc amino acid chelate 50mg.
- Side-effects: nausea, vomiting, metallic taste in mouth. Avoid long-term use and high dosage as this may cause copper deficiency, impair the immune system and cause anaemia.
- Contraindications: sideroblastic anaemia, above normal blood levels of zinc, severe kidney disease.

(NOTE: zinc supplements can inhibit the absorption of copper, therefore it is important to add a copper supplement of 1–3mg/day).

Selenium (sodium selenite, organic selenium found in yeast)

- Indication: may prevent the progression of AMD.
- Dosage: 50–100mcg daily; do not exceed >600mcg daily (health professional supervisionmcg required to avoid toxicity).
- Results: uncertain.
- Side-effects: very mild and rare; nausea, vomiting, rash, sensitivity reactions, toxicity in high doses; nail changes, irritability, fatigue.
- Contraindications: pregnancy, lactation, children <12 years of age; avoid yeast derived selenium if allergic to yeast.

Phytochemicals

Lutein and/or Zeaxanthin

- Indication: may help in retarding the pathophysiology of AMD.
- Dosage: 145mg per day.
- Results: uncertain.
- Side-effects: at the above dose no adverse effects have been reported.
- Contraindications: pregnancy, lactation, children <12 years of age.

References

1 World Health Organization Report. http://www.who.int/blindness/causes/priority/en/print.html (Accessed July 2009).
2 Magnitude and causes of visual impairment, World Health Organization, Fact Sheet No 282.
3 Resnikoff S, Pascolini D, Etya'ale D, et. al. Global data on visual impairment in the year 2002. Bull World Health Organ 2004;82:844–51.
4 Klein R, Peto T, Bird A, Vannewkirk MR. The epidemiology of age-related macular degeneration. Am J Ophthalmol 2004;137:486–95.
5 Friedman DS, O'Colmain BJ, Munoz B, et. al. Prevalence of age-related macular degeneration in the United States. Arch Ophthalmol 2004;122:564–72.
6 Wolfs RC, Borger PH, Ramrattan RS, et. al. Changing views on openangle glaucoma: definitions and prevalences—The Rotterdam Study. Invest Ophthalmol Vis Sci 2000;41:3309–21.
7 Mitchell P, Wang JJ, Foran S, et. al. Five-year incidence of age-related maculopathy lesions: the Blue Mountains Eye Study. Ophthalmology 2002;109:1092–7.
8 Taylor H, Guymer R, Keeffe J. The Impact of Age-Related Macular Degeneration. Access Economics Pty Limited. Melbourne: University of Melbourne, 2006:1–72.
9 Taylor HR, Keeffe JE, Vu HT, et. al. Vision loss in Australia. Med J Aust 2005;182:565–8.
10 Friedman DS, O'Colmain BJ, Munoz B, et. al. Prevalence of age-related macular degeneration in the United States. Arch Ophthalmol 2004;122:564–72.
11 Jonasson F, Arnarsson A, Peto T, et. al. 5-year incidence of age-related maculopathy in the Reykjavik Eye Study. Ophthalmology 2005;112:132–8.
12 Andersen N. Age-related macular degeneration among the Inuit in Greenland. Int J Circumpolar Health 2004;63(Suppl 2):320–3.
13 Vingerling JR, Dielemans I, Hofman A, et. al. The prevalence of age-related maculopathy in the Rotterdam Study. Ophthalmology 1995;102:205–10.
14 Krishnaiah S, Das T, Nirmalan PK, et. al. Risk factors for age-related macular degeneration: findings from the Andhra Pradesh eye disease study in South India. Invest Ophthalmol Vis Sci 2005;46:4442–9.
15 Munoz B, Klein R, Rodriguez J, et. al. Prevalence of age-related macular degeneration in a population-based sample of Hispanic people in Arizona: Proyecto VER. Arch Ophthalmol 2005;123:1575–80.
16 Leske MC, Wu SY, Hennis A, et. al. Nine-year incidence of age-related macular degeneration in the Barbados Eye Studies. Ophthalmology 2006;113:29–35.
17 Wong TY, Loon SC, Saw SM. The epidemiology of age-related eye diseases in Asia. Br J Ophthalmol 2006;90:506–11.
18 Asbell PA, Dualan I, Mindel J, et. al. Age-related cataract. Lancet 2005;365:599–609.
19 Kahn HA, Leibowitz HM, Ganley JP, et. al. The Framingham Eye Study: outline and major prevalence findings. Am J Epidemiol 1977;106:17–32.
20 Klein BE, Klein R, Linton KL. Prevalence of age-related lens opacities in a population. Ophthalmology 1992;99:546–52.

21 Sommer A, Tielsch JM, Katz I, et. al. Racial differences in the cause specific prevalence of blindness in east Baltimore. NEJM 1991;325:1412–17.
22 Asbell PA, Dualan I, Mindel J, et. al. Age-related cataract. Lancet 2005;365(9459):599–609.
23 Hankinson SE. Epidemiology of age-related cataract. In: Albert DM, Jakobiec FA. Principles and Practice of Ophthalmology (2nd edn). WB Saunders, Philadelphia, 2000:511–19.
24 Chou R, Dana T, Bougatsos C. Screening older adults for impaired visual acuity: a review of the evidence for the U.S. Preventive Services Task Force. Ann Intern Med 2009;151(1):44–58.
25 Kaufman SR. Developments in age-related macular degeneration: Diagnosis and treatment. Geriatrics 2009;64(3):16–9.
26 Seddon J, Ajani U, Mitchell B. Familial aggregation of age-related maculopathy. Am J Ophthalmol 1997;123:199–206.
27 Meyers SM, Greene T, Gutman FA. A twin study of age-related macular degeneration. Am J Ophthalmol 1995;120:757–66.
28 Hammond CJ, Webster AR, Snieder H, et. al. Genetic influence on early agerelated maculopathy: a twin study. Ophthalmology 2002;109:730–6.
29 Friedman DS, O'Colmain BJ, Munoz B, et. al. The Eye Diseases Prevalence Research Group. Prevalence of age-related macular degeneration in the United States. Arch Ophthalmol 2004;122(4):564–572.
30 Friedman DS, Katz J, Bressler NM et. al. Racial differences in the prevalence of age-related macular degeneration: The Baltimore Eye Survey Ophthalmology 1999;106(6):1049–1055.
31 Schachat AP, Hyman L, Leske C, et. al. Barbados Eye Study Group. Features of age-related macular degeneration in a black population. Arch Ophthalmol 1995;113(6):728–735.
32 Bressler SB, Muñoz B, Solomon SD, et. al. Salisbury Eye Evaluation (SEE) Study Team. Racial differences in the prevalence of age-related macular degeneration: the Salisbury Eye Evaluation (SEE) Project. Arch Ophthalmol 2008;126(2):241–5.
33 West SK, Munoz B, Schein OD, et. al. Racial differences in lens opacities: the Salisbury Eye Evaluation (SEE) project. Am J Epidemiol 1998;148(11):1033–9.
34 Friedman DS, West SK, Munoz B, et. al. Racial variations in causes of vision loss in nursing homes: The Salisbury Eye Evaluation in Nursing Home Groups (SEEING) Study. Arch Ophthalmol 2004;122(7):1019–24.
35 Cook HL, Patel PJ, Tufail A. Age-related macular degeneration: diagnosis and management. Br Med Bull 2008;85:127–49.
36 Abraham AG, Condon NG, West Gower E. The new epidemiology of cataract. Ophthalmol Clin North Am 2006;19(4):415–25.
37 Seddon JM, George S, Rosner B. Cigarette smoking, fish consumption, omega-3 fatty acid intake, and associations with age-related macular degeneration: the US Twin Study of Age-Related Macular Degeneration. Arch Ophthalmol 2006;124(7):995–1001.
38 Chong EW, Kreis AJ, Wong TY, et. al. Alcohol consumption and the risk of age-related macular degeneration: a systematic review and meta-analysis. Am J Ophthalmol 2008;145(4):707–715.
39 Hiratsuka Y, Li G. Alcohol and eye diseases: a review of epidemiologic studies. J Stud Alcohol 2001;62(3):397–402.
40 Wang S, Wang JJ, Wong TY. Alcohol and eye diseases. Surv Ophthalmol 2008;53(5):512–25.
41 West S. Ocular ultraviolet B exposure and lens opacities: a review. J Epidemiol 1999;9 (6 Suppl):S97–S101.
42 Meyer-Rochow VB. Risks, especially for the eye, emanating from the rise of solar UV-radiation in the Arctic and Antarctic regions. Int J Circumpolar Health 2000;59(1):38–51.
43 McCarty CA, Taylor HR. A review of the epidemiologic evidence linking ultraviolet radiation and cataracts. Dev Ophthalmol 2002;35:21–31.
44 Buch H, Vinding T, Nielsen NV. Prevalence and causes of visual impairment according to World Health Organization and United States criteria in an aged, urban Scandinavian population: the Copenhagen City Eye Study. Ophthalmology 2001;108(12):2347–57.
45 Ryskulova A, Turczyn K, Makuc DM, et. al. Self-reported age-related eye diseases and visual impairment in the United States: results of the 2002 national health interview survey. Am J Public Health 2008;98(3):454–61.
46 Black RL, Ogleby RB, Von Sallmann L, et. al. Posterior subcapsular cataracts induced by corticosteroids in patients with rheumatoid arthritis. JAMA 1960;174:166–71.
47 Dickerson JE Jr, Dotzel E, Clark AF. Steroid-induced cataract: new perspective from in vitro and lens culture studies. Exp Eye Res 1997;65(4):507–16.
48 Jobling AI, Augusteyn RC. What causes steroid cataracts? A review of steroid-induced posterior subcapsular cataracts. Clin Exp Optom 2002;85(2):61–75.
49 James ER. The etiology of steroid cataract. J Ocul Pharmacol Ther 2007;23(5):403–20.
50 Seddon JM, Cote J, Davis N, et. al. Progression of age-related macular degeneration: association with body mass index, waist circumference, and waist-hip ratio. Arch Ophth 2003;121(6):785–92.
51 Peeters A, Magliano DJ, Stevens J, et. al. Changes in abdominal obesity and age-related macular degeneration: the Atherosclerosis Risk in Communities Study. Arch Ophthalmol 2008;126:1554–60.
52 Harris MI. Diabetes in America: epidemiology and scope of the problem. Diabetes Care 1998;21:C11–C14.
53 Kaushik S, Wang JJ, Flood V, et. al. Dietary glycaemic index and the risk of age-related macular degeneration. AJCN 2008;88(4):1104–10.
54 Chiu CJ, Milton RC, Klein R, et. al. Dietary carbohydrate and the progression of age-related macular degeneration: a prospective study from the Age-Related Eye Disease Study. AJCN 2007;86:1210–8.
55 Chiu CJ, Milton RC, Klein R, et. al. Dietary compound score and risk of age-related macular degeneration in the age-related eye disease study. Ophthalmology 2009;116(5):939–46.
56 Tomany SC, Cruickshanks KJ, Klein R, et. al. Sunlight and the 10-year incidence of age-related maculopathy: the Beaver Dam Eye Study. Arch Ophthalmol 2004;122(5):750–7.
57 Cruickshanks KJ, Klein R, Klein BE, et. al. Sunlight and the 5 year incidence of early age-related maculopathy: the Beaver dam eye study. Archives of Ophthalmology 2001;119(2):246–250.
58 Darzins P, Mitchell P, Heller RF. Sun exposure and age-related macular degeneration. An Australian case-control study. Ophthalmology 1997;104(5):770–6.

59 Dementi B. Ocular effects of organophosphates: a historical perspective of Saku disease. J Appl Toxicol 1994;14:119–29.
60 Misra UK, Nag D, Misra NK, et. al. Some observations on the macula of pesticide workers. Hum Toxicol 1985;4:135–45.
61 Knudtson MD, Klein R, Klein BE. Physical activity and the 15-year cumulative incidence of age-related macular degeneration: the Beaver Dam Eye Study. Br J Ophthalmol 2006;90(12):1461–3.
62 Williams PT. Prospective study of incident age-related macular degeneration in relation to vigorous physical activity during a 7-year follow-up. Invest Ophthalmol Vis Sci 2009;50(1):101–6.
63 Williams PT. Prospective epidemiological cohort study of reduced risk for incident cataract with vigorous physical activity and cardiorespiratory fitness during a 7-year follow-up. Invest Ophthalmol Vis Sci 2009;50(1):95–100.
64 Seddon JM, Ajani UA, Sperduto RD, et. al. Dietary carotenoids, vitamins A, C, and E, and advanced age-related macular degeneration. Eye Disease Case-Control Study Group. JAMA 1994;272(18): 1413–20.
65 van Leeuwen R, Boekhoorn S, Vingerling JR, et. al. Dietary intake of antioxidants and risk of age-related macular degeneration. JAMA 2005;294(24): 3101–7.
66 Christen WG, Liu S, Glynn RJ, et. al. Dietary carotenoids, vitamins C and e, and risk of cataract in women: a prospective study. Arch Ophthalmol 2008;126(1):102–9.
67 Chong EW, Simpson JA, Robman LD, et. al. Red meat and chicken consumption and its association with age-related macular degeneration. Am J Epidemiol 2009;169(7):867–76.
68 Smith W, Mitchell P, Leeder SR. Dietary fat and fish intake and age-related maculopathy. Arch Ophthalmol 2000;118(3):401–4.
69 Chong EW, Robman LD, Simpson JA, et. al. Fat consumption and its association with age-related macular degeneration. Arch Ophthalmol 2009;127(5):674–80.
70 Seddon JM, Cote J, Rosner B. Progression of age-related macular degeneration: association with dietary fat, transunsaturated fat, nuts, and fish intake. Arch Ophthalmol 2003;121(12): 1728–37.
71 San Giovanni JP, Chew EY, Agrón E, et. al. The relationship of dietary omega-3 long-chain polyunsaturated fatty acid intake with incident age-related macular degeneration: AREDS report no. 23. Arch Ophthalmol 2008;126(9):1274–9.
72 Chong EW, Kreis AJ, Wong TY, et. al. Dietary omega-3 fatty acid and fish intake in the primary prevention of age-related macular degeneration: a systematic review and meta-analysis. Arch Ophthalmol 2008;126(6):826–33.
73 Tan JS, Wang JJ, Flood V, et. al. Dietary fatty acids and the 10-year incidence of age-related macular degeneration: the Blue Mountains Eye Study. Arch Ophthalmol 2009;127(5):656–65.
74 Cumming RG, Mitchell P, Smith W. Dietary sodium intake and cataract: the Blue Mountains Eye Study. Am J Epidemiol 2000;151(6):624–6.
75 Vanden Langenberg GM, Mares-Perlman JA, Klein R, et. al. Associations between antioxidant and zinc intake and the 5-year incidence of early age-related maculopathy in the Beaver Dam Eye Study. Am J Epidemiol 1998;148:204–14.
76 Age-Related Eye Disease Study Research Group. A randomised, placebo-controlled, clinical trial of high-dose supplementation with vitamins C and E, beta-carotene, and zinc for age-related macular degeneration and vision loss: AREDS report no. 8. Arch Ophthalmol 2001;119(10):1417–36.
77 Evans J. Antioxidant supplements to prevent or slow down the progression of AMD: a systematic review and meta-analysis. Eye 2008;22(6):751–60.
78 Evans JR, Henshaw K. Antioxidant vitamin and mineral supplements for preventing age-related macular degeneration. Cochrane Database Syst Rev. 2008 Jan 23;(1):CD000253.
79 Christen WG, Manson JE, Glynn RJ, et. al. Beta-carotene supplementation and age-related maculopathy in a randomised trial of US physicians. Arch Ophthalmol 2007;125(3):333–9.
80 Chong EW, Wong TY, Kreis AJ, et. al. Dietary antioxidants and primary prevention of age-related macular degeneration: systematic review and meta-analysis. BMJ 2007;335(7623):755.
81 Christen WG, Glynn RJ, Chew EY, et. al. Folic acid, pyridoxine, and cyanocobalamin combination treatment and age-related macular degeneration in women: the Women's Antioxidant and Folic Acid Cardiovascular Study. Arch Intern Med 2009;169(4):335–41.
82 Nowak M, Szapska B, Swietochowska E, et. al. (Blood concentration of homocysteine, vitamin B (12), and folic acid in patients with exudative age-related macular degeneration). Klin Oczna 2004;106(3 Suppl):429–30.
83 Kamburoglu G, Gumus K, Kadayifcilar S, et. al. Plasma homocysteine, vitamin B12 and folate levels in age-related macular degeneration. Graefes Arch Clin Exp Ophthalmol 2006;244(5):565–9.
84 Rochtchina E, Wang JJ, Flood VM, et. al. Elevated serum homocysteine, low serum vitamin B12, folate, and age-related macular degeneration: the Blue Mountains Eye Study. Am J Ophthalmol 2007;143(2):344–6.
85 Parekh N, Chappell RJ, Millen AE, et. al. Association between vitamin D and age-related macular degeneration in the Third National Health and Nutrition Examination Survey, 1988 through 1994. Arch Ophthalmol 2007;125(5):661–9.
86 Mares-Perlman JA, Lyle BJ, Klein R, et. al. Vitamin supplement use and incident cataracts in a population-based study. Arch Ophthalmol 2000;118(11):1556–63.
87 Lyle BJ, Mares-Perlman JA, Klein BE, et. al. Antioxidant intake and risk of incident age-related nuclear cataracts in the Beaver Dam Eye Study. Am J Epidemiol 1999;149(9):801–9.
88 Taylor A, Jacques PF, Chylack LT Jr, et. al. Long-term intake of vitamins and carotenoids and odds of early age-related cortical and posterior subcapsular lens opacities. AJCN 2002;75(3):540–9.
89 Age-Related Eye Disease Study Research Group. A randomised, placebo-controlled, clinical trial of high-dose supplementation with vitamins C and E and beta-carotene for age-related cataract and vision loss: AREDS report no. 9. Arch Ophthalmol. 2001;119(10):1439–52.
90 Christen WG, Glynn RJ, Chew EY, et. al. Vitamin E and age-related cataract in a randomised trial of women. Ophthalmology 2008;115(5):822–829.e1.
91 Vitetta L, Sali A. Omega–3 Fatty Acids PUFA - A Review PART I. Journal of Complementary Medicine 2006;5(6):52–59.

92 SanGiovanni JP, Chew EY. The role of omega-3 long-chain polyunsaturated fatty acids in health and disease of the retina. Prog Retin Eye Res. 2005;24(1):87–138.

93 Nettleton JA. Omega-3 fatty acids: comparison of plant and seafood sources in human nutrition. J Am Diet Assoc. 1991;91(3):331–337.

94 Bazan NG. The metabolism of omega-3 polyunsaturated fatty acids in the eye: the possible role of docosahexaenoic acid and docosanoids in retinal physiology and ocular pathology. Prog Clin Biol Res 1989;312:95–112.

95 Linnane AW, Kios M, Vitetta L. Healthy Ageing: Regulation of the Metabolome by Cellular Redox Modulation and Prooxidant Signaling Systems. The Essential Roles of Superoxide Anion and Nitric Oxide. Biogerontology 2007;8(5):445–67.

96 Kirschfeld K. Carotenoid pigments: their possible role in protecting against photooxidation in eyes and photoreceptor cells. Proc R Soc Lond B Biol Sci 1982;216(1202):71–85.

97 Mares-Perlman JA, Brady WE, Klein R, et. al. Dietary fat and age-related maculopathy. Arch Ophthalmol. 1995;113(6):743–748.

98 Heuberger RA, Mares-Perlman JA, Klein R, et. al. Relationship of dietary fat to age-related maculopathy in the Third National Health and Nutrition Examination Survey. Arch Ophthalmol 2001;119(12):1833–1838.

99 Delcourt C, Carriere I, Cristol JP, et. al. Dietary fat and the risk of age-related maculopathy: the POLANUT Study. Eur J Clin Nutr 2007;61(11):1341–1344.

100 Seddon JM, Rosner B, Sperduto RD, et. al. Dietary fat and risk for advanced age-related macular degeneration. Arch Ophthalmol. 2001;119(8):1191–1199.

101 SanGiovanni JP, Chew EY, Clemons TE, et. al. Age-Related Eye Disease Study Research Group. The relationship of dietary lipid intake and age-related macular degeneration in a case-control study: AREDS report No. 20. Arch Ophthalmol. 2007;125(5):671–679.

102 Chong EW, Kreis AJ, Wong TY, et. al. Dietary omega-3 fatty acid and fish intake in the primary prevention of age-related macular degeneration: a systematic review and meta-analysis. Arch Ophthalmol 2008;126(6):826–33.

103 SanGiovanni JP, Chew EY, Agrón E, et. al. The relationship of dietary omega-3 long-chain polyunsaturated fatty acid intake with incident age-related macular degeneration: AREDS report no. 23. Arch Ophthalmol 2008;126(9):1274–9.

104 Carpentier S, Knaus M, Suh M. Associations between lutein, zeaxanthin, and age-related macular degeneration: an overview. Crit Rev Food Sci Nutr 2009;49(4):313–26.

105 Moeller SM, Parekh N, Tinker L, et. al. CAREDS Research Study Group. Associations between intermediate age-related macular degeneration and lutein and zeaxanthin in the Carotenoids in Age-related Eye Disease Study (CAREDS): ancillary study of the Women's Health Initiative. Arch Ophthalmol 2006;124:1151–1162.

106 Moeller SM, Voland R, Tinker B, et. al. CAREDS Study Group. Women's Health Initiative. Associations between age-related nuclear cataract and lutein and zeaxanthin in the diet and serum in the Carotenoids in the Age-Related Eye Disease Study (CAREDS), an ancillary study of the Women's Health Initiative. Arch Ophthalmol 2008;126(3):354–364.

107 Delcourt C, Carriere I, Delage M, et. al., POL A Study Group. Plasma lutein and zeaxanthin and other carotenoids as modifiable risk factors for age-related maculopathy and cataract: the POLA Study. Invest Ophthalmol Vis Sci 2006;47:2329–2335.

108 Coleman H, Chew E. Nutritional supplementation in age-related macular degeneration. Curr Opin Ophthalmol 2007;18(3):220–3.

109 Bartlett H, Eperjesi F. Age-related macular degeneration and nutritional supplementation: a review of randomised controlled trials. Ophthalmic Physiol Opt 2003;23(5):383–99.

110 Olmedilla B, Granado F, Blanco I, et. al. Serum status of carotenoids and tocopherols in patients with age-related cataracts: a case-control study. J Nutr Health Ageing 2002;6(1):66–8.

111 Bone RA, Landrum JT, Guerra LH, et. al. Lutein and zeaxanthin dietary supplements raise macular pigment density and serum concentrations of these carotenoids in humans. J Nutr 2003;133:992–998.

112 Khachik F, de Moura FF, Chew EY,et. al. The effect of lutein and zeaxanthin supplementation on metabolites of these carotenoids in the serum of persons aged 60 or older. Invest Ophthalmol Vis Sci 2006;47(12):5234–42.

113 Olmedilla B, Granado F, Blanco I, et. al. Lutein, but not alpha-tocopherol, supplementation improves visual function in patients with age-related cataracts: a 2-y double-blind, placebo-controlled pilot study. Nutrition 2003;19(1):21–4.

114 Olmedilla B, Granado F, Blanco I, et. al. Lutein in patients with cataracts and age-related macular degeneration: a long term supplementation study. J Sci Food Agric 2001;81:904–909.

115 Trumbo PR, Ellwood KC. Lutein and zeaxanthin intakes and risk of age-related macular degeneration and cataracts: an evaluation using the Food and Drug Administration's evidence-based review system for health claims. AJCN 2006;84:971–974.

116 Schalch W, Cohn W, Barker FM, et. al. Xanthophyll accumulation in the human retina during supplementation with lutein or zeaxanthin — the LUXEA (Lutein Xanthophyll Eye Accumulation) study. Arch Biochem Biophys. 2007;458:128–135.

117 Rhone M, Basu A. Phytochemicals and age-related eye diseases. Nutr Rev 2008;66(8):465–72.

118 Matsumoto H, Nakamura Y, Iida H, et. al. Comparative assessment of distribution of blackcurrant anthocyanins in rabbit and rat ocular tissues. Exp Eye Res 2006;83:348–356.

119 Rahman I, Biswas SK, Kirkham PA. Regulation of inflammation and redox signaling by dietary polyphenols. Biochem Pharmacol 2006;72:1439–1452.

120 Karlsen A, Retterstol L, Laake P, et. al. Anthocyanins inhibit nuclear factor-kappaB activation in monocytes and reduce plasma concentrations of pro-inflammatory mediators in healthy adults. J Nutr 2007;137:1951–1954.

121 Miura D, Miura Y, Yagasaki K. Resveratrol inhibits hepatoma cell invasion by suppressing gene expression of hepatocyte growth factor via its reactive oxygen species-scavenging property. Clin Exp Metastasis 2004;21:445–451.

122 Sun W, Wang W, Kim J, et. al. Anti-cancer effect of resveratrol is associated with induction of apoptosis via a mitochondrial pathway alignment. Adv Exp Med Biol 2008;614:179–186.

123 King RE, Kent KD, Bomser JA. Resveratrol reduces oxidation and proliferation of human retinal pigment epithelial cells via extracellular signal-regulated kinase inhibition. Chem Biol Interact 2005;151(2):143–9.

124 Doganay S, Borazan M, Iraz M, et. al. The effect of resveratrol in experimental cataract model formed by sodium selenite. Curr Eye Res 2006;31:147–153.

125 Chung HS, Harris A, Kristinsson JK, et. al. *Ginkgo biloba* extract increases ocular blood flow velocity. J Ocul Pharmacol Ther 1999;15:233–240.

126 Quaranta L, Bettelli S, Uva MG, et. al. Effect of *Ginkgo biloba* extract on preexisting visual field damage in normal tension glaucoma. Ophthalmology 2003;110:359–364.

127 Zhang B, Safa R, Rusciano D, et. al. Epigallocatechin gallate, an active ingredient from green tea, attenuates damaging influences to the retina caused by ischemia/reperfusion. Brain Res 2007;1159:40–53.

128 Costa BL, Fawcett R, Li GY, et. al. Orally administered epigallocatechin gallate attenuates light-induced photoreceptor damage. Brain Res Bull 2008;76(4):412–23.

129 Falsini B, Marangoni D, Salgarello T, et. al. Effect of epigallocatechin-gallate on inner retinal function in ocular hypertension and glaucoma: A short-term study by pattern electroretinogram. Graefes Arch Clin Exp Ophthalmol 2009;247(9):1223–33.

130 Cariello AJ, Casanova FH, Lima Filho AA, et. al. Effect of electroacupuncture to prevent selenite-induced cataract in Wistar rats. Arq Bras Oftalmol 2006;69(3):299–303.

131 Gioia L, Cabrini L, Gemma M, et. al. Sedative effect of acupuncture during cataract surgery: prospective randomised double-blind study. J Cataract Refract Surg 2006;32(11):1951–4.

Chapter 4

Anxiety

With contribution from Dr Katherine Sevar

Introduction

Anxiety disorders are amongst the most common disorders suffered by the Australian population, with approximately 7% of men and 12% of women affected each year.[1]

Anxiety disorders are classically under-reported to GPs by the community, with on average only one-fifth of people with anxiety as their primary complaint seeking professional help in 2002.[2] The reasons cited for this include preferring to individually manage the condition and a desire to pursue self-help strategies.[3] Given this finding, it may come as a surprise that anxiety is actually one of the commonest presentations to GPs — when a sub-study of BEACH (Bettering the Evaluation and Care of Health) surveyed a random sample of 379 GPs they discovered that the 3 conditions placing the greatest demand on an individual practitioner's time were anxiety, depression and back pain.[4] Recent statistics suggest 1–2% of the adult population suffer panic disorders — common risk factors include female gender, low socioeconomic status and anxious childhood temperament — and this is associated with significant suicide risk, all-cause mortality and cardiovascular disease.[5]

Sub-classifications of anxiety disorders

There are sub-classifications of anxiety disorders according to DSM-IV criteria, which include generalised anxiety disorder (GAD), panic disorder, agoraphobia, obsessive compulsive disorder (OCD), social anxiety disorder (SAD), and post-traumatic stress disorder (PTSD). There is significant co-morbidity with anxiety disorders and depression and substance abuse.[1]

Generalised anxiety disorder (GAD)

GAD is commonly encountered in general practice and infrequently referred for specialist management. It may be experienced by 5% of the general population at some point in their lives and affects both sexes equally. It is diagnosable when the preoccupation with worry about the present, past and future, begins to interfere with day-to-day functioning and is characterised by hyper-arousal, insomnia, physical symptoms such as chest tightness, over-breathing, tension headache and diarrhoea. Individuals may abuse drugs or alcohol to manage their symptoms. GAD will benefit from psychological intervention with cognitive behaviour therapy (CBT) being the most commonly employed technique. Psychological, behavioural and lifestyle approaches are helpful for alleviating anxiety. Anti-anxiety or antidepressant medication may also be necessary.

Panic disorder and agoraphobia

Panic attacks can be spontaneous or can occur in relation to a specific stimulus. They include somatic features and cognitive features. The somatic features may include palpitations, chest pain, a feeling of choking, nausea, sweating, dizziness. The cognitive features may include acute fear of dying, losing control, going mad and a need to escape from the current situation and there can also a be a feeling of depersonalisation or non-realisation. In up to 90% of cases, these attacks lead to an avoidance of situations where escape may not be possible — agoraphobia.[6] Common associations occur with depression, substance abuse and interpersonal difficulties. Panic disorder is currently treated with anti-anxiety medication and a mix of CBT and exposure therapy. Breathing techniques for the short-term management of panic attacks are advocated and benzodiazepines should only be used in the short-term.

Obsessive compulsive disorder (OCD)

Obsessions can be intrusive thoughts, images or impulses which create anxiety in an individual as they feel unable to control how, when or where these obsessive thoughts may occur. Compulsive behaviour develops as an attempt to relieve the anxiety created by the obsession. Compulsions can include extremely ritualistic behaviours and a need to follow a set routine. Although the compulsions initially relieve anxiety they will over time relieve less anxiety, resulting in them becoming more elaborate and taking up more of the individual's time. OCD becomes a problem when these behaviours interfere with ordinary life. Current treatment strategies include medication with a selective serotonin re-uptake inhibitor (SSRI) or clomipramine (a serotonergic tricyclic antidepressant) in combination with CBT.

Social anxiety disorder (SAD)

Individuals with SAD and/or social phobia describe experiencing extreme anxiety in social scenarios due to a fear they will embarrass themselves and often manifest physical signs of this anxiety by blushing and stuttering if asked to speak in public. They may become avoidant of social situations. They will have typically experienced these problems since childhood and adolescence. Psychological therapies focusing on assertiveness training, CBT, and graded exposure to overcome avoidance behaviour are used in the treatment of SAD and/or social phobia. Pharmacotherapy with SSRIs would be indicated in concurrent depression.

Post-traumatic stress disorder (PTSD)

PTSD may develop months to years after exposure to a situation of extreme traumatic stress. The hallmarks of the condition include re-experiencing the traumatic event, avoidance of the situation in which the event occurred, increased arousal, nightmares related to the event and insomnia. Secondary conditions may develop, such as alcohol dependence or depression, and these may be the first conditions for which people seek help prior to recognising the symptoms of PTSD.

Trends in integrative medicine for anxiety

Research describing long-term trends in complementary medicine (CM) use in the US reported that complementary therapies were used by 57% of people reporting anxiety attacks and 66% of patients consulting a physician for treatment of anxiety. Those surveyed perceived that the efficacy of complementary medicines for anxiety were comparable to conventional drug treatment.[7]

Lifestyle medicine

Lifestyle factors such as chronic stress, poor nutrition, caffeine, smoking, obesity, alcohol and substance abuse may initiate or perpetuate the symptoms of an anxiety disorder[8] and there is an increasing interest among medical and health practitioners to address these lifestyle factors in combination with pharmacotherapy and psychological therapies for anxiety disorders.[9]

Mind-body medicine

Psychological therapies

Counselling for anxiety in general practice

Patient-centred care has also become a major focus in mainstream medicine and is being evaluated and promoted within general practice in particular.[10] Active listening, compassion and empathy are vital factors in the counselling of those patients with an anxiety disorder. Patients who feel their doctors listen to them, and respond with empathy, feel they have greater overall improvement across many conditions.[11] In a study of 309 women seeking psychological support, GPs with good listening skills and those who provided longer consultation times were highly valued.[12] Women who received referral, counselling and relaxation advice from their GP reported a higher degree of satisfaction.

Cognitive behaviour therapy (CBT) and group therapy

CBT is a talking-based therapy arising from the link between thoughts, feelings and behaviour.[13] CBT is a valuable tool for the management of anxiety and it is the first-line treatment for adults and children. The central beliefs of CBT and interventions for anxiety disorders include cognitive restructuring, relaxation, breathing techniques, graded exposure to anxiety provoking situations, problem solving, assertiveness training and social skills development. In an 8-week program,[14] CBT including exposure therapy was better than placebo (supportive, non-directive counselling) or moclobemide for the treatment of panic disorder with agoraphobia. Long-term benefits of CBT occurred when used in combination with moclobemide. Self-help CBT programs available on the internet may also be of help in allaying test anxiety. In a study of 90 university students who were randomised to CBT or a control program, both on the internet,[15] anxiety was rated before and after treatment and 53% of the CBT group showed a significant improvement in anxiety related to the test but only 29% of the control group demonstrated benefit. This study supports the use of CBT on the internet for the treatment of test anxiety.

Research supports the role of CBT for social phobia in both group and individual formats.[16] In this study, symptom measures completed at the beginning and end of group therapy found improvement in group cohesion and social anxiety symptoms over time, as well as

Table 4.1 RANZCP clinical practice guidelines for the treatment of panic disorder and agoraphobia

Education for the patient and significant others	(i) the nature and course of panic disorder and agoraphobia (ii) an explanation of the psychopathology of anxiety, panic and agoraphobia (iii) rationale for the treatment, likelihood of a positive response, and expected timeframe
Cognitive behaviour therapy (CBT)	CBT is more effective and more cost-effective than medication
Pharmaceuticals	Tricyclic antidepressants (TCAs) and serotonin selective reuptake inhibitors (SSRIs) are equal in efficacy and both are to be preferred to benzodiazepines
Treatment choice depends on the skill of the clinician and the patient's circumstances	(i) Drug treatment should be complemented by behaviour therapy (ii) If the response to an adequate trial of a first-line treatment is poor, another evidence-based treatment should be used (iii) A second opinion can be useful *The presence of severe agoraphobia is a negative prognostic indicator, whereas comorbid depression, if properly treated, has no consistent effect on outcome

(Source: RANZCP Guidelines Team for Panic Disorder and Agoraphobia. *Australian and New Zealand Journal of Psychiatry*, 2003;37:641–56)

improvement on measures of general anxiety, depression, and functional impairment.

Clinical guidelines and treatment recommendations by the Royal Australian and New Zealand College of Psychiatrists (RANZCP) are summarised in Table 4.1.[17]

Drugs

Social anxiety disorder (SAD) and lack of family cohesion are known risk factors for drug use such as marijuana and alcohol use.[18] Combination of SAD with either alcohol or drug use is associated with higher comorbidity in anxious individuals and may further aggravate anxiety.[19–22] Patients should be advised to avoid using alcohol and drugs for alleviation of anxiety symptoms.

Mind–body therapies

In general, mind-body therapies, particularly CBT, carry the greatest weight of scientific evidence for the treatment of anxiety. A recent review of the literature exploring various complementary and self-help treatments for anxiety in children and adolescents identified that:

> relevant evidence was available for bibliotherapy, dance and movement therapy, distraction techniques, humour, massage, melatonin, relaxation training, autogenic training, avoiding marijuana, a mineral-vitamin supplement (EMPower+) and music therapy.[23]

The authors concluded these therapies might be useful but warned more trials are recommended.

Autogenic training (AT) and biofeedback

Autogenic training addresses an imbalance between the sympathetic system and parasympathetic system by using a series of relaxation and visualisation techniques which are practised daily.

A systematic review in 2000 evaluated all of the controlled trials investigating AT and identified 8 such trials although the majority of these trials were methodologically flawed.[24] Seven trials reported positive effects of AT in reducing stress and 1 study showed no such benefit. The authors noted no firm conclusion could be drawn from these studies.

However, a recent meta-analysis of AT assessing 7 clinical trials found that 3 trials with control groups showed a positive outcome and that 1 further case controlled trial was also positive but the remaining 3 trials showed no difference. There is encouraging evidence from more recent trials that AT can reduce stress and anxiety in adults, as well as children and adolescents.[25–28]

There are some preliminary results for the use of biofeedback in adults.[29, 30]

Bibliotherapy

Bibliotherapy uses reading as a healing therapy by tailoring the reading material to the patient's current life situation. There have been several meta-analyses completed considering bibliotherapy for the treatment of anxiety and they concluded that bibliotherapy appeared to work best when there was a well-circumscribed problem; that is, a specific phobia,[31] but that it had very little effect on OCD or panic disorder.[32] It appeared to be more effective in highly motivated individuals.

A recent study focusing on social phobia found that a self-help program consisting of an 8-week self-directed CBT with minimal therapist involvement for social phobia based on a widely available self-help book was superior to wait-list on most outcome measures.[33] Benefits were observed with reductions in social anxiety, global severity, general anxiety, and depression following the study and at 3-months follow-up.

Bibliotherapy can also be used in a group setting.[34]

Dance therapy

In a review of complementary therapies for anxiety disorders in 2004, dance therapy was considered to have encouraging evidence for people with self-identified anxiety, test anxiety and other anxiety problems in clinical groups. The authors considered it would be worth exploring whether dance therapy may have a greater anxiolytic effect than physical exercise.[35]

Hypnotherapy

A growing body of research appears to support the role of hypnosis in the treatment of anxiety. In a large prospective, randomised single-centre study published in the *Lancet*,[36] 241 patients undergoing percutaneous vascular and renal procedures were randomised to receive intraoperative standard care (n = 79), structured attention (n = 80) or self-hypnotic relaxation (n = 82). All patients had access to intravenous analgesia (fentanyl and midazolam). Hypnosis had a more pronounced effect on pain and anxiety reduction. Pain increased linearly in both the standard and attention groups, but remained flat in the hypnosis group. With time, anxiety decreased in all 3 groups, but at a higher rate in the hypnosis group. Drug use was twice as likely in the standard group than the attention and hypnosis groups. Only 1 patient became haemodynamically unstable in the hypnosis group compared with 10 and 12 in the attention and standard groups respectively.

In a small RCT[37] of paediatric cancer patients, 45 children aged 6–16 years were randomised into 1 of 3 groups: local aesthetic, local aesthetic plus hypnosis, and local anaesthetic plus attention for the relief of lumbar puncture-induced pain and anxiety. Patients in the local anaesthetic plus hypnosis group reported less anticipatory anxiety and procedure-related pain and anxiety, and they were rated as demonstrating less behavioural distress during the procedure. The magnitude of treatment benefit depended on their level of hypnotisability and this benefit was maintained when patients used hypnosis independently. Another small hospital study,[38] assessing pre-operative anxiety, randomised adult patients into 3 groups: a hypnosis group (n = 26) who received suggestions of wellbeing; an attention-control group (n = 26) who received attentive listening and support without any specific hypnotic suggestions, and a 'standard of care' control group (n = 24). Anxiety was assessed before and after their operation. Patients in the hypnosis group were significantly less anxious following surgery, compared with patients in the attention-control group and the control group. Moreover, the hypnosis group reported a significant decrease of 56% in their anxiety level pre-operatively, whereas, the attention-control group reported an increase of 10% and the control group an increase of 47% in their anxiety. In conclusion, the researchers found that 'hypnosis significantly alleviates preoperative anxiety'. Hypnosis plays a useful role in allaying anxiety for a number of other operative procedures, such as colonoscopy.[39]

A larger well conducted prospective trial published in *Pain* 2006, randomised 236 women for large core needle breast biopsy to receive standard care (n = 76), structured empathic attention (n = 82), or self-hypnotic relaxation (n = 78) during their procedures. Patients were rated for pain and anxiety every 10 minutes during their care.[40]

Women's anxiety increased significantly in the standard group, did not change in the empathy group, and decreased significantly in the hypnosis group. Pain increased significantly in all 3 groups by 50% for standard care, 37% for empathy, and 34% for hypnosis. The researcher concluded that hypnosis 'provides more powerful anxiety relief without undue cost and thus appears attractive for outpatient pain management'.

A systematic review of studies shows that hypnotherapy is highly effective for patients with refractory irritable bowel syndrome (IBS) and alleviating anxiety, but definite efficacy of hypnosis in the treatment of IBS remains unclear due to limited number of controlled trials.[41]

A recent review of the literature identified 60 publications that found hypnotherapy may be useful for a wide range of disorders and problems in children, and is particularly valuable in the treatment of anxiety disorders and trauma-related conditions, especially in conjunction with family therapy and CBT.[42]

School refusal is considered a form of anxiety. A small study increased school attendance by using a form of self-hypnosis on children suffering school refusal.[43]

A review of the research acknowledges the important role of hypnosis in health care, especially for difficult to treat patients and for reducing anxiety.[44] Hypnosis can successfully be used to help alleviate peri-operative anxiety and stress in a hospital setting.[45]

Meditation

A Cochrane review could not conclude from 2 small studies if meditation alone is effective for anxiety.[46] The researchers identified 2 randomised controlled studies of moderate quality that used active control comparisons, meditation, relaxation, or biofeedback. Anti-anxiety drugs were used as standard treatment. The duration of trials ranged from 12 to 18 weeks. In 1 study, transcendental meditation showed a reduction in anxiety symptoms compared with biofeedback and relaxation therapy.[46] Another study compared Kundalini Yoga with relaxation/mindfulness meditation, which showed no statistically significant difference between groups.[46] However, the overall dropout rate in both studies was high (33–44%). Neither study reported on adverse effect of meditation. More studies are warranted.

Relaxation therapies

Patients with an anxiety disorder should be encouraged to learn various relaxation methods as there is strong research demonstrating their benefit. A systematic review of mind–body therapies in 2007 concluded that there was now robust evidence for the use of relaxation therapy in anxiety and insomnia.[47]

A recent meta-analysis of the literature, inclusive of 27 studies, found relaxation training had a significant beneficial effect in the treatment of anxiety.[48] Efficacy was higher for meditation and for longer treatments. Implications and limitations are discussed.

A separate review found that when the different classifications of anxiety disorder were considered separately then relaxation was most effective for GAD, panic disorder, test anxiety and dental phobia, but that it was less effective for PTSD, OCD and specific phobias.[35]

Music therapy

Listening to music may also help alleviate pre-operative anxiety. A randomised controlled trial study of 180 patients having day surgery was conducted to assess anxiety before and after listening to patient-preferred music.[49]

Patients were randomised to either an intervention (n = 60), placebo (n = 60) or control group (n = 60). Statistically, music significantly reduced the state of anxiety level in the music (intervention) group compared with the placebo and control groups, with no differences found between socio-demographic or clinical variables such as gender or type of surgery. Another study on patients undergoing cardiac surgery also demonstrated significant reduction in anxiety and pain levels in those receiving music therapy.[50] Eighty-six patients (69.8% males) were randomised to 1 of 2 groups; 50 patients received 20 minutes of music (intervention), whereas 36 patients had 20 minutes of rest in bed (control). Anxiety, pain, physiologic parameters, and the use of analgesia (opioid) consumption were measured before and after the 20-minute period. The music therapy group demonstrated a significant reduction in anxiety and pain compared with the control group. There was no difference in systolic or diastolic blood pressures, or heart rate. Also, there was no reduction in the use of analgesia (opioid) usage in the 2 groups.

Music therapy may also play a role in palliative care[51] where research demonstrated statistical improvements in mood and anxiety, and in pain control and reducing anxiety in patients during wound dressings.[52]

Religion

Religiosity and spirituality have long been seen as a worthwhile buffer against dealing with life's problems and stresses and a large population study over 9 years showed that all-cause mortality was significantly reduced and life expectancy increased (75 years compared with 82 years) for regular churchgoers. This was not explainable by lifestyle and social variables.[53] However, there has been only 1 randomised trial to date which added a religious component to standard pharmacotherapy for GAD and this showed improvement at 3 months but this did not appear to be sustained at 6 months.[54]

Creativity

Anorexia nervosa (AN) is often associated with distressing, intrusive, anxious preoccupations with control of eating, weight and shape. One study of 38 women with AN admitted to a specialised eating disorder unit were offered knitting lessons and free access to supplies.[55] Of interest, patients reported a significant subjective reduction in anxious preoccupation when knitting, with 74% reporting reduction in the intensity of their fears and thoughts and their minds cleared of eating disorder preoccupations. In addition, 74% reported it had a calming and therapeutic effect and 53% reported it provided satisfaction, pride and a sense of accomplishment. This study demonstrates that creative activities may be of help with anxiety symptoms experienced with AN and more research is required, particularly to see if other creative areas, such as painting and pottery, may also be of help.

Behavioural interventions — summary

The evidence currently suggests using behavioural interventions before considering pharmacotherapy in insomnia. A meta-analysis examining the evidence for behavioural modification CBT, relaxation and behavioural treatment alone, found 23 randomised controlled trials and concluded there were moderate to large effect sizes showing an improvement in sleep for all 3 modalities and the results were the same in both middle-aged adults and older adults (55+).[56] A review of the increasing evidence for mind-body therapies in 2007 concluded that there was now robust evidence for the use of relaxation therapy in anxiety and insomnia.[57]

Sleep

Anxiety and insomnia are highly co-morbid conditions and physiologically anxiety and low mood increase corticotrophin releasing hormone (CRH) and other stress hormones secreted from the adrenal glands which, in turn, have negative impact upon sleep patterns.[58] A large health survey conducted in Germany (n = 4186) found that individuals with anxiety disorder and insomnia experienced significantly worse mental-health related quality of life and increased disability.[59] Most anxiety disorders were moderately associated with reduced sleep quality with GAD (AOR 3.94, 95% CI 1.66-9.34) and SAD (AOR 3.95, 95% CI 1.73-9.04) having the strongest relationship to reduced quality of life scores. For more information see Chapter 22.

Melatonin

In a systematic review of melatonin, 6 RCTs were included which concluded that there was sufficient evidence to show that low dose melatonin improves sleep quality.[60]

Multiple studies have demonstrated that oral melatonin can be an effective premedication for surgery, improves peri-operative analgesia, can act as an anti-anxiolytic, enhances analgesia and promotes better operating conditions under topical anaesthesia, such as in cataract surgery, even reducing the risk of intraocular pressure in eye surgery.[61, 62] In 1 RCT, the anxiolytic effect of 5mg oral melatonin (and clonidine) resulted in reduced postoperative pain, and the need for morphine consumption reduced by more than 30% in patients undergoing abdominal hysterectomy under general anaesthetic; far greater than placebo.[63] The beneficial effects of both melatonin and clonidine were equivalent.

In a recent prospective, double-blind, placebo-controlled, cross-over trial in a community-living population of 22 elderly with a history of sleep disorder complaints of whom 14 were receiving hypnotic drug therapy, participants were randomised to either 2 months of melatonin (5mg/day) and 2 months of placebo. Sleep disorders, mood, behaviour and level of depression and anxiety were evaluated.[64] Melatonin treatment for 2 months significantly improved sleep quality scores and mood levels, especially for depression and anxiety, and facilitated discontinuation of hypnotic drugs compared with placebo.

Acupuncture

A Cochrane review in 2007 reviewed acupuncture as a treatment for insomnia and found that from the small number of RCTs, together with the poor methodological quality and significant clinical heterogeneity, the current evidence is not sufficiently extensive or rigorous to support the use of acupuncture in the treatment of insomnia.[65]

Sunshine

There is increasing evidence pointing to the important role of vitamin D in a multitude of disease processes, from multiple sclerosis to diabetes mellitus. Vitamin D deficiency may be associated with anxiety and depression in those suffering from fibromyalgia and in research from Northern Ireland, patients with vitamin D deficiency (<25 nmol/l) had higher Hamilton Anxiety and Depression Score (HADS), compared with patients with insufficient levels (25–50 nmol/l) or with normal levels (> 50 nmol/l).[66] The exact nature and direction of the causal relationship remains unclear but further research is warranted.

Vitamin D deficiency is prevalent among older adults, and research suggests there may be an association between Vitamin D deficiency and basic and executive cognitive functions, depression, bipolar disorder, and schizophrenia.[67] Vitamin D activates receptors on neurons in regions implicated in the regulation of behaviour, stimulates neurotrophin release, and protects the brain by buffering antioxidant and anti-inflammatory defences against vascular injury and improving metabolic and cardiovascular function.

Although there is currently a lack of evidence for the association of low vitamin D levels with anxiety, given its potential implication in the mood disorders listed above, and already proven health benefits, it would be appropriate to advocate greater monitoring of vitamin D blood levels in the general population, promoting greater safe sun exposure and supplementation in those individuals if needed.

Environment

Smoking

Smoking is well recognised as being a behavioural response to stress and stress management plays an important role in cessation of smoking. Nicotine affects a wide range of neurotransmitters involved in the development of anxiety, including glutamate, GABA, nicotinic acetylcholine receptors and serotonin. It is now widely believed that smoking may increase anxiety levels and that smokers are locked into a cycle where they suffer the short-term anxiety associated with nicotine withdrawal only to relieve that by smoking, therefore perpetuating the problem. There has been some research into the general population suggesting that overall anxiety levels fall after smoking cessation[68] but no RCTs have been conducted in people with anxiety disorders.

Physical activities

Exercise

The beneficial effect of exercise on anxiety disorders has been largely accepted. The most recent meta-analysis conducted in 2008, included only RCTs (n = 49) and came to the overwhelming conclusion that exercise is effective[69] in reducing anxiety compared with no-treatment control groups. Exercise groups also showed greater reductions in anxiety when compared to groups receiving other anxiety reducing treatment.

However, when a large population-based sample of identical twins (n = 5952) was followed between their ages of 18–50, from 1991–2002, in genetically identical twin pairs, the twin who exercised more did not display fewer anxious and depressive symptoms than the co-twin who exercised less.[70] Longitudinal analyses showed that increases in exercise participation did not predict decreases in anxious and depressive symptoms. These researchers concluded that although regular exercise is associated with reduced anxious and depressive symptoms in the population at large, the association does not appear to be because of the causal effects of exercise.

There has been more encouraging evidence in the treatment of anxiety and panic attacks, showing aerobic exercise to be as effective as clomipramine in the treatment of panic disorder.[71]

Yoga

Yoga is gaining in popularity internationally, both for exercise and as a method of relieving stress. There have been several positive RCTs conducted in yoga. An RCT in women with breast cancer undergoing adjuvant radiotherapy and 6 weeks of chemotherapy following surgery (n = 38) were randomised to receive either a weekly 60 minute yoga class or supportive therapy and the women in the yoga group reported an overall decrease in both self-reported state anxiety ($p<0.001$) and trait anxiety ($p = 0.005$).[72] There was also a positive correlation between anxiety states and traits with symptom severity and distress during conventional treatment intervals. Another controlled trial found yoga to be superior to diazepam for generalised anxiety but patients were allowed to choose their allocation of treatment (i.e. yoga or diazepam).[73]

Nutritional influences

Alcohol

Alcohol is a well-known, well-accepted commonly used method to reduce anxiety and there have been several placebo-controlled trials conducted which confirm the short-term anti-anxiolytic effects of alcohol in those with panic disorder,[74] social phobia[75] and GAD.[76] However, in the long-term, anxiety and alcohol abuse can become comorbid conditions as tolerance to alcohol develops and greater amounts are required to produce the same effect. Initially, alcohol affects GABA receptors in the same way as benzodiazepines, but with chronic alcohol use, GABA receptor tone may decrease, which can precipitate anxiety.[77] For individuals with chronic alcohol use, reduced anxiety has been reported from uncontrolled studies following the cessation of alcohol.[78]

Caffeine

Maximal lifetime caffeine intake and caffeine-associated toxicity and dependence are moderately associated with risk for a wide range of psychiatric and substance use disorders.[79] A study of 376 young British adults showed that estimated daily caffeine consumption increased with age, and was associated with smoking and greater alcohol consumption.[80] These researchers found the level of caffeine consumption was not associated with impulsivity, sociability, extraversion or trait anxiety.

Caffeine challenge studies have been conducted as randomised double-blind placebo-controlled trials which uniformly confirm that caffeine exacerbates anxiety in those suffering from GAD,[81] panic disorder[82] and social phobia.[83]

In the community, there is a high rate of discontinuation of caffeine in people with anxiety disorders because of the self-reported increase in symptoms following ingestion of caffeine and this is supported in retrospective analyses[84, 85] and a case series of individuals,[86] who experienced a reduction in anxiety following the cessation of caffeine. Based on the findings of the studies overall, anxiety sufferers should avoid high doses of caffeine. Other symptoms associated with anxiety and high caffeine intake include palpitations and muscle tension. However, there have been no RCTs conducted examining the effect of reduction or abstention from caffeine.

Nutritional supplements

Fish oils (omega-3)

Essential fatty acids help improve neuronal membrane structure and are present in the nervous system and are involved in endocrine and immune functions, hence their potential benefit for various brain-related disorders. Several clinical studies show beneficial effects of omega-3 fatty acids including improved mood profile, increased vigour, reduced anger, and anxiety and depression states.[87]

A recent study demonstrated that a polyunsaturated fatty acid (PUFA) mixture of omega-3 and omega-6 (ratio of 1:4) may improve test anxiety symptoms.[88] Psychologists identified 126 male college students as test anxiety sufferers. Thirty-eight received placebo (mineral oil) and 88 received the PUFA mixture over 3 weeks. Seventy other students who did not suffer test anxiety served as the control group. Behavioural variables associated with test anxiety, such as appetite, mood, mental concentration, fatigue, academic organisation and poor sleep, all significantly improved with the PUFA mixture, as well as lowering elevated cortisol level, with a corresponding reduction of anxiety compared with placebo and control. Another study of 27 untreated, non-depressed patients with social anxiecty disorder (SAD) and 22 controls found lower erythrocyte n-3 PUFA concentrations in the patients.[89] Significant inverse correlations were obtained between levels of n-3 PUFAs and symptom severity in patients with SAD, thereby opening new therapeutic options.

A 3-month double-blind randomised placebo-controlled trial in substance abusers (n = 24) found after supplementation with 3g of n3-PUFA for 3 months their anxiety was significantly improved (p = 0.01) and this was sustained for 6 months after the end of the intervention (p = 0.042).[90] However, a recent systematic review found that inconsistencies still remain in the evidence for fish oil supplementation in anxiety disorders, both in study methodology and findings, so further research is clearly warranted.[91]

Inositol

Inositol is an isomer of glucose and it may theoretically have a psychoactive effect because of its involvement in a second messenger system for some serotonin and noradrenaline receptors. There have been 2 RCTs with small sample sizes (average 20) using inositol 12–18grams/day in panic disorder. Both of these trials showed it to be superior to the placebo,[92] and in 1 trial it was as effective as fluvoxamine.[93] The treatment duration in both trials was 4–6 weeks only. An RCT in PTSD found that it was not effective[94] and in 1 further RCT in OCD it was superior to placebo[95] but not better than an SSRI.[96] It appears that further long-term trials could be warranted.

Magnesium

The rationale for supplementation with magnesium in anxiety is based on the hypothesis that magnesium will be depleted in high stress leading to deficiency which may exacerbate the symptoms of anxiety.[97] There have currently been no RCTs for magnesium alone in the treatment of anxiety but 1 RCT comparing magnesium as an adjunct to anxiolytics in women with a mixed anxiety/depression (n = 20) over a 10-day period found that those in the magnesium group improved more than those in the placebo group.[98] A recent Cochrane report identified a double-blind, placebo-controlled, cross-over study of 44 women with premenstrual syndrome (average age 32 years) randomised to take consecutively all 4 of the following treatments daily for 1 menstrual cycle: (1) 200mg Mg oxide, (2) 50mg vitamin B6, (3) 200mg Magnesium + 50mg vitamin B6 and (4) placebo.[99] The report showed no overall difference between individual treatments, but compared with baseline, a synergistic effect was demonstrated with combined 200mg/day magnesium + 50mg/day vitamin B6 on reducing anxiety-related premenstrual symptoms (nervous tension, mood swings, irritability, or anxiety) during 1 menstrual cycle.[100]

Multivitamins

Whilst a balanced diet containing as many vitamins, minerals and trace elements from food sources as possible would be advocated for anyone with an anxiety disorder, the evidence for specific multivitamin supplementation remains unconvincing. The only RCT to date was conducted using Berroca™, a multivitamin (vitamin B complex, vitamin C, calcium and magnesium) manufactured by Roche, in a group of healthy individuals and whilst those in the intervention group reported increased psychological wellbeing, these results have not been replicated in individuals with an anxiety disorder.[101]

Herbal medicine

A recent systematic review of the literature identified 7 RCTs testing herbal mono-preparations and 1 systematic review of 8 different herbs in alleviating anxiety. It concluded there are a 'lack of rigorous studies in this area and that only kava has been shown beyond reasonable doubt to have anxiolytic effects in humans'.[102]

Kava *Piper methysticum*

Kava, also known as kava kava or Piper methysticum, is a member of the pepper family and traditionally used by Pacific Islanders for social and ceremonial drink. Some Aboriginal communities are also known to use kava. A recent Cochrane review identified 12 double-blind RCTs (n = 700).[103] Only 7 of these studies (n = 380) were included in the meta-analysis using the total score on the Hamilton Anxiety (HAM-A) scale as a common outcome measure. The reviewer's concluded from these results 'a significant effect towards a reduction of the HAM-A total score in patients receiving kava extract compared with patients receiving placebo (weighted mean difference: 3.9)'. They found adverse events were mild, transient and infrequent for short-term treatment (1 to 24 weeks). They also conclude the 'effect lacks robustness and is based on a relatively small sample' and rigorous larger, long term trials are required.[103]

Despite the findings of the reviews, there have been mounting international concerns over reports of hepatotoxicity and deaths from liver failure associated with high doses and ethanolic extracts of kava-containing medicines, including 1 case of a fatality in Australia following acute liver failure, associated with a kava-containing medicine. Following a Therapeutic Goods Administration safety review of kava-containing medicines,[104] there is now a limit on the maximum amount of kava lactones (a group of constituents found in *Piper methysticum*) of 125mgs permitted per dosage form (tablet or a capsule), with a maximum daily dose of no more than 250mg of kava lactones. Also, labels on Australian-made kava products contain warnings that it may harm the liver and to stop using the product if adverse liver symptoms develop.

Sage *Salvia officinalis*

A recent double-blind, placebo, cross-over study of 30 healthy participants aimed to assess the effect of sage (*Salvia officinalis*) to enhance mnemonic performance and mood.[105] Previous studies with sage indicated it possesses in vitro cholinesterase inhibiting properties. The participants were randomised to placebo, 300–600mg dried sage leaf and assessed every 7 days on 3 occasions. Both doses of sage led to improved ratings of mood, with the lower dose improving anxiety and the higher dose increasing alertness, calmness and contentedness compared with placebo.

St John's wort *Hypericum perforatum*

There is high-level evidence that St John's wort is effective in depression and as anxiety is often co-morbid with depression it may have an indirect effect on anxiety. Case reports to date also indicate it may be of help in alleviating anxiety symptoms.[106]

St John's wort is helpful in mild, moderate and severe depression and as anxiety can be a symptom of depression this may explain its observed benefit.[107, 108]

Valerian *Valerian officinalis*

Valerian herb is usually indicated for the treatment of insomnia. Valerian has been investigated as a hypnotic with previously mixed results, but the most recent systematic review found that, overall, although valerian is a safe herb associated with only rare adverse events the evidence does not support the clinical efficacy of valerian as a sleep aid for insomnia.[109] A recent Cochrane review identified 1 small RCT involving 36 patients with GAD.[110] This was a 4-week pilot study of valerian, diazepam and placebo. Whilst there were no significant differences between the valerian and placebo groups in Hamilton Anxiety (HAM-A) total scores, there were also no significant differences in HAM-A scores between the valerian and diazepam groups. However, based on STAI-Trait scores, significantly greater symptom improvement was identified in the diazepam group. Side-effect profile and drop-out rates were similar in all 3 groups. The author's concluded there 'is insufficient evidence to draw any conclusions about the efficacy or safety of valerian compared with placebo or diazepam for anxiety disorders' and 'larger samples and comparing valerian with placebo or other interventions used to treat anxiety disorders, such as antidepressants, are needed'.[110]

Potential but rare side-effects, such as paradoxical hyperactivity and insomnia, have been associated with valerian use and delirium on withdrawal of valerian.[111]

Other herbs

Other herbs with potential anti-anxiolytic effects include passiflora — shown to be equivalent to oxazepam in a small pilot double-blind RCT[112] — *Panax ginseng*,[113] German chamomile,[114] lemon balm[115] and valerian,[116, 117] although research for these are minimal and more research is required.

Herbal combinations

Crataegus oxyacantha, Eschscholtzia californica and magnesium

Two plant extracts Crataegus oxyacantha and Eschscholtzia californica combined with magnesium were assessed for clinical efficacy in mild-to-moderate anxiety disorders under usual general practice prescription conditions.[118] This large scale study of 264 patients (81% female; mean age: 44.6 years) with generalised mild–moderate anxiety were randomised into 2 groups: 130 received the combined herbs and magnesium (Sympathyl) and 134 a placebo for 3 months. The results demonstrated clinical improvement in anxiety scores in the treatment group compared with placebo group. The mean difference between final and pre-treatment scores were, for the treatment group and placebo groups respectively: -10.6 and -8.9 on the total anxiety score; -6.5 and -5.7 on the somatic score; and -38.5 and -29.2 for subjectively assessed anxiety. Adverse events were mostly mild or moderate — digestive or psychopathological disorders in 11.5% of participants in the study group and 9.7% in the placebo group.

A number of herbs have been implicated in possessing sedative effects but to date the evidence for these are minimal and well-performed studies are required to assess their effectiveness.

Homeopathy

A systematic review conducted in 2006 found the evidence for homeopathy in the treatment of anxiety disorders to be inconclusive.[119] They examined 8 RCTs and found them to be contradictory but several uncontrolled and observational studies found positive effects and high levels of patient satisfaction. The authors believed more rigorous trials were warranted given the high level of perceived patient satisfaction and current contradictory results.

Physical therapies

Acupuncture

According to traditional Chinese medicine (TCM), acupuncture is effective by removing blockages to the energy (chi) which travels around the body. A blockage in this energy can lead to an imbalance and, therefore disease; acupuncture works by correcting this imbalance. Research is now beginning to emerge which postulates that the physiological explanations behind the clinical benefits of acupuncture may be due to increases of endomorphin-1, beta endorphin, encephalin, serotonin, and dopamine causing analgesia, and sedation.[120]

In the largest RCT to date, 240 patients diagnosed with anxiety were divided into 3 equal groups and treated accordingly with acupuncture alone, behavioural desensitisation alone, and combined acupuncture and behavioural desensitisation (CABD).[121] The cure rates in the acupuncture, behavioural desensitisation and CABD were 20.0%, 26.3% and 52.5%, respectively. The difference in effectiveness of CABD was statistically significant ($P<0.01$). At 1 year, 60 patients out of the 240 were able to be followed-up and they showed cure rates of 18%, 22% and 48% respectively. That this benefit was largely maintained at 1 year provides a significant rationale for further research into acupuncture for anxiety.

In general, acupuncture is a safe and effective method that can play an important role in managing anxiety associated with difficult to treat conditions such as post-stroke anxiety neurosis where medication side-effect such as sedation can impact on rehabilitation.[122]

In this study, anxiety symptoms of the patients in the acupuncture treatment group demonstrated relief of symptoms by up to 82.35% compared with the control group (Alprazolam) which did not change from baseline.

A recent systematic review of the literature identified 12 controlled trials, of which 10 were randomised controlled trials. Four of these randomised controlled trials focused on acupuncture in generalised anxiety disorder

(GAD) or anxiety neurosis, while the remaining 6 randomised controlled trials focused on anxiety in the perioperative period.[123] Whilst most trials lacked basic methodological details, all trials reported positive findings for acupuncture in the treatment of generalised anxiety disorder or anxiety neurosis, although there is insufficient data for firm conclusions to be drawn. There is limited evidence in favour of auricular acupuncture for peri-operative anxiety.

Aromatherapy

Aromatherapy as a treatment for anxiety has been assessed with most trials using the application of aromatherapy oils through massage. A review of 6 RCTs found that aromatherapy massage had a mild, transient anxiolytic effect, but based on critical assessment of the studies they were unable to recommend aromatherapy as a treatment for anxiety due to inconsistencies in the trials.[124] The length of treatments and number of treatments differed between the studies and also the type of aromatherapy oils used, with 2 studies using lavender oil, 2 studies using chamomile oil, 1 study using orange blossom oil, and a further study using an unspecified aroma.

Massage

A recent Cochrane review found insufficient evidence to draw conclusions about the benefits of massage and aromatherapy massage for cancer patients.[126] The reviewers included 10 studies, of which 8 were RCTs (357 patients). Most of the studies assessed the effect of massage or aromatherapy massage on anxiety. Four trials (207 patients) measuring anxiety detected a reduction following intervention, with benefits of 19–32% reported. It was not clear if there were any added benefits on anxiety conferred with the addition of aromatherapy. The reviewers concluded massage and aromatherapy massage 'confer short-term benefits on psychological wellbeing, with the effect on anxiety supported by limited evidence'.[125]

Reiki/therapeutic touch

A systematic review examining the effectiveness of reiki for any condition conducted in 2008 found 9 randomised clinical trials which met the inclusion criteria.[126] They found 2 trials suggested beneficial effects of reiki compared with sham control on depression and 1 trial which examined pain and anxiety reported inter-group differences in favour of reiki having a positive effect when compared with sham control. One further randomised clinical trial which concentrated on examining stress and hopelessness reported positive effects of reiki and distant reiki compared with distant sham control. They also found 2 randomised clinical trials in women undergoing procedures – amniocentesis, or breast biopsy, where reiki did not reduce anxiety associated with the procedure when compared with conventional care.

Anxiety disorders in children

Anxiety disorders in children can be grouped into the same classifications as adults i.e. generalised anxiety disorder, panic disorder, obsessive compulsive disorder, social anxiety disorder, specific phobias, and specifically separation anxiety. There has been recent research linking the development of anxiety disorders in children with maternal anxiety during pregnancy and post-natal depression. Children with mothers who have suffered post-natal depression appear more likely to develop internalising symptoms of depression and anxiety.[127]

Cognitive behaviour therapy

A Cochrane review in 2006 found CBT to be an effective treatment for anxiety in children and adolescents.[128] Specifically, CBT can be delivered in various formats: individual, group and family/parent and appears effective in just over 50% of cases. They identified 13 studies with 498 subjects and 311 controls involving community or outpatient subjects only, with anxiety of mild to moderate severity. Analyses of the data showed a response rate for remission of any anxiety diagnosis of 56% for CBT versus 28.2% for controls. As an example, in an Australian study surveying the parents of 425 children aged 8 to 11 years, from low income neighbourhoods of Sydney, there were 91 children who demonstrated moderate to severe anxiety symptoms on screening tests.[129] These children were then randomised to a school-based 8-session intervention group, called the 'Cool Kids Program', or a waitlist control group. The intervention group received CBT, education about anxiety, graduated exposure to fear-related stimuli and social skills training in assertiveness and dealing with teasing. Parents were also offered 2 information sessions. The intervention group reported significant reduction in anxiety symptoms compared with children on the waitlist, even at 4 months follow-up. The effects of the intervention were also confirmed by teacher reports.

Exercise

Exercise for anxiety in children and adolescents was also recently considered in a Cochrane review of 16 studies with a total of 1191 participants (aged 11 and 19 years). They concluded that 'there appears to be a small effect in favour of exercise in reducing depression and anxiety scores in the general population of children and adolescents' from a range of clinically diverse studies.[130]

Humour

A randomised prospective study involving humour for pre-operative anxiety for children and their parents found that an intervention lead by 'Clown Doctors' significantly reduced both child and parental anxiety but that the disruption caused by the intervention was such that staff would not have supported the permanent implementation of the intervention.[131]

Massage, relaxation, bibliotherapy, melatonin

There has been relatively little research into complementary therapies in the treatment of childhood anxiety or situational specific anxiety disorders in children; for example, test anxiety, fear of the dark, anxiety related to medical procedures. A systematic review of the literature conducted in 2008[132] concluded that there were few studies of adequate quality that had examined CM in children and adolescents but on the research available there was preliminary evidence that situational-specific anxiety in children could be reduced by massage,[133] relaxation training[134, 135], melatonin supplements,[136] or bibliotherapy[137] instructing parents how to deal with anxious children.

Conclusion

Non-pharmacological therapies can play an important role in the treatment of patients suffering anxiety. They can be used alone in mild-moderate anxiety cases or in combination with pharmaceuticals in severe anxiety. Table 4.2 summarises the current evidence for CM treatments.

Table 4.2 Levels of evidence for lifestyle and complementary medicines/therapies in the management of anxiety disorders

Modality	Level I	Level II	Level IIIa	Level IIIb	Level IIIc	Level IV	Level V
Lifestyle							
Caffeine cessation		x					
Smoking Cessation							x
Sunshine						x	
Physical activity	x						
Creative activities — e.g. knitting						x	
Mind–body medicine							
Autogenic training	x						
Bibliotherapy	x						
CBT	x						
Dance therapy		x					
Hypnotherapy			x				
Meditation		x					
Music therapy		x					
Relaxation therapy	x						
Religion		x					
Reiki	x						
Physical therapies							
Acupuncture	x						
Aromatherapy		x					
Massage		x					
Yoga		x					

Continued

Table 4.2 Levels of evidence for lifestyle and complementary medicines/therapies in the management of anxiety disorders—cont'd

Modality	Level I	Level II	Level IIIa	Level IIIb	Level IIIc	Level IV	Level V
Herbal medicines							
Kava	x						
Passiflora		x					
Sage	x						
St John's wort						x	
Valerian		x					
Combination		x					
Supplements							
Inositol		x					
n–3 fatty acids		x					
Melatonin		x					
Minerals							
Magnesium		x*					
Vitamins		x					
Multivitamin							

*Caution is advocated in interpreting these results as trial conducted in healthy individuals.

Level I — from a systematic review of all relevant randomised controlled trials — meta-analyses.

Level II — from at least 1 properly designed randomised controlled clinical trial.

Level IIIa — from well-designed pseudo-randomised controlled trials (alternate allocation or some other method).

Level IIIb — from comparative studies (including systematic reviews of such studies) with concurrent controls and allocation not randomised, cohort studies, case-control studies, or interrupted time series with a parallel control group.

Level IIIc — from comparative studies with historical control, 2 or more single-arm studies or interrupted time series without a parallel control group.

Level IV — opinions of respected authorities based on clinical experience, descriptive studies or reports of expert committees.

Level V — represents minimal evidence that represents testimonials.

Clinical tips handout for patients — anxiety

1 Lifestyle advice

Sleep

- Restore normal sleep patterns, bed at 9–10 p.m. and rise with the sun.
- Relaxation and counselling, such as cognitive behaviour therapy, are both therapies which are effective in treating anxiety and insomnia.
- Supplementation with low dose melatonin may also be effective for help with sleep difficulties (see Chapter 22 for more advice).

Sunshine

- Everyday — 15 minutes of sunshine in the summer, and 30 minutes in the winter.
- If you have darker skin then more than 30 minutes in summer and winter.
- This ensures adequate vitamin D and melatonin production.
- Sun exposure before 10 a.m. and after 3 p.m. is safest in summer.
- Sunscreen is unnecessary for these short time periods.
- Ensure adequate skin exposure to sun; face, arms, chest.

2 Physical activity/exercise

- Exercise is particularly helpful: 30–60 minutes daily.
- If exercise is not regular, commence with 5 minutes daily and slowly build up to at least 30 minutes. Outdoor exercise, in nature, fresh air and sunshine, is ideal.
- Brisk walking, light jogging, cycling, swimming, stretching, and weight-bearing exercises are all good forms of physical activity/exercise.
- Consider taking dance classes.
- Yoga can be helpful.

3 Mind–body medicine

- Stress management program — for example, six 40 minute sessions for patients to understand the nature of their symptoms, the symptoms' relationship to stress, and the practice of regular relaxation exercises.
- Regular meditation practice at least 10–20 minutes daily.

Rest and stress management

Recurrent stress may cause a return of symptoms. Relaxation is important for a full and lasting recovery.

- Cognitive behaviour therapy and psychotherapy are extremely helpful.
- Hypnotherapy, particularly for specific phobias, autogenic training, and biofeedback may be of help.
- Listening to calming, relaxation music dialy helps.
- Learning to relax is very important. Listen to relaxation tapes regularly, take classes.
- Read positive self-help books.
- Have a massage regularly.
- Meditation — consider trying a class.
- Practice talking kindly to yourself. If you wouldn't give a friend the advice you're currently giving yourself, then stop and re-think how you're talking to yourself.
- Breathing: be aware of breathing at all times.
- Notice if you have a tendency to hold your breath or over-breathe. Always aim to relax the breath and the muscles around your chest wall.
- Stress management — reduce your workload and, where possible, resolve conflicts.
- Supports — family, friends, church or social groups.

Fun

- Joy can be found even in the simplest of tasks.
- Treat yourself by watching funny movies/videos, comedy, hobbies, dancing, playing with pets and children.
- Creative tasks, such as knitting, can help with distressing thoughts.

Focus on wellness, not just the disease.

4 Environment

Avoid:

- alcohol
- caffeine
- smoking
- environmental pollutants, chemicals — at work and in the home
- drug use, such as marijuana.

5 Dietary changes

- Eat regular balanced healthy meals — ideally 3 small meals, and 2 snacks, each containing protein in order to avoid fluctuating blood sugar levels and provide amino acids for nerve transmitters, such as tryptophan.

- Eat more fruit and vegetables — vary colours and aim to eat seasonally.
- Eat 5 or more vegetables daily and 2 or more fruits daily.
- Eat nuts, seeds, sprouts (e.g. alfalfa, mung beans).
- Eat legumes (e.g. beans, lentils, chickpeas).
- Increase fish intake (sardines, tuna, salmon, cod, mackerel), especially deep sea fish, to at least 3 servings per week.
- Reduce red meat intake — preferably use red lean meat (e.g. lamb, kangaroo) and white meat (e.g. free range organic chicken).
- Use cold pressed olive oil and avocado.
- Eat dark chocolate.
- Wholegrains/cereals (variety): rice (brown, basmati, Mahatmi, Doongara), traditional rolled oats, buckwheat flour, wholegrain organic breads (rye bread, Essene, spelt, Kamut), brown pasta, couscous, millet, amaranth etc.
- Reduce dairy intake — use low fat dairy products such as yoghurt and cheeses, unless there is a dairy intolerance.
- Drink more water: 1–2 litres a day.
- Drink teas (e.g. especially organic green tea, black tea). Drink chamomile and peppermint tea: 1 cup of either 30–60 minutes before meals or bed.
- Avoid hydrogenated fats, salt, fast foods, sugar such as in soft drinks, lollies, biscuits, cakes and processed foods (e.g. white bread, white pasta, pastries).
- Minimise coffee as it can cause restlessness and agitation in high doses.
- Avoid chemical additives (e.g. preservatives, colouring and flavours).
- Avoid artificial sweeteners — replace with honey (e.g. manuka, yellow box and stringy bark have lowest GI).

6 Physical therapies

- Acupuncture may help improve general wellbeing.
- Aromatherapy with massage can be useful — lavender, orange blossom oils can be soothing.
- Reiki may help.

7 Supplements

Fish oils

- Indication: could be effective in anxiety and depression, more evidence is needed but given other positive effects, can be recommended.
- Dosage: take with meals. Adult: 1g 1–2 capsules 1–2–3 x daily; Child 500mg 1–2 x daily; can be used during pregnancy or lactation as tolerated.
- Results: 1–4 days.
- Side-effects: often well tolerated, especially if taken with meals. Very mild and rare side-effects; for example, gastrointestinal upset, allergic reactions (e.g. rash, breathing problems if allergic to seafood), blood thinning effects in very high doses > 10g daily (may need to stop fish oil supplements 2 weeks prior to surgery).
- Contraindications: sensitivity reaction to seafood; drug interactions; caution when taking high doses of fish oils > 4g per day together with warfarin (your Doctor will check your INR test).

Inositol

- Indication: could be effective in anxiety; there is some evidence to suggest 12–18g/day could be effective for panic disorder and obsessive compulsive disorder.
- Dosage: 12–18g/day.
- Results: 1–4 days.
- Side-effects: nausea, fatigue, dizziness, diarrhoea.
- Contraindications: pregnancy, breast feeding, reported interactions with carbamazepine, lithium, sodium valproate.

Magnesium and calcium

(best provided together)

- Indication: may be useful in depression, anxiety, restless sleep, cramps and insomnia.
- Dosage: children up to 65–120mg daily in divided doses; adults 350mg daily (including pregnant and lactating women).
- Results: 2–3 days.
- Side-effects: oral magnesium can cause gastrointestinal irritation, nausea, vomiting, and diarrhoea. The dosage varies from person to person. Although rare, toxic levels can cause low blood pressure, thirst, heart arrhythmia, drowsiness and weakness.
- Contraindicated: patients with kidney disease.

Vitamin D (cholecalciferol 1000IU)

Doctors should check blood levels and suggest supplementation if levels are low.

Herbal medicine

Kava

- Indication: may be effective in anxiety.
  - Dosage: 300–400mg/day, in tablet form. Cases of liver damage have been linked to high doses and the ethanolic form (avoid).
- Results: 1–2 weeks.
- Side-effects: most common side-effects are gastrointestinal upset and headaches.
- May cause drowsiness, especially if taken with alcohol or other calmative herbs or medication.
  May slow some individuals reaction times, therefore operating heavy machinery or driving should be approached with caution. In rare cases kava may upset the liver. Stop using kava if you develop liver pains, yellow eyes, itchy skin or dark urine.
  Contraindications: pregnancy, lactation, endogenous depression, caution in the elderly and in those with previous liver problems.

Passiflora

- Indication: effective in anxiety.
- Dosage: 0.25–2 gm/day infusion dried herb.
- Results: 3–4 weeks.
- Side-effects: most common side-effects are gastrointestinal upset and headaches.
- Contraindications: pregnancy, lactation, caution with anticoagulants, benzodiazepines.

St John's wort

- Indication: mild-moderate-severe depression; may help with anxiety symptoms.
- Dosage: 300mg 2–3 x daily.
- Results: 1–3 weeks.
- Side-effects: very mild and rare. May cause: photosensitivity skin rash that is reversible on stopping St John's wort; digestion disturbance; dizziness; fatigue; dry mouth.
- Contraindications: pregnancy, lactation, fertility, drug interaction; avoid use with most pharmaceutical medication such as the oral contraceptive pill, other antidepressants, epileptic medication — check with your doctor.

Melatonin

- Indication: elderly with insomnia and anxiety; may improve anxiety associated with surgery but this must be done under medical supervision; helps insomnia by improving circadian rhythm sleep disorders; reduces the time to fall asleep; jet-lag.
- Dosage: 5–10mg (adult) at 6 p.m. or closer to bedtime; for short-term use.
- Results: within 1–3 hours.
- Side-effects: usually well tolerated. Avoid long-term use. May cause drowsiness, dizziness, depressive symptoms, reduced alertness, irritability, headaches; all these symptoms can be transient.
- Contraindications: young children, pregnant, lactating mothers; epilepsy; taken with alcohol; sedating medication such as benzodiazepines and use with narcotics; depression.

References

1 Andrews G, Hall W. The mental health of Australians. Mental Health branch, Australian government department of health and aged care, Canberra, 1999.

2 Issakadis C, Andrews G. Service utilization for anxiety in an Australian community sample. Soc Psychiatry Psychiatr Epidemiol 2002;37:153–163.

3 Jorm AF, Medway J, Christensen H, et. al. Public beliefs about the helpfulness of interventions for depression: effects on actions taken when experiencing anxiety and depression symptoms. Aust N Z J Psychiatry 2000;34:619–622.

4 The contribution of demographic and morbidity factors to self-reported visit frequency of patients: a cross-sectional study of general practice patients in Australia. BMC Family Practice 2004;5:17 (7 pages).

5 Yates WR. Phenomenology and epidemiology of panic disorder. Ann Clin Psychiatry. 2009 Apr-Jun;21(2):95–102.

6 Bloch S, Singh B. Foundations of Clinical Psychiatry (3rd edn). Melbourne University Publishing, 2007.

7 Kessler RC, Davis RB, Foster DF, et. al. Long-term trends in the use of complementary and alternative medical therapies in the United States. Ann Intern Med 2001;135;262–268.

8 Blashki G, Judd F, Piterman L. General practice psychiatry. McGraw-Hill, Sydney, 2007.

9 Egger G, Binns A, Rossner S. Lifestyle Medicine. McGraw-Hill, Sydney, 2008.

10 Kinnersley P, Stott N, Harvey I. The patient-centredness of consultation and outcome in primary care. Br J Gen Pract 1999;49,711–716.

11 Holism in Primary Care the views of Scotlands general practitioners. Primary Healthcare Research and Development 2005;6:320–328.

12 Outram S, Murphy B, Cockburn J. The role of GPs in treating psychological distress: a study of midlife Australian women. Family Practice 2004;21:276–81.

13 Madden S. Managing anxiety disorders in children and adolescents. Medicine Today. Update: Anxiety and depression today. 2006 supplement August. Pages 6–10.

14 Loerch B, Graf-Morgenstern M, Hautzinger M, et. al. Randomised placebo-controlled trial of moclobemide, cognitive-behavioural therapy and their combination in panic disorder with agoraphobia. British Journal of Psychiatry 1999;174:205–12, 213–18.

15 Orbach G, Linsey S, Grey S. A randomised placebo-controlled trial of a self-help Internet-based intervention for test anxiety. Behav Res Ther 2006 Jun 29.
16 Taube-Schiff M, Suvak MK, Antony MM, et. al. Group cohesion in cognitive-behavioral group therapy for social phobia. Behav Res Ther 2006 Aug 21.
17 Australian and New Zealand clinical practice guidelines for the treatment of panic disorder and agoraphobia. Royal Australian and New Zealand College of Psychiatrists Clinical Practice; Guidelines Team for Panic Disorder and Agoraphobia. Australian and New Zealand Journal of Psychiatry 2003;37:641–656. Online. Available: http://www.ranzcp.org/images/stories/ranzcp-attachments/Resources/Publications/CPG/Clinician/CPG_Clinician%20Full_Panic_Disorder_Agoraphobia.pdf (accessed 28-09-09)
18 Buckner JD, Turner RJ. Social anxiety disorder as a risk factor for alcohol use disorders: a prospective examination of parental and peer influences. Drug Alcohol Depend. 2009 Feb 1;100(1-2):128-37. Epub 2008 Nov 20
19 Morris EP, Stewart SH, Ham LS. The relationship between social anxiety disorder and alcohol use disorders: a critical review. Clin Psychol Rev 2005 Sep;25(6):734–60.
20 Buckner JD, Timpano KR, Zvolensky MJ, et. al. Implications of comorbid alcohol dependence among individuals with social anxiety disorder. Depress Anxiety. 2008;25(12):1028–37.
21 Buckner JD, Schmidt NB. Social anxiety disorder and marijuana use problems: the mediating role of marijuana effect expectancies. Depress Anxiety. 2009 Apr 16. [Epub ahead of print].
22 Buckner JD, Leen-Feldner EW, Zvolensky MJ, et. al. The interactive effect of anxiety sensitivity and frequency of marijuana use in terms of anxious responding to bodily sensations among youth. Psychiatry Res. 2009 Apr 30;166(2–3):238–46. Epub 2009 Mar 10.
23 Parslow R, Morgan AJ, Allen NB, et. al. Effectiveness of complementary and self-help treatments for anxiety in children and adolescents. Med J Aust 2008 Mar 17;188(6):355–9.
24 Ernst E, Kanji N. Autogenic training for stress and anxiety: a systematic review. Complement Ther Med 2000 Jun;8(2):106–10.
25 Stetter F, Kupper S. Autogenic training: a meta-analysis of clinical outcome studies. Appl Psychophysiol Biofeedback 2002;27:45–98.
26 Kanji N, White AR, Ernst E. Autogenic training reduces anxiety after coronary angioplasty:a randomised clinical trial. Am Heart Journal 2004;147:E10.
27 Goldbeck L, Schmid K. Effectiveness of autogenic relaxation training on children and adolescents with behavioural and emotional problems. J Am Acad Child Adolesc Psychiatry 2003;42:1046–1054.
28 Kanji N, White A, Ernst E. Autogenic training to reduce anxiety in nursing students: randomised controlled trial. J Adv Nurs 2006 Mar;53(6):729–35.
29 Reiner R. Integrating a portable biofeedback device into clinical practice for patients with anxiety disorders: results of a pilot study. Appl Psychophysiol Biofeedback. 2008 Mar;33(1):55–61. Epub 2008 Feb 20.
30 Rice KM, Blanchard EB, Purcell M. Biofeedback treatments of generalized anxiety disorder: preliminary results. Biofeedback Self Reg 1993;18:93–105.
31 Marrs RW. A meta-analysis of bibliotherapy studies. Am J Community Psychol 1995; 23:843–870.
32 Gould RA, Clum GA, Shapiro D. The use of bibliotherapy in the treatment of panic: a preliminary investigation. Behav Ther 1993;24:241–252.
33 Abramowitz JS, Moore EL, Braddock AE, et. al. Self-help cognitive-behavioral therapy with minimal therapist contact for social phobia: a controlled trial. J Behav Ther Exp Psychiatry 2009 Mar;40(1):98–105. Epub 2008 Apr 26.
34 Shechtman Z, Nir-Shfrir R. The effect of affective bibliotherapy on clients' functioning in group therapy. Int J Group Psychother 2008 Jan;58(1):103–17.
35 Jorm A, Christensen H, Griffiths K, et. al. Effectiveness of complementary and self-help treatments for anxiety disorders. MJA 2004 October;181(7):4.
36 Lang EV, Bentosch EG, Fick LJ et. al. Adjunctive non-pharmacological analgesia for invasive procedures: a randomised trial. Lancet 2000;355:1486–90.
37 Liossi C, White P, Hatira P. Randomised clinical trial of local anesthetic versus a combination of local anesthetic with self-hypnosis in the management of pediatric procedure-related pain. Health Psychol 2006 May;25(3):307–15.
38 Saadat H, Drummond-Lewis J, Maranets I, et. al. Hypnosis reduces preoperative anxiety in adult patients. Anesth Analg 2006 May;102(5):1394–6.
39 Elkins G, White J, Patel P, et. al. Hypnosis to manage anxiety and pain associated with colonoscopy for colorectal cancer screening: case studies and possible benefits. Int J Clin Exp Hypn 2006 Oct;54(4):416–31.
40 Lang EV, Berbaum KS, Faintuch S, et. al. Adjunctive self-hypnotic relaxation for outpatient medical procedures: A prospective randomised trial with women undergoing large core breast biopsy. Pain 2006 Sep 5; [Epub ahead of print].
41 Gholamrezaei A, Ardestani SK, Emami MH. Where does hypnotherapy stand in the management of irritable bowel syndrome? A systematic review. J Altern Complement Med 2006 Jul-Aug;12(6):517–27.
42 Huynh ME, Vandvik IH, Diseth TH. Hypnotherapy in child psychiatry: the state of the art. Clin Child Psychol Psychiatry 2008 Jul;13(3):377–93.
43 Aviv A. Tele-hypnosis in the treatment of adolescent school refusal. Am J Clin Hypn 2006 Jul;49(1):31–40.
44 Weisberg MB. 50 years of hypnosis in medicine and clinical health psychology: a synthesis of cultural crosscurrents. Am J Clin Hypn 2008 Jul;51(1):13–27.
45 Fern PA. Hypnosis to alleviate perioperative anxiety and stress: a journey to challenge ideas. J Perioper Pract 2008 Jan;18(1):14–6.
46 T Krisanaprakornkit, et. al. Meditation therapy for anxiety disorders. Cochrane Database of Systematic Reviews 2006 Issue 3.
47 Ernst E, Pittler MH, Wider B, et. al. Mind body therapies: are the trial data getting stronger? Altern Ther Health Med 2007 Sep-Oct;13(5):62–4.
48 Manzoni GM, Pagnini F, Castelnuovo G, et. al. Relaxation training for anxiety: a ten-years systematic review with meta-analysis. BMC Psychiatry 2008 Jun 2;8:41.
49 Cooke M, Chaboyer W, Sculter P, et. al. The effect of music on preoperative anxiety in day surgery. Journal Advanced Nursing 2005 Oct;52(1):47–55.
50 Sendelbach SE, Halm MA, Doran KA, et. al. Effects of music therapy on physiological and psychological outcomes for patients undergoing cardiac surgery. J Cardiovasc Nurs 2006 May-Jun;21(3):194–200.

51 Gallagher LM, Lagman R, Walsh D, et. al. The clinical effects of music therapy in palliative medicine. Support Care Cancer 2006 Aug;14(8):859–66.

52 Whitehead-Pleaux AM, Baryza MJ, Sheridan RL. The effects of music therapy on pediatric patients' pain and anxiety during donor site dressing change. J Music Ther 2006 Summer;43(2):136–53.

53 Hummer R, Rogers R, Nam C, et. al. Religious involvement and U.S. adult mortality. Demography 1999;36(2):273–85.

54 Razali SM, Hasanah CI, Aminah K, et. al. Religious sociocultural psychotherapy in patients with anxiety and depression. Aust N Z J Psychiatry 1998;32:867–872.

55 Clave-Brule M, Mazloum A, Park RJ, et. al. Managing anxiety in eating disorders with knitting. Eat Weight Disord 2009 Mar;14(1):e1-e5.

56 Irwin MR, Cole JC, Nicassio PM. Comparative meta-analysis of behaviorual interventions for insomnia and their efficacy in middle-aged adults and older adults 55+ years. Health Psychol 2006 Jan;25(1):3–14.

57 Ernst E, Pittler MH, Wider B, et. al. Mind body therapies: are the trial data getting stronger? Altern Ther Health Med 2007 Sep-Oct;13(5):62–4.

58 Steiger A. Sleep and endocrinology. J Intern Med 2003;254(1):13–22.

59 Ramsawh HJ, Stein MB, Belik SL, et. al. Relationship of anxiety disorders, sleep quality and functional impairment. J Psychiatr Res 2009 Mar;6.

60 Olde Rikert MG. Rigaud AS Melatonin in elderly patients with insomnia. A systematic review. Z Gerontol Geriatr 2001; 34:491–497.

61 Ismail SA, Mowafi HA. Melatonin provides anxiolysis, enhances analgesia, decreases intraocular pressure, and promotes better operating conditions during cataract surgery under topical anesthesia. Anesth Analg 2009 Apr;108(4):1146–51.

62 Mowafi HA, Ismail SA. Melatonin improves tourniquet tolerance and enhances postoperative analgesia in patients receiving intravenous regional anesthesia. Anesth Analg 2008 Oct;107(4): 1422–6.

63 Caumo W, Levandovski R, Hidalgo MP. Preoperative anxiolytic effect of melatonin and clonidine on postoperative pain and morphine consumption in patients undergoing abdominal hysterectomy: a double-blind, randomised, placebo-controlled study. J Pain 2009 Jan;10(1):100–8. Epub 2008 Nov 17.

64 Garzón C, Guerrero JM, Aramburu O, et. al. Effect of melatonin administration on sleep, behavioral disorders and hypnotic drug discontinuation in the elderly: a randomised, double-blind, placebo-controlled study. Aging Clin Exp Res 2009 Feb;21(1):38–42.

65 Cheuk DK, Yeung WF, Chung KF, et. al. Acupuncture for insomnia Cochrane Database Syst Rev 2007 Jul 18;(3):CD005472.

66 Armstrong DJ, Meenagh GK, Bickle I, et. al. Vitamin D deficiency is associated with anxiety and depression in fibromyalgia. Clin Rheumatol. 2007 Apr;26(4):551–4. Epub 2006 Jul 19.

67 Cherniack EP, Troen BR, Florez HJ, et. al. Some new food for thought: the role of vitamin D in the mental health of older adults. Curr Psychiatry Rep 2009 Feb;11(1):12–9.

68 West R, Hajek P. What happens to anxiety levels on giving up smoking? Am J Psychiatry 1997;154: 1589–1592.

69 Wipfli BM, Rethorst CD, Landers DM. The anxiolytic effects of exercise: a meta-analysis of randomised trials and dose-response analysis. J Sport Exerc Psychol 2008 Aug;30(4):392–410.

70 DeMoor MH, Boomsma DI, Stubbe JH, et. al Testing causality in the association between regular exercise and symptoms of anxiety and depression. Arch Gen Psychiatry 65(8):897–905, August 2008.

71 Broocks A, Bandelow B, Pekrun G, et. al. Comparison of aerobic, clomipramine and placebo in the treatment of placebo of panic disorder. Am J Psychiatr 1998;155:603–609.

72 Rao R, Raghuram R, Nagendra HR, et. al. Anxiolytic effects of a yoga program in early breast cancer patients undergoing conventional treatment: a randomised controlled trial. Complement Ther Med 2009 Jan;17(1):1–8. Epub 2008 Oct 14.

73 Sahasi G, Mohan D, Kakcer C. Effectiveness of yogic techniques in the management of anxiety. J Personality Clin Stud 1989; 5:51–55.

74 Kushner MG, Mackenzie TB, Fiszdon J, et. al. The effects of alcohol consumption on laboratory-induced panic and state anxiety. Arch Gen Psychiatry 1996; 53: 264–270.

75 Abrams K, Kushner MG, Medina KL, et. al. The pharmacologic and expectancy effects of alcohol on social anxiety in individuals with social phobia. Drug Alcohol Depend 2001; 64: 219–231.

76 MacDonald AB, Stewart SH, Hutson R, et. al. The roles of alcohol and alcohol expectancy in the dampening of responses to hyperventilation among high anxiety sensitive young adults. Addict Behav 2001;26:841–867.

77 Kushner MG, Abrams K, Borchardt C. The relationship between anxiety disorders and alcohol use disorders: a review of major perspectives and findings. Clin Psychol Rev 2000;20:149–171.

78 Driessen M, Meier S, Hill A, et. al. The course of anxiety, depression and drinking behaviours after completed detoxification in alcoholics with and without comorbid anxiety and depressive disorders. Alcohol 2001;36:249–255.

79 Kendler KS, Myers J, O Gardner C. Caffeine intake, toxicity and dependence and lifetime risk for psychiatric and substance use disorders: an epidemiologic and co-twin control analysis. Psychol Med 2006 Aug 8;1–9.

80 Hewlett P, Smith A. Correlates of daily caffeine consumption. Appetite 2006 Jan;46(1):97–9.

81 Bruce MS, Lader M. Caffeine abstention in the management of anxiety disorders. Psychol Med 1989;19:211–214.

82 Totten GL, France CR. Physiological and subjective anxiety responses to caffeine and stress in nonclinical panic. J Anxiety Disord 1995;9:473–488.

83 Tancer ME, Stein MB, Uhde TW. Lactic acid response to caffeine in panic disorders: comparison of social phobics and normal controls. Anxiety 1994–95;1:138–140.

84 Uhde TW, Boulenger JP, Jimerson DC, et. al. Caffeine: relationship to human anxiety, plasma MHPG and cortisol. Psychopharmacol Bull 1984;20:426–430.

85 Boulenger JP, Uhde TW, Wolff EA, et. al. Increased sensitivity to caffeine in patients with panic disorders: preliminary evidence. Arch Gen Psychiatry 1984;41:1067–1071.

86 Smith GA. Caffeine reduction as an adjunct to anxiety management. Br J Clin Psychol 1988;27: 265–266.

87 Fontani G, et. al. Cognitive and physiological effects of Omega-3 polyunsaturated fatty acid supplementation in healthy subjects. Eur J Clin Invest 2005 Nov;35(11):691–9.

88 Yehuda S, Rabinovitz S, Mostofsky DI. Mixture of essential fatty acids lowers test anxiety. Nutr Neurosci 2005 Aug;8(4):265–7.

89 Green P, Hermesh H, Monselise A, et. al. Red cell membrane omega-3 fatty acids are decreased in nondepressed patients with social anxiety disorder. Eur Neuropsychopharmacol 2006 Feb;16(2): 107–13.

90 Buydens-Branchy L, Branchy M Hibbeln JR. Associations between increases in plasma n-3 polyunsaturated fatty acids following supplementation and decreases in anger and anxiety in substance abusers. Prog Neuropsychopharmacol Biol Psychiatry 2008 Feb 15;32(2):568–75. Epub 2007 No7.

91 Appleton KM, Rogers PJ, Ness AR. Is there a role for n-3 long-chain polyunsaturated fatty acids in the regulation of mood and behaviour? A review of the evidence to date from epidemiological studies, clinical studies and intervention trials. Nutr Res Rev 2008 Jun;21(1):13–41.

92 Benjamin J, Levine J, Fux M, et. al. Double-blind, controlled crossover trial of inositol treatment for panic disorder. Am J Psychiatry 1995;152: 1084–1086.

93 Palatnik A, Frolov K, Fux M, et. al. Double-blind, controlled cross-over trial of inositol versus fluvoxamine for the treatment of panic disorder. J Clin Psychopharmacol 2001;21:335–339.

94 Kaplan Z, Amir M, Swartz M, et. al. Inositol treatment of post-traumatic stress disorder. Anxiety 1996;2:51–52.

95 Fux, Levine J, Aviv A, et. al. Inositol treatment of obsessive compulsive disorder. Am J Psychiatry 1996;153:1219–1221.

96 Fux M, Benjamin J, Belmaker RH. Inositol versus placebo augmentation of serotonin reuptake inhibitor in the treatment of obsessive compulsive disorder: a double blind cross-over study. Int J Neuropsychopharmacol 1999;2:193–195.

97 Kriv GK, Tsachev KN. Magnesium, schizophrenia and manic-depressive disease. Neuropsychobiology 1990,23:79–81.

98 Bockova E, Hronek J, Kolomaznik M, et. al. Potentiation of the effects of anxiolytics with magnesium salts. Cesk Psychiatr 1992;88: 141–144.

99 De Souza MC, Walker AF, Robinson PA, et. al. Cochrane Central Register of Controlled Trials (CENTRAL) 2006 Issue 3 Copyright © 2006. The Cochrane Collaboration. Published by John Wiley & Sons, Ltd. De Souza MC, Walker AF, Robinson PA, Bolland K.

100 De Souza MC, Walker AF, Robinson PA, et. al. A synergistic effect of a daily supplement for 1 month of 200mg magnesium plus 50mg vitamin B6 for the relief of anxiety-related premenstrual symptoms: a randomised, double-blind, crossover study. Journal of Women's Health & Gender-based Medicine 2000 Mar;9(2):131–9.

101 Carroll D, Ring C, Suter M, et. al. The effects of an oral multivitamin combination with calcium, magnesium and zinc on psychological well-being in healthy young male volunteers: a double blind placebo-controlled trial. Psychopahrmacologica 2000;150:220–225.

102 Ernst E. Herbal remedies for anxiety - a systematic review of controlled clinical trials. Phytomedicine 2006 Feb;13(3):205–8.

103 Pittler MH, Ernst E. Kava extract versus placebo for treating anxiety. The Cochrane Database of Systematic Reviews 2006 Issue 3.

104 Therapeutic Goods Administration, Australia. Online. Available: website http://www.tga.gov.au/cm/kavafs0504.htm (accessed 28-09-09)

105 Kennedy DO, Pace S, Haskell et. al. Effects of Cholinesterase Inhibiting Sage (Salvia officinalis) on Mood, Anxiety and Performance on a Psychological Stressor Battery. Neuropsychopharmacology 2006;31:845–52.

106 Davidson Jonathan RT, Connor Kathryn M. Letters To The Editors: *St. John's* Wort in Generalized Anxiety Disorder: Three Case Reports. Journal of Clinical Psychopharmacology 2001 December;21(6):635–636.

107 Linde K, Berner MM, Kriston L. St John's wort for major depression. Cochrane Database of Systematic Reviews 2008, Issue 4. Art. No.: CD000448. DOI: 10.1002/14651858.CD000448.pub3.

108 Ernst E. Herbal remedies for depression and anxiety. Adv Psychiatr Treat 2007;13:312–316.

109 Taibi DM, Landis CA, Petry H, et. al. A systematic review of valerian as a sleep aid: safe but not effective. Sleep Med Rev 2007 Jun;11(3):209–30.

110 Miyasaka LS, Atallah AN, Soares BGO. Valerian for anxiety disorders. The Cochrane Database of Systematic Reviews 2006 Issue 4.

111 Garges HP, Varia I, Doraiswarmy PM. Cardiac Complications and Delirium Associated with Valerian Root Withdrawal. JAMA 1998;280: 1566–1567.

112 Akhondzadeh S, Naghavi HR, Vazirian M, et. al. Passionflower in the treatment of generalized anxiety: a pilot double-blind randomised controlled trial with oxazepam. J.Clin Pharm Ther 2001;26:363–367.

113 Takagi K, Saito H, Tsychiya M. Pharmacological Studies of Panax Ginseng Root: Pharmacological properties of a Crude Saponin Fraction. Japanese Journal of Pharmacology 1972; 2:3339–346.

114 Wong AHC, Smith M, Boon HS. Herbal remedies in psychiatric practice. Arch Gen Psychiatr 1998;55:1033–1044.

115 Kennedy DO, et. al. Attenuation of laborotary-induced stress in humans after acute administration of Melissa officinalis (Lemon Balm). Psychosom Med 2004:66;607–613.

116 Adreatini R, Sartori VA, Seabra ML, et. al. Effect of valepotriates (valerian extract) in generalized anxiety disorder: a randomised placebo-controlled pilot study. Phytother Res 2002;16:650–654.

117 Houghton PJ. The Scientific Basis for Reputed Activity of Valerian. Journal of Pharmacology 1999;5:505–512.

118 Hanus M, Lafon J, Mathieu M. Double-blind, randomised, placebo-controlled study to evaluate the efficacy and safety of a fixed combination containing two plant extracts (Crataegus oxyacantha and Eschscholtzia californica) and magnesium in mild-to-moderate anxiety disorders. Curr Med Res Opin 2004 Jan;20(1):63–71.

119 Pilkington K, Kirkwood G, Rampes H, et. al. Homeopathy for anxiety and anxiety disorders: a systematic review of the research. Homeopathy 2006 Jul;95(3):151–62.

120 Cabyoglu MT, Ergene N, Tan U. The mechanism of acupuncture and clinical applications. Int J Neurosci 2006 Feb;116(2):115–25.

121 Guizhen L, Yunjun Z, Linxiang G, et. al. Comparative study on acupuncture combined with behavioural desensitisation for treatment of anxiety neuroses. Am J Acupunct 1998;26:117–120.

122 Wu P, Liu S. Clinical observation on post-stroke anxiety neurosis treated by acupuncture J Tradit Chin Med 2008 Sep;28(3):186–8.

123 Pilkington K, Kirkwood G, Rampes H, et. al. Acupuncture for anxiety and anxiety disorders--a systematic literature review. Acupunct Med 2007 Jun;25(1–2):1–10.

124 Ernst E, Cooke B. Aromatherapy: a systematic review. British Journal of General Practice 2000 June;493.

125 Fellowes D, Barnes K, Wilkinson S. Aromatherapy and massage for symptom relief in patients with cancer. The Cochrane Database of Systematic Reviews 2006 Issue 3.

126 Lee MS, Pittler MH, Ernst E. Effects of reiki in clinical practice: a systematic review of randomised clinical trials. Int J Clin Pract 2008 Jun;62(6): 947–54. Epub 2008 Apr 10.

127 Essex MJ, Klein MH, Miech R, et. al. Timing of exposure to maternal major depression and children's mental health symptoms in kindergarten. Br J Psychiatry 2001;179:151–56.

128 James A, Soler A, Weatherall R. Cognitive behaviour therapy for anxiety disorders in children and adolescents. The Cochrane Database of Systematic Reviews 2006 Issue 3.

129 Mifsud C, Rapee RM. Early intervention for childhood anxiety in a school setting: outcomes for an economically disadvantaged population. J Am Acad Child Adolesc Psychiatry 2005;44:996–1004.

130 Larun L, Nordheim LV, Ekeland E, et. al. Exercise in prevention and treatment of anxiety and depression among children and young people. The Cochrane Database of Systematic Reviews 2006 Issue 3.

131 Vagnoli L, et. al. Clown Doctors as a Treatment for Preoperative Anxiety in Children: A Randomised, Prospective Study. Pediatrics 2005 October;116(4):e563–e567.

132 Parslow R, Morgan A, Allen N, et. al. Effectiveness of complementary and self-help treatments for anxiety in children and adolescents. MJA 2008;188 (6):355–359.

133 Field T, Seligman S, Scafadi F, et. al. Alleviating post-traumatic in children following Hurricane Andrew. J Appl Dev Psychol 1996;17:37–50.

134 Smead R. A comparison of counsellor administered andtape-recordedrelaxationtrainingondecreasingtarget andnon-targetanxietyinelementaryschoolchildren.Diss Abstr Int B 1981;42:1015–1016.

135 Roque GM. A comparative evaluation of two relaxation strategies with school-aged children. Diss Abstr Int B 1992;53:3165.

136 Samarkandi A, Naguib M, Riad W, et. al. Melatonin vs midazolam premedication in children: a double-blind placebo-controlled study. Eur J Anaesthesiol 2005;22:189–196.

137 Rapee RM, Abbott MJ, Lyneham HJ. Bibliography for children with anxiety disorders using written materials for parents: a randomised controlled trial. J Consult Clin Psychol 2006;74:436–444.

Chapter 5

Asthma

Introduction

The National Asthma Council (NAC) defines asthma as a 'chronic inflammatory disorder of the airways in which many cells and cellular elements play a role, in particular, mast cells, eosinophils, T lymphocytes, macrophages, neutrophils, and epithelial cells' and a 'reversible narrowing of the airways in the lungs'.[1, 2, 3] Asthma is characterised by allergic inflammation that is the major underlying abnormality affecting the airways.[4] This inflammation leads to bronchial hyper-responsiveness to triggers, including infections, allergens and non-specific irritants.

In susceptible individuals, this inflammation causes a variety of respiratory symptoms that include wheezing, coughing (particularly at night or in the early morning), chest tightness, difficulty in breathing and shortness of breath. Asthma is closely linked with allergic rhinitis/ conjunctivitis (hay fever).

Population-based studies indicate the incidence of asthma is more prevalent in Australia than in Europe or North America.[5a] Asthma is a significant health problem in Australia, affecting 10% of the population.[5b] In comparison to international standards, the prevalence of asthma in Australia is high. Studies indicate the prevalence of atopy (a genetic predisposition toward the development of immediate hypersensitivity reactions against common environmental antigens) is increasing worldwide.[6]

Complementary medicine (CM) use in asthma

With the high prevalence of asthma, it is not surprising that the use of CMs is common, with figures indicating more than 50% use in children and adult asthmatics.[7–16] A survey of 48 multicultural parents of children with asthma in the US found up to 81% were using at least 1 form of alternative and complementary treatment for asthma.[17] These included prayer, over-the-counter medications, herbal teas, vitamins, and massage. A review of the literature found the use of CM ranged from 4% to 79% in adults and 33% and 89% in children.[18] Herbal medicine is commonly used in adults (11%) and children (6%) with asthma.[19]

An Australian study identified parental dissatisfaction with conventional therapy and concerns about side-effects from steroid use were the most common reason given by parents of children with asthma for using the complementary medicine (CM) and therapy.[10]

Vitamins and minerals (53.2%) and herbal preparations (29%) were used most commonly and less than 50% of parents had told their doctors about the use of CM. Users of CM and therapies were more likely to have suffered adverse reactions to relieving bronchodilators and were more likely to express dissatisfaction with conventional therapies.

Another study found high CM use amongst children was associated with positive parental beliefs about CM and were significantly associated with greater risks for non-adherence and poorer asthma control.[20] Population-based studies of adults found self-treatment with non-prescription products and CMs such as herbal, tea and coffee products is common [21] and associated with increased risk of reported hospitalisation possibly due to delay in utilisation of more efficacious treatments.[22]

Whilst CM cannot replace drug therapy it may provide a useful adjunct (not alternative), to conventional care by improving quality of life for the asthmatic sufferer. The asthmatic patient still needs monitoring, an action plan, symptomatic relief and should not change their medication dosages without supervision by their doctor. Studies indicate practitioners may help enhance overall wellbeing of the asthma patient by providing advice in improving lifestyle, reducing risk factors and stress levels, appropriate dietary changes, using suitable supplements and changing the environment (see Table 5.1).

However, systematic reviews of the literature note the methodology of clinical trials with many complementary and alternative medicines are frequently inadequate, with positive results described from limited studies for herbals such as *Tylophora indica*, music therapy, buteyko, yoga, magnesium and conflicting evidence for homeopathy remedies.[23, 24]

Aims of asthma treatment should:

- include patient education
- include self management — monitoring and medication

Table 5.1 Key approaches to asthma management

- Identification of relevant allergen triggers
- Allergen avoidance/control
- Appropriate medication
- Written asthma action plan
- Smoking cessation, diet and exercise (including specific management of exercise-induced asthma if required).

adapted from the National Asthma Council 2009[1]

- aim to reduce risk factors
- enhance a healthy lifestyle — diet, exercise, stress management.

Risk factors for asthma

Doctor–patient relationship

The doctor–patient relationship can influence communication about asthma management, health outcomes and compliance with medication. A study found that asthma outcomes improved when patient's physicians encouraged them to participate in decisions about their health care, that contributed to improved quality of life, work disability and need for acute health services.[25] Greater participation occurred most commonly with longer consultations and when the patient had seen the same physician for more than 6 months.

Affluent countries and economic development

A global research study evaluating over 54 000 people using standardised questionnaires identified the link between economic development and risk of asthma and atopic sensitisation.[26] Children in affluent countries were significantly more likely to have an association with current wheeze, allergy-related asthma, and positive skin prick sensitivity compared with children in less affluent settings. Affluent children with allergic sensitisations were 4.0 times as likely to have asthma compared with non-sensitised children, whereas, children in non-affluent countries were only 2.2 times more likely to have an allergic response and asthma compared with non-sensitised children in the non-affluent countries.

Migration

Worldwide figures highlight a significant rise in asthma prevalence and studies amongst migrant populations indicate environmental risk factors may play a role.

A large-scale international study of 7794 Chinese adolescents in China and Hong Kong and 2235 Chinese adolescents living in Vancouver, Canada, found the prevalence of asthma was lowest in residents of mainland China compared with those of Hong Kong and those who immigrated to Canada or were born in Canada.[27] The incidence for 'current wheezing' among boys and girls ranged from 5.9% and 4.3% in Guangzhou (mainland China) respectively, and 11.2% and 9.8% in Canadian-born Chinese adolescents respectively. The prevalence of ever having had asthma ranged from 6.6% (Guangzhou) to 16.6% (Vancouver) for boys and from 2.9% (Gangzhou) to 15.0% (Vancouver) for girls, suggesting asthma symptoms in Chinese adolescents were lowest among residents of mainland China and were greater for those born in Canada. The study also demonstrated that asthma prevalence was higher for Chinese born in Hong Kong and Chinese migrants in Canada. These findings suggest that environmental factors may influence asthma prevalence.

Research involving 211 Australian students who migrated from Asia, the South Pacific, the Middle East, Europe and Africa, demonstrated the prevalence of adolescent migrants living in Australia with asthma was higher compared with similar age groups in their home countries.[28] The risk of developing asthma increased by 11% for every year they lived in Australia.

Travel

Travel is a risk factor for asthma — a study of 203 asthmatics visiting 56 countries found frequent use (> or = 3 times weekly) of inhaled bronchodilators before travel and participation in intensive physical exertion during treks significantly increased the risk of asthma attacks.[29] Asthmatics should avoid intensive trekking.

Low socioeconomic status (SES)

A US twenty year follow-up study of adults and children demonstrated low socioeconomic status had a negative impact on lung function, after adjusting for smoking status, occupational exposures, and race.[30] Researchers reported reductions of forced expiratory volume in 1 second (FEV_1) of greater than 300 mL in men and 200 mL in women of low SES compared with high SES.

There are multiple risk factors that may contribute toward the causation and pathogenesis of asthma. Table 5.2 summarises causes and/or triggers of asthma. These are discussed in detail throughout the chapter.

Table 5.2 Risk factors for asthma

Atopy
Family history
Migration
Low socioeconomic status
Affluent countries
Caesarean section
Lack of breastfeeding, especially first 6 months of life
Serious respiratory infection, especially before age 5
Medical health conditions, for example, viral respiratory infections, gastro-oesophageal reflux disease
More than 3 siblings
Allergic response to internal and external allergens — for example, house dust mite, animal hair, pollens, foods
Environmental — for example, occupational exposure to chemicals, pollution, old mattresses, mould, thunderstorms
Weather and storm patterns, cold air exposure
Stress, depression, anxiety, family issues
Exercise
Travel
Abnormal breathing patterns
Medication — for example, early exposure to antibiotics and beta-blockers in adults
Smoking — active and passive
Diet, chemical additives; lack of fish, vegetable and fruit intake — food intolerances (e.g. wheat) — high polyunsaturated fat intake
Obesity

General risk factors

A study of Australian rural NSW children aged 3–5 years estimated the prevalence of asthma between 18–22%, and identified clear risk factors for asthma.[31] The risk factors which doubled the risk of developing asthma included: atopy; having a parent with a history of asthma; having had a serious respiratory infection in the first 2 years of life; and a high dietary intake of polyunsaturated fats. Protective risk factors include breastfeeding and having 3 or more older siblings.

Other risk factors for asthma include: family history (maternal asthma odds 2.4; paternal 2.1); smoking (1.7 fold); serious respiratory infection before age 5 (2.3 fold); positive skin test to cladosporium (mould), house dust mite (HDM), cat and rye grass pollen; and occupational exposure to allergens.[32] Avoidance to these irritants may be of help (see Table 5.3).

Table 5.3 Possible allergen triggers especially in high risk asthmatics[33]

Ordinary cow's milk-based formula in young infants
Tobacco smoke
Pets e.g. cats, birds, dogs
House dust mite (HDM)
Cladosporium (mould)
Grass pollens — rye
Food — baking flour, wheat, milk, nuts, peanut, soy, egg, some fish and shellfish, polyunsaturated fats
Chemicals and gases — paint fumes, solvents, latex, synthetic bedding, chlorine
Pollution — diesel, wood heater, wood dust

Allergens, allergic triggers

There are a number of preventative methods to help reduce or avoid exposure to allergens or triggers of allergy or asthma. These methods play a more important role particularly in children who are atopic or at risk of developing atopic disease (high-risk infants) and children with early symptoms of allergic disease. This may improve control of asthma and reduce the need of medication.

Asthma patients may benefit from simple avoidance strategies for allergens when and where possible. Advice on effective strategies is an essential part of managing allergic asthma.

Caesarean section

Children born by caesarean section are at a higher risk of developing asthma later in life, and the risk was higher if either or both parents were atopic.[34]

Breastfeeding

Exclusive breastfeeding in the first 3–4 months of life significantly reduces the risk of asthma and atopy. Multiple studies including systematic reviews and meta-analyses have consistently supported this association. [35–39] Also duration of breastfeeding is significant with longer duration greater than 9 months being protective towards risk of asthma and wheeze.[40] Furthermore, a prospective birth-cohort study of over 2000 children from antenatal clinics up to 6 years of age, demonstrated children given non-human breast milk in the first 4 months of life were 40% more susceptible to wheeze 3 or more times since 1 year of age.[41]

The beneficial effect is postulated to be caused by immunomodulatory qualities of breast milk, avoidance of allergens, or a combination of these factors. Interesting, whilst breastfeeding was protective, the association of asthma and breastfeeding was increased in atopic children of asthmatic mothers after 6 years of age.[42] Another study failed to demonstrate protective effects of breastfeeding.[43] A study of the maternal diet of breastfeeding mothers demonstrated that atopic mothers had a higher intake of total fat and saturated fat and a lower intake of carbohydrate as a percentage of total energy intake compared with non-atopic mothers and was associated with atopic sensitisation of the infant which may explain the higher risk.[44] Also higher intake of food allergens may also contribute to this association in atopic mothers.[45]

Breast milk can contain significant numbers of bifidobacteria with studies demonstrating maternal fecal and breast milk bifidobacterial counts impact on the infants' fecal *Bifidobacterium* levels and provide an important source of bacteria in the establishment of infantile intestinal microbiota. A study found allergic mothers had significantly lower amounts of bifidobacteria in breast milk compared with non-allergic mothers and this may impact on the risk of the infant developing allergic disease.[46]

Of 448 children with a parental history of atopy, children put to bed with a bottle in the first year of life were at higher risk of wheezing at 1–5 years of age.[47] The researchers postulated that bronchospasm may be caused by repeated airway irritation due to postprandial reflux.

Antibiotic use and early exposure to respiratory infections

Research indicates that antibiotic use in early infancy (i.e. first 2 years of life) is associated with a 2–3 fold increased risk of developing asthma and hay fever, recognising the role of infections in protecting against asthma.[48] The study found that the number of courses of antibiotics during the first year of life was also associated with significant increased risk of asthma with 1–2 courses, but particularly with 3 or more courses when compared with no antibiotic use in the first year of life. In another study involving 1035 children followed up since birth, young children exposed to older children at home or to other children at day care are at increased risk for infections, which in turn may protect against the development of allergic diseases and asthma later in childhood. [49] Another study also found a significant association between antibiotic use and day care in the first year of life and wheezing at 7 years of age.[50] Similarly antibiotic use in the first year was significantly associated with greater risk of asthma at age 7 years, particularly with the number of antibiotic courses.[51] Compared with children who did not have antibiotics, children who received more than 4 courses of antibiotics were 1.5 times more likely to develop asthma.

Overall, research assessing children who enter day care at an early age, demonstrates exposure to infections in early childhood may prevent and lower the risk of allergy later in life.[52, 53] This supports the theory that exposure to infections early in life determines the way the immune system is stimulated, with T-helper cells geared toward fighting infection rather than produce cytokines that promoted allergy.

However, more recent studies found no association of antibiotic use and asthma prevalence suggesting that the reason that some children who've been given antibiotics appear to develop asthma is because the symptoms of the chest infection in young children can be confused with the start of asthma.[54, 55]

Medication

A retrospective study demonstrated that children medicated with paracetamol in the first year of life, are at higher risk of developing asthma; by up to threefold for frequent use.[56] Similarly another study found regular paracetamol intake in pregnancy has also been associated with greater risk of developing asthma by 60%, and even up to 85%, in offspring.[57] The mechanism behind this finding is not clear. There are many medications known to aggravate asthma such as beta-blockers, non-steroidal anti-inflammatories, aspirin and even the oral contraceptive pill which should be used with caution or avoided in asthmatics.[58]

The modern diet and obesity

The modern diet low in fresh foods such as fruit, vegetables and fish may be responsible for the rise in asthma. Obesity may be a contributor to allergies. Obese children are at greater risk of asthma, especially girls, according to the UK National Study of Health and Growth in London, which surveyed 15 000 children, aged 4 to 11, independent of ethnicity.[59] Obese children are 26% more likely to be more atopic, and sensitivity to milk was at least 50% higher than in normal-weight children.[60] Mean total IgE levels were higher among obese and overweight children than normal-weight children. The risk for atopy (any positive specific IgE measurement) was increased in the obese children largely driven by allergic sensitisation to foods.

Also, abdominal adiposity is known to compromise respiratory lung capacity.[61, 62, 63]

Mattresses

Sleeping on used cot mattress in the first year of life is associated with increased risk of asthma.[37] The study assessed 871 New Zealand children of European descent at birth and ages 12 months, 3.5 years and 7 years. The study found that 24% of children suffered from wheezing at 3.5 years and 18% at 7 years when they had a history of sleeping on a used cot mattress. In this study, other than the use of a used cot mattress for sleeping, asthma was also associated with maternal smoking during pregnancy, being in day care, antibiotic use, and the presence of a dog.

Stressful events

Children born to mothers who suffer chronic stress during their early years have a higher risk of asthma rate compared with their peers according to a cohort study of 14 000 children. This finding was independent of income, gender, maternal asthma, urban location or other known asthma risk factors.[64] The mechanism for how maternal distress causes asthma is not well understood although depressed mothers were more likely to smoke, less likely to breastfeed and less likely to interact with their infants.

Maternal stress and anxiety in pregnancy during fetal life is a risk factor for asthma during childhood. A longitudinal study of 5810 children recruited during pregnancy found a higher incidence of asthma in children at age 7 with mothers who experienced highest levels of anxiety at 32 weeks gestation compared with mothers with lowest levels of anxiety.[65] Poor coping in parenthood is also a known risk factor. Of 150 middle- to upper-class children followed up from birth to 6–8 years of age, one-quarter developed asthma. Both serum IgE levels and parenting difficulties were associated with increased risk of asthma. The researchers concluded that emotional stress may alter both immune and respiratory responses and their results 'should reinforce the importance of providing support and education to new parents and their children'.[65]

Acute stressful events and negative life events increase the risk of asthma exacerbations in a study of 90 primary-school Scottish children, particularly in children suffering multiple chronic stressors.[66] Asthma was self-monitored twice a week for 3 months. Acute negative events, such as family break-up and death of a grandparent increased the risk of suffering asthma. The risk of asthma attacks increased significantly when the acute stress was added to chronic stress such as poverty, family discord, parental substance abuse or being bullied at school.[67]

Stress appears to be a risk factor for asthma.[68]

Post-traumatic stress disorder (PTSD)

A study of 3065 male twin pairs (monozygotic and dizygotic twins), who lived together in childhood and served on active military duty during the Vietnam War, found those who suffered greater PTSD symptoms were 2.3 times as likely to have asthma compared with those who suffered from the least PTSD symptoms.[69] These findings suggest the emotional association between asthma and PTSD occurred despite twins sharing similar genes. The authors postulated that traumatic stress compromises the immune functioning independent of genes.

Mind–body medicine

General

A review of the literature noted psycho-educational self-management programs, relaxation therapy, biofeedback, and family therapy to be particularly useful in improving asthma outcome and significant beneficial effects were found for relaxation therapy. The researchers also identified biofeedback for 'respiratory resistance, trachea sounds, and vagal tone' to show promise.[70]

A Cochrane review of psychological interventions for adults with asthma identified 15 studies, involving 687 participants, aimed at determining the effect of cognitive behaviour therapy (CBT) on quality of life, and biofeedback and relaxation therapy on pulmonary function, FEV_1 and medication use.[71] They found conflicting results but overall quality of life improved with CBT and reduced the use of 'as needed' medications. Relaxation therapy also reduced the need for 'as needed medications' although no significant differences in FEV_1 was found. Biofeedback improved asthma and lung functions such as peak expiratory flow rate and FEV_1 in 2 studies.

Another Cochrane review assessing psychological interventions for children with asthma found conflicting results amongst the 12 studies of 588 children. Two studies examining the effects of relaxation therapy on peak expiratory flow rate (PEFR) significantly favoured the treatment group (32 L/min, 95% CI 13 to 50 L/min).[72]

So, based on the findings of these Cochrane reviews, it appears relaxation therapy, biofeedback and CBT can play a role in asthma management to improve quality of life, pulmonary function and the need for 'as needed' medication in adult and child asthmatics.

Spiritual healing

An innovative study tried to examine if spiritual healing could assist asthma. Spiritual healing was of no benefit for asthma symptoms when compared with sham healing and control.[73]

Psychological counselling

Psychological interventions can help reduce the burden of asthma symptoms and improve the management of disease and compliance with medication.

Depression and anxiety are more prevalent in severe asthmatics and associated with greater morbidity, mortality and non-compliance, requiring close psychological monitoring and the potential role for effective counselling in young asthmatic patients.[74, 75, 76] One study of over 1300 youths aged 11 to 17 years found young people with asthma were twice as likely to suffer depression and anxiety disorders compared with children without asthma.[77]

A population survey of 3010 participants aged 15 years and over found the prevalence of asthma was 9.9% and identified major depression was significantly higher for those who experienced dyspnoea, wakening at night from asthma, morning symptoms of asthma and reduced quality of life compared with those who did not suffer asthmatic symptoms.[78]

A case-controlled study of 21 patients from 8 to 18 years of age with severe asthma who were hospitalised and who died of asthma subsequent to discharge identified psychologic risk factors were prominent, such as conflicts between patients' parents and hospital staff regarding medical management, depressive symptoms and disregard of asthmatic symptoms.[79]

Psychological approaches such as counselling and biofeedback-assisted relaxation therapy were found to be particularly useful in improving mood and asthma.[80, 81, 82]

Family therapy

Asthma can be quite stressful for families and can impact parenting and interaction between family members.[83, 84, 85] Children of parents who experience major depression or panic attacks are also more likely to develop atopic disorders by 67% and 46% respectively.[86] Children with a genetic predisposition to asthma are 3 times more likely to express the illness with domestic stresses and parenting.[87, 88] Research supports the role of family therapy in asthma management.[89]

Relaxation therapy and meditation

Given that stress may exacerbate asthma, there is a role for stress management in the prevention and management of asthma. A review of the literature of variable quality studies demonstrated that stress can produce bronchoconstriction.[90]

Relaxation therapy is associated with respiratory muscle relaxation, reduced panic, reduced airway reactivity, improved lung function, promotion of diaphragmatic breathing, reduction in metabolic rate and may have an anti-inflammatory effect. A study found transcendental meditation (TM) can improve respiratory function.[91] This 6 month study, with cross-over at 3 months, demonstrated TM can be a useful adjunct to asthma treatment.

However, a UK systematic review of the literature found overall, the methodological quality of the 15 randomised clinical trials (RCTs) on relaxation therapy assessed were poor and better quality studies are required.[92]

In addition to the abovementioned research, it was found that music therapy can be particularly helpful for relaxation and asthma.[93]

Despite these findings, generally patients with asthma who practise regular relaxation therapies experience improved quality of life.

Biofeedback

Fear and panic are common emotions experienced by asthmatics.[94, 95, 96]

A review of the literature identified negative emotions such as panic and generalised panic disorder are common in asthmatics. These negative emotions can also affect asthma morbidity.[97] They identified self-regulation strategies as useful adjuncts to asthma treatment such as relaxation therapy, electromyographic (EMG) biofeedback, biofeedback to improve sensitivity in perceiving symptoms, and biofeedback training for increasing respiratory sinus arrhythmia. Relaxation-oriented methods were more beneficial amongst asthmatics with panic symptoms.

A number of studies demonstrated that biofeedback is helpful for dealing with asthma symptoms in children and adults.[98, 99] A 15 month follow up of asthmatics that included a comprehensive multi-behavioural and desensitisation retraining program using EMG and spirometer feedback to encourage slow diaphragmatic breathing in all situations, demonstrated subjects reported reductions in their asthma symptoms, medication use, emergency room visits, and breathless episodes.[100]

Electromyographic feedback methods can also be useful by providing feedback on muscle tension and strain.[101, 102]

Hypnosis

A prospective, randomised, single, blind controlled trial of 39 adults with mild to moderate asthma after a 6-weekly course of hypnotherapy demonstrated a 75% improvement in the degree of bronchial hyper-responsiveness, improved peak expiratory flow rates by 5.5%, and reduction of use of bronchodilators by 26% in the more highly susceptible subjects to hypnosis.[103] Daily home recordings of symptoms also improved.

Another study of severe chronic asthmatics inadequately controlled with medication undergoing relaxation induced hypnotherapy reported: improved asthma symptoms; a significant reduction in hospital admissions, from 44 to 13 a year in total; reduced duration of hospitalisation; and reduction of prednisolone use and side-effects experienced from medication.[104] Air flow tests remained variable among subjects.

Journal writing

A study of patients with mild-moderate asthma or rheumatoid arthritis demonstrated that writing about emotionally traumatic life experiences over a 4-month period can help reduce chronic disease symptoms.[105] With asthma, lung function test forced expiratory volume in 1 second (FEV_1) improved from 63.9% at baseline to 76.3% at the 4 month follow-up period of journal writing, with no change in the control group. The rheumatoid arthritis patients also did well with significant reduction of symptoms and disease activity compared with the control group.

In an RCT 137 adult asthmatic patients were randomly assigned to write for 20 minutes, once per week for 3 weeks, about stressful life experiences (n = 41), positive experiences (n = 37), or neutral experiences (n = 36; control group).[106] The study found only marginal benefit for FEV_1 and for forced vital capacity (FVC) between each group: the stress-writing group demonstrated 4.2% FEV_1 and 3.1% FVC improvement, the positive-writing group 1.3% $FEV_1$and 3.6% FVC, and in the control group 3.0% FEV_1 and 2.4% FVC.

Laughter

Laughter and excitement can also trigger asthma, such as cough and dyspnoea, with cohort studies suggesting the incidence is common, estimated at 32% in young asthmatics.[107] The researchers examined 285 children who had experienced an acute asthma attack and found 'mirth-triggered' asthma, especially cough symptom, occurred within 2 minutes of laughing.

Mirth-triggered asthma is an indication of sub-optimal asthma control and treatment.

Pet ownership

Allergens are a common cause for triggering asthma attacks. Allergens from pet and animal hair can trigger symptoms in an atopic asthmatic.

Pet keeping in early childhood can impact on allergies and asthma depending on the type of pet, the age and the allergic sensitisation of the individual.[108] A review of the literature found recent published studies have produced heterogeneous results.[109] Sensitisation to pets is a risk factor for asthma and can occur in children who live in homes with no pets and with low levels of pet. allergen. The authors of the review conclude 'excluding pets from the home will not necessarily protect children from the development of sensitisation to pets'.

Another systematic review found exposure to pets increases the risk of asthma in children over 6 years of age.[110]

A large international survey of almost 19 000 adults found the effects of having pets during childhood varied according to the type of pet, the allergic sensitisation of each subject and pet prevalence in the community.[111] The survey indicated that keeping a cat doubled the risk of asthma, but only among atopic subjects.

However, dogs kept in early childhood protect against allergic sensitisation and protect against hay fever symptoms in atopic subjects. Those who were not atopic had an increased risk of adult respiratory symptoms with early dog exposure. Having birds in childhood was associated with more adult respiratory symptoms independent of atopic status. These findings confirm that early exposure to animals in early life does influence the development of the immune system and the airways, with the potential to promote or prevent subsequent disease in later adulthood.

Exposure to a dog in early infancy may protect against atopy due to mediation of cytokine response.[106, 112] Further research studying 285 infants demonstrated that children who grow up with a pet dog were less likely to develop allergic sensitisation and atopic dermatitis.[113] The rate of allergic sensitisation was 14% lower and the rate of atopic dermatitis 21% lower in children with a dog compared with children with no dog. Similarly, studies suggest early exposure to pets can be protective towards asthma development.[114, 115]

A recent study of 275 children (3 years of age) at increased risk of developing allergic diseases found exposure to dogs in infancy, and 'especially around the time of birth, is associated with changes in immune development and reductions in wheezing and atopy'.[116]

A community sample of 3181 adults aged 26–82 years found keeping a cat or dog in childhood was associated with increased risk of dyspnoea or breathing difficulties.[117] Based on current evidence there are mixed findings to pet ownership but it appears dogs may offer some benefit in reducing development of asthma risk in atopic children.

Environment

Thunderstorms

Asthma epidemics may be linked with thunderstorms as pollen counts are high during these times. A deluge of grass pollen during thunderstorms may be the cause of epidemic asthma. It may be wise for asthmatics to stay indoors during thunderstorms. The risk of symptoms doubled if asthma patients were outdoors during thunderstorms, according to an analysis of data of 183 patients following a spring storm.[118] Asthmatics sensitive to thunderstorms also tend to suffer hay fever and are allergic to rye grass pollen compared to control groups.[119, 120]

Weather

A change of weather may impact on asthma. Triggers of asthma include changes in temperature; cold windy days; hot humid days; and poor air quality.

Farm children

A study surveyed 1333 farmers' children and a reference group of 566 children aged from 5 to 17 years and found that children with both prenatal and current exposure to farm animals and plants were up to 50% per cent less likely to have allergies such as asthma, eczema and hay fever than the reference group.[121]

House dust mite (HDM)

House dust mite (HDM) is a major allergen found in house dust. There are various methods available to reduce HDM allergens by chemical or physical means, with the aim to reduce asthma symptoms in those who are sensitive to HDM. There are many studies finding links between HDM and allergic and asthma symptoms. Seasonal fluctuations of HDM numbers determined by humidity in children's beds may contribute to fluctuations and influence asthma symptoms.[122]

A large-scale prospective birth-cohort study of 939 newborns, followed up until 7 years of age, cast doubt on the theory of early exposure to HDM allergens as a primary cause of asthma in young children.[123] The study did show that children with asthma were more likely to be sensitised to HDM and cat allergens, but those were not the 'cause' of asthma.

Whilst studies show mixed results, the weight of evidence supports reducing HDM levels in households. Advice to parents to reduce HDM exposure to infants and asthmatics includes: removal of old carpet; use of closely woven dust mite covers on bedding; frequent airing of blankets and mats; keeping indoor humidity low; using hydronic heating instead of central heating; and using damp cloths for wiping surfaces.

Bedding and mattress protectors

Higher HDM antigen levels in bedding appear to be a risk factor for persistent bronchial hyper-reactivity in adolescence.[124] Exposure to HDM in temperate climates is the strongest environmental risk factor for asthma. A study of 616 pregnant women were randomised to HDM intervention by using impermeable mattress covers and an acaricide washing detergent for bedding. When compared with the control group, these methods were effective in reducing HDM allergens.[125]

Mattress covers

A European trial involving 636 highly atopic children aged 1.5 to 5 years, with negative skin tests to HDM, were less likely to be sensitised to HDM with a combination of education and a simple preventive measure (mattress encasement) to reduce mite allergen exposure compared with the control group after 1 year.[126] Sensitisation to mite allergens was tested by skin-prick test or measured by serum specific immunoglobulin E. Another study also demonstrated allergen-impermeable mattress encasings versus placebo mattress encasings were significantly more effective in reducing HDM allergen levels.[127] However, 1 RCT of 47 children found the use of special allergen-occlusive bed covers of little benefit in asthmatic children whose symptoms were triggered by HDM.[128]

One review of the evidence found that in homes of high-risk atopic infants, the current evidence supports measures to reduce the levels of indoor allergens such as HDM and pets by using mattress and pillow encasings.[129] When compared to placebo, semipermeable polyurethane mattress and pillow encasings (allergy control) resulted in a significant perennial reduction of HDM exposure and a significant reduction in the required dose of inhaled steroids by asthmatics.

Synthetic bedding

A number of studies, including cohort studies, demonstrate a clear association between synthetic bedding (e.g. pillow and quilt) and frequent childhood wheeze episodes.[130, 131] Children who sleep with synthetic pillows (foam, sponge, polyester, dacron) and quilts are 5 times more likely to have frequent wheezing according to a Tasmanian study of 900 7-year olds.[123]

A study looking at 758 school children aged 8–10 years demonstrated that those sleeping with synthetic bedding (quilts or pillows) had adverse respiratory outcomes, more asthma and recent wheeze, more than 12 wheezing episodes during the year, and twice the risk of allergic rhino-conjunctivitis if they had a positive skin-prick test than children with a negative test.[132]

Synthetic bedding (e.g. quilts and pillows) should be avoided in atopic individuals and asthmatics.[133]

Feathered pillows

It is best to avoid synthetic pillows and use feather pillows as they are associated with a significantly lower rate of wheezing and sensitisation to HDM according to a number of studies.[134, 135] Synthetic pillows accumulate more HDM than feathered pillows which may account for the benefit of feather pillows.[136–139]

Effective pillow encasings can be useful for reducing HDM numbers.

Laundry washing

Washing laundry at 25 degrees Celsius for at least 5 minutes was sufficient to remove most of the cat and mite allergens, according to an Australian study.[140] There were no distinct differences between which laundry detergents were used and washing at 60 degrees Celsius reduced more allergens, though the benefits were slight.

Physical and chemical methods

A Cochrane review of 54 trials (3002 patients) of which 36 trials assessed physical methods (26 mattress encasings), 10 chemical methods, and 8 a combination of chemical and physical methods, found most trials were of poor quality and the interventions were statistically of no benefit for health outcomes and asthma symptom score.[141] Similarly, a report published in Cochrane PEARLS (Practical Evidence About Real Life Situations) concluded HDM control measures may not reduce asthma symptoms.[142]

A study found successful attempts to reduce environmental allergens such as avoidance of HDMs, pets, tobacco smoke, promoting longer breastfeeding and avoiding early introduction of foods significantly reduced the risk of asthma by 60% and wheeze by 90% in 2-year olds compared with the control group.[143] Table 5.4 provides simple strategies for reducing allergen exposure at home.

Allergen immunotherapy

Allergen immunotherapy also known as ‘desensitisation’ can occur by injection or sublingual.

The National Asthma Council contains good guidelines on injectable allergen-specific immunotherapy which usually occurs subcutaneously in the skin and should be performed by experienced medical practitioners.[144] This is a process that involves gradual increases in quantities of an allergen extract, which modifies the immune response to help reduce airway inflammation and improve asthma control.

A Cochrane review including 75 trials of 3506 participants (3188 with asthma) demonstrated overall immunotherapy significantly reduced asthma symptoms, the use of asthma medications, and improved

Table 5.4 Simple measures for reducing environmental allergens

Measure
Put toys away in cupboards
Wipe surfaces weekly with a damp cloth
Steam clean carpets bi-annually; use built-in vacuum cleaner
Damp mop hard floorboards
Hot wash bedding — add a few drops of Eucalyptus oil to wash
Place bedding in dryer for 15 minutes weekly
Use natural bedding e.g. feathered or cotton pillows and doonas
Dust mite covers for bedding
Allow sun into house and air house out regularly — daily if possible
Avoid smoking inside house
Avoid pets in house

bronchial hyper-reactivity, with 1 study demonstrating effectiveness equal to inhaled steroids.[145] Trials of immunotherapy were tested for HDM allergy, pollen allergy, animal dander, Cladosporium mould allergy, latex and multiple allergens. The authors warned good patient selection was essential as the risk of side-effects included bronchospasm, local reaction, allergic reactions and sometimes anaphylaxis.

A meta-analysis of 9 studies including a total of 441 patients randomised to sublingual immunotherapy (SLIT) or placebo found, overall, there was a significant reduction in both symptoms and medication use following SLIT.[146]

A study of 253 children suffering grass pollen–induced rhinoconjunctivitis with/without asthma, demonstrated significant improvement with grass tablet Grazax compared with placebo.[147] The tablet was generally tolerated, with pruritus the commonest reaction reported by 32% of subjects compared with 2% in the placebo group. Six subjects withdrew due to adverse events.

Damp houses and mould

Dampness in the house is also a risk factor for asthma.

A Munich study of 234 children with asthma, demonstrated that living in damp houses plays a significant risk factor for asthma with increased nocturnal wheeze, shortness of breath and persistence of bronchial hyper-reactivity in adolescence.[148] This risk was not attributed or explained by exposure to HDM antigen.

The Skorge et. al. study also found an association of mould exposure with all the respiratory symptoms such as cough and dyspnoea with 3–5% of the frequency of the respiratory symptoms in the study population attributed to exposure to visible moulds.[117] Of interest, fitted carpet in the bedroom reduced the risk of respiratory symptoms.

A population-based case–control study that involved researchers visiting and assessing the homes of 121 asthmatic children and 241 controls found visible moisture damage and mould growth in the main living quarters (living room or child's bedroom) was significantly associated with the development of asthma in early childhood.[149]

Occupational asthma and chemical exposure

Occupational asthma is caused by reactions to allergens in the workplace.[2] The report, Occupational Asthma in Australia, indicates 9–15% of adult-onset asthma cases can be attributed to exposure to causal agents at work such as wood dust, paint fumes, solvents, latex and baking flour.[150] The commonest causes of occupational asthma in Australia are wood dust from trees such as the Western red cedar, isocyanates (the raw materials used in polyurethane products), paint fumes, solvents, latex, and flour.

One of the largest population studies of occupational asthma that analysed data on 15 637 randomly selected people aged 20–44 from 26 areas of 12 industrial countries estimated the incidence of occupational asthma in young people at 5–10%.[151] A recent population-based study of 13 countries also found that at least 10% of adult onset asthma is related to occupational allergens.[152] Those at greatest risk had a history of atopy or parental asthma. High-risk occupations included farmers, painters, plastic workers, cleaners, spray painters and agricultural workers commonly exposed to chemical substances. Asthma risk was also associated with high exposure to dusts, gases and fumes. People who work in commercial greenhouses are also at risk of occupational asthma if they are sensitised to the flowers they grow, according to German researchers.[153]

Professional and domestic cleaning are also associated with aggravation or inducing asthma due to chemical exposure from cleaning products.[154, 155] A 9-year European study of 3503 adults free of asthma at baseline, found 42% of the sample study who used cleaning sprays at least once weekly increased the risk of asthma symptoms by 49% and wheeze by 39%.[156] The risk increased with increasing use of cleaning sprays but not liquid products. Glass and furniture cleaning sprays and air-refreshers posed the greatest risk to asthma. The overall prevalence of adult onset asthma related to cleaning sprays was estimated at 15% by researchers.

A study of 4500 Spanish women aged 30–65 years found those who had worked in domestic cleaning had a higher rate of all respiratory symptoms, including asthma compared to those who had never worked in domestic cleaning.[157] It was not clear whether exposure to dust mites, cleaning products or other allergens contributed to the increased risk.

Smoking

The association between smoking (passive and active) and asthma is strong and well accepted. The beneficial effects of smoking cessation on lung function are well established. Smoking should be avoided by asthmatics and smoking indoors avoided by other household members (e.g. parental smoking), as even passive smoking may cause or aggravate asthma.[158]

Traffic and air pollution

Air pollution is associated with impaired health, including reduced lung function in adults and children.[159] Air pollution is commonest in major cities and some industrialised areas. Motor vehicles are the main source of air pollution due to particles in suspension, particularly those that use diesel fuel. Air pollution compromises respiratory function. Moving to polluted areas may aggravate lung function in children and adults. A number of studies demonstrate benefit to lung function when children move to cleaner geographic areas.

Epidemiological studies demonstrate an association between the degree of traffic exposure and lung function in asthma. A large-scale study of city school children primarily based in the centre of Oxford (England) demonstrated a statistically significant improvement in peak expiratory flow (PEF) rate and respiratory symptoms among children living where traffic on roads decreased compared to those living where the traffic increased.[160]

Exposure to traffic pollution, particularly diesel exhaust, is associated with impaired lung function in asthmatics and the rise of atopy.[161, 162]

A recent prospective birth cohort study based in Germany of children at the age of 4 and 6 found a strong positive association was found between the distance to the nearest main road and asthmatic bronchitis, hay fever, eczema, and sensitisation, especially in those living less than 50 metres from busy roads.[163]

A study of 460 children in Holland found episodes of wheeze and shortness of breath increased by 140% when exposed to airborne pollutants of small particulate matter and when other pollutants, such as sulphur dioxide and nitrous oxides, were highest.[164] The study found children with bronchial hyper-responsiveness and high concentrations of serum total IgE were more susceptible to health problems from air pollution.

The rise in asthma, allergic rhinitis and atopic eczema may be attributed to a number of combined causes such as air pollution, exposure to diesel exhaust particulates, greater exposure to indoor allergens through adoption of an 'inside' lifestyle, artificial ventilation of buildings and changes to outdoor allergen exposure with climate changes.

Climate change

Climate change gives rise to variations in temperature patterns that impact on plants by varying pollination times and favouring some plant species over others. The presence of high CO^2 concentrations and temperatures can increase pollen counts by plants with the subsequent risk of allergic sensitisation in the human population.[165] For example, an environmentally controlled greenhouse mimicking climate changes by doubling the atmospheric CO^2 concentration stimulated ragweed-pollen production by 61% suggesting significant increases in exposure to allergenic pollen under the scenario of global warming.[166]

A prospective study of 9651 adults (18 to 60 years of age) randomly selected from population registries found an association between indoor and outdoor pollution (particulate air pollution) and decline in lung function, especially of small airway function.[167]

Street trees

Children living in areas with more tree-lined streets have lower rates of asthma and a lesser risk of developing asthma, as trees improve air quality or encourage children to play more outdoors.[168] Street trees were associated with a lower prevalence of early childhood asthma.

Indoor pollution

Indoor pollution may play a role in the pathogenesis of childhood asthma but not as the cause of asthma in childhood.[169] There are potentially multiple indoor allergens that can cause sensitisation such as dust mite, cockroach, pet, rodent allergens, and indoor air pollutants; for example, ozone, particulate matter, nitrogen dioxide, environmental tobacco smoke, sulfur dioxide, and carbon monoxide.[170]

A study of 409 children in 5 New Zealand communities between the ages of 6 and 12 with diagnosed asthma, were assessed before and after more effective heating was installed in their homes.[171] After installing better heating such as heat pumps, flued gas heaters or pellet burners, children demonstrated improved health, less sleep disturbance, reduced asthma symptoms such as wheezing, less coughing at night and overall improved respiratory symptoms. Consequently they had fewer sick days off school and less doctor visits.

A cohort study of children (2–6 years of age) monitored the air in their bedrooms for 3 days to assess the level of indoor pollution specifically for particulate matter, nitrogen dioxide, and ozone.[172] They found the level of bedroom air pollutant concentrations did not differ significantly between asthmatic and non-asthmatic subjects. Whilst these substances may aggravate asthma, the study did not support the causative role of these factors for developing asthma.

Overall a systematic review of the literature supports a link between housing improvement, such as rehousing, refurbishment, and energy efficiency measures and health gains after the intervention.[173]

Of interest, exposure to airborne inhaled allergens released during cooking can provoke asthma in atopic children allergic to foods.[174] The study identified inhaling allergens from foods such as fish, chickpeas, and buckwheat during cooking, and even opening packets of peanuts in a confined space, can provoke an asthma attack. Asthmatics with food allergies need dietary advice and need to be aware of environmental measures that may be required to limit exposure to aerosolised food.

Winter air pollution — wood smoke

High wood smoke for home heating causing indoor air pollution, as measured by particulate matter in smoke, can affect the health of boys with asthma by reducing lung function.[175] The boys who didn't have respiratory problems such as asthma were not affected, although all the students (with and without asthma) coughed slightly more on high pollution nights from wood chips.

Installing non-polluting heating in the homes of children with asthma can significantly reduce symptoms of asthma, days off school, visits to health care workers and chemists without significantly improving lung function.[176]

Swimming pools — chlorine

Swimming offers an excellent way to build up fitness and can improve lung function. However, a number of studies demonstrate exposure to indoor and outdoor chlorinated swimming pools can be detrimental to the airways of swimmers and pool attendants and can be associated with higher risks of asthma, airway inflammation and some respiratory allergies.[177–181]

In addition, case reports describe occupational asthma in swimming pool attendants, due to poor air quality above indoor chlorinated swimming pools.[182] It would appear swimming in non-chlorinated pools such as ozone-treated pools or the beach is preferred for asthmatics.

Exercise

Lack of exercise in Western society, including lack of outdoor activity by children, may contribute to rising incidence of asthma.[183] Exercise improves cardiovascular fitness and quality of life in asthmatics.

Trekking

Young adults with mild to moderate asthma are at risk of aggravating their symptoms with high-altitude trekking due to cold, dry air and exposure to new allergens. Of the 88 high-altitude trekkers surveyed, 45% noted their asthma worsened, 37% experienced the worst attack in their life and 11% experienced a life-threatening attack.[184]

Swimming

While some asthmatics suffer exercise-induced bronchoconstriction, a number of trials have demonstrated the benefits of exercise, such as swimming, that improves aerobic capacity, in the management of asthma particularly.[185] Review of available evidence suggests that swimming induces less severe bronchoconstriction than other sports, due to the high humidity of inspired air at water level. Based on the findings of chlorine induced asthma, it is preferable to swim in non-chlorinated pools, such as ozone-treated pools.

Yoga

A number of yoga studies investigating yoga and breath work for treating asthma have been promising with several randomised controlled trials showing benefit from yoga postures and breathing versus control (usual care).

A double-blind, controlled trial of 56 adult asthmatics on maximum doses of inhaled steroids for poorly controlled asthma were randomised to sessions of Sahaja yoga, a traditional form of 'yoga meditation' or a control group for 2 hours on a weekly basis for 4 months. Yoga provided significant benefits in improving asthma hyper-responsiveness at the end of each treatment.[186]

University students who practised yoga techniques 3 times a week for 16 weeks reported a significant degree of relaxation, positive attitude, better yoga exercise tolerance and lesser usage of beta adrenergic inhalers compared with control groups, but no significant difference in pulmonary function measured with spirometry between the 2 groups.[187]

A study of 53 asthmatic patients compared with 53 control patients practising 65 minutes of daily yoga over 2 weeks resulted in significantly fewer attacks per week, less use of medication and improved PEFR.[188]

Similar findings were demonstrated in a study of 570 asthmatic patients, with those undergoing yoga therapy of 2–4 weeks and followed up at 3 and 54 months experiencing significant improvement in PEFR and at least 66% reduction in asthma medication, especially in those who practised consistently on a daily basis for longer periods of time.[189]

Yoga breathing exercises (pranayama) statistically significantly reduced the dose of histamine needed to provoke a 20% reduction in FEV_1 in patients with mild asthma compared with the placebo device.[190]

Another study demonstrated that a yoga therapy program on 46 indoor patients with chronic bronchial asthma improved exercise tolerance and pulmonary functions, reduced symptom scores and reduced medication requirements, even at 1 year follow-up.[191]

One trial did not find yoga any different to benefits derived from breath-work and stretching alone. This randomised, controlled, double-masked clinical trial of 62 asthmatics compared the active control involving breath-work and stretching with yoga intervention over a 4-week period.[192] Both groups demonstrated significant improvement in post-bronchodilator forced expiratory volume in 1 second and morning symptom scores at 4 and 16 weeks, but no differences were found between the 2 groups.

Yoga clearly has a potential as an adjunct to asthma management as well as improving quality of life, such as reducing stress symptoms.

Qigong

Qigong, part of traditional Chinese medicine (TCM), combines movement, meditation and breathing techniques. It may assist asthmatics according to a pilot study of 30 patients who demonstrated improved lung function tests (peak flow), reduced emergency hospital visits and sick leave.[193]

Alexander technique

Alexander technique, a physical therapy involving a series of movements designed to correct posture and bring the body into natural alignment, may play a role in management of chronic asthma although robust, well-designed RCTs are required in order to test claims by practitioners.[194]

Breathing exercises

Dysfunctional breathing

There is a growing body of research that demonstrates a high prevalence of dysfunctional breathing occurs in asthmatics.[195, 196] Asthma symptoms can be confused with breathing dysfunction and it is important to identify this difference to tailor appropriate treatment.[197] The prevalence of dysfunctional breathing may be as high as one-third of women and one-fifth of men.[198]

A suitably designed questionnaire may help identify dysfunctional breathing patterns even in children.[199, 200] This is an important distinction that should be made as breathing dysfunction can be treated with appropriate breathing exercises.

A cross-sectional study of 219 general practice patients demonstrated that one-third of them, especially young women, diagnosed with asthma have dysfunctional breathing or a combination of both. Treatment for dysfunctional breathing includes relaxation therapy, breathing retraining exercises and reassurance.[201]

An accompanying editorial concludes 'asthma and anxiety with dysfunctional breathing are both common conditions and they often coexist'.[202] This highlights why it is vital to differentiate dysfunctional breathing associated with anxiety from asthma.

Breathing exercises

There is now ample evidence to demonstrate that breathing exercises can help asthma patients. There are different methods of breathing exercises that may be of help. Some breathing exercises may not improve lung function scores but they appear to play a role in managing symptoms of asthma, improving quality of life and reducing the need for medication.

One study aimed to assess 1 breathing exercise focusing on shallow nasal breathing with those of non-specific upper-body exercises and found little benefit favouring 1 technique over the other.[203] Both groups of exercises led to a dramatic reduction in use of reliever medication by 86% and inhaled corticosteroid dose reduced by 50%. The authors recommended breathing exercises be practised twice daily, as a first-line symptom treatment to help reinforce the message of relaxation and self-efficacy. The breathing exercise can be viewed for free online at:

http://www.asthmacrc.org.au/

In a prospective parallel-group single-blinded trial of 183 asthmatics, patients were randomised to breathing training or asthma education.[204] At 6 months following intervention, there was significant improvement in asthma-specific health status, mood scores (anxiety and depression) and quality of life in asthmatics undergoing breathing training compared with the patient education group, but they did not differ for airway physiology, inflammation or hyper-responsiveness.

In another trial, 85 patients were randomised to a control group or to an intervention group of treatment by the Papworth method, an integrated breathing and relaxation technique used by physiotherapists since the 1960s.[205] Both groups received usual medical care. Following 12 months of treatment, there was significant improvement in asthma scores, respiratory function and adverse mood, such as anxiety, for the Papworth group compared with the control group.

A Cochrane review identified 7 studies in total demonstrating that breathing retraining and interventions overall significantly reduced use in rescue bronchodilator, acute exacerbations of asthma and improved quality of life measures.[206] However 5 studies compared breathing retraining with no active control and 2 with asthma education control groups illustrating how difficult it is to draw firm conclusions with trials being considerably different. Nevertheless, the authors conclude, in view of improved quality of life with breathing interventions, more trials are warranted.

Inspiratory muscle training

Inspiratory muscle training to improve inspiratory muscle strength training and endurance, also improved asthma symptoms, reduced hospitalisations for asthma, emergency department visits, absence from school or work, and use of medication in patients with asthma.[207,208] These exercises may also benefit patients with cystic fibrosis.[209]

Buteyko

The buteyko method shows potential but there is still debate until more definitive trials are completed as to whether these benefits are physiological or purely subjective. The high incidence of dysfunctional breathing amongst asthmatics may explain or account for the therapeutic effect of breathing retraining exercises and buteyko method of treating asthma.[195,210]

Those practising the buteyko method reduced hyperventilation and their use of beta 2-agonists, with daily inhaled steroid dosage reduced by 49% and observed better quality of life, despite no change in FEV_1 levels.[211] In another study, buteyko significantly improved quality of life and reduced inhaled bronchodilator use.[212] A study of 69 patients found the buteyko technique improved symptoms and reduced the use of bronchodilator use compared with the pranayama breathing exercises (a yoga breathing technique).[213]

A blinded RCT comparing buteyko breathing with control in 38 people with asthma (18–70 years of age) over 6 months found no significant change in FEV_1 but a significant reduction in inhaled steroid use of 50% and beta2-agonist use of 85% at 6 months from baseline compared with the control group.[214] The control group remained unchanged with steroid use and there was an observed reduction of beta2-agonist by 37%.

A 2-year Scottish study of 600 asthma patients (aged 18–69 years) randomised to receive buteyko breathing therapy, standard asthma management by physiotherapists, or continued standard asthma management with medication, found buteyko considerably improved asthma symptoms.[215] Overall, the buteyko group reduced asthma symptoms by 98%, the need for reliever medications by 98%, preventer medications by 92%, oral preparations by 100%, oral preventers by 96%, and reduced the incidence of colds or viral infections by 20%. This compared with 'no significant change' in the other 2 groups.

Dietary changes

Diet can play a major role in the management of asthma. Traditional advice in many cultures (e.g. Chinese and Indian) includes ensuring 'warm, cooked, spicy foods' for asthmatics as opposed to cold foods from the fridge. A cup of warm chamomile tea with honey may be beneficial for its calmative effect for coughs, although some allergic asthmatics need to avoid chamomile.

Pregnancy

An assessment of 1253 pregnant women's diet during pregnancy demonstrated low intake of foods containing vitamin E (not supplements) was associated with increased risk of infants developing asthma symptoms and wheeze.[216] Mothers with the lowest vitamin E intake were 5 times more likely to have children with asthma compared with mothers with high intake. Foods rich in vitamin E include vegetable oils, nuts, sunflower seeds and green leafy vegetables.

Mediterranean diet

Fruit and vegetables

Data extracted from a large Europe-wide asthma study, the European Community Respiratory Health Survey, using random samples of 20–44 year old subjects, found an inverse association (i.e. a protective effect) with intake of fruit, vitamins A and C, and riboflavin from dietary intake.[217] Research supports the role of high dietary intake of fruits and vegetables as being protective towards asthma.

Adherence to the Mediterranean diet — high in fresh fruit, vegetables, nuts and fish — during childhood appears to be protective towards asthma and rhinitis, reducing the risk by up to 64% compared with low adherence to the diet.[218] Wheeze and rhinitis are rare in Crete and the traditional Mediterranean diet appears to play a role. A cross-sectional survey of 690 children (aged 7–18 years) demonstrated 80% of children ate fresh fruit, namely grapes, oranges, apples, and fresh tomatoes, and 68% ate vegetables at least twice a day. Consumption of nuts was also significantly inversely associated with wheezing. Margarine more than doubled the risk of both wheeze and allergic rhinitis.

Similarly a study of over 18 000 children's diets in Italy found those eating fruit rich in vitamin C up to 5–7 times per week was associated with a reduced incidence of nocturnal cough, chronic cough, non-coryzal rhinitis, shortness of breath and wheeze.[219] In children with a history of asthma, those eating fresh fruit at least once a week experienced a lower 1-year occurrence of wheeze (29.3%) than those eating fruit less than once per week (47.1%).

A major study conducted in 10 English and Welsh towns of 2650 children aged 8–11 demonstrated that eating fresh fruit daily was associated with improved lung function by 4.3% (FEV_1 of 79ml) in asthmatics suffering wheeze, not related to vitamin C levels.[220]

High antioxidants, such as ascorbate, may have a protective effect. In a cross-sectional analysis of 4104 children, after controlling for several confounders (sex, study area, paternal education, household density, maternal smoking, paternal smoking, bedroom dampness or mould, parental asthma), intake of citrus fruit or kiwi fruit was found to be a highly significant protective factor for wheeze, shortness of breath, nocturnal cough, rhinitis and chronic cough in the last 12 months, even among children whose intake of fruit was as little as only 1–2 times per week.[221]

Similar findings were demonstrated in a prospective cohort study of 2512 men aged 45–59 who demonstrated lung function to be 138ml higher in men eating 5 or more apples per week and seemed to be independent of total vitamin E and C intakes.[222] Quercetin found in apples (and onions) may contribute to the observed benefits. Traditionally, onions are thought to be beneficial for the prevention and treatment of colds and respiratory problems.

A study of over 63 000 middle-aged men and women found those who smoked, and ate more fruit and soy, were associated with reduced risk of developing cough and chronic respiratory symptoms.[223]

A diet rich in fish and containing more than 40g a day of 'fruity vegetables' — namely tomatoes, eggplants, cucumber, green beans and zucchini — reduces the risk of asthma and allergies according to a 7-year study of 460 Spanish children.[224] Children who consumed more than 60g of fish a day and mothers who ate fish during pregnancy were also associated with significantly reduced risks of childhood allergies.

Fish intake

Population studies such as in Eskimo communities demonstrate diets high in fish also have low rates of asthma, whereas diets high in polyunsaturated fats are associated with increased risk of asthma. Ecological and temporal data from population and migration studies suggest that dietary factors may play a role in increased prevalence of asthma. The typical Western diet has 20- to 25-fold more omega n-6 polyunsaturated fatty acids (PUFA) than n-3 PUFA, contributing to a more 'pro-inflammatory diet' promoting the release of pro-inflammatory arachidonic acid metabolites (leukotrienes and prostanoids).[225]

School children who eat fish more than once a week have a significantly reduced risk of developing asthma than those who don't eat fish.[226] After adjusting for other risk factors such as ethnicity, country of birth, atopy, parental smoking and family history, fresh, oily fish (>2% fat) was protective against asthma in childhood. Children with a diet rich in omega-3 fatty acids (e.g. fish and flaxseed oil) had less asthma, as these foods are known to inhibit inflammation. Reduced asthma symptoms with n-3 fatty acid ingestion in the asthma patient who responded appear to be related to 5-series leukotriene production, although the mechanism is still not clear. Those who did not benefit from fish oils displayed a different leukotriene picture: '5-series leukotriene excretion with high n-3 PUFA ingestion was significantly greater for responders than for non-responders'.[227]

A large population-based study, the Respiratory Health in Northern Europe (RHINE) study, of 16 187 subjects aged 23–54 years found that, after excluding other confounders such as smoking, a minimum weekly fish intake reduced the incidence of asthma in adults.[228] They found people in Iceland and Norway eat more fish both in childhood and adulthood compared with Sweden, Estonia and Denmark. Fish intake less than once weekly in adults was associated with increased risk of asthma symptoms, while more frequent fish intake did not appear to decrease the risk further as the association was not dose–response related. Those who never ate fish in childhood had the highest risk for asthma and earlier asthma onset. Of interest, daily or no cod oil consumption was associated with asthma, with lowest risk in those taking cod oil some days during the week.

Fast foods and polyunsaturated fat intake

The rise in dietary intake of fast foods in the Western diet may partly explain the rise of asthma incidence in these communities.

High dietary polyunsaturated fats — for example, margarine and frying in polyunsaturated fats — doubled the risk of developing asthma in preschool children.[31]

Frequent consumption of hamburgers increased the risk of asthma and bronchial hyper-responsiveness in children even after excluding other risk factors.[229] This effect was dose-dependent.

Vegan diets

Vegetarian diets may be protective towards asthma. A study of 35 patients demonstrated significantly reduced asthma symptoms, with 71% reporting improvement at 4 months and 92% at 1 year, and reduction of asthma relieving medication on a vegan diet.[230] Part explanation for this observation may also be the increase of intake of fruits and vegetables that are known to help asthma. Patients were also drinking up to 1.5 litres of spring water instead of tap, and there is documentation of the benefits of increasing fluids.

Food allergies versus food intolerances

About 20% of people suffer food-related symptoms but true allergy occurs in about 1–3%, particularly children.[231] These symptoms may manifest in different organ systems of the body; for example, the gut, respiratory system, neurological system etc.

Food allergies are adverse reactions to food resulting from an immune-mediated response to protein in the food which are usually IgE mediated or non-IgE (cell) mediated. Reactions can be immediate, such as urticaria or bronchospasm.

Skin prick tests usually detect the presence of food-specific IgE bound to mast cells in the skin causing inflammation, wheal and flare. Serum blood levels for food-specific IgE are measured using RAST tests.[232] These tests are frequently associated with false positives.

Food intolerance is a non-immune mediated food reaction caused by an inherent characteristic of the patient e.g. lactase intolerance to milk products. Larger quantities of food may cause symptoms and is rarely life threatening.

Skin prick testing is useful to identify IgE mediated food allergies.

A trial exclusion diet carefully formulated to ensure no nutritional deficiencies are occurring may also be of help for some asthmatics to identify any possible food intolerances.[233, 234]

The commonest foods identified that can cause reactions in some asthmatics include: wheat, milk, egg, chocolate, salicylates, soy and legumes. Skin tests for food allergens do not necessarily correlate with the oral challenge results.

A study of 322 children (less than 1 year of age) with respiratory allergy placed on a 6-week hypoallergenic restrictive diet consisting of meat base formula, beef, carrots, broccoli and apricots demonstrated significant improvement in respiratory symptom scores in 91% of infants. Food challenge later reproduced symptoms in only 51% of the children. Most importantly the children were followed up for 5 years and only 6% of the children studied showed any evidence of food sensitivity suggesting 'food allergy tends to be "outgrown" '. The data suggest young infants with respiratory allergy may benefit from a hypoallergenic diet.[235]

Delayed introduction of solid foods past 4–6 months of age did not offer benefit or protection from asthma, eczema or allergic rhinitis.[236]

A randomised, cross-over, double-blind, placebo-controlled trial of 20 subjects with asthma found no statistical correlation between dairy products and bronchoconstriction and no improvement in asthma after exclusion of dairy products.[237] However, most children with known beef allergy are also likely to be allergic to cow's milk and should avoid the consumption of dairy products.[238]

Well-known foods that may cause immediate asthma reactions include wheat, milk, nuts, peanut, soy, egg, some fish and shellfish and may account for approximately 90% of food-allergic reactions in children.

Most children with known beef allergy are also likely to be allergic to cow's milk and should avoid the consumption of dairy products.

However, a randomised, cross-over, double-blind, placebo-controlled trial of 20 subjects with asthma found no statistical correlation between dairy products and bronchoconstriction and no improvement in asthma after exclusion of dairy products. There are conflicting studies in this area that require guidance from a well-trained dietician and/or allergy specialist to help identify any food sensitivities that may contribute to the development or aggravation of asthma symptoms. [239]

Wheat hypersensitivity

A review of the literature notes ingestion of wheat may contribute to food allergies demonstrated in children and is recognised as a cause for food-dependent exercise-induced anaphylaxis.[240] Inhalation of wheat flour can also cause sensitisation known as baker's asthma, an occupational respiratory allergy.

There are numerous proteins and the insoluble gliadins within wheat that have been implicated in the IgE mediated allergy reaction to ingested wheat. Diagnosis is usually based on history and skin prick testing in general is not useful.[241] Wheat allergy may manifest as a myriad of symptoms such as exercise-induced anaphylaxis, occupational asthma and rhinitis or contact urticaria.

If an infant displays respiratory symptoms or asthma during breastfeeding, it is worthwhile for the mother to trial an elimination diet as sensitisation to wheat may occur through maternal milk.[242]

Weight reduction

Obesity and high body mass index is an independent risk factor for atopy, wheeze, and cough, including in children.[243]

Weight loss advice for the obese is important. A study of 19 obese asthmatic patients who undertook a weight-loss program over 8 weeks, found that weight loss significantly improved lung function (FEV_1 and FVC), asthma symptoms, morbidity and health status.[244]

Reduction of body mass index in adult obese patients on average from 37.2 to 32.1 kg/m(2) led to a significant increase mean pulmonary function tests such as FEV_1 and FVC after weight loss.[245] Also functional residual capacity and expiratory reserve volume were significantly higher after weight loss.

A Cochrane review identified 1 trial of 38 patients suffering from chronic asthma and found significant increases in FEV_1 and FVC in the active treatment group of dietary calories restriction compared with the control group.[246] However, the reviewers concluded more studies are required before any firm conclusions can be drawn from this 1 study.

Salt reduction

High salt intake in the Western diet appears to be correlated with asthma incidence and may exacerbate pulmonary function tests in individuals with exercise-induced asthma. A study based on regional mortality data for England and Wales demonstrated a relationship between asthma mortality and regional per-person purchases of table salt for men but not for women.[247]

Increasing fluid intake and reducing salt intake may play an important role for exercise-induced asthmatics. Sodium may aggravate asthma symptoms as there appears to be a strong association between sodium dietary intake and bronchial reactivity as demonstrated with histamine challenge tests.[248, 249] There was a significant increase in bronchial-reactivity to histamine in 90% of asthmatic patients when their salt intake was increased.[247] Also, bronchial reactivity strongly correlated with 24-hour excretion of sodium and was seen as an independent risk factor even after excluding confounders for asthma such as age, family history, atopy and cigarette smoking.

A Cochrane review of the literature found low salt intake is associated with improved pulmonary function but based on the current evidence, including 6 randomised control trials (RCTs), no firm conclusions can be drawn whether salt reduction or exclusion has a place for asthma management. A low sodium diet was associated with significantly lower urine sodium excretion, and less use of reliever bronchodilator than asthmatics on normal or high salt diets.[250]

Caffeine and green tea

Caffeine and green tea intake may be useful for asthma due to their content of methylxanthine (like theophylline) a natural bronchodilator, and antioxidant properties.[251] A Cochrane review of 6 cross-over high-quality trials involving a total of 55 people found, when compared with placebo, caffeine consumption improved lung function for up to 4 hours and FEV_1 for up to 2 hours.[252] They concluded caffeine appears to 'improve airways function modestly in people with asthma for up to 4 hours'.

Honey for cough

Traditionally honey has played a very important role in the treatment of infections, for immune support and for alleviation of cough symptoms, and as well a flavouring agent.

One study aimed to test the benefits of buckwheat honey prior to bed for nocturnal cough in 105 children with upper respiratory tract infection for up to 7 days and found significant differences in symptom improvement, with honey consistently scoring best when compared with Dextromethorphan or no treatment for any outcome including better quality sleep.[253, 254] This may be clinically significant for asthmatics who commonly suffer nocturnal cough, particularly asthma following upper respiratory infections and there is a need to clinically evaluate use of honey in asthmatics.

Food additives

Symptoms related to food additives in atopic individuals appear to involve non-IgE-mediate mechanisms and are usually less severe than food intolerances.[255] Asthmatics should be advised to exclude food additives from the diet as they have the potential to trigger asthma, anaphylactic type reactions, rhinitis, urticaria and angioedema.[256] Diagnosis is usually based on a history of suspected food containing additives and confirmed by specific challenge. Examples of additives to avoid include tatrazines (jams, butters, candies, cakes), metabisulfites recognised as food additive numbers 220 to 228 (white wine, beer, dried fruit, cordial), benzoates and monosodium glutamate MSG (Chinese Restaurant Syndrome).[257, 258]

Wine sensitivity

Studies suggest that allergic reactions such as rhinitis, sneezing and cough, and acute asthmatic reactions to wine may be due to its histamine content or the sulphite additives.[259, 260] Salicylates in wines may also play a role.[261]

Toothpaste flavour

Several case reports describe exacerbation of asthma and bronchospasm in people following use of toothpastes containing additives, including peppermint, spearmint and menthol flavours.[262, 263, 264]

Nutritional medicine

Nutrients may play a complementary, therapeutic role in the management of asthma.

Vitamins

Vitamin B6 Pyridoxine

Pyridoxine is the nutrient best researched for asthma, is often low in asthmatics and may benefit asthma.[265] Double-blind studies suggest vitamin B6 (50–200mgs daily) supplementation may reduce the frequency and severity of asthma attacks, including in patients with steroid-dependent asthma,[266, 267] and lead to reduction in use of bronchodilators and cortisone.[268] However, these doses over 50mg and up to 200mg of vitamin B6 daily is quite concerning as B6 toxicity can cause peripheral neuropathy even in levels up to 50mg daily and with prolonged use in adults.[269, 270] It would be advisable to use vitamin B6 for short periods of time and combined in a multi-B supplement.

The mechanism of action of vitamin B6 in asthma benefit is not clear. Vitamin B6 is a cofactor for the synthesis of all neurotransmitters.

Nicotinic acid may be of benefit although further trials are warranted.[271, 272]

Vitamin C Ascorbic acid

There is debate about the role for vitamin C supplementation and its effect on asthma. What is more certain is that a diet low in vitamin C is a risk factor for asthma and diets high in vitamin C are associated with better pulmonary function (e.g. FEV_1 and FVC, smoking-related respiratory symptoms, reduced cough and wheeze).[273, 274, 275]

In a review of 11 studies on vitamin C, 7 studies showed significant improvement in respiratory function following supplementation with 1–2g of oral vitamin C.[276] Vitamin C is often low in smokers and is replenished with supplementation.[277]

A number of studies have demonstrated vitamin C to be useful for asthma and attenuates exercise-induced bronchoconstriction in patients with asthma.[278–281]

One trial did not show any benefit with vitamin C for asthma.[282]

While it is clear that a diet low in vitamin C is a risk factor for the development of asthma, the effects of supplementation are less certain.

A Cochrane review identified 9 studies, randomising a total of 330 participants, and noted most studies were generally poor quality with only 1 small study showing a significant reduction in FEV_1 post-exercise.[283]

They concluded, based on the data, it is insufficient to draw any firm conclusions about the benefits of vitamin C supplementation on any asthma outcome.

A meta-analyses of 7 studies, comprising 13 653 subjects, demonstrated a higher dietary intake of antioxidants (vitamin C and beta-carotene) was not associated with a lower risk of having asthma.[284]

Vitamin D

A cross-sectional survey of the 14 091 people (20 years of age or over) in the US, after adjusting for other co-factors, found on average the mean FEV_1 was 126 mL and the mean FVC was 172 mL greater for those with the highest quintile of serum 25-hydroxy vitamin D level (> or = 85.7 nmol/L) compared with the lowest quintile.[285] This suggests there is a strong relationship between serum concentrations of 25-hydroxy vitamin D, FEV_1, and FVC and further studies are warranted to determine if vitamin D supplementation is of any benefit in patients with respiratory disease.

Sunshine is the best source of vitamin D (see Chapter 30 on osteoporosis).

Minerals

Magnesium

Magnesium is known for its smooth muscle relaxant properties and research indicates valid use for acute attacks of asthma.

Oral magnesium supplements

Magnesium appears to have a bronchodilating effect due to smooth muscle relaxation. Oral magnesium supplements may be useful for asthma management.

A double-blind placebo-controlled trial of 37 patients (aged 7–19 years) were randomised to either magnesium (300mg/day) or placebo for 2 months.[286] Both patient groups received asthma inhaled fluticasone and salbutamol as needed. After 2 months of treatment, compared with the placebo group, the magnesium group demonstrated better lung function, fewer asthma attacks and used less reliever medication. The skin prick tests for recognised allergens also decreased in the magnesium group.

Oral magnesium in low doses of about 300mg per day may be of benefit in asthma management, although in some people it may cause abdominal discomfort and diarrhoea.

Intravenous (IV) magnesium therapy

Slow IV magnesium is now used in some hospital emergency departments for severe, acute asthma attacks and status asthmaticus. A number of studies demonstrate IV magnesium can help improve lung function in the acute severe asthmatic state.[287–290]

The mechanism of action for magnesium treatment in asthmatics is due to its smooth relaxant and bronchodilating properties and may also be via an anti-inflammatory effect.[291]

Serum magnesium levels need to be carefully monitored during IV infusion.

Potential side-effect is arterial hypotension during the initial high bolus due to its smooth muscle relaxant effect. Consequently, IV magnesium may cause postural hypotension and blood pressure needs to be carefully monitored during its use. This suggests IV magnesium may play a role in hypertensive crisis, although research is required to confirm this.

Thirty-eight patients suffering from acute exacerbations of moderate to severe asthma were randomised to either an intravenous infusion of saline placebo or 1.2 g of magnesium sulfate.[285]

Patients in the IV magnesium treatment group demonstrated an increase in PEFR from 225 to 297 L/min as compared with 208 to 216 L/min seen in the placebo group.

The benefits of IV magnesium sulfate appear to be more effective in the severe asthmatic. A Cochrane review of 7 trials of 665 patients found patients receiving magnesium sulfate demonstrated significant improvements in PEFRs only in those with severe acute asthma.[292] It concluded that whilst IV magnesium appears safe and well tolerated, the current evidence does not support the routine use of intravenous magnesium sulfate in all patients with acute asthma.

Another Cochrane review and systematic review of the literature concluded there is a definite role for nebulised inhaled magnesium sulfate in addition to beta2-agonist in the treatment of an acute asthma exacerbation, by improving pulmonary function in patients with severe asthma.[293, 294]

Selenium

In a double-blinded, controlled study, 24 patients with asthma were randomised to receive either placebo or 100 micrograms of sodium selenite.[295] Whilst there were no changes to the placebo group, the asthmatics in the selenium-supplemented group improved significantly.

A recent study of 197 adult asthmatic patients receiving either a high-selenium yeast preparation of selenium (100μg daily) or placebo (yeast only) for 24 weeks demonstrated whilst there was an increase in plasma selenium in the active treatment group, there was no clinical benefit for asthma symptoms except quality of life score compared with the placebo group.[296]

A Cochrane review concluded there is 'some indication that selenium supplementation may be a useful adjunct to medication for patients with chronic asthma'.[297]

Other supplements

Omega-3 fatty acids; Fish oils

A review of the literature found supporting evidence for the beneficial effects of omega-3 fatty acid supplementation for asthma- and exercise-induced bronchoconstriction due to its anti-inflammatory properties reducing airway narrowing, improving asthma symptoms and reducing medication use. Fish oil capsules containing 3.2g eicosapentaenoic acid and 2.2g docohexaenoic acid were compared with placebo capsules containing olive oil taken daily for 3 weeks.[225] The authors conclude fish oil supplements have a markedly protective effect in suppressing exercise-induced bronchoconstriction in elite athletes, attributed to their anti-inflammatory properties.

A recent study of fish oil capsules containing 3.2g of eicosapentaenoic acid and 2.0g of docohexaenoic acid or placebo capsules taken daily for 3 weeks also demonstrated marked improvement in pulmonary function, concurrent reduction in bronchodilator use, significant reduction in leukotriene B4 and increase in leukotriene B5 generation from activated polymorphonuclear leukocytes and reduced exercise-induced bronchoconstriction in asthma patients.[298] A similar study clearly demonstrated fish oils have a protective effect towards exercise-induced bronchoconstriction, particularly in elite athletes.[299]

A double-blind, controlled trial of 39 asthmatic children (aged 8–12 years) was randomised for participants to receive fish oil capsules plus canola oil and margarine (omega-3 group) or safflower oil capsules plus sunflower oil and margarine (omega-6 group) over a 6 month period.[300] Dietary enrichment of omega-3 fatty acids over 6 months increased plasma levels of nutritional markers such as fatty acids and reduced inflammatory mediators such as stimulated tumour necrosis factor (TNF) alpha production, but had no effect on the clinical severity of asthma in these children compared with baseline results.

However, a Cochrane review identified 9 randomised controlled trials, 8 of which compared fish oil supplements with placebo whilst 1 compared high-dose versus low-dose marine n-3 fatty acid supplementation, and 7 of the 9 studies were conducted in adults. The authors concluded there is 'little evidence to recommend that people with asthma supplement or modify their dietary intake of marine n-3 fatty acids (fish oil) in order to improve their asthma control'.[301]

Perilla seed oil, rich in the omega-3 fatty acids, significantly improved lung function tests (FVC and FEV) and suppressed levels of leukotriene B4 (LTB4 and LTC4) inflammatory markers generated by leucocytes compared with corn oil (rich in oimega-6 fatty acid) after 4 weeks of dietary supplementation and may be useful for asthma.[302]

Herbal medicine

Research for herbs is limited and considering their popularity of use, there is an urgent need for more research. A clinical systematic review of herbs for asthma identified 9 of the 17 trials to be reasonable, well-performed trials reporting clinically relevant improvement in lung function and/or symptom scores. Researchers concluded 'evidence promising in some cases but not yet definitive' and there is an urgent need for more research.[303]

A Cochrane review of herbal interventions for chronic asthma in adults and children identified 27 studies of 21 different herbal preparations randomising a total of 1925 participants.[304] The authors conclude that due to the diversity of trials, treatments and evidence base for the effects of herbal treatments from the available data they only provide a small insight into the long-term efficacy and harm profiles. This is understandable as it is difficult to compare 1 type of herb with another, with different study outcomes and quality of trials.

Garlic *(Allium sativum)*

Garlic was used by the ancient Egyptians, Romans and Greeks for its medicinal properties for asthma and other respiratory related problems. Both onions and garlic are well known for their anti-inflammatory action by inhibiting the lipoxygenase enzyme, and anti-infective effects.

Dried ivy leaf extract

Dried ivy leaf extract, commonly used in Europe, is known for its antispasmolytic and mucolytic effect. A systematic review of the literature identified 5 randomised controlled trials investigating the efficacy of ivy leaf extract preparations in chronic bronchitis, 3 of which were conducted in children and 1 compared ivy leaf extract cough drops to placebo, 1 compared suppositories to drops and 1 tested syrup against drops.[305] The review indicated that ivy leaf extract preparations have positive effects with respect to an improvement of respiratory functions of children with chronic bronchial asthma.

Ginkgo *biloba*

Ginkgo *biloba*, traditionally used by the Chinese for asthma, showed some benefit in a small, placebo-controlled trial of Ginkgo leaf extract.[306]

Ma Huang

Ma Huang is a herbal product derived from plants of the Ephedra species. It is a herb traditionally used by the Chinese for thousands of years for the treatment of asthma. The alkaloid compound ephedrine was derived and used in prescription medicine in the early 1900s. Ma Huang availability is now limited due to its abuse potential and its reported cases of hepatotoxicity, including a report of fulminant hepatic failure requiring liver transplant.[307, 308]

Tsumura Saiboku-To

Tsumura Saiboku-To (or TJ-96) is a mixture of Chinese/Japanese herbs (up to 10 herbs such as ginger, licorice and magnolia) traditionally used for asthma treatment and now approved by the Japanese Government as a treatment for atopic asthma. Several well-performed randomised controlled trials have showed benefit for symptomatic control of asthma when compared with placebo but, unfortunately, no lung function tests were performed other than demonstrating reduced blood and sputum eosinophil count.[309, 310, 311] Saiboku-To was noted to have 'steroid like activity' and 'inhibiting the IgE production by mite allergens'.[309] The dose used in most trials was 2.5g of TJ-96 orally 3 times daily.

Ammi visnaga (Khella)

Ammi visnaga (Khella), traditionally used by the Egyptians for thousands of years for its bronchorelaxant effect, has very little known toxicity. Disodium cromoglygate is a chemical derivative of *Ammi visnaga* and today is used as a prophylactic inhaler to stabilise mast cells.[312, 313]

Petasites hybridus

Petasites hybridus, or Butterbur, historically used by Greeks in the treatment of asthma, this herb resulted in significant improvement of FEV_1 and bronchial reactivity on methacholine challenge in a study of 70 asthma or chronic bronchitis patients.[314]

Lagundi

Lagundi is a Philippine indigenous herb, that contains a smooth muscle relaxant and antihistamine, chrysophenol D, claimed to ease bronchospasm in patients with asthma.[315]

Boswellia serrata

Boswellia serrata, or Boswellia or Frankincense, is a traditional Ayurvedic Indian gum resin, noted to have anti-inflammatory properties, useful for asthma, arthritis and other inflammatory conditions.[316, 317]

In a double-blind, placebo-controlled study, *B. serrata* significantly improved asthma symptoms, dyspnoea and wheezing and lung function tests (FEV_1, FVC, PEF), compared with the placebo group, in up to 70% of asthma sufferers over a 6-week period.[318]

Tylophora indica and Tylophora asthmatica

Tylophora indica and *Tylophora asthmatica* are Ayurvedic Indian indigenous herbs, of which the leaves were used in the treatment of atopic allergy and asthma for their bronchodilation, anti-inflammatory and mucous-reducing effects. *T. indica* has been most widely researched, including a number of double-blind studies.[319–326]

Solanum xanthocarpum and *Solanum trilobatum*

Solanum xanthocarpum (*S. xanthocarpum*) and *Solanum trilobatum* (*S. trilobatum*) are traditional Indian herbs used to treat respiratory diseases. Respiratory functions were assessed prior to, and 2 hours after, oral administration of 300mg of either *S. xanthocarpum* or *S. trilobatum*. Standard bronchodilator drugs salbutamol (4mg) and deriphylline (200mg) were used for comparison.

Coleus

Coleus, or Forskolin, isolated from the Indian plant *Coleus forskohlii,* was tested in double-blind and cross-over studies in healthy volunteers [327] and also in subjects with asthma.[328] It demonstrated bronchodilating effects equal to the effects of the pharmaceutical fenoterol.

Albizia labeck

Albizia labeck has traditionally been in use by Ayurvedic physicians for bronchial asthma and eczema.[329, 330]

Adhatoda vasica

Adhatoda vasica, or Vasicine, is an Indian herb traditionally used for respiratory conditions and is the active alkaloid extracted from vasica.[331, 332] Its properties were utilised in the development of Bisolvon, as it has bronchodilating properties and may increase ciliary movement.[333] Forty asthmatic patients were randomised to receive Bisolvon intravenously which resulted in fewer bronchial aspirations, less fluid secretions and reduction in total mucus. However, several scientific reports attribute the herb to oxytocic and abortifacient effects.[334]

Thyme extract

Thyme extract is clinically as effective in managing cough as the pharmaceutical Bisolvon. It is an effective expectorant, bronchospasmolytic and has anti-inflammatory actions.[335, 336, 337]

Common herbs used as expectorants and for their sympathomimetic effects, yet still not adequately clinically trialled, include *Lobelia* (Indian tobacco), *Euphorbia*, *Grindelia*, *Senega*, *Licorice*, *Ginseng*, *Mullein*, *Zizyphi fructusia* and *Ziziphi jujube*, *Cinnamon*, *Beupleurum*, *Ligusticum wallichii*, *Schisandra chinesis*, *Kan-Lin* preparation, ginger and *Ginkgo biloba*.[338]

Herbs causing systemic reactions and asthma

There are reported cases of systemic reactions, including asthma, to:

- oregano and thyme[339]
- occupational asthma caused by several aromatic herbs: thyme, rosemary, bay leaf, and garlic[340]
- pollen from *Euphorbia fulgens*.[341]

Homeopathy

Homeopathy involves the use of highly diluted substances, which in their undiluted form cause similar symptoms to the disease. Whilst homeopathy may be clinically effective as a placebo, little scientific evidence exists for the use of homeopathy in asthma management.

Two trials published in the *Lancet* found some benefit for homeopathy and asthma.[342, 343]

British investigators conducted a double-blind, randomised, controlled trial of homeopathic doses of HDM in 242 asthmatic adults with positive skin tests for HDM. After 4 weeks they found improvements within both groups in key outcome measures (FEV_1, quality of life and mood), but differences between groups were not statistically significant.[344]

A recent randomised placebo-controlled trial of 96 asthmatic children over 12 months demonstrated no benefits with individualised homeopathic remedies over placebo.[345]

Despite a meta-analysis in the *Lancet* suggesting a positive effect of homeopathy on asthma, a recent Cochrane review identified 6 randomised-placebo-controlled trials of 556 people and found all of variable quality and with conflicting results.[346, 347] Overall the authors concluded there is not enough reliable evidence to support the use of homeopathy for asthma. Another meta-analysis of the literature for homeopathy and asthma and rhinitis noted 'some positive results were described with homeopathy in good-quality trials in rhinitis, but a number of negative studies were also found'.[348]

A *Lancet* review of the literature identified 110 homoeopathy trials in total for various conditions and 110 matched conventional-medicine trials were analysed to compare its effectiveness. They noted biases were present in both placebo-controlled trials of both homoeopathy and conventional medicine and 'there was weak evidence for a specific effect of homoeopathic remedies'.[349] Conventional medicine was more effective.

Manual therapies

A Cochrane review identified a number of manual therapy techniques utilised by chiropractors, osteopaths and physiotherapists and concluded there is insufficient scientific evidence for manual therapies in asthma management and there is a need to conduct well-performed trials.[350]

Acupuncture

A Cochrane review of 12 studies (350 participants) of variable quality concluded there is not enough evidence to make recommendations of acupuncture treatment for chronic asthma.[351] One of the main concerns with acupuncture research is comparing real acupuncture with sham acupuncture which can cause a strong placebo response.

A study comparing the real (laser) acupuncture with placebo acupuncture for exercise-induced asthma found no differences in effects between the 2 methods.[352] Another study compared real acupuncture with sham acupuncture and a control group (no needle acupuncture) and still found no notable differences between the 3 groups.[353]

Despite the Cochrane conclusion and negative findings, a well-performed trial demonstrated real acupuncture to be superior over sham acupuncture for exercise-induced asthmatic children resulting in improved lung function tests FEV_1, FVC and PEFR following exercise when compared with sham acupuncture and the control group.[354] Interesting, sham acupuncture provided some benefit over the control group also, indicating the placebo effect may have a positive response to asthma outcome too.

Massage

Thirty-two asthmatic children of varying ages were randomly assigned to 20 minutes massage therapy by their parents before bed or relaxation therapy for 30 days.[355] In the massage therapy group, the younger children experienced immediate reduction in behavioural anxiety and cortisol levels, improved attitude towards asthma and improved respiratory function (forced expiratory flow from 25 to 75%) compared with the relaxation group.

Massage therapy may also benefit children with other respiratory diseases such as cystic fibrosis by exerting a relaxation effect.[356]

Speleotherapy for asthma

Speleotherapy, the use of subterranean environments such as staying underground (e.g. in caves and mines), is a popular therapy in Central and Eastern European countries used for the treatment of respiratory disorders such as asthma and chronic obstructive airways diseases. A Cochrane review aimed to identify trials with asthma treatment.[357] They identified 3 trials of 124 asthmatic children. Two trials reported short-term benefit of lung function with speleotherapy. The authors concluded that there is still not enough evidence to allow a reliable conclusion as to whether speleotherapy is effective for chronic asthma.

Reflexology

A 10-week study comparing active and placebo reflexology found subjective scores describing symptoms and quality of life, and also bronchial sensitivity to histamine improved in both groups. However, no differences were found between active or placebo reflexology groups.[358] Peak flow increased in asthmatics in 1 study on reflexology.[359]

Conclusion

Asthma can be managed successfully by educating the patient about the condition, and combining pharmaceutical medication with attending to environmental, behavioural and lifestyle factors that promote wellbeing. There are a number of safe complementary medicines and therapies that may be of help. While the science may not be strong for some of these, overall they are generally safe and can improve quality of life for the asthmatic patient. The evidence for lifestyle and complementary medicine and therapies are summarised in Table 5.5.

Table 5.5 Levels of evidence for lifestyle and complementary medicines/therapies in the management of asthma[360]

Modality	Level I	Level II	Level IIIa	Level IIIb	Level IIIc	Level IV	Level V
Lifestyle modification					x		
Mind–body medicine					x		
Counseling/cognitive behaviour therapy	x						
Meditation/relaxation therapy	x						
Music therapy			x				
Biofeedback	x						
Hypnosis			x				
Journal writing			x				
Environment							
Pet ownership — avoid pets	x						
House dust mite allergen reduction	x						
Bedding advice — mattress and pillow covers	x						
Immunotherapy	x						
Chemical exposure				x			
Smoking cessation					x		
Air traffic and pollution					x		
Exercise							
Muscle strength training						x	
Swimming		x					
Physical training	x						
Breathing exercises	x						
Buteyko	x						
Yoga	x						
Qigong						x	
Diet							
Weight management			x				
Vegetables and fruit			x				
Vegetarian diet			x				
Alcohol — wine			x				
Caffeine	x						
Fish intake			x				
Food intolerance — wheat sensitivity			x				
Salt reduction	x						
Food additives					x		
Wine sensitivity					x		
Physical activity	x	x					
Tai chi			x				
Qigong			x				

Continued

Table 5.5 Levels of evidence for lifestyle and complementary medicines/therapies in the management of asthma[360]—cont'd

Modality	Level I	Level II	Level IIIa	Level IIIb	Level IIIc	Level IV	Level V
Nutritional supplements							
Vitamin B6 Pyridoxine		x					
Vitamin C	x						
Magnesium — nebulised, oral, intravenous	x				x		
Vitamin D	x						
Selenium	x						
Fish oils	x						
Herbal medicines							
Garlic							x
Dried ivy leaf extract							x
Ginkgo					x		
Ma Huang					x		
Tsumura Saiboku-To or TJ-96					x		
Ammi visnaga (Khella)					x		
Petasites hybridus or Butterbur		x					
Lagundi is a Philippine indigenous herb							x
Boswellia serrata		x					
Tylophora indica and *Tylophora asthmatica*	x						
Coleus		x					
Albizia						x	
Thyme extract		x					
Chinese herbal medicine					x		
Japanese herbal medicine TJ	x						
Homoeopathy	x						
Physical therapies							
Chiropractic		x					
Massage		x					
Acupuncture		x					
Reflexology					x		

Level I — from a systematic review of all relevant randomised controlled trials, meta–analyses.
Level II — from at least 1 properly designed randomised controlled clinical trial.
Level IIIa — from well-designed pseudo-randomised controlled trials (alternate allocation or some other method).
Level IIIb — from comparative studies (including systematic reviews of such studies) with concurrent controls and allocation not randomised, cohort studies, case-control studies, or interrupted time series with a parallel control group.
Level IIIc — from comparative studies with historical control, 2 or more single-arm studies or interrupted time series without a parallel control group.
Level IV — opinions of respected authorities based on clinical experience, descriptive studies or reports of expert committees.
Level V — represents minimal evidence that represents testimonials.

Clinical tips handout for patients — asthma

1 Lifestyle advice

Sleep

- Restore normal sleep patterns. Most adults require about 7 hours sleep. (See Chapter 22 for more advice.)

Sunshine

- Amount of exposure varies with local climate.
- At least 15 minutes of sunshine needed daily for vitamin D and melatonin production — especially before 10 a.m. and after 3 p.m. when the sun exposure is safest during summer; much more exposure in winter when supplementation needs to be considered.
- Ensure gradual adequate skin exposure to sun; avoid sunscreen and excess clothing to maximise levels of vitamin D.
- More time in the sun is required for dark skinned people.
- Direct exposure to about 10% of body (hands, arms, face), without sunscreen and not through glass.
- Vitamin D is obtained in the diet from fatty fish, eggs, liver and fortified foods (some milks and margarines); it is unlikely that adequate vitamin D concentrations can be obtained from diet alone.

2 Physical activity/exercise

- Exercise for 30 minutes or more daily. Swimming is ideal for asthma, although best in non-chlorinated pools (e.g. ozone-treated pools).
- If exercise is not regular, commence with 5 minutes daily and slowly build up to at least 30 minutes. Outdoor exercise with nature, fresh air and sunshine is ideal (e.g. brisk walking, light jogging, cycling, stretching).
- Physical training and weight-bearing exercises or resistance exercise are beneficial.
- Outdoors — the more time you spend outdoors the better, especially in tree-lined streets. Avoid traffic pollution — this can aggravate asthma.
- Yoga may be particularly helpful; other examples: qi qong, tai chi.
- Alexander technique — a physical therapy involving a series of movements designed to correct posture and bring the body into natural alignment.

3 Mind–body medicine

- Stress management program; for example, initially 6 x 40 minute sessions for patients: to understand the nature of their symptoms, the symptoms' relationship to stress and the practice of regular relaxation exercises.
- Regular meditation practice at least 10-20 minutes daily.

Breathing

- Be aware of breathing from time to time. Notice if tendency to hold breath or over-breathe. Always aim to relax the breath and the muscles around the chest wall.
- Breathing exercises are extremely helpful for asthma; see http://www.asthmacrc.org.au/ for free instructions.
- Buteyko breathing can be helpful for asthma.

Rest and stress management

Relaxation therapy is particularly helpful. Recurrent stress may cause a return of symptoms. Relaxation is important for a full and lasting recovery.

- Reduce workload and resolve conflicts. Contact family, friends, church, social or other groups for support.
- Listening to relaxation music and daily baths can help.
- Meditation is helpful.
- Music therapy is helpful; listen to calming music once daily.
- Massage therapy — massage children 20 minutes every night before bed.
- Hypnotherapy and biofeedback may be particularly helpful.
- Reflexology may help.

Cognitive behaviour therapy, counselling and psychotherapy

- These therapies and counselling are extremely helpful.

Fun

- Laughter can trigger asthma. This may mean asthma needs better control. It is important to have fun in life. Joy can be found even in the simplest tasks, such as being with friends with a sense of humour, funny movies/videos, comedy, hobbies, dancing, playing with pets and children.

4 Environment

- Pollution is linked to asthma; avoid living/exercising near busy roads or near traffic.
- Spend more time in nature.
- Do not smoke.

- A change of weather may impact on asthma. Triggers of asthma include: changes in temperature; cold windy days; hot humid days; poor air quality.
- Walk in parks, but avoid trekking at high altitude.
- Ensure office or home has a view overlooking garden or park.

Precautions

- Avoid smoking, environmental pollutants, traffic, wood smoke, chemicals — at work and in the home.
- Stay indoors during thunderstorms.
- Avoid artificial sweeteners, food additives, chemicals in foods.

Simple measures for reducing triggers/ environmental allergens

Simple measures for reducing triggers/environmental allergens
Put toys away in cupboards
Wipe surfaces with damp cloth weekly
Steam clean carpets bi-annually; in-built vacuum cleaner
Damp mop hard floorboards
Laundry washing of bedding — add a few drops of Eucalyptus oil to wash
Place bedding in dryer and tumble dry for 15 minutes weekly
Use natural bedding (e.g. feathered or cotton pillows and doonas)
Avoid synthetic bedding
Avoid old cot mattresses for newborns
Dust mite covers for bedding — mattresses and pillow Use mattress covers such as semipermeable polyurethane mattress and pillow encasings (allergy control)
Avoid damp houses and mould
Allow sun into house and air house regularly — daily if possible
Avoid smoking inside house or, better still, do not smoke
Avoid pets in the house; dogs may protect against asthma in some children
Occupational asthma is not uncommon: avoid household cleaning sprays, wood dust, chemicals, paint fumes, solvents, latex and wheat flour

Allergen immunotherapy also known as 'desensitisation' can occur by injection or sublingual. This should be done under medical supervision — see National Asthma Council website,

Asthma Information Brochures for consumers:

http://www.nationalasthma.org.au/html/-management/infopapers/consumer/1002.asp#asthma

5 Dietary changes

- Maintain a healthy weight. Being overweight can aggravate asthma.
- Eat more fruit and vegetables — both a variety of colours and those in season.
- Eat at least 5 different vegetables and 1–2 fruit (apples especially) daily.
- Avoid cold foods from the fridge (e.g. ice-cream, cold milk).
- Speak with your practitioner/dietician to exclude any food intolerances, especially to wheat, milk, nuts, peanut, soy, egg, some fish and shellfish, salicylates.
- Increase deep sea fish up to 3 times weekly — canned fish is okay (mackerel, salmon, sardines, cod, tuna, salmon).
- Reduce red meat intake (preferably use red lean meat e.g. lamb, kangaroo) and white meat (e.g. free-range organic chicken).
- Use cold pressed olive oil and avocado.
- Low GI wholegrains/cereals (variety): rice (brown, Basmati, Mahatmi, Doongara), traditional rolled oats, buckwheat flour, wholegrain organic breads (rye bread, essene, spelt, kamut), brown pasta, millet, amaranth etc.
- Reduce dairy intake; low fat dairy products such as yoghurt and occasionally cheeses, such as Greek or Bulgarian fetta made from sheep or goats milk, unless there is a dairy intolerance.
- Drink more water: 1–2 litres a day, and teas (e.g. especially organic green tea; black tea) plus vegetable juices. Black tea and coffee can help asthma.
- Avoid *high* doses of caffeine — can cause restlessness and agitation.
- One teaspoon of honey in tea can help night cough from viral infections.
- For newborns, breastfeeding is best; avoid medication during early infancy unless absolutely necessary.
- In pregnancy, foods rich in Vitamin E (e.g. vegetable oils, nuts, sunflower seeds and green leafy vegetables) may help prevent asthma in the newborn.

Precautions

- Salt — this can aggravate asthma.
- Hydrogenated fats, salt, fast foods, added sugar such as in soft drinks, lollies, biscuits, cakes and processed foods e.g. white bread, white pasta, pastries.
- Minimise alcohol intake. Avoid white wine.
- Avoid chemical additives — preservatives, colouring and flavouring.
- For sweetener try honey (e.g. yellow box and stringy bark have lowest GI).

6 Physical therapies

- Acupuncture may help.
- Speleotherapy (e.g. sitting in cave or mine) may help — this is common in Eastern Europe.

7 Supplements

Vitamin Bs, especially B6

- Indication: vitamin B6 may help asthma.
- Dosage: upper level of intake of vitamin B6 should not exceed 50mg/day. Do not take vitamin B6 alone; use a multi-B vitamin that contains vitamin B6.
- Results: uncertain.
- Side-effects: avoid overuse of single vitamin products (e.g. oral and injectable forms of vitamin B6) or concomitant use of multivitamin products could result in some patients routinely exceeding the upper limit for vitamins associated with severe toxicity. Toxicity in high doses of vitamin B6 includes peripheral neuropathy, such as tingling, burning and numbness of limbs.
- Contraindications: avoid in anemias until assessed by a doctor.

Vitamin C

- Indication: may help asthma although dietary sources are preferred.
- Dosage: 500–1000mg daily or as tolerated.
- Results: unknown.
- Side-effects: with high doses can cause nausea, heartburn, abdominal cramps and diarrhoea.
- Contraindications: can increase iron absorption. Use with caution if glucose-6-phosphate dehydrogenase deficiency.

Note: Vitamin C and Vitamin E are best given together.

Vitamin D3 (cholecalciferol 1000 international units)

Doctors should check blood levels and suggest supplementation if levels are low.

Vitamin D3 (cholecalciferol)

- Indication: may help asthma if levels are low.
- Dosage: adult: 1000IU daily; your doctor should check your blood levels to determine correct dosage to avoid toxicity.
- Results: uncertain.
- Side-effects: very mild and rare; nausea, vomiting, diarrhoea, sensitivity reactions.
- Contraindications: avoid if you suffer high calcium levels, systemic lupus erythematosis, sarcoidosis, hyperparathyroidism as these conditions can impact on calcium levels; pharmaceutical medication such as lipid-lowering drugs, calcium channel blockers for hypertension.

Selenium (sodium selenite, organic selenium found in yeast)

- Indication: may help asthma.
- Dosage: 50–100mcg daily; do not exceed >600 microgram daily (health professional supervision required to avoid toxicity).
- Results: uncertain.
- Side-effects: very mild and rare; nausea, vomiting, rash, sensitivity reactions, toxicity in high doses; nail changes, irritability, fatigue.
- Contraindications: pregnancy, lactation, children <12 years of age; avoid yeast derived selenium if allergic to yeast.

Magnesium and calcium (best provided together)

- Indication: magnesium relaxes bronchial airways, muscle relaxant.
- Dosage: children, 65–120mg daily in divided doses; adults, 350mg daily including pregnant and lactating women.
- Results: 2–3 days.
- Side-effects: oral magnesium especially at a dose greater than 400mg daily can cause gastrointestinal irritation, nausea, vomiting and diarrhoea. The dosage varies from person to person. Although rare, toxic levels can cause low blood pressure, thirst, heart arrhythmia, drowsiness and weakness.
- Contraindications: patients with kidney disease and heart block.

Fish oils

- Indication: may help inflammation, bronchospasm, asthma.

- Dosage: 3–7g daily as tolerated. If consuming fish 2–3 times a week, a 1000mg capsule per day may be sufficient.
- Results: 4–7 days.
- Side-effects: often well tolerated especially if taken with meals. Very mild and rare side-effects; for example, gastrointestinal upset; allergic reactions (e.g. rash, breathing problems if allergic to seafood); blood thinning effects in very high doses > 10g daily (may need to stop fish oil supplements 2 weeks prior to surgery).
- Contraindications: sensitivity reaction to seafood; drug interactions; caution when taking high doses of fish oils >4g per day together with warfarin (your doctor will check your INR test).

Herbs

Some may be effective but need to be dispensed by a trained herbalist. Herbs that may be useful for asthma include:

- Dried ivy leaf extract
- *Ginkgo biloba*
- Ma Huang a Chinese herb
- Tsumura Saiboku-To or TJ-96 is a mixture of Chinese/Japanese herbs (up to 10 herbs such as ginger, licorice and magnolia)
- *Boswellia serrata* or Boswellia or Frankincense is a traditional Ayurvedic Indian gum resin
- *Tylophora indica* and *Tylophora asthmatica* are Ayurvedic Indian indigenous herbs
- Coleus or Forskolin isolated from the Indian plant *Coleus forskohlii*
- Thyme extract.

Note: homeopathy may be effective.

References

1 Asthma Management Handbook. National Asthma Council. Online. Available: http://www.nationalasthma.org.au/cms/index.php?option=com_content&task=view&id=49&Itemid=29 (accessed 7April 2009) Content created 16 November 2006. Last updated 1 June 2007.

2 National Asthma Council. Asthma Information Brochures for Consumers. Online. Available: http://www.nationalasthma.org.au/html/management/infopapers/consumer/1002.asp#asthma (accessed 7 April 2009).

3 Guidelines for the Diagnosis and Management of Asthma. National Heart, Lung, and Blood Institute. Bethesda, Maryland, USA, 1997.

4 National Asthma Council website. Available: http://www.nationalasthma.org.au/html/management/infopapers/health_professionals/1002.asp#facts (accessed 7 April 2009).

5 (a) Determinants of bronchial responsiveness in the European Community Respiratory Health Survey in Italy: evidence of an independent role of atopy, total serum IgE levels, and asthma symptoms. Allergy. 1998 Jul;53(7):673–81.[No authors listed] PMID:9700036.
(b) ACAM 2008. Asthma in Australia 2008. Cat. no. ACM 14.AiHW. Online. Available: www.asthmamonitoring.org. (accessed Jan 2010).

6 Macan J, Varnai VM, Maloča I, et. al. Increasing trend in atopy markers prevalence in a Croatian adult population between 1985 and 1999. Clinical & Experimental Allergy Dec 2007;37(12):1756–63.

7 Blanc PD, Ware GK, Katz PP, et. al. Use of herbal products, coffee or black tea, and over-the-counter medications as self-treatments among adults with asthma. J. Allergy Clin. Immunol 1997;100:789–91.

8 Blanc PD, Trupin L, Earnest G, et. al. Alternative Therapies Among Adults with a Reported Diagnosis of Asthma or Rhinosinusitis: Data from a Population-Based Survey. Chest 2000;120:1461–7.

9 Andrews L, Lokuge S, Sawyer M, et. al. The use of alternative therapies by children with asthma: A brief report. J Paediatrics Child Health 1998;34(2):131–34.

10 Shenfield G, Lim E, Allen H. Survey of the use of complementary medicines and therapies in children with asthma. J Paediatrics Child Health 2002;38(3):252–7.

11 Mazur LJ, De Ybarrondo L, Miller J, et. al. Use of alternative and complementary therapies for pediatric asthma. Tex Med 2001;97:64–8.

12 Ernst E. Use of Complementary therapies in childhood asthma. Pediatric Asthma, Allergy and Immunology 1998;12:29–32.

13 Janson C, Chinn S, Jarvis D, et. al. Physician-diagnosed asthma and drug utilization in the European Community Respiratory Health Survey. Eur Respir J 1997;10:1795–1802.

14 Andrews L, Lokuge S, Sawyer M, et. al. The use of alternative therapies by children with asthma: A brief report. J Paediatrics Child Health 1998;34:131–4.

15 Ernst E. Complementary Therapies for Asthma: What Patients Use. J Asthma 1998;35:667–71.

16 Pachter LM, Cloutier MM, Bernstein BA. Ethnomedical (folk) remedies for childhood asthma in a mainland Puerto Rican community. Archives of Pediatric and Adolescent Medicine 1995;149:982–8.

17 Mazur LJ, De-Ybarrondo L, Miller J, et. al. Use of alternative and complementary therapies for pediatric asthma. Texas-medicine 2001 Jun;97(6):64–8.

18 Slader CA, Reddel HK, Jenkins CR, et. al. Complementary and alternative medicine use in asthma: who is using what? Respirology 2006 Jul;11(4):373–87.

19 Ernst E. Complementary therapies in asthma: what patients use. Journal of Asthma, 1999;36:667–71.

20 Adams SK, Murdock KK, McQuaid EL. Complementary and alternative medication (CAM) use and asthma outcomes in children: an urban perspective. J Asthma 2007 Nov;44(9):775–82.

21 Blanc PD, Trupin L, Earnest G, et. al. Alternative therapies among adults with a reported diagnosis of asthma or rhinosinusitis: data from a population-based survey. Chest 2001 Nov;120(5):1461–7.

22 Blanc PD, Kuschner WG, Katz PP, et. al. Use of herbal products, coffee or black tea, and over-the-counter medications as self-treatments among adults with asthma. J Allergy Clin Immunol 1997 Dec;100(6 Pt 1):789–91.

23 Passalacqua G, Bousquet PJ, Carlsen K-H, et. al. ARIA update: I—Systematic review of complementary and alternative medicine for rhinitis and asthma. J Allergy Clin Immunol 2006;117:1054–62.
24 Marks G, Cohen M, Kotsirilos V, et. al. Asthma and complementary therapies. A guide for health professionals. National Asthma Council Australia. Online. Available: http://www.nationalasthma.org.au/content/view/54/112/ (accessed 8 June 2009).
25 Adams RJ, Smith BJ, Ruffin RE. Impact of the physician's participatory style in asthma outcomes and patient satisfaction. Ann Allergy Asthma Immunol 2001 Mar;86(3):263–71.
26 Weinmayr G, Weiland SK, Björkstén B, et. al. ISAAC Phase Two Study Group. Atopic sensitization and the international variation of asthma symptom prevalence in children. Am J Respir Crit Care Med 2007 Sep 15;176(6):565–74.
27 Wang H-Y, Wong GWK, Chen Y-Z, et. al. Prevalence of asthma among Chinese adolescents living in Canada and in China. CMAJ 2008;179(11). doi:10.1503/cmaj.071797.
28 Gibson PG, Henry RL, Shah S, et. al. Migration to a western country increases asthma symptoms but not eosinophilic airway inflammation. Pediatr Pulmonol 2003 Sep;36(3):209–15.
29 Golan Y, Onn A, Villa Y, et. al. Asthma in adventure travelers: a prospective study evaluating the occurrence and risk factors for acute exacerbations. Arch Intern Med 2002 Nov 25;162(21):2421–6.
30 Hegewald MJ, Crapo RO. Socioeconomic status and lung function. Chest 2007 Nov;132(5):1608–14. Online. Available: http://www.chestjournal.org/cgi/content/abstract/132/5/1608 (accessed 8 June 2009).
31 Haby MM, Peat JK, Marks GB, et. al. Asthma in preschool children: prevalence and risk factors. Thorax 2001 Aug;56(8):589–95.
32 Abramson M, Kutin JJ, Raven J, et. al. Risk factors for asthma among young adults in Melbourne, Australia. Respirology 1996 Dec;1(4):291–7.
33 Halken S. Prevention of allergic disease in childhood: clinical and epidemiological aspects of primary and secondary allergy prevention. Pediatr Allergy Immunol. 2004 June;15(16 suppl.):4–5, 9–32.
34 Roduit C, Scholtens S, de Jongste JC, et. al. Asthma at 8 years of age in children born by caesarean section. Thorax 2009 Feb;64(2):107–13.
35 Gdalevich M, Mimouni D, Mimouni M. Breast-feeding and the risk of bronchial asthma in childhood: a systematic review with meta-analysis of prospective studies. J Pediatr 2001 Aug;139(2):261–6.
36 Peat JK, Allen J, Oddy W, et. al. Breastfeeding and asthma: Appraising the controversy. Pediatr Pulmonol 2003 May;35(5):331–4.
37 Oddy WH. Breastfeeding and asthma in children. A prospective cohort study. Adv Exp Med Biol 2000;478:393–4.
38 Oddy WH, de Klerk NH, Sly PD, et. al. The effects of respiratory infections, atopy, and breastfeeding on childhood asthma. Eur Respir J 2002 May;19(5):899–905.
39 Oddy WH. Breastfeeding and asthma in children: findings from a West Australian study. Breastfeed Rev 2000 Mar;8(1):5–11.
40 Dell S, To T. Breastfeeding and asthma in young children: findings from a population-based study. Arch Pediatr Adolesc Med 2001 Nov;155(11):1261–5.
41 Oddy WH, Holt PG, Sly PD, et. al. Association between breastfeeding and asthma in 6 year old children: findings of a prospective birth cohort study. BMJ 1999 Sep 25;319(7213):815–9.
42 Wright AL, Holberg CJ, Taussig LM, et. al. Factors influencing the relation of infant feeding to asthma and recurrent wheeze in childhood. Thorax 2001 Mar;56(3):192–7.
43 Kramer MS, Matush L, Vanilovich I, et. al. for the Promotion of Breastfeeding Intervention Trial (PROBIT) Study Group. Effect of prolonged and exclusive breastfeeding on risk of allergy and asthma: cluster randomised trial. BMJ 2007;335:815 (20 October).
44 Hoppu U, Kalliomäki M, Isolauri E. Maternal diet rich in saturated fat during breastfeeding is associated with atopic sensitization of the infant. Eur J Clin Nutr 2000 Sep;54(9):702–5.
45 Goldman AS. Association of atopic diseases with breast-feeding: Food allergens, fatty acids, and evolution. The Journal of Pediatrics 1999;134(1):5–7.
46 Grönlund MM, Gueimonde M, Laitinen K, et. al. Maternal breast-milk and intestinal bifidobacteria guide the compositional development of the Bifidobacterium microbiota in infants at risk of allergic disease. Clinical & Experimental Allergy, 2007;37(12):1764–72.
47 Celedón JC, Litonjua AA, Ryan L, et. al. Bottle feeding in the bed or crib before sleep time and wheezing in early childhood. Pediatrics 2002 Dec;110(6):e77.
48 Wickens K, Pearce N, Crane J, et. al. Antibiotic use in early childhood and the development of asthma. Clinical & Experimental Allergy, 1999;29(6):766–71.
49 Ball TM, Castro-Rodriguez JA, Griffith KA, et. al. Siblings, day-care attendance, and the risk of asthma and wheezing during childhood. N Engl J Med 2000 Aug 24;343(8):538–43.
50 Mitchell EA, Robinson E, Black PN, et. al. Risk factors for asthma at 3.5 and 7 years of age. Clinical & Experimental Allergy 2007;37(12):1747–55.
51 Kozyrskyj AL, Ernst P, Becker AB. Increased risk of childhood asthma from antibiotic use in early life. Chest 2007 Jun;131(6):1753–9.
52 Haby MM, Marks GB, Peat JK, et. al. Day-care attendance before the age of two protects against atopy in preschool age children. Pediatr Pulmonol 2000 Nov;30(5):377–84. PMID:11064428.
53 Krämer U, Heinrich J, Wjst M, et. al. Age of entry to day nursery and allergy in later childhood. Lancet 1999 Feb 6;353(9151):450–4.
54 Kusel MMH, de Klerk N, Holt PG, et. al. Clinical & Experimental Allergy 2008;(38):1921–8.
55 Wickens K, Ingham T, Epton M, et. al. The association of early life exposure to antibiotics and the development of asthma, eczema and atopy in a birth cohort: confounding or causality? Clin Exp Allergy 2008;38:1318–24.
56 Beasley R, Clayton T, Crane J, et. al. ISAAC Phase Three Study Group. Association between paracetamol use in infancy and childhood, and risk of asthma, rhinoconjunctivitis, and eczema in children aged 6–7 years: analysis from Phase Three of the ISAAC program. Lancet 2008 Sep 20;372(9643):1039–48.
57 Shaheen SO, Newson RB, Henderson AJ, et. al. ALSPAC Study Team. Prenatal paracetamol exposure and risk of asthma and elevated immunoglobulin E in childhood. Clin Exp Allergy 2005;35(1):18–25.

58 Macsali F, Real FG, Omenaas ER, et. al. Oral contraception, body mass index, and asthma: a cross-sectional Nordic-Baltic population survey. J Allergy Clin Immunol 2009 Feb;123(2):391–7.

59 Figueroa-Muñoz JI, Chinn S, Rona RJ. Association between obesity and asthma in 4–11 year old children in the UK. Thorax 2001 Feb;56(2):133–7.

60 Visness CM, London SJ, Daniels JL, et. al. Association of obesity with IgE levels and allergy symptoms in children and adolescents: Results from the National Health and Nutrition Examination Survey 2005–2006. J Allergy and Clin Immunol 2009 Feb 20.

61 Ochs-Balcom HM, Grant BJ, Muti P, et. al. Pulmonary function and abdominal adiposity in the general population. Chest 2006 Apr;129(4): 853–62.

62 Verhulst SL, Schrauwen N, Haentjens D, et. al. Sleep-disordered breathing: a new risk factor of suspected fatty liver disease in overweight children and adolescents? European Respiratory Review, 2008;17:99–100.

63 Oddy WH, Sherriff JL, de Klerk NH, et. al. The relation of breastfeeding and body mass index to asthma and atopy in children: a prospective cohort study to age 6 years. Am J Public Health 2004 Sep;94(9):1531–7.

64 Kozyrskyj AL, Mai XM, McGrath P, et. al. Continued exposure to maternal distress in early life is associated with an increased risk of childhood asthma. Am J Respir Crit Care Med 2008 Jan 15;177(2):142–7.

65 Cookson H, Granell R, Joinson C, et. al. Mothers' anxiety during pregnancy is associated with asthma in their children. J Allergy Clin Immunol 2009 Apr;123(4):847–53.e11

66 Sandberg S, Paton JY, Ahola S, et. al. The role of acute and chronic stress in asthma attacks in children. Lancet 2000 Dec 2;356(9245):1932.

67 Sandberg S, Järvenpää S, Penttinen A, et. al. Asthma exacerbations in children immediately following stressful life events: a Cox's hierarchical regression. Thorax 2004 Dec;59(12):1046–51. Erratum in: Thorax 2005 Mar;60(3):261. PMID:15563703.

68 Sandberg S, McCann DC, Ahola S, et. al. Positive experiences and the relationship between stress and asthma in children. Acta Paediatr 2002;91(2):152–8. PMID:11952001.

69 Goodwin RD, Fischer FE, Goldberg JA Twin study of post-traumatic stress disorder symptoms and asthma. Am J Respir Crit Care Med 2007 Nov 15;176(10):983–7.

70 Lehrer PM, Sargunaraj D, Hochron S. Psychological approaches to the treatment of asthma. J Consult Clin Psychol 1992 Aug;60(4):639–43.

71 Yorke J, Fleming SL, Shuldham CM. Psychological interventions for adults with asthma. Cochrane Database of Systematic Reviews 2006, Issue 1. Art No:CD002982. doi:10.1002/14651858.CD002982.pub3.

72 Yorke J, Fleming S, Shuldham C. Psychological interventions for children with asthma. Cochrane Database of Systematic Reviews 2005, Issue 4. Art No:CD003272. doi:10.1002/14651858.CD003272.pub2.

73 Cleland JA, Price DB, Lee AJ, et. al. A pragmatic, three-arm randomised controlled trial of spiritual healing for asthma in primary care. Br J Gen Pract 2006 Jun;56(527):444–9.

74 Mrazek DA. Psychiatric complications of pediatric asthma. Ann Allergy 1992 Oct;69(4):285–90.

75 Ettinger A, Reed M, Cramer J. Epilepsy Impact Project Group. Depression and comorbidity in community-based patients with epilepsy or asthma. Neurology 2004 Sep 28;63(6):1008–14. PubMed PMID:15452291.

76 Mrazek DA, Schuman WB, Klinnert M. Early asthma onset: risk of emotional and behavioral difficulties. J Child Psychol Psychiatry 1998 Feb;39(2):247–54. PMID:9669237.

77 Katon W, Lozano P, Russo J, et. al. The prevalence of DSM-IV anxiety and depressive disorders in youth with asthma compared with controls. J Adolesc Health 2007 Nov;41(5):455–63.

78 Goldney RD, Ruffin R, Fisher LJ, et. al. Asthma symptoms associated with depression and lower quality of life: a population survey. Med J Aust 2003 May 5;178(9):437–41.

79 Strunk RC, Mrazek DA, Fuhrmann GS, et. al. Physiologic and psychological characteristics associated with deaths due to asthma in childhood. A case-controlled study. JAMA 1985 Sep 6;254(9):1193–8.

80 Kern-Buell CL, McGrady AV, Conran PB, et. al. Asthma severity, psychophysiological indicators of arousal, and immune function in asthma patients undergoing biofeedback-assisted relaxation. Appl Psychophysiol Biofeedback 2000 Jun;25(2):79–91.

81 Meuret AE, Wilhelm FH, Roth WT. Respiratory biofeedback-assisted therapy in panic disorder. Behav Modif 2001 Sep;25(4):584–605. PMID:11530717.

82 Noeker M, von Rüden U, Staab D, et. al. Processes of body perception and their therapeutic use in pediatrics. From nonspecific relaxation therapy to training to recognize disease-specific symptoms. Klin Padiatr 2000 Sep–Oct;212(5):260–5. Review. German. PMID:11048285.

83 Klinnert MD, Kaugars AS, Strand M, et. al. Family psychological factors in relation to children's asthma status and behavioral adjustment at age 4. Fam Process 2008 Mar;47(1):41–61. PMID:18411829.

84 Miller BD, Wood BL. Emotions and family factors in childhood asthma: psychobiologic mechanisms and pathways of effect. Adv Psychosom Med 2003;24:131–60. Review. PMID:14584352.

85 Klinnert MD, Nelson HS, Price MR, et. al. Onset and persistence of childhood asthma: predictors from infancy. Pediatrics 2001 Oct;108(4):E69. PMID:11581477.

86 Mojtabai R. Parental psychopathology and childhood atopic disorders in the community. Psychosom Med 2005 May–Jun;67(3):448–53.

87 Mrazek DA, Klinnert MD, Mrazek P, et. al. Early asthma onset: consideration of parenting issues. J Am Acad Child Adolesc Psychiatry 1991 Mar;30(2): 277–82.

88 Mrazek D. Psychiatric complications of paediatric asthma. Annals of Allergy 1992;69:285–90.

89 Klinnert MD, Mrazek PJ, Mrazek DA. Early asthma onset: the interaction between family stressors and adaptive parenting. Psychiatry 1994 Feb;57(1): 51–61.

90 Rietveld S, Everaerd W, Creer TL. Stress-induced asthma: a review of research and potential mechanisms. Clin Exp Allergy 2000 Aug;30(8): 1058–66. Review PMID:10931112.

91 Wilson AF, Honsberger R, Chiu JT, et. al. Transcendental meditation and asthma. Respiration 1975;32(1):74–80.

92 Huntley A, White AR, Ernst E. Relaxation therapies for asthma: a systematic review. Thorax 2002 Feb;57(2):127–31.

93 Lehrer PM, Hochron SM, Mayne T, et. al. Relaxation and music therapies for asthma among patients prestabilized on asthma medication. Journal of Behavioral Medicine 1994;17(1):1–24.
94 Carr RE. Panic disorder and asthma: causes, effects and research implications. J Psychosom Res 1998 Jan;44(1):43–52. Review Panic disorder and asthma: causes, effects and research implications. PMID:9483463.
95 Creer TL. Emotions and asthma. J Asthma 1993;30(1):1–3.
96 Lehrer PM, Isenberg S, Hochron SM. Asthma and emotion: a review. J Asthma 1993;30(1):5–21. Review. PMID:8428858.
97 Lehrer PM. Emotionally triggered asthma: a review of research literature and some hypotheses for self-regulation therapies. Appl Psychophysiol Biofeedback 1998 Mar;23(1):13–41.
98 Kern-Buell CL, McGrady AV, Conran PB, et. al. Asthma severity, psychophysiological indicators of arousal, and immune function in asthma patients undergoing biofeedback-assisted relaxation. Appl Psychophysiol Biofeedback 2000 Jun;25(2):79–91. PMID:10932333.
99 Kotses H, Glaus KD. Applications of biofeedback to the treatment of asthma: a critical review. Biofeedback Self Regul 1981 Dec;6(4):573–93. Applications of biofeedback to the treatment of asthma: a critical review. PMID:7034795.
100 Peper E, Tibbetts V. Fifteen-month follow-up with asthmatics utilizing EMG/incentive inspirometer feedback. Biofeedback Self Regul 1992 Jun;17(2):143–51.
101 Jahanshahi M, Sartory G, Marsden CD. EMG biofeedback treatment of torticollis: a controlled outcome study. Biofeedback Self Regul 1991 Dec;16(4):413–48. PMID:1760462.
102 Gallego J, Perez de la Søta A, Vardon G, et. al. Electromyographic feedback for learning to activate thoracic inspiratory muscles. Am J Phys Med Rehabil 1991 Aug;70(4):186–90. PMID:1878176.
103 Ewer TC, Stewart DE. Improvement in bronchial hyper-responsiveness in patients with moderate asthma after treatment with a hypnotic technique: a randomised controlled trial. Br Med J (Clin Res Ed) 1986 Nov 1;293(6555):1129–32.
104 Morrison JB. Chronic asthma and improvement with relaxation induced by hypnotherapy. J R Soc Med 1988 December; 81(12): 701–4.
105 Smyth J, Stone AA, Hurewitz A, et. al. Effects of writing about stressful experiences on symptom reduction in patients with asthma or rheumatoid arthritis: a randomised trial. JAMA 1999;281(14):1304–9.
106 Harris AH, Thoresen CE, Humphreys K, et. al. Does writing affect asthma? A randomized trial. Psychosom Med 2005 Jan–Feb;67(1):130–6.
107 Liangas G, Morton JR, Henry RL. Mirth-triggered asthma: is laughter really the best medicine? Pediatr Pulmonol 2003 Aug;36(2):107–12.
108 Svanes C, Heinrich J, Jarvis D, et. al. Pet-keeping in childhood and adult asthma and hay fever: European community respiratory health survey. J Allergy Clin Immunol 2003 Aug;112(2):289–300.
109 Simpson A, Custovic A. Early pet exposure: friend or foe? Current Opinion in Allergy and Clinical Immunology 2003,3:7–14.
110 Apelberg BJ, Aoki Y, Jaakkola JJK. Systematic review: exposure to pets and risk of asthma and asthma-like symptoms. J Allergy Clin Immunol 2001;107:455–60.
111 Svanes C, Heinrich J, Jarvis D, et. al. Pet-keeping in childhood and adult asthma and hay fever: European community respiratory health survey. J Allergy Clin Immunol 2003 Aug;112(2):289–300.
112 Lau S, Wahn U. Pets—good or bad for individuals with atopic predisposition? J Allergy Clin Immunol 2003 Aug;112(2):263–4.
113 Gern JE, Reardon CL, Hoffjan S, et. al. Effects of dog ownership and genotype on immune development and atopy in infancy. J Allergy Clin Immunol 2004 Feb;113(2):307–14.
114 Marks GB. What should we tell allergic families about pets? J Allergy Clin Immunol 2001;108:500–2.
115 Apter AJ. Early exposure to allergen: Is this the cat's meow or are we barking up the wrong tree. J Allergy Clin Immunol 2003;111:938–46.
116 Bufford JD, Reardon CL, Li Z, et. al. Effects of dog ownership in early childhood on immune development and atopic diseases. Clin Exp Allergy. 2008 Oct;38(10):1635–43.
117 Duelien Skorge T, Eagan TML, Eide GE, et. al. Indoor exposures and respiratory symptoms in a Norwegian community sample. Thorax 2005;60:937–42.
118 Girgis ST, Marks GB, Downs SH, et. al. Thunderstorm-associated asthma in an inland town in south-eastern Australia. Who is at risk? Eur Respir J 2000 Jul;16(1):3–8.
119 Wark PA, Simpson J, Hensley MJ, et. al. Airway inflammation in thunderstorm asthma. Clin Exp Allergy 2002 Dec;32(12):1750–6.
120 D'Amato G, Liccardi G, Frenguelli G. Thunderstorm-asthma and pollen allergy. Allergy. 2007 Jan;62(1):11–6.
121 Douwes J, Cheng S, Travier N, et. al. Eur Respir J 2008 Sep;32(3):603–11.
122 Crisafulli D, Almqvist C, Marks G, et. al. Seasonal trends in house dust mite allergen in children's beds over a 7-year period Allergy 2007 Dec;62(12):1394–400.
123 Lau S, Illi S, Sommerfeld C, et. al. Early exposure to house-dust mite and cat allergens and development of childhood asthma: a cohort study. Multicentre Allergy Study Group. Lancet 2000 Oct 21;356(9239):1392–7.
124 Nicolai T, Illi S, von Mutius E. Effect of dampness at home in childhood on bronchial hyperreactivity in adolescence. Thorax 1998 Dec;53(12):1035–40.
125 Mihrshahi S, Marks GB, Criss S, et. al. CAPS Team. Effectiveness of an intervention to reduce house dust mite allergen levels in children's beds. Allergy. 2003 Aug;58(8):784–9.
126 Tsitoura S, Nestoridou K, Botis P, et. al. Randomized trial to prevent sensitization to mite allergens in toddlers and preschoolers by allergen reduction and education: one-year results. Arch Pediatr Adolesc Med 2002 Oct;156(10):1021–7.
127 van Strien RT, Koopman LP, Kerkhof M, et. al. Prevention and Incidence of Asthma and Mite Allergy Study Mattress encasings and mite allergen levels in the Prevention and Incidence of Asthma and Mite Allergy study. Clin Exp Allergy 2003 Apr;33(4):490–5.
128 Lau S, Illi S, Sommerfeld C, et. al. Early exposure to house-dust mite and cat allergens and development of childhood asthma: a cohort study. Multicentre Allergy Study Group. Lancet 2000 Oct 21;356(9239):1392–7. PubMed PMID:11052581.
129 Halken S. Prevention of allergic disease in childhood: clinical and epidemiological aspects of primary and secondary allergy prevention. Pediatr Allergy Immunol. 2004 Jun;15(suppl.):16:4–5, 9–32.

130 Ponsonby AL, Dwyer T, Kemp A, et. al. Synthetic bedding and wheeze in childhood. Epidemiology. 2003 Jan;14(1):37–44.
131 Synthetic pillows and wheezing in childhood. Child Health Alert. 2003 Feb;21:2 (no authors listed).
132 Ponsonby AL, Gatenby P, Glasgow N, et. al. The association between synthetic bedding and adverse respiratory outcomes among skin-prick test positive and skin-prick test negative children. Allergy 2002 Mar;57(3):247–53.
133 Ponsonby AL, Dwyer T, Trevillian L, et. al. The bedding environment, sleep position, and frequent wheeze in childhood. Pediatrics 2004 May;113(5):1216–22.
134 Ponsonby AL, Kemp A, Dwyer T, et. al. Feather bedding and house dust mite sensitization and airway disease in childhood. J Clin Epidemiol 2002 Jun;55(6):556–62.
135 Strachan D, Carey IM. Reduced risk of wheezing in children using feather pillows is confirmed. BMJ 1997 Feb 15;314(7079):518.
136 Rains N, Siebers R, Crane J, et. al. House dust mite allergen (Der p 1) accumulation on new synthetic and feather pillows. Clin Exp Allergy 1999 Feb;29(2):182–5.
137 Crane J, Kemp T, Siebers R, et. al. Increased house dust mite allergen in synthetic pillows may explain increased wheezing. BMJ 1997 Jun 14;314(7096):1763–4.
138 Mills S, Siebers R, Wickens K, et. al. House dust mite allergen levels in individual bedding components in New Zealand. NZ Med J. 2002 Apr 12;115(1151):151–3.
139 Kemp TJ, Siebers RW, Fishwick D, et. al. House dust mite allergen in pillows. BMJ 1996 Oct 12;313(7062):916.
140 Tovey ER, Taylor DJ, Mitakakis TZ, et. al. Effectiveness of laundry washing agents and conditions in the removal of cat and dust mite allergen from bedding dust. J Allergy Clin Immunol 2001 Sep;108(3):369–74.
141 Gøtzsche PC, Johansen HK. House dust mite control measures for asthma. Cochrane Database of Systematic Reviews 2008, Issue 2. Art. No: CD001187. doi: 10.1002/14651858.CD001187.pub3.
142 McAvoy BR. Cochrane PEARLS (Practical Evidence About Real Life Situations). No. 80, August 2008.
143 Becker A, Watson W, Ferguson A, et. al. The Canadian asthma primary prevention study: outcomes at 2 years of age. Allergy Clin Immunol 2004 Apr;113(4):650–6.
144 National Asthma Council website. Available: http://www.nationalasthma.org.au/html/management/infopapers/health_professionals/1010.asp (accessed 7 April 2009).
145 Abramson MJ, Puy RM, Weiner JM. Allergen immunotherapy for asthma. Cochrane Database of Systematic Reviews 2003, Issue 4. Art No: CD001186. doi: 10.1002/14651858.CD001186.
146 Penagos M, Passalacqua G, Compalati E, et. al. Metaanalysis of the Efficacy of Sublingual Immunotherapy in the Treatment of Allergic Asthma in Pediatric Patients, 3 to 18 Years of Age. Chest 2008; 133:599–609.
147 Bufe A, Eberle P, Franke-Beckmann E, et. al. Safety and efficacy in children of an SQ-standardized grass allergen tablet for sublingual immunotherapy. Journal of Allergy and Clinical Immunology 2009;123(1):167–173.e7.
148 Nicolai T, Illi S, von Mutius E. Effect of dampness at home in childhood on bronchial hyperreactivity in adolescence. Thorax 1998 Dec;53(12):1035–40.
149 Pekkanen J, Hyvärinen A, Haverinen-Shaughnessy U, et. al. Moisture damage and childhood asthma: a population-based incident case–control study. Eur Respir J March 2007; 29:509–15 (doi:10.1183/09031936.00040806).
150 Australian Government. Australian Institute of Health and Welfare (AIHW). Bulletin 59; April 2008 Occupational Asthma in Australia http://www.aihw.gov.au/publications/index.cfm/title/10328 (accessed Jan 2010)
151 Kogevinas M, Antó JM, Sunyer J, et. al. Occupational asthma in Europe and other industrialised areas: a population-based study. European Community Respiratory Health Survey Study Group. Lancet 1999 May 22;353(9166):1750–4.
152 Kogevinas M, Zock JP, Jarvis D, et. al. Exposure to substances in the workplace and new-onset asthma: an international prospective population-based study (ECRHS-II). Lancet 2007 Jul 28;370(9584):336–41.
153 Monsó E, Magarolas R, Badorrey I, et. al. Occupational asthma in greenhouse flower and ornamental plant growers. Am J Respir Crit Care Med 2002 Apr 1;165(7):954–60.
154 Medina-Ramón M, Zock JP, Kogevinas M, et. al. Asthma symptoms in women employed in domestic cleaning: a community based study. Thorax 2003 Nov;58(11):950–4.
155 Jaakkola JJ, Jaakkola MS. Professional cleaning and asthma. Curr Opin Allergy Clin Immunol 2006 Apr;6(2):85–90.
156 Zock JP, Plana E, Jarvis D, et. al. The use of household cleaning sprays and adult asthma: an international longitudinal study. Am J Respir Crit Care Med 2007 Oct 15;176(8):735–41.
157 Medina-Ramón M, Zock JP, Kogevinas M, et. al. Asthma symptoms in women employed in domestic cleaning: a community based study. Thorax 2003 Nov;58(11):950–4.
158 Belousova EG, Toelle BG, Xuan W, et. al. The effect of parental smoking on presence of wheez or airway hyper-responsiveness in New South Wales school children. Aust N Z J Med 1999 Dec;29(6):794–800.
159 Chen E, Schreier HM, Strunk RC, et. al. Chronic traffic-related air pollution and stress interact to predict biologic and clinical outcomes in asthma. Environ Health Perspect 2008 Jul;116(7):970–5. PMID:18629323.
160 MacNeill SJ, Goddard F, Pitman R, et. al. The Oxford Transport Strategy: impact of a traffic intervention on PEF and wheeze among children. European Respiratory Review June 1 2008;17: 88–9.
161 McCreanor J, Cullinan P, Nieuwenhuijsen MJ, et. al. Respiratory Effects of Exposure to Diesel Traffic in Persons with Asthma. N Engl J Med 2007 December 6;357:2348–58.
162 Diaz-Sanchez D, Proietti L, Polosa R. Diesel fumes and the rising prevalence of atopy: an urban legend? Curr Allergy Asthma Rep. 2003 Mar;3(2):146–52.
163 Morgenstern V, Zutavern A, Cyrys J, et. al for the GINI Study Group and the LISA Study Group. Atopic diseases, allergic sensitization, and exposure to traffic-related air pollution in children. Am J of Respiratory and Critical Care Medicine 2008;177:1331–7.
164 Boezen HM, van der Zee SC, Postma DS, et. al. Effects of ambient air pollution on upper and lower respiratory symptoms and peak expiratory flow in children. Lancet 1999 Mar 13;353(9156):874–8.

165 Bartra J, Mullol J, del Cuvillo A, et. al. Air pollution and allergens. J Investig Allergol Clin Immunol. 2007;17(suppl.):2:3–8.
166 Wayne P, Foster S, Connolly J, et. al. Production of allergenic pollen by ragweed (Ambrosia artemisiifolia L.) is increased in CO2–enriched atmospheres. Ann Allergy Asthma Immunol 2002 Mar;88(3):279–82.
167 Downs SH, Schindler C, Liu S, et. al. Reduced Exposure to PM10 and Attenuated Age-Related Decline in Lung Function. NEJM 2007;357:2338–47.
168 Lovasi GS, Quinn JW, Neckerman KM, et. al. Children living in areas with more street trees have lower prevalence of asthma. J Epidemiol Community Health 2008 Jul;62(7):647–9.
169 Lau S, Nickel R, Niggemann B, et. al; MAS Group. The development of childhood asthma: lessons from the German Multicentre Allergy Study (MAS). Paediatr Respir Rev 2002 Sep;3(3):265–72.
170 Sharma HP, Hansel NN, Matsui E, et. al. Indoor environmental influences on children's asthma. Pediatr Clin North Am 2007 Feb;54(1):103–20, ix.
171 Howden-Chapman P, Pierse N, Nicholls S, et. al. Effects of improved home heating on asthma in community dwelling children: randomised controlled trial. BMJ 2008;337:a1411.
172 Diette GB, Hansel NN, Buckley TJ, et. al. Home indoor pollutant exposures among inner-city children with and without asthma. Environ Health Perspect. 2007 Nov;115(11):1665–9.
173 Thomson H, Petticrew M, Morrison D. Health effects of housing improvement: systematic review of intervention studies. BMJ 2008;337:a1411.
174 Roberts G, Golder N, Lack G. Bronchial challenges with aerosolized food in asthmatic, food-allergic children. Allergy 2002 Aug;57(8):713–7.
175 Epton MJ, Dawson RD, Brooks WM, et. al. The effect of ambient air pollution on respiratory health of school children: a panel study. Environmental Health 2008; 7: 16.
176 Howden-Chapman P, Pierse N, Nicholls S, et. al. Effects of improved home heating on asthma in community dwelling children: randomised controlled trial. BMJ 2008;337:a1411.
177 Bernard A, Nickmilder M, Voisin C. Outdoor swimming pools and the risks of asthma and allergies during adolescence. Eur Respir J 2008; 32:979–88.
178 Thickett KM, McCoach JS, Gerber JM, et. al. Occupational asthma caused by chloramines in indoor swimming-pool air. Eur Respir J 2002 May;19(5):827–32. PMID:12030720.
179 Eggleston PA. Chlorinated pools and the risk of asthma. Environ Health Perspect 2007 May;115(5):A240; author reply A240–1. Chlorinated pools and the risk of asthma. PMID:17520032.
180 Carraro S, Pasquale MF, Da Frè M, et. al. Swimming pool attendance and exhaled nitric oxide in children. J Allergy Clin Immunol 2006 Oct;118(4):958–60.
181 Bernard A. Chlorination products: emerging links with allergic diseases. Curr Med Chem 2007;14(16):1771–82. Review. Chlorination products: emerging links with allergic diseases. PMID:17627515.
182 Nemery B, Hoet PH, Nowak D. Indoor swimming pools, water chlorination and respiratory health. Eur Respir J 2002 May;19(5):790–3.
183 Lucas SR, Platts-Mills TA. Physical activity and exercise in asthma: relevance to etiology and treatment. J Allergy Clin Immunol 2005 May;115(5):928–34. Review. Erratum in: J Allergy Clin Immunol 2005 Aug;116(2):298.
184 Golan Y, Onn A, Villa Y, et. al. Asthma in adventure travellers: a prospective study evaluating the occurrence and risk factors for acute exacerbations. Arch Intern Med 2002 Nov 25;162(21):2421–6.
185 Matsumoto I, Araki H, Tsuda K, et. al. Effects of swimming training on aerobic capacity and exercise-induced bronchoconstriction in children with bronchial asthma. Thorax 1999 Mar;54(3): 196–201.
186 Manocha R, Marks GB, Kenchington P, et. al. Sahaja yoga in the management of moderate to severe asthma: a randomised controlled trial. Thorax 2002 Feb;57(2):110–5.
187 Vedanthan PK, Kesavalu LN, Murthy KC, et. al. Clinical study of yoga techniques in university students with asthma: a controlled study. Allergy Asthma Proc 1998 Jan-Feb;19(1):3–9.
188 Nagarathna R, Nagendra HR. Yoga for bronchial asthma: a controlled study. Br Med J (Clin Res Ed) 1985 Oct 19;291(6502):1077–9.
189 Nagendra HR, Nagarathna R. An integrated approach of yoga therapy for bronchial asthma: a 3–54–month prospective study. J Asthma 1986;23(3):123–37.
190 Singh V, Wisniewski A, Britton J, Tattersfield A. Effect of yoga breathing exercises (pranayama) on airway reactivity in subjects with asthma. Lancet 1990 Jun 9;335(8702):1381–3.
191 Jain SC, Talukdar B. Evaluation of yoga therapy program for patients of bronchial asthma. Singapore Med J 1993 Aug;34(4):306–8.
192 Sabina AB, Williams AL, Wall HK, et. al. Yoga intervention for adults with mild-to-moderate asthma: a pilot study. Ann Allergy Asthma Immunol 2005 May;94(5):543–8.
193 Reuther I. Aldridge D. Qigong Yangsheng as a complementary therapy in the management of asthma: a single-case appraisal. Journal of Alternative & Complementary Medicine. 998;4(2):173–83.
194 Dennis J, Cates CJ. Alexander technique for chronic asthma. Cochrane Database of Systematic Reviews 2000, Issue 2. Art No: CD000995. doi: 10.1002/14651858.CD000995.
195 Thomas M, McKinley RK, Freeman E, et. al. The prevalence of dysfunctional breathing in adults in the community with and without asthma. Prim Care Respir J 2005 Apr;14(2):78–82.
196 Stanton AE, Vaughn P, Carter R, et. al. An observational investigation of dysfunctional breathing and breathing control therapy in a problem asthma clinic. J Asthma 2008 Nov;45(9):758–65.
197 Keeley D, Osman L. Dysfunctional breathing and asthma. It is important to tell the difference. BMJ 2001 May 5;322(7294):1075–6.
198 Thomas M, McKinley RK, Freeman E, et. al. Prevalence of dysfunctional breathing in patients treated for asthma in primary care: cross sectional survey. BMJ 2001 May 5;322(7294):1098–100.
199 Thomas M, McKinley RK, Freeman E, et. al. Prevalence of dysfunctional breathing in patients treated for asthma in primary care: cross sectional survey. BMJ 2001 May 5;322(7294):1098–100.
200 Bidat E, Sznajder M, Fermanian C, et. al. A diagnostic questionnaire for the hyperventilation syndrome in children. Rev Mal Respir 2008 Sep;25(7):829–38. French.
201 Thomas M, McKinley RK, Freeman E, et. al. Prevalence of dysfunctional breathing in patients treated for asthma in primary care: cross sectional survey. BMJ 2001 May 5;322(7294):1098–100.

202 Keeley D, Osman L. Dysfunctional breathing and asthma. It is important to tell the difference. BMJ 2001 May 5;322(7294):1075–6.
203 Slader CA, Reddel HK, Spencer LM, et. al. Double-blind randomised controlled trial of two different breathing techniques in the management of asthma. Thorax 2006; 61: 651–6.
204 Thomas M, McKinley RK, Mellor S, et. al. Breathing exercises for asthma: a randomised controlled trial. Thorax 2009 Jan;64(1):55–61.
205 Holloway EA, West RJ. Integrated breathing and relaxation training (the Papworth method) for adults with asthma in primary care: a randomised controlled trial. Thorax 2007;62:1039–42 Dec 2007.
206 Holloway E, Ram FSF. Breathing exercises for asthma. Cochrane Database of Systematic Reviews 2004, Issue 1. Art No: CD001277. doi: 10.1002/14651858.CD001277.pub2.
207 Weiner P. Azgad Y. Ganam R. Weiner M. Inspiratory muscle training in patients with bronchial asthma. Chest 1992;102(5):1357–61.
208 Weiner P, Azgad Y, Ganam R. Inspiratory muscle training for bronchial asthma. Harefuah 1992 Feb 2;122(3):155–9. Hebrew. PMID:1563665.
209 de Jong W, van Aalderen WM, Kraan J, et. al. Inspiratory muscle training in patients with cystic fibrosis. Respir Med 2001 Jan;95(1):31–6. PMID:11207014.
210 Thomas M, McKinley RK, Freeman E, et. al. Breathing retraining for dysfunctional breathing in asthma: a randomised controlled trial. Thorax 2003 Feb;58(2):110–5.
211 Bowler SD, Green A, Mitchell CA. buteyko breathing techniques in asthma: a blinded randomised controlled trial. Med J Aust 1998 Dec 7–21;169(11–12):575–8.
212 Opat AJ, Cohen MM, Bailey MJ, et. al. A clinical trial of the buteyko Breathing Technique in asthma as taught by a video. J Asthma 2000;37(7):557–64.
213 Cooper S, Oborne J, Newton S, et. al. Effect of two breathing exercises (buteyko and pranayama) in asthma: a randomised controlled trial. Thorax. 2003 Aug;58(8):674–9.
214 McHugh P, Aitcheson F, Duncan B, et. al. buteyko Breathing Technique for asthma: an effective intervention. N Z Med J 2003 Dec 12;116(1187):U710.
215 McGowan J. Health Education in Asthma Management. Does 'The buteyko Institute of Method' make a difference? Thorax Medical Journal 2003;58(III).
216 Devereux G, Turner SW, Craig LC, et. al. Low maternal vitamin E intake during pregnancy is associated with asthma in 5–year-old children.Am J Respir Crit Care Med 2006 Sep 1;174(5):499–507.
217 Heinrich J, Hölscher B, Bolte G, et. al. Allergic sensitization and diet: ecological analysis in selected European cities. Eur Respir J 2001 Mar;17(3):395–402.
218 Chatzi L, Apostolaki G, Bibakis I, et. al. Protective effect of fruits, vegetables and the Mediterranean diet on asthma and allergies among children in Crete. Thorax 2007;62:677–83.
219 Forastiere F, Pistelli R, Sestini P, et. al. Consumption of fresh fruit rich in vitamin C and wheezing symptoms in children. SIDRIA Collaborative Group, Italy (Italian Studies on Respiratory Disorders in Children and the Environment. Thorax 2000 Apr;55(4):283–8.
220 Cook DG, Carey IM, Whincup PH, et. al. Effect of fresh fruit consumption on lung function and wheeze in children. Thorax 1997 Jul;52(7):628–33.
221 Forastiere F, Pistelli R, Sestini P, et. al. Consumption of fresh fruit rich in vitamin C and wheezing symptoms in children. SIDRIA Collaborative Group, Italy (Italian Studies on Respiratory Disorders in Children and the Environment). Thorax 2000 Apr;55(4):283–8.
222 Butland BK, Fehily AM, Elwood PC. Diet, lung function, and lung function decline in a cohort of 2512 middle aged men. Thorax 2000 Feb;55(2):102–8.
223 Butler LM, Koh WP, Lee HP, et. al. Dietary fiber and reduced cough with phlegm: a cohort study in Singapore. Am J Respir Crit Care Med. 2004 Aug 1;170(3):279–87.
224 Chatzi L, Torrent M, Romieu I, et. al. Diet, wheeze, and atopy in school children in Menorca, Spain. Pediatric Allergy Immunol 2007: 18: 480–5.
225 Mickleborough TD, Rundell KW. Dietary polyunsaturated fatty acids in asthma- and exercise-induced bronchoconstriction. Eur J Clin Nutr 2005 Dec;59(12):1335–46.
226 Hodge L, Salome CM, Peat JK, et. al. Consumption of oily fish and childhood asthma risk. Medical Journal of Australia 1996;164(3):137–40.
227 Broughton KS, Johnson CS, Pace BK, et. al. Reduced asthma symptoms with n-3 fatty acid ingestion are related to 5–series leukotriene production. Am J Clin Nutr 1997 Apr;65(4):1011–7.
228 Laerum BN, Wentzel-Larsen T, Gulsvik A, et. al. Relationship of fish and cod oil intake with adult asthma. Clinical & Experimental Allergy 2007 Nov;37(11):1616–23. doi: 10.1111/j.1365-2222.2007.02821.x.
229 Wickens K, Barry D, Friezema A, et. al. Fast foods — are they a risk factor for asthma? Allergy. 2005 Dec;60(12):1537–41.
230 Lindahl O, Lindwall L, Spångberg A, et. al. Vegan regimen with reduced medication in the treatment of bronchial asthma. J Asthma 1985;22(1):45–55.
231 Rona RJ, Keil T, Summers C, et. al. The prevalence of food allergy: a metaanalysis. J Allergy Clin Immunol 2007;120:638–46.
232 Ostblom E, Lilja G, Ahlstedt S, et. al. Patterns of quantitative food-specific IgE-antibodies and reported food hypersensitivity in 4–year-old children. Allergy 2008 Apr;63(4):418–24.
233 Bock SA. Food-related asthma and basic nutrition. J Asthma 1983;20(5):377–81.
234 Oehling A. Importance of food allergy in childhood asthma. Allergol Immunopathol (Madr) 1981;(suppl.):9:71–3.
235 Ogle KA, Bullock JD. Children with allergic rhinitis and/or bronchial asthma treated with elimination diet: a five-year follow-up. Ann Allergy 1980 May;44(5):273.
236 Zutavern A, Brockow I, Schaaf B, et. al. LISA Study Group. Timing of solid food introduction in relation to eczema, asthma, allergic rhinitis, and food and inhalant sensitization at the age of 6 years: results from the prospective birth cohort study LISA. Pediatrics 2008 Jan;121(1):e44–e52.
237 Woods RK, Weiner JM, Abramson M, et. al. Do dairy products induce bronchoconstriction in adults with asthma? J Allergy Clin Immunol 1998 Jan;101(1 Pt 1):45–50.
238 Martelli A, De Chiara A, Corvo M, et. al. Beef allergy in children with cow's milk allergy; cow's milk allergy in children with beef allergy. Ann Allergy Asthma Immunol. 2002 Dec;89(6) (suppl.1):38–43.

239 Perry CA, Dwyer J, Gelfand JA, et. al. Health effects of salicylates in foods and drugs. Nutr Rev 1996;54(8):225–40.
240 Palosuo K. Current Opinion in Allergy and Clinical Immunology 2003, 3:205–9.
241 Majamaa H, Moisio P, Holm K, et. al. Wheat allergy: diagnostic accuracy of skin prick and patch tests and specific IgE. Allergy 1999;54:851–6.
242 Linna O. Specific IgE antibodies to uningested cereals. Allergy 1996;51:849–50.
243 Schachter LM, Peat JK, Salome CM. Asthma and atopy in overweight children. Thorax 2003 Dec;58(12):1031–5.
244 Stenius-Aarniala B, Poussa T, Kvarnström J, et. al. Immediate and long term effects of weight reduction in obese people with asthma: randomised controlled study. BMJ 2000 Mar 25;320(7238):827–32.
245 Hakala K, Stenius-Aarniala B, Sovijärvi A. Effects of weight loss on peak flow variability, airways obstruction, and lung volumes in obese patients with asthma. Chest 2000 Nov;118(5):1315–21.
246 Cheng J, Pan T. Calorie controlled diet for chronic asthma. Cochrane Database of Systematic Reviews 2003, Issue 2. Art No: CD004674. doi: 10.1002/14651858.CD004674.pub2.
247 Burney PG, Neild JE, Twort CH, et. al. Effect of changing dietary sodium on the airway response to histamine. Thorax 1989 Jan;44(1):36–41.
248 Burney PG, Britton JR, Chinn S, et. al. Response to inhaled histamine and 24 hour sodium excretion. Br Med J (Clin Res Ed) 1986 Jun 7;292(6534):1483–6.
249 Javaid A, Cushley MJ, Bone MF. Effect of dietary salt on bronchial reactivity to histamine in asthma. BMJ 1988 August 13;297:454.
250 Ardern K. Dietary salt reduction or exclusion for allergic asthma. Cochrane Database of Systematic Reviews 2004, Issue 2. Art No: CD000436. doi: 10.1002/14651858.CD000436.pub2.
251 Blanc PD, Ware GK, Katz PP, et. al. Use of herbal products, coffee or black tea, and over-the-counter medications as self-treatments among adults with asthma. J Allergy Clin Immunol 1997;100:789–91.
252 Bara A, Barley E. Caffeine for asthma. Cochrane Database of Systematic Reviews 2001, Issue 4. Art No: CD001112. doi: 10.1002/14651858.CD001112.
253 Paul IM, Beiler J, McMonagle A, et. al. Effect of Honey, Dextromethorphan, and No Treatment on Nocturnal Cough and Sleep Quality for Coughing Children and Their Parents. Arch Pediatr Adolesc Med 2007;161(12):1140–6.
254 Warren MD, Pont SJ, Barkin SL, et. al. The effect of honey on nocturnal cough and sleep quality for children and their parents. Arch Pediatr Adolesc Med 2007 Dec;161(12):1149–53.
255 Cardinale F, Mangini F, Berardi M, et. al. Intolerance to food additives: an update [Article in Italian]. Minerva Pediatr 2008 Dec;60(6):1401–9.
256 Tarlo SM, Sussman GL. Asthma and anaphylactoid reactions to food additives. Can Fam Physician 1993 May;39:1119–23.
257 Freedman BJ. A dietary free from additives in the management of allergic disease. Clin Allergy 1977 Sep;7(5):417–21.
258 Stevenson DD, Simon RA. Sensitivity to ingested metabisulfites in asthmatic subjects. J Allergy Clin Immunol 1981 Jul;68(1):26–32.
259 Vally H, Thompson PJ. Allergic and asthmatic reactions to alcoholic drinks. Addict Biol 2003 Mar;8(1):3–11.
260 Vally H, Thompson PJ. Role of sulfite additives in wine induced asthma: single dose and cumulative dose studies. Thorax 2001 Oct;56(10):763–9.
261 Vally H, de Klerk N, Thompson PJ. Alcoholic drinks: important triggers for asthma. J Allergy Clin Immunol 2000 Mar;105(3):462–7.
262 Subiza J, Subiza JL, Valdivieso R, et. al. Toothpaste flavor-induced asthma. J Allergy Clin Immunol 1992 Dec;90(6 Pt 1):1004–6.
263 Spurlock BW, Dailey TM. Shortness of (fresh) breath--toothpaste-induced bronchospasm. N Engl J Med. 1990 Dec 27;323(26):1845–6.
264 Baer PN. Toothpaste allergies. J Clin Pediatr Dent 1992 Spring;16(3):230–1.
265 Reynolds RD, Natta CL. Depressed plasma pyridoxal phosphate concentrations in adult asthmatics. Am J Clin Nutr 1985 Apr;41(4):684–8.
266 Kaslow JE. Double-blind trial of pyridoxine (vitamin B6) in the treatment of steroid-dependent asthma. Ann Allergy 1993 Nov;71(5):492. PubMed PMID:8250357.
267 Sur S, Camara M, Buchmeier A, et. al. Double-blind trial of pyridoxine (vitamin B6) in the treatment of steroid-dependent asthma. Ann Allergy 1993 Feb;70(2):147–52. PubMed PMID:8430923.
268 Collipp PJ, Goldzier S III, Weiss N, et. al. Pyridoxine treatment of childhood bronchial asthma. Ann Allergy 1975 Aug;35(2):93–7.
269 Renwick AG. Toxicology of micronutrients: Adverse effects and uncertainty. J. Nutr 2006; 136: 493S–501S.
270 Australian Adverse Drug Reactions Bulletin. Therapeutic Goods Administration 2008 August;27;(4).
271 Maisel FE, Somkin E. Treatment of asthmatic paroxysm with nicotinic acid. J Allergy 13:397–403, 1942.
272 Melton G. Treatment of asthma by nicotinic acid. BMJ 1943, May 15:600–01.
273 Omenaas E, Fluge O, Buist AS, et. al. Dietary vitamin C intake is inversely related to cough and wheeze in young smokers. Respir Med 2003 Feb;97(2):134–42.
274 Grievink L, Smit HA, Ocké MC, et. al. Dietary intake of antioxidant (pro)-vitamins, respiratory symptoms and pulmonary function: the MORGEN study. Thorax 1998 Mar;53(3):166–71.
275 Britton JR, Pavord ID, Richards KA, et. al. Dietary antioxidant vitamin intake and lung function in the general population. Am J Respir Crit Care Med 1995 May;151(5):1383–7.
276 Hatch GE. Asthma, Inhaled Oxidants and Dietary Antioxidants. American Journal of Clinical Nutrition 1995 Mar;61(3)(suppl.):625s–30s.
277 Lykkesfeldt J, Christen S, Wallock LM, et. al. Ascorbate is depleted by smoking and repleted by moderate supplementation: a study in male smokers and non-smokers with matched dietary antioxidant intakes. Am J Clin Nutr 2000 Feb;71(2):530–6.
278 Bucca C, Rolla G, Oliva A, 13. Effect of vitamin C on histamine bronchial responsiveness of patients with allergic rhinitis. Ann Allergy 1990;65:311–14.
279 Anah CO, Jarike LN, Baig HA. High dose ascorbic acid in Nigerian asthmatics. Tropical Geograph. Med 1980;32:132–7.
280 Schachter EN, Schlesinger A. The attenuation of exercise-induced bronchospasm by ascorbic acid. Ann Allergy 1982 Sep;49(3):146–51.
281 Tecklenburg SL, Mickleborough TD, Fly AD, et. al. Ascorbic acid supplementation attenuates exercise-induced bronchoconstriction in patients with asthma. Respir Med 2007 Aug;101(8):1770–8.

282 Malo JL, Cartier A, Pineau L, et. al. Lack of acute effects of ascorbic acid on spirometry and airway responsiveness to histamine in subjects with asthma. J Allergy Clin Immunol 1986;78(6):11532–58.
283 Kaur B, Rowe BH, Arnold E. Vitamin C supplementation for asthma. Cochrane Database of Systematic Reviews 2009, Issue 1. Art No: CD000993. doi:10.1002/14651858.CD000993. pub3.
284 Gao J, Gao X, Li W, et. al. Observational studies on the effect of dietary antioxidants on asthma: a meta-analysis. Respirology 2008 Jun;13(4):528–36.
285 Black PN, Scragg R. Relationship between serum 25–hydroxyvitamin d and pulmonary function in the third national health and nutrition examination survey Chest. 2005 Dec;128(6):3792–8.
286 Gontijo-Amaral C, Ribeiro MA, Gontijo LS, et. al. Oral magnesium supplementation in asthmatic children: a double-blind randomized placebo-controlled trial. Eur J Clin Nutr. 2007 Jan;61(1):54–60.
287 Skobeloff EM, Spivey WH, McNamara RM, Greenspon L. Intravenous magnesium sulfate for the treatment of acute asthma in the emergency department. JAMA 1989 Sep 1;262(9):1210–3.
288 Brunner EH, Delabroise AM, Haddad ZH. Effect of parenteral magnesium on pulmonary function, plasma cAMP, and histamine in bronchial asthma. J Asthma 1985;22(1):3–11.
289 Sydow M, Crozier TA, Zielmann S, et. al. High-dose intravenous magnesium sulfate in the management of life-threatening status asthmaticus. Intensive Care Med 1993;19(8):467–71.
290 Silverman RA, Osborn H, Runge J, et. al. Acute Asthma/Magnesium Study Group. IV magnesium sulfate in the treatment of acute severe asthma: a multicenter randomized controlled trial. Chest 2002 Aug;122(2):489–97.
291 Cairns CB, Kraft M. Magnesium attenuates the neutrophil respiratory burst in adult asthmatic patients. Acad Emerg Med 1996 Dec;3(12):1093–7.
292 Rowe BH, Bretzlaff JA, Bourdon C, et. al. Magnesium sulfate for treating exacerbations of acute asthma in the emergency department. Cochrane Database Syst Rev 2000;(2):CD001490.
293 Blitz M, Blitz S, Beasely R, et. al. Inhaled magnesium sulfate in the treatment of acute asthma. Cochrane Database Syst Rev 2005 Oct 19;(4):CD003898.
294 Blitz M, Blitz S, Hughes R, et. al. Aerosolized magnesium sulfate for acute asthma: a systematic review. Chest 2005 Jul;128(1):337–44.
295 Hasselmark L, Malmgren R, Zetterström O, et. al. Selenium supplementation in intrinsic asthma. Allergy 1993;48:30–6.
296 Shaheen SO, Newson RB, Rayman MP, et. al. Randomised, double-blind, placebo-controlled trial of selenium supplementation in adult asthma. Thorax 2007;62:483–90 June 2007.
297 Allam MF, Lucena RA. Selenium supplementation for asthma. Cochrane Database of Systematic Reviews 2004, Issue 2. Art No: CD003538. doi: 10.1002/14651858.CD003538.
298 Mickleborough TD, Lindley MR, Ionescu AA, et. al. Protective effect of fish oil supplementation on exercise-induced bronchoconstriction in asthma. Chest 2006 Jan;129(1):39–49.
299 Mickleborough TD, Murray RL, Ionescu AA, et. al. Fish oil supplementation reduces severity of exercise-induced bronchoconstriction in elite athletes. Am J Respir Crit Care Med 2003 Nov 15;168(10):1181–9.
300 Hodge L, Salome CM, Hughes JM, et. al. Effect of dietary intake of omega-3 and omega-6 fatty acids on severity of asthma in children. Eur Respir J 1998 Feb;11(2):361–5.
301 Thien FCK, De Luca S, Woods R, et. al. Dietary marine fatty acids (fish oil) for asthma in adults and children. Cochrane Database of Systematic Reviews 2002, Issue 2. Art No: CD001283. doi: 10.1002/14651858.CD001283.
302 Okamoto M, Mitsunobu F, Ashida K, et. al. Effects of dietary supplementation with n-3 fatty acids compared with n-6 fatty acids on bronchial asthma. Intern Med. 2000 Feb;39(2):107–11.
303 Huntley A, Ernst E. Herbal medicines for asthma: a systematic review. Thorax 2000 Nov;55(11):925–9.
304 Arnold E, Clark CE, Lasserson TJ, et. al. Herbal interventions for chronic asthma in adults and children. Cochrane Database of Systematic Reviews 2008, Issue 1. Art No: CD005989. doi: 10.1002/14651858.CD005989.pub2.
305 Hofmann D, Hecker M, Völp A. Efficacy of dry extract of ivy leaves in children with bronchial asthma-a review of randomized controlled trials. Phytomedicine. 2003 Mar;10(2–3):213–20.
306 Li M, Yang B, Yu H, Zhang H. Clinical observation of the therapeutic effect of ginkgo leaf concentrated oral liquor on bronchial asthma. CJIM 1997;3:264–7.
307 Nadir A, Agrawal S, King PD, et. al. Acute hepatitis associated with the use of a Chinese herbal product, ma-huang. Am J Gastroenterol 1996 Jul;91(7):1436–8.
308 Skoulidis F, Alexander GJ, Davies SE. Ma huang associated acute liver failure requiring liver transplantation. Eur J Gastroenterol Hepatol 2005 May;17(5):581–4.
309 Urata Y, Yoshida S, Irie Y, et. al. Treatment of asthma patients with herbal medicine TJ-96: a randomized controlled trial. 82 Respir Med 2002 Jun;96(6):469–74.
310 Egashira Y, Nagano H. A multicenter clinical trial of TJ-96 in patients with steroid-dependent bronchial asthma. A comparison of groups allocated by the envelope method. Ann N Y Acad Sci 1993 Jun 23;685:580–3.
311 Nakajima S, Tohda Y, Ohkawa K, et. al. Effect of saiboku-to (TJ-96) on bronchial asthma. Induction of glucocorticoid receptor, beta-adrenaline receptor, IgE-Fc epsilon receptor expression and its effect on experimental immediate and late asthmatic reaction. Ann N Y Acad Sci 1993 Jun 23;685:549–60.
312 Palecek I. Amni-visnaga, Munchener Medizinische Wochenschrift, 1970, Jan. 30;112(5):199–202.
313 Schindl R. Treatment of asthma with germakellin. Body plethysmographic investigations [Article in German]. Munch Med Wochenschr 1971 Oct 29;113(44):1471–4.
314 Zioglo G, Samochoweic L. Study on Clinical Properties and Mechanisms of Action of Petasites in Bronchial Asthma and Chronic Obstructive Bronchitis. Pharm Acta Helv 1998;72:378–80.
315 Zara P. Dept. Science & technology. Phillipine Council for Health Research 2002.
316 Ammon HP. Boswellic acids (components of frankincense) as the active principle in treatment of chronic inflammatory diseases [Article in German]. Wien Med Wochenschr 2002;152(15–16):373–8.
317 Ammon HP, Safayhi H, Mack T, et. al. Mechanisms of Anti-Inflammatory Actions of Curcumine and Boswellic Acids. Journal of Ethno-Pharmacology 1993;38:113–19.

318 Gupta I, Gupta V, Parihar A, et. al. Effects of Boswellia serata Gum Resin in patients with Bronchial Asthma: Results of a double-blind, placebo-controlled, 6 week clinical study. Eur J Med Res 1998;3(11):511–14.
319 Gupta S, George P, Gupta V, et. al. Tylophora indica in bronchial asthma--a double-blind study. Indian J Med Res 1979 Jun;69:981–9.
320 Mathew KK, Shivpuri DN. Treatment of asthma with alkaloids of Tylophora indica: a double-blind study. Aspects Allergy Appl. Immunol 1974;7: 166–79.
321 Shivpuri DN, Menon MPS, Parkash D. A crossover double-blind study on Tylophora indica in the treatment of asthma and allergic rhinitis. J Allergy 1969:43(3):145–50.
322 Shivpuri DN, Singhal SC, Parkash D. Treatment of asthma with an alcoholic extract of tylophora indica: a cross-over, double-blind study. Annals of Allergy 1972;30(7):407–12.
323 Shivpuri DN, Agarwal MK. Effect of Tylophora indica on bronchial tolerance to inhalation challenge with specific allergens. Ann Allergy 1973;31(2): 87–94.
324 Thiruvengadam KV, Haranath K, Sudarsan S, et. al. Tylophora indica in bronchial asthma. J Indian Med Assoc 1978;71:172–7.
325 Shivpuri DN, Menon MP, Parkash D. Preliminary studies in Tylophora indica in the treatment of asthma and allergic rhinitis. J Assoc Physicians India. 1968 Jan;16(1):9–15.
326 Gore KV, Rao AK, Guruswamy MN. Physiological studies with Tylophora asthmatica in bronchial asthma. Indian J Med Res 1980 Jan;71:144–8.
327 Kaik KG, Witte PU. Protective effect of forskolin in acetylcholine provocation in healthy probands. Comparison doses with fenoterol and placebo. (German, English abstract). Wien Med Wochenschr 1986;136(23–24):637–41.
328 Bauer K, Dietersdorfer F, Sertl K, et. al. Pharmacodynamic effects of inhaled dry powder formulations of fenoterol and colforsin in asthma. Clin Pharmacol Ther 1993 Jan;53(1):76–83.
329 Tripathi RM, Sen PC, Das PK, et. al, Studies on the mechanism of action of Albizia Labbek, an Indian indigenous drug used in the treatment of atopic allergy. J. Ethnopharmacol 1979;1(4):397–400.
330 Tripathi RM, Sen PC, Das PK. Further studies on the mechanism of the anti-anaphylactic action of Albizzia lebbeck, an Indian indigenous drug. J Ethnopharmacol 1979 Dec;1(4):397–400.
331 Cambridge GW, Jansen AB, Jarman DA. Bronchodilating action of vascinone and related compounds. Nature 1962;196:1217.
332 Gupta OP, Sharma ML, Ghatak BJ, et. al. Pharmacological investigations of vasicine and vasicinone- the alkaloids of Adhatoda vasica. Indian J Med. Res 1977;66(4):680–91.
333 Racle JP, Girard M, Delage J, et. al. Clinical and anatomopathological effect of Bisolvon in respiratory resuscitation. Ann Anesthesiol Fr 1976;17(1):51–8.
334 Claeson UP, Malmfors T, Wikman G, et. al. Adhatoda vasica: a critical review of ethnopharmacological and toxicological data. J Ethnopharmacol 2000 Sep;72(1–2):1–20.
335 Meza RA, Bridges-Webb C, Sayer GP, et. al. The management of acute bronchitis in general practice: results from the Australian Morbidity and Treatment Survey, 1990–1991. Aust Fam Physician 1994 Aug;23(8):1550–3.
336 Ernst E, Marz R, Sieder Ch. A controlled multicentre study of herbal versus synthetic secretolytic drugs for acute bronchitis. Phytomedicine 1997;4.287–93.
337 Blumenthal M, Goldberg A, Brinckmann J. Herbal Medicine. Expanded Commission E monographs. Author Affiliation: American Botanical Council, PO Box 144345, Austin, TX 78714–4345, USA. Editors: Blumenthal M, Goldberg A, Brinckmann J. Herbal medicine. Expanded Commission E monographs, IMC, 2000.
338 Bielory L, Lupoli K. Review article. Herbal Interventions in Asthma and Allergy. Journal of Asthma 1999;36(1):1–65.
339 Benito M, Jorro G, Morales C, et. al. Labiatae allergy: systemic reactions due to ingestion of oregano and thyme. Ann Allergy Asthma Immunol 1996 May;76(5):416–8.
340 Lemiere C, Cartier A, Lehrer SB, et. al. Occupational asthma caused by aromatic herbs. Allergy 1996 Sep;51(9):647–9.
341 Hausen BM, Ketels-Harken H, Schulz KH. Berufsbedingte Inhalationsallergie durch Pollen von Euphorbia fulgens Karw [Occupational allergy due to inhalation of pollen from Euphorbia fulgens Karw (author's transl)]. Dtsch Med Wochenschr 1976 Apr 9;101(15):567–70.
342 Reilly DT, Taylor MA, McSharry C, et. al. Is homeopathy a placebo response? Controlled trial of homoeopathic potency with pollen in hayfever as a model. Lancet 1986;2:881–6.
343 Reilly D, Taylor MA, Beattie NGM, et. al. Is evidence for homeopathy reproducible? Lancet 1994; 344: 1601–6.
344 Lewith GT, Watkins AD, Hyland ME, et. al. Use of ultramolecular potencies of allergen to treat asthmatic people allergic to house dust mite: double-blind randomised controlled clinical trial. BMJ 2002 Mar 2;324(7336):520. PubMed PMID:11872551; PubMed Central PMCID:PMC67767.
345 White A, Slade P, Hunt C, et. al. Individualised homeopathy as an adjunct in the treatment of childhood asthma: a randomised placebo-controlled trial. Thorax 2003 Apr;58(4):317–21.
346 Linde K, Clausius N, Ramirez G, et. al. Are the clinical effects of homoeopathy placebo effects? A meta-analysis of placebo-controlled trials. Lancet 1997;350:834–43.
347 McCarney RW, Linde K, Lasserson TJ. Homeopathy for chronic asthma. Cochrane Database of Systematic Reviews 2004, Issue 1. Art No: CD000353. doi: 10.1002/14651858.CD000353.pub2.
348 Passalacqua G, Bousquet PJ, Carlsen KH, et. al. ARIA update: I-Systematic review of complementary and alternative medicine for rhinitis and asthma. J Allergy Clin Immunol 2006 May;117(5):1054–62.
349 Shang A, Huwiler-Muntener K, Nartey L, et. al. Are the clinical effects of homoeopathy placebo effects? Comparative study of placebo-controlled trials of homoeopathy and allopathy. Lancet 2005 Aug 27–2 Sep;366(9487):726–32.
350 Hondras MA, Linde K, Jones AP. Manual therapy for asthma. Cochrane Database of Systematic Reviews 2005, Issue 2. Art No: CD001002. doi: 10.1002/14651858.CD001002.pub2.
351 McCarney RW, Brinkhaus B, Lasserson TJ, et. al. Acupuncture for chronic asthma. The Cochrane Database of Systematic Reviews 2003, Issue 3. Art No: CD000008. doi: 10.1002/14651858.CD000008. pub2.

352 Gruber W, Eber E, Malle-Scheid D, et. al. Laser acupuncture in children and adolescents with exercise-induced asthma. Thorax 2002 Mar;57(3):222–5.
353 Medici TC, Grebski E, Wu J, et. al. Acupuncture and bronchial asthma: a long-term randomized study of the effects of real versus sham acupuncture compared to controls in patients with bronchial asthma. J Altern Complement Med 2002 Dec;8(6):737–50; discussion 751–4.
354 Fung KP, Chow OK, So SY. Attenuation of exercise-induced asthma by acupuncture. Lancet 1986;Dec 20–27;2(8521–22):1419–22.
355 Field T, Henteleff T, Hernandez-Reif M, et. al. Children with asthma have improved pulmonary functions after massage therapy. J Pediatr 1998 May;132(5):854–8.
356 Hernandez-Reif M, Field T, Krasnegor J, et. al. Children with cystic fibrosis benefit from massage therapy. J Pediatr Psychol 1999 Apr;24(2):175–81. PMID:10361400.
357 Beamon S, Falkenbach A, Fainburg G, et. al. Speleotherapy for asthma. Cochrane Database of Systematic Reviews 2001, Issue 2. Art No: CD001741. doi: 10.1002/14651858.CD001741.
358 Brygge T, Heinig JH, Collins P, et. al. No evidence was found that reflexology has a specific effect on asthma beyond placebo influence. Respiratory Medicine 2001 Mar.
359 Petersen LN, Faurschou P, Olsen OT, et. al. Footzone therapy and bronchial asthma — a clinically controlled investigation. Ugeskr Laeger 1992;154:2065–8.
360 National Health and Medical Research Council. A guide to the development, implementation and evaluation of clinical practice guidelines. Commonwealth of Australia, Canberra, 2000.

Chapter 6

Attention deficit hyperactivity disorder (ADHD)

With contribution from Dr Lily Tomas

Introduction

Attention Deficit Hyperactivity Disorder (ADHD) — characterised by attention-deficit, impulsivity and hyperactivity — is one of the most common neurobehavioral disorders affecting children and adolescents today.[1, 2, 3] The incidence of ADHD is rising with the annual prevalence in Australia in 2001 being estimated at 11% (diagnosed by DSM-IV criteria), equating to a 7.5% prevalence in people aged 6–17 years.[4]

There has been a concomitant rise in the use of stimulant medications, namely phenylmethidate and dexamphetamine, despite a lack of studies regarding long-term social and psychological effects, and cardiovascular and neurophysiological clinical effects. Although stimulants are very helpful in 60–70% of patients, many families seek alternatives because of adverse reactions, lack of compliance and the fact that stimulants cannot be given late in the day, limiting the benefits largely to school hours.[5]

The use of complementary and alternative medicines (CAM) for ADHD has increased, both by parents and health care providers.[6] Parents are especially drawn to CAM interventions in order to avoid or decrease the use of psychotropic medications.[7, 8] Because of the wide-ranging disruptive impact on the lives of both patients and their families, an integrative approach to management simply reflects the multifactorial aetiology and nature of this disorder.

A recent Australian survey demonstrated that the most common CAM therapies used include dietary modification, nutritional supplementation, aromatherapy and chiropractic. It has been advised that doctors should always inquire about the use of CAM and use available resources to help guide families in their therapeutic choices.[9]

The exact aetiology of ADHD is unknown and, indeed, may differ from individual to individual. Genetics and genetic polymorphisms certainly play a role, however, major aetiological contributors may also include adverse responses to food additives, intolerances of foods, differing biochemical pathways and nutritional deficiencies, sensitivities to environmental chemicals and exposure to neurodevelopmental toxins such as heavy metals and tobacco smoke.[10–15]

ADHD is a complicated condition that requires multidimensional treatment strategies.[16] It is imperative to understand that the aetiology and hence the management of ADHD may be different for each individual. One must attempt to elucidate all possible contributory factors and eliminate or treat each respectively.

Neuropsychological and imaging studies indicate that ADHD is associated with alterations in the prefrontal cortex (PFC) and its links to the striatum and cerebellum.

The PFC, especially the right hemisphere, is crucial to the regulation of behaviour and attention. It is extremely sensitive to its neurochemical environment, with either too much or too little catecholamine release weakening the individual's cognitive control of both behaviour and attention.[17]

Individuals with ADHD are known to have depleted levels of dopamine and noradrenaline most likely as a result of dysfunctional transporter systems.[18] The role of other neurotransmitters such as histamine, acetylcholine, glutamine and serotonin in modulating catecholamine pathophysiology in ADHD is yet to be elucidated.[19]

Lifestyle

Most of the lifestyle factors associated with ADHD are covered under the appropriate headings below.

Mind–body medicine

Neurobiofeedback

Electroencephalogram (EEG) biofeedback is a promising alternative treatment for patients with ADHD.[20] It is a form of behavioural training aimed at developing skills for the self-regulation of brain activity.[21] Most individuals with ADHD, as compared to matched peers, show abnormal functioning of their anterior cingulate cortex with excess slow-wave (theta) activity and reduced fast-wave (beta) activity during tasks of selection attention.[22, 23]

In particular, it is well documented that hyperactive behaviour in many children with ADHD is due to abnormally enhanced 4-8Hz Theta activity in both frontal and central cortical areas of the brain.[24] In the last decade there has been a multitude of clinical trials and literature reviews that demonstrate the positive effects of biofeedback on these children with clinical improvement being primarily directly related to declining theta/beta ratios and/or amplitudes over the frontal/central cortex.[25–42] These have largely been good quality studies that have tended to overcome the methodological shortcomings of earlier studies.[21]

Research findings published to date indicate a positive clinical response (reduced hyperactivity and impulsivity, improved attention, IQ, processing speed and music performance) in approximately 75% of patients treated in controlled group studies. The Association for Applied Psychophysiology and Biofeedback and the International Society for Neuronal Regulation deem EEG biofeedback to be 'probably efficacious' for the treatment of ADHD, particularly for those patients who do not respond to medications.[30, 36, 38]

During biofeedback, individuals are taught to increase their beta activity and suppress their theta activity over a period of usually 30 or more sessions.[29, 30, 32, 33] This enables the child to become an active agent of their own coping strategies and thus increase their internal locus of control.[43] EEG biofeedback therapy works by rewarding scalp EEG frequencies that are associated with relaxed attention and suppressing those frequencies associated with under or over-arousal.[20] It provides immediate feedback to the individual about his/her brain-wave activity in the form of a video/computer game, the action of which is influenced by the individual meeting predetermined threshold of brain activity.[22] Obviously, the child must be at an age where they are able to play such games — most studies include children aged 6 years and above.[28, 29, 30, 33]

There are many different forms of biofeedback available. The regulation of cortical excitation thresholds are also considered to be impaired in children with ADHD and the training of slow cortical potentials addresses the regulation of cortical excitability. It has been suggested that the regulation of fronto–central negative slow cortical potentials affects the cholinergic-dopaminergic balance, allowing children to adapt to task requirements with more flexibility.[21, 25, 30]

Recently published studies using quantitative EEG (QEEG) techniques indicate that power spectral analysis and event-related cortical potentials may be useful in differentiating ADHD from other disorders, such that QEEGs may be used clinically in the assessment, diagnosis and treatment of ADHD.[25, 35] In particular, a deficit in low frequency wave (approximately 1 Hz) activity associated with levels of hyperactivity and impulsivity has been demonstrated in both children and adolescents with ADHD. This marker is evident across a range of tasks and may, indeed, be specific to ADHD.[25]

Several recent neuro-feedback trials have demonstrated comparable results with Methylphenidate (Ritalin) in terms of increased attention span and reduced problem behaviour (impulsivity and hyperactivity) in children with ADHD without the side-effects often associated with medication.[20, 22, 31, 37, 39, 44]

It is also important to note that in those studies of children using both biofeedback and methylphenidate, only those children who had received biofeedback sustained these gains when reassessed without Ritalin. Furthermore, Quantitative Electroencephalographic Scanning Process (QESP) studies show a significant reduction in persistent cortical slowing only in those patients who underwent EEG biofeedback.[39, 45] This is confirmed by parent and teacher evaluations who report significant behavioural and cognitive improvements for at least 6 months after the cessation of treatment.[29]

Psychosocial and/or cognitive behaviour therapy (CBT)

Although pharmacological treatments have traditionally been considered the first-line therapy for ADHD, many individuals continue to experience major functional impairment or choose not to use such medications. Behavioural school interventions and parent training have been supported by empirical evidence.[1, 46] It is important to note, however, that the children respond to such behavioural interventions only when they are appropriately implemented both at home and in the classroom setting.[47]

Psychosocial therapies, especially behavioural modification techniques, should be considered for children with ADHD and oppositional behaviours whilst cognitive behaviour therapy (CBT) may be useful for adolescents and adults.[48, 49] When behavioural therapies have been combined with medication, improvements in function have been demonstrated and the amount of stimulant reduced.[50]

A recent Cochrane review has confirmed that both behavioural and CBT interventions are highly effective, however, access to these treatments is limited due to length of consultations and expense, with significant behavioural improvements taking up to 2 hours of therapist time.[51]

It has been hypothesised that family therapy without medication may help to develop family structure and may help to manage children's behaviour. A 2005 Cochrane review has deemed that further research is necessary to determine whether family therapy is an effective intervention for children with ADHD.[52]

Available data supports the use of group and individual structured, skills-based psychosocial interventions for adults with ADHD.[53, 54]

Meditation and relaxation training

Mindfulness meditation may also improve behavioural and neurocognitive impairments in adolescents and adults with ADHD. One recent study has demonstrated improved attention and cognition with reduced anxiety and depression after an 8 week mindfulness training program.[55]

A range of studies have suggested that relaxation training can help children with ADHD to learn to relax, thereby decreasing their autonomic activity.[7, 56] Reductions in problem behaviour, increased attention span and greater internal locus of control are other potential benefits of relaxation therapy. It should be noted, however, that these skills need to be practised regularly for continued effect.[57–60]

In the mainstream literature there have been no published studies on the potential application of meditation for ADHD, however, the Royal Hospital for Women, Sydney, has devised a pilot clinic aimed at developing meditative strategies, using Sahaja Yoga Meditation, to help these children (www.sesiahs.health.nsw.gov.au/rhw/). The clinic exclusively accepted children with a formal diagnosis of ADHD and whose usual supervising health professional had permitted their involvement. Both the child and at least 1 parent were required to attend classes and practice daily meditation. The results were very promising. Of the 16 children who completed the program, 6 were able to decrease and 3 were able to stop their medication whilst maintaining completely normal behavioural traits. All parents reported feeling generally better, less stressed and more relaxed and most felt the program had benefited their children.

About half the parents said their child was less restless with improved sleep and that they were experiencing a better relationship with them. Whilst this is not a randomised controlled study, it is at the moment the best available evidence for meditation's potential role in ADHD and clearly suggests that Sahaja Yoga meditation may be particularly beneficial for this condition. More rigorously designed studies are planned in order to achieve a more conclusive understanding of this radically different approach.[3]

Sound therapy

Recent studies have demonstrated that children with ADHD, upon performing visual discrimination tasks, were less attentive than controls when exposed to distracting novel sounds. Event-related brain potentials correspondingly displayed significant differences over the fronto-central left hemisphere and the left parietal scalp region, revealing low control of involuntary attention that may further underlie their abnormal distractibility.[61]

Systems such as the 'Tomatis Method', 'Integrated Listening System' (ILS) and Dr Guy Berard's (ENT physician) Auditory Integration Training (www.integratedlistening.com) have been designed around the brain's ability to form new neural connections throughout life, changing the way the brain processes auditory information. ILS stimulates both cerebellar activity, in order to strengthen these neural connections, and the vestibular system, in order to improve balance, posture and hand/eye coordination. Such therapies are used by many patients who experience auditory processing difficulties and hypersensitivity to specific auditory frequencies. There are currently no well-designed studies in the literature regarding such therapies, however, anecdotal reports are very promising.

The Moderate Brain Arousal model suggests that dopamine levels modulate how much noise is required for optimal cognitive performance. Studies have shown that individuals with low dopamine levels (ADHD) need more background noise than controls for optimal cognitive performance. This positive effect of noise may be explained by the phenomenon of Stochastic Resonance (SR), whereby external noise is relayed as internal noise into the neural network subsequently affecting neurotransmitter levels.[62] This method aims to teach children with ADHD to focus and intently listen to specific sounds, subsequently helping with behaviour modification, cognitive development and concentration.

Normally, high dopamine down-regulates stimuli-evoked phasic dopamine responses through autoreceptors, however, abnormally low extracellular dopamine in ADHD up-regulates these receptors so that stimuli-evoked phasic dopamine is boosted. It is postulated that these boosted phasic responses create hypersensitivity to environmental stimuli in ADHD. Empirical data supports the concept that more noise is required for SR to occur in dopamine-deprived neural systems in ADHD.[17]

There is also some evidence to show that music therapy may contribute to a reduction in a range of ADHD symptoms in the classroom.[43, 63]

Sleep and behaviour

It is important to note that, even in children that do not suffer with ADHD, sleep problems during school transitions are common, and are associated with poor outcomes. Future RCTs could determine if sleep interventions can reduce the prevalence and impact of such detrimental sleep problems.[64]

Sleep restoration/melatonin

There is a clear correlation between ADHD and sleep difficulties with substantial evidence that ADHD psychopathology and sleep/wake regulation share common neurobiological mechanisms. Furthermore, there may even be an overlap between ADHD and sleep disorders such as obstructive sleep apnoea and restless leg syndrome (RLS).[65] Anecdotal evidence strongly suggests that magnesium assists in the treatment of RLS.

Approximately 25% of children suffering with ADHD also experience some form of sleep disorder. Unfortunately, in contrast with adults, these often go undetected. Diagnosis of these patients is critical.[66] Therefore, all children with ADHD should be fully assessed for sleep disturbances because adequate treatment is often associated with improvement of symptoms and a decreased requirement for stimulant medications.[65, 66]

The circadian rhythm of melatonin secretion from the pineal gland is reflective of mechanisms that are in control of the sleep/wake cycle. In those individuals with primary insomnia, nocturnal plasma melatonin levels tend to be lower than in healthy controls. Melatonin has been used successfully to treat insomnia in children with ADHD.[67] Several randomised double-blind placebo-controlled trials using 3–6mg melatonin for 1 month demonstrated enhanced total time asleep in children with ADHD and chronic sleep onset insomnia. Melatonin is shown to be a safe and effective treatment for sleep disorders, however this had no observable effect on other ADHD symptoms.[68, 69]

Environment

Outdoor play

Research on children with ADHD demonstrates significant improvement in symptoms such as inattention and impulsivity after exposure to natural views or settings. Four hundred and fifty-two parents or guardians from across the US with ADHD or Attention Deficit Disorder (ADD) children aged 5–18 years enrolled in a study to assess the benefits of playing outdoors in a natural setting.[70] Compared with baseline results, outdoor activities conducted in natural environments significantly improved ADHD symptoms (difficulty in remaining focused, completing tasks, listening and following directions, and in resisting distractions) compared to activities conducted indoors or those in built outdoor settings, such as parking lots.

While the results of this study need to be verified using a more rigorous study design, these findings are promising as spending more time outdoors in natural environments is an inexpensive accessible treatment that is free of side-effects.

Heavy metals and chemicals

Lead

Lead is a common environmental contaminant such that in the year 2000, nearly 1 million preschool-aged children in the US alone were shown to have elevated blood levels (>10ug/dL).[71]

In 1991, the US Centres for Disease Control and Prevention (CDC) established 10ug/dL as the lowest concern for children's blood lead levels. However, in recent years, there has been a wealth of evidence-based clinical trials demonstrating that levels below 10ug/dL may impair neurological development. In fact, there is now sufficient and compelling scientific evidence to call for the CDC to lower the blood lead action level in children to a level as low as 2ug/dL.[72, 73, 74]

Indeed, no level of lead exposure appears to be safe with multiple studies now demonstrating reduced IQ and academic deficits in otherwise 'healthy' children. There appears to be an inverse relationship between lead levels and IQ levels, particularly at levels <10ug/dL.[75, 76, 77] At lower levels of toxicity, a child may have no specific individual symptoms but may certainly be affected sub-clinically.[78] For this reason, health care practitioners should obtain a thorough environmental history on all children they examine.[74]

Having adjusted for covariates, children with 5–10ug/dL have been shown to have 5 points lower IQ scores compared to children with blood lead levels of 1–2ug/dL. Verbal IQ appears to be more negatively associated than performance IQ, as does reading and maths composite scores. Working memory and attention were also shown to be lowered with increasing lead levels.[79, 80]

In particular, there have been several studies associating ADHD with elevated lead levels. Individuals with ADHD are more likely to have been exposed to lead during childhood, such that ADHD may now be deemed an additional deleterious outcome of lead exposure, even when levels are <10ug/dL.[81] Its effects may be mediated by less effective cognitive control, consistent with a route of influence via striatal-frontal neural circuits.[82]

Chelation therapy is advised for children with blood level concentrations of >44ug/dL, however, there are no evidence-based clinical trials for other gentler chelation treatment options for children with levels less than this. Because lead absorption is partially related to nutritional status, micronutrient supplements may be a possible solution for combating low-level chronic lead exposure.[71, 80] Zinc, in particular, is 1 supplement that has shown some results in effectively reducing oppositional, hyperactive, cognitive problems and other ADHD symptoms in most individuals.[80, 83]

Mercury

Numerous studies report positive correlations between the number of dental amalgams and urinary mercury concentrations in non-occupationally exposed individuals.[84, 85, 86] Experimental evidence consistently demonstrates that mercury is released from dental amalgams and is absorbed by the human body.[87] However, there is much controversy regarding the effects of mercury (from dental amalgams and vaccinations) on neurodevelopment, renal and immune function.

One of the latest randomised controlled studies has confirmed that treatment of children with amalgam restorations leads to increased, albeit low level, exposure to mercury. Amalgam exposure resulted in small, transient immune deficits 5–7 days post treatment, however, it did not cause overt immune defects. The authors concluded that these changes 'most likely did not need to be of concern to practitioners considering the use of this restorative dental material'.[88] It is important to note, however, the history of what initially constituted toxic lead levels and how this has changed in recent years with accumulated evidence-based studies.

In a similar manner, mean urinary mercury concentrations have been found to be greater in children with amalgams rather than composite dental restorations.[89, 90] Children treated with mercury amalgams did not 'on average' have statistically significant differences with respect to neuropsychological function. 'Although it is possible that very small IQ effects cannot be ruled out', thus far evidence-based trials largely demonstrate that dental amalgam is not associated with an increase in children's risk of experiencing neuropsychological dysfunction.[75, 90, 91, 92,]

These results support the concept that some healthy children may, indeed, be out of the bell-curve, being more predisposed to toxic effects of mercury at lower levels than others. This is further highlighted by a recent trial specifically concerning children suffering with ADHD. In this study of Chinese children, a significant difference in blood mercury levels was noted between children with ADHD compared with controls, after adjustments for age, gender and parental occupations. The geometric mean blood mercury level was also significantly higher in children with inattentive and combined subtypes of ADHD. In fact, children with a blood mercury level >29nmol/L were found to have 9.69 times higher risk of having ADHD after adjustment for confounding variables. The researchers concluded that high blood mercury levels were associated with ADHD.[93]

Manganese/aluminium

Manganese (Mn) is an essential trace element, however, it has also been shown to be toxic at high doses. Animal studies have recently shown that intra-nasally administered Mn actually circumvents the Blood-Brain-Barrier and passes directly into the brain via olfactory pathways. Long-term exposure to inhaled Mn from shower water as a significant risk for central nervous system (CNS) neurotoxicity is currently being investigated. Similarly, existing Mn drinking water standards may also need to be revised.[94]

A recent study of Canadian children found that those who were exposed to drinking water that was naturally high in Mn had greater scores of hyperactivity and oppositional behaviour (Revised Connor's Rating Scale) than controls. All children with T scores >65 had hair Mn higher than 3.0ug/g.[95]

It is postulated that both aluminium and Mn toxicity may potentiate oxidative and inflammatory stress, subsequently leading to impaired neurological function.[96]

Industrial chemicals

It is now accepted that antenatal and early childhood exposures to industrial chemicals in the environment can damage the developing brain and can lead to neurodevelopmental disorders, subclinical brain dysfunction and other conditions including ADHD.

Available data up to 2007 show that at least 202 widely-used industrial chemicals, (including lead, methylmercury, polychlorinated biphenyls, arsenic and toluene) can damage the human brain, the researchers concluding that chemical pollution may have harmed the brains of millions of children worldwide.[97, 98] The specific role these chemicals may play in the development of ADHD is not certain, but a detailed environmental history should be taken in all of those with neurodevelopmental disorders.[99]

Tobacco smoke, air pollution, pesticides

Environmental tobacco smoke, air pollution and pesticides have also been shown to have adverse effects on fetal growth and child neurodevelopment.[100, 101, 102]

Tobacco smoke

A recent systematic review has demonstrated that both prenatal and possibly postnatal tobacco smoke exposure are significantly associated with increased rates of behaviour problems and ADHD.[11, 12, 14, 15] If causally linked, it is estimated that prenatal tobacco exposure may account for at least 270 000 excess cases of ADHD in American children today.[13]

Like stimulant medication, nicotine has been shown to lower the availability of the dopamine transporter, a significant factor in dopamine metabolism.[18]

Physical activity

Exercise

Exercise is considered an important part of the management of the child with ADHD as it not only increases coordination skills (that many children with ADHD lack) but it provides opportunities for social interaction.[7] A recent study determining the effects of exercise on children with ADHD suggests that vigorous exercise may provide a dopaminergic adjuvant in the management of behavioural features of ADHD.[103]

It has also been demonstrated that adolescents with ADHD have frontal lobe deficits, particularly on the right sides of their brain. Animal studies were subsequently designed which showed that 'rough-and-tumble' play therapy was able to reduce hyperactivity and excessive playfulness, concluding that this may be a useful new treatment for ADHD.[104]

Another pilot study on Therapeutic Eurythmy — a holistic movement developed by Rudolph Steiner — has also reported shifts in the concentration and motor skills of children with ADHD.[105]

Yoga

Randomised controlled trials (RCTs) on the effectiveness of body-oriented therapies such as yoga for children with ADHD are lacking. The effects of yoga were recently compared to the effects of conventional motor exercises in children with ADHD. It was found that yoga was an effective complementary or concomitant treatment for children with ADHD. It should be noted that the training was especially effective for children also taking medications.[106] Another study of boys with ADHD practicing yoga confirmed this finding, where yoga was particularly effective in the evening when the effects of medication were absent.[107]

Dietary modifications

Food elimination regimes

There has been much discussion over the last 30 years regarding the possible links between diet and behaviour of the individual with ADHD. In 1975, Benjamin Feingold, an allergist, hypothesised that an intake of salicylates in artificial flavours, colours and preservatives and/or natural salicylates may induce hyperactive behaviour and learning disabilities in children. Although Feingold demonstrated that 50% of children with ADHD improved after eliminating these substances from their diet, this has not been successfully repeated until recent years.[43]

The use of food elimination diets in the management of individuals with ADHD is now well documented.[108–112] In fact, a strictly supervised elimination diet is considered to be a valuable instrument in determining whether dietary factors are contributing to ADHD symptoms. In a recent RCT, the number of criteria on the ADHD rating scale showed a scale reduction of 69.4%. Furthermore, comorbid symptoms of oppositional defiant disorder (ODD) also showed a significantly greater decrease in the intervention than the control group.[113]

There is an accumulating body of evidence that many children with behavioural problems, including ADHD, are sensitive to 1 or more food components that can negatively impact upon their behaviour.[114] In 1 study, 19 of 26 children with ADHD improved dramatically after eliminating artificial colours, corn, wheat, milk, soy and oranges from their diet. It is interesting that most of the children who responded to such dietary changes had atopic histories implying that atopic children are more likely to benefit from a restricted diet.[112] Other risk factors associated with a beneficial dietary response were a family history of migraine and young age.[109] Another study also demonstrated a significant improvement in behaviour in 62% of 40 children with ADHD after a 2-week diet based solely on rice, turkey, pear and lettuce.[115] This diet is clearly too restrictive for any child but it does demonstrate that nutrition can influence behaviour.

For children showing behaviour problems such as hyperactivity, the use of dietary manipulation tends to be a more acceptable approach to treatment than the use of drugs.[116] If parents strongly suspect a specific dietary item, a trial of elimination is warranted.[117] However, there are various regimes; usually this would consist of avoiding the item for 3 weeks then reintroducing it in a step-wise fashion — a little the first day, then challenging the body with a higher dose during the second day if no obvious reaction has already occurred. Depending upon the age of the child, multiple foods may be eliminated simultaneously and reintroduced separately in a similar manner under strict supervision. In conducting such dietary modifications, it is mandatory that all practitioners be aware of the dangers potentially associated with unsupervised restriction diets with children.[116, 118]

It is imperative that a food elimination diet be only short-term and the rechallenge process, well structured and clearly documented by the patient/family at the time. A maintenance diet may then be designed by a nutritional practitioner according to the results of the rechallenge process and with optimal levels of both nutritional health and behaviour modification of the child in mind.

In general, dietary modification plays a major role in the management of ADHD and should be routinely considered as part of the treatment protocol.[114] Many children with ADHD have associated digestion problems — including diarrhoea, constipation, abdominal bloating, excess burping and/or flatulence, reflux/indigestion or abdominal pain/discomfort. These are generally symptoms of deficient beneficial gut flora (probiotics) and/or food intolerances which may serve as triggers for abnormal behaviour.

A plethora of studies have now shown that food additives have also been shown to increase hyperactivity symptoms in children.[119, 120] This includes a recent systematic review, which concluded that an additive-free elimination diet was considered Level II evidence with respect to its current level of evidence.[121]

Although the use of single food additives at their regulated concentrations are believed to be relatively safe in terms of their neuronal development, their combined effects remain unclear. Four common food additives, brilliant blue, L-glutamic acid, Quinolone yellow and aspartame were observed in combination. Neurotoxicity (measured as inhibition of neurite outgrowth) was found at concentrations of additives theoretically achievable in plasma by the ingestion of a typical snack and drink.[122]

Symptoms that are due to, or exacerbated by, specific food additives usually involve non-IgE mediated mechanisms that are usually less severe than those induced by food allergy.[123] A recent RCT demonstrated that artificial colours and/or a sodium benzoate preservative in the diet results in increased activity in children aged 3 or 8–9 years old.[124] This confirmed an earlier study where the adverse behaviour of 3-year olds from the same additives was detectable by parents but not by a simple clinical assessment.[125]

Despite a plethora of anecdotal reports that sugar increases hyperactivity and disruptive behaviour in the child with ADHD, there are as yet no consistent clinical trials to support this allegation.[126]

Like most neuropsychiatric disorders, there is evidence that ADHD is associated with increased oxidative stress and therefore increased lipid peroxidation. For this reason, it is postulated that individuals with ADHD may benefit from a whole-food, plant-based diet that is high in antioxidants and devoid of refined carbohydrate products.[127]

Several recent studies have also reported a possible association of coeliac disease with ADHD. In fact, ADHD-like symptomatology is markedly over represented amongst individuals with untreated coeliac disease. A gluten-free diet can result in a significant improvement of such symptoms within a short time period, such that coeliac disease (as well as gluten intolerance) should be included in the list of diseases associated with ADHD-like symptomatology.[128,129] Furthermore, a high frequency (57%) of antigliadin antibodies has been demonstrated in adult patients with neurological dysfunctions of unknown cause. In a study of children with various neurological disorders, including ADHD, 13% (compared with 9% of controls) showed positive for IgG antigliadin antibodies but negative for IgA and endomysial antibodies.[130]

Nutritional supplementation

Nutritional supplementation is widely used to help ameliorate the symptoms of ADHD. Many nutrients, (vitamins, minerals, essential amino acids, essential fatty acids) have direct effects on the structure and function of the human brain.[131] Indeed, the role of nutrition in the prevention and management of ADHD is vital, cost-effective and extremely safe.[132]

Magnesium/vitamin B6

Magnesium deficiency has long been known to cause hyperexcitability with seizures in animal studies, effects that have been successfully reversed by treatment with magnesium. Significantly decreased plasma and red blood cell magnesium with concomitant decreases in Mg(2+) ATPase activity have been identified in children with ADHD.[133–136] Magnesium is required for more than 350 different biochemical metabolism pathways in the human body, including oxidation/reduction and ionic regulation.[131]

Vitamin B6 is essential to the synthesis of many neurotransmitters, particularly dopamine, noradrenaline, GABA, etc (see Figure 6.1).[131]

Several European trials have demonstrated an improvement in the symptoms of ADHD with a combination of magnesium and vitamin B6. Children prescribed a magnesium/B6 regimen (6mg/kg/day Mg, 0.6mg/kg/day B6) for at least 8 weeks displayed a significant reduction in their symptoms of hyperactivity and aggressiveness whilst their attention at school was improved. When the supplementation was ceased, clinical symptoms of the disease reappeared within a few weeks, as did their original lower red blood cell Mg concentrations.[137]

After 1 month of supplementation of magnesium and B6, magnesium homeostasis was again normalised and there were noticeable improvements in behaviour and attention whilst levels of anxiety and aggression were reduced. Thus, it has been postulated that the determination of plasma and red blood cell Mg can be used to detect deficits and monitor the efficiency of treatment.[135,136]

An earlier study found that even though 32 out of 50 children with ADHD demonstrated low red blood cell Mg levels, *all* patients showed an improvement in symptoms (hyperexcitability, physical aggressiveness, instability, attention, hypertony, spasm, myoclony) after 1–6 months of treatment with magnesium.[133] Similarly, children with ADHD receiving 200mg/day magnesium showed a significant decrease in hyperactivity compared to a non-supplemented control group.[138]

Iron

Iron is necessary to ensure oxygenation, produce energy in the cerebral parenchyma (via cytochrome oxidase) and for the synthesis of both neurotransmitters and myelin. Iron concentrations in the umbilical artery are critical for the development of the fetus and are specific to the IQ/cognition of the child, playing a major role in both brain structure and function.[131,132]

Iron deficiency causes abnormal dopaminergic neurotransmission with many studies supporting its contribution to the pathophysiology of ADHD. Serum ferritin levels have consistently been found to be low in children with ADHD compared with controls.

Furthermore, the lower the serum ferritin levels, the more severe the general ADHD (hyperactivity) symptoms.[139] Available data is conflicting as to the relationship of low serum ferritin specifically to cognitive deficits.[140,141]

As stated previously, there is a documented significant comorbidity between ADHD and RLS. Iron is a cofactor in dopamine production and patients with restless legs have lower levels of dopamine in their substantia nigra.[142] Thus iron deficiency may, indeed, be one of the underlying common pathophysiological mechanisms in individuals with both ADHD and RLS. Thus, it is suggested that physicians assess children with ADHD for RLS, a family history of RLS and iron deficiency.[139]

A recent trial of iron supplementation (ferrous sulfate 170mg/day) resulted in an improvement of ADHD symptoms in those children with low serum ferritin levels. Iron therapy was well tolerated with effectiveness comparable to stimulant medication.[143] However, an earlier Cochrane study has demonstrated that there is no clear evidence that iron treatment in children less than 3 years of age with iron deficiency anaemia will improve psychomotor development after 5–11 days of treatment.[144] There is a need for future investigations with larger controlled trials.

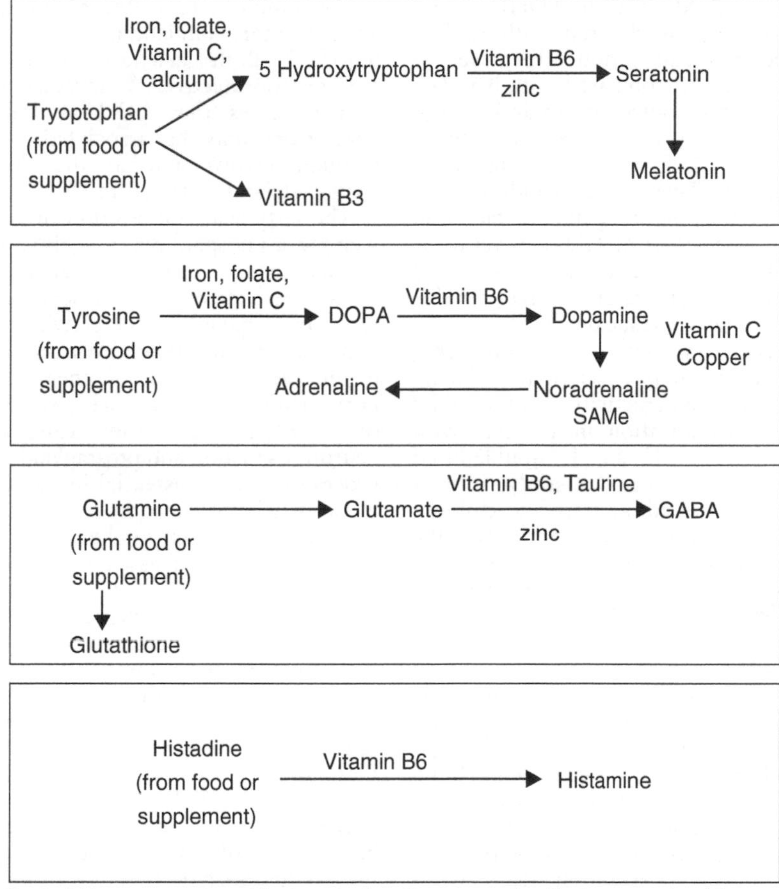

Figure 6.1 Central Nervous system biochemical pathways and cofactors required for neurotransmitter and hormone production[132]

Zinc

Zinc is an important co-factor that is needed for the metabolism of free fatty acids, neurotransmitters, prostaglandins and melatonin. It plays a role in the both the structure and function of the brain and indirectly affects the metabolism of dopamine (by inhibiting the dopamine transporter), known to be intricately involved in ADHD.[18, 132, 145] Furthermore, plasma zinc levels have recently been found to have a direct effect on information processing in children with ADHD through event related potentials. In particular, the latencies of 'N2' waves in both the frontal and parietal regions of children with zinc deficiency and ADHD are significantly longer. N2 wave changes may reflect a different inhibition process and further studies are deemed warranted to investigate the effects of zinc on the inhibitory process in children with low zinc and non-low zinc ADHD.[146]

It is also important to note that zinc has a direct effect on the synthesis of GABA, one of our major inhibitory neurotransmitters that contributes to feelings of calm and relaxation.

Numerous controlled studies report cross-sectional evidence that mean plasma and tissue zinc levels have been found to be significantly lower in children with ADHD than controls suggesting that zinc deficiency may play a substantial role in the aetiopathogenesis of ADHD.[146, 147, 148] Previous reports regarding this have come mainly from countries with differing diets and socioeconomic status, however, recent studies also show that zinc deficiency is common, for example, in middle-class Americans. Although there are mixed results, these studies suggest that inattention symptoms are more prominent with lower zinc levels.[149]

A statistically significant correlation has been found between zinc and serum free fatty acids (FFA) in children with ADHD.[147, 150] A study involving 48 children with ADHD demonstrated a mean serum FFA level of 0.176+/-0.102 mEq/L compared with 0.562+/-0.225 mEq/L in the control group and a mean serum zinc level of 60.6 +/-9.9 microg/dL compared with 105.8 +/-13.2 microg/dL in the control group. These findings indicate that zinc deficiency may be a significant factor in the aetiopathogenesis of ADHD. It is yet to be determined whether FFA deficiency is one of the primary causal factors of ADHD or if this is actually secondary to zinc deficiency.[150]

Several recent trials have demonstrated that zinc supplementation is effective in reducing symptoms of hyperactivity, impulsivity and impaired socialisation in patients with ADHD.[147, 149, 151, 152] In 1 double-blind randomised placebo-controlled study, 150mg/day zinc sulfate was administered to children with ADHD. It was determined that the reduction of the above symptoms were more significant in patients of older age, higher BMI score with low zinc and low free fatty acid levels. Zinc sulfate was well tolerated with a low rate of side-effects.[147]

Several trials have documented a synergistic effect when zinc is used in combination with drug therapy methylphenidate.[149, 153, 154] In a recent 6-week placebo-controlled double-blind RCT children with ADHD were given either medication Methylphenidate plus Zinc sulfate 55mg/day (15mg elemental zinc) or placebo. The parent and teacher rating scale scores improved significantly in the group receiving zinc. There was no difference in side-effects.[153]

A recent double-blind placebo-controlled study determining the relationships between zinc, essential fatty acids and d-amphetamine found that responses to d-amphetamine improved in a linear fashion with zinc levels. [145, 155]

Essential fatty acids (EFAs)

There have been numerous studies of late demonstrating a definitive link between essential fatty acids (EFAs) and neurodevelopment. It has been shown that many children suffering from ADHD have significantly lower concentrations of plasma and red blood cell omega-3 and omega-6 EFAs.[156] Both omega-3 and omega-6 long chain polyunsaturated fatty acids (LCPUFAs) are critical for brain development and function.[157] They function exclusively via cell membranes, in which they are anchored by phospholipids.

Docosahexaenoic acid (DHA, an omega-3 EFA) is a major structural component of neuronal membranes and is essential to pre- and postnatal brain development whereas eicopentanoic acid (EPA, an omega-3 EFA) appears more influential on behaviour and mood.[158] Both generate metabolites that are neuroprotective.[159] Increasing evidence also indicates that LCPUFA imbalance or deficiencies may be associated with ADHD through involvement in the dopaminergic cortico-striatal metabolism.[160]

The fatty acid composition of neuronal cell membrane phospholipids directly reflects dietary intake. Changes in the fatty acid composition of neuronal membranes subsequently leads to functional changes in the activity of receptors and other proteins embedded in the phospholipid membrane.[158] The ratio of omega-3 to omega-6 fatty acids also influences various aspects of serotoninergic and catecholaminergic neurotransmission and prostaglandin formation processes that are essential in the maintenance of normal brain function. This, again, can be modulated by dietary intake.[161]

There is a direct association between EFA deficiency or imbalance with a variety of behavioural disorders including ADHD.[132, 157, 162, 163, 164] Indeed, it has been demonstrated that children with lower concentrations of omega-3 fatty acids display significantly more maladaptive behaviours, hyperactivity, temper tantrums, learning, health and sleep difficulties than those with higher concentrations of omega-3 EFAs.[165, 166]

It is not known exactly why these children have lower concentrations of EFAs, however, several theories have been postulated, including low dietary intake, decreased conversion of EFAs to LCPUFAs and increased metabolism of EFAs.[165] It has also been suggested that deficiencies of DHA may be responsible for abnormal signal transduction associated with learning disabilities and cognitive deficits. Such abnormalities in this signal transduction process have been shown to be partially corrected by supplementation with DHA.[167]

In many randomised placebo-controlled double-blind trials, EPA and DHA combinations have been shown to benefit ADHD, amongst many other neuropsychiatric disorders. [151, 157–160, 168–175]. For instance, 132 Australian children with ADHD recently participated in a 15-week placebo-controlled double-blind RCT where they received PUFAs, PUFAs + micronutrients or placebo. Improvements in hyperactivity, impulsivity and inattention were recorded in both PUFA groups, with no additional effects being found with micronutrient supplementation.[172] Different doses have been used in each study up to a maximum of 16.2g EPA/DHA daily. In this study of high-dose EPA/DHA, there was also a significant correlation between the reduction in the AA:EPA ratio and global severity of illness scores.[172]

Supplementation with omega-6 EFAs has demonstrated mixed results regarding effects on the symptoms of ADHD. Correct dosage may be critical for optimal effectiveness and further studies are warranted.[158, 176, 177]

Given that supplementation with EFAs is safe and well-tolerated compared with existing pharmacological interventions, results from such studies strongly support the case for further investigations.[178, 179]

Essential amino acids

Functional and morphological studies in children with ADHD demonstrate a prefrontal cortex (PFC) dysfunction. This region of the brain is regulated by dopaminergic, noradrenergic, cholinergic, serotonergic, glutamatergic and histaminergic pathways. Currently, there is a wealth of evidence showing that those with ADHD have depleted levels of dopamine and noradrenaline, however, there is still much to be learnt regarding other neurotransmitter systems and how they interact with each other.[180–190]

The pharmaceutical Methylphenidate primarily affects the PFC and striatum, increasing dopamine and noradrenaline release through multiple means.[191, 192, 193] Recent animal studies are now demonstrating that high-dose intranasal dopamine reduces hyperactivity and intermediate-dose improves attention.[194] Likewise, further studies have now indicated that there is an inverse relationship between 5-hydroxytryptophan (5HT) and aggression in adolescents with ADHD.[195, 196, 197] There is also new evidence implicating the glutamatergic prefrontal-striatal pathway in the pathogenesis of ADHD.[190, 191] CNS histamine in the PFC is closely linked with cognition and it has only recently become known that Methylphenidate also enhances cortical histamine in animal studies. The newer non-stimulant drugs primarily work as selective noradrenaline re-uptake inhibitors and by increasing extracellular levels of histamine in the PFC.[198, 199] Modulation of the H3 histamine receptor can affect cognition via the release of several other neurotransmitters, including acetylcholine and noradrenaline.[200, 201, 202]

It is imperative to remember that all neurotransmitters are synthesised from amino acids and all require various vitamins and minerals, primarily zinc and vitamin B6, as cofactors. Deficiencies or imbalances in amino acids, vitamins and minerals can therefore profoundly influence neurotransmitter synthesis and breakdown. Supplements that contain the essential amino acids and nutrients can significantly reduce symptoms by their conversion to specific neurotransmitters.[203]

To date, there is a paucity of studies regarding specific amino acid supplementation and its effects on the symptoms of ADHD. There is increasing evidence for oxidative stress mechanisms underlying the pathophysiology of ADHD, which offers new treatment targets in oxidation biology systems. Of these, the glutathione system has the most favourable theoretical foundation as it is the most generic of all cellular antioxidants. Several studies have shown the efficacy of N-Acetylcysteine, a glutathione precursor, in the treatment of various psychiatric conditions of oxidative stress, indicating that glutathione itself may be a promising therapeutic target.[204]

Carnitine is another amino acid that has been shown to exert positive effects on the symptoms of ADHD. Acetyl-L-Carnitine (ALC) is essential for energy metabolism and essential fatty acid anabolism. A 16-week placebo-controlled RCT demonstrated that 500–1500mg bd L-carnitine was superior to placebo in treating inattention-type symptoms.[205] This confirms earlier studies which have reported significant benefits in ADHD symptoms. Another study has shown significantly reduced attention problems and aggressive behaviour in boys with ADHD supplemented with carnitine.[206] Animal studies have demonstrated that ALC increases noradrenaline and the 5HIAA/5HT ratio in the cingulated cortex, subsequently decreasing behavioural impulsivity.[207] As ALC is safe with no psychostimulant properties, more studies are warranted, particularly for possible significant benefits in the inattentive type.[207]

Homeopathy

An increasing number of parents are turning to homeopathy to treat their hyperactive child.[208] There have been several placebo-controlled double-blind RCTs demonstrating mixed results for the efficacy of homeopathy in the treatment of ADHD.[208–211] A 2007 Cochrane review, however, has deemed that there is currently little evidence to support the use of homeopathy, with the recommendation that optimal treatment protocols be developed prior to further RCT being undertaken.[212]

It is important to note, however, that homeopathy focuses on the individual characteristics of each patient's experience and symptoms and uses this information to determine the appropriate prescription for each patient.[213] For this reason, RCTs are very difficult to conduct and the results, difficult to interpret.[213, 214]

One study of children with ADHD receiving individualised homeopathic treatment demonstrated a 75% response to treatment, reaching a clinical improvement rating of 73% and an amelioration of the Connors Global Index (CGI) of 55%. In comparison, clinical improvement under Methylphenidate was 65% with a lowering of the CGI to 48%. Both treatments appeared to be similar in efficacy and it was concluded that in cases where treatment is not urgent, homeopathy is a valuable alternative to methylphenidate.[215]

Herbal medicines

St John's wort

There has been only 1 recent study on the effects of Hypericum perforatum on the symptoms of ADHD. No differences were observed between St John's wort or placebo.[216]

Ginkgo biloba + ginseng

A pilot study has recently been conducted on a herbal product containing American ginseng extract, panax quinquefolium (200mg) and ginkgo biloba extract (50mg). One capsule administered twice daily for only 1 month resulted in significant improvements in behaviour of many children with ADHD, warranting further research in this area.[217]

Traditional Chinese medicine (TCM)

There have been several clinical trials conducted in China with promising results in the treatment of ADHD. One RCT involving 100 children compared a combination of *Bupleurum chinense*, *Scutellaria baicalensis*, *Astragalus membranaceus*, *Codonopsis pilosula*, *Ligustrum lucidum*, *lophatherum gracile* and *thread of ivory* with 5–15mg Ritalin twice daily administered for 1–3 months. In the TCM group, 23 cases were 'cured' (measured by clinical symptoms disappearing, an increase of 10 IQ units, a normalised EEG and no recurrence of symptoms 6 months post-treatment). Four cases were improved (symptoms and signs markedly improved, an increase of 4 IQ units and normalising EEG) and 11 cases ineffective. In the group taking Ritalin, 6 cases were 'cured', 12 cases improved and 2 cases were ineffective. Although there was no significant difference regarding efficacy between the 2 groups in this study, the side-effects of TCM were considerably less.[218]

Double-blind studies comparing the effects of *Duodongining* (DDN) with Ritalin have also shown similar clinical responses with a marked reduction of side-effects in those taking DDN.[219]

These effects have once again been seen with Tiaoshen liquor. Its therapeutic mechanism is thought to be related to improvements in information transmission through cholinergic neuron synapses and enhancement of hypoxia tolerance of cerebral tissues.[220]

A further randomised controlled study involving 200 children assessed the effects of Ritalin, *Yihzi* mixture (YZM) and a combination of both, for a period of 3 months. By assessment with multiple questionnaires, it was shown that the therapeutic effect of the combined treatment was better than either Ritalin or YZM alone. Furthermore, only the YZM and combined groups showed significant improvement in both soft nerve signs and EEGs, again with less side-effects than Ritalin.[221]

An interesting study of Jiangqian granules (JQG) has also shown significant clinical improvements when compared with Ritalin. In this particular study, blood lead concentrations were measured and found to be significantly higher in the ADHD group compared with the control group. These parameters were remeasured at the end of the 3-month study. Although there were reductions in blood lead concentrations in both groups, the lowering was significantly more in the group treated with JQG and this is believed to be its prime mechanism of action.[222]

Pycnogenol

Oxidative stress has been implicated in the pathogenesis of many chronic diseases, including ADHD, with correspondingly new targets for the development of different therapeutic interventions.[223]

Pycnogenol, an extract from the bark of the French maritime pine, is a potent polyphenol complex that contains phenolic acids, cetechin, taxifolin and procyanidins. It acts as a highly powerful antioxidant and chelating agent that stimulates the activity of other antioxidants such as SOD (superoxide dismutase) and eNOS (endothelial nitric oxide synthase).[224–228]

Concentrations of catecholamines have been found to be higher in the urine of patients with ADHD compared with healthy children. Furthermore, adrenaline and noradrenaline concentrations positively correlate with plasma levels of oxidised glutathione.[224]

Several placebo-controlled, double-blind RCTs have shown that pycnogenol reduces symptoms of hyperactivity and improves attention, visual-motor co-ordination and concentration in children with ADHD. One month of pycnogenol (1mg/kg/day) significantly reduced oxidised glutathione and increased reduced glutathione compared with placebo. Urinary catecholamines (dopamine, adrenaline and noradrenaline) were also decreased. Thus, pycnogenol reduces oxidative damage to DNA, normalising total antioxidant status of ADHD children.[224, 225, 229] At 1 month post-cessation of Pycnogenol, a relapse of ADHD symptoms was noted.[226]

Physical therapies

Massage

Massage intervention is known to benefit childhood mental wellbeing. For instance, a meta-analysis of the literature demonstrated massage intervention can be of benefit in promoting mental and physical wellbeing in any child under the age of 6 months by improving the mother–infant interaction, sleeping and crying, and on hormones influencing stress levels which may impact positively in children's behaviour in later life.[230]

Massage has been shown to increase serotonin levels which may modulate dopamine levels in children with ADHD. One study demonstrated increased concentration and decreased hyperactivity after children with ADHD received 15 minute massages for 10 consecutive school days.[231] More recently, massage for 20 minutes twice weekly for 1 month benefited students with ADHD by improving short-term mood state and longer-term classroom behaviour.[232]

Chiropractic

In 1 small study, chiropractic manipulation has been shown to decrease autonomic nervous system activity and improve behaviour in children with ADHD, thus warranting further investigation in this area.[233]

There is currently a placebo-controlled, double-blind RCT underway in Australia investigating the effects of Neuro Emotional Technique (NET), a branch of chiropractic, on children with ADHD. The control group are continuing their existing medical regime whilst the intervention and placebo group have the addition of NET and sham NET protocols added to their regime, respectively. These NET/sham NET protocols are performed twice weekly for the first month and then monthly for the next 6 months. This study should provide good evidence as to the efficacy of NET as an adjunct therapy to conventional medical therapy.[234]

Conclusion

ADHD is a chronic, complex and multifactorial illness that has become one of the most common cognitive and behavioural disorders diagnosed among children of school age today. Current conventional treatment includes the use of stimulant medications which significantly influence catecholamine concentrations. Not all children respond to these medications and the risk of side-effects combined with concerns regarding the safety of the long-term use of such medications makes CAM therapies an attractive option. There is a wealth of evidence for the use of many of these therapies and an holistic approach to the management of our future generations is well warranted. Management of ADHD should include various behavioural and lifestyle changes that include avoidance of chemicals and smoking, sleep restoration, dietary changes, exercise outdoors in a natural setting and relaxation strategies. Table 6.1 summarises the best evidence for CAM therapies for ADHD.

Table 6.1 Levels of evidence for lifestyle and complementary medicines/therapies in the management of ADHD

Modality	Level I	Level II	Level IIIa	Level IIIb	Level IIIc	Level IV	Level V
Physical activity				x			
Mind–body medicine							
Neurobiofeedback				x			
CBT	x						
Meditation	x			x			
Behaviour modification	x						
Relaxation/meditation	x						
Sound therapy					x		
Music therapy					x		
Family therapy	x						
Sleep restoration					x		
Environment							
Outdoor-play/natural environment			x				
Heavy metals					x		
Lead					x		
Mercury					x		
Manganese					x		
Aluminium					x		
Pesticides					x		
Tobacco smoke					x		
Sunshine					x		
Physical activities		x					
Outdoor play					x		
Yoga				x			
Nutritional influences							
Food sensitivities and trial elimination diet		x					
Additives		x					
Colourings					x		
Nutritional supplements							
Magnesium/B6		x					
Zinc		x					
Iron				x			
Other supplements							
Amino acids (acetyl-L-caratine)		x			x		
n–3 fatty acids/EFA		x					
Tryptophan					x		
Melatonin (sleep)		x					

Continued

Table 6.1 Levels of evidence for lifestyle and complementary medicines/therapies in the management of ADHD—cont'd: TCM herbs)—cont'd

Modality	Level I	Level II	Level IIIa	Level IIIb	Level IIIc	Level IV	Level V
Herbal medicines							
SJW		x(-)					
Ginkgo biloba and/or *Ginseng*				x			
Traditional Chinese medicine mixture:							
[*Bupleurum chinense, Scutellaria baicalensis, Astragalus membranaceus, Codonopsis pilosula, Ligustrum lucidum, lophatherum gracile* and *thread of ivory*]				x			
Duodongining				x			
Yihzi mixture				x			
Pycnogenol		x					
Homeopathy	x(-)						
Physical therapies							
Massage	x						
Chiropractic					x		

Level I — from a systematic review of all relevant randomised controlled trials, meta-analyses.
Level II — from at least 1 properly designed randomised controlled clinical trial.
Level IIIa — from well-designed pseudo-randomised controlled trials (alternate allocation or some other method).
Level IIIb — from comparative studies (including systematic reviews of such studies) with concurrent controls and allocation not randomised, cohort studies, case-control studies, or interrupted time series with a parallel control group.
Level IIIc — from comparative studies with historical control, 2 or more single-arm studies or interrupted time series without a parallel control group.
Level IV — opinions of respected authorities based on clinical experience, descriptive studies or reports of expert committees.
Level V — represents minimal evidence that represents testimonials.

Clinical tips handout for patients — attention deficit hyperactivity disorder (ADHD)

1 Lifestyle advice

Sleep

- All children should be fully assessed and treated for underlying sleep disorders.
- Appropriate amount of physical activity during the day can help sleep.
- Herbal teas such as chamomile can be helpful in some cases.
- Magnesium (up to 350mg elemental) can be used to calm the child during the day and assist sleep at night (3 month trial).
- L-Tryptophan (50–100mg in children and 100–200mg adults) may be trialled for 1 month 1 hour before bedtime (not with antidepressant medications).
- Melatonin (3mg for children and 3–6mg for adults) at bedtime may be trialled for 1 month (not with L-Tryptophan or antidepressant medications).

Sunshine

- At least 15 minutes sunshine is needed daily for vitamin D production. More sun exposure may be required in cooler areas, winter and in people with dark skin.
- Sunscreen can block the conversion to vitamin D so this should be avoided during this specified time period.

2 Physical activity/exercise

- Play outdoors in a natural environment such as a natural park or countryside as much as possible. As little as 30 minutes daily can make a significant difference.
- Vigorous exercise and 'rough-and-tumble' play can help to reduce levels of hyperactivity and assist sleep.
- Yoga practice is a useful adjunct to ADHD medications.

3 Mind–body medicine

- Neurobiofeedback in the form of video games can be very helpful in reducing symptoms of hyperactivity and impulsivity, and can improve attention, IQ, processing speed and music performance.
- The child should be 6 years of age or older.
- Usually 20–30 sessions of biofeedback are required to achieve results comparable to methylphenidate. Significant behavioural and cognitive improvements are reported for at least 6 months after cessation of biofeedback.

Counselling/psychotherapy

- Both behavioural and cognitive behaviour therapy (CBT) interventions are highly effective for children and adults with ADHD.
- Children respond positively to behavioural interventions only when they are appropriately implemented at school and in the home.
- Mindfulness meditation, Sahaja Yoga meditation and relaxation training can all be effective in improving symptoms of ADHD. (see: www.sesighs.health.nsw.gov.au/rhw/)
- Anecdotal evidence strongly supports the use of soothing music and sound therapy (Tomatis Method, integrated listening system eg.www.integratedlistening.com).

4 Environment

- Playing outdoors in a natural environment such as a natural park or countryside as much as possible to avoid air pollution, traffic, and breathe fresh air.
- Lead, mercury, manganese, aluminium, copper and industrial chemicals (PCBs, arsenic) have all been found to be possible contributing factors to ADHD.
- All children with ADHD should ideally be tested for the presence of heavy metals. This can be done by hair mineral analysis or comprehensive urinary element profile through a health practitioner.
- Only with heavy metal toxicity detected: Chelation therapies can range from gentle (Epsom salt/clay baths, coriander, chlorella, chelating foot-pads) to stronger means (zinc supplementation, metallothionine promoting supplements, DMSA, DMPS chelating agents) where necessary. Discuss this with your doctor.
- Avoidance of chemicals, pesticides and tobacco smoke is important.

5 Dietary changes

- Many children have digestion problems ('irritable bowel syndrome') (abdominal bloating/discomfort, diarrhoea, constipation, excess burping/flatulence, reflux) which may adversely affect their behaviour.
- An abdominal X-ray can often reveal hidden constipation.
- Supervised food elimination regimes are extremely important in identifying problem foods that trigger hyperactivity, impulsivity and inattention. There is no point using

other therapies if the child is eating something every day that continues to trigger certain behaviours.
- The most common problem foods include artificial additives, sugar, wheat (gluten), cow's milk (casein) and salicylates.
- Foods may be eliminated for a period of 3 weeks, then each food/component reintroduced separately (e.g. wheat/yeast/gluten; lactose-free, 'A2' milk).

6 Supplementation

Probiotics

- Indication: to aid digestion and reduce 'IBS' symptoms. They should be used in conjunction with dietary modifications.
- Dosage: 1–2 capsules before breakfast.
- Results: 1 month.
- Side-effects: if using wrong probiotic, digestion symptoms may get worse.
- Contraindications: true dairy allergies if dairy in preparation.

Digestive enzymes

- Indication: to aid digestion in the short term and improve quality of life (e.g. at birthday parties) where children are exposed to 'problem foods'.
- Dosage: 1 capsule 10 minutes before 'problem food'.
- Results: immediate.
- Side-effects: very mild and rare.
- Contraindications: nil known.

Gut-healing herbs and nutrients (glutamine, aloe-vera, slippery elm)

- Indication: to assist healing of the digestive system whilst avoiding 'problem foods'.
- Dosage: maximum dose as directed.
- Results: 1–3 months.
- Side-effects: diarrhoea.
- Contraindications: hypersensitivity to ingredients.

Magnesium

- Indication: to reduce hyperactivity, restless legs, teeth grinding, 'growing pains', chocolate cravings and to improve sleep.
- Dosage: up to 350mg elemental milligrams/day until age 12 or equivalent usual weight: 750mg/day for adults.
- Results: 1–3 months.
- Side-effects: diarrhoea, gastric irritation; oral magnesium can cause gastrointestinal irritation, nausea, vomiting, and diarrhoea. The dosage varies from person to person. Although rare, toxic levels can cause low blood pressure, thirst, heart arrhythmia, drowsiness and weakness.
- Contraindications: Renal failure, kidney disease, heart block.

Vitamin B6

- Indication: to reduce hyperactivity/anxiety and increase attention in combination with magnesium.
- Dosage: Pyridoxal-5-Phosphate (Activated B6) up to 20mg/day.
- Results: 1–3 months. Always need to be combined with B complex in long-term use.
- Side-effects: paraesthesia in extremities, bone pain, muscle weakness at high levels. Reversible on cessation of supplement as soon as symptoms develop; may cause long-term problems with long-term use and with very high doses(>50mg/day).
- Contraindications: caution with amiodarone, phenobarbitone, phenytoin.

Zinc

- Indication: to treat zinc deficiency (note white marks on nails, plasma zinc ideally >14). To chelate heavy metals (if evident upon testing). To assist with reducing hyperactivity, impulsivity, impaired socialisation and reducing inattention.
- Dosage: needs to be individualised as some children need very high doses depending upon their biochemistry. Minimum dose 10mg elemental zinc.
- Results:1–3 months.
- Side-effects: nausea and vomiting (if taken in excess), metallic taste in mouth, reduced copper after long-term use.
- Contraindications: sideroblastic anaemia, severe kidney disease, above normal plasma levels of zinc (>18 micromols/litre).

Fish oils (EPA/DHA)

- Indication: To improve attention, IQ, sleep and reduce hyperactivity, and impulsivity.
- Dosage: Ideally DHA>EPA for learning, processing disorders. Doses between 1-9g EPA/DHA daily.
- Results: 1–3 months.
- Side-effects: Fishy burps, diarrhoea, gastrointestinal discomfort.
- Contraindications: Fish allergy. Caution with anticoagulants at very high doses.

L-Tyrosine

- Indication: to reduce hyperactivity and impulsivity.
- Dosage: 500mg up to 3 times daily as required.
- Results: 1–3 months. Can be as early as 1 week.

- Side-effects: migraines, gastrointestinal upset, fatigue, reflux, arthralgia, insomnia, nervousness.
- Contraindications: melanoma. Caution with manic conditions, hyperthyroidism, antidepressants (MAOIs, SSRIs TCAs).

Iron

- Indication: to treat iron deficiency, restless legs at night, reduced hyperactivity.
- Dosage: depending on age and serum levels, between 20mg-40mg/day.
- Results: 3–6 months.
- Side-effects: constipation, dark stools, nausea, diarrhoea, reflux.
- Contraindications: haemachromatosis, haemosiderosis, above normal iron levels.

Carnitine

- Indication: inattention, possibly aggressive behaviour.
- Dosage: 500–1500mg twice daily.
- Results: 1–3 months.
- Side-effects: mild gastrointestinal symptoms-nausea, vomiting, diarrhoea, changes in body odour.
- Contraindications: caution with anticoagulants, epilepsy, chronic liver disease.

References

1 Kaiser NM, Hoza B, Hurt EA. Multimodal treatment for childhood ADHD. Expert Rev Neurother 2008;8(10):1573–83.
2 Hassler F, Duck A, Reis O, et. al. Alternative agents used in ADHD. Z Kinder Jugendpsychiatr Psychother 2009;37(1):13–24.
3 Tomas L. ADHD. J Comp Med 2004;3(2): 24–30.
4 J Am Acad Child Adolesc Psychiatry 2001;40:141–7.
5 Appl Psychophysiology and Biofeedback 2003;28(1):1–12.
6 Weber W, Newmark S. Complementary and alternative medical therapies for ADHD and autism. Pediatr Clin North Am 2007;54(6):983–1006.
7 Chan E. The role of CAM in ADHD. J Dev Behave Pediatr 2002;23(1)(suppl.):S37–45.
8 Sawni A. ADHD and CAM. Adolesc Med State Art Rev 2008;19(2):313–26.
9 Sihna D, Efron D. CAM use in children with ADHD. J Pediatr Child Health 2005;41(1–2):23–6.
10 Kidd PM. ADHD in children: rationale for its integrative management. Altern Med Rev 2000;5:402–28.
11 Herrmann M, King K, Weitzman M. Prenatal tobacco smoke and postnatal second hand smoke exposure and child neurodevelopment. Curr Opin Pediatr 2008;20(2):184–90.
12 Braun JM, Froelich TE, Daniels JL, et. al. Association of environmental toxicants and conduct disorder in US children: NHANES 2001–2004. Environ Health Perspect 2008;116(7):956–62.
13 Braun JM, Kahn RS, Froelich T, et. al. Exposures to environmental toxicants and ADHD in US children. Environ Health Perspect 2006;114(12):1904–9.
14 Banerjee TD, Middleton F, Faraone SV. Environmental risk factors for ADHD. Acta Pediatr 2007;96(9):1269–74.
15 Linnet KM, Dalsgaard S, Obel C, et. al. Maternal lifestyle factors in pregnancy risk of ADHD and associated behaviours: review of the current evidence. Am J Psychiatry 2003;160(6):1028–40.
16 Patel K, Curtis LT. A comprehensive approach to treating autism and ADHD; a prepilot study. J Altern Complement Med 2007;13(10):1091–7.
17 Brennan AR, Arnsten AF. Neuronal mechanisms underlying ADHD: the influence of arousal on prefrontal cortical function. Ann N Y Acad Sci 2008;1129:236–45.
18 Krause J. SPECT and PET of the dopamine transporter in ADHD. Expert Rev Neurother 2008;8(4):611–25.
19 Wilens TE. Effects of Methylphenidateon the catecholaminergic system in ADHD. J Clin Psychopharmacol 2008;28(3)(suppl. 2):S46–S53.
20 Friel PN. EEG biofeedback in the treatment of ADHD. Altern Med Rev 2007;12(2):146–51.
21 Heinrich H, Gevensleben H, Strehl U. Annotation: Neuro-feedback-train your brain to train your behaviour. J Child Psycho Psychiatry 2007;48(1): 3–16.
22 Butnik SM. Neuro-feedback in adolescents and adults with ADHD. J Clin Psychol 2005;61(5):621–5.
23 Levesque J, Beauregard M, Mensour B. Effect of neuro-feedback training on the neural substrates of selective attention in children with ADHD: a functional MRI study. Neurosci Lett 2006;394(3):216–21.
24 Thompson L, Thompson M. Neuro-feedback combined with training in metacognitive strategies; effectiveness in students with ADD. Appl Psychophysiol Biofeedback 1998;23(4):243–63.
25 Monastra VJ. QEEG and ADHD: Implications for clinical practice. Curr Psychiat Rep 2008;10(5): 432–8.
26 Hou JH, Zhang Y, Xu C. EEG Biofeddback for the treatment of ADHD in children. Zhongguo Dang Dai Er Ke Za Zhi 2008;10(6):726–7.
27 Doehnert M, Brandeis D, Straub M, et. al. Slow cortical potential neuro-feedback in ADHD: is there neurophysiological evidence for specific effects? J Neural Transm 2008;115(10):1445–56.
28 Alexander DM, Hermens DF, Keage HA, et. al. Event-related wave activity in the EEG provides new marker of ADHD. Clin Neurophysiol 2008;119(1):163–79.
29 Leins U, Goth G, Hinterberger T, et. al. Neuro-feedback for children with ADHD: a comparison of SCP and Theta/Beta protocols. Appl Psychophysiol Biofeedback 2007;32(2):73–88.
30 Strehl U, Leins U, Goth G, et. al. Self-regulation of slow cortical potentials: a new treatment for children with ADHD. Pediatrics 2006;118(5):e1530-40.
31 Holtmann M, Stadler C. EEG Biofeedback for the treatment of ADHD in children and adolescence. Expert Rev Neurother 2006;6(4):533–40.
32 Beauregard M, Levesque J. Functional MRI investigation of the effects of neuro-feedback training on the neural bases of selective attention and response inhibition in children with ADHD. Appl Psychophysiol Biofeedback 2006;31(1):3–20.
33 Xiong Z, Shi S, Xu H. A controlled study of the effectiveness of EEG biofeedback training on children with ADHD. J Huazhong Univ Sci Technolog Med Sci 2005;25(3):368–70.

34 Fox DJ, Tharp DF, Fox LC. Neuro-feedback: an alternative and efficacious treatment for ADHD. Appl Psychophysiol Biofeedback 2005;30(4): 365–73.
35 Loo SK, Barkley RA. Clinical utility of EEG in ADHD. Appl Neuropsychol 2005;12(2):64–76.
36 Gruzelier J, Wegner T. Critical validation studies of neuro-feedback. Child Adolesc psychiatr Clin N Am 2005;14(1):83–104.
37 Rossiter T. the effectiveness of neuro-feedback and stimulant drugs in treating ADHD: part 11. Replication. Appl Psychophysiol Biofeedback 2004;(2)994:233–43.
38 Monastra VJ. EEG biofeedback as a treatment for ADHD: rationale and empirical foundation. Child Adolesc Psychiatr Clin N Am. 2005;14(1):55–82.
39 Holtmann M, Stadler C, Leins U, et. al. Neuro-feedback for the treatment of ADHD in childhood and adolescence. Z Kinder Jugendpsychiatr Psychother. 2004;32(3):187–200.
40 Nash JK. Treatment of ADHD with Neurotherapy. Clin EEG 2000;31(1):30–7.
41 Linden M, Habib T, Radojevic V. A controlled study of the effects of EEG biofeedback on cognition and behaviour of children with ADD and learning disabilities. Biofeedback and Self-regulation 1996;21:35–49.
42 Lubar JF, Swartwood MO, Swartwood JN, et. al. Evaluation of the effectiveness of EEG neuro-feedback training for ADHD in a clinical setting as measured by changes in T.O.V.A. scores, behavioural ratings and WISC-R performance. Biofeedback and Self-regulation 1995;20(1):83–99.
43 Baumgaertal A. Alternative and controversial treatments for ADHD. Paediatr Clin of North Am 1999; 46(5):977–92.
44 Fuchs T, Birbaumer N, Lutzenberger W, et. al. Neuro-feedback treatment for ADHD in children: a comparison with methylphenidate. Appl Psychophysiology and Biofeedback 2003;28(1):1–12.
45 Monastra VJ, Monastra DM, George S. The effects of stimulant therapy, EEG biofeedback and parenting style of ADHD. Appl Psychopys and Biofeedback 2002;27(4):231–49.
46 Knight LA, Rooney M, Chronis-Tuscano A. Psychosocial treatments for ADHD. Curr Psychiatry Rep 2008;10(5):412–8.
47 Daly BP, Creed T, Xanthpoulos M, et. al. Psychosocial treatments for children with ADHD. Neuropsychol Rev 2007;17(1):73–89.
48 Waxmonsky JG. Non-stimulant therapies for ADHD in children and adults. Essent Psychopharmacol 2005;6(5):262–76.
49 Toplak ME, Connors L, Shuster J, et. al. review of Cognitive, CBT and neural-based interventions for ADHD. Clin Psychol Rev 2008;28(5):801–23.
50 Brown RT, Amler RW, Freeman WS, et. al. Treatment of ADHD: Overview of the evidence. Pediatrics 2005;115(6):e749–57.
51 Montgomery P, Bjornstad G, Dennis J. Media-based behavioural treatments for behavioural problems in children. Cochrane Database Syst Rev 2006;(1):CD002206.
52 Bjornstad G, Montgomery P. Family therapy for ADD or ADHD in children and adolescents. Cochrane Database Syst Rev 2005;(2):CD005042.
53 Knouse LE, Cooper-Vince C, Sprich S, et. al. Recent developments in the psychosocial treatment of ADHD. Expert Rev Neurother 2008;8(10): 1537–48.
54 Ramsay JR. Current status of CBT as a psychosocial treatment for adults with ADHD. Curr Psychiatry Rep 2007;9(5):427–33.
55 Zylowski L, Ackerman DL, Yang MH, et. al. Mindfulness meditation training in adults and adolescents with ADHD: a feasibility study. J Atten Disord 2008;11(6):737–46.
56 Goldbeck L, Schmid K. Effectiveness of autogenic relaxation training in children and adolescents with behavioural and emotional problems. J Am Acad Child Adolesc Psychiatry 2003;42(9):1046–54.
57 Klein SA, Deffenbacher JL. Relaxation and exercise for hyperactive impulsive children. Percept Mot Skills 1977;45:1159–62
58 Donney VK, Poppen R. Teaching parents to conduct behavioural relaxation training with their hyperactive children. J Behav Ther Exp Psychiatry 1989;20:319–25.
59 Raymer R, Poppen R. Behavioural relaxation training with hyperactive children. J Behav Ther Exp Psychiatry 1985;16:309–16.
60 Dunn FM, Howell RJ. Relaxation training and its relationship to hyperactivity in boys. J Clin Psychology 1982;38:92–100.
61 Gumenyuk V, Korzyukov O, Escera C, et. al. Electrophysiological evidence of enhanced distractability in ADHD children. Neurosci Lett 2005;374(3):212–7.
62 Soderlund G, SikstromS, Smart A. Listen to the noise: Noise is beneficial for cognitive performance in ADHD. Child Psychol Psychiatry 2007;48(8):840–7.
63 Rickson DJ. Intstructional and improvisational models of music therapy with adescents who have ADHD: a comparison of the effects on motor impulsivity. J Music Ther 2006;43(1):39–62.
64 Quach J, Hiscock H, Canterfield L, et. al. Outcomes of child sleep problems over the school transition period: Australian Population Longitudinal Study. Pediatrics 2009;123(5):1287–92.
65 Dominguez-Ortega L, de Vincente-Colomina A. ADHD and sleep disorders. Med Clin (Barc) 2006;126(13):500–6.
66 Betancourt-Fursow DE, Jimenez YM, Jimenez-Leon JC, et. al. ADHD and sleep disorders. Rev Neurol 2006;42(suppl.2):S37–51.
67 Pandi-Perumal SR, Srinivasan V, Spence DW, et. al. Role of the Melatonin system in the control of sleep: therapeutic implications. CNS Drugs 2007;21(12):995–1018.
68 Van der Heijden KB, Smits MG, Van Someren EJ, et. al. Effect of melatonin on sleep, behaviour and cognition in ADHD and chronic sleep-onset insomnia. J Am Acad Child Adolesc Psychiatry 2007;46(2):233–41.
69 Weiss MD, Wasdell MB, Bomben MM, et. al. Sleep hygiene and melatonin treatment for children and adolescents with ADHD and initial insomnia. J Am Acad Child Adolesc Psychiatry 2006;45(5):512–9.
70 Kuo FE, Taylor AF. A potential natural treatment for attention-deficit/hyperactivity disorder: evidence from a national study. American Journal of Public Health 2004;94(9):1580–6.
71 Markowitz M. Lead poisoning: a disease for the next millennium. Curr Probl Pediatr 2000;30(3):62–70.
72 Gilbert SG, Weiss B. A Rationale for lowering the blood lead action level from 10 to 2ug/dL. Neurotoxicology 2006;27(5):693–701.
73 Woolf AD, Goldman R, Bellinger DC. Update on the clinical management of childhood lead poisoning. Pediatr Clin North Am 2007;54(2):271–94.

74 Binns HJ, Campbell C, Brown MJ, et. al. Interpreting and managing blood lead levels of <10ug/dL in children and reducing childhood exposure to lead: recommendations of the Centres for Disease Control and Prevention Advisory Committee on Childhood Lead Poisoning Prevention. Pediatrics 2007;120(5):e1285–98.

75 Bellinger DC. Very low lead exposures and children's neurodevelopment. Curr Opin pediatr 2008;20(2):172–7.

76 Lanphear BP, Hornung R, Khoury J, et. al. Low-level environmental lead exposure and children's intellectual function: an international pooled analysis. Environ Health Perspect 2005;113(7):894–9.

77 Canfield RL, Henderson CR Jr, Cory-Slechta DA, et. al. Intellectual impairment in children with blood lead concentrations <10ug/dL. N Engl J Med 2003;348(16):1517–26.

78 Guidotti TL, Ragain L. Protecting children from toxic exposure: 3 strategies. Pediatr Clin North Am 2007;54(2):227–35.

79 Surkan PJ, Zhang A, Trachtenberg F, et. al. Neuropsychological function in children with blood levels <10ug/dL. Neurotoxicology 2007;28(6):1170–7.

80 Rico JA, Kordas K, Lopez P, et. al. Efficacy of iron and/or zinc supplementation on cognitive performance of lead-exposed Mexican school-children: a RCT. Pediatrics 2006;117(3):e518–27.

81 Wang HL, Chen XT, Yang B, et. al. Case-control study of blood lead levels and ADHD in Chinese children. Environ Health Perspect 2008;116910):1401–6.

82 Nigg JT, Knottnerus GM, Martel MM, et. al. Low blood levels associated with clinically diagnosed ADHD and mediated by weak cognitive control. Biol Psychiatry 2008;63(3):325–31.

83 Kordas K, Stoltzfus RJ, Lopez P, et. al. Iron and zinc supplementation does not improve parent or teacher ratings of behaviour in first Grade Mexican children exposed to lead. J Pediatr 2005;147(5):632–9.

84 Dye BA, Schober SE, Dillon CF, et. al. Urinary mercury concentrations assoc with dental restorations in adult women aged 16–49 years: US 1999–2000. Occup Environ Med 2005;62(6):368–75.

85 Nylander M, Friberg L, Lind B. Mercury concentrations in the human brain and kidneys in relation to exposure from dental amalgam fillings. Swed Dent J 1987;11(5):179–87.

86 Kingman A, Albertini T, Rown LJ. Hg concentrations in urine and whole blood assoc with amalgam exposure in a US military population. J Dent Res 1998;77(3):461–71.

87 Brownawell AM, Berent S, Brent RL, et. al. The potential adverse effects of dental amalgam. Toxicol Rev 2005;24(1):1–10.

88 Shenker BJ, Maserejian NN, Zhang A, et. al. Immune function effects of dental amalgam in children: a RCT. J Am Dent Assoc 2008;139(11): 1496–505.

89 DeRouen TA, Martin MD, Leroux BG, et. al. Neurobehavioral effects of dental amalgam in children — a Randomised clinical trial. JAMA 2006;295(15):1784–92.

90 Bellinger DC, Trachtenberg F, Daniel D, et. al. Dental amalgam restorations and children's neuropsychological function: the New England Children's Amalgum Trial. Environ Health Perspect 2007;115(3):440–6.

91 Bellinger DC, Trachtenberg F, Barregard L, et. al. Neuropsychological and renal effects of dental amalgam in children- a Randomised clinical trial. JAMA 2006;295(15):1775–83.

92 Bellinger DC, Trachtenberg F, Daniel D, et. al. A dose-effect analysis of children's exposure to dental amalgam and neuropsychological function: the New England Children's Amalgum Trial. J Am Dent Assoc 2007;138(9):1210–6.

93 Cheuk DK, Wong V. ADHD and blood Mercury level: a case-control study in Chinese children. Neuropediatrics 2006;37(4):234–40.

94 Elsner RJ, Spangler JG. Neurotoxicity of Inhaled Mn: public health danger in the shower? Med Hypotheses 2005;65(3):607–16.

95 Bourchard M, Laforest F, Vandelac L, et. al. Hair Mn and hyperactive behaviours: pilot study of school-age children exposed through tap water. Environ Health Perspect 2007;115(1):122–7.

96 Halatek T, Sinczuk-Walczak H, Rydzynski K. Early neurotoxic effects of inhalation exposure to Al and/or Mn assessed by serum levels of phospholipid-binding Clara cells protein. J Environ Sci Health A Tox Hazard Subst Environ Eng 2008;43(2): 118–24.

97 Labie D. Developmental neurotoxicity of industrial chemicals. Med Sci (Paris) 2007;23(10):868–72.

98 Grandjean P, Landrigan PJ. Developmental neurotoxicity of industrial chemicals. Lancet 2006;368:2167–78.

99 Hussain J, Woolf AD, Sandel M, et. al. Environmental evaluation of a child with developmental disability. Pediatr Clin North Am 2007;54(1):47–62.

100 Perera FP, Rauh V, Whyatt RM, et. al. A summary of recent findings on birth outcomes and development effects of prenatal ETS, PAH and pesticide exposures. Neurotoxicology 2005;26(4):573–87.

101 Landrigan PJ. Pesticides and PCBs: an analysis of the evidence that they impair children's neurobehavioral devt. Mol Genet Metab 2001;73(1):11–7.

102 Brondum J. Environmental exposures and ADHD. Environ Health Perspect 2007;115(8):A398.

103 Tantillo M, Kesick CM, Hynd GW, et. al. The effects of exercise on children with ADHD. Med Sci Sports Exerc 2002;34(2):203–7.

104 Panskepp J, Burgdorf J, Turner C, et. al. Modelling ADHD-type arousal with unilateral cortex damage in rats and beneficial effects of play therapy. Brain Cogn 2003;52(1):97–105.

105 Complement Ther Nurs Midwif 2004;10(1):46–53.

106 Haffner J, Roos J, Goldstein N, et. al. The effectiveness of body-oriented methods in the treatment of ADHD: results of a controlled pilot study. Z Kinder Jugendpsychiatr Psychotherapy 2006;(3)491:37–47.

107 Jensen PS, Kenny DT. The effects of Yoga on the attention and behaviour of boys with ADHD. J Atten Disord 2004;7(4):205–16.

108 Sinn N. Nutritional and dietary influences on ADHD. s.l.: Nutr Rev 2008;66(10):558–68.

109 Breakey J. The role of diet and behaviour in childhood. J Paediatric Clin Health 1997;33:190–4.

110 Bellisle F. Effects of diet on behaviour and cognition in children. s.l.: Br J Nutr 2004;92(suppl.2): S227–32.

111 Chaves-Carbello E. Diet therapy in the treatment of neuropaediatric disorders. s.l.: Rev Neurol 2003;37(3):267–74.

112 Boris M, Mandel FS. Foods and additives are common causes of ADHD in children. Ann Allergy 1994;72(5):462–8.
113 Peisser LM, Frankena K, Toorman J, et. al. A RCT into the effects of food on ADHD. Eur Child Adolesc Psychiatry 2009;18(1):12–19.
114 Schnoll R, Burshteyn D, Cea-Aravena J. Nutrition in the treatment of ADHD: a neglected but important aspect. s.l.: Appl Psychophysiol Biofeedback 2003:28(1):63–75.
115 Pelsser LM, Buitelaar JK. Favourable effect of a standard elimination diet on the behaviour of young children with ADHD: A pilot study. Nederlands Tijdschrift voor Geneeskunde 2002. 146(52):2543–47.
116 Stevenson J. Dietary influences on cognitive development and behaviour in children. s.l.: Proc Nutr Soc 2006;65(4):361–5.
117 Cruz NV, Bahna SL. Do food or additives cause behaviour disorders? s.l.: Pediatr Ann 2006;35(10):744–5,748–54.
118 Lees of MH. Food Intolerances and Allergy — a review. QJ Med 1983;52(206):111–9.
119 Silfverdal SA, Hernall O. Food additives can increase hyperactivity in children. Results from a British study confirm the connection t. s.l.: Lakartidningen 2008;105(6):354–5.
120 Wallis C. Hyper kids? Check their diet. Reserach confirms a long-suspected link between hypcrectivity and food additives. s.l.: Time 2007;170(13):68.
121 Ghuman JK, Arnold LE, Anthony BJ. Psychopharmacological and other treatments in preschool children with ADHD: Current evidence and practice. s.l.: J Child Adolesc Psychopharmacol 2008;18(5):413–47.
122 Lau K, McLean WG, Williams DP, et. al. Synergistic interactions between community used food additives in a developmental neurotoxicity test. s.l.: Toxicol Sci 2006;90(1):178–87.
123 Cardinale F, Mangini F, Berardi M, et. al. Intolerance to food additives: an update. s.l.: Minerve Pediatr 2008:60(6):1401–9.
124 McCann D, Barrett A, Cooper A, et. al. Food additives and hyperactive behaviour in 3 year old and 8/9 year old children in the community: a Randomised Double Blinded Placebo-controlled Trial. s.l.: Lancet 2007;370(9598):1560–7.
125 Batemen B, Warner JO, Hutchinson E, et. al. The effects of a double-blind,placeb-controlled, artificial food colourings and benzoate preservatives challenge on hyperactivity in a general population sample of preschool children. s.l.: Arch Dis Child 2004;89(6):506–11.
126 Krummel D, Seligson FH, Guthrie HA. Hyperactivity: Is candy causal? Critical Reviews in Food Science and Nutrition 1996;36(1, 2):31–47.
127 Tsaluchidu S, Cocchi M, Tonello L, et. al. Fatty acids and oxidative stress in psychiatric disorders. s.l.: BMC Psychiatry 2008;8(suppl.)1:S5.
128 Niederhofer H, Pittschieler K. A preliminary investigation of ADHD symptoms in persons with coeliac disease. s.l.: J Atten Disord 2006;10(2):200–4.
129 Pynnonen PA, Isometsa ET, Verkasalo MA, et. al. Gluten-free diet mey alleviate depressive and behavioural symptoms in adolescents with coeliac disease: a prospective follow-up acse-series. s.l.: BMC Psychiatry 2005:5:14.
130 Lahlat E, Broide E, Leshem M, et. al. Prevalence of coeliac antibodies in children with neurological disorders. s.l.: Pediatr Neurol 2000;22(5):393–6.
131 Bourre JM. Effects of nutrients (food) on the structure and function of the nervous system: update on dietary requirements for brain. Part 1: micronutrients. J Nutr Health Ageing 2006;10(5):377–85.
132 Ramakrishnan U, Imhoff-Kunsch B, DiGirolamo AM. Role of DHA in maternal and child health. Am J Clin Nutr 2009;89(3):958S–62S.
133 Mousain-Bosc M, Roche M, Rapin J, et. al. M6 / Vit B6 intake reduces CNS hyperexcitability in children. s.l.: J Am Coll Nutr 2004;23(5):545S–48S.
134 Nogovitsina OR, Levitina EV. Neurological aspects of the clinical features, pathophysiology and corrections of impairments in ADHD. Neurosci Behav Physiol 2007;37(3):199–202.
135 Nogovitsina OR, Levitina EV. Effect of MAGNE-B6 on the clinical and biochemical manifestations of the syndrome of attention deficit and hyperactivity in children. Eksp Klin Farmacol 2006;69(1):74–7.
136 Nogovitsina OR, Levitina AV. Diagnostic value of examination of ther Mg homeostasis in children with ADHD. Klin Lab Diagn 2005;(5):P17–9.
137 Mousain-Bosc M, Roche M, Polge A, et. al. Improvement of neurobehavioral disorders in children supplemented with magnesium-Vitamin B6. ADHD. Magnes Res 2006; 19(1):46–52.
138 Starobrat-Hermilin B, Kozielec T. The effects of Mg physiological suppl on hyperactivity in children with ADHD. Positive response to Mg oral loading test. Magnes Res 1997;10(2):149–56.
139 Konofal E, Lecendreux M, Arnulf I, et. al. Iron deficiency in children with ADHD. Arch Pediatr Adolesc Med 2004;158(12):1113–5.
140 Oner O, Alkar OY, Oner P. Relation of ferritin levels with symptom ratings and cognitive performance in children with ADHD. Pediatr Int 2008;50(1):40–4.
141 Burden M, Westerlund A, Armony-Sivan R, et. al. An event-related potential study of attention and recognition memory in infants with iron deficiency anaemia. Pediatrics 2007; !20(2):336–345.
142 Patrick LR. Restless legs syndrome: pathophysiology and the role of iron and folate. Altern Med Rev 2007;12(2):101–12.
143 Konofal E, Lecendreux M, Deron J, et. al. Effects of iron suppl on ADHD in children. Pediatr Neurol 2008;38(1):20–6.
144 Martins S, Logan S, Gilbert R. Cochrane Database of Syst Rev 2006; CD001444.
145 Arnold LE, Pinkham SM, Votolato N. Does zinc moderate essential fatty acid and amphetamine treatment for ADHD? J Child & Adolescent Psychopharmacology 2000. 10(2):111–17.
146 Yorbik O, Ozdag MF, Olgun A, et. al. Potential effects of zinc on information processing in boys with ADHD. Prog Neuropsychopharmacol Biol Psychiatry 2008;32(3):662–7.
147 Bilici M, Yildrim F, Kandil S, et. al. Double-blind, placebo-controlled study of zinc sulfate in the treatment of ADHD. Prog Neuropsychopharmacol Biol Psychiatry 2004;28(1):181–90.
148 Arnold LE, DiSilvestro RA. Zinc in ADHD. J Child Adolesc Psychopharmacol 2005;15(4):619–27.
149 Arnold LE, Bozzolo H, Hollway J, et. al. Serum zinc correlates with parent and teacher-rated inattention in children with ADHD. J Child Adolesc Psychopharmacol 2005;15(4):628–36.
150 Bekaroglu M, Aslan Y, Gedik Y, et. al. Relationships between serum free fatty acids and zinc, and ADHD: A research note. J Child Psychology & Psychiatry & Allied Disciplines.1996; 37(2):225–7.

151 Rucklodge JJ, Johnstone J, Kaplan BJ. Nutrient supplementation approaches in the treatment of ADHD. s.l.: Expert Rev Neurother 2009:9(4): 461–76.
152 Uckardes Y, Ozmert EN, Unal F, et. al. Effects of zinc supplementation on parent and teacher behaviour rating scores in low socioeconomic level Turkish primary school children. Acta Paediatr 2009;98(4):731–6.
153 Akhondzadeh S, Mohammadi MR, Khademi M. Zinc sulfate as an adjunct to Methylphenidate for the treatment of ADHD in children: a double-blind and randomized trial. BMC Psychiatry 2004;4:9.
154 DiGirolamo AM, Ramirez-Zea M. Role of zinc in maternal and child mental health. Am J Clin Nutr 2009;89(3):940S–45S.
155 Arnold LE, Votolato NA, Kleykamp D, et. al. Does hair zinc improve amphetamine improvement of ADD/Hyperactivity? Int J Neuros ci.,1990.50(1–2):103–7.
156 Stevens LJ, Zentall SS, Deck JL, et. al. Essential fatty acid metabolism in boys with ADHD. Am J Clin Nut 1995.62(4):761–8.
157 Germano M, Meleleo D, Montorfano G, et. al. Plasma, RBC phospholipids and clinical evaluation after long chain n-3 supp. in children with ADHD. Nutr Neurosci 2007;10(1–2):1–9.
158 Peet M, Stokes C. Omega-3 fatty acids in the treatment of psychiatric disorders. Drugs 2005;65(8):1051–9.
159 Kidd PM. Omega-3 DHA and EPA for cognition, behaviour and mood: clinical findings and structural functional synergies with cell membrane phospholipids. Altern Med Rev 2007;12(3): 207–27.
160 Frohlich J, Dopfner M. The treatment of ADHD with PUFAs-an effective treatment alternative? Z Kinder Jugendpsychiatr Psychother 2008;36(2): 109–16.
161 Haag M. Essential fatty acids and the brain. Can J Psychiatry 2003. 48(3):195–203.
162 Antalis CJ, Stevens LJ, Campbell M, et. al. Omega-3 fatty acids in ADHD. Prostaglandins Leuko essent Fatty acids 2006;75(4–5):299–308.
163 Richardson AJ. LCPUFAs in childhood developmental and psychiatric disorders. Lipids 2004;39(12):1215–22.
164 Young GS, Conquer JA, Thomas R. Effect of randomized supplementation with high dose olive, flax or fish oil on serum phospholipid fatty acid levels in adults with ADHD. Reprod Nutr Rev 2005;45(5):549–58.
165 Burgess JR, Stevens L, Zhang W, et. al. Long chain polyunsaturated fatty acids in children with ADHD. Am J Clin Nut 2000. 71(1)(suppl.): 327S–30S.
166 Mitchell EA, Aman MG, Turbott SH, et. al. Clinical characteristics and serum EFA levels in hyperactive children. Clin Paediatr 1987. 26(8):406–411.
167 Farooqu AA, Horrocks LA. Plasmalogens, phospholipase A2 and DHA turnover in brain tissue. J Mol Neurosci 2001. 16(2–3):263–272;discussion 279–284.
168 Riediger ND, Othman RA, Suh M, et. al. A systemic review of the roles of n-3 fatty acids in health and disease. J Am Diet Assoc 2009;109(4):668–79.
169 Sinn N, Bryan J, Wilson C. Cognitive effects of PUFAs in children with ADHD symptoms: a RCT. Prostaglandins Leukot Essent Fatty Acids 2008;7894–5):311–26.
170 Vaisman N, Kaysar N, Zaruk-Adasha Y, et. al. correlation between changes in blood fatty acid composition and visual sustained attention performance in children with inattention: effect of dietary n-3 fatty acids containing phospholipids. Am J Clin Nutr 2008;87(5):1170–80.
171 Sinn N, Bryan J. Effect of supplementation with PUFAs and micronutrients on learning and behaviour problems associated with child ADHD. J Dev Behav Pediatr 2007;28(2):82–91.
172 Sorgi PJ, Hallowell EM, Hutchins HL, et. al. Effects of an open-label pilot study with high dose EPA/DHA concentrates on plasma phospholipids and behaviour in children with ADHD. Nutr J 2007;6:16.
173 Ross BM, Seguin J, Sieswerda LE. Omega-3 fatty acids as treatments for mental illness: which disorder and which fatty acid? Lipids Health Dis 2007;6:21.
174 Richardson AJ. Omega-3 fatty acids in ADHD and related neurodevelopmental disorders. Int Rev Psychiatry 2006;18(2):155–72.
175 Richardson AJ, Montgomery P. The Oxford-Durham study: a RCT of dietary supp with fatty acids in children with development coordination disorder. Pediatrics 2005;115(5):1360–6.
176 Arnold LE, Kleykamp D, Votolato NA, et. al. Gamma-linolenic acid for ADHD: Placebo-controlled comparison to D-Amphetamine. Biol Psychiatry 1989.15;25(2):222–8.
177 Aman MG, Mitchell EA, Turbott SH. The effects of EFA supplementation in hyperactive children. J Abnorm Child Psychology 1987;15(1):75–90.
178 Richardson AJ, Puri BK. A Randomised double-blind, placebo-controlled study of the effects of supplementation with highly unsaturated fatty acids on ADHD-related symptoms in children with specific learning difficulties. Prog Neuropsychopharmacol Biol Psychiatry 2002.26(2):233–9.
179 Richardson AJ, Puri BK. The Potential role of fatty acids in ADHD. Prostaglandins, Leukotrienes and EFA's,2000. 63(1–2):79–87.
180 Viggiano D, Ruocco LA, Arcieri S, et. al. Involvement of NAd in the control of activity and attention processes in animal models of ADHD. Neural Plast 2004;11(1–2):133–49.
181 Prince J. Catecholamine dysfunction in ADHD: an update. J Clin Psychopharmacol. 2008;28(3)(suppl. 2): S39–45.
182 Spencer TJ, Biederman J, Madras BK, et. al. Further evidence of dopamine transporter in ADHD: a controlled PET imaging study using altropane. Biol Psychiatry 2007;62(9):1059–61.
183 Levy F. What do dopamine transporter and COMT tell us about ADHD? Pharmacogenomic implications. Aust NZ J Psychiatry 2007;41(1):10–6.
184 Staller JA, Faraone SV. Targeting the dopamine system in the treatment of ADHD. Expert Rev Neurother 2007;7(4):351–62.
185 Walitza S, Melfson S, Herhaus G, et. al. Association of Parkinson's disease with symptoms of ADHD in childhood. J Neural Transm (suppl.):2007;(72):311–5.
186 Spencer TJ, Biederman J, Madras BK, et. al. In vivo neuroreceptor imaging in ADHD: a focus on the dopamine transporter. Biol Psychiatry 2005;57(11):1293–300.
187 Juciate A, Fernell E, Halldin C, et. al. Reduced midbrain dopamine transporter binding in male adolescents with ADHD: association between striatal dopamine markers and motor hyperactivity. Bio psychiatry 2005;57(3):229–38.

188 Bellgrove MA, Domachke K, Hawi Z, et. al. The methionine allele of the COMT polymorphism impairs prefrontal cognition in children and adolescents with ADHD. Exp Brain Res 2005;163(3):352–60.
189 Perlov E, Philipsen A, Hesslinger B, et. al. Reduced cingulated glutamate/glutamine to creatine ratios in adult patients with ADHD — a magnet resonance spectroscopy study. J Psychiat Res 2007;41:934–41.
190 Carrey NJ, MacMaster FP, Gaudet L, et. al. Striatal creatine and glutamate/glutamine in ADHD. J Child Adolesc Psychopharmacol 2007;17(1):11–7.
191 Pliszka SR. The neuropsychopharmacology of ADHD. Biol Psychiatry 2005;57(11):1385–90.
192 Arnsten AF. Stimulants: Therapeutic actions in ADHD. Neuropsychopharmacol 2006;31(11): 2376–83.
193 Madras BK, Miller GM, Fischman AJ. The dopamine transporter and ADHD. Biol Psychiatry 2005;57(11):1397–409.
194 Ruocco LA, de Souza Silva MA, Topic B, et. al. Intranasal application of dopamine reduces activity and improves attention in Naples High Excitability rats that feature the mesocortical variant of ADHD. Eur Neuropsychopharmacol 2009 Mar 27 [Epub ahead of print].
195 Stadler C, Zepf FD, Demisch L, et. al. Influence of rapid tryptophan depletion on laboratory-provoked aggression in children with ADHD. Neuropsychobiology 2007;56(2–3):104–10.
196 Zepf FD, Stadler C, Demisch L, et. al. Serotonergic functioning and trait-impulsivity in ADHD boys: influence of rapid tryptophan depletion. Hum Psychopharmacol 2008;23(1):43–51.
197 Zepf FD, Wockel L, Poustka F, et. al. Diminished 5–HT functioning in CBCL pediatric bipolar disorder-profiled ADHD patients versus normal ADHD: susceptibility to rapid tryptophan depletion influences reaction time performance. Hum Psychopharmacol 2008;23(4):291–9.
198 Liu LL, Yang J, Lei GF, et. al. Atomoxetine increases histamine release and improves learning deficits in an animal model of ADHD: the spontaneously hypertensive rat. Basic Clin Pharmacol Toxicol 2008;102(6):527–32.
199 Prasad S, Steer C. Switching from neurostimulant therapy to atomoxetine in children and adolescents with ADHD: clinical approaches and review of current available evidence. Paediatr Drugs 2008;10:39–47.
200 Stocking EM, Letavic MA. Histamine H3 antagonists as wake-promoting and pro-cognitive agents. Curr Top Med Chem 2008;8(11):988–1002.
201 Esbenshade TA, Browman KE, Bitner RS, et. al. The histamine H3 receptor: an attractive target for the treatment of cognitive disorders. Br J Pharmacol 2008;154(6):1166–81.
202 Esbenshade TA, Fox GB, Cowart MD. Histamine H3 receptor antagonists: preclinical promise for treating obesity and cognitive disorders. Mol Interv 2006;6(2):77–88, 59.
203 Lakhan SE, Vleira KF. Nutritional therapies for mental disorders. s.l.: Nutr J 2008;7:2.
204 Berk M, Ng F, Dean O, et. al. Glutathione: a novel treatment target in psychiatry. Trends Pharmacol Sci 2008;29(7):346–51.
205 Arnold LE, Amato A, Bozzolo H, et. al. ALC in ADHD: a multi-site, placebo-controlled pilot trial. s.l.: J Child Adolesc Psychopharmacol 2007 17(16):791–902.
206 Van Oudheusden LJ, Scholte HR. Efficacy of carnitine in the treatment of children with ADHD. Prostaglandins Leukot Essental fatty Acids 2002;67(1):33–8.
207 Adriana W, Rea M, Baviera M, et. al. ALC reduces impulsive behaviour in adolescent rats. Psychopharmacology (Berl.) 2004;176(3–4): 296–304.
208 Frei H, Everts R, von Ammon K, et. al. Homeopathic treatment of children with ADHD: a randomized, double-blind, placebo-controlled trial. Eur J Pediatr 2005;164(12):758–67.
209 Altunc U, Pittler MH, Ernst E. Homeopathy for childhood and adolescence ailments: systematic review of RCTs. Mayo Clin Proc 2007;82(1):69–75.
210 Jacobs J, Williams AL, Girard C, et. al. Homeopathy for ADHD: a pilot RCT. J Altern Complement Med 2005;11(5):799–806.
211 Pintov S, Hochman M, Livne A, et. al. Bach flower remedies used for ADHD in children- a prospective double-blind controlled study. Eur J Paediatr Neurol 2005;9(6):395–8.
212 Coulter MK, Dean ME. Homeopathy for ADHD or hyperkinetic disorder. Cochrane Database Syst Rev 2007;(4):CD005648.
213 Frei H, Everts R, von Ammon K, et. al. RCTs of homeopathy in hyperactive children: Treatment procedure leads to an unconventional study design. Experience with open-label homeopathic treatment preceding the Swiss ADHD placebo- controlled, randomized, double-blind cross-over trial. Homeopathy 2007;96(1):35–41.
214 Frei H, von Ammon K, Thurneyson A. Treatment of hyperactive children: increased efficacy through modifications of homeopathic diagnostic procedure. Homeopathy 2006;95(3):163–70.
215 Frei H, Thurneysen A. Treatment for hyperactive children: homeopathy and Methylphenidate compared in a family setting. Br Homeopath J 2001;90(4):183–8.
216 Weber W, Vander Stoep A, McCarty RL, et. al. Hypericum perforatum for ADHD in children and adolescents: a RCT. JAMA 2008;(299922):2633–41.
217 Lyon MR, Cline JC, Totosy de Zepetnek J, et. al. Effect of the Herbal Extract combination Panax quinquefolium and Ginkgo biloba on ADHD: A Pilot study. J Psychiatry Neurosci 2001;26(3):221–3.
218 Zhang H, Huang J. Preliminary study of TCM treatment of minimal brain dysfunction: analysis of 100 cases. Zhong Xi Yi He Za Zhi 1990;10(5):260, 278–9.
219 Li X, Chen Z. Clinical comparative observation on Duodongining and Ritalin in treating child hyperkinetic syndrome. Zhongguo Zhong Xi Yi Jie He Za Zhi 1999;19(7):410–11.
220 Wang LH, Li CS, Li GZ. Clinical and experimental studies on tiaoshen liquor for infantile hyperkinetic syndrome. Zhongguo Zhong Xi Yi Jie He Za Zhi 1995;15(6):337–40.
221 Ding GA, Yu GH, Chen SF. Assessment on effect of treatmentforchildrenhyperkineticsyndromebycombined therapyYizhimixtureandRitalin.ZhongguoZhongXiYi Jie He Za Zhi 2002; 22(4):255–7.
222 Chen J, Chen YY, Wang XM. Clinical study on treatment of children ADHD by Jiangqian granules. Zhongguo Zhong Xi Yi Jie He Za Zhi 2002;22(4):258–60.
223 Ng F, Berk M, Dean O, et. al. Oxidative stress in psychiatric disorders: evidence base and therapeutic implications. Int J Neuropsychopharmacol 2008;11(6):851–76.

224 Dvorakova M, Jezova D, Blazicek P, et. al. Urinary catecholamines in children with ADHD: modulation by a polyphenolic extract from pine bark (Pycnogenol). Nutr Neurosci 2007;10(3–4):151–7.
225 Dvorakova M, Sivonova M, Trebaticki J, et. al. The effect of polyphenolic extract from pine bark, Pycnogenol on the level of glutathione in children suffering from ADHD. Redox Rep 2006;11(4): 163–72.
226 Trebaticka J, Kopasova S, Hradecna Z, et. al. treatment of ADHD with French maritime pine bark extract, Pycnogenol Eur Child Adolesc Psychiatry 2006;15(6):329–35.
227 Rohdewald P. A Review of the French maritime pine bark extract, Pycnogenol, a herbal medication with a diverse clinical pharmacology. Int J Clin Pharmacol Ther 2002;40(4):158–68.
228 Packer L, Rimbach G, Virgili F. Antioxidant activity and biologic properties of a procyanidin-rich extract from pine (Pinus maritime) bark, Pycnogenol. Free Radic Biol Med 1999;27(5–6):704–24.
229 Chovanova Z, Muchova J, Sivonova M, et. al. Effect of polyphenolic, Pycnogenol, on the level of 8–oxoguanine in children suffering from ADHD. Free Radic Res 2006;40(9):1003–10.
230 Underdown A, Barlow J, Chung V, Stewart-Brown S. Massage intervention for promoting mental and physical health in infants aged under six months. The Cochrane Database of Systematic Reviews 2006:(4).
231 Field T, Quintino O, Hernandez-Reif M, et. al. Adolescents with ADHD benefit from massage therapy. Adolescence 1998;33(129):103–8.
232 Khilnani S, Field T, Hernandez-Reif M, et. al. Massage therapy improves mood and behaviour of students with ADHD. Adolescence 2003;38(152):623–38.
233 Giesen JM, Center DB, Leach RA. An evaluation of chiropractic manipulation as a treatment of hyperactivity in children. J Manipulative Physiol Ther 1989;12(5):353–63.
234 Karpouzis F, Pollard H, Bonello R. A RCT of NET for ADHD: a protocol. Trials 2009;10:6.

Chapter 7

Autism

With contribution from Dr Jenny Altermatt

Introduction

Autism is a lifelong complex neurodevelopmental disorder that has its onset in infancy. It has a wide range of clinical presentations, mostly heralded by impairments in social interaction, and communication, and repetitive, stereotyped behaviours.[1, 2] This spectrum of disorders dramatically affects the lives of patients and their families and the broader community.[3]

Children with Autism Spectrum Disorder (ASD) continue to have problems as adults, and experience challenges with independent living, mental health and social relationships, regardless of their intellectual capacity.[4]

Autism Spectrum Disorders is classified in the DSM-IV as 1 of 5 related pervasive developmental disorders, of which Asperger's syndrome, Pervasive Developmental Disorder Not Otherwise Specified (PDD-NOS), Rett's syndrome, and Disintegrative Disorder are the other 4 and these have different ages of onset and presentations.[5, 1]

Definition/diagnosis

A child may be brought into a general practice with the parents complaining that something is wrong. Listed below are established 'red flags' that alert the GP to possible concerns:[5]

- a plateau or regression in development (particularly language or social skills) not typically associated with a regression in physical development
- speech and language delay (i.e. no single words by 2 years), or stereotypical use of language such as repetition or jargon
- a lack of, or reduced, social eye contact
- failure to orient to name
- failure to 'cuddle in' or lift their arms up to be picked up by parent or caregiver
- failure to point or use gestures, such as showing, to engage parent (or caregiver) to share an experience or an object of interest
- lack of interactive and/or functional play — that is, the child does not use toys as they should be used but focuses on a particular part of the toy
- lack of interest in peers
- unusual preoccupations; may be with parts of objects or interests such as trains or water
- resistance to change
- unusual body movements such as hand flapping or twisting, rocking, spinning, pacing, toe walking, unusual sensory interests (e.g. over- or under-reacting to sound and pain, mouthing objects, feeling textures).

The Checklist for Autism in Toddlers (CHAT) screening test is used by the Royal Children's Hospital (Australia) and can be easily used by both parent and clinician to decide whether further, more involved testing is required. Figure 7.1 shows the CHAT screening test designed to be used in children from 18 months to 36 months to help identify autism.[6, 7, 8]

Overall the more 'NOs' in the CHAT test the higher the chance of autism.

In the Baron Cohen studies:

- failing all questions with shaded boxes — risk of autism 80–85%
- passing all questions with shaded boxes — risk of autism 0%.

While a diagnosis of Autism is generally formally made between the ages of 2 and 3 years[1], recent published research (2008) using home video observations and parental interview have found anomalies in eye contact, smiling, sharing and interaction initiation on video as early as 12 months and reported by parents as early as 6 months.[9]

This has implications for age of surveillance screening and Australian researchers, including Professor Cheryl Dissanayake, developmental psychologist, who heads the newly established Olga Tennison Autism Research Centre at Latrobe University Melbourne (Australia), now believe that intense intervention should commence as soon as these children are detected. Research is suggesting that children detected early can make huge strides in improving connection, language and behaviour.[10, 11] This early detection is supported by the American Academy of Paediatrics.[4] Care can be coordinated with paediatricians and a large, hopefully integrated, team of psychologists, occupational therapists, speech therapists, and

CHAT Section A — Questions for parents

	Yes or No
Does your child enjoy being swung, bounced on your knee, etc?	
Does your child take an interest in other children?	
Does your child like climbing on things, such as up/on chairs?	
Does your child enjoy playing peek-a-boo and/or hide & seek?	
Does your child ever pretend, for example, to make a cup of tea using a toy cup and teapot, or pretend other things (pouring juice)? **[pretend play (PP)]**	
Does your child ever use his or her index finger to point, to ask for something?	
Does your child ever use his or her index finger to point, to indicate interest in something? **[protodeclarative pointing (PDP)]**	
Can your child play properly with small toys (e.g. cars or blocks) without just mouthing, fiddling, or dropping them?	
Does your child ever bring objects over to you (parent), to show you something?	
Shaded boxes indicate critical questions most indicative of autistic characteristics.	

CHAT Section B — Paediatrician's questions and/or observations

	Yes or No
Eye contact: During the appointment, has the child made eye contact with you?	
Gaze monitoring(GM): Get the child's attention, then point across the room at an interesting object and say, 'Oh Look! There's a (name of a toy)!' Watch the child's face. Does the child look across to see what you are pointing at? (To record a YES, make sure the child does not just look at your hand, but at the object you are pointing at.)	
Pretend play (PP): Get the child's attention, then give the child a miniature toy cup and teapot and say, 'Can you make a cup of tea?' Does the child pretend to pour out tea and drink it? (If you can elicit an example of pretending in some other game, score a YES on this item.)	
Protodeclarative pointing (PDP): Say to the child, 'Where's the light?' or 'Show me the light.' Does the child point with their index finger at the light? (Repeat this with, 'Where's the bear?' or some other unreachable object if the child does not understand the word light. To record a YES on this item, the child must have looked up at your face around the time of pointing.)	
Block tower: Can the child build a tower of blocks? (If so how many?)	
Shaded boxes indicate critical questions most indicative of autistic characteristics.	

Figure 7.1 Checklist for Autism in Toddlers (CHAT) screening test, 18–36 months
(Source: Royal Children's Hospital. Online: www.rch.au/genmed/clinical.cfm?doc_id=2497)

teachers to provide intense therapy and care and achieve improved outcomes.

Intense behavioural, developmental, or structured teaching interventions applied at least 25 hours a week throughout the year can provide documented improvements in IQ, language, academic performance and behaviour. These should be commenced as early as possible for the best gains.

Medical issues should be attended to concurrently, including childhood illnesses, sleep dysfunction, challenging behaviours and psychiatric conditions that these children may suffer. Bowel dysfunction has been found to be more common in autistic children, although this needs further research due to a lack of controls in studies.[4]

Incidence/prevalence

The number of people with ASD has dramatically increased over the past decade, and problem behaviours in autism are an increasing challenge to families, schools, physicians and other health care professionals.[12, 13]

Researchers are not certain whether this increase is due to broader diagnostic criteria, better detection or a true increase.[14] This is likely to be the result of more precise diagnosis, better service availability and improved awareness of autism.[15] Many studies have confirmed this increased incidence, but have reported differences in incidence depending on the study. It has been reported at 6.7 per 10 000 for autism[16] and 25 per 10 000 for

ASD[17], but also as high as 13 per 10 000 for autism and 60–65 per 10 000 for ASD.[18]

US epidemiological data suggest that this increased rise in incidence is slowing in recent years.[17] Prevalence in Australia is difficult to determine as there are inconsistencies in existing data. There is a need to improve data systems across the country.[19]

Autism rates were measured to be as low as 4–5 per 10 000 in WA and NSW in 2000.[20]

Risk factors and causes of autism

Genetic susceptibility, health, nutritional status, and environmental exposures might all contribute to the causation of this complex of disorders.[5] There is unprecedented pressure for autism researchers to find a cause. This is difficult because of the multitude of brain deficits and genetic variants, and no integrated theory has emerged. Research going forward should assume that autism is an aggregation of myriad independent disorders of impaired sociality, social cognition, communication, and motor and cognitive skills.[21]

Genetic predisposition

Multiple genes are involved in inheritance, which demonstrate great phenotypic variation. If 1 sibling already has an ASD, there is approximately a 5–6% risk of a subsequent sibling having the disorder, and this is higher still with subsequent children.[22]

Monozygotic twin studies also show 60% concordance for Autism and 92% for ASD.[5]

Possible involved chromosomes are 2q, 7q, 16p and 19p, and cytogenetic abnormalities have also been found on chromosome 15 and in Fragile X Syndrome.[1]

New groundbreaking research published in *Nature* in March 2009 as an association study of 2 large cohorts (n = 3100 and 1200) of affected children and 6500 controls, found a genome-wide significant association of variants on chromosome 5 for susceptibility for ASD.[23] Especially significant were genes coding for 'neuronal cell adhesion molecules', responsible for neuron to neuron communication. These abnormalities are especially seen in the areas of the brain that are structurally abnormal in autism and ASD: namely the frontal, temporal lobes and the amygdala (which is larger than normal in autistic children in the first 2 years of life). Crucially, this work was replicated in 2 other independent cohorts, and has implications for further research.

Genetic screening of at-risk newborns — that is, those with parents or siblings with the disorder — is an emerging science.

Medical causes

A specific medical cause is only found in 6–10% of cases. These include prenatal causes such as congenital rubella, untreated metabolic disorders, anticonvulsants during pregnancy, tuberous sclerosis and severe postnatal infections.[1]

Epilepsy

Epilepsy may be associated with autistic regression and impaired mental functioning in childhood autism.[24] The incidence of seizures has been estimated to be between 11–39%, and is associated with severe global developmental delay, where the incidence is higher at 42%. With children with ASD and no mental retardation, the incidence is only 6–8%. There are 2 peaks, 1 in children less than 5 years of age, and another peak in adolescence. Electroencephalogram (EEG) abnormalities occur in 10–72% of affected children.[25]

Immune malfunction

Immune dysfunction has been associated with autism, and further research in this area might be productive. Antenatal levels of fetal protein IgG were found in some mothers who carried children who went on to develop ASD.[26]

While immune malfunction, deficiency and auto immunity also has some evidence to support causality, no theory is unified and complete.[5]

Nutritional deficiencies

Many nutrients play a role in behavioural and cognitive development. Deficiency of nutrients, such as iron, zinc, calcium, magnesium and iodine may impact on the child's neurodevelopment and possibly increase the risk of ASD.

One study of 45 children found lower levels of blood and red cell zinc in autistic children compared with controls.[27] More research is required to test this hypothesis.

Environmental exposure to metals and chemicals

Research demonstrates biochemical abnormalities can occur in autism and include liver detoxification impairment via impaired sulfation pathways, mineral imbalances such as reduced zinc/excess copper,[28] environmental insults such as heavy metal and organochlorine pesticide exposure,[29, 30, 31] and gastro intestinal disturbances which are theorised to lead to excessive intestinal permeability and excessive absorption of breakdown products of certain foods leading to opioids intoxicating the brain.

It is well recognised that some industrial chemicals such as lead, methylmercury, polychlorinated biphenyls (PCBs), arsenic and toluene are toxic to brain development and lead to impaired brain function. A further 200 chemicals are neurotoxic to adults, and many more are toxic to laboratory animals.[32] More careful precautionary regulation is required to protect fetal brains from possible exposure causing damage at far lower levels than adults.

Lead, mercury and PCBs have proven effects in attention, memory, learning, social behaviour and IQ at only background-population levels.[33] Testing is usually lacking and not carried out for patients with neurodevelopmental problems.

Organochlorines and organophosphate exposure

Researchers in USA, California have identified a possible link between antenatal organochlorine pesticide exposure and increased risk of autism spectrum disorders.[34] The study compared all births in the area (over 200 000) and compared these with all cases of ASD (465). They found that children had a 6-fold increased risk of ASD if their mothers lived within 500m of a field sprayed with organochlorines. Limitations to the study were that only a small proportion of mothers living in proximity to spraying in the critical early gestational period of neural development were found to be associated with increased risk (29 mothers, of whom 8 of their children had ASD). The authors comment that more studies are needed to confirm this hypothesis.

A review in 2008 confirmed these findings, reporting on in-utero organochlorine and organophosphate exposure and impaired neurodevelopment.[35] It thus is logical to advise mothers to avoid exposure to these harmful substances if possible.

The incidence of ASD has been positively linked in the Pacific North West of the US to times of precipitation, implying possible fallout from airborne pollutants with rain.[36]

Research centering on the San Francisco Bay (USA) area studied 284 children with ASD and 657 controls and hazardous air pollutant concentrations.[37] They found an increased association between autism and exposure to estimated airborne metal concentrations and possibly solvents, namely mercury, nickel, cadmium, trichloroethylene and vinyl chloride. They conclude that more refined exposure studies are required.

Mercury

Mercury is a heavy metal that has also been studied to identify any associations with ASD. A recent population study in Texas found that ASD incidence rises 2.6% per 1000lbs of industrial exposure release, and rises 3.7% with power plant emissions.[38] These risks reduced with increasing distance from exposure, reducing to 2% and 1.6% respectively at 10 miles.

A prospective blinded study evaluating 28 children with severe ASD demonstrated that they had higher mercury intoxication-associated urinary porphyrins compared with less severe sufferers, and decreased plasma levels of reduced glutathione, cysteine and sulfate.[39] They also had higher oxidised glutathione levels and there was an association with increased autism severity scores with these levels, and also the mercury associated porphyrins. The researchers implied from this that mercury intoxication is significantly associated with autistic symptoms, and that transsulfuration abnormalities observed indicate that this is associated with increased oxidative stress and decreased detoxification capacity.[39]

A small study from Arizona, USA, measuring levels of mercury, lead, and zinc in baby teeth of children with ASD compared with normal controls, found that autistic children had significantly higher levels of mercury only.[40] They also had a higher use of oral antibiotics, which in rats inhibits excretion of mercury due to gut flora alteration. This is proposed as a possible mechanism for the higher mercury, and also for the increased incidence of chronic gastrointestinal problems in autistic children.

However, a case controlled study of 400 children compared with 410 controls that explored a possible association with risk of ASD and administration of anti-D globulin during pregnancy, which contains thimerosal, to Rh negative mothers. It showed no increased incidence.[41]

This lack of association was further confirmed in another US study conducted in Missouri.[42]

Clearly, more research into the vexed issue of mercury exposure as a risk factor for autism is needed with larger trials of excellent standard and replicated results.

Environmental climate factors

Researchers in Louisiana have found that the prevalence of autism in offspring is related to exposure of mothers to severe hurricanes and electrical storms during middle and late gestation ($p<0.001$), complementing other research suggesting that antenatal events predispose children to having autism.[43]

Sunshine

There is currently an enormous interest in vitamin D as an important area of health research. Vitamin D supplementation is postulated to potentially reduce the risk of all-cause mortality by up to 7%.[44]

Research postulates that the apparent increase in autism is coincidental with widespread lowered vitamin D levels as a result of advice to avoid sun exposure to reduce risk of skin malignancies.[45] This hypothesis needs to be supported by solid research. However, animal studies demonstrate that severe vitamin D deficiency during gestation leads to protein dysregulation and abnormal neurodevelopment and similar anatomical changes found to that of autistic children. Children with rickets have autistic markers that disappear with supplementation. Calcitriol is also involved, reducing inflammatory cytokines in the brain, which are increased in autism disorders. Calcitriol responds more to testosterone than oestrogen, so potentially explaining the differences in incidence in males. Dark skinned people also have a higher incidence of autism, and autism-related disorders increase with distance from the equator. This theory and hypothesis is worthy of more research.

Researchers describe 2 cases of scurvy and vitamin D deficiency in children who also had cognitive disorders, highlighting the importance of adequate good quality nutrition and exercise, and dietary histories in at-risk children.[46]

Maternal smoking

A single cross-sectional survey of 546 children and their mothers found that maternal smoking during pregnancy was associated with high fetal testosterone levels, and a low ratio of the length of the 2nd and 4th fingers, which is thought to be related to increased incidence of autism. The observation only held for boys.[47]

Obviously more research is required to make any claims, but due to other known negative effects of maternal smoking, abstinence in pregnancy is strongly recommended.

Fetal testosterone and autism traits

Professor Baron-Cohen has undertaken much work in the area of high fetal testosterone levels being related to an increased incidence of autism later on. He presents recent research to support this linking high fetal amniotic testosterone levels with autistic traits as determined by written tests completed by mothers about their children (n = 74).[48]

This supports earlier work identifying a link between high fetal testosterone and abnormal social development and the concept of an 'extreme male brain'. Animal research studies have also identified an association.[49] More prospective work is required in this controversial area.

Pregnancy

A review of articles on epidemiological studies of pre- and perinatal risk factors for ASD demonstrated increased paternal[50] and maternal age, maternal place of birth outside of Europe or North America, low birth weight, duration of gestation, and intra partum hypoxia were associated with ASD.[51] Further prospective studies were recommended.

Danish researchers found that maternal age and 'medicine' use during pregnancy, but not birth interventions or fetal distress, was associated with an increased risk of autism in offspring. Low birth weight babies and congenital malformations were also positively associated.[52]

Examination of obstetric data of mothers who have given birth to children with ASD found an association with a wide range of complications: threatened abortion, epidural anaesthesia use, induction of labour, precipitate labours of less than 1 hour, fetal distress, low Apgars of less than 6 at 1 minute and caesarean section were all positive risk factors.[53] Because there is no single causal association the conclusion is that underlying genetic factors interact with the environment.

Prenatal stress

Researchers in Ohio tried to correlate prenatal stressors for mothers and subsequent incidence of autism, and found a positive correlation from stressors occurring between 21–32 weeks and an increase in ASD.[54] It is thought to cause pathological changes in the cerebellum consistent with autism. Prospective studies are recommended.

Alcohol during pregnancy

Excessive alcohol exposure during pregnancy can increase the risk of ASD as well as other neurodevelopmental disorders.[55]

Pre-term infants

A study of 91 pre-term infants who were found to have a 26% rate for development of autism, and risk factors included low birth weight, male gender, chorioamnionitis, acute intra partum haemorrhage, illness severity on admission, and abnormal MRI studies.[56]

A population-based case-control study found that mothers who had assisted reproduction had offspring with a lower incidence of autism than matched controls.[57] This could be due to their generally better health, and warrants further research and bigger studies.

Pregnancy and folic acid

A hypothesis put forward by researchers is that the increased incidence in autism is related to the supplementation of pregnant mothers with folic acid, due to the survival of fetuses who would otherwise miscarry, with a combination of polymorphism of 5-methylenetetrahydrofolate reductase and consequent high homocysteine levels.[58] They are now surviving in the presence of high folate levels but then after delivery are suffering neurodevelopmental disorders including autism, when the folate levels are not maintained, due to lack of methylation during this critical period. They suggest that detection of these polymorphisms as well as other methionine cycle enzymes would be helpful in detection of at risk infants.

Exercise

Two small studies have found that children with ASD are less active compared with their more 'normal' counterparts.[59] There was no consistency to their exercise pattern.[60]

Table 7.1 provides a summary of the possible risk factors for autism.

Vaccination and autism

MMR Vaccine

Wakefield and his team achieved great notoriety when they suggested an association between the MMR vaccine and inflammatory bowel disease in 1993, and again in 1998 when they described a type of inflammatory bowel disease that was associated with developmental disorders such as autism.[61] Criticisms of their work have been discredited worldwide and attributed to studies being of small sample size, unblinded, lacking no controls, and conducted on highly selected patients with gastrointestinal disease.[62]

The link between behavioural change and vaccination was based on parental recall, and the timing of vaccination coincides with the age at which parents became concerned about their child's development anyway. Criticisms also included lack of scientific evidence of any benefit in giving the individual components separately and that it would in fact cause a resurgence of these childhood illnesses because of reduction in vaccination uptake. Any possible link between MMR vaccine and an increased risk of ASD has been refuted by many large epidemiological studies; for example, from the UK (n = 498)[63] and France (n = 6100).[64] A retrospective study of all children vaccinated in Denmark[65] from 1991 to 1998 showed less risk if any of ASD in vaccinated children, similarly supported by a lack of increased incidence of autism with MMR vaccine coverage over time in California[66] and in UK general practices.[67] Finland failed to find 1 serious adverse event from MMR vaccination over 14 years.[68]

This supports other research published in 2001, again refuting a link with the MMR vaccine, and also refuting the link between MMR and gastric enterocolitis, as there is no proven increased incidence of this colitis in the face of almost universal vaccination.[69]

Thimerosal, which was the preservative in the MMR vaccine in these studies, is therefore not implicated as being associated with an increased risk of autism.

Complementary therapies

Parents are presenting to their doctors armed with a myriad of complementary treatment suggestions and doctors should have an open mind to discussing and knowing about these treatments to encourage objectiveness about what works and what doesn't and the safety of the various therapies and treatment modalities. It is vital the medical practitioner coordinates care with the various health practitioners for the autistic child and families concerned.[70]

The use of complementary medicine (CM) administered by parents for their autistic child is widespread, but trials have been small and limited in number, lacking sound clinical evidence. There have been anecdotes of benefit, especially if coupled with intensive behavioural and education intervention.[71, 2]

A review of 3 private paediatrician practices in the eastern US demonstrated a ubiquitous use of CM and delay in diagnosis of 18 months amongst sample patients. Causes attributed to autism as thought by the parents included genetic risk, immunisations and environmental exposure. Fifty percent of the parents of autistic children interviewed thought the child had at least 1 gastrointestinal, neurological and/or allergic symptom, and one-third had immunological symtoms.[72]

Mind–body medicine

Cognitive behaviour therapy (CBT)

Cognitive behaviour therapy (CBT) should be considered and offered to autistic children and family members in addition to a comprehensive integrated behavioural program, which includes applied behaviour analysis, cognitive approaches, developmental therapy, and structured teaching.[4]

A study of 47 children with high functioning ASD and anxiety responded well to family based CBT after 12 weekly group sessions with significant reductions in symptoms of anxiety

Table 7.1 Possible risk factors for autism*

Genetic susceptibility	Male gender
Medical causes	Congenital rubella (maternal) Untreated metabolic disorders (maternal) Anticonvulsants during pregnancy Tuberous sclerosis (maternal) Severe postnatal infections (maternal) Liver detoxification impairment Gastrointestinal disturbances (child) Immune deficiency; auto-immunity
Nutritional status	Mineral imbalance such as reduced zinc/excess copper ratio Iron deficiency Zinc deficiency
Environmental exposures	Heavy metal exposure; e.g. mercury, lead Organochlorine and organophosphate pesticide exposure
Climate factors	Hurricanes and tropical storms
Sunshine	Vitamin D deficiency Lack of sun exposure
Maternal smoking	Fetal testosterone — high
Pregnancy	Paternal and maternal age Maternal place of birth outside of Europe or North America Low birth weight Duration of gestation Intra partum hypoxia Alcohol during pregnancy Chorioamnionitis Acute intra-partum haemorrhage Illness severity on admission during pregnancy Abnormal MRI studies Folic acid supplementation Prenatal stress
Labour	Complications in labour and association with ASD: • threatened abortion • epidural anaesthesia use • induction of labour • precipitate labours of less than 1 hour • fetal distress • low Apgars of less than 6 at 1 minute • caesarean section
Hormonal factors	Fetal testosterone — high
Exercise and physical activity	Lack of exercise

*Care must be taken with how these findings are interpreted as more research is required to validate these findings.

and 71% no longer suffering from an anxiety disorder as such compared with a control group.[73]

A small pilot study (n = 16) in Singapore showed that a CBT program over 16 sessions improved symptoms of anxiety in children with high functioning ASD or Asperger's syndrome (mean age 11.5 years), and reduced parental and teacher stress.[74]

A small study of high functioning adults with ASD responded well to CBT compared with controls that had treatment as usual.[75]

Israeli researchers examined cognitive improvement in children (n = 81) with autism, and found that improvement is not predictable from the baseline severity of autism, but that with cognitive improvement comes improvement in social behaviour and communication.[76]

Music and sound therapy

A Cochrane systematic review published in 2004 identified 6 randomised controlled trials (RCTs) with 1 cross-over trial, of which half showed improvement in features of ASD, auditory processing, quality of life and adverse events after 3 months (n = 171) with sound therapy.[77] The technique used was Auditory Integration Therapy to reduce abnormal sound sensitivity in sufferers of ASD. There is still insufficient evidence for its use but warrants further research.

An update of the 2004 Cochrane review in 2006 included 3 small studies (n = 24) and found that after 1 week of daily sessions of music therapy that verbal and gestural communication skills improved, but not behaviour.[78]

In a recent randomised control study, Californian researchers investigated the use of a specific sound therapy called 'Tomatis Sound Method' and showed that although there was improvement in language development, it was unrelated to autism itself.[79]

In 2009, a small (n = 12) controlled trial on 11-year old autistic students was conducted, and found that background music was helpful in helping these children understand their emotions, so crucial to social interactions.[80]

Considering the safety of music therapy, more research is warranted using bigger trials to discover if the effects are enduring and to what extent.

Animals

An innovative pilot study in the US showed that occupational therapy for autistic children which incorporated animals revealed significantly improved language and social interaction skills.[81] It may be that the animals offer a way of modelling behaviour using non-verbal stimulus cues.

Sleep

Sleep disturbance is common in autistic children and can negatively impact behaviour. Poor sleep patterns are associated with impaired behaviour and social interaction in these children.[82] Furthermore, sleep disturbance is also associated with impaired health such as vision problems, upper respiratory tract infections, poor appetite and poor growth.[83]

Numerous studies, both large and small, have documented sleep disturbances in children with autism and ASD with longer duration of getting to sleep and increased night-time waking than the control groups.[84–88] Concurrent factors such as younger age, bedtime rituals, asthma, ADHD, medication use, co-sleeping, and family history of sleep problems were also contributory. Epilepsy contributed to daytime sleepiness.[89]

Canadian researchers found that sleep disturbances may be related to abnormal organisation of neural networks interfering with the microstructure of sleep in ASD sufferers.[90]

Understandably, parents reported marked increased stress levels when their children had sleep difficulties.[91]

Behavioural strategies for sleep

Intervention behavioural strategies to improve sleep can improve daytime functioning and behaviour enormously in autistic children.[92–95] Strategies include bedtime routines, reinforcement, effective instructions, partner support and extinction (removing reinforcement to reduce a specific behaviour) maintained consistently over time.[96]

Sleep apnoea

Concurrent sleep apnoea also requires attention and treatment in children with autism.[4]

A case report of a 5-year old female with ASD described significant improvement of sleep patterns and daytime functioning such as social communication, attention, and repetitive behaviours following adenotonsillectomy for the treatment of the sleep apnoea.[97]

Melatonin

Melatonin is a pineal hormone that plays a central part in regulating bodily rhythms and sleep. Studies suggest melatonin treatment may be helpful for sleep problems in children with ASD and Fragile X Syndrome.

In a very small trial of 7 children with ASD, the children were randomised to melatonin or placebo. Sleep improved significantly with melatonin supplementation resulting in reduced wakings per night, earlier onset of sleep and increased duration of sleep.[98]

A 4-week randomised placebo-controlled cross-over trial included 12 children with ASD and/or Fragile X Syndrome (11 males; mean age 5.47 years) demonstrated when compared with placebo children taking melatonin 3mgs nocte, overall mean night sleep duration was longer by 21 minutes, sleep-onset patency was shorter by 28 minutes and sleep-onset time was earlier by 42 minutes.[99]

Researchers in Europe have found that autistic children have a defect in melatonin synthesis due to reduced activity of aceylserotonin methyltransferase, the final enzyme in the melatonin biosynthetic pathway, and may be a risk factor for ASD. Mutation abnormalities in gene coding for this were found on the autosomal region on the sex chromosome.[100] This highlights the crucial function of melatonin in human cognition and behaviour.

This is an important area for ongoing research, with larger trials necessary before any firm conclusions are made or recommendations given.

Sunshine

Lack of sunshine exposure and vitamin D deficiency may be a risk factor for autism (see section under risk factors). Sunshine is the main source of vitamin D produced by the body in response to direct skin exposure to ultraviolet B (UVB). This means that no or minimal exposure to sun can contribute to vitamin D deficiency, as seen in community groups with dress codes (e.g. wearing veils), and those living in geographically prone areas, especially over winter (southern or northern latitudes), working indoors (e.g. office work), institutionalised patients, and those who are bed-bound and requiring prolonged hospitalisation, particularly in dark skinned people who need longer sun exposure for adequate vitamin D absorption. (See also Chapter 30, Osteoporosis.) Vitamin D deficiency is likely to be the commonest nutritional deficiency in Australia and many other countries worldwide. Vitamin D has a multiplicity of roles involving virtually every body system.

Meanwhile, sensible advice for appropriate moderate sun exposure at appropriate times of the day, depending on skin colour, is recommended.

Physical activity

Physical activity/exercise

US researchers found that youths with ASD benefited from a 9-month treadmill walking program resulting in positive reductions in Body Mass Index.[101]

There were no studies linking exercise to behavioural or cognitive improvement, but it makes sense to recommend exercise for the usual reasons of improved mood, health, sleep and wellbeing, particularly outdoor exercise for fresh air and sun exposure.

Environmental

Heavy metal detoxification

Chelation therapy

This form of heavy metal detoxification has been used by many quarters claiming benefit.

An RCT of chelation therapy using dimercaptosuccinic acid to treat lead-exposed children failed to show any benefit.[102]

Tetrahydrofurfuryl disulfide has been used as a chelating agent in children with autism, due to its mechanism of enhancing excretion of mercury, cadmium, arsenic and lead. An open pilot study claimed benefits, but requires more rigorous trials before its use can be supported.

Hepatotoxicity and anaphylaxis have been reported as a side-effect of chelation,[103] including reports of cardiac arrests as a result of hypocalcaemia from the wrong chelating agent being used (Na EDTA).[104] Its use therefore is not recommended.

Redox and metallothioneins

Redox active metals, such as copper and zinc can play an important role in the healthy functioning of the nervous system.[105] Metallothioneins are physiological proteins that naturally help to regulate the levels of redox active metals within the body and they form the first line of defence against toxic heavy metals as their structure incorporates multiple sulfhydryl groups. Consequently, the use of 'metallothionein promoters' could be of benefit to autistic children, although there is a lack of solid evidence to support their use.

Of interest, a study of 66 people from families with autistic children found a 30% incidence of anti-metallothionein IgG; however these antibodies did not correlate with the autistic children in these families.[106]

Zinc and copper ratios were measured retrospectively in 230 children with ASD and found to be much lower than normal controls, implying that this might indicate metallothionein enzyme dysfunction, and also be a biomarker of heavy metal toxicity.[107]

Glutathione has been implicated with this, an antioxidant tripeptide involved in DNA and protein synthesis, enzyme and immune system function. Glutathione is theorised to reduce oxidative stress implicated in autism, but there is no research to confirm this.[2]

A clinical trial involving combined anti-androgen and anti-heavy metal therapy over a 4-month period demonstrated significant improvements in sociability, cognitive awareness, behaviour, and clinical symptoms/ behaviours of hyperandrogenemia observed in children with ASDs, resulting in significant decreases in blood androgens and increases in urinary heavy metal concentrations compared with the baseline.[108] Minimal drug adverse effects were identified with this treatment, warranting additional studies in this area.

Nutritional influences

Gastrointestinal symptoms

Gastrointestinal symptoms are also exceedingly common in children with autism and ASD. A prevalence of 24% of at least 1 gastrointestinal (GI) symptom was found in a sample size of 137 children in a specialised clinic in the US.[109] However there was no association between GI symptoms and developmental regression.

A lack of case controls limits the validity of these studies. However a cross-sectional study of structured interviews asking about a lifetime history of gastrointestinal symptoms have found that 70% of ASD sufferers complain of abnormal stools, constipation, vomiting and abdominal pain, compared with 42% of children with other developmental disorders and 28% of normal controls.[110]

Gastroscopies found lymphoid nodular hyperplasia, oesophagitis, gastritis, duodenitis, and colitis in a high number of ASD sufferers, and unique inflammatory immunohistochemical features (seen only in ASD children).

If children with ASD present with gastrointestinal symptoms, it is reasonable for appropriate further investigation and, if necessary, for endoscopy.

Diet

Gluten and casein free diets

Casein and gluten free diets are among the most popular interventions for children with ASD. The theory is that opioid peptides form from incomplete breakdown of gluten and casein in the gut, and increased gut permeability seen in these children allows absorption of these to the bloodstream and then across the blood brain barrier to affect neurotransmission and contribute to the typical behavioural and social disorders seen in autism.

A recent Cochrane review explored the efficacy of gluten and casein free diets for ASD.[111] It found only 1 trial of adequate quality for assessment, and found that it helped in the important area in reduction in autistic traits, though there was huge variation in the cognition, linguistic and motor skills. This has been cited as an important area of research.

A small randomised control prospective trial found no change in urinary casein and gliadin peptide levels of children on such a diet compared with the controls, refuting the increased gut permeability or 'leaky gut' theory, and also demonstrated no statistically significant change in behavioural markers in these children.[112]

Care is required with dietary restrictions and elimination of food groups in autistic children as this may lead to further micronutrient deficiencies, as autistic children are prone to poor nutritional intake and deficiencies due to self-restriction of food intake, especially for fibre, calcium, iron, vitamin E and vitamin D.[113, 114]

Two further rigorous studies are being conducted with bigger numbers and for at least 12 weeks: a single-blind trial in Norway[115] and a double-blind trial in the US[116] to assess dietary interventions on children's behaviour with autism. Results are awaited with interest.

A study of 109 children with ASD found an association between gastrointestinal symptoms and ingestion of cow's milk protein, but not for casein or soy, and demonstrated marked production and elevated levels of pro inflammatory cytokines TNF-alpha and IL-12.[117] However, biochemical abnormalities do not equate to clinical effects, and more research is needed.

Probiotics

Probiotics may help ASD children, especially if they have a history of multiple courses of antibiotics and suffer entercolitis.[118, 119]

Clostridium histolyticum has been found in larger numbers in these children than normal controls and Vancomycin has been found to help gastrointestinal symptoms in children with severe regressive symptoms of ASD.[4,120] It may help limit any toxic effects of abnormal bacteria on the bowel and production of a so-called 'leaky gut'.

Nutritional supplements

Vitamins

Multivitamins

One trial showed improvement in sleep and gastrointestinal symptoms in children with ASD (n = 20) supplemented with a multi-mineral and vitamin supplement.[121]

Vitamin B6

Pyridoxine is involved in the synthesis of several neurotransmitters. Nutritional supplementation is very popular for children with autism.[2]

Small trials have demonstrated that children with autism have high serum vitamin B6 levels and low levels of the active form of the vitamin, pyridoxal 5 phosphate. They have also shown that these children have low pyridoxal kinase activity, which is necessary for neurotransmitter formation and over 100 other enzymatic reactions.[122, 123]

Interestingly, a trial demonstrated children with autism have abnormally high plasma levels of vitamin B6 even when not taking supplements compared to controls not taking supplements.[119]

Despite the findings above a small trial (n = 8) found an increase in verbal IQ with B6 supplementation compared with placebo, with 2 other trials failing to show an effect (n = 10 and 15).[124, 125]

However, high dose vitamin B6 can cause side-effects, including a dose-related sensory neuropathy. It is recommended not to exceed the safe upper limit of 50mg/day in adults, so based on weight, proportionally much lower doses are required in children.

More rigorous research is needed before blanket recommendations can be given.

Folic acid

Researchers identified a subgroup of autistic patients who demonstrated folate receptor autoimmunity with consequent blocking of folate binding to choroid epithelial cells, thereby reducing folate transport across the blood brain barrier into the CSF. These patients had low 5-methyltetrahydrofolate levels, despite normal serum folate. Supplementing this group with folate led to 'partial or complete clinical recovery after 12 months'.[126]

Further to this, researchers have found preliminary evidence for genetic polymorphisms of dihydrofolate reductase leading to possible interactions between folate and glutamate and abnormal neural excitation.[127]

A case report of a 6-year old girl with autistic features had documented low CSF levels of 5-methyltetrahydrofolate, normal peripheral blood folate and serum vitamin B12 levels.[128] Treatment with folinic acid corrected low CSF abnormalities and improved motor skills.

Vitamin B12

An open label trial of autistic children (n = 40) demonstrated that methylcobalamin and folinic acid treatment resulted in improved levels of glutathione, cysteinyl-glycine, cysteine, and reduced oxidised disulfide form of glutathione, and an increased glutathione redox ratio.[129] No mention in the trial was made of clinical improvement in these children, and more research is warranted to ascertain whether this intervention is indeed to be recommended.

Vitamin C

Vitamin C may play an important role in fetal brain development and neurohormonal production. It is a cofactor in the conversion of tyrosine to dopamine and tryptophan to serotonin, which is an antioxidant, important for moods and also an immune function regulator.[130]

A double-blind, placebo-controlled trial (1993) of a small number of English autistic children (n = 18) of megadose vitamin C therapy (8g/70kg/day) demonstrated a significant improvement in behaviour in the ascorbic acid arm compared with the placebo arm.[131]

Minerals

Magnesium and Vitamin B6

An update of a systematic review from 2002 of combined vitamin B6-magnesium supplementation for treating children with ASD, has found that only 3 studies could be included, and that due to the small size of the studies, and poor methodological quality, no recommendation could be given.[132]

Research published a year after the Cochrane review, of 33 children with ASD and 36 controls, measured baseline red blood cell magnesium (Mg) levels and supplemented with a Mg-vitamin B6 combined supplement.[133] Children with ASD demonstrated significantly lower red blood cell magnesium levels, and following supplementation for 6 months, demonstrated improved social interaction, communication, stereotyped restricted behaviour and abnormal/delayed functioning compared with controls. After cessation of supplements the behaviours deteriorated after a few weeks.

More research is warranted in this area.

Iron and zinc

If deficient, supplementation with iron or zinc may improve cognitive development and behaviour in children with ASD.

A small (n = 33) controlled clinical trial found a correlation between low iron intake and sleep disturbance, which improved with supplementation, and also noted a high incidence of iron deficiency (69% of preschoolers and 35% of school age) in children with autism and related disorders.[134]

More research in this important area is needed.

Other supplements

Omega-3 fatty acids

Omega-3 and omega-6 fatty acids are vital for neurodevelopmental growth.[2]

A review of randomised double-blind control trials demonstrated that DHA and EPA supplementation improved symptoms in autism disorder.[135]

Apart from this review, 4 small trials had mixed results, and 1 small double-blind placebo controlled-trial of 13 adolescents showed preliminary behavioural benefit especially in hyperactivity after 6 weeks of 1.5gram/day EFA supplementation.[136] However, 2 small trials could not replicate these findings and demonstrate any benefit with omega-3 supplementation.[137, 138]

In fact, a very small study of 16 male children with high functioning autism showed a naturally occurring significant increase in DHA fatty acids, with an increase in the 3:6 ratio.[139] The researchers hypothesise that 3-polyunsaturated fatty acids (PUFAs) may cause alterations in serotonin turnover and the immune response system, and advise caution regarding omega-3 supplementation.

A study of children with autism and Asperger's syndrome demonstrated significant fatty acid deficiency but the children responded to supplementation in those with larger increases in blood levels of EPA and DHA than supplemented controls.[140] Supplemented autistic children also had reduced pro-inflammatory phospholipase A2 levels than non-supplemented autistic children.

More research is warranted in this area.

Physical therapies

Acupuncture

A small pilot study of 2 cases of autistic children administered intensive electroacupuncture over 8 weeks and found variable responses in certain aspects of social functioning and relatedness, but much more investigation is obviously required.[141]

Hyperbaric oxygen therapy

A recent multi-centre randomised control trial (RCT) of 62 children used hyperbaric oxygen therapy and found that 30% of children were 'very much improved' or 'much improved' compared with 8% of controls. Treated children had improved language, social skills and eye contact.[142] The therapy used a pressure of 1.3 atmospheres and 24% oxygen for an hour and was administered 40 times over a month, and was very well tolerated. The authors speculated that hyperbaric oxygen works by decreasing brain inflammation and therefore swelling and improving function via increased oxygen delivery. PET scans confirmed this improved perfusion of oxygen supply and brain activity in these children.

The study has drawn wide criticism from neurologists as 8 out of the 10 physicians involved in the study had received funding from the International Hyperbarics Association. Also the science is unclear as autism is not a vascular deficiency disorder but a complex genetic one, and that there is not a case for improvement in brain metabolism with oxygen.

More well-performed research is required to confirm these findings.

Massage

An open exploratory study of 14 parents and children involved in a 'Training and Support Program' demonstrated improvement in children's' sleep patterns, openness to being touched and relaxation.[143] They were also able to undertake routine tasks such as dressing more easily. At the end of 16 weeks they were actually asking for further massage. This has implications for helping enhance the emotional bonds between parent and child.[144, 145]

An open design US study (n = 20) comparing autistic children who were massaged for 15 minutes every evening to another group being read Dr Seuss stories found that massage therapy improved social interactions, better sleep and less stereotyped behaviour compared with the reading group.[146]

One controlled study of 13 young autistic children in China treated with a form of qigong massage daily for 5 months showed that they had significantly improved socialisation, basic living skills, bowel and sleep normalisation, and reduction in sensory impairment.[147]

Conclusion

In view of the rising global trend in autism worldwide, it would appear that there is an urgent need for well-performed studies to explore risk factors, lifestyle factors and treatment options for children with autism and ASD. There are no lifestyle and complementary treatments that can effectively cure autism but many may be of benefit for improving social skills and behaviour patterns in an autistic child.

For example, exercise, restoring adequate sleep, treating sleep apnoea if necessary, sunshine exposure and dietary changes may show clinical benefit on behaviour patterns associated with ASD. Counselling and cognitive therapy for the high functioning child with ASD and for the parents who need substantial emotional support may be of benefit. Music and massage therapy, whilst not demonstrating high level evidence, are relatively safe and can help with sleep and behaviour patterns. Table 7.2 summarises the level of evidence for some CM therapies for ASD.

ASD is a condition that is difficult to treat, and challenges parents, family members, any health practitioner and teachers. The parents require support on many levels. The child with ASD requires coordinated care from a team of carers.

Table 7.2 Levels of evidence for lifestyle and complementary medicines/therapies in the management of Autism Spectrum Disorder (ASD)

Modality	Level I	Level II	Level IIIa	Level IIIb	Level IIIc	Level IV	Level V
Mind–body medicine							
CBT				x			
Music therapy	x						
Sound therapy		x					
Sleep restoration							
Behavioural therapy					x		
Sleep apnoea treatment				x			
Melatonin		x					
Environment							
Heavy metals					x		
Lead					x		
Mercury					x		
Physical activity							
Outdoor play					x		
Yoga		x					
Sunshine					x		
Nutrition/diet							
Food sensitivities and trial Elimination diet					x		
Casein and gluten		x					
Nutritional supplements							
Magnesium/vitaminB6		x					
Iron		x					
Zinc			x				
Multivitamin				x			

Continued

Table 7.2 Levels of evidence for lifestyle and complementary medicines/therapies in the management of Autism Spectrum Disorder (ASD)—cont'd

Modality	Level I	Level II	Level IIIa	Level IIIb	Level IIIc	Level IV	Level V
Other supplements							
n–3 fatty acids			x				
Physical therapies							
Acupuncture						x	
Hyperbaric oxygen therapy		x					
Massage					x		

Level I — from a systematic review of all relevant randomised controlled trials, meta-analyses.
Level II — from at least 1 properly designed randomised controlled clinical trial.
Level IIIa — from well-designed pseudo-randomised controlled trials (alternate allocation or some other method).
Level IIIb — from comparative studies (including systematic reviews of such studies) with concurrent controls and allocation not randomised, cohort studies, case-control studies, or interrupted time series with a parallel control group.
Level IIIc — from comparative studies with historical control, 2 or more single-arm studies or interrupted time series without a parallel control group.
Level IV — opinions of respected authorities based on clinical experience, descriptive studies or reports of expert committees.
Level V — represents minimal evidence that represents testimonials.

Clinical tips handout for patients — Autistic Spectrum Disorder (ASD)

1 Lifestyle advice

Sleep

- All children should be fully assessed and treated for underlying sleep disorders.
- The appropriate amount of physical activity during the day can help sleep.
- Massage the child before bed.
- Develop a consistent routine.
- Calming music may help.
- Herbal teas such as chamomile can be helpful in some cases.
- Magnesium can be used to calm the child during the day and assist sleep at night.

Sunshine

- At least 15 minutes sunshine is needed daily for vitamin D and melatonin production:
  - especially before 10am and after 3pm when the sun exposure is safest during summer
  - much more exposure is required in winter, and supplementation needs to be considered.
- Ensure gradual, adequate skin exposure to sun; avoid sunscreen and excess clothing to maximise levels of vitamin D.
- More time in the sun is required for dark skinned people and people with vitamin D deficiency.
- Directly expose about 10% of the body (hands, arms, face), without sunscreen and not through glass.
- Vitamin D is obtained in the diet from fatty fish, eggs, liver and fortified foods (some milks and margarines); diet alone is not a sufficient source of vitamin D.

2 Physical activity/exercise

Play outdoors in a natural environment such as a natural park or country-side as much as possible. As little as 30 minutes daily can make a significant difference to settling hyperactive behaviour.

3 Mind–body medicine

Counselling/psychotherapy

- Both behavioural and cognitive behaviour therapy interventions are effective for children and adults with ASD.
- Children respond positively to behavioural interventions only when they are appropriately implemented at school and in the home.
- Anecdotal evidence strongly supports the use of soothing music and sound therapy (Tomatis Sound Method, integrated listening system; auditory integration therapy).

4 Environment

- Play outdoors as much as possible in a natural environment, such as parks or the countryside, to avoid air pollution, traffic, and breathe fresh air.
- Lead, mercury, manganese, aluminium, copper and industrial chemicals (PCBs, arsenic) have all been found to be possible contributing factors to autism.
- All children with autism should ideally be tested for the presence of heavy metals. This can be done by hair mineral analysis or comprehensive urinary element profile.
- Chelation therapies for heavy metal toxicity can range from gentle (Epsom salt/clay baths, coriander, chlorella, chelating foot-pads) to stronger means (zinc supplementation, metallothionine promoting supplements, DMSA, DMPS chelating agents) where necessary. Discuss this with your doctor.
- Avoidance of chemicals, pesticides and tobacco smoke is important.

5 Dietary changes

- Many children have digestion problems ('Irritable Bowel Syndrome') (abdominal bloating/discomfort, diarrhoea, constipation, excess burping/flatulence, reflux) which may adversely affect their behaviour.
- An abdominal X-ray can often reveal hidden constipation.
- Supervised food elimination regimes are extremely important in identifying problem foods that trigger hyperactivity, impulsivity and inattention. There is no point using other therapies if the child is eating something every day that continues to trigger certain behaviours.
- The most common problem foods include artificial additives, sugar, yeast, wheat (gluten), cow's milk (casein) and salicylates.

- Foods may be eliminated for a period of 3 weeks, then each food/component reintroduced separately (e.g. wheat/yeast/gluten; lactose-free, 'A2' milk). This should be done under the supervision of a dietician.

6 Nutritional supplementation

Probiotics

Indication: to aid digestion and reduce 'IBS' symptoms. They should be used in conjunction with dietary modifications.

Dosage: 1–2 capsules before breakfast.

Results: 1 month.

Side-effects: if using wrong probiotic, digestion symptoms may get worse.

Contra-indications: true dairy allergies if dairy in preparation.

Vitamin D3

Indication: correct vitamin D deficiency; improve bone density, prevent osteoporosis, fractures and falls; reduce muscle and whole body pain.

The following drugs may reduce vitamin D levels: carbamazepine, cholestyramine, colestipol, phenobarbitol, phenytoin, rifampin, orlistat, stimulant laxatives, sunscreens. Corticosteroids increase need for vitamin D.

Dosage: safe sunshine exposure of skin is the safest source of vitamin D.

Vitamin D (cholecalciferol 1000 international units).

Doctors should check blood levels and suggest supplementation if levels are low.

Adults: 400–1000IU daily, for maintenance; 3000–5000IU daily for 1 month then 1000IU daily if vitamin D level below normal.

Children at risk: 200–400IU daily under medical supervision.

Pregnant and lactating women at risk: under medical supervision.

Results: 3 to 6 to 12 months.

Side-effects: very high doses can cause toxicity vitamin D toxicity; raised calcium levels in the blood.

Contraindications: can increase aluminium and magnesium absorption; prolonged heparin therapy can increase resorption and reduce formation of bone and hence more vitamin D and calcium required; thiazide diuretics decrease urinary calcium and hence hypercalcaemia possible with vitamin D supplementation; high levels of vitamin D can reduce effectiveness of verapamil.

Use vitamin D with caution in those with artery disease, hyperparathyroidism, lymphoma, renal disease and sarcoidosis.

Vitamin B6

Do not provide as a single nutrient.

Indication: to reduce hyperactivity/anxiety and increase attention in combination with magnesium.

Dosage: up to 20mg Pyridoxal-5-Phosphate (Activated B6).

Results: 1–3 months: always needs to be combined with B complex in long-term e.g. multi B complex.

Side-effects: parasthesia in extremities, bone pain, muscle weakness at high levels — reversible on cessation of supplement as soon as symptoms develop; may cause long-term problems with long-term use and with very high doses.

Contraindications: caution with amiodarone, phenobarbitone, phenytoin.

Multivitamins, especially B-group and minerals

Vitamin supplement containing low doses of B1, B3, B5, B6, folate and the minerals zinc, iron, calcium and magnesium may be of help in the production of melatonin.

Proteins

Peptic HCl ↓ Zinc, B_1, B_6

L–Tryptophan

Tryptophan hydroxylase ↓ Folate, Fe, Ca, B3

5–Hydroxytryptophan

Dopa Decarboxylase ↓ B_6, Zn, Mg, Vit C

5–Hydroxytryptamine (serotonin)

Protein → Methionine SAMe ↓ B_5

Melatonin

Magnesium

Best combined with calcium.

- Indication: may assist abnormal behaviour patterns associated with ASD; reduce hyperactivity, restless legs, teeth grinding, 'growing pains', chocolate cravings and to improve sleep.
- Dosage: 350mg up to 750mg/day for adults. Children less than 12 years: 30–350mg/day.
- Results: 1–3 months.
- Side-effects: diarrhoea, gastric irritation; oral magnesium can cause gastrointestinal irritation, nausea, vomiting, and diarrhoea. The dosage varies from person to person. Although rare, toxic levels can cause low blood pressure, thirst, heart arrhythmia, drowsiness and weakness.

- Contraindications: renal failure, kidney disease, heart block.

Zinc

- Indication: to treat zinc deficiency; to chelate heavy metals; may assist with reducing hyperactivity, impulsivity, impaired socialisation and reducing inattention (see ADHD chapter).
- Dosage: needs to be individualised as some children need very high doses depending upon their biochemistry. Minimum dose 10mg elemental zinc.
- Results: 1–3 months.
- Side-effects: nausea and vomiting (if taken in excess), metallic taste in mouth, reduced copper after long-term use.
- Contraindications: sideroblastic anaemia, severe kidney disease, above normal plasma levels of zinc for age.

Iron

- Indication: restless legs at night, reduced hyperactivity.
- Dosage: depending on age and serum levels, between 20–40mg/day.
- Results: 3–6 months.
- Side-effects: constipation, dark stools, nausea, diarrhoea, reflux.
- Contraindications: haemachromatosis, haemosiderosis.

Fish Oils (EPA/DHA)

- Indication: to improve attention, IQ, sleep and reduce hyperactivity, and impulsivity.
- Dosage: ideally DHA>EPA for learning, processing disorders. Doses between 1–9g EPA/DHA daily.
- Results: 1–3 months.
- Side-effects: fishy burps, diarrhoea, gastrointestinal discomfort.
- Contraindications: fish allergy. Caution with anticoagulants at very high doses.

Supplements that may be of assistance for children with digestive problems

Digestive enzymes

- Indication: to aid digestion in the short term and improve quality of life (e.g. at birthday parties) where children are exposed to 'problem foods'.
- Dosage: 1 capsule 10 minutes before 'problem food'.
- Results: immediate.
- Side-effects: very mild and rare.
- Contraindications: nil known.

Gut-healing herbs and nutrients (glutamine, aloe-vera, slippery elm)

- Indication: to assist healing of the digestive system whilst avoiding 'problem foods'.
- Dosage: maximum dose as directed.
- Results: 1–3 months.
- Side-effects: diarrhoea.
- Contraindications: hypersensitivity to ingredients.

Sleep disturbance

Melatonin

Melatonin is naturally produced by the body from tryptophan and requires various minerals and vitamins for its production (see 'multivitamins' above). Use only under medical supervision.

- Indication: helps insomnia by improving circadian rhythm sleep disorders; reduces the time to fall asleep; jet-lag.
- Dosage: 0.3–5mg at 6pm or closer to bedtime; for short-term use.
- Results: within 1–3 hours.
- Side-effects: usually well tolerated. Avoid long-term use. May cause drowsiness, dizziness, depressive symptoms, reduced alertness, irritability, headaches; all these symptoms can be transient.
- Contraindications: very young children, pregnant, lactating mothers; epilepsy; taken with alcohol, sedating medication such as benzodiazepines and use with narcotics; depression.

References

1 Baird G, Cass H, Slonims V. Diagnosis of autism BMJ 2003;327:488–93.

2 Angley M, Semple S, Hewton C, et. al. Children with Autism. Part 2–Management with Complementary Medicines and Dietary Interventions. Australian Family Physician 2007 October;36(10):827–829.

3 Altevogt BM, Hanson SL, Leshner AI. Autism and the environment: challenges and opportunities for research. Institute of Medicine, Forum on Neuroscience and Nervous System Disorders, Washington, DC 2001, USA. Online. Available: baltevogt@nas.edu (accessed 27-08-09).

4 Myers SM, Johnson CP, the Council on Children With Disabilities. Management of Children With Autism Spectrum Disorders. Pediatrics 2007 November;120(5):1162–1182. (doi:10.1542/peds.2007–2362).

5 Angley M, Ellis D, Chan W. Children with Autism. Part 1-Recognition and Pharmacological Management. Australian Family Physician 2007 September;36(9):741–4.

6 Baron Cohen S, Allen J, Gillberg C. Can autism be detected at 18 months? The needle the haystack and the CHAT. British Journal of Psychiatry 1992;161:839–843.

7 Baron Cohen S, Wheelwright S, Cox A, et. al. Early identification of autism by the Checklist for Autism in Toddlers (CHAT). J R Soc Med 2000;93:521–525.

8 Baird G. et. al. A screening instrument for autism at 18 months of age: a 6 year follow up study. Am.Acad. Child and Adolesc. Psychiatry 2000;39:694–702.

9 Clifford SM, Dissanayake C. The early development of joint attention in infants with autistic disorder using home video observations and parental interview. J Autism Dev Disord. 2008 May;38(5):791–805.

10 Clifford SM, Dissanayake C. The early development of Joint Attention in Infants with Autistic Disorder Using Home Video Observations and Parental Interview. Journal of Autism and Development Disorders 2008 May;38(5):791–805. Online. Available: http://www.ncbi.nlm.nih.gov/pubmed/17917803 (accessed 27–08–09).

11 Barbaro J, Dissanayake C Autism Spectrum Disorders in infancy and toddlerhood: A review of evidence on early signs, early identification tools, and early diagnosis. Publisher: (Forthcoming, 2009) Journal of Developmental and Behavioral Pediatrics. Online. Available: http://journals.lww.com/jrnldbp/pages/default.aspx (accessed 27-08-09).

12 Hollander E, Phillips AT, Yeh C-C. Targeted treatments for symptom domains in child and adolescent autism. Lancet 2003 Aug 30;362(9385):732–4.

13 Barbaresi WJ, Katusic SK, Colligan RC, et. al. The incidence of autism in Olmsted County, Minnesota, 1976–1997: results from a population-based study. Arch Pediatr Adolesc Med 2005 Jan;159(1):37–44.

14 Baird G, Simonoff E, Pickles A, et. al. Prevalence of disorders of the autism spectrum in a population cohort of children in South Thames: the Special Needs and Autism Project (SNAP). Lancet 2006 Jul 15;368(9531):210–5.

15 Barbaresi WJ, Katusic SK, Colligan RC, et. al. The incidence of autism in Olmsted County, Minnesota, 1976–1997: results from a population-based study. Arch Pediatr Adolesc Med 2005 Jan;159(1):37–44.

16 Autism and Developmental Disabilities Monitoring Network Surveillance Year 2000 Principal Investigators; Centers for Disease Control and Prevention. Prevalence of autism spectrum disorders–autism and developmental disabilities monitoring network, six sites, United States, 2000. MMWR Surveill Summ 2007 Feb 9;56(1):1–11.

17 Newschaffer CJ, Falb MD, Gurney JG. National Autism Prevalence Trends From United States. Special Education Data. Pediatrics 2005 Mar;115(3):e277–82.

18 Fombonne E. Epidemiology of autistic disorder and other pervasive developmental disorders. J Clin Psychiatry 2005;66:3–8.

19 Williams K, MacDermott S, Ridley G, et. al. The prevalence of autism in Australia. Can it be established from existing data? J Paediatr Child Health 2008 Sep;44(9):504–10. Epub 2008 Jun 28.

20 Williams K, Glasson EJ, Wray J, et. al. Incidence of autism spectrum disorders in children in two Australian states. Med J Aust 2005 Feb 7;182(3):108–11.

21 Waterhouse L. Autism overflows: increasing prevalence and proliferating theories. Neuropsychol Rev 2008 Dec;18(4):273–86. Epub 2008 Nov 18.

22 Johnson CP, Myers SM, and the Council on Children with Disabilities. Identification and Evaluation of Children With Autism Spectrum Disorders. Pediatrics 2007;120:1183–1215. (doi:10.1542/peds. 2007–2361).

23 Wang K, Zhang H, Ma D, et. al. Common genetic variants on 5p14.1 associate with autism spectrum disorders Nature advance online publication 28 April 2009 doi:10.1038/nature07999; Received 28 November 2008; Accepted 18 March 2009; Published online 28 April 2009.

24 Hrdlicka M, Komarek V, Propper L, Kulisek R, Zumrova A, Faladova L, Havlovicova M, Sedlacek Z, Blatny M, Urbanek T. Eur Child Adolesc Psychiatry. 2004 Aug;13(4):209–13.

25 Myers SM, Johnson CP, and the Council on Children With Disabilities. Management of Children With Autism Spectrum Disorders. Pediatrics 2007 November;120(5):1162–1182. (doi:10.1542/peds.2007–2362).

26 Croen LA, Braunschweig D, Haapanen L, et. al. Maternal mid-pregnancy autoantibodies to fetal brain protein: the early markers for autism study. Biol Psychiatry. 2008 Oct 1;64(7):583–8. Epub 2008 Jun 20.

27 Yorbik O, Akay C, Sayal A, et. al. Zinc status in autistic children. The Journal of Trace Elements in Experimental Medicine 2004;17:101–7.

28 Angley M, Ellis D, Chan W, et. al. Children with Autism. Part 1-Recognition and Pharmacological Management. Australian Family Physician 2007 Setember;36(9):741–744.

29 Roberts E, et. al. Maternal Residence Near Agricultural Pesticide Applications and Autism Specrum Disorders amond Children in the California Central Valley. Environ Health Perspect. 2008 Apr;116(4):A155.

30 Windham GC, Zhang L, Gunier R, et. al. Autism Spectrum Disorders in Relation to Distribution of Hazardous Air Pollutants in the San Francisco Bay Area. Environmental Health Perspectives. Research Triangle Park 2006 Sep;114(9):1438–44 (7 pp.).

31 Fitzpatrick M. Autism and environmental toxicity. The Lancet Neurology. London: 2007 Apr;6(4):297(1 pg).

32 Grandjean P, Landrigan PJ. Developmental neurotoxicity of industrial chemicals. The Lancet. London: 2006 Dec 16–22;368(9553):2167–78 (12 pp.).

33 Stein J, Schettler T, Wallinga D, et. al. In harm's way: toxic threats to child development. J Dev Behav Pediatr. 2002 Feb;23(1 Suppl):S13–S22.

34 Roberts E, et. al. Maternal Residence Near Agricultural Pesticide Applications and Autism Specrum Disorders amond Children in the California Central Valley. Environ Health Perspect 2008 Apr;116(4):A155.

35 Rosas LG, Eskenazi B. Pesticides and Child Neurodevelopment. Current Opinion Pediatric 2008 April;20(2):191–7.

36 Waldman M, Nicholson S, Adilov N, et. al. Autism prevalence and precipitation rates in California, Oregon, and Washington counties. Arch Pediatr Adolesc Med 2008 Nov;162(11):1026–34.

37 Gayle C Windham, Lixia Zhang, Robert Gunier, et. al. Autism Spectrum Disorders in Relation to Distribution of Hazardous Air Pollutants in the San Francisco Bay Area. Environmental Health Perspectives. Research Triangle Park 2006 Sep;114(9):1438–44 (7 pp.).

38 Palmer RF, Blanchard S, Wood R. Proximity to point sources of environmental mercury release as a predictor of autism prevalence. Health Place 2009 Mar;15(1):18–24.

39 Geier DA, Kern JK, Garver CR, et. al. Biomarkers of environmental toxicity and susceptibility in autism. J Neurol Sci 2009 May 15;280(1–2):101–8. Epub 2008 Sep 25.

40 Adams JB, Romdalvik J, Ramanujam VM, et. al. Mercury, lead, and zinc in baby teeth of children with autism versus controls. J Toxicol Environ Health A 2007 Jun;70(12):1046–51.
41 Croen LA, Matevia M, Yoshida CK, et. al. Maternal Rh D status, anti-D immune globulin exposure during pregnancy, and risk of autism spectrum disorders. Am J Obstet Gynecol 2008 Sep;199(3):234.e1–e6. Epub 2008 Jun 13.
42 Miles JH, Takahashi TN. Lack of association between Rh status, Rh immune globulin in pregnancy and autism. Am J Med Genet A 2007 Jul 1;143A(13):1397–407.
43 Kinney DK, Miller AM, Crowley DJ, et. al. Autism prevalence following prenatal exposure to hurricanes and tropical storms in Louisiana. J Autism Dev Disord 2008 Mar;38(3):481–8. Epub 2007 Jul 6.
44 Cannell JJ, Hollis BW. Use of vitamin D in clinical practice. Altern Med Rev 2008 Mar;13(1):6–20.
45 Cannell JJ. Autism and vitamin D. Med Hypotheses 2008;70(4):750–9. Epub 2007 Oct 24.
46 Noble JM, Mandel A, Patterson MC. Scurvy and rickets masked by chronic neurologic illness: revisiting 'psychologic malnutrition'. Pediatrics 2007 Mar;119(3):e783–90.
47 Rizwan S, Manning JT, Brabin BJ. Maternal smoking during pregnancy and possible effects of in utero testosterone: evidence from the 2D:4D finger length ratio. Early Hum Dev 2007 Feb;83(2):87–90. Epub 2006 Jun 30.
48 Auyeung B, Baron-Cohen S, Ashwin E, et. al. Fetal testosterone and autistic traits. Br J Psychol 2009 Feb;100(Pt 1):1–22. Epub 2008 Jun 10.
49 Knickmeyer RC, Baron-Cohen S. Fetal testosterone and sex differences in typical social development and in autism. J Child Neurol 2006 Oct;21(10):825–45.
50 Reichenberg A, Gross R, Weiser M, et. al. Advancing paternal age and autism. Arch Gen Psychiatry 2006;63:1026–32.
51 Kolevzon A, Gross R, Reichenberg A. Prenatal and perinatal risk factors for autism: a review and integration of findings. Arch Pediatr Adolesc Med 2007 Apr;161(4):326–33.
52 Maimburg RD, Vaeth M. Perinatal risk factors and infantile autism. Acta Psychiatr Scand. 2006 Oct;114(4):257–61.
53 Glasson EJ, Bower C, Petterson B, et. al. Perinatal factors and the development of autism: a population study. Arch Gen Psychiatry 2004 Jun;61(6):618–27.
54 Kinney DK, Munir KM, Crowley DJ, et. al. Prenatal stress and risk for autism. Neurosci Biobehav Rev 2008 Oct;32(8):1519–32. Epub 2008 Jun 13.
55 Aronson M, Hagberg B, Gillberg C. Attention deficits and autistic spectrum problems in children exposed to alcohol during gestation: a follow-up study. Dev Med Child Neurol 1997;39:583 –587.
56 Limperopoulos C, Bassan H, Sullivan NR, et. al. Positive screening for autism in ex-pre-term infants: prevalence and risk factors. Pediatrics 2008 Apr;121(4):758–65.
57 Maimburg RD, Vaeth M. Do children born after assisted conception have less risk of developing infantile autism? Hum Reprod 2007 Jul;22(7): 1841–3. Epub 2007 Apr 24.
58 Rogers EJ. Has enhanced folate status during pregnancy altered natural selection and possibly Autism prevalence? A closer look at a possible link. Med Hypotheses 2008 Sep;71(3):406–10. Epub 2008 Jun 2.
59 Pan CY, Frey GC. Physical activity patterns in youth with autism spectrum disorders. J Autism Dev Disord 2006 Jul;36(5):597–606.
60 Pan CY.Objectively measured physical activity between children with autism spectrum disorders and children without disabilities during inclusive recess settings in Taiwan. J Autism Dev Disord 2008 Aug;38(7):1292–301. Epub 2007 Dec 18.
61 Wakefield AJ, Anthony A, Murch SH, et. al. Enterocolitis in Children With Developmental Disorders. Am J Gastroenterol 2000;95:2285–2295.
62 McIntyre P, and McIntyre CR. Editorial: MMR, autism and inflammatory bowel disease: responding to patient concerns using an evidence-based framework. There is no convincing evidence that the MMR vaccine is associated with autism or IBD. MJA 2001;175:129–132.
63 Taylor B, Miller E, Farrington CP, et. al. Autism and measles, mumps, and rubella vaccine: no epidemiological evidence for a causal association. Lancet 1999;353:2026–2029.
64 Fombonne E, Du Mazaubrun C, Cans C, et. al. Autism and associated medical disorders in a French epidemiological survey. J Am Acad Child Adolesc Psychiatry 1997;36:1561–1569.
65 Madsen KM, Hviid A, Vestergaard M, et. al. A population-based study of measles, mumps, and rubella vaccination and autism. N Engl J Med 2002;347:1477–82.
66 Dales L, Hammer SJ, Smith NJ. Time trends in autism and in MMR immunization coverage in California. JAMA 2001;285:1183–1185.
67 Kaye JA, del Mar Melero-Montes M, Jick H. Mumps, measles, and rubella vaccine and the incidence of autism recorded by general practitioners: a time trend analysis. BMJ 2001;322:460–463.
68 Patja A, Davidkin I, Kurki T, et. al. Serious adverse events after measles-mumps-rubella vaccination during a fourteen-year prospective follow-up. Pediatr Infect Dis J 2000;19:1127–1134.
69 Fombonne E, Chakrabarti S. No Evidence for a New Variant of Measles-Mumps-Rubella–Induced Autism. Pediatrics 2001 October;108(4):1–8.
70 Levy SE, Hyman SL. Use of complementary and alternative treatments for children with autistic spectrum disorders is increasing. Pediatr Ann 2003 Oct;32(10):685–91.
71 Hanson E, Kalish LA, Bunce E, et. al. Use of complementary and alternative medicine among children diagnosed with autism spectrum disorder. J Autism Dev Disord 2007 Apr;37(4):628–36.
72 Harrington JW, Rosen L, Garnecho A, et. al. Parental perceptions and use of complementary and alternative medicine practices for children with autistic spectrum disorders in private practice. J Dev Behav Pediatr 2006 Apr;27(2 Suppl):S156–61.
73 Chalfant AM, Rapee R, Carroll L. Treating anxiety disorders in children with high functioning autism spectrum disorders: a controlled trial. J Autism Dev Disord 2007 Nov;37(10):1842–57. Epub 2006 Dec 15.
74 Ooi YP, Lam CM, Sung M, et. al. Effects of cognitive-behavioural therapy on anxiety for children with high-functioning autistic spectrum disorders. Singapore Med J 2008 Mar;49(3):215–20.
75 Turner-Brown LM, Perry TD, Dichter GS, et. al. Brief report: feasibility of social cognition and interaction training for adults with high functioning autism. J Autism Dev Disord 2008 Oct;38(9): 1777–84. Epub 2008 Feb 2.
76 Ben Itzchak E, Lahat E, Burgin R, et. al. Cognitive, behavior and intervention outcome in young children with autism. Res Dev Disabil 2008 Sep-Oct;29(5):447–58. Epub 2007 Oct 17.

77 Sinha Y, Silove N, Wheeler D, et. al. Auditory integration training and other sound therapies for autism spectrum disorders. Cochrane Database Syst Rev 2004;(1):CD003681.

78 Gold C, Wigram T, Elefant C. Music therapy for autistic spectrum disorder. Cochrane Database Syst Rev 2006 Apr 19;(2):CD004381.

79 Corbett BA, Shickman K, Ferrer E. Brief report: the effects of Tomatis sound therapy on language in children with autism. J Autism Dev Disord 2008 Mar;38(3):562–6.

80 Katagiri J. The effect of background music and song texts on the emotional understanding of children with autism. J Music Ther 2009 Spring;46(1):15–31.

81 Sams MJ, Fortney EV, Willenbring S. Occupational therapy incorporating animals for children with autism: A pilot investigation. Am J Occup Ther 2006 May-Jun;60(3):268–74.

82 Malow BA, Marzec ML, McGrew SG, et. al. Characterizing sleep in children with autism spectrum disorders: a multidimensional approach. Sleep 2006 Dec 1;29(12):1563–71.

83 Gail Williams P, Sears LL, Allard A. Sleep problems in children with autism. J Sleep Res 2004 Sep;13(3):265–8.

84 Allik H, Larsson JO, Smedje H. Sleep patterns in school-age children with Asperger syndrome or high-functioning autism: a follow-up study. J Autism Dev Disord 2008 Oct;38(9):1625–33. Epub 2008 Feb 22.

85 Goodlin-Jones BL, Tang K, Liu J, et. al. Sleep patterns in preschool-age children with autism, developmental delay, and typical development. J Am Acad Child Adolesc Psychiatry 2008 Aug;47(8):930–8.

86 Krakowiak P, Goodlin-Jones B, Hertz-Picciotto I, et. al. Sleep problems in children with autism spectrum disorders, developmental delays, and typical development: a population-based study. J Sleep Res 2008 Jun;17(2):197–206.

87 Bruni O, Ferri R, Vittori E, et. al. Sleep architecture and NREM alterations in children and adolescents with Asperger syndrome. Sleep 2007 Nov 1; 30(11):1577–85.

88 Miano S, Bruni O, Elia M, et. al. Sleep in children with autistic spectrum disorder: a questionnaire and polysomnographic study. Sleep Med 2007 Dec;9(1):64–70. Epub 2007 Aug 28.

89 Liu X, Hubbard JA, Fabes RA, et. al. Sleep disturbances and correlates of children with autism spectrum disorders. Child Psychiatry Hum Dev 2006 Winter;37(2):179–91.

90 Limoges E, Mottron L, Bolduc C, et. al. Atypical sleep architecture and the autism phenotype. Brain 2005 May;128(Pt 5):1049–61. Epub 2005 Feb 10.

91 Goodlin-Jones BL, Tang K, Liu J, Anders TF. Sleep patterns in preschool-age children with autism, developmental delay, and typical development. J Am Acad Child Adolesc Psychiatry 2008 Aug;47(8):930–8.

92 Johnson KP, Malow BA. Assessment and pharmacologic treatment of sleep disturbance in autism. Child Adolesc Psychiatr Clin N Am 2008 Oct;17(4):773–85, viii.

93 Polimeni MA, Richdale AL, Francis AJ. A survey of sleep problems in autism, Asperger's disorder and typically developing children. J Intellect Disabil Res 2005 Apr;49(Pt 4):260–8.

94 Johnson KP, Malow BA. Sleep in children with autism spectrum disorders. Curr Neurol Neurosci Rep 2008 Mar;8(2):155–61.

95 Polimeni MA, Richdale AL, Francis AJ. A survey of sleep problems in autism, Asperger's disorder and typically developing children. J Intellect Disabil Res 2005 Apr;49(Pt 4):260–8.

96 Weiskop S, Richdale A, Matthews J. Behavioural treatment to reduce sleep problems in children with autism or fragile X syndrome. Dev Med Child Neurol 2005 Feb;47(2):94–104.

97 Malow BA, McGrew SG, Harvey M, et. al. Impact of treating sleep apnea in a child with autism spectrum disorder. Pediatr Neurol 2006 Apr;34(4):325–8.

98 Garstang J, Wallis M. Randomized controlled trial of melatonin for children with autistic spectrum disorders and sleep problems. Child Care Health Dev 2006 Sep;32(5):585–9.

99 Wirojanan J, Jacquemont S, Diaz R, et. al. The Efficacy of Melatonin for Sleep Problems in Children with Autism, Fragile X Syndrome, or Autism and Fragile X Syndrome. Journal of Clinical Sleep Medicine 2009;5(2)145–150

100 Melke J, Botros HG, Chaste P, et. al. Abnormal melatonin synthesis in autism spectrum disorders. Molecular Psychiatry 2008;13:90–98. doi:10.1038/sj.mp.4002016; published online 15 May 2007.

101 Pitetti KH, Rendoff AD, Grover T, et. al. The efficacy of a 9–month treadmill walking program on the exercise capacity and weight reduction for adolescents with severe autism. J Autism Dev Disord 2007 Jul;37(6):997–1006.

102 Dietrich KN, Ware JH, Salganik M, et. al. Effect of chelation therapy on the neuropsychological and behavioral development of lead exposed children after school entry. Pediatrics 2004;114: 19–26.

103 Angley M, Semple S, Hewton C, et. al. Children and Autism. Part 2– Management with Complementary Medicines and Dietary Interventions Aust Fam Physician 2007 Oct;36(10):827–30.

104 Beauchamp RA, Willis TM, Betz TG, et. al. Deaths Associated With Hypocalcemia From Chelation Therapy-Texas, Pennsylvania, and Oregon, 2003–2005. JAMA Chicago 2006 May 10;295(18): 2131–2133 (3 pp.).

105 Angley M, Semple S, Hewton C, et. al. Children and Autism. Part 2–Management with Complementary Medicines and Dietary Interventions. Aust Fam Physician 2007 Oct;36(10):827–30.

106 Russo AF. Anti-metallothionein IgG and levels of metallothionein in autistic families. Swiss Med Wkly 2008 Feb 9;138(5–6):70–7.

107 Faber S, Zinn GM, Kern JC 2nd, et. al. The plasma zinc/serum copper ratio as a biomarker in children with autism spectrum disorders. Biomarkers 2009 May;14(3):171–80.

108 Geier DA, Geier MR. A clinical trial of combined anti-androgen and anti-heavy metal therapy in autistic disorders. Neuro Endocrinol Lett 2006 Dec;27(6):833–8.

109 Molloy CA, Manning-Courtney P.Prevalence of chronic gastrointestinal symptoms in children with autism and autistic spectrum disorders. Autism 2003 Jun;7(2):165–71.

110 Scott M. Myers, Chris Plauché Johnson, the Council on Children With Disabilities. Management of Children With Autism Spectrum Disorders. Pediatrics 2007 November;120(5):1162–1182. (doi:10.1542/peds.2007–2362).

111 Millward C, Ferriter M, Calver S, et. al. Gluten- and casein-free diets for autistic spectrum disorder. Cochrane Database Syst Rev 2004;(2):CD003498. Update in: Cochrane Database Syst Rev 2008;(2):CD003498.

112 Elder JH. The gluten-free, casein-free diet in autism: an overview with clinical implications. Nutr Clin Pract 2008 Dec-2009 Jan;23(6):583–8.

113 Herndon AC, DiGuiseppi C, Johnson SL, et. al. Does nutritional intake differ between children with autism spectrum disorders and children with typical development? J Autism Dev Disord 2009 Feb;39(2):212–22. Epub 2008 Jul 4.

114 Goday P.Whey Watchers and Wheat Watchers: The Case Against Gluten and Casein in Autism. Nutrition in Clinical Practice 2008 Dec;23(6): 581–582.

115 Clinical Trails Registry. Scan Brit. Dietary Intervention in Autism. http://clinicaltrials.gov/ct2/show/NCT00614198 Accessed Aug 8 2008.

116 Clinical Trials Registry. Diet and Behaviour in Young Children with Autism. http://clinicaltrials.gov/ct/show/NCT00090428 Accessed Aug 8 2008.

117 Jyonouchi H, Geng L, Ruby A, et. al. Evaluation of an association between gastrointestinal symptoms and cytokine production against common dietary proteins in children with autism spectrum disorders. J Pediatr 2005 May;146(5):605–10.

118 Garvey J. Diet in autism and associated disorders. J Fam Health Care 2002;12:34–8.

119 Horvath K, Perman JA. Autism and gastrointestinal symptoms. Curr Gastroenterol Rep 2002;4:251–8.

120 Finegold SM, Molitoris D, Song Y, et. al. Gastrointestinal microflora studies in late-onset autism. Clin Infect Dis 2002 Sep 1;35(Suppl 1):S6–S16.

121 Adams JB, Holloway C. Pilot study of a moderate dose multivitamin/mineral supplement for children with autistic spectrum disorder. J Altern Complement Med 2004 Dec;10(6):1033–9.

122 Adams JB, Holloway C. Pilot study of a moderate dose multivitamin/mineral supplement for children with autistic spectrum disorder. J Altern Complement Med 2004 Dec;10(6):1033–9.

123 Adams JB, George F, Audhya T. Abnormally high plasma levels of vitamin B6 in children with autism not taking supplements compared to controls not taking supplements. J Altern Complement Med 2006 Jan-Feb;12(1):59–63.

124 Kuriyama S, Kamiyama M, Watanabe M, et. al. Pyridoxine treatment in a subgroup of children with pervasive developmental disorders. Dev Med Child Neurol 2002;44:284–6.

125 Angley M, Semple S, Hewton C, et. al. Children and Autism Part 1–Recognition and Pharmacological Management. Aust Fam Physician 2007 Oct;36(10):827–30.

126 Ramaekers VT, Blau N, Sequeira JM, et. al. Folate receptor autoimmunity and cerebral folate deficiency in low-functioning autism with neurological deficits. Neuropediatrics 2007 Dec;38(6):276–81.

127 Adams M, Lucock M, Stuart J, et. al. Preliminary evidence for involvement of the folate gene polymorphism 19bp deletion-DHFR in occurrence of autism.Med Hypotheses 2008;70(4):750–9. Epub 2007 Oct 24.

128 Moretti P, Sahoo T, Hyland K, et. al. Cerebral folate deficiency with developmental delay, autism, and response to folinic acid. Neurology 2005 Mar 22;64(6):1088–90.

129 James SJ, Melnyk S, Fuchs G, et. al. Efficacy of methylcobalamin and folinic acid treatment on glutathione redox status in children with autism. Am J Clin Nutr 2009 Jan;89(1):425–30. Epub 2008 Dec 3.

130 McEachin JJ, Smith T, Lovaas OI. Long term outcomes for children with autism who received early intensive behavioral treatment. Am J Ment Retard 1993;97:359–72.

131 Dolske MC, Spollen J, McKay S, et. al. A preliminary trial of ascorbic acid as supplemental therapy for autism. Prog Neuropsychopharmacol Biol Psychiatry 1993 Sep;17(5):765–74.

132 Nye C, Brice A. Combined vitamin B6–magnesium treatment in autism spectrum disorder. Cochrane Database Syst Rev 2005 Oct 19;(4):CD003497.Update of: Cochrane Database Syst Rev. 2002;(4):CD003497.

133 Mousain-Bosc M, Roche M, Polge A, et. al. Improvement of neurobehavioral disorders in children supplemented with magnesium-vitamin B6. II. Pervasive developmental disorder-autism. Magnes Res 2006 Mar;19(1):53–62.

134 Dosman CF, Brian JA, Drmic IE, et. al. Children with autism: effect of iron supplementation on sleep and ferritin. Pediatr Neurol 2007 Mar;36(3):152–8.

135 Kidd PM. Omega-3 DHA and EPA for cognition, behavior, and mood: clinical findings and structural-functional synergies with cell membrane phospholipids. Altern Med Rev 2007 Sep;12(3):207–27.

136 Amminger GP, Berger GE, Schäfer MR, et. al. Omega-3 fatty acids supplementation in children with autism: a double-blind randomized, placebo-controlled pilot study. Biol Psychiatry 2007 Feb 15;61(4):551–3. Epub 2006 Aug 22.

137 Peregrin T. Registered dietitians' insights in treating autistic children. J Am Diet Assoc 2007 May;107(5):727–30.

138 Politi P, Cena H, Comelli M, et. al. Behavioral effects of omega-3 fatty acid supplementation in young adults with severe autism: an open label study. Arch Med Res 2008 Oct;39(7):682–5.

139 Sliwinski S, Croonenberghs J, Christophe A, et. al. Polyunsaturated fatty acids: do they have a role in the pathophysiology of autism? Neuro Endocrinol Lett 2006 Aug;27(4):465–71.

140 Bell JG, MacKinlay EE, Dick JR, et. al. Essential fatty acids and phospholipase A2 in autistic spectrum disorders. Prostaglandins Leukot Essent Fatty Acids 2004 Oct;71(4):201–4.

141 Chen WX, Wu-Li L, Wong VC. Electroacupuncture for children with autism spectrum disorder: pilot study of 2 cases. J Altern Complement Med 2008 Oct;14(8):1057–65.

142 Rossignol DA, Rossignol LW, Smith S, et. al. Hyperbaric treatment for children with autism: a multicenter, randomized, double-blind, controlled trial. BMC Pediatr 2009 Mar 13;9:21.

143 Cullen LA, Barlow JH, Cushway D. Positive touch, the implications for parents and their children with autism: an exploratory study. Complement Ther Clin Pract 2005 Aug;11(3):182–9.

144 Williams TI. Evaluating effects of aromatherapy massage on sleep in children with autism: a pilot study. Evid Based Complement Alternat Med 2006 Sep;3(3):373–7. Epub 2006 Apr 19.

145 Cullen L, Barlow J. Kiss, cuddle, squeeze': the experiences and meaning of touch among parents of children with autism attending a Touch Therapy Program. J Child Health Care 2002 Sep;6(3):171–81.

146 Escalona A, Field T, Singer-Strunck R, Cullen C, Hartshorn K. Brief report: improvements in the behavior of children with autism following massage therapy. J Autism Dev Disord 2001 Oct;31(5):513–6.

147 Silva LM, Cignolini A, Warren R, et. al. Improvement in sensory impairment and social interaction in young children with autism following treatment with an original qigong massage methodology. Am J Chin Med 2007;35(3): 393–406.

Chapter 8

Breast disease and breast cancer

Introduction

When many women think of breast disease, they think of breast cancer. However, there are many other diseases and conditions, both benign and malignant, that affect women's breasts.

Benign breast diseases

The phrase *benign breast diseases* encompasses a heterogeneous group of lesions that may present a wide range of symptoms or may be detected as attendant microscopic findings. The incidence of benign breast lesions begins to rise during the second decade of life and peaks in the 4th and 5th decades, as opposed to malignant diseases, for which the incidence continues to increase after menopause, although at a significant less rapid pace[1, 2, 3]

The majority of the lesions that occur in the breast are benign[4] and are far more frequent than malignant ones[5, 6, 7] With the advent of screening techniques such as mammography, ultrasound, and magnetic resonance imaging of the breast and the extensive use of needle biopsies, the diagnosis of a benign breast disease can be accomplished without surgery in the majority of patients.

The most frequently seen benign lesions of the breast have been summarised as developmental abnormalities, inflammatory lesions, fibrocystic changes, stromal lesions, and neoplasms (see Table 8.1).

Benign breast conditions — fibrocystic breast changes

Fibrocystic breast conditions (FBC) are the most common benign breast problem encountered in women. The following characteristics have been reported:[8]

- most common of benign breast conditions
- multiple tender breast masses
- may be cyclic in nature
- may have exaggerated response to hormones
- usually present as cyclic, bilateral pain and engorgement
- pain diffuse, often radiates to shoulders or upper arms
- prominent thickened plaques of breast tissue, often in upper outer quadrants.

Treatment (or management) of FBC

Lifestyle

Lifestyle changes that may be helpful include exercise, which may decrease breast tenderness. In 1study, women who walked approximately 30 minutes on most days reported less breast tenderness as well as improvement in other symptoms, such as anxiety.[8]

Diets

Some studies have reported that women with FBC drink more coffee than women without the disease,[9, 10] whereas other studies do not.[11, 12] Eliminating caffeine for less than 6 months does not appear to be effective at reducing symptoms of FBC.[13, 14] However, long-term and complete avoidance of caffeine does reduce symptoms of FBC.[15, 16] Some women are more sensitive to effects of caffeine than others, so benefits of restricting caffeine are likely to vary from woman to woman. Caffeine is found in coffee, black tea, green tea, cola drinks, chocolate, and many over-the-counter drugs. A decrease in breast tenderness can take 6 months or more to occur after caffeine is eliminated. Breast lumpiness may not go away, but the pain often decreases.

FBC has been linked to excess oestrogen. When women with FBC were put on a low-fat diet, their oestrogen levels decreased.[17, 18] After 3–6 months, the pain and lumpiness also decreased.[19,20] The link between dietary fat and symptoms appears to be most strongly related to saturated fat.[21] Foods high in saturated fat include meat and dairy products. Fish, non-fat dairy, and tofu are replacements to consider.

A recent study from the Women's Health Initiative Dietary Modification trial

Table 8.1 Benign and malignant conditions of the breast[4]

Benign breast conditions
Inflammatory and related lesions • Mastitis • Acute mastitis • Granulomatous mastitis • Foreign body reactions • Recurring subareolar abscess
Fibrocystic changes • Mammary duct ectasia • Fat necrosis • Cysts • Adenosis • Metaplasia • Epithelial hyperplasia • Ductal lesions • Lobular lesions • Columnar cell lesions • Radial scar and complex sclerosing lesion • Intraductal papilloma and papillomatosis
Malignant breast conditions
Proliferative stromal lesions • Diabetic fibrous mastopathy • Pseudoangiomatous stromal • Hyperplasia of the breast
Benign Neoplasms • Fibroadenoma • Lipoma • Adenoma • Nipple adenoma • Harmatoma • Granular cell tumour

investigated a total of 48 835 post-menopausal women, aged 50–79 years, without prior breast cancer.[22] Participants were randomly assigned to the dietary modification intervention group or to the comparison group. The intervention was designed to reduce total dietary fat intake to 20% of total energy intake, and to increase fruit and vegetable intake to ≥5 servings per day and intake of grain products to ≥6 servings per day. Risk for developing benign breast disease varied by levels of baseline total vitamin D intake but it varied little by levels of other baseline variables. Hence, the results suggested that a modest reduction in fat intake and increase in fruit, vegetable, and grain intake do not alter the risk of benign proliferative breast disease. It is difficult to conclude about the importance of diet in such a study without knowing details relating to other lifestyle factors, such as behavioural and exercise habits.

Supplements

Omega-6 fatty acids

In a double-blind research trial, evening primrose oil (EPO) reduced symptoms of FBC,[23] though only moderately. One group of researchers reported that EPO normalises blood levels of fatty acids in women with FBC.[24] However, even these scientists had difficulty linking the improvement in lab tests with an actual reduction in symptoms. Nonetheless, most reports continue to show at least some reduction in symptoms resulting from EPO supplementation with doses of 3g/day of EPO for at least 6 months to alleviate symptoms of FBC.[25, 26]

Vitamins

While several studies report that 200–600IU of vitamin E per day, taken for several months, reduces symptoms of FBD,[27, 28] most double-blind trials have found that vitamin E does not relieve FBC symptoms.[29, 30]

Vitamin B6

As with vitamin E, the effectiveness of vitamin B6 remains uncertain. The reduction of symptoms by vitamin B6 supplementation is controversial.[31, 32] Since vitamin B6 supplementation is effective for relieving the symptoms of premenstrual syndrome (PMS), in addition to breast tenderness, women should discuss the use of vitamin B6 with their health care provider.

Iodine

Laboratory animal studies demonstrate that iodine deficiency can cause symptoms similar to of FBC.[33] There are no clinical studies that recommend the use of iodine for FBC.

Herbal medicines

Since many women with FBD and cyclical breast tenderness also suffer from PMS, there is often an overlap in herbal recommendations for these 2 conditions despite a lack of research dealing directly with FBC.

Vitex agnus castus (Chasteberry)

In 1 double-blind trial, a liquid preparation containing 32.4mg of *Vitex agnus castus* (VAC) and homeopathic ingredients was found to successfully reduce breast tenderness associated with the menstrual cycle (e.g. cyclic mastalgia).[34] VAC is thought to reduce breast tenderness at menses because of its ability to reduce elevated levels of the hormone prolactin.[35]

Breast cancer — risk modification for prevention

Weight control and energy intake

There are numerous studies that report that controlling weight gain by reducing energy intake is associated with prevention of breast cancer.[36, 37] Weight gain in adult life is an important risk factor for breast cancer. Observational studies indicate that pre-menopausal or post-menopausal weight loss is associated with a reduction in risk of post-menopausal breast cancer.[38] On current scientific evidence the overall perception is that epidemiologic studies provide sufficient evidence that obesity is a risk factor for both cancer incidence and mortality.[39] Moreover, the evidence supports strong links of obesity with the risk for cancer of the breast (in post-menopausal women) as well as numerous other malignancies.[40]

Environmental factors

An increasing body of scientific evidence from both human and animal models indicates that exposure of fetuses, young children and adolescents to radiation and or environmental chemicals puts them at considerably higher risk for developing breast cancer in later life.[41] These data are consistent with the role of environmental exposures, especially at young ages, in affecting the later incidence of breast cancer in women who have immigrated to relatively industrialised areas from regions of the world with lower risks of breast cancer. There are numerous environmental chemicals that have been associated with breast cancer (see Table 8.2).

The increasing incidence of breast cancer in the decades following World War II paralleled the proliferation of synthetic chemicals. An estimated 80 000 synthetic chemicals have been documented to be in use today in the US, and another 1000 or more are added each year.[42] A recent survey indicated that 216 chemicals and radiation sources have been registered by international and national regulatory agencies as being experimentally implicated in breast cancer causation.[43, 44] Many of the chemicals (i.e. that include common fuels, solvents and industrial processes) can persist in the environment[45] and can accumulate in body fat and may remain in breast tissue for decades.[46, 47]

Nutritional influences

Soy and phytoestrogens

Phytoestrogens present in soy are structurally and functionally similar to oestrogen and have hence received significant attention as potential dietary modifiers of breast cancer risk. A meta-analysis of published studies on soy intake and breast cancer noted a significant protective effect of high soy intake on risk of breast cancer.[49] The comparatively high dietary intake of soy in Asian countries has been hypothesised to at least partly explain the lower breast cancer incidence patterns in these countries as compared with the Western world. The hypothesis is however contentious.[50, 51]

A variety of health benefits, including protection against breast cancer, have been attributed to soy food consumption, primarily because of the soybean isoflavones (genistein, daidzein, glycitein).[52] Isoflavones are considered to be possible selective oestrogen receptor modulators but possess non-hormonal properties that also may contribute to their effects.

A recent RCT study did not support the hypothesis however, that soy intake reduced breast cancer risk.[53] A diet high in soy protein among post-menopausal women did not decrease mammographic density. A further recent study from Japan supports this notion.[54] This prospective study suggested that consumption of soy food had no protective effects against breast cancer and that large-scale investigations eliciting genetic factors may clarify different roles of various soybean-ingredient foods on the risk of breast cancer.

Moreover, no effect on menopausal symptoms was reported in a RCT that investigated oral soy supplements versus placebo for the treatment of menopausal symptoms in patients with early breast cancer.[55]

It has been proposed though that intake of soy in early life and or in adolescence may be protective for the later development of breast cancer.[56] In most Asian countries where the incidence of breast cancer is exceptionally low, soy is consumed 2–3 times daily, and hence it is likely that it is protective.[57]

Dairy foods

There have been 3 meta-analysis published that have investigated the relationship between dairy food consumption and the risk of breast cancers. The first meta-analysis to combine the results of 5 cohort and 12 case-control studies about dairy product consumption and breast cancer risk found a small increased risk of breast cancer in women with greater intakes of milk.[58]

In 2002, and forming part of the Pooling Project, a pooled analysis of 8 cohort studies was published.[59] For this pooled analysis, 8 prospective studies with at least 200 cases of breast cancers each were included, thus bringing a total of 351041 healthy women and 7379 invasive breast cancer cases to

Table 8.2 A selection of compounds linked to breast cancer

Hormones and endocrine disrupting compounds	Link to breast cancer			Designated as endocrine disrupting
	Confirmed	Probable	Possible	
Oestrogens and progestins				
• Hormone replacement therapy	✓			
• Oral contraceptives	✓			
• Diethylstilbestrol	✓			
• Oestrogens and placental hormones (progestins) in personal care products	✓			
Xenoestrogens and other endocrine disrupting compounds				
• Dioxins	✓			✓
Persistent organochlorines DDT/ DDE and PCBs				✓
• DDT/DDE			✓	✓
• PCBs		✓		✓
Pesticides				
• Triazine herbicides— Atrazine				✓
• Heptachlor				✓
• Dieldrin and Aldrin				✓
• Other pesticides				✓
Polycyclic aromatic hydrocarbons				✓
Tobacco smoke — active and passive exposures	✓			✓
Bisphenol A				✓
Alkylphenols				✓
Some metals (e.g. mercury, lead)	✓			✓
Phthalates				✓
Parabens				✓
Sunscreens (UV filters)				✓
Growth promoters used in food production				
• Recombinant Bovine Growth Hormone / Recombinant Bovine				Inconclusive as at 2009
• Somatotropin				✓
• Zeranol				✓
Other chemicals that are of concern				
• Benzene	✓			
• Other organic solvents		✓		
• Vinyl Chloride	✓			
• 1,3–Butadiene		✓		
• Ethylene Oxide	✓			
• Aromatic Amines		✓		✓

(Source: adapted and modified from Gray et. al. 2009)[48]

the analysis. With respect to dairy products, different food groups were considered. Dairy products were divided into solids (butter and cheese) or liquids (milk, yoghurt, ice cream, etc.). Subgroups were also considered (whole, semi-skimmed or skimmed milk). Thus, ten different subgroups of dairy products were considered. Dairy product intake was analysed as a continuous variable (incrementally of 100g daily consumption for all products except butter and cream, and 10g for cream) and as categorical variable comparing higher versus lower quartiles of consumption. Other dietary and non-dietary factors associated with breast cancer were also considered, such as total energy, alcohol intake, parity, menopausal status and body mass index (BMI; i.e. level of obesity). Women in the 4th quartile of liquid dairy products consumed almost 630g of this kind of dairy product daily, whereas women in the first quartile consumed only 360g daily. No relationship was found between dairy product intake and breast cancer risk, neither treating dairy products as a continuous variable nor treating it as a categorical one. The research did not find statistically significant associations in any of the 10 subgroups of dairy products considered. The analysis concluded that, taking into account data of more than 350 000 women, there was no evidence that a diet rich in dairy products during middle or advanced age could increase or modify the risk of breast cancer in North American or European women.[59]

A more recent review about consumption of dairy products and risk of breast cancer concluded that published epidemiological data do not provide consistent evidence for an association between the consumption of dairy products and breast cancer risk.[60] This study pointed out limitations that must be considered. Namely the moderate reliability of the methods used to assess dairy product intake, which could lead to some misclassifications. Also that consumption of dairy products may be associated with other dietary habits or other variable nutrient content of dairy products (such as vitamin D consumption through food fortifications) that could also influence breast cancer risk.[59]

What makes this conclusion relevant from these studies is that in Asian countries where there is an exceptionally low incidence of breast cancer, dairy products are almost completely absent as part of the routine diet.

Meat consumption

A hypothesis has been advanced that links red meat consumption to the induction of carcinogenesis through it's highly bio-available iron content, growth-promoting hormones used in animal production, carcinogenic heterocyclic amines formed in cooking, and its specific fatty acid content.[61, 62]

A meta-analysis of case-control and cohort studies reported that there was a modest association of red meat intake with breast cancer incidence,[63] but no association was noted in a pooled analysis of prospective studies.[64] More recent reports from 2 large prospective cohorts noted an elevated risk with higher red meat consumption. In an analysis of the NHS II (n = 1021 cases that were predominantly pre-menopausal), a positive association between red meat and breast cancer risk was observed, especially for oestrogen receptor-negative and progesterone receptor-positive cancers,[65] comparing more than 1.5 servings per day to 3 or fewer servings per week. In the UK Women's Cohort Study (n = 678 cases), an increased risk of breast cancer was observed among women with a high red meat intake, with a 12% increase in risk per 50g increment of meat each day.[66] A study of post-menopausal Danish women (n = 378 cases) showed an elevated risk of breast cancer in those women consuming red meat and processed meat (≥25g per day). This association was confined to women genetically susceptible to carcinogenic aromatic amines due to polymorphisms in N-acetyl transferase.[67]

Carbohydrates

A number of prospective cohort studies have not shown any consistent associations between total carbohydrate, glycaemic index, glycaemic load, and breast cancer risk, and most results have not been significant.[68] However, these findings are not consistent with the association of refined carbohydrates and obesity in Western societies and the link to breast cancer which is opposite to findings in Asian countries (see under 'Weight control and energy intake' in this chapter).

Alcohol

Moderate alcohol consumption has been reported to increase sex steroid hormone levels and may interfere with folate metabolism, both of which are potential mechanisms for the observed associations of moderate alcohol intake with several forms of cancer, particularly breast and colorectal.[69, 70]

A meta-analysis of pooled cohort studies showed that there was a 10% increase in breast cancer risk for every 10g of alcohol consumed per day.[71] A similar magnitude of association was noted in 2 pooled analyses.[72] A dose-response relationship without a threshold effect has been reported, such that with even 1 drink per day was predictive of a modestly elevated risk for breast cancer.[73, 74] Menopausal status and type of alcoholic drink do not seem to modify this association. However, an interaction between folate and alcohol intake suggests that an adequate folate intake (most commonly achieved by taking a multiple vitamin or folate supplement) appears to reduce or eliminate the excess risk due to alcohol consumption.[75, 76]

A recent descriptive study has reported that alcohol and breast cancer risk may be defined by oestrogen and progesterone receptor status.[77] Moreover, the study supported the notion that alcohol was more strongly related to oestrogen positive than to oestrogen negative breast tumours. Furthermore, a further study concluded that although smoking was not related to asynchronous contralateral breast cancer, this study, the largest study of asynchronous contralateral breast cancer to date, demonstrated that alcohol was a risk factor for the disease, as it was for a first primary breast cancer.[78]

Diets

Mediterranean diet

An early review has pointed out that a number of cancers, such as cancer of the large bowel, breast and other hormonal dependent organs, are less frequent in Mediterranean countries than in northern Europe.[79] It has been put forward that a low dietary intake of saturated fat, accompanied by a higher intake of unrefined carbohydrates, and possibly other protective nutrients (phytochemicals in fruits and vegetables) could be the cause of such risk differences.

Recent studies suggested that adherence to a Mediterranean diet may be protective against breast cancer. An Italian study reported that a traditional Mediterranean diet significantly reduced endogenous oestrogen.[80] The results of this important study could eventually lead to identifying selected dietary components that more effectively can decrease oestrogen levels and, hence, provide a basis to develop dietary preventive measures for breast cancer. A US study confirms such notions by reporting that in their study, selected dietary patterns (such as those found in the Mediterranean diet) may be protective primarily in the presence of pro-carcinogenic compounds such as those found in tobacco smoke.[81]

Moreover, Western lifestyles, characterised by reduced physical activity and a diet rich in fat, refined carbohydrates, and animal protein is associated with high prevalence of overweight, metabolic syndrome, insulin resistance, and high plasma levels of several growth factors and sex hormones. Most of these factors are associated with breast cancer risk and, in breast cancer patients, with increased risk of recurrences. Such metabolic and endocrine imbalances can be favourably modified through comprehensive dietary modification, shifting from a Western to Mediterranean and macrobiotic diets.[82]

It is also important to note that a key factor associated with the Mediterranean diet is the Mediterranean lifestyle and unless this is included in the study the research recommendations would be incomplete.

Vegetarian diets

A recent study strongly suggests that a diet characterised by a low intake of meat and/or starches and a high intake of legumes is associated with a reduced risk of breast cancer in Asian Americans.[83]

Further, a recent study investigated the associations of different dietary patterns (Western, Prudent, Native Mexican, Mediterranean, and Dieter) with the risk for breast cancer in Hispanic women (757 cases and 867 controls) and non-Hispanic white women (1524 cases and 1598 controls) from the Four-Corners Breast Cancer Study.[84] The results showed that the Western (odds ratio for highest versus lowest quartile) and Prudent dietary patterns were associated with greater risk for breast cancer, and the Native Mexican and Mediterranean dietary patterns were associated with lower risk of breast cancer. Body mass index modified the associations of the Western diet and breast cancer among post-menopausal women and those of the Native Mexican diet among pre-menopausal women. Associations of dietary patterns with breast cancer risk varied by menopausal and body mass index status, but there was little difference in associations between non-Hispanic white and Hispanic women.

It has also been reported that nutrition for primary prevention of breast cancer by dietary means therefore relies on an individually tailored mixed diet, rich in basic foods and traditional manufacturing and cooking methods.[85]

Nutritional supplements

Multivitamins and/or minerals

The relationship between breast cancer and micronutrients is complex. It includes folate, vitamins, and carotenoids, and has been investigated in large prospective studies using biomarkers of intake. Two recent meta-analyses noted a possible protective effect by folate, especially among women who drank alcohol.[86, 87]

A recent systematic review of vitamin and mineral supplement use among US adults after cancer diagnosis reported that breast cancer survivors had the highest use.[88]

A recent double-blinded, randomly controlled, cross-over trial of multivitamins versus placebo in patients with breast cancer undergoing radiation therapy was undertaken to evaluate fatigue and quality of life.[89] The study results showed that no significant changes were elicited with the use of multivitamins. Hence, multivitamins supplementation did not improve radiation-related fatigue in patients with breast cancer. Moreover, a recent report on multivitamin use and risk of cancer in the Women's Health Initiative (WHI) cohorts showed that following a median follow-up of 8.0 and 7.9 years in the clinical trial and observational study cohorts, respectively, the WHI study provided convincing evidence that multivitamin use had no influence on the risk of common cancers, cardiovascular disease (CVD), or total mortality in post-menopausal women.[90] However, this study did not include lifestyle factors such as behaviour and exercise and, hence, it is difficult to see how its findings could be conclusive. Moreover, the recent Framingham study found that elevated homocystine was the most important risk factor for CVD which is usually normalised by a multivitamin supplement.[91]

Vitamin D

Vitamin D, a fat-soluble pro-hormone, is synthesised in response to sunlight. It has been documented that experimental evidence suggests that vitamin D may reduce the risk of cancer through regulation of cellular proliferation and differentiation as well as inhibition of angiogenesis.[92]

There have been 10 descriptive studies that have investigated the relationship between vitamin D intake and breast cancer risk. Namely, 5 cohort studies [93–97] and 5 case control studies.[98–102] Overall, the case control study of Knight et. al.[99] examined sunlight exposure and intake of vitamin D-rich foods as well as vitamin D supplements at various ages (10–19, 20–29, 45–54 years). Sun exposure and use of vitamin D supplements or multivitamins between the ages of 10–19 and 20–29 were associated with reduced risk of breast cancer. Of the hospital-based case-control studies, Nunez et. al.[96] and the cohort studies of John et. al.,[90] Shin et. al.,[91] and McCullough et. al.[94] provided some evidence for inverse associations, while the results of most of the remaining studies were essentially null.

Vitamins E

Pre-menopausal women with breast cancer often experience early menopause as a result of the therapy for their malignant disease. The abrupt occurrence of menopause resulting from such treatments as chemotherapy, oophorectomy, radiation therapy, or gonadal dysgenesis frequently results in hot flushes that begin at a relatively younger age and may occur with greater frequency and intensity than hot flushes associated with natural menopause.

A double-blind, placebo-controlled, cross-over randomised clinical trial reported a marginal statistical effect of vitamin E (dose used 800IU/day) in the treatment of hot flashes. The treatment duration was for 4 weeks of daily vitamin E consumption and was compared with placebo in 120 breast cancer patients.[103] Vitamin E was associated with 1 less hot flash per person per day and did not induce any significant toxicity. A cross-over analysis showed that vitamin E was associated with a minimal decrease in hot flashes. There was no preference for use of vitamin E over placebo when participants were assessed at the end of the study. The study hence suggested that vitamin E at a dose of 800IU daily can be used because it is inexpensive and non-toxic and it might result in a slightly better relief of hot flashes than placebo. The scientific evidence is therefore limited. Thus, more clinical data are warranted and caution is advocated as vitamin E is not registered for this use. However, these studies did not elucidate whether the synthetic or the natural form of vitamin E was used and hence the conclusions reached may be controversial.

Vitamin A and/or vitamin a-analogs

Studies on specific carotenoid intake and breast cancer risk modulation are limited.[104] The roles that carotenoids, retinol, and tocopherols may have in breast cancer aetiology remain complex and largely inconclusive.[105] It has been suggested though that consumption of fruits and vegetables high in specific carotenoids and vitamins may be the best option that could reduce pre-menopausal breast cancer risk.[101, 106] Recently the relationship between plasma carotenoids at enrolment and 1, 2 or 3, 4 and 6 years and breast cancer-free survival in the Women's Healthy Eating and Living (WHEL) Study participants (N = 3043), who had been diagnosed with early-stage breast cancer, concluded that higher biological exposure to carotenoids, when assessed over the timeframe of the study, was associated with greater likelihood of breast cancer-free survival regardless of study group assignment.[107]

An early study administered vitamin A to randomly allocated patients (n = 100) with metastatic breast carcinoma treated by chemotherapy.[108] The daily doses employed indefinitely ranged from 350 000 to 500 000IU according to body weight. There was noted a significant increase in the complete response rate. When subgroups determined by menopausal status were considered in the analysis of the data, it was observed that serum retinol levels were only significantly increased in the post-menopausal group on high dose Vitamin A. Response rates, duration of response and projected survival were only significantly increased in this subgroup.

Chemotherapy, which is fundamental for the treatment of metastatic breast cancer, is reported to rarely cure due to the presence of minimal residual disease that has spread to other organs. A pilot study was designed to test whether vitamin A (as retinyl palmitate) in combination with interferon and tamoxifen could improve overall survival in metastatic breast cancer patients.[109] The results showed that the combination was feasible and showed activity in metastatic breast cancer with an acceptable level of toxicity.

Preclinical models suggest that synthetic retinoids can inhibit mammary carcinogenesis.[110] In a recent review of clinical trials with synthetic retinoids for breast cancer chemo prevention it was reported that a phase III breast cancer prevention trial, investigating fenretinide (a synthetic retinoid derivative of vitamin A), showed a durable trend to a reduction of second breast malignancies in pre-menopausal women. This pattern was associated with a favourable modulation of circulating IGF-I and its main binding protein IGFBP-3, which have been associated with breast cancer risk in pre-menopausal women in different prospective studies.[111] Moreover, a recent study showed that fenretinide positively balanced the metabolic profile in overweight pre-menopausal women at high risk for breast cancer, and this was postulated to perhaps favourably affect breast cancer risk.[112]

All trans retinoic acid (ATRA) (also known as Tretinoin) is the acid form of vitamin A. A phase II trial employed all trans retinoic acid so as to evaluate its tumour cytoreduction in patients with metastatic breast cancer and to characterise the initial pharmacokinetics of the compound.[113] The study concluded that ATRA did not have any significant activity in patients with hormone refractory metastatic breast cancer.

A phase I–phase II combination clinical trial with tamoxifen and ATRA in patients with advanced breast cancer investigated their additive antitumor effects.[114] The study showed that declines in serum IGF-I concentrations observed in patients treated with tamoxifen and ATRA were similar to those observed in patients treated with tamoxifen alone. Additional studies are warranted to further investigate these data.

Lycopene

The epidemiologic literature regarding intake of tomatoes and tomato-based products and blood lycopene (a compound derived predominantly from tomatoes) level in relation to the risk of various cancers was reviewed. The outcome suggested strongly that there was a consistently lower risk of cancer for a variety of anatomic sites (including breast) that was associated with higher consumption of tomatoes and tomato-based products adding further support for current dietary recommendations to increase fruit and vegetable consumptions.[115]

A recent review concluded that the emerging area of health-derived benefits from food sources such as lycopene requires additional investigations into its effects on breast cancer.[116]

Integrative management of malignant breast disease

Lifestyle

Breast cancer can spread insidiously. The prevalence in the US during the years 2000–2004 in women aged 20–24 years had the lowest breast cancer incidence rate of 1.4 cases per 100 000 women, and women aged 75–79 years had the highest incidence rate of 464.8 cases per 100 000. The decrease in age-specific incidence rates that occurs in women aged 80 years and older may reflect lower rates of screening, the detection of cancers by mammography before age 80, and incomplete detection.[117]

An early investigation of approximately 25 000 women diagnosed with breast cancers reported that at diagnosis, 5–15% of patients had metastatic disease and almost 40% had regional spread of the disease.[118]

Promotion of behaviour patterns that optimise energy balance (i.e. weight control and increasing physical activity) may be viable options for the prevention of breast cancer. Researchers from the US and Peoples Republic of China (PRC) have evaluated the hypothesis that a pattern of behavioural exposures indicating positive energy balance (i.e. less physical activity/sport activity, high BMI, or high energy food intake) would be associated with an increased risk for breast cancer in the Shanghai

Breast Cancer Study.[119] This population-based study comprised 1459 incident breast cancer cases and 1556 age frequency-matched controls. Participants completed in-person interviews that collected information on breast cancer risk factors, usual dietary intake and physical activity in adulthood. Anthropometric indices were also measured. The study concluded that lack of physical activity/sport activity, low occupational activity, and high BMI were all individually associated with an increased risk for breast cancer (odds ratios [OR] 1.49 to 1.86).

In general, the study documented that women with lower physical activity/sport activity level and higher BMI, or those with higher energy food intake, were at an increased risk compared with women who reported participation in more physical activity/sport activities, had lower BMIs, or reported less energy food intake. There was a significant multiplicative interaction (P = 0.02) between adult physical activity/sport activity and BMI, with inactive women in the upper BMI quartile being at increased risk (OR, 2.16) compared with their active and lean counterparts. This association was stronger in post-menopausal than in pre-menopausal women, and non-participation in physical activity in post-menopausal women with higher BMIs had a significantly increased risk (OR, 4.74) for breast cancer. Hence, it was concluded that promoting behavioural changes that optimise energy balance (weight control and increasing physical activity) may be a viable option for breast cancer prevention.

A recent study has summarised that lifestyle changes including continuous or intermittent energy restriction and/or physical activity may be significantly beneficial for preventing breast cancer.[120]

Mind–body medicine

Cancer is a profoundly stressful experience. A cancer diagnosis is full of trepidation by most people because of its life-threatening implications and the potentially serious side-effects of the treatments. Hence, mind–body therapies have become more popular within cancer populations as methods to treat physical and psychiatric symptoms in conjunction with conventional allopathic care. Interventions such as support groups, educational programs, guided imagery, and expressive writing have been studied and are now frequently incorporated into plans of care for all types of cancer patients.[121, 122, 123]

Psychotherapeutic and social support interventions provide emotional and other psychological benefits to cancer patients.[124] Group, individual and family interventions have been shown to reduce depression and anxiety, improve coping and mobilise social support.[125, 126] However, what is more controversial are findings that psychosocial interventions may affect the course of the disease as well as the adjustment to it. Most people are ready to accept that changes in physical status influence cognition and affect.[127] In the context of a holistic approach to health that includes the concept of unity of mind and body, it makes sense that intervention at a mental level might have physical consequences.[128]

Research by a number of investigators has reported that patients who underwent psychological intervention lived longer than the national average.[129–132] Some researchers have analysed the psychological attributes associated with patients who survive what is thought to be terminal cancer. Roud[133] noted that all long-term survivors believed that there was a direct relationship between the outcomes experienced and their psychological states. They remained confident that they would not die, and felt that these positive expectations were critical to the healing process. They assumed responsibility for all aspects of their lives, including recovery and established relationships with physicians described as trusting, meaningful, and healing.

The key components of effective interventions appear to be:

- A supportive, stable and consistent environment.
- Intervention clearly delineated and implemented by trained professionals — important for having the patient feel confident in the treatment and therefore willing to participate fully.
- Groups homogeneous to disease and stage — a natural bonding may occur when patients share a similar disease and prognosis. This is important for undoing a commonly felt sense of isolation in cancer patients. It is possible to successfully lead homogeneous groups[134] but this is more challenging and requires greater skill. Leaders need to facilitate an understanding among group members. To date, no evidence to suggest that homogeneous groups affect survival time.
- Educational component — serves to diminish uncertainty and boost a sense of mastery and control.
- Teaching stress management and coping strategies.

These interventions help cancer patients prepare for the worst but hope for the best.

All have the goal of living better, and improve prognosis.

Mindfulness meditation

Mindfulness meditation is a form of mind–body therapy that is gaining credibility and interest for use in oncology patients.[135] It has been reported that the primary emphasis of mindfulness meditation is experiencing life fully and being in touch with the full range of human emotions and sensory experiences. Rather than a method to control or change unpleasant or unwanted emotions, thoughts, or sensations, mindfulness meditation is a way of being engaged in the complete experience of what is happening in the present moment without getting entangled in reflections about previous experiences or an anticipated future.[136, 137] Mindfulness meditation will often elicit relaxation, and as a result, offers individuals a way to alleviate suffering that often accompanies pain or emotional discomfort.[138]

Mindfulness Based Stress Reduction (MBSR)

MBSR is a well-defined, systematic, educational, patient-focused intervention with formal training in mindfulness meditation and its applications in everyday life, which includes managing physical and emotional pain for cancer patients.[136]

A recent study demonstrated that MBSR is a significantly effective program that is feasible for women recently diagnosed with early stage breast cancer and the results provided preliminary evidence for beneficial effects of MBSR on immune function, quality of life and coping.[139] A further study utilising MBSR to investigate a 1-year pre-post intervention follow-up of psychological, immune, endocrine and blood pressure outcomes demonstrated that MBSR program participation was associated with enhanced quality of life and decreased stress symptoms, altered cortisol and immune patterns.[140] These results were consistent with less stress and mood disturbances, and decreased blood pressure. The pilot data represented a preliminary investigation of the longer-term relationships between MBSR program participation and a range of potentially important biomarkers in patients with breast cancer.

Overall recent reviews conclude that from all the current available scientific evidence, MBSR may be a potentially beneficial intervention.[141, 142] Moreover, a recent clinician's guide to MBSR concluded that it was a safe, effective, integrative approach for reducing stress. Also both patients and health care providers experiencing stress or stress-related symptoms may benefit from MBSR programs.[143] MBSR interventions can be safely and effectively used in a variety of patient populations.

Cognitive behaviour therapy (CBT)

CBT is a psychotherapeutic approach that aims to influence dysfunctional emotions, behaviours and cognitions through a goal-oriented, systematic procedure in, for example, cancer patients. Behavioural symptoms are a common adverse effect of breast cancer diagnosis and treatment and include disturbances in energy, sleep, mood, and cognition.

CBT was found to be helpful for survivors of breast cancer who reported cognitive impairment after chemotherapy in a single-arm pilot study.[144] Ferguson et. al. reported that a specialised intervention using CBT principles called 'memory and attention adaptation training' was delivered to 29 survivors of breast cancer. The study concluded that participants reported high treatment satisfaction and rated the memory and attention adaptation training as helpful in improving ability to compensate for memory problems. Given these results, the CBT treatment appears to be a feasible and practical cognitive behaviour program that necessitates continued evaluation among cancer survivors who experience persistent cognitive dysfunction.

Few studies have examined the experience of cognitive impairment and how it affects day-to-day life. A small interview-based study with 10 survivors of breast cancer who reported cognitive impairment after chemotherapy showed that the women who reported the most disruption from cognitive impairment were those with high-stress occupations and coping with professional and family commitments.[145]

A recent Cochrane review that assessed the effects of psychological interventions (educational, individual cognitive behavioural, psychotherapeutic, or group support) on psychological and survival outcomes for women with metastatic breast cancer reported that there was insufficient evidence to advocate that group psychological therapies be recommended to women with metastatic breast cancer.[146] However, this review did not analyse the results of other studies that showed benefit for psychological therapies.[147]

Hypnosis

A recent review has investigated the potential use of hypnosis in reducing the frequency and intensity of hot flashes in women with breast cancer.[148] The study concluded that hypnosis may be a preferred treatment because of the few side-effects it elicits and the preference of many women for a non-hormonal therapy. Two recent randomised trials have confirmed this notion.[149, 150]

In the first study, 60 female breast cancer survivors with hot flashes were randomly assigned to receive hypnosis intervention (5-weekly sessions) or no treatment.[147] The study concluded that hypnosis appeared to reduce perceived hot flashes in breast cancer survivors and may have additional benefits, such as reduced anxiety and depression, and improved sleep. In the second trial 150 women with primary breast cancer who experienced hot flashes were randomised to either the intervention group, who received a single relaxation training session and were instructed to use practice tapes on a daily basis at home for 1 month, or to the control group who received no intervention.[43] This study concluded that relaxation may be a useful component of a program of measures to relieve hot flashes in women with primary breast cancer.

Environment

Studies have investigated the combined effects of 11 different environmental contaminants — all added at levels so low that they did not have any effects in isolation — and found the various chemicals had additive effects with each other and also with naturally occurring oestradiol.[151] Likewise, at concentrations found in the environment, the ubiquitous plasticiser bisphenol A has been reported to significantly increase the effects of oestradiol.[152] These combined experimental results show that even at low concentrations, environmental chemicals may exacerbate some of the biological effects of natural oestrogens.

Recent large clinical studies of women with breast cancer have investigated the effects of exposures to environmental chemicals and radiation in combination with other factors. The data from these studies illustrate how complex the interactions among breast cancer risk factors may be (Figure 8.1). The data also help clarify why large epidemiological studies examining the effects of different chemicals on breast cancer risk in women may have contradictory results.

In a study examining the possible link between organochlorin pesticide residues and breast cancer among African American and white women in North Carolina, higher blood (plasma) levels of the chemicals did not match to a diagnosis of breast cancer.[153] However, the data did suggest that race/ethnicity, body mass, reproductive history and social factors might make some women more susceptible to the carcinogenic effects of the organochlorin pesticides. Several other studies suggest that specific combinations of genes may make some women more susceptible to specific environmental carcinogens.[150, 154, 155]

Physical activity

Physical activity is a critical component of energy balance. The daily adherence to physical activity has a significant impact on preventing chronic diseases such as cancer.[156] Moreover, current reports clearly support the beneficial role that physical activity and exercise play in

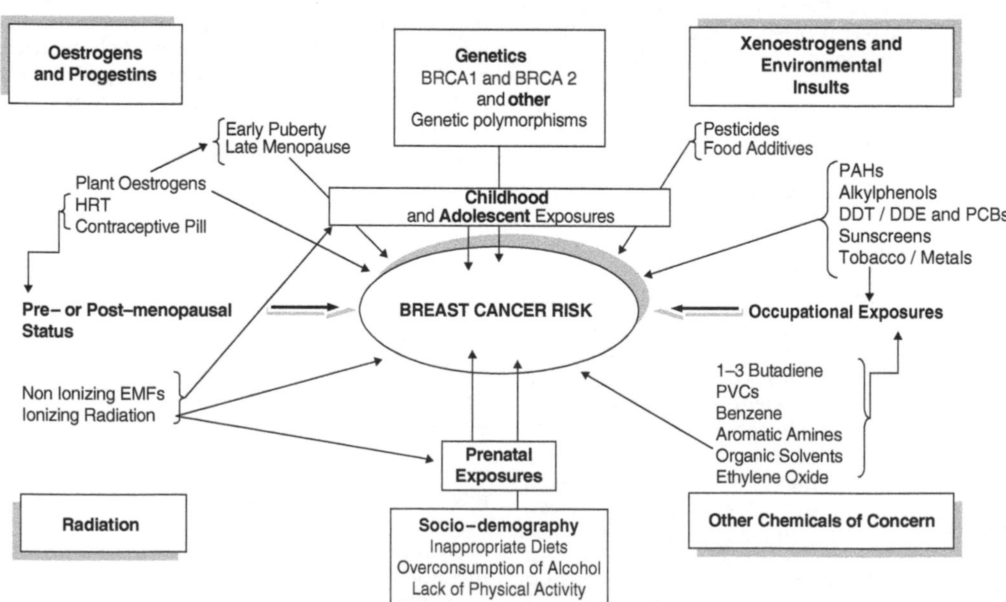

Figure 8.1 The complexity of breast cancer causation (examples)

reducing the risk for developing breast cancer and preventing or attenuating disease and treatment-related impairments.[157]

A recent systematic review has reported on 9 randomised clinical trials and the effects of exercise on quality of life in women living with breast cancer.[158] The systematic review reported that there was strong evidence that exercise positively influences quality of life in women living with breast cancer. Moreover, a large study with a follow-up of 18 years reported that women who participated in physical activity had half the chance of death as compared with those that did not exercise.[159]

Adherence to a physical activity program may have additional benefits for women undergoing conventional treatments for breast cancer. A recent small placebo-controlled RCT demonstrated that an exercise intervention administered to breast cancer patients undergoing medical treatment assisted in the alleviation of some treatment side-effects, including decreased total caloric intake, increased fatigue, and negative changes in body composition.[160]

The mechanism that may assist women in managing breast cancer symptoms due to treatment regimens as well as delaying disease progression when participating in physical activity may include the down regulation of pro-growth factors such as insulin-like growth factor, IGF-I, and its main binding protein, IGFBP-3.

Recently it was reported in a systematic review that IGF-I and IGFBP-3, can modulate cell growth and survival, and are thought to have important attributes in tumour development.[161] The adherence to a prudent physical activity regime may extend survival from cancer through interactions with the IGF–1 axis and in particular IGFBP-3.

A recent RCT demonstrated that moderate-intensity aerobic exercise, such as brisk walking, decreased IGF-I and IGFBP-3. The exercise-induced decreases in IGF may mediate the observed association between higher levels of physical activity and improved survival in women diagnosed with breast cancer.[162] A further study did not support a protective effect of physical activity on breast cancer recurrence or mortality but did suggest that the regular implementation of physical activity was beneficial for breast cancer survivors in terms of total mortality.[163]

Recently in a study of physical activity and post-menopausal breast cancer patients, it was concluded that only BMI and oestrone were convincingly associated with both post-menopausal breast cancer risk and physical activity. However, it was also reported that aetiologic studies should consider interactions among biomarkers, whereas exercise trials should explore exercise effects independently of weight loss, different exercise prescriptions, and effects on central adiposity.[164]

Overall, the scientific data is strong for the protective effects associated with physical activity. A study that investigated the associations between recreational physical activity and quality of life in a multiethnic cohort of breast cancer survivors, specifically testing whether associations are consistent across racial and/or ethnic groups after accounting for relevant medical and demographic factors that might explain disparities in quality of life outcomes, showed that meeting recommended levels of physical activity is associated with improved quality of life in non-Hispanic white and black breast cancer survivors.[165] These findings may help support future interventions among breast cancer survivors and promote supportive care that includes physical activity.

Yoga

There are not many studies on the efficacy of yoga in women with breast cancer.

Two recent trials have demonstrated benefit in women with breast cancer in abrogating disease and treatment side-effects. The earlier pilot study showed that a home-based yoga program provided participants with significantly lower levels of pain and fatigue, and higher levels of invigoration, acceptance, and relaxation.[166] The more recent study, a small RCT carried out by the same research group also showed that women with breast cancer that participated in yoga experienced significantly lower levels of pain and fatigue, and higher levels of invigoration, acceptance, and relaxation.[167]

Tai chi

There are few studies investigating the efficacy of tai chi as an adjunct intervention in patients with breast cancer as treatment for breast cancer produces side-effects that diminish functional capacity and quality of life. Three studies from the same research group has reported that tai chi can be beneficial and may enhance functional capacity and quality of life among breast cancer survivors.[168, 169, 170]

However, a recent systematic review has concluded that there is not enough evidence to recommend it as a useful adjunct intervention for women with breast cancer.[171]

Nutrition

Epidemiological studies show that populations which consume a typical Asian diet have lower incidences of a number of cancers, including breast cancer, than those consuming a Western diet.[172] The Asian diet includes mostly plant foods, including legumes, fruits, and vegetables, and is low in fat. The Japanese have the highest consumption of soy foods. The typical Western diet includes large amounts of animal foods, is lower in fibre and complex carbohydrates, and is high in fat. Soy foods are dietary staples in Asia, but are not commonly included in the Western diet.[173] The epidemiological data reports that there are a number of food groups that have an association with breast cancer risk in both pre- and post-menopausal women and an overview is presented in Table 8.3.

Dietary fat

The relationship between saturated fat consumption and breast cancer incidence and survival remains controversial. Early descriptive studies have reported that the 5-year survival of women with breast cancer in Tokyo, where dietary fat intake is low, was about 15% greater than that of women from Western countries.[175, 176, 177] A recent study supported this premise.[178] However, additional recent studies do not support this concept.[179, 180]

The Women's Healthy Eating and Living (WHEL) Study was a large, multi-institutional, randomised trial designed to test if noticeably increasing the consumption of vegetables, fruit, fibre and carotenoids and with concomitant decreases in total and saturated fat consumption (a study design as a putative cancer-preventive dietary guide) would lower the risk of breast cancer events such as recurrences and new primaries for women who had been recently diagnosed (within 4 years of diagnosis) with early-stage breast cancer.[181] The recent WHEL report concluded that the difference between study groups of the RECT was significant only in upper baseline quartiles of intake of vegetables, fruit, and fibre and in the lowest quartile of fat. A significant trend for fewer breast cancer events was observed across quartiles of vegetable, fruit and fibre consumption.[182]

Together with previously reported efficacy results, the WHEL study data suggests that a lifestyle intervention that reduces dietary fat intake and is associated with modest weight loss may favourably influence breast cancer recurrence.[183, 184] The WHEL low-fat eating plan can serve as a model for implementing long-term dietary interventions in clinical practice.

Herbal medicines

Traditional Chinese medicine (TCM)

Despite a quite extensive series of laboratory investigations detailing many biological effects of herbal medicine compounds, there are only a few clinical trials that have been completed to test specific hypotheses regarding the mode of action of TCM.[185]

Juzentaiho–to is a mixture of extracts from 10 medicinal herbs and has been used traditionally to treat patients with anaemia, anorexia or fatigue.[186] An early RCT study from Japan demonstrated that *Juzentaiho–to* supportive therapy improved quality of life in patients with advanced breast cancer.[187]

Immuno-stimulating polysaccharides extracted from the Chinese medicinal plant *Yun Zhi* (*Coriolus versicolor*) have been found to enhance various immunological functions, and *Danshen* (*Salvia miltiorrhiza*) to show beneficial effects on the circulatory system.[188] A recent study has demonstrated that the regular oral consumption of *Yunzhi–Danshen* capsules could be beneficial for promoting immunological function in post-treatment of breast cancer patients.[189]

A recent double-blind RCT of a Chinese herbal medicine as complementary therapy for reduction of chemotherapy-induced toxicity reported that the TCM did not reduce the hematologic toxicity associated with chemotherapy. However, supplementally the TCM did have a significant impact on control of nausea.[190] The herbs in this study consisted of 225 types of the commonly used herbs stocked in packaged form. Each package contained 3–10g of water-soluble herbal granules (see: http://annonc.oxfordjournals.org/cgi/reprint/18/4/768).[191]

Ruyiping is a TCM compound/herbal medicine composed of 5 Chinese herbs for removing toxic materials and dissipating nodules from *Runing II*, another traditional Chinese compound/herbal medicine for treating breast cancer, and in preventing recidivation and metastasis in breast cancer patients post surgery. The effect of *Ruyiping* in preventing recidivation and metastasis was similar to that of *Runing II*.[192] *Ruyiping* is reported as being the essential component of *Runing II* for preventing recidivation and metastasis. The result provides some clinical evidence for the theory that *Yudu Pangcuan* (vestigial poison invasion elsewhere) is the essential pathogenesis of breast cancer's recidivation and metastasis and the utilisation of *Sanjie Jiedu* (dispersing accumulation and detoxification) is the important therapeutic principle in preventing recidivation and metastasis after breast cancer surgery.

The TCM *Shenqi Fuzheng* (radix ginseng rubra; radix aconiti lateralis preparata) has traditional immune enhancement activity.[193] A study investigating *Shenqi Fuzheng* injections in combination with chemotherapy in treating metastatic cancer could reduce the occurrence

Table 8.3 Epidemiological associations — foods and nutrient groups and breast cancer risk in women

Food and/or nutrient group	Effect on pre-menopausal women	Effect on post-menopausal Women	Level of evidence based upon selected references
Alcohol	5–10% ↑ in risk at 10g alcohol/day	5–10% ↑ in risk at 10g alcohol/day	Pooled analysis of 6 prospective studies
Total fat	NA	Ambiguous	• Observational cohort, Nurses' Health Study • Randomised study, Women's Health Initiative • Pooled analysis of 8 studies • Observational cohort, AARP Diet and Health Study
Animal fat	• Inconsistent associations • Overall trend of risk ↑ animal fat intake	• Weak positive association for saturated fat intake • Mixed results for unsaturated fats	• Observational cohort, Nurses' Health Study • Pooled analysis of 8 studies • Observational cohort, AARP Diet and Health Study
Total carbohydrates	NA	NA	• Observational cohort, Nurses' Health Study
Carbohydrate quality (glycaemic index and glycaemic load)	NA	NA	• Observational cohort, Cancer prevention Study II, Nurses' Health Study • Women's Health Study
Fibre	NA	NA	• Observational cohort, Nurses' Health Study
Red meat	Inconsistent association ↑risk with ↑meat consumption may be restricted to hormone-sensitive breast malignancies	Inconsistent association overall	• Observational cohort, Nurses' Health Study • UK Women's Health Study • Pooled analysis of 8 prospective studies
Dairy milk	NA	NA	• Pooled analysis of 8 prospective studies • Observational cohort, Nurses' Health Study
Fruits and vegetables	NA	NA	• Pooled analysis of 8 prospective studies
Soy and/or phytoestrogens	Approximately 30% ↓ risk among those reported highest intakes	Approximately 20–25% reduced risk among those reporting the highest intakes	• Meta-analysis • Review

Continued

Table 8.3 Epidemiological associations — foods and nutrient groups and breast cancer risk in women—cont'd

Food and/or nutrient group	Effect on pre-menopausal women	Effect on post-menopausal Women	Level of evidence based upon selected references
Coffee and/or caffeine	NA	NA	• Observational cohort, Swedish Mammography Screening
Vitamin D	• Reduced risk among women with high serum vitamin D	• Possible reduced risk among women with high plasma vitamin D	• Observational cohort, Nurses' Health • Study
Vitamins E, A and C	• Weak association for ↓ risk • with ↑ intake, which may be modified among women with a family history of breast cancer	NA	• Observational cohort, Nurses' Health Study • Reviews
Folic acid	• NA • ↑ intake may moderate breast cancer risk due to alcohol consumption	• NA • ↑ intake may reduce excess breast cancer risk due to alcohol consumption	• Observational cohort, Nurses' Health Study
Carotenoids	• Trend favouring ↓risk among highest quintiles of carotenoid consumption • may vary by carotenoid class	• Trend favouring ↓risk among highest quintiles of carotenoid consumption • may vary by carotenoid class	• Observational cohort, Nurses' Health Study

NA = no association
(Source: adapted and modified from Mahoney et. al. 2008)[174]

of adverse reactions to chemotherapy, improve clinical symptoms, elevate quality of life and enhance immunity in patients with metastatic disease.[194]

In a further study investigating the treatment of advanced breast cancer, *Shenqi Fuzheng* injections alleviated the bone marrow inhibition caused by chemotherapy, improved clinical symptoms and quality of life and prolonged the survival period by regulating cellular immune function of the patients, so as to enhance the therapeutic effect of chemotherapy.[195]

A recent randomised phase II study using mitomycin/cisplatin regimen with or without *Kanglaite* (a TCM extracted from a tropical Asian grass called Coix) as salvage treatment was conducted to exploit the herb's potential effects on patients with advanced breast cancer.[196] The study reported no additional benefit when the TCM herb was added to the regimen doublet in the management of advanced breast cancer.

A recent systematic Cochrane review does not support the use of TCM herbs in the management of breast cancer patients.[197] This review provides limited evidence of the effectiveness and safety of TCM medicinal herbs in alleviating chemotherapy induced short-term side-effects. TCM medicinal herbs, when used together with chemotherapy, may offer some benefit to breast cancer patients in terms of bone marrow improvement and quality of life, but the evidence is very limited to make any confident conclusions. The requisite is for well-designed clinical trials before any conclusions can be drawn about the effectiveness and safety of TCM in the management of breast cancer patients.

Other herbs

There are a number of herbal therapies available for the management of hot flashes in women without breast cancer (see Chapter 25, menopause) that could be useful for those women diagnosed with breast cancer. In this section we have included only those published studies that were specifically investigating the efficacy of herbal remedies in patients diagnosed with breast cancer.

Black cohosh

Black cohosh (*Cimicifuga racemosa*) is a herb that has a long history of traditional use in North American Indian medicine and has been used widely in Western cultures since the early 1800s. It is generally used for the relief of the symptoms of menopause. Hot flushes are the most frequent adverse reaction to tamoxifen adjuvant therapy in breast cancer survivors.

A study with black cohosh was not significantly more efficacious than placebo against most menopausal symptoms, including number and intensity of hot flashes.[198] However, a more recent study with a preparation of black cohosh designated as CR BNO 1055 reported that the combined administration of tamoxifen plus CR BNO 1055 for a period of 12 months allowed satisfactory reduction in the number and severity of hot flushes.[199]

Femal

A RCT investigating Femal, a herbal remedy elaborated from pollen extracts, demonstrated that the pollen extract significantly reduced hot flushes and certain other menopausal symptoms when compared to placebo.[200] Hence this may be useful in breast cancer patients with this symptom.

Ginseng

The scientific literature suggests that fatigue is commonly reported by women during and after breast cancer treatment, where treatment options are often limited. A small 8-week randomised, double-blind, placebo-controlled trial evaluated the feasibility of a larger clinical trial to investigate the efficacy of ginseng for treating breast cancer-related fatigue.[201] The study encountered numerous methodological problems, which made efficacy reporting impossible to assess. There is a literature though that stipulates that ginseng is widely used in Asian countries as a tonic to increase energy.[202]

Green and/or black tea polyphenols

Experimental studies have shown that tea and tea polyphenols have anti-carcinogenic properties against breast cancer.[203] A number of epidemiologic studies, both case-control and cohort in design, have examined the possible association between tea intake and breast cancer development in humans.[204, 205, 206]

Recent meta-analytic systematic reviews reporting on the current epidemiologic literature supports the hypothesis that green tea protects against breast cancer.[207, 208] Given the relative paucity of human data, prospective cohort studies with a wide range of green tea exposure and longer duration of follow-up are needed to affirm the protective effect of green tea on human breast cancer development. Current epidemiological data do not support a role for black tea in protection against breast cancer in humans. Cohort studies with longer duration of follow-up are also needed to elucidate the effect of black tea on different stages of breast cancer development. Since genetic intertwined with lifestyle and/or dietary cofactors could influence the effect of green and/or black tea on breast carcinogenesis additional studies may have to address the possible interaction effects between tea and other dietary and/or genetic cofactors.[209, 210]

Aloe vera

Erythema is an effect produced by radiotherapy treatment in breast cancer patients. A recent trial investigating aloe vera for the amelioration of erythema in radiotherapy-treated patients with breast cancer, included 50 women who were selected consecutively to participate in the study.[211] All of the participants were subjected to treatment with high-energy electrons (9–20 MeV) after mastectomy, 2 Gy per day to a total dose of 50 Gy. Measurements were performed before the start of radiotherapy and thereafter once a week during the course of treatment. Aloe vera and Essex lotion were applied twice every radiation day in selected sites. The study concluded that there was no additional benefit with the use of aloe vera. An earlier phase III study also concluded that an aloe vera gel did not significantly reduce radiation-induced skin side-effects.[212] However, an aqueous cream was useful in reducing dry desquamation and pain related to radiation therapy.

Other supplements

Omega-3 fatty acids (n-3 FA)

A review that examined the scientific evidence on biological mechanisms which may be involved in the inhibition of mammary carcinogenesis by long-chain n-3 FAs, focused on an apoptotic effect by its lipid peroxidation products. It viewed dietary supplements of fish oil rich in n-3 FA as viable alternative supplements for pre-menopausal women over the age of 40 years who are shown to be at increased breast cancer risk.[213] A recent review that investigated a large body of literature spanning numerous cohorts from many countries and with different demographic characteristics does not provide evidence to suggest a significant association between omega-3 fatty acids and cancer incidence. The review concluded that dietary supplementation with omega-3 fatty acids was unlikely to prevent cancer.[214]

The methodology of the systematic review may have a population selection bias. It has been proposed though that intake of fish in early life and/or in adolescence may be protective for the later development of breast cancer.

In countries such as Japan, where the population consumes fish 2 to 3 times daily, and where the incidence of breast cancer is almost negligible, daily seafood consumption is likely to be protective.

Some potential mechanisms for the activity of n-3 fatty acids against cancer include modulation of eicosanoid production and inflammation, angiogenesis, proliferation, susceptibility for apoptosis, and oestrogen signalling. In humans, n-3 PUFA have also been used to suppress cancer-associated cachexia and to improve the quality of life. Moreover, the efficacy of chemotherapy drugs, such as doxorubicin, epirubicin and tamoxifen, and radiation therapy has been improved when the diet included n-3 PUFA.[215] A current recommendation is that cancer patients supplement with n-3 fatty acids EPA/DHA at a dose of 8–10 g/day, with good results observed consistently concerning body-weight maintenance, immune function and appetite.[216]

Physical therapies

Acupuncture

Acupuncture has been studied in breast cancer patients primarily with the intention of reducing chemotherapy-induced nausea and vomiting, menopausal symptoms and pain perception.[217, 218, 219] Investigational data supports the efficacy of acupuncture for cancer-related pain[220] and reducing the frequency of vomiting.[221] These effects, however, were of limited duration.

A review on CAM modalities concludes, though, that the available data on CAMs that includes acupuncture in the treatment of early-stage breast cancer does not support their application.[222]

A small trial with 38 post-menopausal breast cancer patients who were treated for 12 weeks with electro-acupuncture, reported reducing hot flashes significantly.[223]

There is an emerging consensus that between one-fifth and one-half of breast cancer patients experience chemotherapy-associated cognitive dysfunction.[224] Research shows that patients with cancer are often interested in acupuncture for symptom relief. It has been suggested that a skilled practitioner could use acupuncture to relieve a substantial variety of chemotherapy-induced side-effects, including pain, fatigue, nausea and/or vomiting, xerostomia, and mood disorders.[225] A recent review supports this notion.[226] There is evidence that acupuncture may be effectively used to manage a range of psychoneurological issues in breast cancer patients, some of which are similar to those experienced by patients with chemotherapy-associated cognitive dysfunction.

However, the general use of acupuncture in its treatment of pain and vomiting, which are common symptoms in cancer patients, is beneficial and can be repeated whenever needed without any significant side-effects.

Massage therapy

The improvement in the life expectancy of women with breast cancer raises important questions about how to improve the quality of life for women sustaining complications of breast cancer treatment.

Massage therapy in combination with aromatherapy has been shown to be beneficial for cancer patients in the management of disease and treatment-related symptoms.[227]

A Cochrane review investigated only 3 studies involving 150 randomised patients. Since none studied the same intervention it was not possible to combine the data. In summary the review documented the following:[228]

- One cross-over study consisted of manual lymph drainage followed by self-administered massage versus no treatment. It concluded that improvements seen in both groups were attributable to the use of compression sleeves and that manual lymph drainage provided no extra benefit at any point during the trial.
- A further trial looked at hosiery versus no treatment and had a very high dropout rate, with only 3 out of 14 participants in the intervention group finishing the trial and only 1 out of 11 in the control group. Wearing a compression sleeve was beneficial.
- The bandage plus hosiery versus hosiery alone trial concluded that in this mixed group of participants bandage plus hosiery resulted in a greater reduction in

excess limb volume than hosiery alone and this difference in reduction was maintained long-term.

A recent nursing review reported on the various approaches for treating lymphoedema that included skin care, elevation of the affected arm, the use of compression hosiery, multi-layer bandaging, massage (manual lymphatic drainage), and surgery.[229] Bandage plus hosiery, massage and compression hosiery were concluded to be effective.

Conclusion

Three decades of intensive experimental and clinical research on cancer prevention have yielded an impressive body of scientific knowledge about cancer epidemiology, causation, and preventative measures. The complexity of the aetiology of breast cancer is significant though (see Figure 8.1, page 178).

Despite our increased understanding in these critical areas, this knowledge is not being translated adequately into initiatives that will impact upon public health. The recent release of the World Cancer Research Fund / American Institute for Cancer Research report on diet and lifestyle strategies for cancer prevention — grounded in an evidence-based systematic review of the published literature — is a strong acknowledgment of the benefits of a lifestyle approach to reduce cancer risk.[230]

The apparent lack of association between diet and breast cancer may reflect a true absence of association between diet and breast cancer incidence or may be due to measurement error exceeding the variation in the diet studied, lack of sufficient follow-up, and focus on an age range of low susceptibility, or the lack of consideration of lifestyle factors as described earlier.

The risk of breast cancer can be reduced by avoidance of weight gain in adulthood and limiting the consumption of alcohol and adherence to a more prudent diet consisting of fish, vegetables and fruit daily, along with physical activity. Table 8.4 summarises the current evidence for CM treatments.

Table 8.4 Levels of evidence for lifestyle and complementary medicines/therapies in the management of breast cancer

Modality	Level I	Level II	Level IIIa	Level IIIb	Level IIIc	Level IV	Level V
Lifestyle modification							
Weight management / BMI		x					
Energy intake		x					
Mind–body medicine							
Mindfulness-based stress reduction	x						
Cognitive behaviour therapy		x					
Hypnosis		x					
Nutrition							
Dietary fat (↑ risk)		x					
Dairy foods (↑ risk)		x					
Meat consumption (↑ risk)		x					
Soy and phytoestorgens (↓ risk)			x				
Diets							
Mediterranean diet (↓ risk)		x					
Vegetarian diet (↓ risk)			x				
Alcohol reduction (↓ risk)		x					
Environmental factors							
(increased risk, see Table 8.2)		x					
Physical activity							
Yoga				x			
Tai chi				x			

Continued

Table 8.4 Levels of evidence for lifestyle and complementary medicines/therapies in the management of breast cancer—cont'd

Modality	Level I	Level II	Level IIIa	Level IIIb	Level IIIc	Level IV	Level V
Supplements							
Vitamin E				x			
Vitamin A and/or Vitamin A Analogs		x					
Vitamin D				x			
Multivitamins and/or minerals				x			
Traditional Chinese medicines							
Juzentaiho–to					x		
Shenqi Fuzheng					x		
Ruyiping					x		
Kanglaite					x		
Other herbal medicines							
Black cohosh			x				
Femal				x			
Ginseng					x		
Green and/or black tea polyphenolics					x		
Aloe vera					x		
Physical therapies							
Acupuncture				x			
Massage therapy				x			

Level I — from a systematic review of all relevant randomised controlled trials — meta-analyses.
Level II — from at least 1 properly designed randomised controlled clinical trial.
Level IIIa — from well-designed pseudo-randomised controlled trials (alternate allocation or some other method).
Level IIIb — from comparative studies (including systematic reviews of such studies) with concurrent controls and allocation not randomised, cohort studies, case-control studies, or interrupted time series with a parallel control group.
Level IIIc — from comparative studies with historical control, 2 or more single-arm studies or interrupted time series without a parallel control group.
Level IV — opinions of respected authorities based on clinical experience, descriptive studies or reports of expert committees.
Level V — represents minimal evidence that represents testimonials.

Clinical tips handout for patients — breast disease

1 Lifestyle advice

Sleep

- Ensure 7–8 hours sleep and regular sleep pattern. Avoid shift work at night, it can be a risk for cancer. (See Chapter 22 for more advice.)

Sunshine

- Amount of exposure varies with local climate.
- At least 15 minutes of sunshine needed daily for vitamin D and melatonin production — especially before 10 a.m. and after 3 p.m. when the sun exposure is safest during summer. Much more exposure required in winter when supplementation needs to be considered.
- Ensure gradual, adequate skin exposure to sun; avoid sunscreen and excess clothing to maximise levels of vitamin D.
- More time in the sun is required for dark skinned people and people with vitamin D deficiency.
- Direct exposure to about 10% of the body (hands, arms, face), without sunscreen and not through glass.
- Vitamin D is obtained in the diet from fatty fish, eggs, liver and fortified foods (some milks and margarines); diet alone is not a sufficient source of vitamin D.

2 Physical activity/exercise

- Exercise 30–60 minutes daily.
- If exercise is not regular, commence with 5 minutes daily and slowly build up to at least 30 minutes. Outdoor exercise with nature, fresh air (avoid polluted air) and sunshine is ideal (e.g. brisk walking, light jogging, cycling, swimming, stretching, resistance or weight-bearing exercises).
- Tai chi, qigong and yoga may be particularly helpful.

3 Mind–body medicine (most helpful)

- Stress management program — for example, six 40 minute sessions for patients to understand the nature of their symptoms, the symptoms' relationship to stress, and the practice of regular relaxation exercises.
- Regular meditation practice at least 10–20 minutes daily, especially transcendental, mindfulness meditation and autogenic training.
- Anger management may be of help.
- Psychological therapy may help to deal with stressors.

Breathing

- Be aware of breathing from time to time. Notice if tendency to hold breath or over-breathe.
- Snoring and irregular breathing during sleep needs to be reported and investigated further.
- Avoid exposure to polluted air as much as possible.

Rest and stress management

Recurrent stress may cause a return of symptoms in those with cyclical and non-cyclical breast pain. Relaxation is important for a full and lasting recovery.

- Reduce workload and resolve conflicts. Contact family, friends, church or social groups for support. Full-time work can increase breast cancer risk whereas part-time work does not.
- Listening to relaxation music helps.
- Relaxation massage therapy helps.
- Hypnotherapy, biofeedback, cognitive behaviour therapy, and psychotherapy may be of help.

Fun

- It is important to have fun in life. Joy can be found even in the simplest tasks, such as funny movies/videos, comedy, hobbies, dancing, playing with pets and children.

4 Environment

- Don't smoke.
- Avoid smoking environments, environmental pollutants, chemicals — at work and in the home, especially from plastic food containers.
- Don't microwave with plastic cling wrap.
- Avoid chemicals (phthalates) in cosmetics (e.g. in lipstick and hair spray) are of concern.
- Some sunscreens may also increase cancer risk.
- Avoid artificial sweeteners.

5 Dietary changes

- Do not rush your meals; relax before meals; chew your food thoroughly before swallowing as this aids digestion and regular, relaxed eating patterns.
- Aim to lose weight if you or your medical advisor believe you are overweight. Eating slowly can help with weight loss.
- Eat more fruit and vegetables — a variety of colours and those in season.
- Eat more fish especially deep sea fish (e.g. mackerel, sardines, salmon, cod, tuna).
- A vegetarian diet high in legumes (e.g. soy), vegetables, garlic, nuts and fruit is particularly helpful.
- Lean towards the Mediterranean diet.
- Increase fibre; for example, add psyllium fibre (husks) to your cereal.
- Fresh garlic and other members of the onion family offer protection. Cruciferous or brassica group of vegetables, which include broccoli, cabbage, brussels sprouts, cauliflower and bok choy are protective.
- Eat more nuts and seeds (especially flax seeds — best if ground just before use, refrigerate if ground), beans sprouts (e.g. alfalfa, mung beans, lentils), soy (best if fermented, e.g. miso, soy sauce, natto and tempah).
- Reduce red meat intake (preferably use lean red meat e.g. lamb, kangaroo) — no more than twice weekly and not well done — and white meat (e.g. free range organic chicken fillets).
- Use cold pressed olive oil (4 teaspoons daily) and avocado oil.
- Can consume dark chocolate, 25–50g daily, unless not tolerated.
- Eat a variety of wholegrains/cereals (best if not toasted). Cooked traditional rolled oats for breakfast are particularly helpful, as is rice (brown, basmati, Mahatma, Dongara), buckwheat flour, wholegrain organic breads (rye bread, Essene, spelt, kamut) — when toasting make hot and crisp, not brown, to avoid acrylamide — brown pasta, couscous, millet, amaranth, etc.
- Consume low-fat dairy products, such as low-fat yoghurt, unless there is a dairy intolerance. Soy milk (organic) is an alternative.
- Drink more water, 1–2 litres a day, and teas, especially green tea, chamomile, peppermint and black tea (best if organic).
- For alternative sweetener try honey (e.g. yellow box, and stringy bark have lowest GI).
- Minimise alcohol intake to no more than 1–2 glasses daily; red wine may be best.
- Avoid sea salt.
- Avoid hydrogenated, saturated fats and trans-fatty acids such as butter, margarines, crispy potato chips, dairy fat (e.g. yellow cheeses and cream), fat in meat and poultry, commercial biscuits, most cakes, pastries and takeaway foods, fast foods, sugar such as in soft drinks, lollies and processed foods (e.g. white bread, white pasta, pastries).
- Avoid chemical additives — preservatives, colouring and flavours.

6 Physical therapies

Acupuncture may help with breast pain and symptoms of PMS: chemotherapy induced nausea; vomiting; fatigue and moodiness; and can help with alleviation of cancer pain and back pain.

7 Supplements

Fish oils

- Indication: may reduce breast inflammation and breast cancer. Can reduce chemotherapy toxicity and normalise immunity.
- Dosage: 4–10g of 1000mg capsules daily as tolerated (e.g. EPA 180/DHA 120mg/1000mg capsule).
- Results: 4–7 days.
- Side-effects: Often well tolerated especially if taken with meals. Very mild and rare side-effects (e.g. gastrointestinal upset; allergic reactions such as rash, breathing problems if allergic to seafood; blood thinning effects in very high doses > 10g daily (may need to stop fish oil supplements 2 weeks prior to surgery).
- Contraindications: sensitivity reaction to seafood; drug interactions; caution when taking high doses of fish oils >4g per day together with warfarin (your doctor will check your INR test).

Vitamins and minerals

Multivitamin/mineral

- Indication: folate may offer protection from alcohol; beta-carotene may be of value in reducing recurrence. The effect of folate is likely to be enhanced by vitamins B6 and B12.

- Dosage: once or twice daily.
- Result: variable.
- Side-effects: very mild and rare; gastrointestinal irritation can be avoided if taken after meals. Avoid vitamin B6>50mg/day for long periods of time.
- Contraindications: avoid any vitamin A content greater than 2000IU daily and also those with synthetic vitamin E and beta-carotene. Avoid beta-carotene supplements in smokers and for lung cancer. Avoid high-dose folate (75mg) in bowel cancer.

Vitamin D3

- Indication: low levels are a risk factor for breast cancer.
- Dosage: safe sunshine exposure of skin is the safest source of vitamin D. Vitamin D (cholecalciferol 1000 international units). Doctors should check blood levels and suggest supplementation if levels are low.

  Adults: 400–1000IU daily, for maintenance; 3000–5000IU daily for 1 month then 1000IU daily if vitamin D level below normal. If unsure, repeat blood measurement.

  Children at risk: 200–400IU daily under medical supervision.

  Pregnant and lactating women at risk: under medical supervision.
- Results: 6–12 months.
- Side-effects: very high doses can cause vitamin D toxicity; raised calcium levels in the blood. Can increase aluminium and magnesium absorption; prolonged heparin therapy can increase resorption and reduce formation of bone and hence more vitamin D and calcium required.
- Contraindications: thiazide diuretics decrease urinary calcium and hence hypercalcaemia possible with vitamin D supplementation.

Vitamin C

- Indication: may reduce risk of thrombosis and improve immunity when combined with natural Vitamin E and selenium by reducing blood stickiness.
- Dosage: 500–1000mg daily.
- Results: can reduce blood stickiness in 1 week.
- Side-effects: with high doses can cause nausea, heartburn, abdominal cramps and diarrhoea.
- Contraindications: can increase iron absorption. Use with caution if glucose-6-phosphate dehydrogenase deficiency.

Natural vitamin E

- Indication: may reduce risk of thrombosis plus improve immunity, when combined with vitamin C and selenium. Can help prevent venous thromboembolism.
- Dosage: 400–800IU daily.
- Results: can reduce blood stickiness in 1 week.
- Side–effects: doses below 1500IU daily are very unlikely to result in haemorrhage, rarely causes diarrhoea, flatulence, nausea, heart palpitations.
- Contraindications: Use with caution if bleeding disorder or if taking with blood thinning medication. If using very high dose, reduce dose before surgery. Pregnancy. Can reduce effectiveness of thyroid hormone replacement.

Herbal medicines

Evening primrose oil (*Oenothera biennis*)

- Indication: cyclical mastalgia.
- Dosage: take with meals. Adult, 1–2 x 3–4g capsules 1–2 times daily. Child, 500mg capsule 1–2 x daily. Can be used in lactation as tolerated; avoid high doses in pregnancy.
- Results: 1–2 years.
- Side-effects: often well tolerated, especially if taken with meals. Very mild and rare side-effects; for example, gastrointestinal upset; allergic reactions (e.g. rash, breathing problems).
- Contraindications: avoid if you suffer epilepsy or seizures.

Ginger (Zingiber officinale)

- Indication: useful for treating nausea and vomiting related to chemotherapy for breast cancer.
- Dosage: 1–2g dried ginger daily.
- Side-effects: heartburn and bloating plus stomach irritation. Theoretical risk of bleeding increased with warfarin and antiplatelet drugs. Side-effects are rare with doses less than 6g/day.
- Contraindications: use with caution if heartburn or gastric ulcers present. Can increase bleeding risk with warfarin or antiplatelet drugs.

References

1. London SJ, Connolly JL, Schnitt SJ, et. al. A prospective study of benign breast disease and the risk of breast cancer. JAMA 1992;267:941–944.
2. Pfeifer JD, Barr RJ, Wick MR. Ectopic breast tissue and breast-like sweat gland metaplasias: an overlapping spectrum of lesions. J Cutan Pathol 1999;26:190–196.

3 McDivitt RW, Stevens JA, Lee NC, et. al. Histologic types of benign breast disease and the risk for breast cancer. Cancer 1992;69:1408–1414.
4 Guray M, Sahin AA. Benign breast diseases: classification, diagnosis, and management. Oncologist 2006;11(5):435–49.
5 Sarnelli R, Squartini F. Fibrocystic condition and "at risk" lesions in asymptomatic breasts: a morphologic study of post-menopausal women. Clin Exp Obstet Gynecol 1991;18:271–279.
6 Fitzgibbons PL, Henson DE, Hutter RV. Benign breast changes and the risk for subsequent breast cancer: an update of the 1985 consensus statement. Cancer Committee of the College of American Pathologists. Arch Pathol Lab Med 1998;122: 1053–1055.
7 Kelsey JL, Gammon MD. Epidemiology of breast cancer. Epidemiol Rev 1990;12:228–240.
8 Meisner AL, Fekrazad MH, Royce ME. Breast disease: benign and malignant. Med Clin North Am 2008;92(5):1115–41
9 Marshall JM, Graham S, Swanson M. Caffeine consumption and benign breast disease: a case-control comparison. Am J Publ Health1982;72(6):610–2.
10 Lubin F, Ron E, Wax Y, et. al. A case-control study of caffeine and methylxanthines in benign breast disease. JAMA 1985;253(16):2388–92.
11 Boyle CA, Berkowitz GS, LiVoisi VA, et. al. Caffeine consumption and fibrocystic breast disease: a case-control epidemiologic study. JNCI 1984;72:1015–9.
12 Vecchia C, Franceschi S, Parazzini F, et. al. Benign breast disease and consumption of beverages containing methylxanthines. JNCI 1985;74:995–1000.
13 Ernster VL, Mason L, Goodson WH, et. al. Effects of a caffeine-free diet on benign breast disease: a randomised trial. Surgery 1982;91:263.
14 Allen S, Froberg DG. The effect of decreased caffeine consumption on benign proliferative breast disease: a randomized clinical trial. Surgery 1987;101:720–30.
15 Minton JP, Foecking MK, Webster DJT, et. al. Caffeine, cyclic nucleotides, and breast disease. Surgery 1979;86:105–8.
16 Minton JP, Abou-Issa H, Reiches N, et. al. Clinical and biochemical studies on methylxanthine-related fibrocystic breast disease. Surgery 1981;90:299–304.
17 Rose DP, Boyar AP, Cohen C, et. al. Effect of a low-fat diet on hormone levels in women with cystic breast disease. I. Serum steroids and gonadotropins. JNCI 1987;78:623–6.
18 Woods MN, Gorbach S, Longcope C, et. al. Low-fat, high-fiber diet and serum estrone sulfate in pre-menopausal women. AJCN 1989;49:1179–83.
19 Rose DP, Boyar A, Haley N, et. al. Low fat diet in fibrocystic disease of the breast with cyclic mastalgia: a feasibility study. AJCN 1985;41(4):856 (abstract).
20 Boyd NF, McGuire V, Shannon P, et. al. Effect of a low-fat high-carbohydrate diet on symptoms of cyclical mastopathy. Lancet 1988;ii:128–32.
21 Lubin F, Wax Y, Ron E, et. al. Nutritional factors associated with benign breast disease etiology: a case-control study. AJCN 1989;50:551–6.
22 Rohan TE, Negassa A, Caan B, et. al. Low-fat dietary pattern and risk of benign proliferative breast disease: a randomized, controlled dietary modification trial. Cancer Prev Res 2008;1(4):275–84.
23 Mansel RE, Harrison BJ, Melhuish J, et. al. A randomized trial of dietary intervention with essential fatty acids in patients with categorized cysts. Ann NY Acad Sci 1990;586:288–94.
24 Gateley CA, Maddox PR, Pritchard GA, et. al. Plasma fatty acid profiles in benign breast disorders. Br J Surg 1992;79:407–9.
25 Harding C, Harvey J, Kirkman R, et. al. Hormone replacement therapyinduced mastalgia responds to evening primrose oil. Br J Surg 1996;83(Suppl 1):24 (abstract # Breast 012).
26 Pye JK, Mansel RE, Hughes LE. Clinical experience of drug treatments for mastalgia. Lancet 1985;ii:373–7.
27 Abrams AA. Use of vitamin E in chronic cystic mastitis. NEJM 1965;272(20):1080–1.
28 London RS, Sundaram GS, Schultz M, et. al. Endocrine parameters and alpha-tocopherol therapy of patients with mammary dysplasia. Cancer Res 1981;41:3811–3.
29 Ernster VL, Goodson WH, Hunt TK, et. al. Vitamin E and benign breast "disease": a double-blind, randomized clinical trial. Surgery 1985;97:490–4.
30 London RS, Sundaram GS, Murphy L, et. al. The effect of vitamin E on mammary dysplasia: a double-blind study. Obstet Gynecol 1985;65:104–6.
31 Brush MG, Perry M. Pyridoxine and the premenstrual syndrome. Lancet 1985;i:1399.
32 Smallwood J, Ah-Kye D, Taylor I. Vitamin B6 in the treatment of pre-menstrual mastalgia. Br J Clin Pract 1986;40:532–3.
33 Krouse TB, Eskin BA, Mobini J. Age-related changes resembling fibrocystic disease in iodine-blocked rat breasts. Arch Pathol Lab Med 1979;103:631–4.
34 Halaška M, Beles P, Gorkow C, et. al. Treatment of cyclical mastalgia with a solution containing Vitex agnus extract: results of a placebo-controlled double-blind study. The Breast 1999;8:175–81.
35 Böhnert KJ. The use of Vitex agnus castus for hyperprolactinemia. Quar Rev Nat Med 1997;Sprg:19–21.
36 Chang SC, Ziegler RG, Dunn B, et. al. Association of energy intake and energy balance with post-menopausal breast cancer in the prostate, lung, colorectal, and ovarian cancer screening trial. Cancer Epidemiol Biomarkers Prev 2006;15(2):334–41.
37 Silvera SA, Jain M, Howe GR, et. al. Energy balance and breast cancer risk: a prospective cohort study. Breast Cancer Res Treat 2006;97(1):97–106.
38 Harvie M, Howell A. Energy balance adiposity and breast cancer - energy restriction strategies for breast cancer prevention. Obes Rev 2006;7(1):33–47.
39 Fair AM, Montgomery K. Energy balance, physical activity, and cancer risk. Methods Mol Biol 2009;472:57–88.
40 Pan SY, DesMeules M. Energy intake, physical activity, energy balance, and cancer: epidemiologic evidence. Methods Mol Biol 2009;472:191–215.
41 Birnbaum LS, Fenton SE. Cancer and developmental exposure to endocrine disruptors. Environ Health Persp 2003;111:389–94.
42 Environmental Protection Agency, Office of Pollution Prevention and Toxics. Overview: Office of Pollution Prevention and Toxics Programs (Internet) 2007. www.epa.gov/oppt/pubs/oppt101c2.pdf (accessed 12 April 2009)
43 Brody JG, Moysich KB, Humblet O, et. al. Environmental pollutants and breast cancer: epidemiologic studies. Cancer 2007;109(Suppl 12): 2667–711.
44 Rudel RA, Attfield KA, Schifano JN, Brody JG. Chemicals causing mammary gland tumors in animals signal new directions for epidemiology, chemicals testing, and risk assessment for breast cancer prevention. Cancer 2007;109(Suppl 12):2635–66.

45 Rudel RA, Camann DE, Spengler JD, et. al. Phthalates, alkylphenols, pesticides, polybrominated diphenyl ethers, and other endocrine-disrupting compounds in air and dust. Environ Sci Technol 2003;37: 4543–53.

46 Siddiqui MK, Anand M, Mehrotra PK, et. al. Biomonitoring of organochlorines in women with benign and malignant breast disease. Environ Res 2004;98:250–7.

47 Nickerson K. Environmental contaminants in breast milk. J Midwifery Women's Health 2006;51:26–34.

48 Gray J, Evans N, Taylor B, et. al. State of the evidence: the connection between breast cancer and the environment. Int J Occup Environ Health 2009;15(1):43–78.

49 Trock BJ, Hilakivi-Clarke L, Clarke R. Metaanalysis of soy intake and breast cancer risk. JNCI 2006;98:459–471.

50 Van Patten CL, Olivotto IA, Chambers GK, et. al. Effect of soy phytoestrogens on hot flashes in post-menopausal women with breast cancer: a randomized, controlled clinical trial. J Clin Oncol 2002;20(6):1449–55.

51 Messina MJ, Loprinzi CL. Soy for breast cancer survivors: a critical review of the literature. J Nutr 2001;131(11 Suppl):3095S-108S.

52 Messina MJ, Wood CE. Soy isoflavones, estrogen therapy, and breast cancer risk: analysis and commentary. Nutr J 2008;7:17.

53 Verheus M, van Gils CH, Kreijkamp-Kaspers S, et. al. Soy protein containing isoflavones and mammographic density in a randomized controlled trial in post-menopausal women. Cancer Epidemiol Biomarkers Prev 2008;17(10):2632–8.

54 Nishio K, Niwa Y, Toyoshima H, Tamakoshi K, et. al. Consumption of soy foods and the risk of breast cancer: findings from the Japan Collaborative Cohort (JACC) Study. Cancer Causes Control 2007;18(8):801–8.

55 MacGregor CA, Canney PA, Patterson G, et. al. A randomised double-blind controlled trial of oral soy supplements versus placebo for treatment of menopausal symptoms in patients with early breast cancer. Eur J Cancer 2005;41:708–14.

56 Duffy C, Perez K, Partridge A. Implications of phytoestrogen intake for breast cancer. CA Cancer J Clin 2007;57:260–277.

57 Quak SH, Tan SP. Use of soy-protein formulas and soyfood for feeding infants and children in Asia. AJCN 1998;68(6 Suppl):1444S-1446S.

58 Boyd NF, Martin LJ, Noffel M, et. al. A meta-analysis of studies of dietary fat and breast cancer risk. Br J Cancer 1993;68: 627–636.

59 Missmer SA, Smith-Warner SA, Spiegelman D, et. al. Meat and dairy food consumption and breast cancer: a pooled analysis of cohort studies. Int J Epidemiol 2002;31:78–85.

60 Moorman PG, Terry PD. Consumption of dairy products and the risk of breast cancer: a review of the literature. AJCN 2004;80:5–14.

61 Mignone LI, Giovannucci E, Newcomb PA, et. al. Meat consumption, heterocyclic amines, NAT2, and the risk of breast cancer. Nutr Cancer 2009;61(1):36–46.

62 Hanf V, Gonder U. Nutrition and primary prevention of breast cancer: foods, nutrients and breast cancer risk. Eur J Obstet Gynecol Reprod Biol 2005;123(2):139–49.

63 Boyd NF, Stone J, Vogt KN, et. al. Dietary fat and breast cancer risk revisited: a meta-analysis of the published literature. Br J Cancer 2003;89:1672–85.

64 Missmer SA, Smith-Warner SA, Spiegelman D, et. al. Meat and dairy food consumption and breast cancer: a pooled analysis of cohort studies. Int J Epidemiol 2002;31:78–85.

65 Cho E, Chen WY, Hunter DJ, et. al. Red meat intake and risk of breast cancer among pre-menopausal women. Arch Intern Med 2006;166:2253–2259.

66 Taylor EF, Burley VJ, Greenwood DC, Cade JE. Meat consumption and risk of breast cancer in the UK Women's Cohort Study. Br J Cancer 2007;96:1139–1146.

67 Egeberg R, Olsen A, Autrup H, et. al. Meat consumption, N-acetyl transferase 1 and 2 polymorphism and risk of breast cancer in Danish post-menopausal women. Eur J Cancer Prev 2008;17: 39–47.

68 Michels KB, Mohllajee AP, Roset-Bahmanyar E, et. al. Diet and breast cancer: a review of the prospective observational studies. Cancer 2007;109(suppl):2712–2749.

69 Mukamal KJ, Rimm EB. Alcohol consumption: risks and benefits. Curr Atherosc Rep 2008;10:536–43.

70 Kune GA, Vitetta L. Alcohol consumption and the etiology of colorectal cancer: a review of the scientific evidence from 1957 to 1991. Nutr Cancer 1992;18(2):97–111.

71 Smith-Warner SA, Spiegelman D, Yaun SS, et. al. Alcohol and breast cancer in women: a pooled analysis of cohort studies. JAMA 1998;279:535–540.

72 Hamajima N, Hirose K, Tajima K, et. al. Alcohol, tobacco and breast cancer—collaborative reanalysis of individual data from 53 epidemiological studies, including 58,515 women with breast cancer and 95,067 women without the disease. Br J Cancer 2002;87:1234–1245.

73 Chen WY, Willett WC, Rosner B, et. al. Moderate alcohol consumption and breast cancer (abstract). J Clin Oncol 2005;23(suppl):7s. Abstract 515.

74 Zhang SM, Lee IM, Manson JE, et. al. Alcohol consumption and breast cancer risk in the Women's Health Study. Am J Epidemiol 2007;165:667–676.

75 Zhang SM, Willett WC, Selhub J, et. al. Plasma folate, vitamin B6, vitamin B12, homocysteine, and risk of breast cancer. JNCI 2003;95:373–380.

76 Zhang S, Hunter DJ, Hankinson SE, et. al. A prospective study of folate intake and the risk of breast cancer. JAMA 1999;281:1632–1637.

77 Deandrea S, Talamini R, Foschi R, et. al. Alcohol and breast cancer risk defined by estrogen and progesterone receptor status: a case-control study. Cancer Epidemiol Biomarkers Prev 2008;17:2025–8.

78 Knight JA, Bernstein L, Largent J, et. al. Alcohol intake and cigarette smoking and risk of a contralateral breast cancer: The Women's Environmental Cancer and Radiation Epidemiology Study. Am J Epidemiol 2009;169(8):962–8.

79 Berrino F, Muti P. Mediterranean diet and cancer. Eur J Clin Nutr 1989;43(Suppl 2):49–55.

80 Carruba G, Granata OM, Pala V, et. al. A traditional Mediterranean diet decreases endogenous estrogens in healthy post-menopausal women. Nutr Cancer 2006;56(2):253–9.

81 Tseng M, Sellers TA, Vierkant RA, et. al. Mediterranean diet and breast density in the Minnesota Breast Cancer Family Study. Nutr Cancer 2008;60(6):703–9.

82 Berrino F, Villarini A, De Petris M, et. al. Adjuvant diet to improve hormonal and metabolic factors affecting breast cancer prognosis. Ann N Y Acad Sci 2006;1089:110–8.

83 Wu AH, Yu MC, Tseng CC, et. al. Dietary patterns and breast cancer risk in Asian American women. AJCN 2009;89(4):1145–54.

84 Murtaugh MA, Sweeney C, Giuliano AR, et. al. Diet patterns and breast cancer risk in Hispanic and non-Hispanic white women: the Four-Corners Breast Cancer Study. AJCN 2008;87(4):978–84.

85 Hanf V, Gonder U. Nutrition and primary prevention of breast cancer: foods, nutrients and breast cancer risk. Eur J Obstet Gynecol Reprod Biol 2005;123(2):139–49.

86 Larsson SC, Giovannucci E, Wolk A. Folate and risk of breast cancer: a meta-analysis. JNCI 2007;99:64–76.

87 Lewis SJ, Harbord RM, Harris R, et. al. Meta-analyses of observational and genetic association studies of folate intakes or levels and breast cancer risk. JNCI 2006;98:1607–1622.

88 Velicer CM, Ulrich CM. Vitamin and mineral supplement use among US adults after cancer diagnosis: a systematic review. J Clin Oncol 2008;26(4):665–73.

89 de Souza Fêde AB, Bensi CG, et. al. Multivitamins do not improve radiation therapy-related fatigue: results of a double-blind randomized cross-over trial. Am J Clin Oncol 2007;30(4):432–6.

90 Neuhouser ML, Wassertheil-Smoller S, Thomson C, et. al. Multivitamin use and risk of cancer and cardiovascular disease in the Women's Health Initiative cohorts. Arch Intern Med 2009;169(3):294–304.

91 de Ruijter W, Westendorp RG, Assendelft WJ. Use of Framingham risk score and new biomarkers to predict cardiovascular mortality in older people: population based observational cohort study. BMJ 2009;338:a3083. doi: 10.1136/bmj.a3083.

92 Ali MM, Vaidya V. Vitamin D and cancer. J Cancer Res Ther 2007;3(4):225–30.

93 John EM, Schwartz GG, Dreon DM, et. al. Vitamin D and breast cancer risk: the NHANES I epidemiologic follow-up study, 1971–1975 to 1992. National Health and Nutrition Examination Survey. Cancer Epidemiol Biomarkers Prev 1999;8:399–406.

94 Shin MH, Holmes MD, Hankinson SE, et. al. Intake of dairy products, calcium, and vitamin D and risk of breast cancer. JNCI 2002;94:1301–1311.

95 Frazier AL, Li L, Cho E, et. al. Adolescent diet and risk of breast cancer. Cancer Causes Control 2004;15:73–82.

96 Frazier AL, Ryan CT, Rockett H, et. al. Adolescent diet and risk of breast cancer. Breast Cancer Res 2003;5:R59–R64.

97 McCullough ML, Rodriguez C, Diver WR, et. al. Dairy, calcium, and vitamin D intake and post-menopausalbreast cancer risk in the Cancer Prevention Study II Nutrition Cohort. Cancer Epidemiol Biomarkers Prev 2005;14:2898–2904.

98 Simard A, Vobecky J, Vobecky JS. Vitamin D deficiency and cancer of the breast: an unprovocative ecological hypothesis. Can J Public Health. 1991;82:300–303.

99 Nunez C, Carbajal A, Belmonte S, Moreiras O, Varela G. A case-control study of the relationship between diet and breast cancer in a sample from 3 Spanish hospital populations. Effects of food, energy and nutrient intake. Rev Clin Esp 1996;196:75–81.

100 Witte JS, Ursin G, Siemiatycki J, et. al. Diet and pre-menopausal bilateral breast cancer: a case-control study. Breast Cancer Res Treat 1997;42:243–251.

101 Levi F, Pasche C, Lucchini F, et. al. Dietary intake of selected micronutrients and breast-cancer risk. Int J Cancer 2001;91:260–263.

102 Knight JA, Lesosky M, Barnett H, et. al. Vitamin D and reduced risk of breast cancer: a population-based case-control study. Cancer Epidemiol Biomarkers Prev 2007;16:422–429.

103 Barton DL, Loprinzi CL, Quella SK et. al. Prospective evaluation of vitamin E for hot flashes in breast cancer survivors. J Clin Oncol 1998;16:495–500.

104 Zhang S, Hunter DJ, Forman MR, et. al. Dietary carotenoids and vitamins A,C, and E and risk of breast cancer. J Natl Cancer Inst 1999;91: 547–556.

105 Tamimi RM, Hankinson SE, Campos H, et. al. Plasma carotenoids, retinol, and tocopherols. and risk of breast cancer. Am J Epidemiol 2005;161:153–160.

106 Sato R, Helzlsouer KJ, Alberg AJ, et. al. Prospective study of carotenoids, tocopherols, and retinoid concentrations and the risk of breast cancer. Cancer Epidemiol Biomarkers Prev 2002;11(5):451–7.

107 Rock CL, Natarajan L, Pu M, et. al. Longitudinal biological exposure to carotenoids is associated with breast cancer-free survival in the Women's Healthy Eating and Living Study. Cancer Epidemiol Biomarkers Prev 2009;18(2):486–94

108 Israël L, Hajji O, Grefft-Alami A, et. al. (Vitamin A augmentation of the effects of chemotherapy in metastatic breast cancers after menopause. Randomized trial in 100 patients) Ann Med Interne (Paris) 1985;136(7):551–4.

109 Recchia F, Rea S, Pompili P, et. al. Beta-interferon, retinoids and tamoxifen as maintenance therapy in metastatic breast cancer. A pilot study. Clin Ter 1995;146(10):603–10.

110 Bonanni B, Lazzeroni M. Retinoids and breast cancer prevention. Recent Results Cancer Res 2009;181:77–82.

111 Zanardi S, Serrano D, Argusti A, et. al. Clinical trials with retinoids for breast cancer chemoprevention. Endocr Relat Cancer 2006;13(1):51–68.

112 Johansson H, Gandini S, Guerrieri-Gonzaga A, et. al. Effect of fenretinide and low-dose tamoxifen on insulin sensitivity in pre-menopausal women at high risk for breast cancer. Cancer Res 2008;68:9512–8.

113 Sutton LM, Warmuth MA, Petros WP, et. al. Pharmacokinetics and clinical impact of all-trans retinoic acid in metastatic breast cancer: a phase II trial. Cancer Chemother Pharmacol 1997;40(4):335–41.

114 Budd GT, Adamson PC, Gupta M, et. al. Phase I/II trial of all-trans retinoic acid and tamoxifen in patients with advanced breast cancer. Clin Cancer Res 1998;4:635–42.

115 Giovannucci E. Tomatoes, tomato-based products, lycopene, and cancer: review of the epidemiologic literature. JNCI 1999;91(4):317–31.

116 Wane D, Lengacher CA. Integrative review of lycopene and breast cancer. Oncol Nurs Forum 2006;33(1):127–37.

117 American Cancer Society. Online. Available: http://www.cancer.org/downloads/STT/BCFF-Final.pdf (accessed 25 February 2010).

118 Carter CL, Allen C, Henson DE. Relation of tumor size, lymph no de status, and survival in 24,740 breast cancer cases. Cancer 1989;63:181–187.

119 Malin A, Matthews CE, Shu XO, et. al. Energy balance and breast cancer risk. Cancer Epidemiol Biomarkers Prev 2005;14(6):1496–501.

120 Howell A, Chapman M, Harvie M. Energy restriction for breast cancer prevention. Recent Results Cancer Res 2009;181:97–111.

121 Astin J, Shapiro S, Eisenberg D, et. al. Mind-body medicine: state of the science, implications for practice. J Am Board Fam Pract 2003;16:131–147.

122 Ernst E, Cassileth BR. The prevalence of complementary/alternative medicine in cancer: a systematic review. Cancer 1998;83:777–782.

123 Andersen B, Farrar W, Golden-Kreutz D, et. al. Psychological, behavioural, and immune changes after a psychological intervention: a clinical trial. J Clin Oncol 2004;22:3570–3580.

124 Kissane D. Beyond the psychotherapy and survival debate: the challenge of social disparity, depression and treatment adherence in psychosocial cancer care. Psychooncology 2009;18(1):1–5.

125 Biegler KA, Chaoul MA, Cohen L. Cancer, cognitive impairment, and meditation. Acta Oncol 2009;48(1):18–26.

126 Pardue SF, Fenton MV, Rounds LR. The social impact of cancer. Dimens Oncol Nurs 1989 Spring;3(1):5–13.

127 Bower JE. Behavioural symptoms in patients with breast cancer and survivors. J Clin Oncol 2008;26(5):768–77.

128 McGregor BA, Antoni MH. Psychological intervention and health outcomes among women treated for breast cancer: a review of stress pathways and biological mediators. Brain Behav Imm 2009;23:159–66.

129 Meares A. What can the cancer patient expect from intensive meditation? Aust Fam Physician. 1980;9(5):322–5.

130 Simonton OC, Matthews-Simonton S, Sparks TF. Psychological intervention in the treatment of cancer. Psychosomatics 1980;21(3):226–7.

131 Carlsson M, Hamrin E. Psychological and psychosocial aspects of breast cancer and breast cancer treatment. A literature review. Cancer Nurs 1994;17(5):418–28.

132 van der Pompe G, Antoni M, et. al. Adjustment to breast cancer: the psychobiological effects of psychosocial interventions. Patient Educ Couns 1996;28(2):209–19.

133 Roud PC. Psychosocial variables associated with the exceptional survival of patients with advanced malignant disease. J Natl Med Assoc 1987;79(1):97–102.

134 Fawzy FI, Kemeny ME, Fawzy NW, et. al. A structured psychiatric intervention for cancer patients, II. Changes over time in immunological measures. Archives of General Psychiatry 1990;47:729–735.

135 Ott MJ, Norris RL, Bauer-Wu SM. Mindfulness meditation for oncology patients: a discussion and critical review. Integr Cancer Ther 2006;5(2): 98–108.

136 Kabat-Zinn J. Full Catastrophe Living. Delacorte, New York, NY, 1990.

137 Carlson LE, Speca M, Patel KD, et. al. Mindfulness-based stress reduction in relation to quality of life, mood, symptoms of stress and levels of cortisol, dehydroepiandrosterone sulfate (DHEAS) and melatonin in breast and prostate cancer outpatients. Psychoneuroendocrinology 2004;29(4):448–74.

138 Matchim Y, Armer JM. Measuring the psychological impact of mindfulness meditation on health among patients with cancer: a literature review. Oncol Nurs Forum 2007;34(5):1059–66.

139 Witek-Janusek L, Albuquerque K, Chroniak KR, et. al. Effect of mindfulness based stress reduction on immune function, quality of life and coping in women newly diagnosed with early stage breast cancer. Brain Behav Immun 2008;22(6):969–81.

140 Carlson LE, Speca M, Faris P, et. al. One year pre-post intervention follow-up of psychological, immune, endocrine and blood pressure outcomes of mindfulness-based stress reduction (MBSR) in breast and prostate cancer outpatients. Brain Behav Immun 2007;21(8):1038–49.

141 Bower JE. Behavioural symptoms in patients with breast cancer and survivors. J Clin Oncol 2008;26(5):768–77.

142 Winbush NY, Gross CR, Kreitzer MJ. The effects of mindfulness-based stress reduction on sleep disturbance: a systematic review. Explore (NY) 2007;3(6):585–91.

143 Praissman S. Mindfulness-based stress reduction: a literature review and clinician's guide. J Am Acad Nurse Pract 2008;20(4):212–6.

144 Ferguson RJ, Ahles TA, Saykin AJ, et. al. Cognitive-behavioural management of chemotherapy-related cognitive change. Psychooncology 2007;16(8):772–7.

145 Mulrooney T. Cognitive impairment after breast cancer treatment. Clin J Oncol Nurs 2008;12(4):678–80.

146 Edwards AG, Hulbert-Williams N, Neal RD. Psychological interventions for women with metastatic breast cancer. Cochrane Database Syst Rev 2008;(3):CD004253.

147 McGregor BA, Antoni MH. Psychological intervention and health outcomes among women treated for breast cancer: a review of stress pathways and biological mediators. Brn Behav Imm 2009;23(2):159–66.

148 Elkins G, Marcus J, Palamara L, et. al. Can hypnosis reduce hot flashes in breast cancer survivors? A literature review. Am J Clin Hypn 2004;47(1):29–42.

149 Elkins G, Marcus J, Stearns V, et. al. Randomized trial of a hypnosis intervention for treatment of hot flashes among breast cancer survivors. J Clin Oncol 2008;26(31):5022–6.

150 Fenlon DR, Corner JL, Haviland JS. A randomized controlled trial of relaxation training to reduce hot flashes in women with primary breast cancer. J Pain Symptom Manage 2008;35(4):397–405.

151 Rajapakse N, Silva E, Kortenkamp A. Combining xenoestrogens at levels below individual no-observed-effect concentrations dramatically enhances steroid hormone action. Env Health Persp 2002;110:917–21.

152 Rajapakse N, Ong D, Kortenkamp A. Defining the impact of weakly estrogenic chemicals on the action of steroidal chemicals. Toxicol Sci 2001;60:296–304.

153 Millikan R, DeVoto E, Duell EJ, et. al. Dichloro-diphenyldichloroethene, polychlorinated biphenyls and breast cancer among African-American and white women in North Carolina. Cancer Epidemiol Biomarkers Prev 2000;9:1233–40.

154 Laden F, Ishibe N, Hankinson SE, et. al. Polychlorinated biphenyls, cytochrome P450 1A1, and breast cancer risk in the Nurses' Health Study. Cancer Epidemiol Biomarkers Prev 2002;11:1560–5.

155 Olivier M, Hainaut P. TP53 mutation patterns in breast cancers: searching for clues of environmental carcinogenesis. Sem Cancer Biol 2001;11:353–60.

156 Pan SY, DesMeules M. Energy intake, physical activity, energy balance, and cancer: epidemiologic evidence. Methods Mol Biol 2009;472:191–215.

157 Reigle BS, Wonders K. Breast cancer and the role of exercise in women. Methods Mol Biol 2009;472:169–89.

158 Bicego D, Brown K, Ruddick M, et. al. Effects of exercise on quality of life in women living with breast cancer: a systematic review. Breast J 2009;15(1):45–51.

159 Holmes MD, Chen WY, Feskanich D, et. al. Physical activity and survival after breast cancer diagnosis. JAMA 2005;293(20):2479–86.
160 Battaglini CL, Mihalik JP, Bottaro M, et. al. Effect of exercise on the caloric intake of breast cancer patients undergoing treatment. Braz J Med Biol Res 2008;41(8):709–15.
161 Renehan AG, Zwahlen M, Minder C, et. al. Insulin-like growth factor (IGF)-I, IGF binding protein-3, and cancer risk:systematic review and meta-regression analysis. Lancet 2004;363(9418): 1346–53.
162 Irwin ML, Varma K, Alvarez-Reeves M, et. al. Randomized controlled trial of aerobic exercise on insulin and insulin-like growth factors in breast cancer survivors: the Yale Exercise and Survivorship study. Cancer Epidemiol Biomark Prev 2009;18(1):306–13.
163 Sternfeld B, Weltzien E, Quesenberry CP Jr, et. al. Physical activity and risk of recurrence and mortality in breast cancer survivors: findings from the LACE study. Cancer Epidemiol Biomarkers Prev 2009;18(1):87–95.
164 Neilson HK, Friedenreich CM, Brockton NT, Millikan RC. Physical activity and post-menopausal breast cancer: proposed biologic mechanisms and areas for future research. Cancer Epidemiol Biomarkers Prev 2009;18(1):11–27.
165 Smith AW, Alfano CM, Reeve BB, et. al. Race/ethnicity, physical activity, and quality of life in breast cancer survivors. Cancer Epidemiol Biomarkers Prev 2009;18(2):656–63.
166 Carson JW, Carson KM, Porter LS, et. al. Yoga for women with metastatic breast cancer: results from a pilot study. J Pain Symptom Manage 2007;33(3):331–41.
167 Carson JW, Carson KM, Porter LS, et. al. Yoga of Awareness program for menopausal symptoms in breast cancer survivors: results from a randomized trial. Support Care Cancer. 2009 Feb 12. (Epub ahead of print)
168 Mustian KM, Katula JA, Gill DL, et. al. Tai Chi Chuan, health-related quality of life and self-esteem: a randomized trial with breast cancer survivors. Support Care Cancer 2004;12(12):871–6.
169 Mustian KM, Katula JA, Zhao H. A pilot study to assess the influence of tai chi chuan on functional capacity among breast cancer survivors. J Support Oncol 2006;4(3):139–45.
170 Mustian KM, Palesh OG, Flecksteiner SA. Tai Chi Chuan for breast cancer survivors. Med Sport Sci 2008;52:209–17.
171 Lee MS, Pittler MH, Ernst E. Is Tai Chi an effective adjunct in cancer care? A systematic review of controlled clinical trials. Support Care Cancer 2007;15(6):597–601.
172 Wu AH, Yu MC, Tseng CC, et. al. Dietary patterns and breast cancer risk in Asian American women. AJCN 2009;89(4):1145–54.
173 Wu AH, Yu MC, Tseng CC, et. al. Epidemiology of soy exposures and breast cancer risk. Br J Cancer 2008;98(1):9–14.
174 Mahoney MC, Bevers T, Linos E, et. al. Opportunities and strategies for breast cancer prevention through risk reduction. CA Cancer J Clin 2008;58(6):347–71.
175 Wynder EL, Kajitani T, Kuno J, et. al. A comparison of survival rates between American and Japanese patients with breast cancer. Surg Gynecol Obstet 1963; 117:196–200.
176 Morrison AS, Lowe CR, MacMahon B, et. al. Some international differences in treatment and survival in breast cancer. Int J Cancer 1976;18:269–273.
177 Morrison AS, Lowe CR, MacMahon B, et. al. Incidence risk factors and survival in breast cancer: Report on five years of followup observation. Eur J Cancer 1977;13:209–214.
178 Freedman LS, Potischman N, Kipnis V, et. al. A comparison of two dietary instruments for evaluating the fatbreast cancer relationship. Int J Epidemiol 2006;35:1011–21.
179 Prentice RL, Caan B, Chlebowski RT, et. al. Low-fat dietary pattern and risk of invasive breast cancer: the Women's Health Initiative Randomized Controlled Dietary Modification Trial. JAMA 2006;295:629–42.
180 Kim EH, Willett WC, Colditz GA, et. al. Dietary fat and risk of post-menopausal breast cancer in a 20-year follow-up. Am J Epidemiol 2006;164:990–7.
181 Pierce JP, Faerber S, Wright FA, et. al. A randomized trial of the effect of a plant-based dietary pattern on additional breast cancer events and survival: the Women's Healthy Eating and Living (WHEL) Study. Control Clin Trials 2002;23:728–56.
182 Pierce JP, Natarajan L, Caan BJ, et. al. Dietary change and reduced breast cancer events among women without hot flashes after treatment of early-stage breast cancer: subgroup analysis of the Women's Healthy Eating and Living Study. AJCN 2009;89(5):1565S-1571S.
183 Hoy MK, Winters BL, Chlebowski RT, et. al. Implementing a low-fat eating plan in the Women's Intervention Nutrition Study. J Am Diet Assoc 2009;109(4):688–96.
184 Hyder JA, Thomson CA, Natarajan L, et. al. WHEL Study Group. Adopting a Plant-Based Diet Minimally Increased Food Costs in WHEL Study. Am J Health Behav 2009;33(5):530–9.
185 Cohen I, Tagliaferri M, Tripathy D. Traditional Chinese medicine in the treatment of breast cancer. Semin Oncol 2002;29(6):563–74.
186 Kogure T, Ltoh K, Tatsumi T, et. al. The effect of Juzen-taiho-to/TJ-48 on the expression of killer-cell immunoglobulin-like receptors (CD158a/b) on peripheral lymphocytes in vitro experiment. Phytomedicine 2005;12(5):327–32.
187 Adachi I, Watanabe T. (Role of supporting therapy of Juzentaiho-to (JTT) in advanced breast cancer patients) Gan To Kagaku Ryoho 1989;16(4 Pt 2-2):1538–43.
188 Wong CK, Tse PS, Wong EL, et. al. Immunomodulatory effects of yun zhi and danshen capsules in health subjects—a randomized, double-blind, placebo-controlled, cross-over study. Int Immunopharmacol 2004;4(2):201–11.
189 Wong CK, Bao YX, Wong EL, et. al. Immunomodulatory activities of Yunzhi and Danshen in post-treatment breast cancer patients. Am J Chin Med 2005;33(3):381–95.
190 Mok TS, Yeo W, Johnson PJ, et. al. A double-blind placebo-controlled randomized study of Chinese herbal medicine as complementary therapy for reduction of chemotherapy-induced toxicity. Ann Oncol 2007;18(4):768–74.
191 See the appendix in the article which is available free at: http://annonc.oxfordjournals.org/cgi/reprint/18/4/768, accessed April 2009.
192 Liu S, Hua YQ, Sun ZP,et. al. (Clinical observation of Ruyiping in preventing recidivation and metastasis of breast cancer) Zhong Xi Yi Jie He Xue Bao 2007;5(2):147–9.

193 Ling Xu, Li Xing Lao, Adeline Ge, et. al. Chinese Herbal Medicine for Cancer Pain. Integr Cancer Ther 2007; 6; 208–234.
194 Bo Y, Li HS, Qi YC, et. al. Clinical study on treatment of mammary cancer by shenqi fuzheng injection in cooperation with chemotherapy. Chin J Integr Med 2007;13(1):37–40.
195 Huang ZF, Wei JS, et. al. Effect of Shenqi Fuzheng injection combined with chemotherapy on thirty patients with advanced breast cancer. Zhongguo Zhong Xi Yi Jie He Za Zhi 2008;28(2):152–4.
196 Guo HY, Cai Y, Yang XM, et. al. Randomized phase II trial on mitomycin-C/cisplatin +/- KLT in heavily pretreated advanced breast cancer. Am J Chin Med 2008;36(4):665–74.
197 Zhang M, Liu X, Li J, et. al. Chinese medicinal herbs to treat the side-effects of chemotherapy in breast cancer patients. Cochrane Database Syst Rev 2007 Apr 18;(2):CD004921.
198 Jacobson JS, Troxel AB, Evans J, et. al. Randomized trial of black cohosh for the treatment of hot flashes among women with a history of breast cancer. J Clin Oncol 2001;19(10):2739–45.
199 Hernández Muñoz G, Pluchino S. Cimicifuga racemosa for the treatment of hot flushes in women surviving breast cancer. Maturitas 2003;44 Suppl 1:S59–S65.
200 Winther K, Rein E, Hedman C. Femal, a herbal remedy made from pollen extracts, reduces hot flushes and improves quality of life in menopausal women: a randomized, placebo-controlled, parallel study. Climacteric 2005;8(2):162–70.
201 Elam JL, Carpenter JS, Shu XO, et. al. Methodological issues in the investigation of ginseng as an intervention for fatigue. Clin Nurse Spec 2006;20(4):183–9.
202 Coleman CI, Hebert JH, Reddy P. The effects of Panax ginseng on quality of life. J Clin Pharm Ther 2003;28(1):5–15.
203 Vergote D, Cren-Olive C, Chopin V, et. al. Epigallocatechin (EGC) of green tea induces apoptosis of human breast cancer cells but not of their normal counterparts. Breast Can Res Tre 2002; 76:195–201.
204 Ewertz M. Breast cancer in Denmark. Incidence, risk factors, and characteristics of survival. Acta Oncol 1993;32:595–615.
205 Franceschi S, Favero A, La Vecchia C, et. al. Influence of food groups and food diversity on breast cancer risk in Italy. Int J Cancer 1995;63:785–789.
206 Goldbohm RA, Hertog MG, Brants HA, et. al. Consumption of black tea and cancer risk: a prospective cohort study. JNCI 1996; 88:93–100.
207 Sun CL, Yuan JM, Koh WP, et. al. Green tea, black tea and breast cancer risk: a meta-analysis of epidemiological studies. Carcinogenesis 2006;27(7):1310–5.
208 Seely D, Mills EJ, Wu P, et. al. The effects of green tea consumption on incidence of breast cancer and recurrence of breast cancer: a systematic review and meta-analysis. Integr Canc Ther 2005;4(2):144–55.
209 Wu AH, Tseng CC, Van Den Berg D, et. al. Tea intake, COMT genotype, and breast cancer in Asian American women. Cancer Res 2003;63:7526–7529.
210 Wu AH, Yu MC, Tseng CC, et. al. (2003) Green tea and risk of breast cancer in Asian Americans. Int J Cancer 2003:106:574–579.
211 Nyström J, Svensk AC, Lindholm-Sethson B, et. al. Comparison of three instrumental methods for the objective evaluation of radiotherapy induced erythema in breast cancer patients and a study of the effect of skin lotions. Acta Oncol 2007;46(7):893–9.
212 Heggie S, Bryant GP, Tripcony L, et. al. A Phase III study on the efficacy of topical aloe vera gel on irradiated breast tissue. Cancer Nurs 2002;25(6):442–51.
213 Stoll BA. N-3 fatty acids and lipid peroxidation in breast cancer inhibition. Br J Nutr 2002;87(3): 193–8.
214 MacLean CH, Newberry SJ, Mojica WA, et. al. Effects of omega-3 fatty acids on cancer risk: a systematic review. JAMA 2006;295(4):403–15.
215 Hardman WE. (n-3) fatty acids and cancer therapy. J Nutr 2004;12(Suppl):3427S-3430S.
216 Sali A. Personal communication, Melbourne, September 2009.
217 Pan CX, Morrison RS, Ness J, et. al. Complementary and alternative medicine in the management of pain, dyspnea, and nausea and vomiting near the end of life A systematic review. J Pain Symptom Manage 2000;20:374–387.
218 Harris PF, Remington PL, Trentham-Dietz A, et. al. Prevalence and treatment of menopausal symptoms among breast cancer survivors. J Pain Symp Mang 2002;23:501–509.
219 Cui Y, Shu XO, Gao Y, et. al. Use of complementary, alternative medicine by Chinese women with breast cancer. Breast Cancer Res Treat 2004;85: 263–270.
220 Alimi D, Rubino C, Pichard-Leandri E, et. al. Analgesic effect of auricular acupuncture for cancer pain: a randomized, blinded, controlled trial. J Clin Oncol 2003;21:4120–4126.
221 Shen J, Wenger N, Glaspy J, et. al. Electroacupuncture for control of myeloablative chemotherapy-induced emesis: A randomized controlled trial. JAMA 2000;284:2755–2761.
222 Gerber B, Scholz C, Reimer T, et. al. Complementary and alternative therapeutic approaches in patients with early breast cancer: a systematic review. Breast Cancer Res Treat 2006;95(3):199–209.
223 Nedstrand E, Wijma K, Wyon Y, et. al. Vasomotor symptoms decrease in women with breast cancer randomized to treatment with applied relaxation or electro-acupuncture: a preliminary study. Climacteric 2005;8:243–250.
224 Phillips KA, Bernhard J. Adjuvant breast cancer treatment and cognitive function: current knowledge and research directions. JNCI 2003;95: 190–197.
225 Cohen AJ, Mentor A, Hale L. Acupuncture: role in comprehensive cancer care—a primer for the oncologist and review of the literature. Integr Cancer Ther 2005;4:131–143.
226 Johnston MF, Yang C, Hui KK, et. al. Acupuncture for chemotherapy-associated cognitive dysfunction: a hypothesis-generating literature review to inform clinical advice. Integr Cancer Ther 2007;6(1): 36–41.
227 Kite SM, Maher EJ, Anderson K, et. al. Development of an aromatherapy service at a Cancer Centre. Palliat Med 1998;12(3):171–80.
228 Badger C, Preston N, Seers K, et. al. Physical therapies for reducing and controlling lymphoedema of the limbs. Cochrane Database Syst Rev 2004 Oct 18;(4):CD003141.
229 Harmer V. Breast cancer-related lymphoedema: risk factors and treatment. Br J Nurs 2009;18:166–72.
230 Greenwald P, Dunn BK. Do we make optimal use of the potential of cancer prevention? Recent Results Cancer Res 2009;181:3–17.

Chapter 9

Cancer

Cancer — what is it?

Various other terms, apart from cancer, are used to describe this family of diseases that include malignancy and neoplasia. The difference between a malignant and benign tumour is summarised in Table 9.1.

Cancers can be divided primarily into 2 groups: solid and blood-borne malignancies. Solid cancers form masses, whereas blood cancers such as leukaemia form in bone marrow or lymph nodes. The latter can lead to masses also. Cancer cells display uncontrollable growth that can divide at a rapid rate without the usual hormonal and other controls exhibited by normal cells.

Cancer cells are invasive and are not restricted to normal boundaries, therefore they destroy adjacent tissues. These cells survive beyond the limitations of normal cells. The telomere shortening that occurs at the end of chromosomes in normal cells is not seen in cancerous cells.[1]

Cancer cells can either be differentiated (Grade 1) or undifferentiated (Grade 3). In general, the differentiated cells are associated with normal immunity, whereas the undifferentiated ones are associated with poor immunity and, hence, the latter spread (metastases) more rapidly throughout the body.[2]

Cancer cells not only utilise lots of energy (a marked increase in glycolytic capacity) but also have a negative influence on metabolism, especially increased protein metabolism.[3] Cancer cachexia, which is a loss of weight, muscle atrophy and loss of appetite, is not only due to poor intake, but also changes in metabolism.

How common is cancer?

Cancer can affect people of all ages. Over the course of a lifetime about every 1:2 males and 1:3 females in Australia and most Westernised countries will develop an invasive cancer.[4, 5] The commonest internal cancer in males in 2005 in Australia was prostate cancer, and in females, breast cancer.[4]

The commonest cancers in males (in a descending order of frequency) are:

- prostate
- colorectal
- melanoma
- lung
- lymphoma
- bladder.

The commonest cancers in females (in a descending order of frequency) are:

- breast
- colorectal
- melanoma
- lung
- lymphoma
- uterus.

The total numbers of cancers is increasing, this growth is due mainly to the ageing population.[4] In males the top 5 cancers accounted for over 67% of all diagnoses, whereas in females, the top 5 cancers accounted for 63% of all diagnoses. When sexes are combined, the commonest cancer is prostate cancer.[4] The 5 top cancers accounted for over 61% of all diagnoses.

The commonest cancers, sexes combined (in a descending order of frequency) are:

- prostate
- colorectal
- breast
- melanoma
- lung
- lymphoma.

Almost all cancers occur at higher rates in males than females. The male rate is 1.4 times the female rate.[4]

As a cause of death, cancer is closing in on cardiovascular disease. The rate of the latter has been decreasing, whereas death from cancer has been increasing in Australia.

There are many different types of cancer which vary in their rate of spread. A number of the common cancers have been extensively studied compared to the majority of the uncommon cancers. It is likely that, in general, the principles to do with management of either common or uncommon cancers are similar.

Risk factors

In general, it is reasonable to assume that there is not 1 particular factor that is completely responsible for the cause of cancer, although

Table 9.1 Differences between benign and malignant tumours

Benign	Malignant
Non-invasive	Invasive
Slow growth	Rapid growth
Not metastatic	Metastatic

1 factor is likely to be more important than the others. It is most probable that cancer cells are formed on a regular basis, but they are destroyed when important mechanisms, such as immunity, are functioning normally and there are not excessive stimulatory hormones and other chemical insults that can destabilise immune and metabolic control.

The risk factors for cancer are:

- genetic (family history and age)
- behavioural and social factors
- inflammation and infection
- dietary factors
- smoking
- sleep patterns
- lack of exercise
- obesity
- lack of sunlight
- environmental factors
- occupational exposure
- poor immunity
- other.

Genetics (family history and ageing)

Most cancers are sporadic and have no strong hereditary basis. A large number of cancers have now been found to have a genetic link, but this is not the key factor leading to the development of the cancer.[6] Genetic cancer research is being very actively researched with the hope of detecting those individuals who are at risk, and then being able to provide additional protection through lifestyle changes. Hopefully in the future, it may be possible to genetically engineer these genes with the aim of preventing cancer.

A number of cancers are recognised as syndromes of cancer that have a defective tumour suppressor allele.[7] The following are examples: mutations in genes, BRCA1 and BRCA2 which are associated with an elevated risk of breast and ovarian cancers, and hereditary non-polyposis colorectal cancer (HNPCC), also known as the Lynch syndrome. Several genes are involved and include cancers of the colorectum, uterine, gastric and ovarian sites without preponderance of colorectal polyps. A range of genetic mutations and switches are activated which can initiate cancer.

Age

Most developed countries have an increased ageing population, and with it there is an increase in cancer. Ageing is the largest risk factor for most of the common cancers in humans.

Behavioural and social factors

Psycho-oncology is the scientific field that describes the links between psychological and social factors with cancer. Depression is the key emotional factor that can influence immunity (psychoneuroimmunology (PNI)), as well as numerous hormones (psychoneuroendocrinology (PNE)). Depression can also influence lifestyle factors, including smoking, excess alcohol, physical activity and excess weight.[8]

The general overview of the key mechanisms involved in cancer are shown in Figure 9.1

An extensive review by David Spiegel concluded that chronic and severe depression is probably associated with an increased risk of developing cancer and the evidence was strong that depression predicts a poor prognosis, with more rapid progression of cancer.[9] Risk of developing cancer due to depression is nearly doubled, independent of other lifestyle factors, and it is not related to any particular cancer.[10, 11, 12]

The longer the duration of depression the greater the risk for developing cancer.[13] Depression and stress depress immunity and also increase levels of cortisol, growth hormone, prolactin and epinephrine, all of which are known to stimulate cancer growth.[14–17]

Insulin plus insulin-like growth factors (IGFs) have been shown in numerous epidemiological studies to be involved in increasing cancer risk.[18, 19, 20] Stress can suppress natural killer cells leading to poor cancer surveillance in some cancers.[21] There is increasing evidence that behaviour can influence our genes. Stress can damage DNA and impair genetic mutation repair.[22, 23, 24]

Personality factors, as well as sexual differences, are important relating to DNA damage.[25] DNA damage is related to tension, anxiety and self-blame coping strategy in males, and in females, depression and rejection. The worst factor was the lack of subjective closeness to parents in childhood. DNA damage was also higher in subjects who had experienced the loss of a close family member within the last 3 years.

Immune cells have less ability to initiate genetically programmed cancer cell suicide with psychological stress.[26] The repair of DNA is often depressed in cancer patients, which is a possible marker of cancer susceptibility.[27]

Shift work is associated with an increased risk of cancer which may be due to depleted melatonin levels.[27] Melatonin is known to have

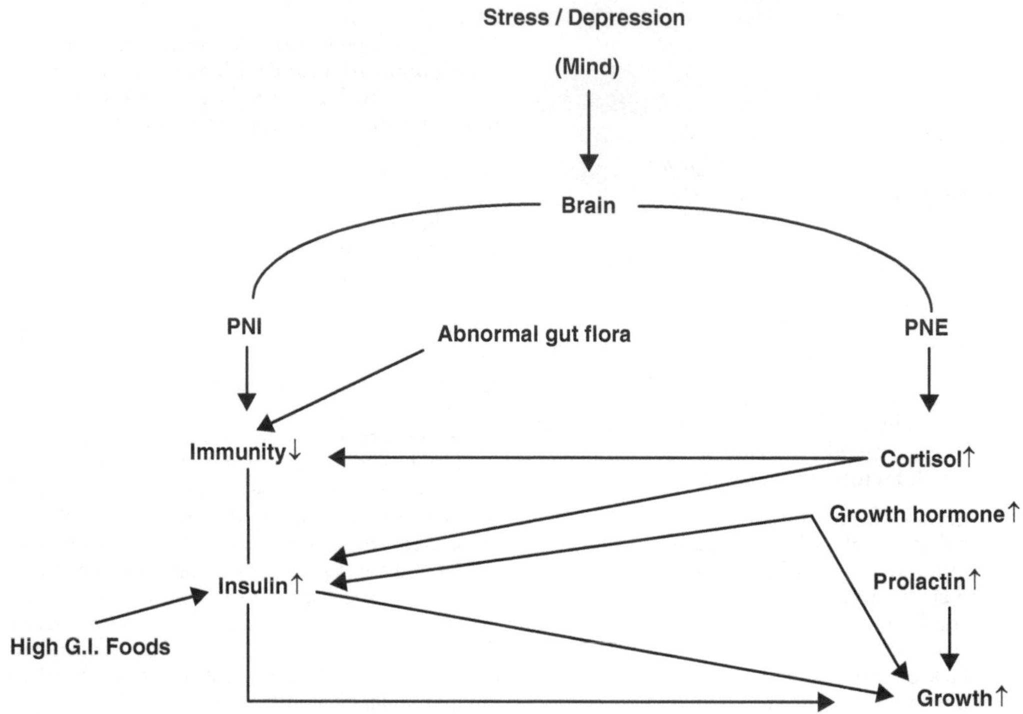

Figure 9.1 Mind–body medicine connections

a positive influence on immunity and also has anti-cancer effects.[28, 29]

Melatonin can inactivate cancer genes plus inhibits cancer growth factors.[30]

Inflammation and infection

Chronic inflammation is a central event that is closely associated with cancer development. Under normal circumstances, insulin has an anti-inflammatory action but this can be reversed with insulin resistance.[31, 32]

A recent study found that people with the highest blood levels of C-reactive protein were about 3 times more likely to develop colorectal cancer, as those with the lowest ranges.[33] Elevated serum interleukin-6, which is another inflammatory marker, is also linked to cancer.[34] The interesting chemo-prevention of cancer with COX-2 inhibitors is partially to do with this inflammatory process.[35, 36, 37]

Selective COX-2 inhibitors (Clecoxib and Rofecoxib) were used to prevent cancer with reasonable success, but withdrawn for this use because of serious side-effects.[38, 39, 40]

Curcumin, which is found in ginger and turmeric, is a COX-2 inhibitor and also has anti-cancer activity.[41, 42] It is possible that the anti-inflammatory action of vitamin D is an important reason why it can protect from cancer.[43, 44, 45] Inflammation associated with surgery can increase the size of metastases.[46]

Men with periodontal disease have been found to have 63% higher risk of pancreatic cancer compared to those with no sign of the disease.[47] Inflammation is thought to be a key factor, but also higher levels of oral bacteria and higher levels of nitrosamines might also play a role. Other studies have shown that periodontal disease is a risk factor for other cancers.[48, 49]

Helicobacter pylori (*H. pylori*)

Stomach cancer is the second leading cause of cancer death worldwide, and approximately half of the world's population is infected with *H. pylori*.[50] Conventional triple therapy is now involved with a 20% failure. In addition to being expensive, it has significant side-effects.[51, 52]

On a global basis, there is geographic correlation between areas with high stomach mortality rates and high prevalence of *H. pylori* infection.[53]

Studies have reported an inverse association between vitamin C intake and gastric cancer risk.[54] A randomised double-blind study from China was designed to reduce the prevalence of precancerous stomach lesions. This study had 3 groups, namely 3365 eligible participants that were randomly assigned in a factorial design to 3 interventions or placebos: amoxicillin and omeprazole for 2 weeks in 1995, (*H. pylori* treatment); vitamin C, vitamin E, and selenium for 7.3 years (vitamin supplement); and aged garlic extract and steam-distilled garlic oil for 7.3 years (garlic supplement). The study concluded that the drug treatment group showed a protective effect against pre-malignancy and malignancy. The supplement groups did not show a positive response. The authors of this study agree that the quality and doses of supplements may have been inadequate.[55]

There have been numerous studies using *in vitro*, animal and human groups dealing with *H. pylori* and probiotics, which have been summarised by Vitetta and Sali.[56] *In vitro* probiotics inhibit *H. pylori* infection and all studies show that probiotics can reduce *H. pylori* gastritis and reduce the number of *H. pylori*.[56]

Seven of 9 human studies showed an improvement of *H. pylori*-induced gastritis and a decrease of *H. pylori* density following administration of probiotics.[56] The addition of probiotics to standard antibiotic treatment improved *H. pylori* eradication and *H. pylori* therapy-associated side-effects.[57]

Olive oil polyphenols have *in vitro* activity against *H. pylori* and hence have the potential of being a chemo-preventive agent for peptic ulcer or gastric cancer.[58]

Viruses and cancer

Hepatitis virus B and C (HBV and HCV)

Several epidemiologic and experimental studies have established a causal role for HBV and HCV in the development of hepatocellular carcinoma.[50, 59, 60]

Patients with cirrhosis develop nutritional deficiencies and subsequent immunologic problems. These factors could be part of the reason why these patients are at an increased risk to develop liver cancer.[61] Specific nutrient deficiencies have also been found in those with liver cirrhosis such as impaired vitamin E status, reduced carotenoids and lipid soluble vitamins.[62, 63, 64]

Vegetable, fruit and antioxidant nutrient consumption has been found to be associated with decreased subsequent risk of hepatocellular carcinoma.[65] This group found that consumption of vegetables, green-yellow and green leafy vegetables were inversely associated with the risk of hepatocellular cancer.

Curcumin has been found to inhibit hepatic fibrosis in the rodent model, and may offer protection from subsequent hepatocellular carcinoma development.[66]

Sho-saiko-to, a traditional Japanese herbal formula, has been shown to play a chemo-preventive role in the prevention of hepatocellular carcinoma in cirrhotic patients.[67]

Human papilloma viruses (HPVs)

HPVs are DNA viruses that have been causally linked to cancers of the cervix and are suspected to be causally related to anal cancers and cancers of the aerodigestive tract.[50, 68, 69]

Apart from smoking, dietary factors appear to modulate cervical cancer.[70] Women consuming low levels of vitamin C and carotenoids are at increased risk of cervical neoplasia, vitamin E and folate may also provide protection. Another study found that a diet high in folate, riboflavin, thiamine and vitamin B12 may play a protective role in cervical carcinogenesis.[71] It is possible that these nutrients may help reverse cervical dysplasia.

Elevated serum homocysteine levels are strongly significantly predictive of invasive cervical cancer risk; folate, B6 and B12 are known to reduce homocysteine.[72] Vegetable consumption and an increase in circulating cis-lycopene were protective against HPV persistence in another study.[73]

Dietary factors

It is now understood that the development of most cancers is clearly a result of an intimate interaction between endogenous and lifestyle factors, the most notable of these lifestyle factors is diet. Estimates suggest that approximately 30% of cancers are a consequence of suboptimal diet.[74, 75, 76] In developing countries, the contribution of diet to cancer is estimated to be lower (20%) based mainly on higher tobacco consumption.[77]

Our food and drink contain mutagens and carcinogens in addition to a variety of chemicals that may be able to block carcinogenesis.[78] Epidemiological investigations have been very helpful in defining the general profile of the diet which is protective: one which is low in red meat and various fats, modest in calories and alcohol, and high in fruit, vegetables and fibre. It is quite clear that a diet high in fresh fruits and vegetables is highly protective against colorectal cancer.[79, 80]

It is important to note that nutrition plays a role in influencing the body in many ways (e.g. immunity, behaviour) and, hence, it is likely that it plays some part in the development of all cancers, even where there is no data available. Most of the data relating to cancer and nutrition is for the more common cancers, and it is likely that a food that is good or bad for 1 cancer will be good or bad for another cancer.

Additives

Thousands of substances are added to foods; for example, sugar, artificial sweeteners, colouring agents, etc. Very little epidemiological research exists to do with food additives with respect to cancer.

Carcinogens in food

The importance of dietary acrylamide and its association with human cancers remains controversial.[81, 82, 83]

In 2002, Swedish scientists reported the presence of acrylamide in carbohydrate-rich foods that were produced at high temperatures, such as French fries, potato chips, breakfast cereals and toasted bread.[84] Studies have shown positive dose-response relations to acrylamide exposure and cancer in multiple organs in both mice and rats.[85, 86]

Xenoestrogens

Xenoestrogens are defined as chemicals that mimic some structural parts of the physiological oestrogen compounds, therefore may act as oestrogens or could interfere with the actions of endogenous oestrogens. Organochlorine chemicals — pesticides, polychlorinated biphenyl compounds and other members of the Dioxin family are regarded as xenoestrogens or 'endocrine disruptors'. These chemicals are capable of modulating hormonally unregulated processes including changes in growth factors that may be responsible for carcinogenesis, as well as congenital defects plus infertility in males.[87, 88, 89]

There is still controversy as to how significant the role of xenoestrogens are in humans.[90]

Chlorine

In population-based case-controlled studies, chlorine in water, which is the most important and the most common disinfectant, has been linked to several cancers including bladder, colorectal and possibly brain cancer.[91, 92, 93] The risk is higher with more tap water that is consumed. Another group found that drinking chlorinated water disinfection by-products increased the risk of chronic myeloid leukaemia with increasing years of exposure.[94]

It was unusual that a protective effect was noted for chronic lymphoid leukaemia.[93]

Arsenic

Ingestion of inorganic arsenic from drinking water has emerged as an important factor in the cause of lung, bladder and non-melanoma skin cancers and possibly other cancers.[95, 96] High levels of inorganic arsenic are found in the drinking water of many countries, including China, Argentina, Finland, Hungary and the US.[95, 96]

For a summary of dietary factors in cancer risk see Table 9.2.

Environmental factors

Air pollution

Long-term exposure to combustion-related air pollution is known to increase the risk of lung cancer, being higher in the more polluted cities.[98] The cancer risks of organic hazardous air pollutants in the US have been ranked.[99] Most of the polycyclic aromatic hydrocarbon, benzene, acetaldehyde and 1,3-butadiene risk was found to come from outdoor sources, whereas indoor sources were primarily responsible for chloroform, formaldehyde, and naphthalene risks.[99]

Electromagnetic fields (EMFs)

An advisory panel to the US and National Institutes of Science challenged a 1996 panel from the same institutes which said they *found no conclusive evidence that EMFs generated by power lines and appliances were a threat to humans.*[100]

The more recent panel found that children living near power lines appeared to have a 50% risk of leukaemia and adults had a similar increased risk of leukaemia if they were exposed to high levels of EMFs from utilities in their work places.[100]

A Tasmanian study has investigated residential exposure to electric transmission lines and risk of cancer.[101] This case-controlled study found that there is a possibility that residents close to high voltage power lines, especially early in life, may increase the risk of myeloproliferative and lymphoproliferative disorders. Further larger, independent studies are required to be more conclusive about this issue.

In developed countries, people are constantly being irradiated from numerous sources including phones, internet, wireless, various kitchen appliances (e.g. microwave ovens and electric blankets), and it remains controversial as to whether this exposure produces adverse health effects. It is possible that EMFs may interfere with melatonin secretion.[102, 103]

A case-controlled study of 1700 workers employed as electricians and exposed to electric fields showed no increase in leukaemia, but there was an increase in brain tumours (no specific type), as well as colorectal cancer.[104]

Genetically modified foods (GM foods)

Current research in GM foods is contradictory and inconclusive, and includes much evidence showing potential health risks.[105] Compass

Table 9.2 Dietary constituents reported to raise or lower the risk of cancer[74, 97]

Dietary constituents in cancer		
Additives?	Fat ↑	Tea ↓
Agricultural chemicals?	Fibre ↓	Herbs and spices ↓
Antioxidants ↓	Fish oils ↓	Alcohol ↑
Calcium ↓	Folic acid ↓	Bio-engineered foods?
Cholesterol?	Irradiated foods?	Fluorides?
Coffee?	Nitrites ↑	Garlic ↓
Energy intake↑	Salt ↑	Vitamin D↓

cases of adverse reactions to GM crops in humans have been recorded ranging from allergies following skin contact to an outbreak of unprecedented disease affecting thousands and dubbed eoseniamyalgia.[106, 107]

It is controversial whether GM crops can produce higher yields. There is also evidence showing that non-GM crops using natural matters can increase crop yield.[108] There is insufficient data to do with the long-term effects of GM foods on human health.

Ionising radiation

Most people are unaware that the greatest source of exposure to ionising radiation is background radiation in the environment, which constitutes 82% of all exposure (see Figure 9.2).[109]

Medical radiation is the largest source of human-made radiation and exposure is continuing to increase with time.[110] X-ray treatment for ankylosing spondylitis increases the risk of leukaemia, radiation for menorrhagia leads to a threefold risk of leukaemia, and radiotherapy to cancer patients has been clearly shown to increase the risk of developing secondary cancers.[111, 112, 113] The thyroid is particularly sensitive to ionising radiation, especially when given to children.[114]

A recent retrospective study found that thyroid cancer patients with exposure to radiation from health care work places, or treatments for conditions such as breast cancer and acne, appeared to have worse outcomes than patients with the disease and no exposure.[115] The use of computer tomography (CT) scans is of real concern, as studies demonstrate that radiation exposure from CT coronary angiography is a risk for cancer.[116] Melbourne radiologists have called for a curb on CT scans unless completely essential.[117]

Toxic chemicals

Pesticides, weed-killers

It is estimated that there are about 80 000 toxic chemicals in use at present, with about 5000 used extensively.[118, 119, 120]

An environmental history from a patient investigates the following areas of exposure:

- household
- community
- hobbies
- occupation
- parents' occupation.

Some examples of toxic chemicals include dioxins and bisphenol-A (BPA).

Dioxins

A number of disorders are associated with exposure to dioxins including learning disabilities, infertility, endometriosis, immune dysfunction, endocrine disruption and carcinogen. High levels are found in large fish such as sharks, marlin and swordfish, as well as in breastmilk.[120]

Bisphenol-A (BPA)

Recent investigations have shown that BPA has oestrogenic activity which can lead to miscarriage, birth defects, disruption of beta cells of the pancreas, thyroid hormone disruption, liver damage plus obesity-promoting effects.[121] This study also found an association of elevated urinary BPA with cardiovascular disease, diabetes and abnormal liver function tests. BPA is commonly used to line baby's milk bottles, as well as food cans.[121]

Occupational exposure

Diesel exhaust fumes in trucking industry workers

Trucking industry workers who have regular exposure to diesel vehicle exhaust and other types of vehicles on highways, city streets, and loading docks have an elevated risk of lung cancer with increasing years of work.[122]

Exposure to pesticides

Brain tumours have been associated with several occupational and environmental exposures.[123, 124, 125]

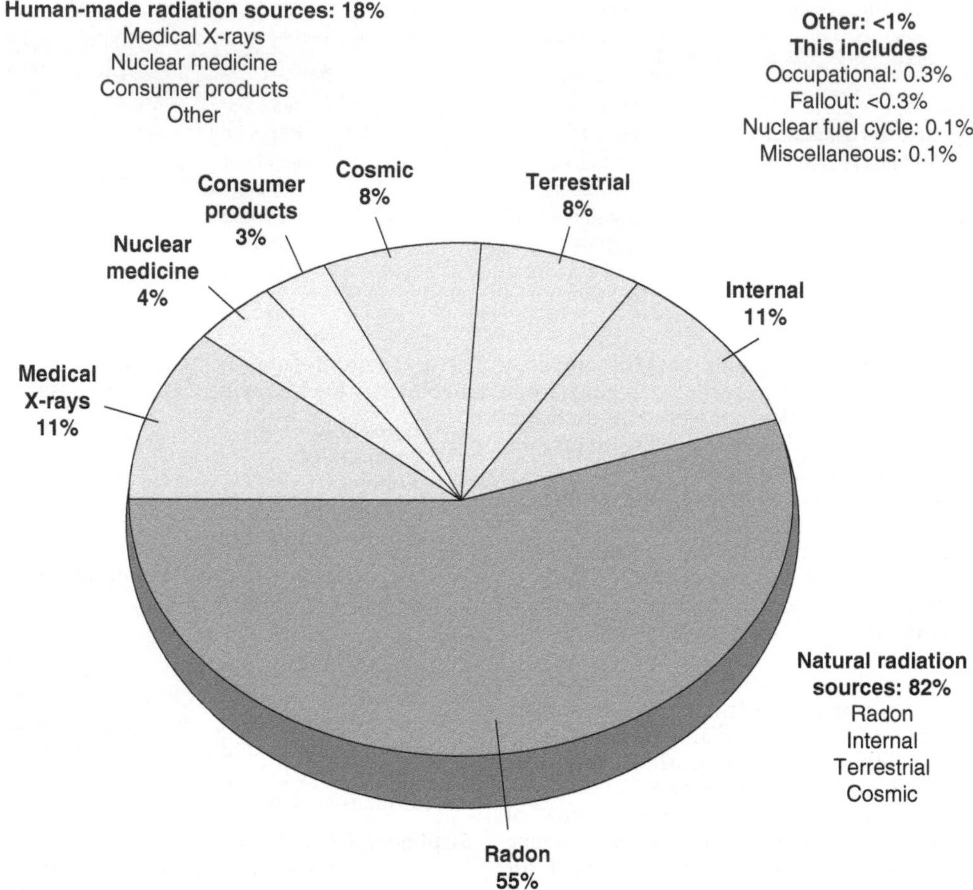

Figure 9.2 Ionising radiation exposure to the public
(Source: Nasca PC, Pastides H 2008 *Fundamentals of Cancer Epidemiology*. Jones and Bartlett Publishers, Boston)

Some pesticides contain alkylureas or amines that metabolise to nitroso compounds which have been associated with neurogenic tumours.[126] However, a more recent study investigating exposure to pesticides and risk of adult brain tumours did not find an association between herbicide or insecticide exposure among men.[123] Women with occupational exposure to herbicides had an increased risk of meningioma.[123]

Exposure to the styrene-butadiene rubber industry

An epidemiological study of 17 000 workers in the rubber industry found an increased risk of chronic lymphocytic and myelogenous leukaemia in the most highly exposed workers.[127] Furthermore, in a study of workers involved in butadiene-monomer production, an association with non-Hodgkin's lymphoma was found.[128]

Ethylene oxide

This chemical is used in the production of other chemicals although most human exposure occurs from its use in sterilisation of medical equipment. An increase in breast cancer occurs with a significant exposure-response relationship between ethylene oxide exposure and breast cancer incidence.[129]

Vinyl chloride exposure

Two large multi-centre cohort studies in facilities that manufactured vinyl chloride, polyvinyl chloride or polyvinyl chloride products showed a substantial increase in the relative risk for liver and gliosarcoma with risk increasing with duration of exposure or total exposure.[130, 131]

Hair dyes

Personal use of hair dyes may play a role in the risk of follicular lymphoma and chronic lymphatic leukaemia plus small lymphocytic leukaemia.[132] A meta-analysis of epidemiological data has found that personal use of hair dyes is associated with an increased risk of bladder cancer.[133]

Cooking oil fumes

Fumes from 6 different oils: safflower, olive, coconut, mustard, vegetable and corn have been collected and polycyclic aromatic hydrocarbons (PAHS) were extracted from air samples.[134] Fumes from safflower oil, vegetable oil and corn oil were found to have PAHS. It is thought that PAHS fumes are linked to lung cancer.

Risks to fire fighters

A review of 32 studies on fire fighters, which was to determine cancer risk using a meta-analysis, has found that there is an elevated risk of multiple myeloma.[135] In addition, a probable association with non-Hodgkin's lymphoma, prostate and testicular cancer was demonstrated.

Sleep patterns

Both short and long sleep duration have been associated with increased mortality from all causes for both sexes, yielding a u-shaped relationship with total mortality and a nadir at 7 hours of sleep.[136] It is also of significance that usage of hypnotics is associated with an increased all-cause mortality and cause a specific mortality in regular users of hypnotics.[137]

It is not surprising that lack of sleep disturbance can influence mortality, as it is closely associated with stress and depression which, in turn, are linked to cancer and cardiovascular disease. Short sleep duration is also associated independently with weight gain and the latter is a risk factor for a number of cancers.[138, 139, 140]

Studies have found that increased sleep duration is associated with a decreased risk of breast cancer.[141, 142]

The frequent occurrence of disturbed sleep in cancer patients is of great concern, as many of these patients may already be suffering from fatigue due to psychological factors, chemotherapy, cancer pain or general debilitation.[143] It is essential to enquire about sleep in cancer patients and to ensure that sleep disturbance is managed properly. The patient's quality of life and their tolerance to treatment, as well as the development of mood disorders is dependent on adequate sleep.[143]

It is controversial whether the level of melatonin is strongly associated with the risk of breast cancer.[141, 144]

Exercise and cancer

Cancer prevention

The protective effect of regular exercise has been demonstrated in a number of cancers including breast, colorectal, prostate, testicular and lung cancer.[145, 146, 147] There is also evidence that exercise may offer protection against endometrial, ovarian and also other forms of cancer.[145, 148, 149]

Exercise is known to improve immunity in the following ways:

- Activation of natural killer cells (NK) whose destructive effects on cancer cells are significantly improved, as well as activation of macrophages.[145, 150, 151]
- Pscyhoneuro immunological exercise has an antidepressant effect.[152]
- Exercise can also help prevent obesity, which is a cancer risk factor.[153, 154]
- Exercise can help reduce insulin resistance which in turn is likely to influence cancer development.[155, 156]

A large study of 30 000 men found that unless they were extremely obese, cardiorespiratory fitness can abolish the risk of dying of cancer associated with being overweight.[157]

In the US, the surgeon general recommends 30 minutes a day of exercise most days of the week, which is generally accepted as 5 days of the week for a total of 150 minutes a week.[158, 159]

Resistance exercise may also be protective, as it can reduce insulin resistance in a similar way to aerobic exercise.[160, 161]

Cancer survival

Regular exercise can improve survival in colorectal and breast cancer patients, 50–60%.[162, 163]

A study of 3000 women with various stages of breast cancer were followed for 18 years and those who walked 3–5 hours per week had twice the survival than those who did not exercise.[163] A further study in women with breast cancer, followed up for a period of 9 years, who exercised regularly had a 44% reduction in mortality.[164] A group of 500 colorectal cancer patients were found to have half the mortality if they exercised regularly.[162]

In a very large prospective study of nearly 48 000 men, of the men over 65 years of age 3000 developed prostate cancer. Those who exercised regularly had reduced their chance of developing an aggressive cancer by two-thirds compared to the men who did not exercise.[165]

A meta-analysis of cancer survival following chemotherapy in cancer patients by Morgan and others, found that survival was improved by 2% in 5 years, which is minimal compared to the benefits of exercise.[166]

Exercise used during cancer treatment can counteract side-effects of disease and treatments.[167] Twice weekly resistant training appears to be safe and well-tolerated, resulting in increased muscle mass and decreased body fat.[168] Resistance exercise, particularly useful in men receiving androgen deprivation therapy for prostate cancer, resulted in improved quality of life and muscular fitness.[160]

Cancer fatigue

Exercise may also reduce fatigue resulting from chemotherapy, in cancer patients. Regular exercise can increase the fitness in breast cancer patients treated with conventional chemotherapy.[169]

The relative importance of cancer fatigue has been compared with other patient symptoms and concerns over 9 cancer types, and emerged as the top-rated symptom.[170] To explore this issue, the author surveyed 534 patients and 91 physician experts from 5 institutions and community support agencies. It was thought by most that fatigue was attributable to both disease and treatments. Sleep disorders and difficulty falling asleep, problems maintaining sleep, poor sleep efficacy, early awakening and excessive daytime sleep are prevalent in cancer patients.[171] Cancer fatigue can be modified by ensuring optimum sleep quality.[172] Exercise and counselling may help to reduce fatigue.[173]

Overweight and obesity

The increasing incidence of obesity throughout most Western countries is said to impose a major additional cancer burden at a time when population ageing is projected to cause unprecedented growth in cancer incidence.[174, 175]

While obesity is frequently associated with type 2 diabetes, hypertension, lipids abnormalities and death from heart disease and stroke, there is growing evidence of its role in causing cancer. A systematic review and meta-analysis, which included the Million Women Study, investigated the link between body mass index (BMI; calculated by dividing weight in kilograms by height in metres squared) and types of cancer.[176, 177]

In men, a 5 kg per metre squared increase in BMI was strongly associated with adenocarcinoma of the oesophagus, thyroid, colon and renal cancers, and in women with adenocarcinoma of the oesophagus, endometrial, gall bladder and renal cancers. There were weaker associations for melanoma and rectal cancer in men, and post-menopausal breast, thyroid and colon cancer in women. Leukaemia, myeloma and Hodgkin's disease were associated in both sexes. Another study found higher risks of oesophageal and gastric cardia adenocarcinoma with increasing BMI.[178]

It is uncertain if obesity is related to prostate cancer.[179] Recent evidence suggests that obesity increases risk of advanced prostate cancer and prostate cancer mortality, but not the risk of less aggressive disease.[179]

Many nutritional factors are also associated with aggressive and fatal prostate cancer.[196] Furthermore, greater plasma insulin-like growth factor, 1 level (IGF-1), is associated with a fivefold increased risk of advanced stage prostate cancer, but was not associated with early-stage prostate cancer.[180] It is of interest that insulin receptors are present on primary human prostate cancers.[181]

A possible mechanism for the association of obesity and cancer is that chronic insulinaemia results in raised levels of 3 IGF-1, with higher mean concentration in men compared to women. The raised level of free IGF-1 alters the environment of cells to favour cancers developing.[182]

Autocrine stimulation of the growth factor receptor (IGF-IR) by IGF-22 is 1 mechanism that allows cancer cells to maintain unregulated growth and to resist program cell death (PCD).[183] Obesity and type 2 diabetes are generally independently associated with an increased risk of developing cancer and a worse prognosis.[184] The etiology is yet to be determined, but insulin resistance and hyperinsulinaemia may be important factors. Hyperglycaemia, hyperlipidaemia and inflammatory cytokines in addition to IGFs are also possible factors involved in the process.

A study has found that patients with elevated insulin or glucose at the time of colorectal adenoma removal are at increased risk of recurrent adenoma.[185] Those with an increased glucose and an increased risk for recurrence of advanced adenomas, however a systematic review meta-analysis investigating the association of glycaemic index (GI) and glycaemic load (GL) intakes with the risk of digestive tract neoplasms found that neither GI or GL intakes were associated with colorectal or pancreatic cancers.[186] In contrast, results from the very large Nurses Health Study showed that high GL and insulin resistance combined to increase pancreatic cancer risk.[187]

It is known that diabetes diagnosed 5 or more years prior to cancer detection was associated with a twofold increasing risk of pancreatic cancer; another study found a 50% increase for diabetes diagnosed 10 or more years prior to cancer detection.[188, 189] Numerous studies show that overweight individuals are consistently at high risk of pancreatic cancer compared to leaner individuals.[190, 191]

The association between body weight and diabetes suggests that insulin resistance may play a role in pancreatic carcinogenesis. A systematic review and meta-analysis of dietary GI, GL and breast cancer by the same group did not provide strong support of an association between dietary GI and GL and breast cancer risk.[192] Another meta-analysis found that low GI and/or low GL diets were independently associated with reduced risk for heart disease and diabetes.[193]

A Cochrane review demonstrated a low GI and GL diet reduced body mass and improved lipids profiles.[194]

In comparison, a large Swedish study of more than 60 000 women over a 20-year period found that when women were overweight they had signs of insulin resistance — such as elevated blood glucose or insulin levels, they were about 50% more likely to be diagnosed with an advanced breast cancer.[195]

In contrast, another meta-analysis of dietary GI, GL and endometrial plus ovarian cancer showed that a high GI, but not a high GL diet, is positively associated with a risk of endometrial cancer, particularly among obese women.[190]

A retrospective study found that diabetes is a significant predictor of tumour recurrence after potentially curative therapy for hepatocellular carcinoma.[196]

Obesity appears to not be associated with prostate cancer, but studies have suggested that obese men are more likely to develop aggressive and fatal prostate cancer.[197, 198] Beneficial effects of exercise in reducing colorectal, breast and prostate cancer may be through reducing hyperinsulinaemia and via IGF access.[199, 200]

Methological issues might explain the failure to detect differences between high and low GI diets.[201] There are always difficulties in collecting accurate dietary information which would allow for the accurate calculation of GI and GL, which in turn influences the results of these studies.

Adiponectin and cancer

The mechanisms underlying malignancies are not fully understood. Adiponectin, and adipocyte secreted protein hormone is an andogenous insulin sensitiser, appears to play an important role not only in glucose and lipid metabolism, but also in the development and progression of several obesity-related malignancies.[202, 203]

Adiponectin is also anti-angiogenic and anti-inflammatory, inversely correlated with BMI, found in higher concentration in men than in women and, in some studies, its level is inversely associated with cancer risk.[204] In adipocytes, androgens are converted to oestradiol, and chronic hyperinsulinaemia, also reduces sex hormone-binding globulin, leaving more oestrogen to impact on oestrogen-sensitive tissues.[202, 203] Adiponectin is considered a link between obesity, insulin resistance and cancer. Levels of adiponectin are lower in obese than lean subjects.[202]

There is a negative relation between obesity, especially central obesity, insulin resistance and circulating adiponectin.[205, 206] Adiponectin concentrations increase with weight loss, but are decreased in obesity, cardiovascular disease, hypertension and metabolic syndrome.[204, 207] Circulating levels of adiponectin are inversely associated with the risk of malignancies associated with obesity and insulin resistance.[201]

Cancer screening

Prevention is the most important and reliable cancer-fighting tool that exists today. Cancer cannot be prevented entirely, and hence it is critical to detect it early. One of the hallmarks of an integrative treatment approach is to detect signs of cancer as early as possible, obtain appropriated treatment, and then take practical pro-active steps to avoid recurrence, which is known as secondary prevention.

The 2 common statistical measures of the usefulness of a screening test are sensitivity and specificity. Sensitivity refers to the probability that a test will show a positive result when cancer exists, specificity is the probability that a negative test result occurs when cancer is absent.

Breast screening

In Australia the government recommends recruiting and screening women aged 50–69 years for early detection of cancer. Women aged 40–49, and 70 years and older are able to attend for screening.[208]

There can be differences in the results of screening when comparing different countries. A comparison of screening mammography in the US and the UK found that open surgical biopsy rates are twice as high in the US than in the UK, but the cancer detection rates were similar.[209]

Efforts to improve US mammographic screening should target lowering the recall rate without reducing the cancer detection rate. Recently MRI has been used to detect breast cancers that cannot be detected by mammography and ultrasonography.[210]

Russian equipment utilising a microwave imaging technique which detects heat at depths of 6cm may be able to detect breast cancer earlier than mammography especially in younger women with dense breasts.[211,212] An advantage of this technology is that is does not involve radiation.

Early diagnosis of breast cancer is associated with better prognosis, especially when implemented with lifestyle improvements, as well as psychosocial change.[213]

A recent Norwegian study found that it is likely that some breast cancers detected by mammography would not persist to be detectable at the end of 6 years by mammography, raising the possibility that the natural course of some screen-detected invasive breast cancers is to spontaneously regress.[214]

A screening mammography can result in 33% more surgery, 20% more mastectomies and more use of radiotherapy because of over-diagnosis and others argue that the information provided to the patient about screening mammography is incomplete.[215, 216] Keen and Keen, from the US, found after an extensive analysis, that less than 5% of women with screen-detectable cancers have their lives saved.[217] Both of these studies are reviewed by a *Lancet* editorial which points out that there are problems with screening in mammography, and also that there are vested interests that make screening a business.[218]

Cervical screening

Cervical screening is one of the oldest and most successful forms of screening to prevent cancer. The PAP smear can detect both cervical dysplasia and carcinoma, and is now thought that about 80% of high-grade dyskaryosis and high-grade dysplasia will not progress to cancer.[219]

Human papilloma virus (HPV) can cause cervical cancer and the majority of the HPV involved can be eradicated by vaccination against HPV if used before being infected by the virus.[220] There has been concern about the potential effect of decreased cervical cancer screening participation after HPV vaccination.[221] Like most other cancers, cervical cancer is strongly associated with lifestyle factors and diet. Risk factors include unsafe sex, smoking (even second-hand smoke), being overweight and an unhealthy diet.[222]

The following nutrient supplements can be protective or prevent dysplasia from progressing:

- folic acid (supplements)[223, 224]
- vitamin C and E (diet)[225, 226]
- vitamin A[225]
- riboflavin and thiamine (diet)[225, 223]
- vitamin B12[223, 224]
- carotene[226]
- coenzyme Q_{10} (diet)[227]
- selenium.[226]

The role of nutrients and cervical cancer has been summarised by Sali and Vitetta.[224]

It is uncertain whether particular nutrients can reduce the rate of acquisition of a high risk HPV or whether they facilitate the clearance of high risk HPV. Women with higher folate blood levels are inversely associated with a positive high risk HPV test when compared to lower folate status.[228] A large case-controlled study has found that serum homocysteine was strongly and significantly predictive of cervical cancer risk.[229]

Chemotherapy and survival

Despite widespread optimism with the introduction of chemotherapy that it would significantly improve cancer survival, this has not been the case for the overwhelming majority. In a literature search of randomised clinical trials reporting a 5-year survival benefit attributed solely to curative and adjuvant cytotoxic chemotherapy in adult malignancies, the survival was estimated to be 2.3% in Australia and 2.1% in the US.[230] Even the role of anti-angiogenic drugs, which have been shown to shrink tumours initially but can then show an unexpected surge in growth spreading both locally and to distant organs, has been disappointing.[231]

Chemotherapy has numerous side-effects and it is hoped that the further development of biological therapies such as the angiostatic and antibody drugs would produce better results and less side-effects. There are also concerns about the conflicts of interest in published clinical cancer research.[232, 233, 234]

Nearly 1 in 5 oncology articles to do with oncology research is published in prestigious journals and are funded by the pharmaceutical industry.[233]

Mind–body medicine

A cancer diagnosis is often life threatening to the patient. Not only do they have to deal with a grave illness, but the patient also often has to deal with toxicity related to chemotherapy and radiotherapy, and then they also often have to deal with difficulties following surgical procedures.[235–238] Even adjuvant treatment can be given over a year and be associated with problems. There is also considerable stress for the families of the cancer patient.

Earlier in this chapter, the basic mechanisms of mind–body medicine were discussed (see Figure 9.1, page 199). It is difficult to meet the enormous emotional needs of the cancer patient. Proper care starts with the consultation. Even the words used can be important during the consultations, not just telling the patient they have 'a cancer' rather than 'cancer'. The former can arouse less suspicion according to results of an Australian study.[239]

The psychological adaptation to cancer is influenced by various disease, demographic and psychosocial factors, including personality factors, coping abilities and social support.[240] There are a number of mind–body therapies available which have predominantly evolved because of the documented negative psychosocial consequences of cancer.

Psychosocial support and mental relaxation

There are a number of modalities that have been found to benefit cancer patients including cognitive behavioural interventions, supportive psychotherapy, informational and educational treatments, social support, as well as exercise therapy, art therapy, music therapy plus other therapies. In general, it is agreed that psychosocial support for cancer patients is therapeutic.[241 242]

Even chatting, ideally with a confidante, helps in influencing mortality related to cancer. Research shows that 7 years after initial breast cancer treatment, a patient with 1 confidante can improve life expectancy by 15%, whereas 2 confidantes can lead to an improvement of 25%.[243]

Various treatment programs have also been established to help cancer patients to cope with the various psychosocial problems that are associated with this disease; programs such as the Gawler Foundation in Melbourne.[244]

Mental relaxation techniques

Meditation is one of the most popular and most commonly used mind–body therapies. The value of meditation and hypnosis, in the management of cancer patients, is well-documented.[245, 246, 247]

There are a number of meditation techniques. Basically they can be divided into either passive or physical types. In addition, they can also be divided into those that are based around spirituality and religion, and non-spiritual practices. Most of the research relates to passive meditation and yoga. Common forms of passive meditation include mindfulness, guided imagery and those that include breathing techniques. Relaxation techniques are often used as part of the psychosocial support program.

Meditation can reduce pain, anxiety, depression and in addition, help with sleep disturbance and fatigue.[248–251]

Quality of life was improved in breast and prostate cancer patients with meditation.[252] The combination of mindfulness-based art therapy, which is mindfulness meditation and art therapy combined, reduced stress, distress and improved health-related quality of life.[252]

The benefits of mindfulness-based mood disturbance can also be maintained 6 months later, and stress reduction more than 12 months later.[250, 253]

Six studies have found improvement in survival and mental health[8]. Spiegel's group was the first to show that psychosocial intervention over a 1-year period could improve quality of life and survival in metastatic breast cancer patients when followed up over a 10-year period.[245] In another study, Fawzy was able to reduce recurrence and death in melanoma patients with a 6-week management program, and they were followed up for 6 years.[246] In the Fawzy study, it was also shown that immunity improved 6 months after the 6 week management program. An improvement in survival has also been recorded with cancers of liver, gastrointestinal tract and lymphoma, plus a further study on breast cancer patients.[254, 255, 256]

Not all studies offering mental and social health programs have shown improved survival.[8] Of these 6 studies with no improvement in survival, 3 did show improvement in quality of life. The lack of improved survival may be related to the quality of psychosocial support being offered, and whether the patient was fully involved.[257, 258]

Hypnosis

Breast cancer patients undergoing surgery reported less anxiety and less analgesic if they used hypnosis.[259] It is likely that there would be cost reduction in the care of surgical patients who have less pain and less anxiety. Mental wellbeing was also improved with the use of hypnosis in patients undergoing radiotherapy.[260]

Hypnotherapy has also been beneficial for children being treated with chemotherapy; they have less nausea prior to and after chemotherapy.[261]

Tai chi

Tai chi is a mixture of various physical movements and synchronised breathing with meditation. The physical demands of tai chi need not be great and can be suitable for most cancer patients. A clinical trial on breast cancer patients found that tai chi performed for 60 minutes, 3 times per week, can improve quality of life and self-esteem.[262] A recent study has shown that tai chi can improve immunity.[263]

Qigong

Qigong is a mind–body integrative exercise, or intervention, from Chinese medicine used to prevent and cure ailments, and to improve health and energy levels through regular practice.[264] One study has reported decreased leukopaenia and platelet count, as well as decreased anaemia resulting from chemotherapy in the qigong group.[265] Several reviews claim that qigong offers therapeutic benefits for cancer patients.[266, 267, 268]

Nine studies, 4 randomised and 5 non-randomised, were examined. The methodology was regarded as being poor. Two trials suggested effectiveness in prolonging life of cancer patients. The reviewers concluded that the evidence supporting qigong was incomplete based on the studies that were analysed.[265]

Another study showed decreased psychological distress with qigong.[269]

Psychological improvements occurred in an experimental group of participants after 1 month of practicing qigong.[270]

Reiki and/or therapeutic touch

Reiki is classified as an energy medicine, as is qigong, in the US CAM classification. A number of small clinical studies generally show some benefit in cancer patients in reducing pain and fatigue.

A study on cancer patients has used an evidence-based approach to examine research regarding the effectiveness of therapeutic touch.[271] This review examined 12 clinical studies involving cancer patients. All studies had experimental control groups. Eleven of the studies reported benefit from therapeutic touch.

Massage therapy

Massage therapy differs to reiki or therapeutic touch, as it involves application of varying degrees of pressure to the body. Benefits of massage in palliative care are found later in this chapter.

Massage can reduce pain in cancer patients.[272] It has also been shown to be useful for postoperative pain.[273] Massage was effective in controlling nausea in breast cancer patients.[273]

Biofeedback

Biofeedback involves measurement of muscle tension with electrobiography and also temperature or measurement of brain waves (electroencephalography).

It is possible with biofeedback to control processes that are normally voluntary. The measurements are visible on a monitor to the patient. It has been beneficial in treating cancer pain, and also helping to regain both urinary and faecal competence after surgery.[274]

Music therapy

Music therapy is provided by musicians who also receive training as counsellors. In cancer patients it has been shown to treat anxiety related to radiotherapy.[275] Music therapy can also reduce pain plus nausea and vomiting related to chemotherapy.[275]

Music therapy has been found to be beneficial in the treatment of blood pressure, insomnia, depression, pain and stress in those without cancer.

Aromatherapy

Aromatherapy is discussed later in this chapter under palliative care. A few studies have demonstrated that aromatherapy can reduce stress, pain, depression and also can improve quality of life.[276, 277, 278]

Nutritional influences

Carotenoids

Dietary lycopene are carotenoids that are found in tomatoes and other red-coloured foods and has been shown in clinical studies to protect against cancer, including prostate, pancreas, ovary, breast, CRC and bladder cancer.[279–285]

Lycopene can inhibit IGF-1 in rat prostate.[286] Lycopene supplement can also suppress prostate cancer growth.[231]

An extensive survey found that 57 of 72 studies reported an inverse association between tomato intake or blood lycopene level and cancer risk.[287] Evidence for benefit was strongest for cancers of the prostate, lung and stomach. There was also benefit for pancreas, CRC, oesophagus, oral cavity, breast and cervix.

In addition to preventing cancer, vitamin A derivatives have been used to cure promyelocytic leukaemia.[288]

Curcumin

Curcumin is an active ingredient in the spice turmeric, and has been shown to prevent cancer and also have therapeutic properties. Curcumin can suppress tumour initiation, promotion and metastases.[289]

Curcumin can decrease PGE-2 substantially and this may be 1 of its actions in antagonising cancer.[290] Curcumin can inhibit *in vitro* growth of cancers of prostate, colon and animal breast cancer.[291, 292, 293]

A small study using curcumin in pancreas cancer patients showed improvement in some patients.[294] In animal experiments, curcumin circumvents chemo-resistance *in vitro* and potentiates the effect of Thalidomide and Bortezomib against multiple myeloma.[295] Curcumin can inhibit the growth of cancer cells and enhances the anti-tumour effects of Gemcitabine and radiation.[296] In another study, curcumin was found to sensitise ovarian and breast cancer cell lines to cisplatin through apoptotic cell death.[297]

Teas

Teas have protective effect against cancer, but the unfermented green tea offers the best protection with the catechins and theaflavins being the active ingredients.[298]

Consuming 5 or more cups of green tea a day reduced the risk of developing breast, lung, leukaemia and prostate cancer and could help reduce recurrence in breast and ovarian cancer.[299–303] It is possible that tea may protect from squamous cell skin cancers also.[304]

In an *in vitro* study, tea polyphenols plus retinoic acid inhibited cervical cell growth and promoted apoptosis. Polyphenol by itself was inactive.[305] A nutrient formulation which includes green tea, lysine, proline, arginine and ascorbic acid inhibits *in vitro* renal carcinoma growth and invasion.[306, 307]

A recent study found that hot tea was associated with squamous cell carcinoma of the oesophagus.[308] The mechanisms for this are not understood. It is controversial if milk, added to tea, can impair the bioavailability of tea catechins.[309, 310]

Allium vegetables

Garlic and/or onions

Garlic and onion consumption in a series of case-controlled studies have been shown to be protective against cancers of the oral cavity, pharynx, oesophagus, CRC, larynx, breast, ovary, prostate and renal cell.[311]

Allium vegetables can suppress growth of cancer cells *in vitro* and *in vivo* by causing apoptosis, and can also suppress angiogenesis.[312] Another study found that garlic caused apoptosis of human glioblastoma cells *in vitro*.[313] Garlic has been known to have anti-cancer properties because it can disrupt the action of cancer-causing agents.[308, 314]

Cruciferous vegetables

Cruciferous vegetables include cabbage, cauliflower, broccoli, bok choy, and brussel sprouts. Although a vegetable intake has been shown to be protective against cancer, results can be inconsistent. It is thought that this inconsistency can be explained by specific sub-groups of vegetables such as the cruciferous vegetables which are more strongly related to cancer risk.[315]

In the Health Professional Study (HPFS), cruciferous vegetables were associated with decreased risk of bladder cancer.[316] These vegetables are also protective for prostate and lung cancer.[317, 318, 319]

It is possible that these vegetables may decrease breast cancer risk due to the action of indole-3-carbinol which is found in cruciferous vegetables.[320]

The 16 alpha-hydroxyestrone plus 4-hydroxyestrone are thought to be responsible for the carcinogenic effect of oestrogen. On the other hand, the oestrogen metabolite 2-hydroxyestrone has been found to be protective against several types of cancer, including breast cancer.[321] Indole-3-carbinol can increase the ratio of 2-hydroxyestrone to 16 alpha-hydroxyestrone, and also to inhibit the 4-hydroxalation of oestradiol.[322]

There is controversy whether microwave cooking can destroy active ingredients of the cruciferous vegetables with 1 group finding that it does, and the other finding the opposite.[323, 324] It is thought that the addition of water to these vegetables at the time of microwaving may be critical.[319] If cooking does influence the active ingredients in the cruciferous vegetables, this could also explain discrepancy of findings.[325]

Mushrooms

Medicinal properties have been attributed to mushrooms for thousands of years. Mushrooms can exert tumour-inhibitory effects by influencing T cells and macrophages, and it is thought that the glucans (lentinans) from mushrooms mediate these effects.[326]

Glycoproteins (lectins) present in mushrooms, broad beans, seeds and nuts have been shown *in vitro* experiments to increase the differentiation of cancer cells indicating that the cancer processes are either halted or reversed, as well as inhibiting cell multiplication.[327] Inhibition of colon cancer and lymphoma by lentinan from shitake mushrooms has also been documented in animal experiments.[328]

Another mushroom (*Phellinus linteus*), has been shown to suppress breast, melanoma and prostate cancer growth, and also angiogenesis. The active substances are thought to be polysaccharides.[329, 330] The *Phellinus linteus* mushroom has been found to have a synergistic effect with Doxorubicin and prostate cancer cell lines.[331]

Anticancer effect of *Ganoderma lucidum* on *in vitro* breast cancer cells is increased by green tea extract.[332] A large case-controlled study in China revealed that high dietary intake of mushrooms decreased breast cancer risk in pre- and post-menopausal women, and there was an additional decreased risk of breast cancer from the joint effect of mushrooms and green tea.[333]

In vitro studies demonstrate that both mushrooms and green tea suppress invasive behaviour of cancer cells.[334] Mushroom extracts increase the activity of natural killer cells in gynaecological cancer patients undergoing chemotherapy.[335]

Polysaccharide extract of *Ganoderma lucidum*, when given 1800mg, 3 times daily for 12 weeks improved the natural killer cell numbers in advanced stage cancer patients.[336]

Polysaccharide peptides (PSP) isolated from a mushroom *Coriolus versicolor* significantly improved leukocyte and neutrophil count in a randomised, double-blind, placebo-controlled study of patients with advance non-small cell lung cancer.[337] Another clinical study which included patients with various cancers treated with maitake mushroom showed a significant improvement, especially in those patients with breast, lung and liver cancer.[338]

Soy

Epidemiological studies have demonstrated the role of soy in cancer prevention of breast, prostate, endometrium and stomach.[339–342] Soy intake is most protective against breast cancer when consumed during childhood as found in a recent case-controlled study.[334]

Early Genistein exposure from soy promotes cell differentiation in breast tissue which suppresses the development of breast cancer in adulthood by decreasing the activity of the epidermal growth signal pathway. It has been observed that soy isoflavone Genistein induces apoptosis and inhibits growth of both androgen sensitive and androgen independent prostate cancer cells *in vitro*.[343]

The isoflavones, Genistein and Diadzein stimulate the synthesis of serum hormone-binding globulin (SHBG) in the liver which results in a fall of testosterone levels.[344, 345]

Isoflavones can also reduce free androgens.[346] A combination of soy phytochemical concentrate in green tea can reduce serum IGF and testosterone concentrations in mice.[347] Soy and tea combinations have the potential of preventing breast and prostate cancers.[342] Genistein can inhibit colonic cancer cells *in vitro*.[348]

Colon cancer can be hormonally influenced.[349] A Japanese case-controlled study investigating the association between dietary isoflavone intake and risk of colorectal adenoma revealed a significant inverse association between dietary isoflavone intake and risk of colorectal adenoma.[350]

Genistein can inhibit human stomach cancer cell growth *in vitro*.[351] Genistein has also been shown to inhibit the growth of leukaemia *in vitro*.[352] This finding has led to the development of ipriflavone, a phenyl isoflavone, a derivative used as a treatment of leukaemia.[347]

Bladder cancer cells are also inhibited *in vitro* by soy isoflavones.[353] A study from Singapore found an increased risk of bladder cancer linked to dietary soy intake.[354] Consideration should be given to the chemical modification of isoflavones in soy foods during cooking and processing.[355]

Soy isoflavone Genistein in mouse models of melanoma has an anti-tumour and anti-angiogenic activity.[356] Similar anti-angiogenic effects were obtained with soy food based diet. Another study found that soybean isoflavones reduced the experimental metastases in mice.[357] Genistein has been demonstrated to be a radio-sensitiser for prostate cancer *in vitro* and animal experiments.[358]

Citrus fruits

Citrus fruits are thought to offer protection from cancer through their flavonoid content. Their high vitamin C content may also be important.[359] The flavonoids can control cancer cells by suppression, blockage and transformation.[354] Citrus fruits can have anti-proliferative, anti-invasive and anti-angiogenic effects.[354] Citrus flavonoids have anti-proliferative effects on the following cancer cells: squamous, meningioma, leukaemia, breast, lung, melanoma and hepatoma.[354]

A systematic review has investigated the association between dietary intake of citrus fruits and gastric cancer risk.[360] High citrus fruit intake is protective against stomach cancer. Citrus fruits have also been found to have a possible protective effect on bladder cancer.[361]

There is an inverse association between intake of citrus fruits and the risk of pancreatic cancer, and squamous cell oesophageal cancers.[362, 363]

Grapefruit

A study showed that grapefruit intake was associated with an increase in breast cancer risk and it was hypothesised that this may be mediated by an effect on oestrogen levels.[364] However, the researchers were unable to examine grapefruit juice intake. An examination of grapefruit juice intake and breast cancer risk in the Nurses' Health Study showed a significant decrease in risk of breast cancer with a greater intake of grapefruit in women.[365]

Interactions with various drugs

Grapefruit juice is an inhibitor of intestinal cytocrome P-453A4 system which is responsible for the first-pass metabolism of many drugs leading to elevation of their serum concentrations: in particular are its effects on the calcium channel antagonists and the statin group of drugs.[366]

Folic acid and cancer risk

The association with folic acid and CRC has been previously discussed. Dietary folate deficiency has also been associated with an increased risk of other cancers including prostate, breast, bladder, oral, pharyngeal, ovary, pancreas and lung cancer.[367–373]

It is thought that the key role of folate is that it can guard against DNA damage and promote gene stability.[374]

Pomegranate and ellagic acid

Pomegranate shows both antioxidant and anti-atherosclerotic properties attributed to the high content of polyphenols including ellagic acid in its free and bound forms, gallotamins and anthocyanins and other flavonoids. The most abundant of these polyphenols is punicalagin, a potent antioxidant which is hydralised to ellagic acid.[375, 376]

Ellagic acid, which is also found in berries and other plant foods, has been shown to exhibit anticarcinogenic properties *in vitro* and in animal experiments.[377, 378]

Pomegranate juice was found to have greater anti-proliferative action against human oral, colon and prostate tumour cells compared to purified polyphenols punicalagin and ellagic acid.[379] Pomegranate juice has been found to have *in vitro* and *in vivo* anti-cancer properties against human breast cancer, human promyelocytic leukaemia cells, lung, liver, oesophageal and pancreas cancer.[379, 380, 381] Ellagic acid can significantly potentiate the anti-carcinogenic potential of quercetin *in vitro* human leukaemia cells.[382]

A study on humans with rising PSA after surgery or radiotherapy for prostate cancer with a Gleeson score = /< than 7, who were treated with pomegranate juice significantly reduced the rate of PSA increase.[383]

Patients' use of nutritional and herbal supplements

A growing number of the public, both young and old, are using nutritional and herbal supplements.[384–389] It is therefore not surprising that cancer patients are even more likely to take supplements.[390, 391, 392]

Supplements are taken by cancer patients to help improve prognosis or to deal with physical or psychosocial issues and report positive responses to do with stress, depression, lack of sleep, nausea, poor immunity, pain and dyspnoea.[393, 394, 395]

Communication problems with medical practitioners

Due to the lack of education of medical practitioners in nutritional medicine, patients are frequently unable to receive relevant nutritional medicine information.[396] Patients fear discussing issues relating to supplements because they often receive a negative response from their medical practitioner. There are a number of communication problems between the oncologist and patient. A recent study found that oncologists and thoracic surgeons rarely responded empathically to the concerns raised by patients with lung cancer.[397] Empathic responses that did occur were frequently in the last third of the encounter.

Another study has also found that the oncologists encountered a few empathic opportunities and responded with empathic statements infrequently.[398]

Previous research has shown that the physicians responded to empathic opportunities in 38% of surgical cases, and in 15–21% of primary care cases.[399, 400]

Empathy is associated with improved patient satisfaction and compliance with recommended treatment.[390, 401] Patients who are satisfied with their consultation, have improved understanding of their condition with less anxiety, and improved mental functioning.[402]

Cancer specialists also struggle if they are discussing the high costs of drugs with patients. Surprisingly, the oncologists surveyed reported the least difficulty with disclosing cancer diagnosis and being honest about the patient's prognosis.[403]

A study has found that nearly all oncologists disclose to their patients that they will die, although there is a wealth of data concerning advanced-cancer patients who do not understand their prognosis.[404] Fostering of hope, even in terminally ill patients, is essential.[405]

A cross-sectional nationwide survey was conducted with 714 (56%) members of the Clinical Oncology Society of Australia.[406] Results show that Australian cancer care workers experience considerable occupational distress and regular screening for burnout is recommended.

Nutritional status of cancer patients

Malnutrition in cancer patients is common and an inverse prognostic indicator of survival with up to 80% of patients with cancer being malnourished on presentation.[407, 408, 409]

Malnutrition is a significant contributor to death in up to 20% of patients.[410] Those that have lost weight have a poorer response to treatment, reduced quality of life and increased risk of death.[411, 412] The NICE guidelines state that patients should undergo nutritional assessment.[413] Unfortunately few doctors deal with malnutrition adequately.[414, 415]

A UK survey found that 72% of specialist oncological trainees were incapable of identifying patients with malnutrition.[416] A Swedish study also found that doctors had inadequate nutritional knowledge.

Why cancer patients use complementary therapies

The widespread use of complementary medicine by cancer patients is in the hope of improving survival, reducing recurrence, reducing side-effects of surgery and chemotherapy, and also treating physical and psychosocial issues.

Complementary medicine is used to treat nausea and vomiting, fatigue, pain and other symptoms.

Anxiety, depression and fear are very common in cancer patients and can be treated effectively with complementary medicine. Most people are happy to use complementary medicine currently with conventional medicine, and not instead of it.[386, 399]

Nutritional supplements

Selenium / vitamin E

Selenium supplements can protect from cancer especially with CRC, lung, oesophageal, gastric and prostate cancer.[417, 418] It is likely that dietary selenium is protective against breast cancer, but other studies have not supported this finding.[371, 419] Selenium levels decline with age and therefore it is possible that selenium supplementation may be of benefit, in particular in the elderly.[371] Selenium supplementation does not benefit nor protect basal and squamous cell carcinomas of the skin.[420]

The result of the Selenium and Vitamin E Cancer Prevention Trial (SELECT) and Vitamins and Lifestyle (VITAL) studies does not support a role for vitamin E, either alone or in combination with selenium for prostate and other cancers.[421, 422] A series of other studies do not support this finding.[423–429]

Reasons for failure of the SELECT study include the use of a vitamin E supplement that reduces gamma-tocopherol which offers major protection against prostate cancer.[382, 383] The problems of using synthetic forms of vitamin E, as used in this study, have been highlighted previously. It is suggested that future supplement studies should combine alpha and gamma-tocopherol together.[382] Selenium can sensitise human prostate cancer cells to TRAIL, a cytotoxic agent indicating that selenium may help overcome resistance to cytotoxic drugs.[430, 431]

Tamoxifen is widely used for the treatment of oestrogen-sensitive breast cancer, but the subsequent development of resistance is a key problem. Studies on breast cancer lines show that selenium synergises with Tamoxifen to improve its efficacy and help overcome resistance.[432, 433]

Vitamin E can reduce the risk of developing breast, lung, prostate, gastrointestinal and ovarian cancers.[434, 435, 436]

Vitamin E supplements may also be able to reduce the risk of breast cancer recurrence among breast cancer survivors.[427] Long-term use of vitamin E protected against bladder cancer.[437] In animal studies, vitamin E has been shown to be protective against melanoma.[438] Vitamin E analogues can induce apoptosis in malignant cell lines and inhibit tumourogenesis *in vivo*.[439] Vitamin E analogues, epitomised by alpha-tocopherol succinate are pro-apoptotic agents with selective neoplastic activity.[440, 441]

Flavonoids combined with vitamin E can reduce angiogenic peptide vascular endothelial growth factor from human breast cancer cells, and the inhibitory effect was greatest from the flavonoid naringen and alpha-tocopherol succinate.[442] Another major defect with these negative studies is the lack of an integrative approach which would consider behavioural, dietary, exercise and the importance of vitamin D levels.

Vitamin C

A number of case control studies have investigated the role of vitamin C in cancer prevention, and most have shown that higher intakes of dietary vitamin C are associated with decreased incidence of cancers of the mouth, throat, vocal chords, oesophagus, stomach, CRC and lung.[443, 444]

Combinations of vitamin C and other micronutrients generally show a positive result. Vitamin C and retinoic acid can inhibit the proliferation of human breast cancer cells by altering their gene expression.[445]

Lipoic acid can synergistically enhance ascorbate cytotoxicity *in vitro* experiments.[446]

Ascorbate efficacy was also enhanced in an additive fashion with vitamin K_3.[437]

The dose of micronutrients used in this latter study could be achieved *in vivo*. Dietary vitamin C, E and beta-carotene have been shown to be protective against uterine cancer in a systematic literature review and meta-analysis.[447] A case control study also found that dietary vitamin C and E showed an inverse association with prostate cancer incidence.[448]

In the double-blind placebo-controlled Women's Antioxidant and Cardiovascular Study, women were supplemented with vitamin C, vitamin E (600IU every other day) and beta-carotene 50mg (every other day). Supplements with vitamins C, E and beta-carotene either individually or in combination did not reduce cancer incidence or reduce cancer mortality.[449]

The Males Physicians' Health Study II was a randomised double-blind placebo-controlled trial of vitamin E, 400IU (every other day) and vitamin C, 500mg daily.[450]

Neither vitamin E nor C supplementation reduced the risk of prostate cancer or total cancer in this large trial.

A large randomised placebo-controlled trial (SELECT) investigated the role of selenium (200mcg/day selenium methionine), and vitamin E (400IU synthetic form). Selenium or vitamin E, alone or in combination, did not prevent prostate cancer.[379]

In all of these randomised placebo-controlled trials, the alpha-tocopherol form of vitamin E was used. In 2 of the studies, it was the synthetic form of vitamin E, in none of these studies was gamma-tocopherol used which is the predominant form in foods.[451]

The doses of the type of vitamin E used in these studies are known to reduce the absorption of the gamma form of vitamin E. In SELECT, gamma-tocopherol was measured and showed nearly a 50% decline.[452, 453]

Gamma-tocopherol form of vitamin E is the most protective against prostate cancer.[445] Hence the lowering of gamma-tocopherol in SELECT is likely to have been a factor in the lack of cancer risk reduction. In the Physicians' Health Study, synthetic form of vitamin E was used; the natural form has proven to be better.[454]

When Japanese researchers gave natural and synthetic vitamin E and measured blood levels, 100mg (149IU) of natural vitamin E produced levels that required 300mg (448IU) of synthetic vitamin E to achieve.[455]

Most studies show that the synthetic vitamin E is only half as active in the body as the natural form.[456] The doses of vitamin E used in all of these studies are inadequate and also the incorrect form is being used. It is unknown if a higher dose of vitamin C may be more protective. Vitamin C is a water-soluble vitamin, and it is more possible to maintain elevated serum levels if it is taken at least twice daily. It is not consistent with an integrative approach towards cancer prevention to be relying on 1 or 2 supplements.

The integrative approach involves stress reduction, relaxation techniques, regular exercise, healthy food with adequate sunlight exposure plus the use of supplements to support healthy lifestyle and diets. Integrative doctors seldom use single or double nutrients as they are used in clinical studies.

Use of vitamin C for the treatment of cancer

Numerous studies have investigated the possibility of vitamin C being used in the treatment of cancer.[457]

Early studies by Cameron et. al., reported that it was possible to improve survival and quality of life of cancer patients using high dose intravenous vitamin C.[458] Cameron was supported by Pauling to research the role of intravenous vitamin C and cancer therapy. Moertel et. al. from the Mayo Clinic reported that a high dose of oral C (10gm) was ineffective against advanced cancer.[459]

A clear difference in the 2 studies was the plasma concentration of vitamin C which was much lower with the oral dose. More recent studies have shown that vitamin C acts as a toxic agent against cancer cells when given intravenously. A 10gm intravenous dose of ascorbate produces plasma concentrations greater than 25-fold higher than concentrates from a similar oral dose.[379]

Levine's group have shown in animal experiments that it has been possible to kill cancer cells, but not normal cells.[380] These researchers have traced ascorbate's anti-cancer effect to the formation of hydrogen peroxide in the extracellular fluid surrounding the tumours.[415] They were able to significantly decrease growth rates of ovarian, pancreatic and glioblastoma established tumours. Similar pharmacological concentrations were readily achieved in humans given ascorbate intravenously.

Case reports of patients with advanced cancers have been documented. Unexpectedly long survival times after receiving high dose intravenous vitamin C therapy have been noted.[460, 461]

In another report, large doses of vitamin C used in combination with oral antioxidants (vitamin E, beta-carotene, coenzyme Q_{10} and multivitamin/

mineral complex) and chemotherapy led to patients having a positive response.[462]

A randomised controlled trial (RCT) is necessary before conclusion can be drawn about high dose intravenous vitamin C and cancer therapy.

Intravenous vitamin C for pain control

A South Korean group have investigated the effects of intravenous vitamin C on terminal cancer patients and health-related quality of life.[463] All patients were given an intravenous administration of 10gm vitamin C twice with a 3-day interval and an oral intake of 4gm vitamin C daily for a week. There was a significant improvement in the quality of life after administration of vitamin C.

Vitamin D

Vitamin D plays a role in the prevention of numerous cancers including breast, CRC, prostate, pancreas, ovary, skin, non-Hodgkin's lymphoma and other sites.[464–467]

It is also known that those that live near the equator have higher vitamin D levels and are less likely to die from cancer than people in northern latitudes.[468]

Data from the Third National Health and Nutrition Examination Survey in the US showed that serum vitamin D deficiency exists in the US and it has major public health implications.[469] Studies relating to vitamin D and cancer have been inconsistent, but researchers agree that deficiency should be prevented and vitamin D supplemented as necessary depending on blood levels.[470]

There is also some evidence showing that cancer survival is linked to vitamin D levels. A large study in England found that cancer survival was dependant on season of diagnosis and sunlight exposure with diagnosis in summer and autumn associated with improved survival compared to that in winter.[471]

Other studies have shown that exposure to sunlight was associated with reduced mortality from breast, ovarian, prostate, colon and lung cancers.[466, 472, 473] Further evidence is warranted to examine the link between vitamin D and cancer incidence, survival and mortality.

Multivitamin use and risk of cancer

The role of multivitamins in isolation from an integrative approach remains controversial. In 2002, *JAMA* published a review supporting the role of vitamin use, especially as there are groups of patients who are at higher risk for vitamin deficiency and suboptimal vitamin status.[474] Another review came to the conclusion that multivitamin and mineral supplement use may prevent cancer in individuals with poor or suboptimal nutritional status.[475] It is suspected that common micronutrient deficiencies are likely to damage DNA which is likely to be a major factor in cancer development.[476, 477]

A Women's Health Initiative study collected data on multivitamin use at baseline and follow-up time for a 7.9 year period.[478] This study showed that multivitamin use had little or no influence on the risk of common cancers. Criticism of this study include that it was not a prospective placebo-controlled double-blind study which could avoid bias, little detail is given about the composition of the multivitamin, and there was no verification of dose taken or if the supplement was taken at all.

Individuals who used dietary supplements generally report higher dietary nutrient intakes and healthier diets, and also have healthier lifestyles.[479, 480, 481]

Antioxidants, vitamin E and selenium for cancer prevention

The National Prevention of Cancer Trial, recorded a 65% reduction in prostate cancer incidence in men receiving selenium supplementation.[474] This study came only 2 years after the ATBC (alpha-tocopherol, beta-carotene) Cancer Prevention Trial reported a 35% reduction in prostate cancer recurrence among men taking vitamin E supplementation.[482]

The selenium and vitamin E cancer prevention trial (SELECT) was established to examine the effects of L-selenomethionine and racemic alpha-tocopherol acetate, alone or in combination, on the risk of prostate cancer and other health outcomes in relatively healthy men.[475] This placebo-controlled study included 35 533 men (with a planned minimum follow-up of 7 years). There were 1 of 4 interventions: L-selenomethionine (200mcg/day); vitamin E placebo or racemic alpha-tocopherol acetate (400IU/day) and selenium placebo; L-selenomethionine plus or racemic alpha-tocopherol acetate or a placebo. This trial found that neither selenium nor vitamin E supplementation, alone or in combination, produced any reduction in prostate cancer or cancer of any type.

A key problem to do with SELECT or any other antioxidant supplement intervention trials is that they are not part of any integrative approach to a medical problem.[405, 445] These trials are consistent with reductionist-type medicine.[483]

There are other problems with the SELECT study: it was expected that 75–100 prostate cancer deaths would occur, but there was only1 prostate cancer death in this trial. A major flaw of this study is also that racemic alpha-tocopherol led to decreasing gamma-tocopherol which has been found to increase the incidence of prostate cancer.[382]

The importance of nutrients like vitamin D, as well as individual's diets are clearly important but were not measured in this study. Supplements should be used to supplement a healthy diet and lifestyle, and not as substitutes.

Mega-dose supplements for bladder cancer

An RCT of 65 patients with transitional cell bladder cancer, were given intravesical Bacillus Calmette-Guérin (BCG) with or without percutaneous BCG administration.

They were then randomised to high-dose multiple supplements (40 000IU vitamin A, 100mg vitamin B6, 2000mg vitamin C, 400IU vitamin E and 900mg zinc) or the same supplements in the recommended daily allowance (RDA).[484]

Additional percutaneous BCG did not influence recurrence, but it was markedly reduced in the patients receiving mega-dose of supplements after 10 months. It is possible that vitamin D could also help reduce bladder cancer, as *in vitro* bladder experiments with human bladder cancer cell lines show that it inhibits proliferation and induces apoptosis.[485]

Herbal and dietary supplements during chemotherapy and radiotherapy

The role of nutritional and mineral supplements, particularly when used in conjunction with chemotherapy and radiation therapy, is an issue of considerable controversy.[486–491]

It is difficult to be conclusive about potential interactions between supplement use and chemotherapy plus radiotherapy, but based on clinical experience, their use appears to be safe and may help improve prognosis, but further clinical studies are needed.

A study of lung cancer patients with supplements — vitamin C, vitamin E and beta-carotene — did not show interference with the effectiveness of chemotherapy.[492] There was a better response and survival in those who received the supplement although the difference did not reach statistical significance.

Breast cancer patients were treated with 5-fluorouracil (5-FU) plus folic acid. It was possible to improve 5-FU effectiveness.[493] Survival in the group receiving 5-FU plus folic acid was 47% greater than the group receiving 5-FU alone.

Two prescription antioxidants, amifostine and dexrazoxane, have been used concurrently with chemotherapy and radiotherapy.[491]

According to 29 studies, amifostine reduces side-effects and increases response rates of chemotherapy and radiation therapy. In 21 studies, dexrazoxane has been shown to protect the heart from Adriamycin toxicity without interfering with anti-tumour effect by chelating iron that would otherwise form free radicals.[491]

Common nutrient deficiencies in cancer patients include folic acid, vitamin C, pyridoxine and other nutrients.[494] Chemotherapy and radiotherapy reduce serum levels of antioxidants, vitamins and minerals due to lipid peroxidation and fast produce higher levels of oxidative stress.[491–499]

Fifty human studies using either single or multiple nutrients in combination with chemotherapy and/or radiation treatment found that nutrients do not interfere with treatment.[500–502] Side-effects were decreased in 47 of these 50 studies, and the other 3 studies showed no differences.

Simone and others have analysed all evidence from 1965 to November 2003 concerning antioxidant and other nutrients used together with radiotherapy and/or chemotherapy.[492] Fifty clinical randomised or observational trials involving 8521 patients have been conducted using: beta-carotene; vitamin D_3; vitamin K_3; vitamins A, C, and E, selenium; cysteine; B vitamins; and glucothione, as single agents or in combination. Also included were 62 *in vitro* and 218 *in vivo* studies published in peer reviewed journals. The results of the human studies show that nutritional supplements do not interfere with chemotherapy or radiotherapy. The efficacy of the therapeutic modalities was enhanced, decreasing side-effects and protecting normal cells. In 15 of the 50 human studies, those who took supplements had increased survival.

The above findings are not too surprising, as from a theoretical perspective, many of the chemotherapy drugs are not cytotoxic because of oxidative mechanisms nor do hormonal and biological agents, anti-metabolites plus other drugs work in this way.[503]

Antioxidants and cisplatin

Cisplatin can be used effectively in the treatment of solid tumours, utilising free radical damage, but unfortunately it has a number of undesirable side-effects including neurotoxicity leading to deafness and peripheral neuropathy and nephrotoxicity.

The use of nutritional and herbal antioxidants with cisplatin in human and animal experiments reduces side-effects and increase efficacy of treatment in some studies.[504–508]

Foods and hormonal influence

The enormous diversity of foods available, theoretically, can influence tumour growth or influence hormonal treatments. Foods with high flavonoid content (e.g. vegetables, fruit, cocoa, red wine) and herbs such as St John's wort and St Mary's thistle may have theoretical positive effects.[509]

The role of soy in breast cancer patients who are hormone positive is conflicting, but it is likely to enhance the antagonism of oestrogen-binding agents such as Tamoxifen.[510]

Pharmokinetic interactions

Preliminary data exists indicating that P-glycoprotein can force a number of drugs out of cells.[510]

St. John's wort can influence P-glycoprotein, but the clinical data is limited. This herb can also influence metabolism of drugs by inducing enzymes.[510–512]

A similar influence on metabolism of drugs has been found for St Mary's thistle, but no clinically significant effects have been described.[513–516]

Integrative approach

If a patient is to use nutritional or herbal supplements then a clinician with expertise in these supplements should be involved during concurrent chemotherapy and radiotherapy, as it is not only about providing a supplement, but caring for the patient with an integrative approach.

Does lifestyle and diet influence recurrence?

A number of studies have shown that lifestyle and diet influence longevity, and hence, it would be reasonable to assume that they would also influence survival in cancer patients. Several studies have found that the Mediterranean lifestyle and diet helps to prevent cancer and illness in general, as well as a reduction in cancer and overall mortality.[517–519]

Major scientific associations strongly encourage people to consume a Mediterranean-style dietary pattern to reduce their risk of disease.[517, 518, 519] Studies show that a healthier diet and lifestyle can reduce the risk of mortality of cardiovascular disease and cancer.[520–522]

A number of recent studies have found that diet and lifestyle factors influence survival of cancer patients. A study was established to see whether a telephone counselling and mailed print material-based diet and exercise intervention was effective in reorientating functional decline in older, overweight cancer survivors.[523]

Long-term survivors of colorectal, breast, and prostate cancer found diet and exercise intervention reduced the rate of self-reported functional decline compared with no intervention.

Pre–treatment health behaviours which included smoking, diet and physical activity predict survival among patients with head and neck squamous cell carcinoma.[524]

A systematic review of the effect of diet on prostate cancer prevention and treatment found that dietary recommendations for patients diagnosed with prostate cancer was similar to those aiming to reduce the risk of prostate cancer.[525]

A multi–centred prospective study investigating the interaction between physical activity, diet and obesity to breast cancer survival has concluded that those who consume a healthy diet and are physically active may increase their years of survival after diagnosis.[526] They further stated that the combination of these 2 variables appears to attenuate the increased risk of cancer death observed among obese cancer survivors.

A report describing longitudinal changes in lifestyle behaviours and death status among colon cancer survivors and population-based controls, examined demographic and psychosocial correlates of healthy lifestyle changes following a colon cancer diagnosis.[527]

Colon cancer survivors reported significant increases in vegetable intake, physical activity and supplement use, and a non-statistically significant increase in fruit/fruit juice consumption. The pre-diagnosis of patients undergoing potentially curative colorectal cancer surgery influenced 5-year survival.

Another study investigated the association of dietary patterns with cancer recurrences and mortality of colon cancer survivors.[528] During a median follow-up of 5.3 years, a higher intake of a Western dietary pattern was associated with a higher risk of recurrence and mortality among patients with stage 3 colon cancer treated with surgery and adjuvant chemotherapy.

It is surprising that a meta-analysis of 59 trials published earlier found little evidence that diet is associated with survival or prognosis of cancer patients.[529] In an accompanying editorial examining the study it is suggested that errors in study design may have led to the wrong conclusions.[530]

Herbal medicines

Plant products have been used for centuries as medicine. In the developing world, plant remedies are the most common treatments.

Many oncology drugs are derived from plant products; for example, Taxol and Taxotere from the Western yew tree *(Taxus brevifolia)*.[531]

Although examples of traditional usage of herbal medicines are available, there have been limited, more organised clinical studies. In traditional Chinese medicine, multiple herbs are generally used and hence it is difficult to understand the role of individual herbs. In traditional use of these herbs, other factors are also likely to be important, such as positive support by practitioners and dietary changes.

There are many herbal medicines that have been investigated regarding their role against cancer. It is only possible to include some examples of these herbs in this chapter.

St Mary's thistle (SMT) and Silibilin (*Silybum marianum*)

This herb is most commonly known because of its hepato-protective effect, but there is increasing evidence about its effects on cancer. In animal studies, SMT has been found to inhibit chemically induced urinary bladder tumour growth and progression, possibly by inhibiting cell proliferation, and enhancing apoptosis.[532]

SMT has been shown to induce cell cycle arrest in different human prostate cancer cells.[533] Silibinin can suppress proliferation of other cancers *in vitro* including breast, ovary, colon, glioma and lung.[534] SMT has also been shown to influence prostate, lung and ovarian cancer growth in animal experiments.[535] There is an emerging role for SMT in providing protection from chemotherapy toxicity including protection from nephrotoxicity *in vivo* against cisplatin.[536, 537] Combining SMT with cisplatin *in vitro* and *in vivo* can potentiate anti-cancer activity.[538, 539]

Polysaccharide Krestin (PSK)

Polysaccharide Krestin (PSK) is isolated from a mushroom, *coriolus versicolor*, and is also mentioned in the chapter relating to CRC. PSK has been studied *in vitro*, in animal studies and also in controlled clinical human trials.[540, 541]

PSK has been used as adjunct therapy for colon cancer and found to be better than the control group.[542] When combined with radiotherapy for stage 3 non-small-cell lung cancer, it was possible to significantly improve survival.[543] PSK combined with chemotherapy in breast cancer with vascular invasion improved survival compared to chemotherapy alone.[544] When used as adjuvant treatment for gastric cancer with chemotherapy it improved survival compared to chemotherapy alone.[545]

Essiac

Essiac is usually consumed as a herbal tea and consists of 4 herbs (burdock root, slippery elm, sheep sorrel, and Indian or Turkish rhubarb root). Two systematic reviews have not found a single published clinical trial.[546, 547]

Black cohosh (*Cimicifuga racemosa*)

Extracts of black cohosh have been shown to inhibit the growth of breast cancer cells.[548] Other laboratory studies have confirmed this finding.[549, 550] A systematic review of the safety of black cohosh in breast cancer patients has found no risk for liver disease.[551]

Mistletoe (*Viscum album*)

Mistletoe is the most widely used cancer drug in Germany where it was introduced by Rudolph Steiner, founder of anthroposophy.[552] Mistletoe preparations contain several biologically active substances and have immunomodulating cytotoxic and antiviral effects.[553] Three independent systematic reviews of RCTs of mistletoe did not demonstrate benefits.[553, 554, 555] As is often the case in systematic reviews, a number of the studies with a positive response to mistletoe were excluded.

A more recent and comprehensive Cochrane review found that the majority of the included trials reported benefits for patients treated with mistletoe extracts in1 or more outcome measures.[553]

However, there were methodological drawbacks that raised doubts about the findings. Safety data showed that mistletoe extracts are generally safe. It is likely that mistletoe extracts may be more useful in those cancers that are associated with poor immunity, as an important action is to improve immunity.[553] Immuno-stimulation is likely to improve immunity in cancer patients with poor immunity whereas those patients with cancer who had normal immunity did not appear to benefit from immuno-stimulation.[556]

Mistletoe lectins are cytotoxic to breast cancer cells and, therefore, this may be another therapeutic mechanism.[557] Further research with well-designed clinical trials is necessary to obtain more conclusive results.

Korean ginseng (*Panax ginseng*)

Ginseng has anti-tumour, anti-proliferative, anti-metastatic and apoptosis-inducing actions which have been demonstrated *in vitro* and animal studies.[558, 559] Extracts of ginseng have been shown to be cytotoxic to the following cancers: hepatocellular, prostate and ovarian.[560–562]

In animal experiments, ginseng extracts can influence melanoma growth and metastases which is thought to be due to immune stimulation plus anti-angiogenesis.[563, 564] Ginseng can prevent lung, hepatoma and head and neck cancers demonstrated in human studies reducing the relative risk by 40–50%.[565, 566]

Extracts of ginseng can sensitise cancer cells by chemotherapeutic agents *in vitro* such as multi-drug resistant breast cancer cells.[559, 567, 568, 569]

Ginseng extracts in cancer have been shown to reduce toxicity of chemotherapy use for ovarian cancer.[559] It can reduce nausea and vomiting due to chemotherapy or radiotherapy plus general anaesthetics.[570]

Chlorella (*Chlorella pyrenoidosa*) and Spirulina (*Spirulina platensis*)

Chlorella and Spirulina are blue-green algae. They are high in all of the essential amino acids (around 60%), beta-carotene and other vitamins. Chlorophyll and nucleic acids, anti-cancer and immuno-stimulatory activity have been identified.[571, 572, 573] Chlorella has been shown to improve survival in a study of glioblastoma patients.[574]

Modified citrus pectin (MCP)

Pectin is a soluble complex polysaccharide (carbohydrate) formed as part of the fibrous structure of many plants especially citrus fruits. MCP is a chemically modified form of pectin. *In vitro* experiments have shown that MCP is able to inhibit adhesion of cancer cells.[575] In animal experiments, oral MCP can inhibit the growth and metastases of rat prostate cells, human breast cancer and melanoma cells.[576–579]

Further studies with human breast and colon cancer cells plus multiple myeloma and haemangiosarcoma have found that MCP inhibits tumour growth, angiogenesis and metastases.[580] MCP can significantly increase prostatic specific antigen doubling time in patients with recurrent prostate cancer.[581] MCP also increases the sensitivity of cancer cells to various chemotherapeutic agents such as cisplatin, etoposide, botezomib, dexamethasone and doxirubicin. [560] It has been demonstrated that MCP can reverse multiple myelomas and cell resistance to Bortezomib and enhance their response to apoptosis induced by Dexamethasone.[582] In another study MCP dramatically increased sensitivity of haemangiosarcoma to Doxorubicin.[583]

Garlic *(Allium sativum)*/ Allium species

Garlic has long been known to have anti-cancer properties due to its ability to disrupt the function of cancer causing agents.[584, 585] Several cancers are less likely to occur with garlic consumption including stomach, colon, breast, cervix and prostate.[586, 587]

A systematic review of 20 epidemiological studies to do with allium vegetables found that 19 of the studies showed protection against cancer especially of the gastrointestinal tract.[588, 589]

A garlic extract when given to patients with colorectal adenomas, suppressed both the size and number of adenomas after a year of use compared to the control group where there was an increase in adenomas.[590]

Garlic supplementation improves immunity in cancer patients.[591, 592]

Ginger (*Zingiber officinale*)

Ginger has been found to be very useful in the control of nausea and vomiting associated with chemotherapy.[593, 594] Ginger was able to treat nausea and vomiting from Cyclophosphamide and was as effective as Metoclopramide in a double-blind cross-over study.[595] Nausea and vomiting due to cisplatin was also treated effectively with ginger.[592]

Liquorice (*Glycyrrhiza glabra*)

Liquorice has been shown *in vitro* and animal studies to reduce recurrence of cancer.[596, 597] Licorice can induce apoptosis and can enhance the effect of Paclitaxel and Vinblastine.[598] Liquorice can inhibit prostate and breast cancer cell lines.[599] Liquorice extract *in vitro* and in most experiments reduces tumour COX-2 activity, tumour growth and metastases *in vitro*.[600, 601]

Modulators of immunity

Numerous herbs have been shown to improve immunity and examples include olive leaf *(Olea europea L)*, astragalus *(Astragalus membranaceus)*, Echinacea *(Echinacea purpurea)* and various mushroom extracts, plus others.[602, 603, 604]

Chinese herbal medicines

There are numerous Chinese herbs that have potential for the use in the treatment of cancer. A number of controlled clinical studies have reported responses to numerous cancers when treated by various herbal therapies. Some of the larger studies are seen in Table 9.3.

A Cochrane review of medicinal herbs for oesophageal cancer was performed to assess the benefit of Chinese herbal medicines by comparing chemotherapy or radiotherapy with or without concurrent medicines.[605] This review found that there were no RCTs in the field and, hence, they were not able to make

Table 9.3 Cancer treatments and responses

Cancer	Treatment	Response	Author
Nasopharyngeal	Destagnation compared to radiotherapy	Destagnation better	Xu[606]
Lung	Various herbs	Better than chemotherapy	Liu[607]
Gastric	Shenqui Fuzhing	Better than chemotherapy	Zhou[608]
Hepatic	Sho Saiao-to	Better than chemotherapy	Oka[609]

any recommendations. Another Cochrane review investigated the role of Chinese medicinal herbs in the treatment of side-effects of chemotherapy in breast cancer patients.[610] Seven randomised studies were identified involving 542 patients using various herbs. The results suggested that Chinese herbal medicine improved marrow suppression, the immune system and may improve quality of life. There was no evidence of toxicity from Chinese herbal medicine. However, there were concerns about the quality of trials and that they were unable to draw any conclusions.

The role of Chinese medical herbs for chemotherapy side-effects in colorectal cancer patients have also been the subject of a Cochrane review.[602]

Four relevant studies which included 442 patients were found to have adequate data. It was concluded that decoctions of Huang Qi compounds provided some benefit compared to patients that were treated with chemotherapy alone. Patients receiving the Huang Qi decoctions were less likely to experience nausea and vomiting, plus white cell counts increased and there is also some evidence of immune stimulation. No toxicity was found from the Huang Qi decoctions. The reviewers suggest further large scale trials with Huang Qi decoctions and the prevention of chemotherapy-related side-effects.[602]

Prostate cancer formula (PC–SPES)

A prostate cancer herbal formula is based on a traditional Chinese medicine formula, PC-SPES, which contained *Chrysthanthemum morifolium*, *Ganodermia lucidium*, *Glycyrrhiza glabra*, *Isatio indigeotica*, *Panax pseudoginseng*, *Robdosia rubescens*, *Scutellaria baicalensis* and *Serenoa repens*.

Several studies found that PC-SPES could lower PSA, cause regression of prostate cancer *in vitro*, as well as in humans even when androgen suppression therapies no longer worked.[611, 612, 613] Unfortunately this formula had to be withdrawn because of contamination with warfarin, diethylstilboestrol and indomethacin plus variable other substances.[614]

A new formula, initially called Prostasol and now called Quercetin Plus, has become available with a similar composition of herbs, and no clinical trial has been published so far.

Naltrexone

Naltrexone is a drug for treating addiction by blocking opioid receptors in the brain. Almost all immune cells have receptors for the opioids, endorphins and enkefalins. Naltrexone can inhibit secretion of endorphins and enkefalins. A study has shown that the use of Naltrexone to blockade the brain opioid system which plays a physiological immunosuppressive role, may improve anti-cancer effects of IL-2 in humans.[615]

Research has shown that low dose Naltrexone (LDN) can have a therapeutic effect on lymphoma, pancreatic cancer and autoimmune disorders.[616, 617]

In vitro experiments have demonstrated that Naltrexone can inhibit growth of the following cancer cells: pancreatic; colon; head and neck; and ovarian.[618–621]

Similar findings have been found with animal experiments with the following cancers: pancreatic; colon; head and neck; and neuroblastoma. Bilhari first used LDN to treat cancer and has treated 450 patients with cancer, most of whom had failed standard treatment.[622] He noted that at least 86 of these patients had at least 75% reduction of tumour bulk, and at least 125 stabilised and were moving towards remission.

Berkson and others have reported 2 patients who have responded to LDN — a patient with metastatic pancreas cancer alive 4 years later, and also another patient with B-cell lymphoma who had reversal of enlarged lymph nodes and was well a year later.[616, 617] Until now, there has not been a report of a controlled clinical trial with LDN in the treatment of cancer.

Physical therapies

Acupuncture

There is no scientific evidence that acupuncture is effective in the treatment of cancer itself. Beta-endorphins and neuropeptides are increased with acupuncture, which increases interleukin-2 (IL-2) levels and natural killer cell activity. It is possible that these changes could have a positive influence on prognosis of some cancers.[623]

Based on systematic reviews, acupuncture and acupressure reduce chemotherapy nausea-induced symptoms.[624, 625, 626]

The role of acupuncture for control of cancer pain remains controversial. A systematic review of 6 clinical trials did not show an advantage over 'sham' acupuncture.[627]

A recent systematic review of RCTs of acupuncture, placebo acupuncture and no acupuncture was unable to conclude about the role of acupuncture and whether pain was reduced because of the treatment ritual. There is now evidence that 'sham' acupuncture has a significant placebo effect.[628] The role of acupuncture in the treatment of hot flushes in breast cancer patients is controversial.[629, 630] It is possible that acupuncture may be useful in reducing flushing symptoms in prostate cancer patients on hormone therapy.[631]

Acupuncture was useful in the treatment of cancer-related fatigue after chemotherapy in a preliminary study.[632] A study has also found that it can help with xerostomia resulting from radiotherapy.[633]

Palliative care

The main role of palliative care is to provide palliation for the terminally ill and their families.[634, 635, 636]

Hypnosis may improve symptoms in the terminally ill cancer patient, especially in relieving pain.[637] Of the 27 publications to do with hypnotherapy in palliative care of cancer patients, only 1 was an RCT, and hence, further research is required. Acupuncture, as discussed previously, and reiki can also be helpful in palliative care of cancer patients. One RCT to do with the use of reiki for cancer pain suggested that it improved pain.[638]

Listening to patients

There is increasing evidence that just listening to patients with untreatable diseases can help relieve their distress.[639] Psychological stress is likely to be an important factor leading to disease. Listening to patients is likely to improve their health as a result of reducing psychological stress.[640]

Cancer-related anxiety

Massage therapy and aromatherapy was found to benefit cancer patients with anxiety in 4 out of 8 RCTs.[640]

Music therapy

A number of studies have demonstrated that music benefits palliative cancer care.[641] Music therapy can reduce anxiety and pain in a number of situations in palliative care cancer patients.[642]

Fatigue

Fatigue is common in terminally ill patients and has high distress impact.[636]

Acupuncture, massage, aromatherapy, foot soak and reflexology can alleviate fatigue in palliative care of cancer patients.[642, 643, 644]

Nausea and vomiting

Nausea and vomiting have a strong influence in reducing quality of life.[636] Acupuncture and acupressure are useful treatments.[645]

Ginger and Huang Qi decoctions can help with chemotherapy, nausea and vomiting.[646–649]

Mind–body medicine

Varying relaxation techniques can help with the management of anxiety, nausea and vomiting.[650–653]

Nutrition and supplementation

A common cause of reduced quality of life in palliative care patients is malnutrition and cachexia.[636]

Nutritional support in patients improves quality of life.[654] L-carnitine can treat fatigue which is a common problem in palliative care patients, especially in those that have had chemotherapy.[655] Trace elements and vitamins that support nutrition are safe and may be associated with reduction in mortality in critically ill patients.[656]

Omega-3 fish oil supplementation can modulate immunity and prolong survival of malnourished patients with generalised malignancy.[657] Another more recent study did not support the latter finding, but called for further research to clarify the potential benefits of fish oil supplementation.[658]

Safety of integrative medicine in cancer patients

There is concern about the interaction of nutritional and herbal supplements with drugs, and hence the importance of being aware of what drugs and supplements the patient is taking.

Drug-to-drug interactions are far more likely to be a problem, but it is possible to have interactions with nutritional and herbal supplements. Acupuncture generally has a very good safety record with the most frequent complications being only minor, such as bleeding and/or bruising and minor pain.[659]

Conclusion

The management of the patient diagnosed with cancer is conducive to an integrative management approach, whether it be to manage the cancer-related symptoms and/or those new symptoms that ensue due to the treatments that are employed.

The best recommendations for the patient are those that are grounded in scientific evidence, based on the individual's family situation, ethnic origins, gender, previous health and nutritional habits as well as physical activity regimens. Moreover, any integrative management strategy would also be best based on past medical history that would incorporate his or her social history.

In so doing, by making recommendations for specific therapeutic interventions (disease related and/or directed or totally supported) to the patient diagnosed with a malignancy, the clinician thus establishes a complete patient profile — this is the role of the integrative clinician. Table 9.4 summarises the current evidence for CAM treatments.

Table 9.4 Levels of evidence for lifestyle and complementary medicines/therapies in the management of cancer

Modality	Level I	Level II	Level IIIa	Level IIIb	Level IIIc	Level IV	Level V
Life risks							
Genetic (family history and/or age)			x				
Behavioural and social factors			x				
Inflammation and infection			x				
Western diet			x				
Obesity			x				
Smoking			x				
Lack of exercise			x				
Lack of sunlight			x				
Environmental factors			x				
Occupational exposure			x				
Poor immunity			x				
Lifestyle management reduced risk							
Weight management / BMI ↓			x				
Energy intake ↓			x				
Mind–body medicine							
Mindfulness-based stress reduction		x					
Cognitive behavioural therapy		x					
Hypnosis		x					
Nutrition							
• ↓Dietary fat (↓risk)				x			
• ↓Processed meat consumption (↓ risk)				x			
• ↑ Soy and phytoestorgens (↓ risk)				x			
Diets							
↑ Mediterranean diet (↓ risk)				x			
↑ Vegetarian diet (↓ risk)				x			
Alcohol reduction (↓ risk)				x			

Continued

Table 9.4 Levels of evidence for lifestyle and complementary medicines/therapies in the management of cancer—cont'd

Modality	Level I	Level II	Level IIIa	Level IIIb	Level IIIc	Level IV	Level V
Physical activity							
Exercise (prudent activity)				x			
Reiki and/or therapeutic touch				x			
Tai chi				x			
Qigong				x			
Nutritional supplements							
Multivitamins and/or minerals				x			
Folate					x		
Selenium and/or vitamin E					x		
Vitamin C					x		
Vitamin D					x		
Herbal medicines and/or supplements							
Black cohosh					x		
Korean ginseng					x		
Green tea, black teas, polyphenolics					x		
Garlic and/or allium					x		
Curcumin					x		
Mushrooms					x		
Soy					x		
Citrus fruits					x		
Grapefruit					x		
Pomegranate and/or ellagic acid					x		
St Mary's Thistle					x		
Polysaccharide Kristin					x		
Essiac					x		
Mistletoe					x		
Chlorella and/or spirulina					x		
Modified citrus pectin					x		
Ginger			x				
Licorice					x		
Traditional Chinese medicines	x						
PC–SPES			x				
Physical therapies							
Acupuncture			x				
Massage therapy				x			
Music therapy					x		
Biofeedback					x		
Aromatherapy					x		

Level I — from a systematic review of all relevant randomised controlled trials, meta–analyses.
Level II — from at least 1 properly designed randomised controlled clinical trial.
Level IIIa — from well-designed pseudo-randomised controlled trials (alternate allocation or some other method).
Level IIIb — from comparative studies (including systematic reviews of such studies) with concurrent controls and allocation not randomised, cohort studies, case-control studies, or interrupted time series with a parallel control group.
Level IIIc — from comparative studies with historical control, 2 or more single-arm studies or interrupted time series without a parallel control group.
Level IV — opinions of respected authorities based on clinical experience, descriptive studies or reports of expert committees.
Level V — represents minimal evidence that represents testimonials.

Clinical tips handout for patients — cancer

1 Lifestyle advice

Sleep

- Ensure 7–8 hours sleep and a regular sleep pattern. Avoid shift work at night as it can be a risk factor for cancer. (See Chapter 22 for more advice.)

Sunshine

- Amount of exposure varies with local climate.
- At least 15 minutes of sunshine needed daily for vitamin D and melatonin production — especially before 10 a.m. and after 3 p.m. when sun exposure is safest during summer. Much more exposure required in winter when supplementation needs to be considered.
- Ensure gradual, adequate skin exposure to sun; avoid sunscreen and excess clothing to maximise levels of vitamin D.
- More time in the sun is required for dark skinned people and people with vitamin D deficiency.
- Direct exposure to about 10% of the body (hands, arms, face), without sunscreen and not through glass.
- Vitamin D is obtained in the diet from fatty fish, eggs, outdoor mushrooms, liver and fortified foods (some milks and margarines), however diet alone is not a sufficient source of vitamin D.

2 Physical activity/exercise

- Exercise is important for cancer prevention and during treatment (if in treatment discuss appropriate exercise regimens with your doctor).
- Exercise for 30–60 minutes daily. If exercise is not regular, commence with 5 minutes daily and slowly build up to at least 30 minutes. Outdoor exercise, in nature, fresh air (avoid polluted air) and sunshine is ideal.
- Brisk walking, light jogging, cycling, swimming, stretching, and weight-bearing exercises are all good forms of physical activity/exercise.
- Tai chi, qigong and yoga may be particularly helpful.

3 Mind–body medicine (most helpful)

- Stress management program — for example, 6 x 40 minute sessions for patients to understand the nature of their symptoms, the symptoms' relationship to stress, and the practice of regular relaxation exercises.
- Regular meditation practice at least 10–20 minutes daily, especially transcendental, mindfulness meditation and autogenic training.
- Anger management may be of help.
- Psychological therapy may help to deal with stressors.

Breathing

- Be aware of breathing from time to time. Notice if tendency to hold breath or over-breathe.
- Snoring and irregular breathing during sleep needs to be reported, treated and further investigated.
- Avoid exposure to polluted air as much as possible.

Rest and stress management

Recurrent stress may cause a return of symptoms. Relaxation is important for a full and lasting recovery.

- Reduce workload and resolve conflicts. Contact family, friends, church or social groups for support. Full-time work can increase breast cancer risk whereas part-time work does not.
- Listening to relaxation music helps.
- Relaxation massage therapy helps.
- Hypnotherapy, biofeedback, cognitive behavioural therapy, and psychotherapy may be of help.

Fun

- It is important to have fun in life.
- Joy can be found even in the simplest of tasks.
- Treat yourself by watching funny movies/videos, comedy, hobbies, dancing, playing with pets and children.
- Creative tasks, such as knitting, can help with distressing thoughts.

Focus on wellness, not just the disease.

4 Environment

- Avoid smoking, environmental pollutants, chemicals — at work and in the home, especially from plastic food containers.
- Don't microwave with plastic cling wrap.
- Avoid chemicals (phthalates) in cosmetics (e.g. in lipstick and hair spray) are of concern.
- Some sunscreens may also increase cancer risk.

5 Dietary changes

- Do not rush your meals; relax before meals; chew your food thoroughly before swallowing as this aids digestion; have regular relaxed eating patterns.
- Aim to lose weight if you or your medical advisor believe you are overweight. Eating slowly can help with weight loss.
- Eat more fruit (>2 daily) and vegetables (>5 daily) — a variety of colours and those in season.
- A vegetarian diet high in legumes (e.g. soy), fish (e.g. sardines) vegetables, garlic, nuts and fruit is particularly helpful (Mediterranean diet).
- Increase fibre; for example, add psyllium fibre (husks) to your cereal.
- Fresh garlic and other members of the onion family offer protection.
- The Cruciferous or brassica group of vegetables, which include broccoli, cabbage, brussels sprouts, cauliflower and bok choy, are protective.
- Eat more nuts, seeds, especially flax seeds (best if ground just before use; refrigerate if ground), beans, sprouts (e.g. alfalfa, mung, bean, lentil), soy (best if fermented e.g. miso, soy sauce, natto and tempah).
- Eat more fish (mackerel, sardines, salmon, cod, tuna), especially deep sea fish.
- Reduce red meat intake (preferably use red lean meat e.g. lamb, kangaroo) — no more than twice weekly and not well done — and white meat (e.g. free range organic chicken fillets).
- Use cold pressed olive oil (4 teaspoons daily) and avocado.
- Use only dark Chocolate (25–50g daily) unless not tolerated.
- Eat a variety of wholegrains/cereals (best if not toasted). Cooked traditional rolled oats for breakfast are particularly helpful, as is rice (brown, basmati, Mahatma, Dongara), buckwheat flour, wholegrain organic breads (rye bread, Essene, spelt, kamut) — when toasting make hot and crisp, not brown, to avoid acrylamide — brown pasta, couscous, millet, amaranth, etc.
- Use low-fat dairy products, such as low-fat yoghurt, unless there is a dairy intolerance. Soy (organic) milk is an alternative.
- Drink more water (1–2 litres a day) and teas, especially green tea, chamomile, peppermint and black teas (best if organic).
- Avoid sea salt.
- Avoid hydrogenated, saturated fats and trans-fatty acids such as butter, margarines, crispy potato chips, dairy fat (e.g. yellow cheeses and cream), fat in meat and poultry, commercial biscuits, most cakes, pastries and takeaway foods, fast foods, sugar such as in soft drinks, lollies and processed foods (e.g. white bread, white pasta, pastries).
- Avoid chemical additives — preservatives, colourings and flavourings.
- Minimise alcohol intake — limit to no more than 1–2 glasses daily; red wine may be best.
- Avoid artificial sweeteners — replace with honey (e.g. manuka, yellow box and stringy bark have lowest GI).

6 Physical therapies

- Acupuncture may help with pain associated with cancer and nausea from chemotherapy.

7 Supplements

Fish oils

- Indication: may reduce inflammation. Can reduce chemotherapy toxicity and normalise immunity.
- Dosage: 4–10g of 1000mg capsules daily as tolerated (e.g. EPA 180/DHA 120mg / 1000mg capsule).
- Results: 4–7 days.
- Side-effects: often well tolerated especially if taken with meals. Very mild and rare side-effects; for example, gastrointestinal upset; allergic reactions (e.g. rash, breathing problems if allergic to seafood); blood thinning effects in very high doses > 10g daily (may need to stop fish oil supplements 2 weeks prior to surgery).
- Contraindications: sensitivity reaction to seafood; drug interactions; caution when taking high doses of fish oils >4g per day together with warfarin (your doctor will check your INR test).

Vitamins and minerals

Vitamins B6, B12, Folate (best given together as a multivitamin + mineral)

- Indication: can reduce homocysteine.
- Dosage: Vitamin B6: best if dosage is no more than 50mg daily.
  Vitamin B12: 600mcg daily.
  Folate: 0.5–1mg daily.
- Result: 1 month.

- Side-effects: no toxicity with this group (within dosage); vitamin B6 toxicity with doses above the recommended dose.
- Contraindications: generally safe when used in combination. If anaemia present, cause must be found.

Vitamin D3 (Cholecalciferol)

- Indication: low levels are a risk factor for any cancer.
- Dosage: safe sunshine exposure of skin is the safest source of vitamin D. Vitamin D (cholecalciferol 1000 international units). Doctors should check blood levels and suggest supplementation if levels are low. Adults: 400–1000IU daily, for maintenance; 3000–5000IU daily for 1 month then 1000IU daily if vitamin D level below normal; ensure repeat blood measurement. Children at risk: 200–400IU daily under medical supervision.
  Pregnant and lactating women at risk: under medical supervision.
- Results: 6–9–12 months.
- Side-effects: very high doses can cause vitamin D toxicity; raised calcium levels in the blood. Can increase aluminium and magnesium absorption; prolonged heparin therapy can increase resorption and reduce formation of bone and hence more vitamin D and calcium required.
- Contraindications: Thiazide and diuretics decrease urinary calcium, hence hypercalcaemia possible with vitamin D supplementation.

Vitamin C

- Indication: when combined with natural Vitamin E and selenium reduces blood stickiness. Useful also as an anti bacterial.
- Dosage: 500–1000mg daily.
- Results: can reduce blood stickiness in 1 week.
- Side-effects: with high doses can cause nausea, heartburn, abdominal cramps and diarrhoea.
- Contraindications: can increase iron absorption. Use with caution if glucose-6-phosphate dehydrogenase deficiency.

Natural vitamin E

- Indication: may reduce blood stickiness and immunity when combined with vitamin C and selenium. Can help prevent venous thromboembolism.
- Dosage: 400–800IU daily.
- Results: can reduce blood stickiness in 1 week.
- Side-effects: doses below 1500IU daily are very unlikely to result in haemorrhage, rarely cause diarrhoea, flatulence, nausea, heart palpitations.
- Contraindications: use with caution if bleeding disorder or if taking with blood thinning medication. If using very high dose, reduce dose before surgery.

Selenium

- Indication: selenium helps to prevent tissue damage caused by free radicals. Some studies suggest that selenium may be inversely associated with prostate cancer and colorectal cancer.
  Dosage: less than 200mcg daily given together with vitamin E and vitamin C.
- Result: 1 month.
- Side-effects: no risk at this dose; toxicity in high doses.
- Contraindications: safe even during pregnancy at this dose.

Chromium Picolinate

- Indication: can reduce blood glucose.
- Dosage: 50–200mcg/day.
- Results: unknown.
- Side-effects: doses less than 1000mcg are safe; can reduce hypoglycaemic drug requirement. Very high doses linked to kidney and liver disease.
- Contradictions: kidney and liver disease, high serum levels.

Coenzyme Q_{10} (CoQ_{10})

- Indication: may protect from chemotherapy toxicity.
- Dosage: adults: 100–200mg in divided doses, 2–3 times per day.
- Results: 7–14 days.
- Side-effects: generally well tolerated. May cause gastrointestinal side-effects such as nausea, vomiting, diarrhoea.
- Contraindications: avoid in pregnant and lactating women and if allergic.

L-Carnitine

- Indication: can improve function of heart muscle and could help with heart failure. Assist in maintaining energy.
- Dosage: 2–4g/day.
- Result: unknown.
- Side-effects: rare, but can cause nausea, vomiting, abdominal pain, heartburn and diarrhoea.
- Contraindications: pregnancy — insufficient evidence. Can reduce effectiveness of thyroid hormone replacement.

Herbal medicines

Garlic (*Allium sativum*)

- Indication: may prevent artery occlusion, a possible mechanism may be improvement of blood stickiness plus improvement of cholesterol levels.
- Dosage 600–900mg/day (3.6–5.4mg of allicin).
- Results: 4–7 days.
- Side-effects: breath and body odour; mouth, stomach and gastrointestinal burning or irritation, heartburn, flatulence, nausea, vomiting and diarrhoea. May increase risk of bleeding as garlic can affect platelet function. Some people are allergic to garlic (by ingestion or even topically) and may cause asthma, runny nose, skin irritation and in rare cases severe allergic reactions.
- Contraindications: avoid if allergic to garlic; beware if taking any blood thinning medication such as warfarin; avoid at least 2 weeks prior to any surgery to minimise risk of bleeding; avoid high doses in pregnancy and lactation.

Probiotics

- Indications: to enhance Gut Associated Lymphoid Tissue (GALT), thereby providing balance between Th1 and Th2 cytokines in order to prevent and treat infectious diseases. Can assist in preventing radiation therapy induced diarrhoea.
- Dosage: depending upon condition, different probiotics may be required. Generalised treatment dose before breakfast (multi-strain formula is best):
  - *Lactobacillus rhamnosus* 12 billion CFU
  - *Lactobacillus acidophilus* 4 billion CFU
  - *Lactobacillus casei* 2 billion CFU
  - *Bifidobacterium bifidum* 1 billion CFU
  - *Bifidobacterium longum* 1 billion CFU.
- Results: from a few days to a few weeks depending on condition.
- Side-effects: gastrointestinal disturbance if wrong probiotics.
- Contraindications: true cow's milk allergy if contained in product.

Prebiotics and/or fibre Oligofructose and inulin to increase bifidobacteria in the distal part of the gastrointestinal tract

- Indications: prebiotics promote the growth and activity of specific strains of bacteria (e.g. bifidobacetrium) in the gut. Oligofructose is used for constipation, traveller's diarrhoea, increasing faecal mass. Inulin is used for constipation.
- Dosage: 20g twice daily mixed with water before meals.
- Results: 15–20 days.
- Side-effects: often well tolerated. Very mild and rare side-effects; transient abdominal discomfort (e.g. bloating; flatulence).
- Contraindications: severely ill and/or immunocompromised patients. Allergies to any of the food sources from which inulin and Oligofructose are derived.

  Inulin is derived from wheat, onions, bananas, leaks, artichokes, asparagus, and hot water extraction from chicory root.

  Oligofructose are plant sugars from a wide variety of fruits, vegetables, and cereals.

References

1 Shay JW, Zou Y, Hiyama E. Telomerase and cancer. Hum Mol Genet 2001;10:677–85.
2 Sali A (Editorial). Cancer treatment is dependant on histological classification. Int Clin Nutr Rev 1989;9:113–15.
3 Tisdale MJ. Catabolism of skeletal muscle proteins and its reversal in cancer cachexia. In: Mason JB, Nitenberg G. Basel, Karger AG, 2000.
4 Australian Institute of Health and Welfare (AIHW). Online. Available: http://www.aihw.gov.au/publications/index.cfm/title/10585 (accessed June 2008)
5 Pastides H. The descriptive epidemiology of cancer. In: Nasca PC, Pastides H. Fundamentals of Cancer Epidemiology. Jones and Bartlett Publishers, Boston, 2008.
6 Pumiglia KM, McSharry J, Higgins PJ. Biology of normal cells. Chapter 3 and 4. In: Nasca PC, Pastides H. Fundamentals of Cancer Epidemiology. Jones and Bartlett Publishers, Boston, 2008.
7 Zheng W, Long Jirong. Epidemiological studies of genetic factors for cancer. Chapter 7. In: Nasca PC, Pastides H. Fundamentals of Cancer Epidemiology. Jones and Bartlett Publishers, Boston, 2008.
8 Hassed C. The essence of health: the seven pillars of wellbeing. Ebury Press, Random House, North Sydney NSW, 2008.
9 Spiegel D, Giese-Davis J. Depression and cancer: mechanisms in disease progression. Biol Psychiat 2003;54:269–82.
10 Brown KW, Levy R, Rosenberger Z, et. al. Psychological distress in cancer survival: a follow-up 10 years after diagnosis. Psychosom Med 2003;65: 636–43.
11 Penninx BW, Guralnik JM, Pahor M, et. al. Chronically depressed mood and cancer risk in older persons. J Natl Cancer Inst 1998;90:1888–93.
12 Serraino D, Pezzotti P, Fratino L, et. al. Chronically depressed mood and cancer risk in older persons. J Natl Cancer Inst 1999;91:1080–81.
13 Oerlemans M, van den Akker M, Schuurman AG, et. al. A meta-analysis on depression and subsequent cancer risk. Clin Pract Epidemiol Ment Health 2007;3:29–35.
14 Selye Hans. Stress in Health and Disease. Butterworths, Boston, 1976.

15 Sali A. Psychoneuroimmunology: fact or fiction? Aust Fam Am Physician 1997;11:1291–99.
16 Nemeroff CB. Psychoneuroimmunology. Psych Clin North America 1998;21:259–506.
17 Vitetta L, Sali A. Mind Body Medicine: the key to health and longevity. In: De Luca BD. Mind Body and Relaxation Research Focus. Nova Press Scientific Publications. ISBN-10: 1600218199 ISBN-13: 978-1600218194.
18 Pollak M. Insulin and insulin-like growth factors signalling in neoplasia. Nat Rev Can 2008;8:915–28.
19 Wolpin BM, Michaud DS, Giovannucci EL,et. al. Circulating insulin-like growth factor axis and the risk of pancreatic cancer in four prospective cohorts. Br J Cancer 2007;97:98–104.
20 Colao A, Pivonello R, Auriemma RS, et. al. The association of fasting insulin concentrations and colonic neoplasms in acromegaly: a colonoscopy-based study in 210 patients. J Clin Endocrinol Metab 2007;92:3854–60.
21 Whiteside TL, Herberman RB. The role of natural killer cells in immune surveillance of cancer. Curr Opin Immunol 1995;7:704–10.
22 Kiecolt-Glaser JK, Stephens R, Lipetz P, et. al. Distress and DNA repair in human lymphocytes. J Behav Med 1985;8:311–20.
23 Irie M, Asami S, Nagata S, et. al. Relationships between perceived workload, stress and oxidative DNA damage. Int Arch Occup Environ Health 2001;74:153–57.
24 Irie M, Asami S, Nagata S, et. al. Psychological factors as a potential trigger of oxidative DNA damage in human leukocytes. Jpn J Cancer Res 2001;92:367–76.
25 Irie M, Asami S, Nagata S, et. al. Psychological mediation of a type of oxidative DNA damage, 8-hydroxydeoxyguanosine, in peripheral blood leukocytes of non-smoking and non-drinking workers. Psychother Psychosom 2002;71:90–96.
26 Tomei ID, Kiecolt-Glaser JK, Kennedy S. Psychological stress and phorbol ester inhibition of radiation-induced apoptosis in human peripheral blood leukocytes. Psychi Res 1990;5:59–71.
27 Pero RW, Roush GC, Markowitz MM, et. al. Oxidative stress, DNA repair and cancer susceptibility. Cancer Detect Prev 1990;14:555–61.
28 Maestroni GJ, Conti A, Pierpaoli W. Role of the pineal gland in immunity. J Neuroimmunol 1986;13:19–30.
29 Pierpaoli W. Neuroimmunomodulation of ageing. A program in the pineal gland. Ann NY Acad Sci 1998;840:491–97.
30 Panzer A, Viljoen M. The validity of melatonin as an oncostatic agent. J Pineal Res 1997;22:184–202.
31 Grimble RF. Inflammatory status and insulin resistance. Curr Opin Clin Nutr Metab Care 2002;5:551–59.
32 Jee SH, Kim HJ, Lee J. Obesity, insulin resistance and cancer risk. Yonsei Med J 2005;46:449–55.
33 Heikkilä K, Ebrahim S, Lawlor DA. A systematic review of the association between circulating concentrations of C reactive protein in cancer. J Epidemiol Community Health 2007;61:824–33.
34 Groblewska M, Mroczko B, Wereszczyńska-Siemiatkowska U, et. al. Serum interleukin-6 (IL-6) and C-reactive protein (CRP) levels in colorectal adenoma and cancer patients. Clin Chem Lab Med 2008;46:1423–8.
35 Herschman HR. Prostaglandin synthase 2. Biochim Biophys Acta 1996;1299:124–40.
36 Elwood PC, Gallagher AM, Duthie GG, et. al. Aspirin, salicylates, and cancer. Lancet 2009;373:1301–09.
37 Howe LR, Dannenberg AJ. A role for cyclooxygenase-2 inhibitors in the prevention and treatment of cancer. Semin Oncol 2002;29:111–9.
38 Harris RE, Beebe-Donk J, Alshafie GA. Reduction in the risk of human breast cancer by selective cyclooxygenase-2 (COX-2) inhibitors. BMC Cancer 2006;6:27.
39 Bresalier RS, Sandler RS, Quan H, et. al. Adenomatous Polyp Prevention of Vioxx (APPROVe) Trial Investigators. Cardiovascular events associated with Rofecoxib in a colorectal adenoma chemoprevention trial. N Engl J Med 2005;35:1092–1102.
40 Dubois RN. New, long term insights from the Adenoma Prevention with Celecoxib Trial on a promising but troubled class of drugs. Cancer Prev Res 2009;2:285–87.
41 Adams BK, Ferstl EM, Davis MC, et. al. Synthesis and biological evaluation of novel curcumin analogs as anti-cancer and anti-angiogenesis agents. Bioorg Med Chem 2004;12:3871–83.
42 Jagetia GC, Aggarwal BB. 'Spicing up' of the immune system by curcumin. J Clin Immunol 2007;27:19–35.
43 Peterson CA, Heffernan ME. Serum tumor necrosis factor-alpha concentrations are negatively correlated with serum 25(OH)D concentrations in healthy women. J Inflamm 2008;5:10.
44 Grant WB. An estimate of premature cancer mortality in the US due to inadequate doses of solar ultraviolet-B radiation. Cancer 2002;94:1867–75.
45 Tuohimaa B, Pukkala E, Scélo G, et. al. Does solar exposure, as indicated by the non-melanoma skin cancers, protect from solid cancers: vitamin D as a possible explanation. Eur J Cancer 2007;43:1701–12.
46 Oliver R. Does surgery disseminate or accelerate cancer? Lancet 1995;346–1506.
47 Michaud DS, Joshipura K, Giovannucci E, et. al. A prospective study of periodontal disease and pancreatic cancer in US male health professionals. J Natl Cancer Inst 2007;99:738–9.
48 Meyer MS, Joshipura K, Giovannucci E, et. al. A review of the relationship between tooth loss, periodontal disease, and cancer. Cancer Causes Control 2008;19:895–907.
49 Michaud DS, Liu Y, Meyer M, et. al. Periodontal disease, tooth loss and cancer risk in male health professionals: a prospective cohort study. Lancet Oncol 2008;9:550–8.
50 Nasca PC. Infectious agents and cancer. In: Nasca PC, Pastides H. Fundamentals of Cancer Epidemiology. Jones and Bartlett, Boston, 2008.
51 Marshall B. Sequential therapy for helicobacter pylori: a worthwhile effort for your patients. Ann Int Med 2008;148:962–63.
52 Perri F, Qasim A, Marras L, et. al. Treatment of helicobacter pylori infection. Helicobacter 2003;8(Suppl 1):53–60.
53 Crew KD, Neugut AI. Epidemiology of gastric cancer. World J Gastroenterol 2006;12:354–62.
54 Correa P, Fontham ETH. Gastric juice ascorbic acid after intravenous injection: effect of ethnicity, pH and helicobacter pylori infection. J Natl Cancer Inst 1995;87:52–53.
55 You WC, Brown LM, Zhang L, et. al. Randomized double-blind factorial trial of three treatments to reduce the prevalence of precancerous gastric lesions. JNCI 2006;98(14):974–83.

56 Vitetta L, Sali A. Probiotics and prebiotics–gastrointestinal health and longevity. In: Cohen M. Integrative Medicine Perspectives, Melbourne, 2007.
57 de Bortoli N, Leonardi G, Ciancia E. Helicobacter pylori eradication: a randomized prospective study of triple therapy versus triple therapy plus lactoferrin and probiotics. Am J Gastroenterol 2007;102:951–6.
58 Romero C, Medina E, Vargas J. *In vitro* activity of olive oil polyphenols against Helicobacter pylori. J Agric Food Chem 2007;55:680–86.
59 Blumberg BS, London WT. Hepatitis B virus and the prevention of primary cancer of the liver. J Natl Cancer Inst 1985;74:267–73.
60 zur Hausen H. Viruses in human cancer. Science 1991;254:1167–73.
61 Sobhonslidsuk A, Roongpisuthipong C, Nantiruj K, et. al. Impact of liver cirrhosis on nutritional and immunological status. J Med Assoc Thai 2001;84:982–8.
62 Ferré N, Camps J, Prats E, et. al. Impaired vitamin E status in patients with parenchymal liver cirrhosis: relationships with lipoprotein compositional alterations, nutritional factors and oxidative susceptibility of plasma. Metabolism 2002;51: 609–15.
63 Rocchi E, Borghi A, Paolillo F, et. al. Carotenoids and liposoluble vitamins in liver cirrhosis. J Lab Clin Med 1991;118:176–85.
64 Teran JC. Nutrition and liver disease. Curr Gastroenterol Rep 1999;1:335–40.
65 Kurahashi N, Inoue M, Iwaski M, et. al. Vegetable, fruit and antioxidant nutrient consumption is subsequent risk of hepatocellular carcinoma: a prospective cohort study in Japan. Br J Cancer 2009;100:181–84.
66 O'Connell MA, Rushworth SA. Curcumin: potential for hepatic fibrosis therapy? Br J Pharmacol 2008;153:403–05.
67 Shimizu I. Sho-saiko-to: Japanese herbal medicine for protection against hepatic fibrosis and carcinoma. J Gastroenterol Hepatol 2000;15(Suppl):D84–D90.
68 Schiffman MH, Brinton LA. The epidemiology of cervical carcinogenesis. Cancer 1995; 76(10 Suppl):1888–1901.
69 Franceschi S, Muñoz N, Bosch XF, et. al. Human papillomavirus in cancers of the upper aerodigestive tract: a review of epidemiological and experimental evidence. Cancer Epidemiol Biomarkers Prev 1996;5:567–75.
70 Potischman N, Brinton LA. Nutrition and cervical neoplasia. Canc Caus Cont 1996;7:113–26.
71 Hermandez BY, McDuffie K, Wilkens LR, et. al. Biomed Life Sci 2003;149:859–70.
72 Weinstein SJ, Ziegler RG, Selhub J, et. al. Elevated serum homocysteine levels and increased risk of invasive cervical cancer in US women. Cancer Causes Control 2001;12:317.
73 Sedjo RL, Roe DJ, Abrahamsen M, et. al. Vitamin A, carotenoids, and risk of persistent oncogenic human papillomavirus infection. Cancer Epidemiol Biomarkers Prev 2002;11:876–84.
74 Pastides H. Diet and Cancer. In: Nasca PC and Pastides H. Fundamentals of Cancer Epidemiology. Boston, Jones and Bartlett Publishers 2008.
75 Doll R, Peto R. The causes of cancer: quantitative estimates of avoidable risks of cancer in the United States today. J Natl Cancer Inst 1981;66:1191–1308.
76 Willett WC. Diet, nutrition and avoidable cancer. Environ Health Perspect 1995;103:165–70.
77 Key TJ, Schatzkin A, Willett WC, et. al. Diet, nutrition and the prevention of cancer. Public Health Nutr 2004;7:187–200.
78 Prochaska HJ, Santamaria AB, Talalay P. Rapid detection of inducers of enzymes that protect against carcinogens. Proc Natl Acad Sci USA1992;89:2394–99.
79 Bostick RN. Nutrition and colon cancer prevention. In: Mason JB, Nitenberg G. Cancer and Nutrition. Prevention and Treatment, Basel Karger, 2000.
80 Kune GA. Causes and Control of Colorectal Cancer. Kluwer, Norwell, 1996.
81 Hogervorst JG, Schouten LJ, Konings EJ, et. al. Dietary acrylamide intake and the risk of renal, bladder and prostate cancer. Am J Clin Nurt 2008;87:428–38.
82 Pelucchi C, Galeone C, Levi F, et. al. Dietary acrylamide and human cancer. Int J Cancer 2006;118:467–71.
83 Klaunig JE. Acrylamide carcinogenicity. J Agric Food Chem 2008;56:5984–88.
84 Konings EJ, Baars AJ, van Klaveren JD, et. al. Acrylamide exposure from foods of the Dutch population and an assessment of the consequent risks. Food Chem Toxicol 2003;41:1569–79.
85 Bull RJ, Robinson M, Laurie RD, et. al. Carcinogenic effects of acrylamide in Sencar and A/J mice. Cancer Res 1984;44:107–11.
86 Bull RJ, Robinson M, Stober JA. Carcinogenic activity of acrylamide in the skin and lung of Swiss-ICR mice. Cancer Lett 1984;24:209–12.
87 Starek A. Estrogens and organochlorine xenoestrogens and breast cancer risk. Int J Accup Med Environ Health 2003;16:113–24.
88 Fisch H, Hyun G, Golden R. The possibility of environmental estrogen disruptors on reproductive health. Curr Urol Rep 2000;1:253–61.
89 Daston GP, Gooch JW, Breslin WJ, et. al. Environmental estrogens and reproductive health: a discussion of the human and environmental data. Reprod Toxicol 1997;11:465–81.
90 Golden RJ, Noller KL, Titus-Ernstoff L, et. al. Environmental endocrine modulators in human health: an assessment to the biological evidence. Crit Rev Toxicol 1998;28:109–27.
91 Cantor KP, Lynch CF, Hildesheim ME, et. al. Drinking water source and chlorination byproducts in Iowa III. Risk of brain cancer. Am J Epidemiol 1999;150:5522–560.
92 Cantor KP, Hoover R, Hartg P, et. al. Drinking water source, and tap water consumption: a case-control study. J Natl Cancer Inst 1987;79:1269–79.
93 Hildesheim ME, Cantor KP, Lynch CF, et. al. Drinking water source and chlorinated byproducts in Iowa II. Risk of colon and rectal cancers. Epidemiol 1998;9:29–35.
94 Kasim K, Levallois P, Johnson KC, et. al. Chlorination disinfection by-products in drinking water and the risk of adult leukaemia in Canada. Am J Epidemiol 2006;163:116–26.
95 Lubin JH, Beane Freeman LE, Cantor KP. Inorganic arsenic in drinking water: an evolving public health concern. J Natl Cancer Inst 2007;99:906–07.
96 Marshall G, Ferreccio C, Yuan Y, et. al. Fifty-year study of lung and bladder cancer mortality in Chile relate to arsenic in drinking water. J Natl Cancer Inst 2007;99:920–28.
97 Willett WC. Diet and Nutrition. In: Schottenfeld D, Fraumeni JF Jr. Cancer Epidemiology and Prevention (3rd edn).Oxford University Press, New York, 2006:405–21.

98 Pope CA, Burnett RT, Thun MJ. Lung cancer, cardiopulmonary mortality and long-term exposure to fine particulate air pollution. JAMA 2002;287:1132–41.

99 Loh NN, Levy JI, Spengler JD, et. al. Ranking cancer risks of organic hazardous air pollutants in the United States. Environ Health Perspect 2007;115:1160–68.

100 Kaiser J. NIH panel revives EMF-cancer link. Science 1998;281:21.

101 Lowenthal RM, Tuck DM, Bray IC. Residential exposure to electric power transmission lines and risk of lymphoproliferative and myeloproliferative disorders: a case-control study. Int ern Med J 2007;37:614–19.

102 Brainard GC, Kavet R, Kheifets LI. The relationship between a electromagnetic field and light exposures to melatonin and breast cancer risk: a review of the relevant literature. J Pineal Res 1999;26:65–100.

103 Graham C, Cook MR, Gerkovich MM, et. al. Examination of the melatonin hypothesis in women exposed at night to EMF or bright light. Environ Health Perspect 2001;109:501–7.

104 Guénel P, Nicolau J, Imbernon E, et. al. Exposure to 50-Hz electric field and incidence of leukaemia, brain tumors, and other cancers among French electric utility workers. Am J Epidemiol 1996;144:1107–21.

105 Sali A. Health and Agriculture: GM food risks. Online. Available: www.niim.com.au (accessed 10 March 2008)

106 Gupta A. Impact of Bt cotton on farmer's health (in Barwani and Dhar district of Madhya Pradesh). Investigation Report Oct-Dec 2005.

107 Mayeno AN, Gleich GJ. Eosinophilia-myalgia syndrome and tryptophan production: a cautionary tale. Trends Biotechnol 1994;12:119–27.

108 Pearce F. Focused bigger harvests, without pesticides or genetically modified crops, farmers can let it happen by making weeds do the work. New Scientist 2001;169:16–17.

109 Pastides H. Ionizing, non ionizing, and solar radiation in cancer. In: Nasca PC, Pastides H. Fundamentals of Cancer Epidemiology. Jones and Bartlett Publishers, Boston, 2008.

110 Ron E. Cancer risk from medical radiation. Health Phys 2003;85:47–59.

111 Smith PG, Doll R. Late effects of x-irradiation in patients treated for metropathia haemorrhagica. Br J Radiol 1976;39:24–232.

112 Greenwald ED, Greenwald S. Cancer epidemiology. Medical Examination Publishing Co, New Hyde Park, NY,1983.

113 Boice JE. Ionizing radiation. In: Schottenfeld D, Fraumeni Jr. Cancer Epidemiology and Prevention (3rd edn).Oxford University Press, New York, 2006.

114 Wakabayashi T, Kato H, Ikeda T, et. al. Studies of the mortality of A-bomb survivors, report 7. Part III. Incidence of cancer in 1959–1978, based on the tumor registry, Nagasaki. Radiat Res 1983;93: 112–46.

115 Seaberg RM, Eski S, Freeman JL. Influence of previous radiation exposure on pathological features and clinical outcome in patients with thyroid cancer. Arch Otolaryngol Head Neck Surg 2009;135:355–9.

116 Einstein AJ, Henzlova MJ, Rajagopalan S. Estimating risk of cancer associated with radiation exposure from 64-sliced computed tomography coronary angiography. JAMA 2007;298:317–23.

117 Thomson KR, Street M, Every BV, et. al. Radiation exposure and the justification of CT scanning in an Australian hospital emergency department. Int Med J 2009 Mar 23. (Epub ahead of print).

118 Scorecard: The pollution information site. Online. Available: www.scorecard.org (accessed 10 March 2009)

119 Agency for toxic substances and disease registry: finalised toxicological profiles. Online. Available: www.atsdr.cdc.gov/toxprofiles (accessed 10 March 2009)

120 Sudak N, Harvie J. Reducing toxic exposures. In: Rakel D. Integrative Medicine (2nd edn). Saunders Elsevier, Philadelphia, 2007.

121 Lang IA, Galloway TS, Scarlett A. Association of urinary bisphenol A concentration with medical disorders and laboratory abnormalities in adults. JAMA 2008;300:1303–10.

122 Garshick E, Laden F, Hart JE, et. al. Lung cancer and vehicle exhaust in trucking industry workers. Environ Health Perspect 2008;116:1327–32.

123 Samanic CM, De Roos AJ, Stewart PA, et. al. Occupational exposure to pesticides and risk of adult brain tumours. Am J Epidemiol 2008;167:976–85.

124 De Roos AJ, Stewart PA, Linet MS, et. al. Occupation and the risk of adult glioma in the United States. Cancer Causes Control 2003;14: 139–50.

125 Khuder SA, Mutgi IV, Schaub EA. Meta-analysis of brain cancer and farming. Am J Ind Med 1988;38:252–60.

126 Musicco M, Sant M, Molinari S, et. al. A case-control study of brain gliomas and occupational exposure to chemical carcinogens: the risk to farmers. Am J Epidemiol 1988;128:778–85.

127 Graff JJ, Sathiakumar N, Macaluso M, et. al. Chemical exposures in the synthetic rubber industry and lymphohematopoietic cancer mortality. J Occup Environ Med 2005;47:916–32.

128 Ward EM, Fajen JM, Ruder AM, et. al. Mortality study of workers in 1,3-butadiene production units identified from a chemical workers cohort. Environ Health Perspect 1995;103:598–03.

129 Steenland K, Whelan E, Deddens J. Ethylene oxide and breast cancer incidence in a cohort study of 7576 women (United States). Cancer Causes Control 2003;14:531–39.

130 Mundt KA, Dell LD, Austin RP, et. al. Historical cohort study of 10 109 men in the North American vinyl chloride industry, 1942–72: update of cancer mortality to 31st December 1995. Occup Environ Med 2000;57:174–781.

131 Ward E, Boffetta P, Andersen A, et. al. Update of a follow-up mortality and cancer incidence among European workers employed in the vinyl chloride industry. Epidemiology 2001;12:710–18.

132 Zhang Y, Sanjose SD, Bracci PM, et. al. Personal use of hair dye and the risk of certain subtypes of non-Hodgkin lymphoma. Am J Epidemiol 2008;167: 130–31.

133 Huncharek M, Kupelnick B. Personal use of hair dyes and the risk of bladder cancer: results of a meta-analysis. Public Heatlh Rep 2005;120:31–8.

134 Chiang TA, Wu PF, Ko YC. Identification of carcinogens in cooking oil fumes. Environ Res 1999;81:18–22.

135 LeMasters GK, Genaidy AM, Succop P, et. al. Cancer risk among firefighters: a review and meta-analysis of 32 studies. J Occup Environ Med 2006;48: 1189–202.

136 Ikehara S, Iso H, Date C, et. al. Association of sleep duration with mortality from cardiovascular disease and other causes for Japanese men and women: the JACC study. Sleep 2009;32:295–301.
137 Mallon L, Broman JE, Hetta J. Is usage of hypnotics associated with mortality? Sleep Med 2009;10; 279–86.
138 Cappuccio FP, Taggart FM, Kandala NB, et. al. Meta-analysis of short sleep duration and obesity in children and adults. Sleep 2008;31:619–26.
139 Chaput JP, Després JP, Bouchard C, et. al. The association between sleep duration and weight gain in adults: a 6-year prospective study from the Quebec Family Study. Sleep 2008;31:517–23.
140 Patel SR, Hu FB. Short sleep duration and weight gain: a systemic review. Obes 2008;16:643–53.
141 Wu AH, Wang R, Koh P, et. al. Sleep duration, melatonin and breast cancer among Chinese women in Singapore. Carcinogenesis 2008;29:1244–8.
142 Kakizaki M, Kuriyama S, Sone T, et. al. Sleep duration and the risk of breast cancer: the Ohsaki Cohort Study. Br J Cancer 2008;99:1502–05.
143 Ancoli-Israel S, Moore PG, Jones V. The relationship between fatigue and sleep in cancer patients: a review. Eur J Cancer Care 2001;10:245–55.
144 Travis RC, Allen DS, Fentiman IS, et. al. Melatonin and breast cancer: a prospective study. J Natl Cancer Inst 2004;17:475–82.
145 Uhlenbruck G, Ledvina I. Exercise in cancer prevention and followup. In: Buth J, Moss RW. Complementary Oncology, Stuttgart Thieme, 2006.
146 Nieman DC. The exercise-health connection. Shambaign, 2, Human Kinetics 998.
147 Parkin J, Cohen B. An overview of the immune system. Lancet 2001;3571:1777–89.
148 MacKinnon IT. Advances in exercise immunology. Human Kinetics 1999.
149 Thune I, Furberg AS. Physical activity in cancer risk: dose-response and cancer, all sites and site-specific. Med Sci Sports Exercise 2001;33:530–50.
150 Lötzerich H, Peters C. Krebs and Sport. Cologne, Germany Verlag Sport, Buch Strauss 1997.
151 Peters C, Lötzerich H, Niemeier B, et. al. Influence of a moderate exercise training on natural killer cytotoxicity and personality traits in cancer patients. Anticancer Res 1994;14:1033–36.
152 Craft LL, Landers DM. The effect of exercise on clinical depression and depression resulting from mental illness: a meta-analysis. J Sport Exercise Psychol 1998;20:339–57.
153 Kushi L, Giovannucci E. Dietary fat and cancer. Am J Med 2002;113(Suppl 9B):63S-70S.
154 Weisburger JH. Dietary fat and risk of chronic disease: mechanistic insights from experimental studies. J Am Diet Assoc 1997;97(Suppl 7): S16–S23.
155 Davidson LE, Hudson R, Kilpatrick K, et. al. Effects of exercise modality on insulin resistance and functional limitation in older adults: a randomised controlled trial. Arch Int Med 2009;169: 122–31.
156 Schiel R, Beltschikow W, Steiner T. Diabetes, insulin, and risk of cancer. Methods Find Exp Clin Pharmacol 2006;28:169–75.
157 Farrell SW, Cortese GM, LaMonte MJ, et. al. Cardiorespiratory fitness, different measures of adiposity, and cancer mortality in men. Obesity 2007;15:3140–9.
158 Lee IM. Dose-response relation between physical activity and fitness: even a little is good: more is better. JAMA 2007;297:2137–39.
159 US Department of Health and Human Services. Physical activity and health: a report of the Surgeon General. Atlanta, GA:US Department of Health and Human Services, Centers for Disease Control and Prevention, National Center for Disease Control and Prevention, Health Promotion 1996.
160 Segal RJ, Reid RD, Courneya KS, et. al. Randomised controlled trial of resistance or aerobic exercise in men receiving radiation therapy for prostate cancer. J Clin Oncol 2009;27:344–51.
161 Rice B, Janssen I, Hudson R, et. al. The effects of aerobic or resistance exercise and/or diet on glucose tolerance and plasma insulin levels in obese men. Diabetes Care 1999;22:684–91.
162 Haydon AM, Macinnis RJ, English DR, et. al. The effect of physical activity and body size on survival after diagnosis with colorectal cancer. Gut 2006;55:62–7.
163 Holmes MD, Chen WY, Feskanich D et. al. Physical activity and survival after breast cancer diagnosis. JAMA 2005;293:2479–86.
164 Pierce JP, Stefanick ML, Flatt SW, et. al. Greater survival after breast cancer and physically active women with high vegetable-fruit intake regardless of obesity. J Clin Oncol 2007;25:2345–51.
165 Giovannucci EL, Liu Y, Leitzmann MF, et. al. A prospective study of physical activity and incident and fatal prostate cancer. Arch Intern Med 2005;165:1005–10.
166 Morgan G, Ward R, Barton M. The contribution of cytotoxic chemotherapy to 5-year survival in adult malignancies. Clin Oncol 2004;16:549–60.
167 Galvão DA, Newton RU. Review of exercise intervention studies in cancer patients. J Clin Oncol 2005;23:899–909.
168 Ruiz JR, Sui X, Lobelo F, et. al. Muscular strength and adiposity as predictors of adulthood cancer mortality in men. Cancer Epidemiol Biomarkers Prev 2009;18:1468–76 1055–9965. epi-08-1075v1.
169 Mock V, Frangakis C, Davidson NE, et. al. Exercise manages fatigue in breast cancer treatment: a randomised controlled trial. Psychooncology 2005;14:464–77.
170 Butt Z, Rosenboom SK, Abernethy AP, et. al. Fatigue is the most important symptom for advanced cancer patients who have had chemotherapy. J Natl Compr Canc Netw 2008;6:448–55.
171 Roscoe JA, Kaufman ME, Matteson-Rusby SE, et. al. Cancer-related fatigue and sleep disorders. Oncologist 2007;12(Suppl 1):35–42.
172 Berger AM, Mitchell SA. Modifying cancer-related fatigue by optimising sleep quality. J Natl Compr Canc Netw 2008;6:3–13.
173 Barsevick AM, Newhall T, Brown S. Management of cancer-related fatigue. Clin J Oncol Nurs 2008;12(Suppl 5):21–5.
174 Murthy NS, Mukherjee S, Ray G, et. al. Dietary factors and cancer chemoprevention: an overview of obesity-related malignancies. J Postgrad Med 2009;55:45–54.
175 Olver IN, Grogan PB. Cancer adds further urgency to prioritising obesity control. (Editorial) Med J Aust 2008;189:191–92.
176 Renehan AG, Tyson M, Egger M, et. al. Body-mass index and incidence of cancer: a systematic review and meta-analysis of prospective observational studies. Lancet 2008;371:569–78.
177 Reeves GK, Pirie K, Beral B, et. al. Cancer incidence and mortality in relation to body mass in the Million Women Study: cohort study. BMJ 2007;335:1134–44.

178 Kubo A, Corley DA. Body mass index and adenocarcinoma of the oesophagus or gastric cardia: a systematic review and meta-analysis. Cancer Epidemiol Biomarkers Prev 2006;15:872–8.
179 Skolarus TA, Wolin KY, Grubb RL. The effect of body mass index on PSA levels and the development, screening and treatment of prostate cancer. Nat Clin Pract Urol 2007;4:605–14.
180 Chang JM, Stampfer MJ, Ma J, et. al. Insulin-like growth factor-1(IGF-1) and IGF binding protein-3 as predictors of advanced stage prostate cancer. J Natl Cancer Inst 2002;94:1099–06.
181 Cox ME, Gleave ME, Zakikhani M, et. al. Insulin receptor expression by human prostate cancers. Prostate 2009;69:33–40.
182 Renehan AG, Frystyk J, Flyvbjerg J. Obesity and cancer: the role of insulin-IGF access. Trends Endocrinol Tab 2006;17:328–36.
183 Singleton JR, Randolf AE, Feldman EL. Insulin-like growth factor one receptor prevents apoptosis and enhances neuroblastoma tumorigenesis. Cancer Res 1996;56:4522–29.
184 LeRoith D, Novosyadlyy R, Gallagher EJ, et. al. Obesity and type 2 diabetes are associated with an increased risk of developing cancer and a worse prognosis: epidemiological mechanistic evidence. Exp Clin Endocrinol Diabetes 2008;116(Suppl 1):S4–S6.
185 Flood A, Mai V, Pfeiffer R, et. al. Elevated serum concentrations of insulin and glucose increase risk of colorectal adenomas. Gastroenterology 2007;133:1423–9.
186 Mulholland HG, Murray IJ, Cardwell CR, et. al. Glycaemic index, glycaemic load, and risk of digestive tract neoplasms: a systematic review and meta-analysis. Am J Clin Nutr 2009;89:568–76.
187 Michaeud DS, Liu S, Giovannucci E, et. al. Dietary sugar, glycaemic load, and pancreatic cancer risk in a prospective study. J Natl Cancer Inst 2002;94: 1293–1300.
188 Everhart J, Right D. Diabetes mellitus as a risk factor for pancreatic cancer. A meta-analysis. JAMA 1995;273:1605–9.
189 Silverman DT. Risk factors for pancreatic cancer: a controlled study based on direct interviews. Teratog Carcinog Nutagen 2001;21:7–25.
190 Coughlin SS, Calle EE, Patel AV, et. al. Predictors of pancreatic cancer mortality among large cohort of United States adults.Cancer Causes Control 2000;11:15–23.
191 Friedman GD, van den Eeden SK. Risk factors for pancreatic cancer: an exploratory study. Int J Epidemiol 1993;22:32–7.
192 Mulholland HG, Murray IJ, Cardwell CR, et. al. Dietary glycaemic index, glycaemic load and endometrial and ovarian cancer risk: a systematic review and meta-analysis. Br J Cancer 2008;99: 434–41.
193 Barclay AW, Petocz P, McMillan-Price J, et. al. Glycaemic index, glycaemic load and chronic disease risk — a meta-analysis of observational studies. Am J Clin Nutr 2008;87:627–37.
194 Thomas DE, Elliot EJ, Bour L. Low glycaemic index or low glycaemic load diets for overweight and obesity. Cochrane Database of Systematic Reviews 2007, Issue 3. Art. Number.:CD005105 .D01:10.1002/14651858. CD005105. pub2.
195 Cust AE. The influence of overweight and insulin resistance on breast cancer risk and tumour stage at diagnosis: a prospective study. Breast Cancer Res and Treat 2009;113:567–76.
196 Kawamura Y, Ikedea K, Arase Y, et. al. Diabetes mellitus worsens the recurrence rate after potentially curative therapy in patients with hepatocellular carcinoma associated with nonviral hepatitis. J Gastroenterol Hepatol 2008;23:1739–46.
197 Wright ME, Chang SC, Schatzkin A, et. al. Prospective study of adiposity and weight change in relation to prostate cancer incidence and mortality. Cancer 2007;109:675–84.
198 Giovannucci E, Liu Y, Platz EA, et. al. Risk factors for prostate cancer incidence and progression in the Health Professionals follow-up study. Int J Cancer 2007;121:1571–78.
199 Haydon AM, Macinnis RJ, English DR, et. al. Physical activity, insulin-like growth factor 1, insulin-like growth factor binding protein 3, and survival from colorectal cancer. GUT 2006;55: 689–94.
200 McTiernan A, Ulrich C, Slate S, et. al. Physical activity and cancer etiology: associations and mechanisms. Cancer Causes Control 1998;9: 487–509.
201 McMillan-Price J, Brand-Miller J. Low-glycaemic index diets and body weight regulation. Intl J Obesity 2006:30:S40-S46.
202 Kelesidis I, Kelesidis T, Mantzoros CS. Adeponectin and cancer: a systematic review. Br J Cancer 2006;94:1221–25.
203 Murthy NS, Mukherjee S, Ray G, et. al. Dietary factors and chemoprevention: an overview of obesity-related malignancies. J Postgrad Med 2009;55: 45–54.
204 Rose DP, Komninou D, Stephenson GD. Obesity, adipocytokines, and insulin resistance in breast cancer. Obes Rev 2004;5:153–65.
205 Chandran M, Phillips SA, Ciaraldi T, et. al. Adiponectin: more than just another fat cell hormone? Diabetes Care 2003;26:2442–50.
206 Barb D, Williams CJ, Neuwirth AK, et. al. Adiponectin in relation to malignancies: a review of existing basic research and clinical evidence. Am J Clin Nutr 2007;86:S858–66.
207 Trujillo ME, Scherer PE. Adiponectin-journey from a adipocyte secretory protein to biomarker of the metabolic syndrome. J Int Med 2005;257:167–75.
208 Breastscreen Australian Government Department of Health and Ageing. Online. Available: www.cancerscreening.gov.au/internet/screening/publishing.nsf/content/breastsc (accessed 17 May 2009)
209 Smith-Bindman R, Chu PW, Miglioretti DL, et. al. Comparison of screening mammorgrapy in the United States and the United Kingdom. JAMA 2003;290:2129–37.
210 Lehman CD, Gatsonis C, Kuhl CK, et. al. MRI evaluation of the contralateral breast in women with recently diagnosed breast cancer. N Eng J Med 2007;356:1295–1303.
211 Avramenko GV. Use of radiothermometry in the screening of nonpalpable breast neoplasms. Vestn Rentgenol Radiol 2007;5:9–12.
212 Sdvigkof AM, Vesnin SG, Kartashova AF, et. al. On the place of radiothermometry in mammological practice. Aktualnyie Problemy Mammalogeii 2000;28–40.
213 Thomas BC, Bultz BD. The future in psychosocial oncology: screening for emotional distress–the sixth vital sign. Future Oncol 2008;4:779–84.
214 Zahl T, Maehlen J, Welch HG. The natural history of the invasive breast cancers detected by screening mammography. Arch Int Med 2008;168:2311–16.

215 Gotzsche PC, Hartling OJ, Nielsen M et. al. Breast screening: the facts–or maybe not. BMJ 2009;338: doi:10.1136/bmj.b86.
216 Smith-Bindman R, Chu PW, Miglioretti DL, et. al. Comparison of screening mammorgrapy in the United States and the United Kingdom. JAMA 2003;290:2129–37.
217 Keen JD, Keen JE. What is the point: will screening mammography save my life? BMC Medform DECIS MAK 2009;9:18. doi:10.1186/1472-6947-9-18.
218 Editorial: The trouble with screening. Lancet 2009;373:1223.
219 Raffle AE, Alden B, Quinn M, et. al. Outcomes of screening to prevent cancer: analysis of cumulative incidences of cervical abnormality and modelling of cases and deaths prevented. BMJ 2003;326:901–06.
220 Sasieni P. Cervical cancer prevention and hormonal contraception. Lancet 2007;370:1591–2.
221 Kulasingam SL, Pagliusi S, Myers E. Potential effects of decreased cervical cancer screening participation after HPV vaccination: an example from the US. Vaccine 2007;25:8110–13.
222 National Cancer Institute: What you need to know about cancer of the cervix. Online. Available: www.cancer.gov/cancertopics/wyntk/cervix/ (accessed July 20, 2006)
223 Hernandez BW, McDuffie K, Wilkens LR, et. al. Diet and premalignant lesions of the cervix: evidence of a protective role for folate, riboflavin, thiamine and vitamin B12. Cancer Causes Control 2003;14: 859–70.
224 Sali A, Vitetta L. Integrative Medicine in Gynaecological Cancers. Aust Fam Physician 2007;36:135–36.
225 Liu T, Soong SJ, Wilson NP, et. al. A case controlled study of nutritional factors in cervical dysplasia. Cancer Epidemiol Biomarkers Prev 1993;2:525–30.
226 Byers T, Perry G. Dietary carotenes, vitamin C, and vitamin E as protective antioxidants in human cancers. Ann Rev Nutr 1992;12:139–59.
227 Palan PR, Mikhail MS, Shaban DW, et. al. Plasma concentration of coenzyme Q10 and tocopherols in cervical intraepithelial neoplasia and cervical cancer. Eur J Cancer Prev 2003;12:321–6.
228 Piyathilake CJ, Henao OL, Macaluso M, et. al. Folate is associated with a natural history of high-risk of human papillomaviruses. Cancer Res 2004;64:8788–93.
229 Weinstein SJ, Ziegler RG, Selhub J, et. al. Elevated serum homocysteine levels increase risk of invasive cervical cancer in US women. Cancer Causes Control 2001;12:317–24.
230 Morgan G, Wood R, Barton M. The contribution of cytotoxic chemotherapy to 5-years survival in adult malignancies. Clin Oncol 2004;16:459–560.
231 Casanovas O, Hicklin DJ, Bergers G, et. al. Drug resistance by evasion of antiangiogenic targeting of VEGF signalling in late-stage pancreatic islet tumors. Cancer Cell 2005;8:299–309.
232 Bekelman JE, Li Y, Gross CP. Scope and impact of financial conflicts of interest in biomedical research: a systematic review. JAMA 2003;289:454–65.
233 Jaqsi R, Sheets N, Jankovic A, et. al. Frequency, nature, effects, and correlates of conflicts of interest in published clinical cancer research. Cancer 2009;115:2783–91.
234 Riechelmann RP, Wang L, O'Carroll A. Disclosure of conflict of interest by authors of clinical trials and editorials in oncology. J Clin Oncol 2007;25:4642–7.
235 Reavley N, Pallant JF, Sali A. Evaluation of the effects of a psychosocial intervention on mood, coping, and quality of life in cancer patients. Integr Cancer Ther 2009 Mar;8:47–55.
236 Glas R, Reavley N, Mrazek L, et. al. Psychosocial interventions and cancer patients: psychological and immune responses may depend on cancer type. Med Hypotheses 2001;56:480–82.
237 Kissane DW, Clarke DM, Ikin J, et. al. Psychological morbidity and quality of life in Australian women with early-stage breast cancer: a cross-sectional survey. Med J Aust 1998;169:192–196.
238 Zabor JR, Blanchard CG, Smith ED, et. al. Prevalence of psychological distress among cancer patients across the disease continuum. J Psychosoc Oncol 1997;15:73–87.
239 Donovan RJ, Jalleh G, Jones SC. The word 'cancer': reframing the context to reduce anxiety arousal. Aust N Z J Public Health 2003;27:291–3.
240 Shapiro SL, Lopez AM, Schwartz GE, et. al. Quality of life and breast cancer: relationship to psychosocial variables. J Clin Psychol 2001;57:501–519.
241 Meyer TJ, Mark MM. Effects of psychosocial interventions with adult cancer patients: a meta-analysis of randomized experiments. Health Psychol 1995;14:101–8.
242 Sheard T, Maguire P. The effect of psychological interventions on anxiety and depression in cancer patients: results of two meta-analyses. Br J Cancer 1999;80:1770–80.
243 Maunsel E, Brisson J, Deschenes L. Social support and survival among women with breast cancer. Cancer 1995;76:631–37.
244 Gawler Foundation in Melbourne. Online. Available: http://www.gawler.org (accessed 11 Feb 2010)
245 Spiegel D, Bloom JR, Kraemer HC, et. al. Effect of psychosocial treatment on survival of patients with metastatic breast cancer. Lancet 1989;2:888–91.
246 Fawzy F, Fawzy NW, Hyun CS, et. al. Malignant melanoma. Effects of an early structured psychiatric intervention, coping, and affective state on recurrence and survival 6 years later. Arch Gen Psychiatry 1993;50:681–89.
247 Meares A. What can the cancer patient expect from intensive meditation? Aust Fam Physician 1980;9:322–5.
248 Smith JE, Richardson J, Hoffman C, et. al. Mindfulness-Based Stress Reduction as supportive therapy in cancer care: systematic review. J Adv Nurs 2005;52:315–27.
249 Carlson LE, Ursuliak Z, Goodey E, et. al. The effects of a mindfulness meditation-based stress reduction program on mood and symptoms of stress in cancer outpatients: 6-month follow-up. Support Care Cancer 2001;9:112–23.
250 Shapiro SL, Bootzin RR, Figueredo AJ, et. al. The efficacy of mindfulness-based stress reduction in the treatment of sleep disturbance in women with breast cancer: an exploratory study. J Psychosom Res 2003;54:85–91.
251 Carlson LE, Speca M, Patel KD, et. al. Mindfulness-based stress reduction in relation to quality of life, mood, symptoms of stress, and immune parameters in breast and prostate cancer outpatients. Psychosom Med 2003;65:571–81.
252 Monti DA, Peterson C, Kunkel EJ, et. al. A randomized, controlled trial of mindfulness-based art therapy (MBAT) for women with cancer. Psychooncology 2006;15:363–73.

253 Carlson LE, Speca M, Patel KD, et. al. Mindfulness-based stress reduction in relation to quality of life, mood, symptoms of stress and levels of cortisol, dehydroepiandrosterone sulfate (DHEAS) and melatonin in breast and prostate cancer outpatients. Psychoneuroendocrinology 2004;29:448–74.
254 Richardson JL, Shelton DR, Krailo M, et. al. The effect of compliance with treatment on survival among patients with hematologic malignancies. J Clin Oncol 1990;8:356–64.
255 Kuchler T, Henne-Bruns D, Rappat S, et. al. Impact of psychotherapeutic support on gastrointestinal cancer patients undergoing surgery: survival results of a trial. Hepatogastroenterology 1999;46:322–35.
256 Andersen BL, Yang HC, Farrar WB, et. al. Psychologic intervention improves survival for breast cancer patients: a randomized clinical trial. Cancer 2008;113:3450–8.
257 Fawzy FI. Psychosocial interventions for patients with cancer: what works and what doesn't. Eur J Cancer 1999;35:1559–64.
258 Cunningham A, Philips C, Lockwood G, et. al. Association of involvement in psychological self-regulation with longer survival in patients with metastatic cancer: an exploratory study. Adv Mind Body Med 2000;16:276–87.
259 Schnur JB, Bovbjerg DH, David D, et. al. Hypnosis decreases presurgical distress in excisional breast biopsy patients. Anesth Analg 2008;106:440–4.
260 Stalpers LJ, da Costa HC, Merbis MA, et. al. Hypnotherapy in radiotherapy patients: a randomized trial. Int J Radiat Oncol Biol Phys 2005;61:499–506.
261 Zeltzer LK, Dolgerin MJ, LeBarron S, et. al. A randomized, controlled study of behavioural intervention for chemotherapy distress in children with cancer. Pediatrics 1991;88:34–42.
262 Musteia KM, Katula JA, Gill DL, et. al. Tai Chi Chuan, health-related quality of life and self-esteem: a randomized trial with breast cancer survivors. Support Care Cancer 2004;12:871–76.
263 Irwin MR, Olmstead R, Oxman MN. Augmenting immune responses to varicella zoster virus in older adults: a randomized, controlled trial of Tai Chi. J Am Geriatr Soc 2007;55:511–7.
264 Lee MS, Chen KW, Sancier KM, et. al. Qigong for cancer treatment: a systematic review of controlled clinical trials. Acta Oncol 2007;46:717–22.
265 Yeh ML, Lee TI, Chen HH, et. al. The influences of Chan-Chuang qi-gong therapy on complete blood cell counts in breast cancer patients treated with chemotherapy. Cancer Nurs 2006;29:149–55.
266 Sancier KM. Medical applications of qigong. Altern Ther Health Med 1996;2:40–6.
267 Chen K, Yeung R. Exploratory studies of qigong therapy for cancer in China. Integr Cancer Ther 2002;1:345–70.
268 Sancier KM. Therapeutic benefits of qigong exercises in combination with drugs. J Altern Complement Med 1999;5:383–9.
269 Lee TI, Chen HH, Yeh ML. Effects of chan-chuang qigong on improving symptom and psychological distress in chemotherapy patients. Am J Chin Med 2006;34:37–46.
270 Manzaneque JM, Vera FM, Maldonado EF, et. al. Assessment of immunological parameters following a qigong training program. Med Sci Monit 2004;10:264–70.
271 Jackson E, Kelley M, McNeil P, et. al. Does therapeutic touch help reduce pain and anxiety in patients with cancer? Clin J Oncol Nurs 2008;12:113–20.
272 Ferrell-Torry AT, Glick OJ. The use of therapeutic massage as a nursing intervention to modify anxiety and the perception of cancer pain. Cancer Nurs 1993;16:93–101.
273 Billhult A, Bergebom I, Stener-Victorin E. Massage relieves nausea in women with breast cancer who are undergoing chemotherapy. J Altern Complement Med 2007;13:53–57.
274 Spencer JW, Jacobs JJ. Complementary and Alternative Medicine: an evidence based approach. Mosby, St Louis, 2003.
275 Smith M, Casey L, Johnson D, et. al. Music as a therapeutic intervention for anxiety in patients receiving radiation therapy. Oncol Nurs Forum 2001;28:855–62.
276 Cooke B, Ernst E. Aromatherapy: a systematic review. Br J Gen Pract 2000;50:493–6.
277 Kite SM, Maher EJ, Anderson K, et. al. Development of an aromatherapy service at a Cancer Centre. Palliat Med 1998;12:171–76.
278 Rosenthal DS. American Cancer Societies guide to complementary and alternative cancer methods. American Cancer Society, Atlanta, 2000.
279 Campbell JK, Canene-Adams K, Lindshield BL, et. al. Tomato phytochemicals and prostate cancer risk. J Nutr 2004;34:3486S-3492S.
280 Kucuk O, Sarkar FH, Djuric Z, et. al. Effects of lycopene supplementation in patients with localised prostate cancer. Exp Biol Med (Maywood) 2000;227:881–5.
281 Nkondjock A, Ghadirian P, Johnson KC. Dietary intake of lycopene is associated with reduced pancreatic cancer risk. J Nutr 2005;135:592–7.
282 Huncharek M, Klassen H, Kupelnick B. Dietary beta-carotene intake and risk of epithelial ovarian cancer: a meta-analysis of 3,782 subjects from five observational studies. *In vivo* 2001;15:339–43.
283 Toniolo P, Van Kappel AL, Akhmedkhanov A, et. al. Serum carotenoids and breast cancer. Am J Epidemiol 2001;153:1142–7.
284 Nair S, Norkus EP, Hertan H, et. al. Serum and colon mucosa micronutrient antioxidants: difference between adenomatous polyp patients and controls. Am J Gastroenterol 2001;96:3400–5.
285 Schabath MB, Grossman HB, Delclos GL, et. al. Dietary carotenoids and genetic instability modified bladder cancer risk. J Nutr 2004;134:3362–69.
286 Liu X, Allen JD, Arnold JT, et. al. Lycopene inhibits IGF-1signal transduction and growth in normal prostate epithelial cells by decreasing DHT-modulated IGF-1production in co-cultured reactive stromal cells. Carcinogenesis 2008;29:816–23.
287 Giovannucci E. Tomatoes, tomato-based products, lycopene, and cancer: review of the epidemiologic literature. J Natl Cancer Inst 1999;91:217–331.
288 Clarke N, Germain P, Altucci L, et. al. Retinoids: potential in cancer prevention and therapy. Exp Rev Mol Med 2004;6:1–23.
289 Aggarwal BB, Kumar A, Bharti AC. Anticancer potential of curcumin: preclinical and clinical studies. Anticancer Res 2003;23:363–98.
290 Shama RA, Euden SA, Platton SL, et. al. Phase 1 clinical trial of oral curcumin: biomarkers of systemic activity and compliance. Clin Cancer Res 2009;10:6847–54.

291 Dorai T, Dutcher JP, Dempster DW, et. al. Therapeutic potential of curcumin in prostate cancer--V: Interference with the osteomimetic properties of hormone refractory C4-2B prostate cancer cells. Prostate 2004;60:1–17.
292 Narayan S. Curcumin, a multi-functional chemopreventive agent, blocks growth of colon cancer cells by targeting beta-catenin-mediated transactivation and cell- cell adhesion pathways. J Mol Histol 2004;35:371–7.
293 Inano H, Onoda M, Inafuku N, et. al. Potent preventive action of curcumin on radiation-induced initiation of mammary tumorigenesis in rats. Carcinogenesis 2000;21:1835–41.
294 Dhillon N, Aggarwal B, Newman RA, et. al. Phase II trial of curcumin in patients with advanced pancreatic cancer. Clin Cancer Res 2008;14:4491–9. doi:10.1158/1078-0432.CCR-08-0024.
295 Sung B, Kunnumakkara AB, Sethi G, et. al. Curcumin circumvents chemoresistance *in vitro* and potentiates the effect of thalidomide and bortezomib against human multiple myeloma in nude mice model. Mol Cancer Ther 2009;8:959–70.
296 Li M, Zhang Z, Hill DL, et. al. Curcumin, dietary component, has anticancer, chemosensitisation, and radiosensitisation effects by down-regulating the MDM2 oncogene through the P13K/mTOR/ET S2 pathway. Cancer Res 2007;67:1988–96.
297 Chirnomas D, Taniguchi T, de la Vega M, et. al. Chemosensitisation to cisplatin by inhibitors of the Fanconi anemia/BRCA pathway. Mol Cancer Ther 2006;5:592–61.
298 Yang CS, Liao J, Yang GY, et. al. Inhibition of lung tumorigenesis by tea. Exp Lung Res 2005;31: 135–44.
299 Seely D, Mills EJ, Wu P, et. al. The effects of green tea consumption on incidence of breast cancer and recurrence of breast cancer: a systematic review and meta-analysis. Integr Cancer Ther 2005;4:144–55.
300 Bonner MR, Rothman N, Mumford J, et. al. Green tea consumption, genetic susceptibility, PAH-rich smoky coal, and the risk of lung cancer. Mutat Res 2005;582:53–60.
301 Zhang SM. Role of vitamins in the risk, prevention, and treatment of breast cancer. Curr Opin Obstet Gynecol 2004;16:19–25.
302 Doss MX, Potta SP, Hescheler J, et. al. Trapping of growth factors by catechins: a possible therapeutical target for prevention of proliferative diseases. J Nutr Biochem 2005;16:259–66.
303 Zhang M, Lee AH, Binns CW, et. al. Green tea consumption enhances survival of epithelial ovarian cancer. Int J Cancer 2004;112:465–9.
304 Bickers DR, Athar M. Novel approaches to chemoprevention of skin cancer. J Dematol 2000;27:691–5.
305 Yokoyama M, Noguchi M, Nakao Y, et. al. Anti-proliferative effects of the major tea polyphenol, (-) – epigallocatechin gallate and retinoic acid in cervical adenocarcinoma. Gyn Oncol 2008;108:326–31.
306 Roomi MW, Ivanov V, Kalinovsky T, et. al. Anticancer effect of lysine, proline, arginine, ascorbic acid and green tea extract on human renal adenocarcinoma. Line 786-0. Oncol Rep 2006;16:943–7.
307 The 3rd International Kidney Cancer Symposium Proceedings. Abstract #39 p-39, 2004.
308 Islami F, Pourshams A, Nasrollahzadeh D, et. al. Tea drinking habits and oesophageal cancer in a high risk area in northern Iran: population based case-control study. BMJ 2009;338:b929. doi:10.1136./bmj.b929.
309 Pfeuffer M, Schrezenmeir J. Addition of milk prevents vascular protective effects of tea. Eur Heart J 2007;28:1265–66.
310 van het Hof KH, Kivits GA, Weststrate JA, et. al. Bioavailability of catechins from tea: effect of milk. Eur J Clin Nutr 1998;52:356–359.
311 Galleone C, Pelucchi C, Levi F, et. al. Onion and garlic use and human cancer. Am J Clin Nutr 2006;84:1027–32.
312 Powolny AA, Singh SV. Multi-targeted prevention and therapy of cancer by diallyl trisulfide and related Allium vegetable-derived organosulfur compounds. Cancer Lett 2008;269:205–14.
313 Das A, Banik NL, Ray SK. Garlic compounds generate reactive oxygen species leading to activation of stress kinases and cysteine proteases for apoptosis in human glioblastoma T98G and U87MG cells. Cancer 2007;110:1083–95.
314 Kahnum F, Anilakumar KR, Viswanathan KR. Anticarcinogenic properties of garlic: a review. Crit Rev Food Sci Nutr 2004;44:479–88.
315 Ambrosone CB. Epidemiological evidence for haemopreventive effects of cruciferous vegetables on cancer risk. Proc Amer Assoc Cancer Res 2006;47.
316 Tang L, Zirpoli GR, Guru K, et. al. Consumption of raw cruciferous vegetables are inversely associated with bladder cancer risk. Cancer Epidemiol Biomarkers Prev 2008;17:938–44.
317 Kirsh DA, Peters U, Mayne ST, et. al. Prospective study of fruit and vegetable intake and risk of prostate cancer. J Natl Cancer Inst 2007;99:1200–9.
318 Lam TK, Gallicchio L, Lindesley K, et. al. Cruciferous vegetable consumption and lung cancer risk: a systematic review. Cancer Epidemiol Biomarkers Prev 2009;18:184–95.
319 Brennan P, Hsu CC, Moullan N, et. al. Effect of cruciferous vegetables on lung cancer in patients stratified by genetic status: a mendelian randomisation approach. Lancet 2005;366:1558–60.
320 Wong GWC, Bradlow HL, Sepkovic DW, et. al. A dose-ranging study of indole-3-carbinol for breast cancer prevention. J Cell Biol 1988;28:1100–06.
321 Bradlow HL, Sepkovic DW, Telang NT, et. al. Multifunctional aspects of the action of indole-3-carbinol as an antitumor agent. Ann NY Acad Sci 1999;889:204–13.
322 Grubbs CJ, Steele VE, Casebolt T, et. al. Chemoprevention of chemically-induced mammary carcinogenesis by indole-3-carbinol. Anticancer Res 1995;15:709–16.
323 Vallejo F, Tomás-Barberán FA, Garcia-Viguera C. Phenolic compound contents in edible parts of broccoli inflorescences after domestic cooking. J Sci Food Agric 2003;83:1511–16.
324 Oerlemans K, Barrett DM, Suades CM, et. al. Thermal degradation of glucosinolates in red cabbage. Food Chem 2006;95:19–29.
325 Giovannucci E, Rimm EB, Liu Y, et. al. A prospective study of cruciferous vegetables and prostate cancer. Cancer Epidemiol Biomarkers Prev 2003;12:1403–09.
326 Borchers AT, Stern JS, Hackman RN, et. al. Mushrooms, tumors, and immunity. Proc Soc Exp Biol Med 1999;221:281–93.
327 Jordinson M, El-Hariry I, Calnan D, et. al. Vicia faba, agglutinin, the lectin present in broad beans, stimulates the differentiation of undifferentiated colon cancer cells. Gut 1999;54:709–14.
328 Ng ML, Yap AT. Inhibition of human colon carcinoma development by lentinan from shitake mushrooms (Lentinus edodes). J Altern Complement Med 2002;8:581–89.

329 Sliva D, Jedinak A, Kawasaki J, et. al. Phellinus linteus suppresses growth, angiogenesis and invasive behaviour of breast cancer cells through the inhibition of AKT signalling. Br J Cancer 2008;98:1348–56.
330 Zaidman BZ, Yassin M, Mahajna J, et. al. Medicinal mushroom modulators of molecular targets as cancer therapeutics. Appl Microbiol Biotechnol 2005:67:453–68.
331 Collins L, Zhu T, Guo J, et. al. Phellinus linteus sensitizes apoptosis induced by doxorubicin in prostate cancer. Br J Cancer 2006;95:282–88.
332 Thyagarajan A, Zhu J, Sliva D. Combined effect of green tea and Ganoderma lucidum on invasive behaviour of breast cancer cells. Int J Oncol 2007;39:63–9.
333 Zhang M, Huang J, Xie X, et. al. Dietary intakes of mushrooms and green tea combined to reduce the risk of breast cancer in Chinese women. Int J Cancer 2009;124:1404–8.
334 Sliva D. Suppression of cancer invasiveness by dietary compounds. Mini Rev Med Chem 2008;8:677–88.
335 Ahn WS, Kim DJ, Chae GT, et. al. Natural killer cell activity and quality of life were improved by consumption of a mushroom extract, Agaricus blazel Murill Kyowa, in gynecological cancer patients undergoing chemotherapy. Int J Gynecol Cancer 2004;14:589–94.
336 Gao Y, Zhou S, Jiang W, et. al. Effects of ganopoly (Ganoderma lucidum polysaccharide extract) on the immune functions in advanced-stage cancer patients. Immunol Invest 2003;32:201–15.
337 Tsang KW, Lam CL, Yan C. Coriolus versicolor polysaccharide peptide slows progression of advanced non-small cell lung cancer. Respir Med 2003;97:618–24.
338 Kodama N, Komuta K, Nanba H. Can maitake MD-fraction aid cancer patients? Altern Med Rev 2002;7:236–39.
339 Korde LA, Wu AH, Fears T, et. al. Childhood soy intake and breast cancer risk in Asian American women. Cancer Epidemiol Biomarkers Prev 2009;18:1050–9.
340 Messina MJ. Emerging evidence on the role of soy and reducing prostate cancer risk. Nutr Rev 2003;61:117–31.
341 Xu W, Zheng W, Xiang Y, et. al. Soya food intake and risk of endometrial cancer among Chinese women in Shanghai: population based case-controlled study. BMJ 2004;328:1285. doi:10.1136/bmj.38093.646215.ae2006.
342 Nagata C, Takatsuka N, Kawakami N, et. al. A prospective cohort study of soy protein intake and stomach cancer death. Br J Cancer 2002;87:31–36.
343 Hussain M, Banerjee M, Sarkar FH, et. al. Soy isoflavones in the treatment of prostate cancer. Nutr Cancer 2003;47:111–17.
344 Vermeulen A. Metabolic effects of obesity in men. Verh K Acad Geneeskd Belg 1993;55:383–93.
345 Adlercruetz H, Höckerstedt K, Bannwart C, et. al. Effects of dietary components, including lignans and phytoestrogens on enterohepatic circulation and liver metabolism of estrogens and on sex hormone-binding globulin (SHGB). J Steroid Biochem 1987;27: 1135–44.
346 Evans BA, Griffiths K, Morton MS. Inhibition of 5 alpha-reductase in genital skin fibroblasts by dietary lignans and isoflavonoids. J Endocrinol 1995;147:295–302.
347 Zhou J, Li L, Pan W. Dietary soy and tea combinations for prevention of breast and prostate cancers by targeting metabolic syndrome elements in mice. AJCN 2007;86: s882–8.
348 Kuo SM, Morehouse HFJr, Lin CP. Effects of anti-proliferative flavonoids on ascorbic acid accumulation in human colon adenocarcinoma cells. Cancer Lett 1997;116:131–37.
349 Messina M, Bennick M. Soy foods, isoflavones and risk of colonic cancer: a review of the *in vitro* and *in vivo* data. Bailliere's Clin Endocrinol Metab 1998;12:707–25.
350 Akhter M, Iwasaki M, Yamaji T, et. al. Dietary isoflavone and the risk of colorectal adenoma: a case-control study in Japan. Br J Cancer 2009;100: 1812–16.
351 Yanagihara K, Ito A, Toge T, et. al. Anti-proliferative effects of isoflavones on human cancer cell lines established from the gastrointestinal tract. Cancer Res 1993;53:5815–21.
352 Uckun FM, Evans WE, Forsyth CJ, et. al. Biotherapy of beta-cell precursor leukemia by targeting genistein to CD19-associated tyrosine kinases. Sci 1995;267:886–91.
353 Su SJ, Yeh TM, Lei HY, et. al. The potential of soybean foods as a chemoprevention approach for human urinary tract cancer. Clin Cancer Res 2000;6:230–36.
354 Sun CL, Yuan JM, Arakawa K, et. al. Dietary soy an increased risk of bladder cancer: the Singapore Chinese Health Study. Cancer Epidemiol Biomarkers Prev 2002;11:1674–77.
355 Coward L, Smith M, Kirk M, et. al. Chemical modification of isoflavones is soy foods during cooking and processing. Am J Clin Nutr 1998; 68 (6 Suppl):1486S–1491S.
356 Farina HG, Pomies M, Alonso DF, et. al. Antitumor and antiangiogenic activity of soy isoflavone genistein in mouse models of melanoma and breast cancer. Oncol Rep 2006;16:885–91.
357 Li D, Yee JA, McGuire MH, et. al. Soybean isoflavones reduced experimental metastases in mice. J Nutr 1999;129:1075–78.
358 Raffoul JJ, Baneerjee S, Che M, et. al. Soy isoflavones enhance radiotherapy in a metastatic prostate cancer model. Int J Cancer 2007;120:2491–8.
359 Benavente-Garcia O, Castillo J. Update on uses and properties on citrus flavonoids: new findings in anticancer, cardiovascular, and anti-inflammatory activity. J Agric Food Chem 2008;56:6185–6205.
360 Bae JM, Lee EJ, Guyatt G. Citrus fruit intake and stomach cancer risk: a quantitative systematic review. Gastric Cancer 2008;11:23–32.
361 Brinkman M, Zeegers MP. Nutrition, total fluid and bladder cancer. Scand J Urol Nephrol Suppl 2008 Sep:25–36.
362 Bae JM, Lee EJ, Guyatt G. Citrus fruit intake and pancreatic cancer risk: a quantitative systematic review. Pancreas 2009;38:168–74.
363 Rossi M, Garavello W, Talamini R, et. al. Flavonoids and risk of squamous cell oesophageal cancer. Int J Cancer 2007;120:1560–4.
364 Monroe KR, Murphy SP, Kolonel LN. Prospective study of grapefruit intake and risk of breast cancer in post-menopausal women: the Multiethnic Cohort Study. Br J Cancer 2007;97:440–45.
365 Kim EH, Hankinson SE, Eliassen AH, et. al. A prospective study of grapefruit and grapefruit juice intake and breast cancer risk. Br J Cancer 2008;98:240–41.

366 Kane GC, Lipsky JJ. Drug- grapefruit juice interactions. Mayo Clin Proc 2000;75:933–42.
367 Palucchi C, Galeone C, Talamini R, et. al. Dietary folate and risk of prostate cancer in Italy. Cancer Epidemiol Biomarkers Prev 2005;14:944–8.
368 Shrubsole MJ, Jin F, Dai Q, et. al. Dietary folate intake and breast cancer risk: results from the Shanghai Breast Cancer Study. Cancer Res 2001;61:7136–41.
369 Chabath MB, Spitz MR, Lerner SP, et. al. Case-control analysis of dietary folate and risk of bladder cancer. Nutr Cancer 2005;53:144–51.
370 Palucchi C, Talamini R, Negri E, et. al. Folate intake and risk of oral and pharyngeal cancer. Ann Oncol 2003;14:1677–81.
371 Larsson SC, Giovannucci E, Wolk A. Dietary folate intake and the incidence of ovarian cancer: the Swedish Mammographic Cohort. J Natl Cancer Inst 2004;96:396–402.
372 Larsson SC, Håkansson N, Giovannucci E, et. al. Folate intake and pancreatic cancer incidence: a prospective study of Swedish women and men. J Natl Cancer Inst 2006;15:404–13.
373 Shen H, Wei Q, Pillow PC. Dietary folate intake and lung cancer risk in former smokers: a case control analysis. Cancer Epidemiol Biomarkers Prev 2003;12:980–6.
374 Strohle A, Wolters M, Hahn A. Folic acid and colorectal cancer prevention: a molecular mechanisms and epidemiologic evidence (Review). Int J Oncol 2005;26:1449–64.
375 Khanduja KL, Gandhi RK, Pathania V, et. al. Prevention of n- nitrosodiethylamine -induced lung tumorigenesis by ellagic acid and quercetin in mice. Food Chem Toxicol 1999;37:313–8.
376 Seeram NP, Adams LS, Henning SM, et. al. *In vitro* anti-proliferative, apoptotic and antioxidant activities of punicalagin, ellagic acid and a total pomegranate tannin extract are enhanced in combination with other polyphenols as found in pomegranate juice. J Nutr Biochem 2005;16:360–67.
377 Chen Q, Espey MG, Sun AY, et. al. Pharmacologic doses of ascorbate act as a prooxidant and decrease growth of aggressive tumor xenografts in mice. Proc Natl Acad Sci 2008;105:11105–9.
378 Padayatty SJ, Sun H, Wang Y. Vitamin C pharmacokinetics: implications for oral and intravenous use. Ann Intern Med 2004; 145:533–7.
379 Lippman SM, Klein EA, Goodman PJ, et. al. Effect of selenium and vitamin E on risk of prostate cancer and other cancers. The Selenium and Vitamin E Cancer Prevention Trial (SELECT). JAMA 2009;301:30–61. doi:10.1001/jama.2008.864.
380 Stoner GD, Mukhtar H. Polyphenols as chemopreventive agents. J Cell Biochem 1995;22(Suppl):169–80.
381 Edderkaoui M, Odianokova I, Ohno I, et. al. Ellagic acid induces apoptosis through inhibition of nuclear factor kappa B in pancreatic cancer cells. World J Gastroenterol 2008;14:3672–80.
382 Mertens-Talcott SU, Talcott S, Percival SS. Low concentrations of quercetin and ellagic acid synergistically influence proliferation, cytotoxicity and apoptosis in MOLT-4 human leukemia cells. J Nutr 2003;133:2669–74.
383 Pantuck AJ, Leppert JT, Zomorodian N, et. al. Phase II study of pomegranate juice for men with rising prostate-specific antigen following surgery or radiation for prostate cancer. Clin Cancer Res 2006;12:4018–26.
384 Xue CCL, Zhang AL, Lin B, et. al. Complementary and alternative medicine use in Australia: a national population-based survey. J Altern Complement Med 2007;13:643–650.
385 Yu SM, Kogan MD, Gergen P. Vitamin-mineral supplement use among preschool children in the United States. Pediatrics 1997;100:E4.
386 MacLennan AH, Myers SP, Taylor AW. Continuing use of complementary and alternative medicine in South Australia: cost and beliefs in 2004. Med J Aust 2006;184:27–31.
387 Shaikh U, Byrd RS, Auinger P. Vitamins and mineral supplement use by children and adolescents in 1999-2004. National Health and Nutrition Examination Survey: relationship with nutrition, food security, physical activity, health care access. Arch Pediatr Adolesc Med 2009;163:150–7.
388 Ishihara J, Sobue T, Yamamoto S, et. al. Demographics, lifestyles, characteristics, dietary intake among dietary supplement users in Japan. Int J Epidemiol 2003;32:546–53.
389 Ritchie MR. Use of herbal supplements and nutritional supplements in the UK: what do we know about there pattern of usage? Proc Nutr Soc 2007;66:479–82.
390 Michaud LB, Karpinski JP, Jones KL, et. al. Dietary supplements in patients with cancer: risks and key concepts, part 1. Am J Health Syst Pharm 2007;64:369–81.
391 Richardson MA, Sanders T, Palmer JL, et. al. Complementary/alternative medicine use in a comprehensive cancer center and the implications for oncology. J Clin Oncol 2000;18:2505–14.
392 Bernstein BJ, Grasso T. Prevalence of complementary and alternative medicine use in cancer patients. Oncology 2001;15:1267–72.
393 Molassiotis A, Cubbin D. 'Thinking outside the box': complementary and alternative therapies using pediatric oncology patients. Eur J Oncol Nurs 2004;8:50–60.
394 Ponholzer A, Struhal G, Madersbacher S. Frequent use of complementary medicine by prostate cancer patients. Eur Urol 2003;453:604–8.
395 Michaud LB, Karpinski JP, Jones KL, et. al. Dietary supplements in patients with cancer: risks and key concepts, part 2. Am J Health Syst Pharm 2007;64:467–80.
396 Ernst E. The current position of complementary/alternative medicine in cancer. Eur J Cancer 2003;39:2273–7.
397 Morse DS, Edwardsen EA, Gordon HS, et. al. Missed opportunities for interval empathy in lung cancer communication. Arch Intern Med 2008;168:1853–58.
398 Pollak KI, Arnold RM, Jeffreys AS, et. al. Oncologists communication about emotion during visits with patients with advanced cancer. J Clin Oncol 2007;25:5748–52.
399 Levinson W, Gorawara-Bhat R, Lamb J. A study of patient clues and physician responses in primary care and surgical settings. JAMA 2000;284:1021–27.
400 Epstein RM, Hadee T, Carroll J, et. al. 'Could this be something serious?' Reassurance, uncertainty, an empathy in response to patients' expressions of worry. J Gen Intern Med 2007;22:1731–39.
401 Stewart MA. What is a successful doctor-patient interview? Study of interactions and outcomes. Soc Sci Med 1984;19:167–75.
402 Fallowfield L, Jenkins F, Farewell V, et. al. Efficacy of a Cancer Research UK communication skills training model for oncologists: a randomised controlled trial. Lancet 2002;359:650–56.

403 Dimoska A, Girgis A, Hansen V, et. al. Perceived difficulties in consulting with patients and families: a survey of Australian cancer specialists. Med J Aust 2008;189:612–15.

404 Daugherty CK, Hlubocky FJ. What are terminally ill cancer patients told about their expected deaths? A study of cancer physicians' self- reports of prognosis disclosure. J Clin Oncol 2008;26:5988–93.

405 Clayton JM, Hancock K, Parker S, et. al. Sustaining hope when communicating with terminally ill patients and their families: a systematic review. Psychooncology 2008;17:641–59.

406 Girgis A, Hansen V, Goldstein D. Are Australian oncology health professionals burning out? A view from the trenches. Eur J Cancer 2009;45:93–99.

407 Warren S. The immediate cause of death in cancer. Am J Med Sci 1932;184:610–16.

408 Dewys WD, Begg C, Lavin PT, et. al. Prognostic effect of weight loss prior to chemotherapy in cancer patients. Eastern Cooperative Oncology Group. Am J Med 1986;69:491–97.

409 O'Gorman P, McMillan DC, McArdle CS. Impact of weight loss, appetite, and the inflammatory response and quality of life in gastrointestinal cancer patients. Nutr Cancer 1998;32:76–80.

410 Ottery FD. Definition of standardised nutritional assessment and interventional pathways in oncology nutrition. Nutrition1996;12:S15-S19.

411 Ovesen L, Hannibal J, Mortensen EL. The interrelationship of weight loss, dietary intake and quality of life in ambulatory patients with cancer of the lung, breast and ovary. Nutr Cancer 1993;19:159–67.

412 Andereyev HJ, Norman AR, Oates J, et. al. Why do patients with weight loss have worse outcome when undergoing chemotherapy for gastrointestinal malignancies? Eur J Cancer 1998;34:503–09.

413 National Institute for Clinical Excellence. Nutrition support in adults. Clinical guideline 32. NICE, London, 2006.

414 McWhirter JP, Pennington CR. Incidence and recognition of malnutrition in hospital. BMJ 1994;308:945–48.

415 Kelly IE, Tessier S, Cahill A, et. al. Still hungry in hospital: identifying malnutrition in acute hospital admissions. QJM 2000;93:93–8.

416 Spiro A, Baldwin C, Patterson A, et. al. The views and practice of oncologists toward nutritional support in patients receiving chemotherapy. Br J Cancer 2006;95:431–34.

417 Combs GF Jr. Current evidence and research and needs to support a health claim for selenium in cancer prevention. J Nutr 2005;135:343–7.

418 Mark SD, Qiao YL, Dawsey SM, et. al. Prospective study of serum selenium levels and incident oesophageal and gastric cancers. J Natl Cancer Inst 2000;92:1753–63.

419 Patrick L. Selenium biochemistry and cancer: a review of the literature. Altern Med Rev 2004;9: 239–58.

420 Clark LC, Combs GFJr, Turnbull BW, et. al. Effects of selenium supplementation for cancer prevention in patients with carcinoma of the skin. A randomised controlled trial. Nutritional Prevention of Cancer Study Group. JAMA 1996;276:1957–63.

421 Lippman SM, Klein EA, Goodman PJ, et. al. Effect of selenium and vitamin E on risk of prostate cancer and other cancers. The Selenium and Vitamin E Cancer Prevention Trial (SELECT). JAMA 2009;301:30–61. doi:10.1001/jama.2008.864.

422 Peters U, Littman AJ, Kristal AR. Vitamin E and selenium supplementation and risk of prostate cancer in the Vitamins and lifestyle (VITAL) study cohort. Cancer Causes Control 2008;19:75–87.

423 Combs JF Jr, Clark LC, Turnbull BW. Reduction of cancer risk with an oral supplement of selenium. Biomed Environ Sci 1997;10:227–34.

424 Myer F, Galan P, Douville P, et. al. Antioxidant, vitamin and mineral supplementation and prostate cancer prevention. SU.V1.MAX trial. Int J Cancer 2005;116:182–6.

425 Kim J, Sun P, Lam YW, et. al. Changes in serum proteomic patterns by presurgical alpha-tocopherol and L-selenomethionine supplementation in prostate cancer. Cancer Epidemiol Biomarkers Prev 2005;14:1697–702.

426 Yu SW, Mao BL, Xiao P, et. al. Intervention trial with selenium for the prevention of lung cancer among tin miners in Yunnan, China. A pilot study. Biol Trace Elem Res 1990;24:105–8.

427 Reid ME, Duffield-Lillico AJ, Garland L, et. al. Selenium supplementation and lung cancer incidence: an update of the nutritional prevention of cancer trial. Cancer Epidemiol Biomarkers Prev 2002;11:1285–91.

428 Helzlsouer KJ, Huang HY, Alberg AJ, et. al. Association between alpha-tocopherol, gamma-tocoperol, selenium and subsequent prostate cancer. J Natl Cancer Inst 2000;92:2018–23.

429 Huang HY, Alberg AJ, Norkus EP, et. al. Prospective study of antioxidant micronutrients in the blood and the risk of developing prostate cancer. Am J Epidemiol 2003;157:335–44.

430 Yamaguchi K, Uzzo RG, Pimkina J, et. al. Methylseleninic acid sensitizes prostate cancer cells to TRAIL-meditated apoptosis. Oncogene 2005;24:5868–77.

431 Hu H, Jiang C, Schuster T, et. al. Inorganic selenium sensitizes prostate cancer cells to TRAIL-induced apoptosis through superoxide/p53/Bax-mediated activation of mitochondrial pathway. Mol Cancer Ther 2006;5:1873–82.

432 Li Z, Carrier L, Rowan BG. Methylseleninic acid synergizes with taxmoifen to induce caspase-mediated apoptosis in breast cancer cells. Mol Cancer Ther 2008;7:3056–63.

433 Shah YM, L-Dhaheri M, Dong Y, et. al. Selenium disrupts estrogen receptor (alpha) signalling and potentiates tamoxifen antagonism in endometrial cancer cells in tamoxifen-resistant breast cancer cells. Mol Cancer Ther 2005;4:1239–49.

434 Sung L, Greenberg ML, Koren N, et. al. Vitamin E: the evidence for multiple roles in cancer. Nutr Cancer 2003;46:1–14.

435 Fleischauer AT, Simonsen N, Arab L. Antioxidants supplements and risk of breast cancer recurrence and breast cancer-related mortality among post-menopausal women. Nutr Cancer 2003;46:15–22.

436 Fleischauer AT, Olson SH, Mignone L, et. al. Dietary antioxidants, supplements, and risk of epithelial ovarian cancer. Nutr Cancer 2001;40:92–8.

437 Jacobs EJ, Henion AK, Briggs PJ. Vitamin C and vitamin E supplement use and bladder cancer mortality in a large cohort of US men and women. Am J Epidemiol 2002;156:1002–10.

438 Malafa MP, Fokum FB, Mowlavi A, et. al. Vitamin E inhibits melanoma growth in mice. Surgery 2002;131:85–91.

439 Neuzil J, Zhao M, Ostermann G, et. al. Alpha-tocopherol succinate, an agent with *in vivo* antitumor activity, uses apoptosis by causing lysosomal instability. Biochem J 2002;363:709–15.

440 Neuzil J, Weber T, Terman A. Vitamin E analogues as induces of apoptosis: implications for their potential antineoplastic role. Redox Rep 2001;6:143–51.

441 Tomic-Vatic A, Eytina J, Chapman J, et. al. Vitamin E amides, a new class of vitamin E analogues with enhanced proapoptotic activity. Int J Cancer 2005;117:188–93.

442 Schindler R, Mentlein R. Flavonoids and vitamin E induced the release of angiogenic peptide vascular endothelial growth factor from human tumor cells. J Nutr 2006;136:1477–82.

443 Carr AC, Frei B. Toward a new recommended dietary allowance for vitamin C based on antioxidant and health effects in humans. Am J Clin Nutr 1999;69:1086–07.

444 Hensen DE, Block G, Levine M. Ascorbic acid: biologic functions and relation to cancer. J Natl Cancer Inst 1991;83:547–52.

445 Kim KM, Pie JE, Park JH. Retinoic acid and ascorbic acid acts synergistically in inhibiting human breast cancer cell proliferation. J Nutr Biochem 2006;17:454–62.

446 Casciari JJ, Riordon NH, Schmidt TL et. al. Cytotoxicity of ascorbate, lipoic acid, and other antioxidants in hollow fibre *in vitro* tumours. Br J Cancer 2001;84:1544–50.

447 Bandera EV, Gifkins DM, Moore DF, et. al. Antioxidant vitamins and the risk of endometrial cancer: a dose-response meta-analysis. Cancer Causes Control 2009;20:699–711.

448 Bidoli E, Talamini R, Zucchetto A, et. al. Dietary vitamins E and C and prostate cancer risk. Acta Oncol 2009;18:1–5.

449 Lin J, Cook NR, Albert C, et. al. Vitamin C and E and beta-carotene supplementation and cancer risk: a randomised controlled trial. J Natl Cancer Inst 2009;101:14–23.

450 Gaziano JM, Glynn RJ, Christen WG, et. al. Vitamins E and C in the prevention of prostate and total cancer in men: the Physicians' Health Study II randomised controlled trial. JAMA 2009;301:52–62. doi:10.1001/jama.2008.862.

451 Block KI. Antioxidants: SELECTed out? Integr Cancer Ther 2009;8:5–8.

452 Dietrich M, Traber MG, Jacques PF, et. al. Does gamma-tocopherol play a role in the primary prevention of heart disease and cancer? A review. J Am Coll Nutr 2006;25:292–99.

453 Handelman GJ, Machlin LJ, Fitch K, et. al. Oral alpha-tocopherol supplements decrease plasma gamma-tocopherol levels in humans. J Nutr 1985;115:807–13.

454 Lodge JK. Vitamin E bioavailability in humans. J Plant Physiol 2005;162:790–6.

455 Kiyose C, Muramatsu R, Kameyama Y, et. al. Biodiscrimination of alpha-tocopherol stereoisomers in humans after oral administration. Am J Clin Nutr 1997;65:785–9.

456 Burton GW, Traber MG, Acuff RF, et. al. Human plasma and tissue alpha-tocopherol concentrations in response to supplementation with deuterated natural and synthetic vitamin E. Am J Clin Nutr 1998;67:669–84.

457 González MJ, Miranda-Massari JR, Mora EM, et. al. Orthomolecular oncology review: ascorbic acid in cancer 25 years later. Integr Cancer Ther 2005; 4:32–44.

458 Cameron E, Pauling L, Leibovitz B. Ascorbic acid in cancer: a review. Cancer Res 1979;39:663–81.

459 Moertel CG, Fleming TR, Creagan ET, et. al. High-dose vitamin C versus placebo in the treatment of patients with advanced cancer who have had no prior chemotherapy. A randomised double-blind comparison. N Eng J Med 1985;312:137–41.

460 Padayatty SJ, Riordon HD, Hewitt SM, et. al. Intravenously administered vitamin C as cancer therapy: three cases. CMAJ 2006;174:937–42.

461 Riordan HD, Riordan NH, Jackson JA, et. al. Intravenous vitamin C as a chemotherapy agent: a report on clinical cases. P R Health Sci J 2004:23:115–8.

462 Drisko JA, Chapman J, Hunter VJ. The use of antioxidants with first-line chemotherapy in two cases of ovarian cancer. J Am Coll Nutr 2003;22:118–23.

463 Yeom CH, Jung GC, Song KJ. Changes of terminal cancer patients' health-related quality of life after high dose vitamin C administration. J Korean Med Sci 2007:22:7–11.

464 Studzinski GP, Moore DC. Sunlight – can it prevent as well as cause cancer? Cancer Res 1995;55:4014–22.

465 Garland CF, Frank PH, Garland C, et. al. Dealing with innovation and uncertainty, the role of vitamin D in cancer prevention. Am J Public Health 2006;96:252–61.

466 Hughes AM, Armstrong PK, Vajdic CM, et. al. Sun exposure may protect against non-Hodgkin lymphoma: a case-control study. Int J Cancer 2004;112:865–71.

467 Grant WB. How strong is the evidence that ultraviolet B and vitamin D reduce the risk of cancer? Dermato Endocrinol 2009;1:17–24.

468 Moan J, Porojnicu AC, Dahlback A, et. al. Addressing the health benefits and risk, involving vitamin D or skin cancer, of increased sun exposure. Proc Natl Acad Sci USA 2008;105:668–73.

469 Ginde AA, Liu MC, Camargo CA Jr. Demographic differences and trends of vitamin D insufficiency in the US population, 1988-2004. Arch Intern Med 2009;23:626–32.

470 Goodwin PJ. Vitamin D in cancer patients: above all, do no harm. J Clin Oncol 2009;27:2117–19.

471 Lim HS, Roychoudhuri R, Peto J, et. al. Cancer survival is dependant on season of diagnosis and sunlight exposure. Int J Cancer 2006;119:1530–36.

472 Freedman DM, Dosemeci M, McGlynn K, et. al. Sunlight and mortality from breast, ovarian, colon, prostate and non-melanoma skin cancer: a composite death certificate based case-control study. Occup Environ Med 2002;59:257–62.

473 Zhou W, Heist RS, Liu G, et. al. Circulating 25-hydroxyvitamin D levels predicts survival in early-stage non-small-cell lung cancer patients. J Clin Oncol 2007;25:479–85.

474 Fairfield KM, Fletcher RH. Vitamins for chronic disease prevention in adults. JAMA 2002;287:3116–26.

475 Huang HY, Caballero B, Chang S, et. al. Multivitamin/mineral supplements and prevention of chronic disease. Evid Rep Technol Assess (Full Rep) 2006;139:1–117.

476 Ames BN. DNA damage from micronutrient deficiencies is likely to be a major cause of cancer. Mutat Res 2001;475:7–20.

477 Xu Q, Parks CG, DeRoo LA, et. al. Multivitamin use and telomere length in women. Am J Clin Nutr 2009;89:1857–63.

478 Neuhouser ML, Wassertheil-Smoller S, Thomson C, et. al. Multivitamin use and risk of cancer and cardiovascular disease in the Women's Health Initiative cohorts. Arch Intern Med 2009;169:294–304.

479 Block G, Jensen CD, Norkus EP, et. al. Usage patterns, health, and nutritional status of long-term multiple dietary supplement users: a cross- sectional study. Nutr J 2007;6:30. doi:10.1186/1475-2891-6-30.

480 Sebastian RS, Cleveland LE, Goldman JD, et. al. Older adults who use vitamin/mineral supplements differ from non-users in nutrient intake adequacy and dietary attitudes. J Am Diet Assoc 2007;107: 1322–32.

481 Rock CL. Multivitamin-multimineral supplements: who uses them? Am J Clin Nutr 2007;85: 277S-279S.

482 The Alpha-Tocopherol, Beta-Carotene Cancer Prevention Study Group. The effect of vitamin E and beta-carotene on the incidence of lung cancer and other cancers in male smokers. N Eng. J Med 1994;330:1029–35.

483 Gann PH. Randomised trials of antioxidant supplementation for cancer prevention. JAMA 2009;301:102–103.

484 Lamm DL, Riggs DR, Shriver JS, et. al. Megadose vitamins in bladder cancer: a double-blind clinical trial. J Urol 1994;151:21–6.

485 Konety BR, Lavelle JP, Pirtskalaishvili G, et. al. Effects of vitamin D (calcitriol) on transitional cell carcinoma of the bladder in vitro and in vivo. Journal of Urology 2001;165:253–8.

486 Block KI, Koch AC, Mead MN, et. al. Impact of antioxidant supplementation on chemotherapeutic toxicity: a systematic review of the evidence from randomised controlled trials. Int J Cancer 2008;123:177–239.

487 Lawenda BD, Kelly KM, Ladas EJ. Should supplemental antioxidant administration be avoided during chemotherapy and radiation therapy? J Natl Cancer Inst 2008;100:773–83.

488 Moss RW. Should patients undergoing chemotherapy and radiotherapy be prescribed antioxidants? Integr Cancer Ther 2006;5:63–82.

489 Drisko JA, Chapman J, Hunter VJ. The use of antioxidant therapies during chemotherapy. Gynecol Oncol 2003;88:434–39.

490 Simone CB, Simone NL, Simone V, et. al. Antioxidants and other nutrients do not interfere with chemotherapy or radiation therapy and can increase kill and increase survival, part 1. Altern Ther 2007;13:22–28.

491 Simone CB 2nd, Simone NL, Simone V, et. al. Antioxidants and other nutrients do not interfere with chemotherapy or radiation therapy and can increase kill and increase survival, Part 2. Altern Ther Health Med 2007;13:40–7.

492 Pathak AK, Bhutani M, Guleria R, et. al. Chemotherapy alone vs. chemotherapy plus high dose multiple antioxidants in patients with advanced non-small cell lung cancer. JACN 2005;24:16–21.

493 Kreienberg R. Therapy of anthracycline-resistant metastatic breast carcinoma. Schweiz Rundsch Med Prax1998;87:573–7.

494 Clemens MR, Ladner C, Ehninger G, et. al. Plasma vitamin E and beta-carotene concentrations during radiochemotherapy preceeding bone marrow transplantation. Am J Clin Nutr 1990;51:216–219.

495 Bhuvarahamurthy V, Balasubramanian N, Govindasamy S. Effect of radiotherapy and chemoradiotherapy on the circulating antioxidants system of human uterine cervical carcinoma. Mol Cell Biochem 1996;158:7–23.

496 Clemens MR, Ladner C, Schmidt H, et. al. Decreased essential antioxidants and increased lipid hydroperoxides following high-dose radiochemotherapy. Free Radic Res Commun1989;7:227–232.

497 Clemens MR, Ladner C, Schmidt H, et. al. Decreased essential antioxidants and increased lipid hydroperoxides following high-dose radiochemotherapy. Free Radic Res Comm 1989; 7(3-6):227–32.

498 Dreizen S, McCredie KB, Keating MJ, et. al. Nutritional deficiencies in patients receiving cancer chemotherapy. Postgrad Med 1990;87:163–67.

499 Weijl NI, Hopman GD, Wipkink-Bakker A, et. al. Cisplatin combination chemotherapy induces a fall in plasma antioxidants of cancer patients. Ann Oncol 1998;9:1331–37.

500 Concato J, Shah N, Horowitz RI. Randomised, controlled trials, observational studies and the hierarchy of research designs. Eng J Med 2000;342:1887–92.

501 Recchia F, Rea S, Pompili P, et. al. Beta-interferon, retinoids and tamoxifen as maintenance therapy in metastatic breast cancer. A pilot study. Clin Ter 1995;146:603–61.

502 Wood LA. Possible prevention of adriamycin-induced alopecia by tocopherol. NEJM 1985;312:1060.

503 Labriola D, Livingston R. Possible interactions in dietary antioxidants and chemotherapy. Oncology 1999;13:1003–8.

504 Ali BH, Al Moundhri MS. Agents ameliorating or augmenting nephrotoxicity of cisplatin and other platinum compounds. A review of some recent research. Food Chem Toxicol 2006;44:1173–83.

505 Lamson DW, Brignall MS. Antioxidants in cancer therapy; there actions and interactions with oncologic therapies. Altern Med Rev 1999;4: 304–29.

506 Ohkawa K, Tsukada Y, Dohzono H, et. al. The effects of co-administration of selenium and cis-platin (CDDP) on CDDP-induced toxicity and antitumour activity. Br J Cancer 1988;58:38–41.

507 Seifried HE, McDonald SS, Anderson D, et. al. The antioxidant conundrum in cancer. Cancer Res 2003;63:4295–8.

508 Pace A, Savarese A, Picardo M, et. al. Neuroprotective effect of vitamin E supplementation in patients treated with cisplatin chemotherapy. J Clin Oncol 2003;21:927–31.

509 Braun L, Cohen M. Herbs and natural supplements, an evidence-based guide. Marrickville Elsevier 2007.

510 Constantinou AI, White BE, Tonetti D, et. al. The soy isoflavone diadzein improves the capacity of tamoxifen to prevent mammary tumours. Eur J Cancer 2005;41:647–54.

511 Dürr D, Stieger B, Kullak-Ublick GA, et. al. St. John's wort induces intestinal P-glycoprotein/MDR1 and intestinal and hepatic CYP3A 4. Clin Pharmacol Ther 2000;68:598–604.

512 Roby CA, Anderson GD, Kantor E, et. al. St. John's Wort: effect on CYP3A4 activity. Clin Pharmacol Ther 2000;67:451–7.

513 Gurley BJ, Gardner SF, Hubbard MA, et. al. *In vivo* assessment of botanical supplementation on human cytochrome P450 phentypes: Citrus aurantium, Echinacea purpurea, milk thistle and saw palmetto. Clin Pharmacol Ther 2004;76:428–40.

514 DiCenzo R, Shelton M, Jordan K, et. al. Coadministration of milk thistle and indinavir in healthy subjects. Pharmacotherapy 2003;23:866–70.

515 Leber HW, Knauff S. Influence of silymarin on drug metabolising enzymes in rat and man. Arznemittelforschung 1976;26:1603–5.
516 Piscitelli SC, Formentini E, Burstein AH, et. al. The effect of milk thistle on the pharmacokinetics on indinavir in healthy volunteers. Pharmacotherapy 2002;22:551–6.
517 Sofi F, Cesari F, Abbate R, et. al. Adherence to Mediterranean diet and health status: meta-analysis. BMJ 2008;337. doi:10.1136/bmj.a1344.
518 Knoops KT, de Groot LC, Kromhout D, et. al. Mediterranean diet, lifestyle factors, and 10-year mortality in elderly European men and women: the Hale project. JAMA 2004;292:1433–9.
519 Mitrou PN, Kipnis V, Thiebaut AC, et. al. Mediterranean dietary pattern in prediction in all-cause mortality in a US population. Arch Intern Med 2007,167:2461–68.
520 Heidemann C, Schulze MB, Franco OH, et. al. Dietary patterns and risk of mortality from cardiovascular disease, cancer, and all cause in a prospective cohort of women. Circulation 2008;118:230–37.
521 van Dam RM, Li T, Spiegelman D, et. al. Combined impact of lifestyle factors on mortality: prospective cohort study in US women. BMJ 2008;337:a1440.
522 Cant AK, Leitzmann MF, Park Y, et. al. Patterns of recommended dietary behaviours predicts subsequent risk of mortality in a large cohort of men and women in the United States. J Nutr 2009;27 (epub ahead of print)
523 Morey MC, Snyder DC, Sloane R, et. al. Effects of home-based diet and exercise on functional outcomes among older overweight long-term cancer survivors. JAMA 2009;301:1883–91.
524 Duffy SA, Ronis DL, McLean S, et. al. Pretreatment health behaviours predict survival among patients with head and neck squamous cell carcinoma. J Clin Oncol 2009;27:1930–2.
525 Ma RW, Chapman K. A systematic review of the effect of diet in prostate cancer prevention and treatment. J Hum Nutr Diet 2009;22:187–99.
526 Pierce JP, Stefanick ML, Flatt SW, et. al. Greater survival after breast cancer in physically active women with high vegetable intake regardless of obesity. J Clin Oncol 2007;25:2345–51.
527 Dray X, Boutron-Ruault MC, Bertrais S, et. al. Influence of dietary factors on colorectal cancer survival. Gut 2003;352:868–73.
528 Meyerhardt JA, Niedzwiecki D, Hollis D, et. al. Association of dietary patterns with cancer recurrence and survival in patients with stage III colon cancer. JAMA 2007;298:754–64.
529 Davies A, Smith GD, Harbord R, et. al. Nutritional interventions and outcome in patients with cancer or pre-invasive lesions: systematic review. J Natl Cancer Inst 2006;98:961–73.
530 Baron JA. (Nutritional) Chemoprevention of cancer:What's up? JNCI 2006;98:945–46.
531 Petterson M. The camptothecin tree: harvesting a Chinese anticancer compound in the US Altern Ther Health Med 1996;2:23–24.
532 Tyagi A, Raina K, Singh RP, et. al. Chemopreventive effects of silymarin and silybilin on N-butyl-N-(4-hydroxybutyl) nitrosamine induced urinary bladder carcinogenesis in male ICR mice. Mol Cancer Ther 2007;6:3248–55.
533 Roy S, Kaur M, Agarwal C, et. al. P21 and P27 induction by silibilin is essential for its cell cycle arrest in prostate carcinoma cells. Mol Cancer Ther 2007;6:2696–707.
534 Agarwal R, Agarwal C, Ichikawa H, et. al. Anticancer potential of silymarin: from bench to bed side. Anticancer Res 2006;26:4457–98.
535 Singh RP, Deep G, Chittezhath M, et. al. Effect of silibinin on the growth and progression of primary lung tumours in mice. J Natl Cancer Inst 2006;98:846–55.
536 Gaedke J, Fels LM, Bokemeyer C, et. al. Cisplatin nephrotoxicity and protection by silibinin. Nephrol Dial Transplant 1996;11:55–62.
537 Ladas EJ, Kelly KM. Milk thistle is there a role for its use as an adjunct therapy in patients with cancer. J Altern Complement Med 2003;9:411–16.
538 Scamdia G, De Vincenzo R, Ranelletti FO, et. al. Anti-proliferative effect of silybin on gynaecological malignancies: synergism with cisplatin and doxyrubicin. Eur J Cancer 1996;32:877–82.
539 Giacomelli S, Gallo D, Apollonio P, et. al. Silybin and its bioavailable phospholipid complex (1dB1016) potentiate *in vitro* and *in vivo* the activity of cisplatin. Life Sci 2002;70:1447–59.
540 Chung CH, Go P, Chang KH. PSK immunotherapy in cancer patients: a preliminary report. Zhonghua Min Guo Wei Sheng Wu Ji Mian Yi Xue Za Zhi 1987;20:210–17.
541 Nio Y, Tsubono M, Tseng CC, et. al. Immunomodulation orally administered protein-bound polysaccharide PSK in patients with gastrointestinal cancer. Biotherapy 1992;4:117–20.
542 Ohwada S, Ikeya T, Yokomori T, et. al. Adjuvant immunochemotherapy with oral Tegafur/Uracil plus PSK in patients with stage II or III colorectal cancer: a randomised controlled study. Br J Cancer 2004;90:1003–10.
543 Hayakawa K, Mitsuhashi N, Saito Y, et. al. Effect of krestin (PSK) as adjuvant treatment on prognosis after radical radiotherapy in patients with non- small cell lung cancer. Anticancer Res 1993;13:1815–20.
544 Leino Y, et. al. 8-year results of adjuvant chemotherapies versus chemotherapy in the treatment of operable breast cancer. Proceedings 18th International Congress of Chemotherapy. Stockholm Sweden p. 162, 1993.
545 Nakazato H, Koike O, Saji S, et. al. Efficacy of immunochemotherapy as adjuvant treatment after the curative resection of gastric cancer. Study Group of Immunochemotherapy with PSK for gastric cancer. Lancet 1994;343:1122–26.
546 Boon H, Wong J. Botanical medicine and cancer: a review of the safety and efficacy. Expert Opin Pharmacother 2004;5:2485–2501.
547 Kaegi E. Unconventional therapies for cancer 1. Essiak. CMAJ 1998:158:897–902.
548 Rice S, Amon A, Whitehead SA. Ethanolic extracts of black cohosh (Actacea racemosa) inhibit growth and oestradiol synthesis from oestrone sulfate in breast cancer cells. Maturitas 2007;56:359–67.
549 Einbond LS, Su T, Wu HA, et. al. The growth inhibitory effect of actein on human breast cancer cells is associated with activation of stress response pathways. Int J Cancer 2007;121:2073–83.
550 Einbond LS, Su T, Wu HA, et. al. Gene expression analysis of the mechanisms whereby black cohosh inhibits human breast cancer cell growth. Anticancer Res 2007;27:697–712.
551 Walji R, Boon H, Guns E, et. al. Black cohosh (Cimicifuga racemosa (L.) Nutt): safety and efficacy for cancer patients. Support Care Cancer 2007;15:913–91.

552 Horneber M, Bueschel G, Huber R, et. al. Mistletoe therapy in oncology. Cochrane Database Syst Rev 2008, Issue 2. Art. No:CD003297. doi:10.1002/14651858.CD003297.pub2.
553 Kaegi E. Unconventional therapies for cancer. 3. Iscador CMAJ 1998;158:1157–59.
554 Cleijnen J, Knipschild P. Mistletoe treatment for cancer: review of controlled trials in humans. Phytomedicine 1994;1:255–60.
555 Ernst E, Schmidt K, Steuer-Vogt MK. Mistletoe for cancer? A systematic review of randomised clinical trials. Int J Cancer 2003;107: 262–67.
556 Sali A. (Editorial) Cancer treatment on dependent on histological classification. Int Clin Nutr Rev 1989;9:113–5.
557 Schumacher U, Stamouli A, Adam E, et. al. Biochemical, histochemical and cell biological investigations on the actions of mistletoe lectins I, II and III with human breast cancer cell lines. Glycoconj J 1995;12:250–7.
558 Shin HJ, Kim YS, Kwak YS, et. al. Enhancement of antitumour effects of paclitaxel (taxol) in combination with red ginseng acidic polysaccharide (RGAP). Planta Med 2004;70:1033–8.
559 Helms S. Cancer prevention and therapeutics: Panax ginseng. Altern Med Rev 2004;9:259–74.
560 Park IH, Piao LZ, Kwon SW, et. al. Cytotoxic dammarane glycosides from processed ginseng. Chem Pharm Bull (Tokyo) 2002;50:538–40.
561 Liu WK, Xu SX, Che CT. Anti-proliferative effect of ginseng saponins on human prostate cancer cell line. Life Sci 2000;67:1297–306.
562 Nakata H, Kikuchi Y, Tode T, et. al. Inhibitory effects of ginsenoside Rh2 on tumour growth in nude mice bearing ovarian cancer cells. Jpn J Cancer Res 1998;89:733–40.
563 Hasegawa H, Suzuki R, Nagaoka T, et. al. Prevention of growth and metastases of murine melanoma through enhanced natural-killer cytotoxicity by fatty acid-conjugate of protopanaxatriol. Biol Pharm Bull 2002:25: 861–66.
564 Sato K, Mochizuki M, Saiki I, et. al. Inhibition of tumour angiogenesis and metastases by a saponin of Panax ginseng, ginsenoside-Rb2. Biol Pharm Bull 1994;17:635–9.
565 Yun TK. Experimental and epidemiological evidence on non-organ specific cancer preventive effect of Korean ginseng and identification of active compounds. Mutat Res 2003;523:63–74.
566 Yun TK, Choi SY. A case-control study of ginseng intake in cancer. Int J Epidemiol 1990;90:871–6.
567 Choi CH, Kang G, Min YD. Reversal of P-glycoprotein-mediated multidrug resistance by protopanaxatriol ginsenosides from Korean red ginseng. Planta Med 2003;79:235–40.
568 Kim JY, Lee KW, Kim SH, et. al. Inhibitory effect of tumour cell proliferation and induction of G2/M cell cycle arrest by panaxytriol. Planta Med 2002;68:119–22.
569 Jia WW, Bu X, Philips D, et. al. Rh2, a compound extracted from ginseng, hypersensitises multidrug-resistant tumour cells to chemotherapy. Can J Physiol Pharmacol 2004;82:431–7.
570 Min KT, Koo BN, Kang JW, et. al. The effect of ginseng saponins on the recombinant serotonin type 3A receptor expressed in xenopus oocytes: implication of possible application as an anti-emetic. J Altern Complement Med 2003;9:505–10.
571 Konishi F, Tanaka K, Himeno K, et. al. Antitumour effect induced by a hot water extract of Chlorella vulgaris (CV): resistance to Meth-A tumour growth mediated by CE-induced polymorphonuclear leukocytes. Cancer Immunol Immunother 1985;19:73–8.
572 Tanaka K, Tomita Y, Tsuruta M, et. al. Oral administration of Chlorella vulgaris augments concomitant antitumour immunity. Immunopharmacol Immunotoxicol 1990;12:277–91.
573 Pugh N, Ross S, Elsohly HN, et. al. Isolation of three high molecular weight polysaccharide preparations with potent immuno-stimulatory activity from Spirulina platensis, aphanizomenon flos-aquae and Chlorella pyrenoidosa. Planta Med 2001;67:737–742.
574 Merchant RE, Wright CD, Young HF. Dietary chlorella pyrenoidosa for patients with malignant glioama: effects on immuno-competence, quality of life, and survival. Phytother Res 1994;220–28.
575 Inohara H, Raz A. Effects of natural complex carbohydrate (citrus pectin) on murine melanoma cell properties related to galectin-3 functions. Glycoconj J 1994;11:527–32.
576 Pienta KJ, Naik H, Akhtar A, et. al. Inhibition of spontaneous metastasis in a rat prostate cancer model by oral administration of modified citrus pectin. J Natl Cancer Inst 1995;87:348–53.
577 Nangia-Makker P, Hogan V, Honjo Y, et. al. Inhibition of human cancer cell growth and metastasis in nude mice by oral intake of modified citrus pectin. J Natl Cancer Inst 2002;94:1854–62.
578 Liu HY, Huang ZL, Yang GH, et. al. Inhibitory effect of modified citrus pectin on liver metastases in a mouse colon cancer model. World J Gastroenterol 2008;14:7386–91.
579 Glinsky VV, Raz A. Modified citrus pectin anti-metastatic properties: one bullet, multiple targets. Carbohydr Res 2008 Sep 26. doi:10.1016/j.resaas.2008.08.038.
580 Nangia-Makker P, Hogan V, Honjo Y, et. al. Inhibition of human cancer cell growth and metastasis in nude mice by oral intake of modified citrus pectin. J Natl Cancer Inst 2002;18:1854–62.
581 Guess BW, Scholz MC, Strum SB, et. al. Modified citrus pectin (MCP) increases the prostate-specific antigen doubling time in men with prostate cancer: a phase II pilot study. Prostate Cancer Prostatic Dis 2003;6:301–4.
582 Chauhan D, Li G, Podar K, et. al. A novel carbohydrate-based therapeutic GCS-100 overcomes bortezomib resistance and enhances dexamethasone-induced apoptosis in multiple myeloma cells. Cancer Res 2005;65:8350–58.
583 Johnson KD, Glinskii OV, Mossine VV, et. al. Galectin-3 as a potential therapeutic target in tumors arising from malignant endothelia. Neoplasia 2007;9:662–70.
584 Das S. Garlic — A Natural Source of Cancer Preventive Compounds. Asian Pac J Cancer Prev 2002;3:305–11.
585 Khanum F, Anilakumar KR, Viswanathan KR. Anticarcinogenic properties of garlic: a review. Crit Rev Food Sci Nutr 2004;44:479–88.
586 Sengupta A, Ghosh S, Bhattacharjee S. Allium vegetables in cancer prevention: an overview. Asian Pac J Cancer Prev 2004;5:237–45.
587 Hsing AW, Chokkalingam AP, Gao YT, et. al. Allium vegetables and risk of prostate cancer: a population-based study. J Natl Cancer Inst 2002;94:1648–51.

588 Ernst E. Can allium vegetables prevent cancer? Phytomedicine 1997;4:79–83.
589 Fleischauer AT, Poole C, Arab L. Garlic consumption and cancer prevention: meta-analyses of colorectal and stomach cancers. Am J Clin Nutr 2000;72:1047–52.
590 Tanaka S, Haruma K, Yoshihara M, et. al. Aged garlic extract has potential suppressive effect on colorectal adenomas in humans. J Nutr 2006;136:821–27.
591 Patyia M, Zahjlka MA, Vanichkin A, et. al. Allicin stimulates lymphocytes and elicits an antitumor effect: a possible role of p21ras. Int Immunol 2004;16:275–81.
592 Hassan ZM, Yaraee R, Zare N, et. al. Immunomodulatory affect of R10 fraction of garlic extract on natural killer activity. Int Immunopharmacol 2003;3:1483–9.
593 Manusrivithayaa S, Srieramote M, Tangjitgamol S, et. al. Antiemetic effect of ginger in gynecologic oncology patients receiving cisplatin. Int J Gynecol Cancer 2004;14:1063–9.
594 Myer K, Schwartz J, Crater D, et. al. Zingiber officinale (ginger) used to prevent 8-Mop associated nausea. Dermatol Nurs 1995;7:242–4.
595 Sontakke S, Thawani V, Naik MS. Ginger as an anti-emetic in nausea and vomiting induced by chemotherapy: a randomised cross-over double-blind study. Indian J Pharmacol 2003;35:32–6.
596 Shibata S. A drug over the millennia: pharmacognosy, chemistry and pharmacology of licorice. Yakugaku Zasshi 2000;120:849–62.
597 Wang ZY, Nixon DW. Licorice and cancer. Nutr Cancer 2001;39:1–11.
598 Rafi MM, Vastano BC, Zhu N, et. al. Novel polyphenol a molecule isolated from licorice root (Glycrrhiza glabra) induces apoptosis, G2/M cell arrest, and Bci-2 phosphorylation in tumor cell lines. J Agric Food Chem 2002;50:677–84.
599 Kanazawa M, Satomi Y, Mizutani Y, et. al. Isoliquiritigenin inhibits the growth of prostate cancer. Eur Urol 2003;43:580–6.
600 Zhang Z, Xu J, Yao B, et. al. Inhibition of 11beta-hydroxysteroid dehydrogenase type II selectively blocks the tumor COX-2 pathway and suppresses colon carcinogenesis in mice and humans. J Clin Invest 2009;119:876–85.
601 Stewart PM, Prescott SM. Can licorice lick colon cancer? J Clin Invest 2009;119:760–3.
602 Taixiang W, Munro AJ, Guanjian L. Chinese medical herbs for chemotherapy side-effects in colorectal cancer patients. Cochrane Database Syst Rev 2005;(1):CD004540.
603 Melchart D, Clemm C, Weber B, et. al. Polysaccharides isolated from Echinacea purpurea herbal cell cultures to counteract undesired effects of chemotherapy–a pilot study. Phytother Res 2002;16:138–42.
604 Ahn WS, Kim DJ, Chae GT, et. al. Natural killer cell activity and quality of life were improved by consumption of a mushroom extract, Agaricus blazei Murill Kyowa, in gynecological cancer patients undergoing chemotherapy. Int J Gynecol Cancer 2004;14:589–94.
605 Wei X, Chen Z, Yang X, et. al. Medicinal herbs for esophageal cancer. Cochrane Database Syst Rev 2007;(2) Art.No:CD004520. doi:10.1002/14651858.CD004520.pub5.
606 Xu Z, Cai WM, Qin DX, et. al. 'Chinese herb destagnation' series 1:combination of radiation with destagnation in the treatment of nasopharyngeal carcinoma. (NPC): a prospective randomised trial on 188 cases. Int J Rad Oncol Biol Phys 1989;16:297–300.
607 Liu CL, Wang YD, Jin XJ. Clinical observation on treatment of non-small cell lung cancer with Chinese herbal medicine combined with bronchial arterial infusion chemotherapy. (Chinese) Zhongguo Zhong Xi Yi Jie He Za Zhi 2001;21:579–81.
608 Zhou K, Wang J, Liu B. Clinical study on effect of shenqi fuzheng injection combined with chemotherapy in treating gastric cancer. (Chin) Zhongguo Zhong Xi Yi Jie He Za Zhi 1999;19: 11–13.
609 Oka H, Yamamoto S, Kuroki T, et. al. Prospective study of chemoprevention of hepatocellular carcinoma with Sho-saiko-to (TJ-9). Cancer 1995;76:743–49.
610 Zhang M, Liu X, Li J, et. al. Chinese medicinal herbs treat the side-effects of chemotherapy in breast cancer patients. Cochrane Database Syst Rev 2007;(2):Art. No.CD004921. doi:10.1002/14651858.CD004921. pub2.
611 de la Taille A, Hayek OR, Buttyan R, et. al. Effects of a phytotherapeutic agent, PC-SPES, on prostate cancer: a preliminary investigation on human cell lines and patients. Br J Urol Int 1999;84:845–50.
612 Pandha HS, Kirby RS. PC-SPES: phytotherapy for prostate cancer. Lancet 2002;359:2213–5.
613 Di Paola RS, Zhang H, Lambert JH, et. al. Clinical and biological activity of an oestrogenic herbal combination (PC-SPES) in prostate cancer. N Eng J Med 1998;339:785–91.
614 White J. PC-SPES- a lesson for future dietary supplement research. J Natl Cancer Inst 2002;94: 1261–63.
615 Lissoni P, Malugani F, Bordin V, et. al. A new neuroimmunotherapeutic strategy of subcutaneous low-dose interleukin-2 plus the long-acting opioid antagonist naltrexone in metastatic cancer patients progressing on interleukin-2 alone. Neuro Endocrinol Lett 2002;23:255–8.
616 Berkson BM, Rubin DM, Berkson AJ. The long-term survival of a patient with pancreatic cancer with metastases to the liver after treatment with the intravenous alpha-lipoic acid/low-dose naltrexone protocol. Integr Cancer Ther 2006;5:83–9.
617 Berkson BM, Rubin DM, Berkson AJ. Reversal of signs and symptoms of a B-cell lymphoma in a patient using only low-dose naltrexone. Integr Cancer Ther 2007;6:293–6.
618 Zagon IN, McLaughlin PJ. Opioid antagonists inhibit the growth of metastatic murine neuroblastoma. Cancer Lett 1983;21:89–94.
619 McLaughlin PJ, Levin RJ, Zagon IS. Opioid growth factor (OGF) inhibits the progression of human squamous cell carcinoma of the head and neck transplanted into nude mice. Cancer Lett 2003;199:209–17.
620 Hytrek SD, McLaughlin PJ, Lang CM, et. al. Inhibition of human colon cancer by intermittent opioid receptor blockade with naltrexone. Cancer Lett 1996;101:159–64.
621 Donahue RN, McLaughlin PJ, Zagon IS. Cell proliferation of human ovarian cancer is regulated by the opioid growth factor-opioid growth factor receptor axis. Am J Physiol Regul Integr Comp Physiol 2009;296:R1716–25.
622 Bilhari B, Keynote Address. Presented at: 1st Annual Low Dose Naltrexone Conference, New York Academy of Sciences. June, 11, New York. NW 2005.
623 Wu B. The effect of acupuncture on the regulation of cell-mediated immunity in the patients with malignant tumours. Zhen Ci Yan Jiu 1995;20: 67–71.

624 Vickers AJ. Can acupuncture have specific effects on health- a systematic review of acupuncture trials. J Roy Soc Med 1996;89:303–11.
625 Klein J, Griffith D. Acupressure for nausea and vomiting in cancer patients receiving chemotherapy. Br J Comm Nurs 2004;9:383–88.
626 Roscoe JA, Morrow GR, Hickok JT. The efficacy of acupressure and acustimulation wrist bandsfor the relief of chemotherapy-induced nausea and vomiting. A University of Rochester Cancer Center Community Clinical Oncology Program multicenter study. J Pain Symptom Manage 2003;26:731–42.
627 Lee H, Schmidt K, Ernst E. Acupuncture for the relief of cancer-related pain--a systematic review. Eur J Pain 2005;9:437–44.
628 White A, Cummings M. Does acupuncture relieve pain? Interpreting the effects of sham acupuncture holds the answer. BMJ 2009;338:a2760. doi:10.1136/bmj.a2760.
629 Deng G, Vickers A, Yeung S, et. al. Randomized, controlled trial of acupuncture for the treatment of hot flashes in breast cancer patients. J Clin Oncol 2007;25:5584–90.
630 Lee MS, Kim KH, Choi SM, et. al. Acupuncture for treating hot flashes in breast cancer patients: a systematic review. Breast Cancer Res Treat 2009;115:497–503.
631 Hammar M, Frisk J, Grimas O. Acupuncture treatment of vasomotor symptoms in men with prostatic carcinoma: a pilot study. J Urol 1999;161:853–6.
632 Molassiotis A, Sylt B, Diggins H. The management of cancer-related fatigue after chemotherapy with acupuncture and acupressure: a randomised controlled trial. Complement Ther Med 2007;15:228–37.
633 Rydholm N, Strang P. Acupuncture for patients in hospital–based homecare suffering from xerostomia. J Palliat Care 1999;15:20–23.
634 VitettaL, Sali A. Palliative care. J Complement Med 2007;6:16–26.
635 Vitetta L, Sali A. Complementary and alternative medicine and palliative care. Aust Fam Phys 2006;35:783.
636 Kenner D, Kissane D, Sali A. Clinical outcomes in terminally ill patients admitted to hospice care: diagnostic and therapeutic interventions. J Palliat Care 2001;17:69–77.
637 Rajasaekaran M, Edmonds PM, Higginson I. Systematic review of hypnotherapy for treating symptoms in terminally ill adult cancer patients. Palliat Med 2005;19:418–26.
638 Syrjala KL, Donaldson GW, Davis MW, et. al. Relaxation and imagery and cognitive-behavioural training reduce pain during cancer treatment: a controlled clinical trial. Pain 1995;63:189–98.K
639 Kiser AK, Pronovost PJ. Management of diseases without current treatment options: something can be done. JAMA 2009;301:1708–09.
640 Liossi C, Hatira P. Clinical hypnosis versus cognitive behavioural training for pain management with pediatric cancer patients undergoing bone marrow aspirations. Int J Clin Exp Hypn 1999;47:104–16.
641 Lewis CR, De Vedia A, Reuer B, et. al. Integrating complementary and alternative medicine (CAM) into standard hospice and palliative care. Am J Hosp Palliat Care 2003;20:221–8.
642 Vickers AJ, Straus DJ, Fearon B, et. al. Acupuncture for postchemotherapy fatigue: a phase II study. J Clin Oncol 2004;22:1731–35.
643 Cassileth BR, Vickers AJ. Massage therapy for symptom control: outcome study at a major cancer center. J Pain Symptom Manage 2004;28:244–49.
644 Kohara H, Miyauchi T, Suehiro Y, et. al. Combined modality treatment of aromatherapy, footsoak, and reflexology relieves fatigue in patients with cancer. J Palliat Med 2004;7:791–6.
645 Mansky PJ, Wallerstedt DB. Complementary medicine in palliative care and cancer symptom management. Cancer J 2006;12:425–31.
646 Boon H, Wong J. Botanical medicine and cancer: a review of the safety and efficacy. Expert Opin Pharmacother 2004;5:2485–5201.
647 Mok T, Yeo W, Johnson P. A double-blind placebo-controlled randomized study of Chinese herbal medicine as complementary therapy for reduction of chemotherapy-induced toxicity. Ann Oncol 2007;18:768–74.
648 Pan CX, Morrison RS, Ness J, et. al. Complementary and alternative medicine in the management of pain, dyspnea, and nausea and vomiting near the end of life. A systematic review. J Pain Symptom Manage 2000;20:374–87.
649 Corner J, Plant H, A'Hern R, et. al. Non-pharmacological intervention for breathlessness in lung cancer. Palliat Med 1996;10:299–305.
650 Meyer TJ, Mark MM. Effects of psychosocial interventions with adult cancer patients: a meta-analysis of randomized experiments. Health Psychol 1995;14:101–8.
651 Canter PH. The therapeutic effects of meditation. BMJ 2003;326:1049–50.
652 Cabat-Zinn J. An outpatient program in behavioural medicine for chronic pain patients based on the practice of mindfulness meditation: theoretical considerations and preliminary results. Gen Hosp Psychiatry 1982;4:33–47.
653 McDonald A, Burjan E, Martin S. Yoga for patients and carers in a palliative day care setting. Int J Palliat Nurs 2006;12:519–23.
654 Davidson W, Ash S, Capra S, et. al. Weight stabilisation is associated with improved survival duration and quality of life in unresectable pancreatic cancer. Clin Nutr 2004;23:239–47.
655 Cruciani RA, Dvorkin E, Homel B, et. al. L-carnitine supplementation for the treatment of fatigue and depressed mood in cancer patients with carnitine deficiency: a preliminary analysis. Ann N Y Acad Sci 2004;1033:168–76.
656 Heyland DK, Dhaliwar R, Suchner U, et. al. Antioxidant nutrients: a systematic review of trace elements and vitamins in the critically ill patient. Intensive Care Med 2005;31:327–37.
657 Gogos CA, Ginopoulos P, Salsa B, et. al. Dietary omega-3 polyunsaturated fatty acids plus vitamin E restore immunodeficiency and prolong survival for severely ill patients with generalized malignancy: a randomized control trial. Cancer 1998;82:395–402.
658 Elia M, Van Bokhorst-de van der Schueren MA, et. al. Enteral (oral or tube administration) nutritional support and eicosapentaenoic acid in patients with cancer: a systematic review. Int J Oncol 2006;28:5–23.
659 MacPherson H, Thomas K, Walters S, et. al. The York acupuncture safety study: prospective survey of 34 000 treatments by traditional acupuncturists. BMJ 2001;323:486–87.

Chapter 10

Cardiovascular disease (CVD)

Introduction

Estimates from the World Health Organization (WHO) show that cardiovascular disease (CVD) accounted for approximately 17 million deaths in 2001, this being approximately 30% of the total 57 million deaths due to chronic diseases.[1] As of the mid-1990s, CVD is also the leading cause of death in developing countries. In Australia, for instance, CVD represented 34% of deaths registered in 2006.[2] The leading underlying cause of death for all Australians was ischaemic heart diseases, contributing to 18% of all male deaths and 17% for all female deaths registered.

In fact, a global CVD epidemic has been predicted based on the epidemiologic transition in which control of infectious, parasitic, and nutritional diseases allows most of the population to reach the ages in which CVD manifests itself. Moreover, diet and lifestyle changes contribute to an increase in over weight and obesity and in the incidence of type 2 diabetes in Western countries, both of which are risk factors for CVD.[1] CVD is currently the leading cause of morbidity and mortality in the world.[3]

Risk factors

The risk factors for CVD are:

- depression and/or anxiety
- social isolation
- stress
- anger and/or hostility
- inadequate exercise
- lack of sunlight
- poor sleep
- hypertension
- poor diet and/or overweight and/or obesity
- abnormal serum lipids and/or homocysteine
- smoking.

Reducing risk factors

In the management of all of these risk factors an integrated approach to the treatment of CVD is required, which includes mind–body medicine, nutrition, supplements and exercise.

For treatment and prevention of hyperlipidaemia see Chapter 18.

For treatment and prevention of hypertension see Chapter 19.

Obesity

A distinct relationship between body weight, blood pressure and CVD have been well documented, and the relative risk of developing hypertension, a risk factor for CVD, increases as body mass index (BMI) increases.[4] Modest weight loss of approximately 10% of body weight can normalise blood pressure. A recent review of the Trials Of Hypertension Prevention (TOHP) phase II revealed that a weight loss of approximately 5 kg can result in a significant reduction in blood pressure.[5] Advice about weight loss is essential. Maintaining weight loss is the greatest difficulty faced by patients. A healthy diet and regular exercise are essential for maintaining ideal BMI.

Recently it has been reported that people lose weight by just eating fewer calories, regardless of where those calories come from.[6, 7] In this US study it was reported that after 2 years, 811 overweight adults randomised to 1 of 4 heart-healthy diets, each emphasising different levels of fat, protein, and carbohydrates, showed similar degrees of weight loss. On average, participants in the study lost 6 kg in 6 months, but gradually began to regain weight after 12 months, regardless of diet group. Briefly, the diets tested in the study included the same types of foods, but in different proportions, and were tailored to patients such that overall calorie consumption was reduced by approximately 750 calories per day, with each diet including a different macronutrient composition:

- high fat, average protein: 40% fat, 15% protein, 45% carbohydrate
- high fat, high protein: 40% fat, 25% protein, 35% carbohydrate
- low fat, average protein: 20% fat, 15% protein, 65% carbohydrate
- low fat, high protein: 20% fat, 25% protein, 55% carbohydrate.

Prevention

The public and health professionals must implement comprehensive preventative programs that address lifestyle and nutritional issues if it is to achieve a significant reversal of the increasing incidence of CVD worldwide.[1] The major focus is currently on treatment of CVD, however, there is increasing interest in dealing with the factors responsible for this disease, but more needs to be done. More is known about the factors responsible for CVD than most other diseases and hence it lends itself well to interventions with primary and secondary prevention.

The Australian Heart Foundation website provides extensive public and health professional information on risk factors, prevention and lifestyle strategies for hypertension and CVD.[8]

Lifestyle

Many studies consistently demonstrate greater reduction of cardiac risk factors by implementing positive lifestyle behavioural changes such as avoiding smoking, stress management, dietary changes, and physical activity.[9, 10]

Combining a low-risk diet and healthy lifestyle behaviour, such as moderate amounts of alcohol, being physically active, not smoking, and maintaining a healthy weight, can significantly reduce the risk of myocardial infarction according to a population-based prospective study of 24 444 post-menopausal women diagnosed with cancer, CVD and diabetes mellitus.[11] Specifically the protective lifestyle factors included: not smoking, waist-hip ratio less than the 75th percentile (< 0.85), being physically active (at least 40 minutes of daily walking or bicycling and 1 hour of weekly exercise) and a dietary pattern characterised by a high intake of vegetables, fruit, wholegrains, fish, and legumes, in combination with moderate alcohol consumption (no more than 5 g of alcohol per day; a standard glass of wine contains 11g of alcohol). The authors concluded that most myocardial infarctions are preventable through lifestyle changes.

The Ornish program has shown that it is possible to reverse CVD in selected patients using a program that incorporates aspects to do with the causes of this disease, namely, psychological factors, nutritional factors and exercise.[12] The Ornish program includes a very low fat, whole food, vegetarian diet rich in complex carbohydrates and low in simple sugars (supplemented with vitamin B12) along with regular walking, smoking cessation and stress management techniques. This program produced a 91% reduction in the frequency of angina and there was regression of coronary atherosclerosis after only 1 year and even more regression after 5 years in select patients.[3] The control group had increased coronary atherosclerosis and increased angina after 1 year and even more stenosis after 5 years. This program has been criticised because patients can have difficulty in maintaining such a low-fat diet, plus tended to have increased serum triglycerides and decreased high density lipoprotein (HDL). Dietary fish or fish oil supplementation can be used to normalise triglycerides and have been demonstrated to improve survival in patients with coronary artery disease and hypercholoesterolaemia.[13, 14]

Despite an increasing interest by various public health authorities to recommend lifestyle and dietary changes to population groups, the general health of those groups is deteriorating as reflected by a decrease in physical activity and a massive increase in the problem of overweight and obesity.[2]

In recent reviews it has been shown that people in developed countries just do not consume the recommended daily allowance of 6–8 helpings of fruit and vegetables.[15, 16] Hence the recommendations have included supplementation with good multivitamin and mineral preparations.[5] In an article in the *Heart Lung* journal, Lewis encourages doctors to utilise nutritional supplements to assist in the management of patients with CVD.[17] In his article he cites the benefits that are to be gained from patients adopting lifestyle–nutritional changes that can easily be annexed to traditional treatment options, and explains why it is necessary. A unique part of this article is how he describes the 3 distinct morphological processes of CVD and explains the difference between primary and secondary prevention. The 3 distinct pathological processes are plaque growth, which begins in adolescence and involves oxidation of low-density lipoprotein (LDL) cholesterol, plaque rupture, and clot formation which leads to immediate coronary artery occlusion and arrhythmias which result from myocardial ischemia. Understanding the timing of the distinct pathological processes allows for the most appropriate use of certain nutritional supplements.

Certainly the inappropriate timing of nutritional supplement use could explain why supplements may not be effective in some CVD studies. Despite this there is increasing evidence that supplements such as vitamins, minerals and omega-3 fats are useful in the prevention and management of CVD.

Family lifestyle intervention for children

Obesity in children and adolescence is a growing problem in virtually every developed country and the prevalence is rising. Extrapolation from current US data found adolescent overweight is projected to increase the prevalence of obesity in adulthood (35-year-olds) in 2020 to 30–37% in men and 34–44% in women, which will consequently increase the incidence and risk of coronary heart disease (CHD), cardiac events and deaths in young adults and the middle aged.[18] Management of the child to lose weight needs to focus on lifestyle interventions such as modifying diet, physical activity and behavioural therapies within the whole family. A recent Cochrane review evaluated the efficacy of lifestyle, drug, and surgical interventions to treat obesity in childhood.[19] A total of 12 studies were directed at lifestyle interventions (physical activity and sedentary behaviour), 6 studies addressed diet and 36 evaluated behaviourally oriented treatment programs. This review concluded that family-based lifestyle interventions that modify diet and physical activity and include behavioural therapy can significantly help obese children lose weight and maintain that loss for at least 6 months compared to standard care or self-help alone.

Breast-feeding

A recent study investigated the relationship between duration of lactation and maternal incident myocardial infarction.[20] It was reported that compared with parous women who had never breastfed, women who had breastfed for a lifetime total of 2 years or longer had 37% lower risk of CHD, adjusting for age, parity, and stillbirth history.

Mind–body medicine

Participants of a large prospective population-based cohort study of 6025 adults without CHD followed for a mean of 15 years demonstrated a dose-response relationship between emotional vitality (defined as a positive state associated with feelings of enthusiasm, energy, and interest) and reduced risk of CHD.[21] The authors concluded: emotional vitality may protect against risk of CHD in men and women.

Depression and social isolation

Depression and social isolation are strongly associated with CVD and can have a major influence on prognosis.[22] The impact of depression and social isolation is of a similar order to conventional risk factors such as smoking. A study of up to 500 patients hospitalised for acute coronary syndrome found that the onset of depression immediately following an acute cardiac event significantly influenced the long-term survival and illness severity of the patient.[23]

The Heart and Soul Study is a prospective cohort study of 1017 outpatients with stable CHD followed for an average period of 4.8 years.[24] After adjustment for co-morbid conditions and disease severity, depressive symptoms were associated with a significant 31% higher rate of cardiovascular events compared with those with no depression, which was largely explained by negative behaviour patterns such as physical inactivity.

Worrying and mental stress are also a risk factor for cardiac events, CHD and accelerates atherosclerosis according to studies.[25,26]

Social isolation is a difficult problem to deal with and requires taking an extensive family history about family and friends and usually assistance and support from other health professionals and support groups.

A cohort of 13 000 women and men demonstrated a doubling of the coronary risk factor with social deprivation over a 10-year period.[27] Having a close friend for regular support when needed can reduce the risk of subsequent myocardial infarction by 50%.[28]

An expert working group for the National Heart Foundation of Australia did a systematic review of the literature and found strong and consistent evidence to indicate depression, social isolation and lack of quality social support is associated with the causes and prognosis of CHD.[29]

Owning a pet may help pet owners survive longer after a heart attack and reduces heart rate variability according to a US study of 100 patients following a myocardial infarction when compared with non-pet owners.[30]

Social support

The Framingham Heart Study social network followed up 4739 individuals over a 10-year period and found that people's degree of happiness was determined by the happiness of others whom they are connected with, being surrounded by happy people and geographical proximity in close range.[31] For example, a happy friend who lives within 1.6 km increases the probability that a person is happy by 25%. Similar effects were seen with partners, siblings who live close and next door neighbours, but not seen between co-workers. Effects are not seen between co-workers and happiness declined with time and geographical separation.

Unhappy marriage

An interesting 5-year follow-up study found that women with CHD had a 3-times higher chance of major cardiac events and death over the 5 years if they had a stressful marital or cohabiting relationship.[32] Negative relationships can increase the likelihood of cardiac events and in 1 study this risk was estimated to be as high as 34% compared with low level negativity.[33, 34] A good marriage also improved survival in women with heart failure.[35]

Anxiety

Anxiety and panic disorder are known risk factors for CHD and sudden death in both men and women. The Nurses Health Study of over 72 000 female nurses with no history of CHD or cancers, followed up over 12 years, found that high levels of anxiety raised the risk of fatal CHD by 1.6 times and sudden cardiac death by 1.8 times compared with women with lowest scores for anxiety. Of interest, the data on all women found that up to 28% had severe phobic anxiety scores, who demonstrated highest baseline cardiovascular risk, particularly in women who did not exercise, were more likely to smoke, have a history of diabetes, high cholesterol or hypertension.

Cognitive behaviour therapy (CBT) and counselling

As emotional problems such as depression and anxiety can contribute to increased risk of heart disease, it would appear CBT and counselling play an important role in the management of patients with heart disease and/or psychological symptoms to help reduce risk factors.[36]

Stress

Stress has been identified as a causative factor in hypertension.[37] Stress is also known to precipitate cardiac events and is considered a more important marker of myocardial infarction than hypertension and diabetes. For example, viewing a stressful soccer match doubles the risk of an acute cardiovascular event such as risk of angina, myocardial infarction or arrhythmia.[38] A sudden emotional shock such as the loss of a loved one can cause symptoms of myocardial infarction even in patients with no clinically significant coronary disease[39], including in young people by triggering coronary vasospasm.[40]

A review of the literature has found stress impacts adversely on health and on longevity and can increase the risk of stroke.[41, 42] A study found that for women who are content with their lives at home and at work, atherosclerosis can actually regress, but progresses in those experiencing ongoing stress, independent of other CVD risk factors such as age, smoking, hypertension and HDL levels at baseline.[43] A *Lancet* review found a strong and consistent association between stress and CVD.[44]

Work stress

A prospective cohort of almost 1000 middle-aged patients following a myocardial infarction demonstrated chronic work stress was associated with a twofold increased risk of CVD 2–6 years after returning to work compared with low job stress.[45] In another study of London civil servants, being in a 'just' or fair workplace reduced the risk of CHD by 35% compared to employees who described their work as being 'unjust'.[46] Also, a sense of 'lack of control' at work can increase the risk of CHD.[47]

Hostility/anger

Hostility is now also recognised as a risk factor for CHD, raised blood pressure and heart rate and can increase risk of death by up to fivefold in men with a history of heart disease.[48] Anger can also increase risk of CHD equivalent to hypertension as a risk factor.[49] Anger management should be offered to patients who display hostile behaviour.

Managing anger also helps prevent atrial fibrillation (AF) according to a study of 4000 people aged 18–77 years involved in the Framingham Heart Study. The risk of AF was up to 30% higher in the people with very high hostility scores compared with low hostility.[50]

A number of mind–body approaches including biofeedback, meditation, yoga and hypnosis have all been shown to have a modest effect on lowering blood pressure.[11]

Transcendental meditation and stress management

A controlled trial of 138 hypertensive African American men and women (aged >20 years) assessed over a 6 to 9 month period, were randomised to a transcendental meditation group or control group and were monitored for carotid wall thickness to assess atherosclerosis.[51] The transcendental meditation group showed a significant reduction in carotid atherosclerosis compared with an increase in the control group.

Heart disease patients who were taught stress management significantly reduced their risk of a repeat cardiac event by 25% compared with those receiving routine care.[52]

Music

A small study of 24 people, half of whom were musicians, found that faster music and more complex rhythms accelerated breathing and heart rate, whilst slower and more meditative music, especially reggae music, reduced breathing rates and heart rate. The researchers concluded that appropriate music can be cardio-protective by inducing relaxation, particularly during a pause.[53] The pause reduced the heart rate, blood pressure, and minute ventilation below baseline.

Sleep

Siesta (afternoon nap)

Greek researchers demonstrated a daily siesta is protective towards CVD and coronary mortality according to a large scale cohort study of 23 681 individuals.[54] After excluding confounders, occasional napping reduced risk of coronary mortality by 12%, and systematic napping by up to 37%, particularly in working men, compared with non-nappers. However, a recent report warns that excessive daytime sleepiness is an independent risk factor for total and cardiovascular-related mortality in elderly individuals.[55]

Sleep deprivation

Lack of sleep is being identified as a new risk factor for coronary artery disease, including calcification of the arteries. A US study of 500 healthy middle-aged men and women found that just 1 hour of extra sleep per night reduced the risk of calcification of the arteries (coronary artery calcification was measured by computed tomography) by an average of 33%.[56] This association was more pronounced in women. The study adjusted for all other risk factors such as age, sex and BMI. The researchers postulated that blood pressure drops during sleep, so insufficient or poor quality sleep may interfere with the decline in blood pressure, increasing the risk of CVD.

A Japanese study of hypertensive patients also found after adjusting for confounders, short sleep duration significantly increases the risk of CVD compared with normal sleep duration.[57] The researchers' conclude that lack of sleep is an independent predictor of cardiovascular events.

Snoring and obstructive sleep apnoea (OSA)

OSA is a well-recognised risk factor for CVD and mortality, including nocturnal sudden cardiac death.[58, 59] Sleep units are now well established in a number of hospitals, especially in developed countries, to help identify this problem and provide nocturnal oxygen inhalation therapy for those with confirmed sleep apnoea. Researchers found that sudden cardiac death occurred overnight significantly more in subjects with severe OSA (46%) than those without OSA (21%) or compared with sudden cardiac death victims in the general population (16%).[60] An observational cohort study of 110 subjects who underwent bilateral carotid and femoral artery ultrasounds to quantify atherosclerosis, demonstrated snoring is a significant independent risk factor for carotid (not femoral) artery atherosclerosis; the risk factor increasing with degree of severity of snoring.[61]

Sunshine and vitamin D

Sunshine exposure, specifically solar ultraviolet B, is the major source for vitamin D production by the human body. Epidemiological studies indicate lack of ultraviolet light exposure may contribute to geographic and racial blood pressure differences, CVD and CVD mortality.[62–66] Deaths due to CVD are more common in the winter and at higher or lower latitudes.[67] Vitamin D deficiency is common worldwide and epidemiological evidence is associated with increased risk of CVD, hypertension, metabolic syndrome, heart disease, congestive heart failure, myopathy, chronic vascular inflammation, peripheral artery disease, hyperparathyroidism, autoimmune diseases, diabetes, cancer and all-cause mortality as well as many other diseases (see also Chapter 30, osteoporosis).[68–76] The proposed mechanisms include an increase in parathyroid hormone and activation of the rennin-angiotensin-aldosterone system. The hormone 1,25 hydroxy-vitamin D is involved in the production of renin which regulates blood pressure.

In a large prospective study the researchers demonstrated that deficiency in either 25-hydroxyvitamin D and 1,25-hydroxyvitamin D were equally associated with increase in all-cause mortality and CVD mortality.[77] Serum parathyroid (PTH) levels increase when vitamin D levels fall below 75mmol/L. Slightly enhanced PTH levels are associated with CVD morbidity and mortality, as seen in renal patients and peripheral artery disease.[78–80]

Also, studies demonstrate vitamin D deficiency is linked with elevated C-reactive protein levels which are associated with increased cardiovascular events.[81] Whilst an observation study did not demonstrate an association of CVD and low levels of 1,25 hydroxy-vitamin D in patients with myocardial infarction,[82] community-based studies have shown a strongly positive correlation with low vitamin D contributing to the pathogenesis of congestive cardiac failure and myocardial infarction.[83, 84] A recent study of over 3200 patients referred for coronary angiogram and assessed over an 8-year period, found a strong independent correlation with low serum 25(OH)vitamin D (7.6–13.3ng/ml) and double risk of cardiovascular mortality.[85] Overall the weight of evidence points strongly towards an association of CVD and lack of sunshine and vitamin D deficiency. Due to its widespread benefit in many areas of health, safe sunshine exposure of at least 30 minutes daily, with walking, would appear to be of great benefit to anyone to ensure normal vitamin D levels and for the prevention and management of CVD.

Environment

Chemicals

Air pollution

Many studies consistently demonstrate an association between air pollution and CHD.[86]

The Women's Health Initiative Observational Study analysing up to 66 000 participants over a 6-year period who were free of CVD at baseline, found each 10mcg/cubic metre rise in air particulate matter (<2.5mcg in diameter) of air pollution led to significant increased risks for cardiovascular events and death linked to CHD, stroke and death from stroke.[87, 88] These findings strengthen previous studies focusing on city areas linking CVD and air pollution.[89, 90]

Exposure to particulate air pollution also increases the risk of Deep Vein Thrombosis (DVT), estimated by up to 70% in a high polluted area compared with a control group and more pronounced in men than in women.[91]

Diesel and/or carbon emissions

Exposure to air traffic pollution is known to increase the risk of CVD. In a double-blind, randomised, cross-over study of men with a history of myocardial infarction, brief exposure to dilute diesel exhaust caused exercise-induced ST-segment depression

significantly more profound during exposure to polluted air than in the control group who used clean air, and also reduced the acute release of endothelial tissue plasminogen activator, thereby increasing the thrombotic effect.[92] These factors may explain the mechanism for increased CVD risk with combustion-derived air pollution.

Smoking

Smoking is clearly a major risk factor for arterial disease and large cohort studies demonstrate that smoking cessation is one of the most important factors that can modify risk of arterial disease. Various conventional approaches for smoking cessations are available.

Smoking can reduce all-cause mortality after smokers quit smoking. The Nurses Health Study, a prospective observational study of nearly 105 000 women over a 20-year period, found significant reduction in all-cause mortality in the first 5 years of smoking cessation by 13% and returned to the same level as non-smokers at 20 years compared with those who continued smoking during these periods.[93] Risk of death from vascular disease declined to non-smoking levels in 20 years. Smoking cessation can substantially improve health outcome, reduce CVD and reduce health care costs.[94]

Physical activity

Exercise

A sedentary lifestyle may increase the risk for depression, hypertension, excess weight, abnormal lipids and CVD. It is well established that regular exercise for 30 minutes on most days can help prevent hypertension.[95] Exercise of this magnitude is important in maintaining an ideal weight and helping to normalise abnormal lipids.

A 15-year, prospective longitudinal study of up to 5000 men and women (aged 18–30 years), found walking throughout adulthood attenuates the long-term weight gain that occurs in most adults.[96]

The National Heart Foundation and Medical Journal of Australia guidelines for clinically stable CVD recommend 30 minutes of low-moderate exercise most days which helps to reduce cardiovascular symptoms, augment physiological functioning, improve coronary risk profile and improve muscular fitness.[97] They also recommend for those who have suffered a recent cardiovascular event to have supervised exercise rehabilitation.

A study reporting on non-pharmacologic treatments for depression in patients with CHD reported that of the psychological therapies, such as cognitive behaviour therapy (CBT) and interpersonal therapy (IPT), aerobic exercise, St John's wort, essential fatty acids, S-Adenosylmethionine (SAMe), acupuncture, and chromium picolinate, it was aerobic exercise that offered more promise to improve both mental and physical health due to its effect on cardiovascular risk factors and outcomes, however, future trials are warranted.[98]

Yoga

Yoga has been recommended as efficacious in the primary and secondary prevention of ischaemic heart disease and post-myocardial infarction patient rehabilitation.[99] There are several studies that demonstrate yoga can reduce cardiovascular reactivity to stress, a factor that is strongly associated with cardiovascular risk.[100] Controlled studies have demonstrated that yoga can reduce blood pressure (see also Chapter 19, hypertension) and hence cardiovascular risk.[101–105]

Tai chi

Tai chi promotes balance and flexibility, and can improve cardiovascular fitness and have substantial emotional benefits according to a control study.[106, 107]

Qigong

Several randomised controlled trials have evaluated qigong interventions from multiple perspectives, specifically targeting older adults.[101] In adults, particularly the aged, this form of physical activity can lead to significant improvements in physical functioning, mood, weight, and in the reduction of cardiovascular risk factors.[101] Improvements in cardiovascular factors such as systolic and diastolic blood pressure, increased pre-ejection fraction and heart rate variability have been documented.[108–111]

Physical therapies

Musculoskeletal therapy

Some complementary and alternative physical therapies show promise in cardiac rehabilitation.[112] A recent study with stroke patients reported that single-modality exercises targeted at existing impairments do not optimally address the functional deficits of walking but did ameliorate the underlying impairments.[113] Also the study reported that the underlying cardiovascular and musculoskeletal impairments were significantly modifiable years after stroke with targeted robust exercise. In another recent study it was reported that regular arm aerobic exercise lead to a marked reduction in systolic and diastolic blood pressures and an improvement in small artery compliance.[114] The study further concluded that arm-cycling was a logical option for hypertensive patients who choose to support blood pressure control by sports despite having coxarthrosis, gonarthrosis, or intermittent claudication.

Acupuncture

An early report concluded that there were sufficient clinical studies in humans that demonstrate acupuncture can exert significant effects on the cardiovascular system and provide effective therapy for a variety of cardiovascular ailments.[115] In a recent study of acupuncture and cardiac arrhythmias; the 8 eligible studies reviewed demonstrated that 87–100% of participants converted to normal sinus rhythm after acupuncture. Hence it was concluded that acupuncture seemed to be effective in treating several cardiac arrhythmias, but limited methodological quality of the studies necessitates better-controlled clinical trials to be performed.[116]

Nutritional influences

Diet

Dietary regimens that increase obesity and raise blood lipid levels and inflammatory markers (i.e. C–reactive protein) have an important role in increasing the risk for the development of chronic diseases such as myocardial infarction and stroke. It has been recently reported that vegetarians have a decreased prevalence of ischemic heart disease mortality that is probably due to lower total serum cholesterol levels, lower prevalence of obesity and higher consumption of antioxidant-type compounds in foods.[117]

Worldwide dietary patterns

Diet is a modifiable risk factor for CVD. The INTERHEART study involving 52 countries identified 3 major dietary patterns: Oriental (high intake of tofu, soy and other sauces), Western (high in fried foods, salty snacks, eggs, and meat), and prudent (high in fruit and vegetables).[118] The study demonstrated an inverse association between the prudent pattern and acute myocardial infarction (AMI); the Western pattern showed a U–shaped association with AMI; the Oriental pattern demonstrated no relationship with AMI. The researchers concluded that the unhealthy dietary intake increases the risk of AMI globally and accounts for about 30% of the population-attributable risk.

The INTERGENE population study of 3452 participants (aged 25–74 years) identified dietary patterns associated with CVD risk factors, obesity and metabolic syndrome.[119] Unhealthy food patterns were characterised by high consumption of energy-dense drinks and white bread, and low consumption of fruit and vegetables. Healthy food patterns was distinguished by more frequent consumption of high-fibre and low–fat foods and lower consumption of products rich in fat and sugar.

A recent Cochrane review of the literature also demonstrates dietary advice lowers prevalence and incidence of CVD.[120]

The Seven Countries study demonstrated that population-related factors significantly affect the risk of CVD and that diet was directly related to the risk of developing coronary artery thrombosis that lead to heart attacks.[120] Dietary factors were far more significant than other risk factors, as variations in cholesterol and incidence of smoking in men from one country to another did not account for the differences seen in CVD. This study also demonstrated lower levels of many cancers, dementia and all-cause mortality in people who adhered closely to their traditional Mediterranean or Japanese diets.

Obesity

Weight management can significantly reduce cholesterol and other known risk factors, and slow progression of coronary artery disease that is associated with calcium deposition as with atherosclerotic plaque disease and coronary events in a cohort of patients with type 1 diabetes.[122]

(See also the section on obesity earlier in this chapter.)

Mediterranean and Japanese diets

Vast quantities of research, including epidemiological studies, have demonstrated the value of the Mediterranean and Japanese diet in the prevention and management of CVD. Their dietary patterns feature high intakes of seafood, vegetables, nuts (e.g. walnuts) and seeds, cereals, fruit (usually for dessert) and legumes. The Mediterranean diet is also rich in olive oil intake. Both diets have some chicken, are low in red meat and dairy, and are mostly vegetarian and high in fish. The saturated fat content of egg and dairy products in the Mediterranean and Japanese diets (e.g. goats or sheep products such as yoghurt and cheeses, which forage on wild greens) differs from Western dairy intake in that they have higher content levels of omega-3 fatty acid (alpha linolenic acid).[123]

Interestingly, a recent Japanese study found that high intake for fruit and vegetables was protective for CVD in women but not men.[124] High dietary soy may be cardio-protective according to a study of post-menopausal women by reducing blood pressure and lowering lipid levels.[125]

A recent study that investigated the Mediterranean diet and the incidence of mortality from CHD and stroke in women reported that a greater adherence to the Mediterranean diet, as reflected by a higher alternate Mediterranean diet score, was associated with a lower risk of incident CHD and stroke in women.[126]

Olive oil

A study of patients with stable CHD aimed to identify the effects of olive oil on cardiac risk factor blood parameters.[127] The placebo-controlled, cross-over, trial randomised patients with either raw daily dose of 50ml of virgin olive oil or refined olive oil over a total 6-week period and found reduction in the inflammatory markers interleukin-6 and C-reactive protein with virgin olive oil intervention compared with refined olive oil group, but no changes observed with glucose and lipid profile.

The polymeal

The polymeal, as opposed to the polypill, are the foods identified to be cardio-protective. The polymeal is far safer and more natural and can reduce the risk of CVD by more than 75% (see Table 10.1).[128] Taking the polymeal daily significantly increased total life expectancy far greater in men than in women.

A recent meta-analysis of 12 prospective cohort studies of over 1.5 million participants over a 3–18 year period affirms the health benefits of the Mediterranean diet.[129] Stricter adherence to the diet conferred significant cardiac protection, and led to further reductions in risk of all cause-mortality, death from CVD, as well as cancer and degenerative diseases compared with low adherence. Adherence to the Mediterranean diet can also significantly reduce the risk for type 2 diabetes.[130]

Table 10.1 Effect of ingredients of polymeal in reducing risk of CVD

Ingredients	Average percentage reduction (95% CI) in risk of CVD source	NHMRC level of evidence MA = meta-analysis; RCT = randomised controlled trial
Wine (150ml/day)	32 %	MA
Fish (114g x 4 times/week)	14%	MA
Dark chocolate (100g/day)	21%	RCT
Fruit and vegetables (400g/day)	21%	RCT
Garlic (2.7g/day)	25%	MA
Almonds (68g/day)	12.5%	RCTs
Combined effect	76% (63 to 84%)	

(Source: adapted from Franco et. al. 2005)[128]

The dietary approaches to stop hypertension (DASH) diet

The DASH diet is high in plant proteins, fruit and vegetables, with moderate amounts of low-fat dairy products and is low in animal proteins.

The DASH trial, which was an 11-week multi-centre feeding trial, tested the effects of dietary patterns on blood pressure. Participants (459) were divided into 3 groups; control, increased fruit and vegetables and a combination diet (rich in fruits, vegetable, low fat dairy and reduced saturated fat). In hypertensive subjects, the combination diet led to a mean reduction of blood pressure of −11.4 mmHg systolic and −5.5mmHg diastolic.[131] It was also found to lower homocysteine.[132]

Furthermore, the DASH diet also reduces the risk of heart disease and stroke among women independent of lowering hypertension.[133] An analysis of the Women's Health Study involving over 88 000 women demonstrated adherence to the DASH diet significantly reduced the incidence of cardiac mortality or myocardial infarction by 24% and reduced the risk of stroke by 18% compared with a diet high in salt or fat during 24 years follow-up. It also reduced plasma levels of C-reactive protein and interleukin, both inflammatory markers.

High fibre diet

Total dietary fibre (cereal, fruit, and vegetable) is associated with a 14% reduction in the risk of all coronary events and a 27% decrease in the risk of coronary death.[134] Further research confirms its protective role towards CVD according to analysis of the Physicians Health Study I, that demonstrated consumption of wholegrain cereal at breakfast and high dietary fibre are associated with less prevalence of hypertension, lower risk of heart failure and reduced incidence of myocardial infarction.[135] Intakes of wholegrain fibre are inversely associated with progression of atherosclerosis, according to a study on post-menopausal women with coronary artery disease.[136] Oatmeal for breakfast also reduces the risk of CHD.[137]

Dietary fibre also improves glycaemic control in diabetics, as well as lowering cholesterol/ low-density lipoprotein LDL.

Low-fat diet

In the Mediterranean diet, Cardiovascular Risks and Gene Polymorphisms (Medi-RIVAGE) study from France, both the Mediterranean-type diet and the low-fat diet significantly reduced the risk factors for CVD equally for total cholesterol, triglycerides and insulinemia after adjustment for BMI during the 3-month intervention.[138]

Vegetarian diet

A vegetarian diet has been reviewed for its beneficial and adverse effects in various medical conditions.[139] It was concluded in that study that the beneficial effects may be due to the diet (consisting of monounsaturated and polyunsaturated fatty acids, minerals, fibre, complex carbohydrates, antioxidant vitamins, flavanoids, folic acid and phytoestrogens) as well as the associated healthy lifestyle that vegetarians pursue. There were few adverse effects reported and these consisted of increased intestinal gas production and a small risk of vitamin B12 deficiency.

A more recent report conducted over a mean of 8.1 years suggested a dietary intervention that reduced total fat intake and increased intakes of vegetables, fruits and grains did not significantly reduce the risk of CHD, stroke, or CVD in post-menopausal women and achieved only modest effects on CVD risk factors, suggesting that more focused dietary and lifestyle interventions may be needed to improve risk factors and reduce CVD risk.[140]

Fish and omega-3 polyunsaturated fatty acids

The benefits of eating just 1–2 servings of fish weekly can significantly reduce the risk of coronary death, which outweighs harm from contaminant exposure from mercury and dioxins from fish intake.[141] Modest intake of fish consumption compared with eating fish only once weekly substantially reduced the risk of CHD amongst middle-aged persons.[142] This prospective study of nearly 42 000 Japanese people demonstrated the more fish intake the lower the risk of CVD. The group with the highest fish intake, equivalent to 180g daily, reduced the CVD risk by 40%.

A number of cohort studies demonstrate that regular consumption of fish, even just 1–2 servings weekly, is associated with reduced risk of sudden death, cardiac arrest, heart failure and atrial fibrillation, compared with those who only eat fish once monthly.[143, 144, 145]

Nuts

It is well recognised that nut consumption (e.g. 30–65g or 6–13 walnuts), which are high in monounsaturated fatty acids (MUFAs) and alpha-linolenic acid, is important for a healthy heart, improves vascular health and lowers lipid levels.[146, 147] The Mediterranean diet usually consists of regular nut consumption. Of interest, pistachio nuts have a dose-response beneficial effect in reducing risk of CVD.[148] Just 2 doses of pistachios added to a low-fat diet can significantly reduce cholesterol levels in a dose-dependent manner. Pistachios have a high amount of phytosterol which may be contributing to the health benefits as well as lowering cholesterol levels. Another study demonstrated that sunflower seeds may also have the same benefit on CVD due to high phytosterol levels also.[149]

Diet high in vitamin K

A diet high in vitamin K, particularly K2, is known to be protective for not only bones but also vascular health[150, 151]

The Dutch Rotterdam study of over 4800 participants with no history of heart attacks found that a high dietary vitamin K2 intake in the upper third was associated with a 57% lower risk of dying from fatal cardiac disease and 52% reduction in severe aortic calcification compared with those in the lower third of total vitamin K2 intake.[152] Furthermore, all-cause mortality reduced by 26%.

Vitamin K2 is important for activating matrix Gla-protein (MGP) — a strong inhibitor of vascular calcification that prevents build up of calcium in blood vessel walls.

Only 10% of dietary vitamin K intake is in the K2 form, the other 90% being the more common K1. Vitamin K2 is obtained mainly from the 'good' bacteria produced in the digestive tract and is also found in certain fermented foods. The ideal dietary source of K2 is natto, Japanese fermented soybeans.[154] vitamin K2 dietary sources also include butter, eggs, cow liver, fermented products and hard white cheese.

Salt/sodium restriction

Data from 2 randomised trials, TOHP I and TOHP II, involved a total of 3126 participants assessed over a 10–15 year period who were randomised to a sodium reduction intervention or control for 18 months (TOHP I) or 36-48 months (TOHP II).[155] The researchers found a significant reduction in risk of a cardiovascular event by up to 30% among those in the low-sodium diet intervention group compared with control group. The researchers concluded: 'Sodium reduction, previously shown to lower blood pressure, may also reduce long-term risk of cardiovascular events'. [154]

A low-salt diet is also cardio-protective in normotensive patients, as well as effectively lowering blood pressure in hypertensives. A recent study of normotensive overweight and obese adults were randomised to low or standard diet groups.[155] Within 2 weeks the low-salt diet group (50nmol sodium per day) demonstrated 30% less brachial artery flow-mediated dilatation, lower systolic blood pressure and reduced 24 hour sodium excretion compared with the standard diet group. This study highlights the need to remove salt from many prepared foods and in the diet to prevent the onset of hypertension.

Cocoa and/or dark chocolate

Several studies have shown that cocoa can decrease blood pressure to a similar extent to that of pharmaceuticals.[156] New research suggests 1 serving of dark chocolate (20g; not milk chocolate) every 3 days significantly reduces the levels of the inflammatory marker C-reactive protein which may help to reduce inflammation, a known risk factor for many diseases, including CVD and cancer.[157] A 30-day trial demonstrated drinking a cup of cocoa daily can improve flow-mediated dilation and combat blood vessel dysfunction linked to diabetes.[158] Daily consumption of 46g of dark chocolate increased blood levels of flavonoid epicatechin and significantly improved arterial function in a group of healthy volunteers.[159]

Alcohol

Whilst the cardio-protective properties of moderate alcohol consumption, compared with abstinence or heavy drinking, are widely recognised, this interesting study, a longitudinal-based cohort study, aimed to identify whether the benefits are experienced equally by all moderate drinkers.[160] The study found a significant benefit of moderate drinking was identified amongst those with poor health behaviours (little exercise, poor diet and smokers) compared with abstinence or heavy drinking. There was no additional benefit from alcohol amongst those with the healthiest behaviour profile (>3 hours vigorous exercise per week, daily fruit or vegetable consumption and non-smokers). The authors concluded the cardio-protective benefit from moderate alcohol drinking 'does not apply equally to all drinkers, and this variability should be emphasised in public health messages'.[160] However, another large-scale US study of a cohort of 8867 men over 16 years found after adjusting for confounders, moderate levels of alcohol (5–30g per day) reduced the risk of myocardial infarction by up to 50%.[161]

Red wine

Moderate red wine consumption, but not white wine, has been shown to be protective towards CVD, although this may be influenced by grape variety, the content of resveratrol, regional factors (e.g. climate) and wine-making practises.[162, 163]

Green and black tea

A large prospective cohort study involving 40 000 Japanese adults (aged 40–79 years) over an 11-year follow-up, after adjusting for demographics, lifestyle and medical risk factors, found that green tea consumption was associated with significant reduction of all-cause and cardiac mortality, but not for cancer mortality. The inverse association was particularly in those drinking more than 5 cups of tea daily, compared with less than one, and was stronger in women than men.[165]

Similarly, drinking at least 3–4 cups of black tea a day was also protective for cardiac disease and reduced the risk of developing MI, according to a review of the literature.[165]

Coffee and energy caffeinated beverages

There is increasing consumption of energy caffeinated drinks by young people. A published case report described an otherwise healthy 28-year old man who developed a cardiac arrest due to an ischaemic event from vasoconstriction, even though angiogram did not show significant coronary lesions, and arrhythmia triggered by the excessive ingestion of caffeine- and taurine-containing energy drinks and strenuous activity.[166] Caffeine before exercise might be more significant as it may impede blood flow during exercise. According to a study of young regular coffee drinkers, just 200mg caffeine dose (equivalent to 2 cups of coffee daily), significantly reduces exercise-induced myocardial flow reserve and this effect is more pronounced at high altitude.[167]

A large US study of over 125 000 adults found even drinking in excess of 6 cups of coffee (mostly filtered coffee) per day did not increase risk of CHD, even in those with type 2 diabetes or who were obese; however, they were more likely to take aspirin, possibly for caffeine withdrawal symptoms![168]

A 3.5 year follow–up study of over 11 000 men who had had a myocardial infarction in the previous 3 months, demonstrated that moderate caffeine consumption (2–4 cups daily) did not increase cardiovascular events. [169]

Pomegranate juice

An RCT demonstrated drinking daily pomegranate juice for 3 months compared with placebo can improve myocardial perfusion in patients with CHD and ischaemic disease.[170] Pomegranate can also improve serum lipids.

Phytonutrient juice powder

A recent pilot study suggests that a phytonutrient concentrate consisting primarily of fruits, vegetables and berries — including acerola cherry, apple, beet, bilberry, blackberry, black currant, blueberry, broccoli, cabbage, carrot, cranberry, Concord grape, elderberry, kale, orange, papaya, parsley, peach, pineapple, raspberry, red currant, spinach and tomato — induced several favourable modifications of markers of vascular health in the study participants. The study supported the concept that plant nutrients are important components of a heart-healthy diet.[171]

Nutritional supplements

Antioxidants

A US cross-sectional study assessed users of a broad range of daily nutritional, herbal and dietary supplements.[172] After adjustment for age, gender, income, education and BMI, supplement use was associated with optimal levels of chronic disease biomarkers (serum homocysteine, C-reactive protein) and high-density lipoprotein cholesterol and triglycerides, less likely to have sub-optimal blood nutrient levels, elevated blood pressure, high BMI and diabetes compared with non-users or multivitamin/mineral users alone.

A trial of 13 017 French adults (7876 women aged 35–60 years and 5141 men aged 45–60 years) randomised to either a single daily capsule of antioxidants (120mg of ascorbic acid, 30mg of vitamin E, 6mg of beta-carotene, 100mcg of selenium and 20mg of zinc) or a placebo over a 7.5 year period. The study found the antioxidant supplement reduced the risk of cancer and all-cause mortality in men, but not in women.[173] The researchers postulated that men are more likely to have lower baseline status of certain antioxidants, especially of beta-carotene.

Vitamins E and C

There is increasing biological plausibility for the use of vitamin supplements for the prevention of CVD. Oxidised LDL cholesterol attracts and interacts with monocytes, macrophages and platelets to promote atherogenesis and also causes endothelial necrosis plus interferes with vaso-relaxation. vitamins E and C have been shown to inhibit LDL oxidation and vitamin E reduces endothelial monocyte adhesion, as well as inhibiting platelet activation.[174–176] Angiographic and ultrasonographic studies in humans suggest that vitamin E also inhibits the progression of atherosclerosis.[8, 9, 177] Often researchers do not distinguish between the synthetic and natural forms of vitamin E which have different structures and functions. Studies in general that utilise natural vitamin E and at doses of 500IU or above have shown a benefit.[178] Whereas, studies that employed a lower dose or the synthetic form of the vitamin were found to be ineffective.[11] There is a known synergy between vitamin E and vitamin C plus selenium that allows for a maximum benefit.

Vitamin E is synergistic also with aspirin as they are both cyclooxygenase inhibitors which significantly increases the efficacy of aspirin therapy.[179] Unfortunately, there are no primary prevention studies that have evaluated the role of natural vitamin E. Vitamin C, in addition to regenerating the antioxidant properties of vitamin E, has an anti-inflammatory action which is thought to be important in the prevention of arterial disease.[180]

According to the Physician's Health Study II, a double-blind, placebo-controlled trial of high doses of synthetic vitamin E (400IU 2nd daily) with vitamin C (500mg daily), or provided alone, compared with placebo over an 8-year period was not cardio-protective and did not reduce total mortality.[181] It was also concerning that the vitamin E treatment group had a marginally significant increased risk of hemorrhagic stroke, which is plausible as vitamin E is known to prolong bleeding times. It is likely the benefits of vitamin E witnessed in other trials are found with the natural forms (not synthetic).

Findings from the Women's Antioxidant Cardiovascular study of 1450 women also demonstrated no overall benefit of either ascorbic acid (500mg/d), vitamin E (600IU every other day) and beta-carotene (50mg every other day) for CVD, although there was a marginally significant reduction in the vitamin E group in women with prior history of CVD and those randomised to both active ascorbic acid and vitamin E experienced fewer strokes.[182] There are concerns with the use of synthetic vitamin E.

Vitamin B

Nicotinic acid (Niacin)

Niacin lowers LDL cholesterol as well as triglycerides plus raising HDL and lowering total cholesterol. The major drawback is that it causes flushing at high doses and can cause liver toxicity.[183] A slowly released form of niacin is generally better tolerated. Further, a meta-analysis of niacin has shown that it is a safe and an effective option for dyslipidemia.[184]

Folate, vitamin B12, vitamin B6 and Homoceysteine

Previously only very high levels of homocystine were thought to be related to coronary artery disease. More recent data suggests that levels as low as 12mol/L may increase the risk of vascular disease.[185] There is a relationship between homocysteine levels and vascular disease that is supported by epidemiological data. However, there are also negative studies. Homocysteine is an amino acid product of normal protein metabolism. Folate, vitamin B12 and vitamin B6 are all involved in the metabolism of homocysteine. Deficiencies of 1 or more of these vitamins can lead to hyperhomocysteinemia.[15, 186] Folic acid in combination with vitamin B12 and vitamin B6 have emerged as potentially valuable nutrients for the prevention and treatment of atherosclerosis.[16]

Since the voluntary fortification of foods in Australia with folate, serum folate levels have risen and there has been a corresponding reduction of homocysteine levels in a group of 468 adults in Western Australia over a 4-year period.[187]

Moreover, it is of relevance that elevated homocysteine levels have also been linked with Alzheimer's disease and hence normalisation of homocysteine levels through the use of folic acid may also provide protection from this disease.[188] Further, folic acid has been shown to be extremely useful for the prevention of most congenital abnormalities,[189, 190] as well as multiple cancer sites that include the cervix, large bowel and breast.[18, 19, 191, 192, 193]

However, there are mixed results for any cardiovascular benefit with folate and vitamin B12 supplementation even where homocysteine levels have dropped. For example, a large US study of 5442 women with CVD or with 3 or more risk factors for CVD was randomised to a daily combined pill of folate (2.5mg) and vitamins B6 (50mg) and B12 (1mg) or placebo.[195] Whilst homocysteine serum levels significantly dropped by 18%, there was no reduction in deaths or cardiovascular events observed in the treatment group compared with placebo. A second large study of 3046 patients over an 8-year period, also demonstrated no preventative effect of intervention with folic acid with vitamin B6 or B12 despite significantly reducing homocysteine levels by 30% after 1 year supplementation with folic acid and vitamin B12.[195] The study groups received daily oral treatment with folic acid (0.8mg) plus vitamin B12 (0.4mg) plus vitamin B6, (40mg) (n = 772); or folic acid plus vitamin B12 (n = 772); or vitamin B6 alone (n = 772); or placebo. These findings did not support the use of B vitamins as secondary prevention in patients with CAD. B group vitamins may be more appropriately indicated for primary prevention.

Vitamin D

Trials demonstrate vitamin D supplementation can help lower blood pressure through the production of the hormone renin which affects the renin-angiotensin system and has a direct effect on blood pressure.[78, 196] Also studies demonstrate vitamin D supplementation can reduce elevated C-reactive protein levels which are associated with increased cardiovascular events.[197]

Consequently, there is a good rationale for supplemental vitamin D which is simple and safe for the prevention of vascular events in those with vitamin D deficiency and risk factors for or established CVD, such as the elderly and those institutionalised.[198]

Vitamin K

Low dose vitamin K (K1 and K2) supplementation may protect against atherosclerosis and heart disease, including in patients taking warfarin.[199, 200]

According to several animal studies, patients taking warfarin are susceptible to developing atherosclerosis from calcification of the arterial walls. vitamin K2, not K1, inhibits warfarin-induced arterial calcification in animal studies.[201, 202] Very low dose vitamin K2 supplementation (50–70mcg/day) may help stabilise INR fluctuations in patients with vitamin K deficiency, although this needs great care under medical supervision and dietary sources are safer.[203–207] vitamin K (oral or intravenous) is used to reduce excessively high INR in patients on warfarin.

Minerals

Magnesium

There has been increasing attention given to the role of magnesium and selenium in CVD. Magnesium deficiency has been shown to produce coronary artery spasm which is thought to be a cause of non-occlusive heart attacks.[208] Furthermore, it has been observed that men who die suddenly of heart attacks have significantly lower levels of myocardial magnesium as well as potassium than matched controls.[23]

It has been suggested that magnesium should become the treatment of choice for angina that is due to coronary artery spasm. Magnesium has also been found to be helpful in the management of arrhythmias and in angina due to artherosclerosis.[209] Oral magnesium therapy improves endothelial function, exercise tolerance, reduces exercise-induced chest pain and quality of life in patients with coronary artery disease.[210, 211] Magnesium is known to be an effective smooth muscle relaxant. It is likely it could even have benefit for angina in the acute setting.

The Paris Prospective Study 2, a cohort of 4035 men (age 30–60 years) during an 18-year follow-up based on baseline serum mineral levels, demonstrated low serum magnesium and high serum copper, and concomitance of low serum zinc with high serum copper or low serum magnesium, contributed significantly to an increased all-cause mortality, mortality cancer risk and cardiovascular deaths in middle-aged men.[212]

Magnesium also helps lower blood pressure which has a favourable effect on CVD (see Chapter 19, hypertension). There is a significant inverse relationship between serum magnesium and both systolic and diastolic blood pressure.[213] Meta-analysis of RCTs demonstrates it is effective for hypertension.[214]

Intravenous magnesium

Over the last 20 years there have been over 17 well-designed studies demonstrating that intravenous magnesium during the first hour of admission into hospital for an acute myocardial infarct (MI) can produce a favourable effect in reducing death rates.[215] Magnesium infusion in 250 patients with suspected MI, resulted in a 54% reduction in mortality from cardiac disease compared with placebo.[216] Its benefit in this situation relates to many properties including dilatation of the coronary arteries, reduction in peripheral vascular resistance, improving cardiac energy production, inhibiting platelet aggregation and probably most importantly improving heart rate and arrhythmia.[217] Key factors in the use of intravenous magnesium are timing after onset of symptoms and timing in relation to thrombolysis, and giving the correct rate of magnesium infusion.[218] Controversy surrounds the use of intravenous magnesium in acute myocardial infarction because the 2 large negative trials (ISIS-4 and MAGIC)[219, 220] involving more than 64 000 patients, and therefore with stronger statistical power calculations, used a higher dose of intravenous magnesium in the first 24 hours than any of the prior positive studies. There has as yet been no published dose-related meta-analysis of intravenous magnesium in acute myocardial infarction.

Calcium

A large trial of 1471 healthy post-menopausal women (mean age 74), were randomised to either calcium supplementation alone or placebo over a 5-year period.[221] Myocardial infarction, stroke and sudden death were significantly higher in the calcium group by over 50% compared with the placebo group. The researchers note the detrimental effect on CVD could outweigh any benefits on bone from calcium supplements. More studies are warranted to assess if calcium combined with magnesium and vitamin D, may offset these effects.

Selenium

Some epidemiological studies have shown an inverse relationship between the incidence of CVD and selenium intake.[222] The possible anti-artherogenic activity of selenium may in part be due to its antioxidant activity.[223]

Selenium also decreases platelet aggregation by preventing lipoperoxide accumulation. Lipoperoxides impair prostaglandin synthesis and promote thromboxane synthesis which can increase platelet aggregation. The selenium content of foods is very much linked to its content in soil and it is very much dependant on the region where the food has been produced.[224]

It is of significance that low selenium levels have been found to be associated with several cancers such as prostate and bladder cancer and that selenium supplementation appears to be highly protective against cancer development.[30, 225] (For more information see Chapter 9.)

Chromium

Chromium is necessary for insulin utilisation and therefore glucose and lipid metabolism, and manganese and copper can also influence myocardial electrical stability, and the influence of these minerals on the development of CVD could be explored further.

Fish oils / omega-3 fats

Fish oil supplements are generally well tolerated and safe. Due to the overwhelming weight of scientific evidence including meta-analyses, high dietary fish intake and fish oil supplements are now recommended for adults with cardiovascular risk factors.

Research including a meta-analysis of the literature, suggest taking just 1 capsule of fish oil supplements (1g daily) can lower resting heart rate, stabilise heart rate variability and reduce risk of fatal dysrhythmias which may explain its cardio-protective properties.[226–229]

United States recommendations

The American Heart Association recommends that fish oil be considered for all patients who have recovered from MI.[230] Moreover, the Nutrition Committee of the American Heart Association has also recommended that fish oil needs to be considered in all patients following a heart attack due to its proven benefit for reducing sudden death.[231]

Further, recently the American Heart Foundation carried out an extensive review of the scientific literature regarding omega-6 fatty acids and risk for CVD.[232] The advisory committee concluded that based on the current evidence, from aggregate data from randomised trials, case-control and cohort studies, and long-term animal feeding experiments indicate that the consumption of at least 5–10% of energy from omega-6 PUFAs significantly reduces the risk of CHD relative to lower intakes. The data also suggested that higher intakes appear to be safe and may be even more beneficial (as part of a low-saturated-fat, low-cholesterol diet regimen).

Australian recommendations

The Australian Heart Foundation has prepared an extensive review of the literature that includes meta-analyses on the value of omega-3 PUFAs and fish in the prevention of CVD that includes cardiac disease, heart failure, myocardial infarction and stroke.[233] For established CVD in an adult, the Heart Foundation recommends fish oil supplementation be strengthened to include consumption of approximately 1g Eicosapentaenoic acid (EPA) plus Docosahexaenoic acid (DHA) and >2g Alpha Linolenic Acid (ALA) daily. Other studies recommend dosage of EPA and DHA in the combined range of 800–1000mg daily for both primary and secondary prevention of CVD.[234] The authors have concerns about the recommendation of linseed in bread because of the potential for damage to linseed ALA with heat. (See Table 10.2.)

Lipid profiles

Omega-3 fish oils have been shown to favourably affect lipid profiles, platelet aggregation and arrhythmia and may reduce plaque rupture and clot formation hence its potential for reducing cardiac events as well as reducing sudden death.[235] Docosahexaenoic acid decreases vascular adhesion and eicosapentaenoic acid increases nitric oxide production.

Evidence from a clinical trial suggests that dietary supplementation with omega-3 fatty acids using a dosage of 900mg per day over 3.5 years leads to a clinically important and statistically significant cardiovascular benefit.[222]

Furthermore, in diabetics a larger dose of 4g of omega-3 fatty acids daily improved endothelium function.[236] It is highly recommended diabetics consider fish oil supplementation for the prevention of diabetic related CVD.

Other nutritional supplements

Coenzyme Q_{10} (Ubiquinone)

CoQ_{10} is a vitamin-like nutrient. Its primary role relates to the production of energy (ATP) in the mitochondria and it also acts as an antioxidant. CoQ_{10} is known to have anti-hypertensive

Table 10.2 Australian Heart Foundation recommendations

To lower their risk of CHD, all adult Australians should:	Health professionals should advise adult Australians with documented CHD to:
1 Consume about 500mg per day of combined DHA and EPA through a combination of the following: • 2–3 serves (150g serve) of oily fish per week • fish oil capsules or liquid • food and drinks enriched with marine n-3 PUFA. 2 Consume at least 2g per day of ALA such as walnut, soy linseed bread soybean oil, lean lamb meat, mushrooms, spinach and lettuce. 3 Follow government advice on fish consumption regarding local safety issues.	1 Consume about 1000mg per day of combined DHA and EPA through a combination of the following: • 2–3 serves (150g serve) of oily fish per week • fish oil capsules or liquid • food and drinks enriched with marine n-3 PUFA. 2 Consume at least 2g per day of ALA such as walnut, soy linseed bread soybean oil, lean lamb meat, mushrooms, spinach and lettuce. 3 Follow government advice on fish consumption regarding local safety issues.

(Source: adapted from Australian Heart Foundation recommendations)[233]

properties by normalising peripheral resistance (see Chapter 19, hypertension).

A large body of growing data supports the potential use of CoQ_{10} for mitochondrial diseases with heart involvement, heart failure and cardiomyopathy in both adults and children.[237–240]

The ENDOTACT study demonstrated a positive influence of CoQ_{10} supplementation on human endothelial function independent of lipid lowering .[241] In a study of 38 patients with coronary artery disease, they were randomised to either oral CoQ_{10} (300mg daily divided into 3 doses) or placebo for 1 month.[242] All patients were assessed for brachial artery endothelium-dependent assessment, cardiopulmonary exercise test, and the measurement of endothelium-bound ecSOD activity (baseline and post-study). All parameters, such as endothelium-dependent dilatation and improved peak ventilation oxygen levels, statistically improved in the CoQ_{10} group compared with placebo.

CoQ_{10} can also play a role in angina treatment. CoQ_{10} (150mgs 3 times daily for 4 weeks) reduced the frequency of anginal episodes by over 50% and the need for nitroglycerine medication compared with patients receiving placebo.[243]

Statin drugs are known to adversely interact and reduce levels of CoQ_{10}. The statins inhibit the enzyme HMG CoA reductase required for the manufacture of cholesterol in the liver, but by doing so, this blocks the substances required to produce CoQ_{10}. Consequently this may explain the adverse effect of statins such as fatigue and muscle pain which correlates with lowering of CoQ_{10} levels.[244] Supplementation of CoQ_{10} together with statins may help reduce the risk of these side-effects.

L-carnitine

L-carnitine is an endogenous molecule that is an important contributor to cellular energy metabolism. The concept of modulating the energy metabolism of the heart so as to ameliorate the performance of the dysfunctional myocardium is a firmly established notion.[245] Cardiac muscle contains high levels of carnitine and many patients with CVD demonstrate low levels of carnitine.[246] A recent review concluded that L-carnitine could prevent apoptosis of skeletal muscle cells and that it has a role in the treatment of congestive heart failure-associated myopathy.[247] This has evolved from an emergent literature describing the clinical efficacy of L-carnitine in patients affected by heart disease[248, 249, 250] albeit with some controversy.[251]

Further, cardiovascular function has an intimate relationship with cognition in the ageing process. Recently it has been demonstrated that oral administration of levocarnitine produces a reduction of total fat mass, increases total muscular mass, and facilitates an increased capacity for physical and cognitive activity by reducing fatigue and improving cognitive functions.[252]

Herbal medicines

A number of supplements including garlic, ginseng, flavonoids plus herbs are likely to have a role in the prevention and treatment of CVD. Interactions may occur when herbal remedies are utilised with prescription cardiovascular medications, however, CAM used alone specifically to treat cardiovascular conditions is a less common occurrence.[253] Therefore it is scientifically plausible that, as the evidence becomes available, an integrative approach to the treatment of CVDs should be adopted.

Garlic (Allium sativum)

A double-blind randomised controlled trial of garlic over a 4-year period showed that garlic reduced the development of atherosclerosis, supporting the role of garlic in overall cardiovascular care.[254, 255] A recent review found garlic to benefit CVD.[256] Garlic can maintain the elastic properties of arteries.[257]

Garlic can also reduce cholesterol levels and can have a direct beneficial effect on endothelial function, but the data is conflicting.[258, 259] Garlic can also inhibit platelet activation, adhesion and aggregation through various mechanisms.[46, 260]

Ginseng (Panax ginseng)

Ginseng (*Panax*) has saponins which could act as selective calcium antagonists and enhance release of nitric oxide from endothelial cells, thus providing protection during ischemia or reperfusion.[261]

Flavonoids

Flavonoids are chemical compounds that are found in the pulp of many plant foods, such as those in blueberries, prunes and cocoa, which have exceptionally high antioxidant activity. Flavonoids have numerous other positive functions including protection from various malignancies and have been reported to delay the development of dementia.[262] It is of interest that the phytochemicals present in antioxidant-rich foods such as blueberries may be beneficial in reversing the course of neuronal and behavioural ageing.[263]

Hawthorn berries (Crataegus oxycantha)

The herb hawthorn, which is rich in flavonoids, has been shown to have a number of beneficial actions, including coronary vasodilation, protection against ischemia-induced arrhythmia as well as high antioxidant and anti-inflammatory effects.[264] Hawthorn has been shown to improve exercise tolerance and decrease the incidence of angina.[265] The evidence for hawthorn berries is particularly convincing for the treatment of congestive heart failure according to a recent Cochrane meta-analysis of the literature.[266]

Red yeast rice extracts (Monascus purpureus)

Red rice has a similar biochemical action to statins where it inhibits HMG CoA reductase and helps to normalise abnormal serum lipids according to a meta-analysis of randomised control trials (RCTs).[267] A high dose could cause liver enzyme abnormality similar to statins.[47]

Red yeast rice extracts have been documented to improve lipid profiles[268] and 1 study reported that it was as effective as simvastatin.[269] It is interesting to note that simvastatin is also derived from the fungus *Aspergillus terreus.*

Chinese herb Suxiao jiuxin wan

A Cochrane review of 15 trials involving 1776 people concluded that whilst *Suxiao jiuxin wan* appears to be effective in the treatment of angina pectoris, the evidence remains weak due to poor methodological quality of the studies.[270]

Other heart and vascular diseases

Atrial fibrillation (AF)

Exercise

Regular daily leisurely, light to moderate-paced walking reduces the risk of new-onset AF compared with no exercise, although vigorous, strenuous exercise may increase AF risk especially in young athletes and middle-aged adults.[273]

Massage therapy

Lymphoedema

Massage therapies such as compression therapy provide a means to treat venous stasis, venous hypertension, and venous oedema. Different methods of compression therapy have been described periodically over the last 2000 years.[274] Compression techniques can be static or those utilising specialised compression pumps. The technique of massage called manual lymphatic drainage has emerged to treat primary and secondary lymphoedema.[272] Recent reviews have emphasised that there is a need for large controlled trials of the whole range of physical therapies.[275]

Fish oil supplements

Numerous epidemiological studies, case-control series, and randomised trials have demonstrated the ability of fish oil to reduce major cardiovascular events, particularly sudden cardiac death and all-cause mortality.[276] In a study of fish and AF it was demonstrated that in an elderly group of adults, consumption of tuna or other broiled or baked fish, but not fried fish or fish sandwiches, is associated with lower incidence of AF. It was noted that the consumption of fish could influence risk of arrhythmia.[277]

A review of the evidence suggests fish oils and vitamin C may be useful for the treatment of atrial fibrillation due to their antioxidant and anti-inflammatory qualities by modulating inflammatory pathways.[278, 279]

A 3-month study randomised 65 obese sedentary volunteers to tuna fish oil supplements (1·56 g/day of DHA and 0·36 g/day of EPA) and compared them to placebo (sunflower oil).[280] The fish oil supplement group reduced heart rate variability and significantly attenuated heart rate responses to exercise, and resting heart rate, thereby reducing cardiovascular risk. According to the researchers, the effects are mediated by modulating parasympathetic activity.

A recent systematic review of the literature of 12 studies inclusive of 32 779 patients for fish oils, found most of the studies reported a significant reduction risk for sudden cardiac death, all-cause mortality and a reduction in deaths from cardiac causes that was dose responsive, but interestingly had no effect on arrhythmias or all-cause mortality.[281] No conclusion could be drawn from the studies about the optimal formulation of EPA or DHA.

Fish oil supplements can also help regulate heart rate and are recommended for prevention of both atrial and ventricular arrhythmias.[246]

Alcohol

Alcohol consumption and risk and prognosis of AF among older adults has been reported from the Cardiovascular Health Study.[282] Furthermore, recently in patients with CHD, moderate wine drinking was associated with higher marine omega-3 concentrations than no alcohol use. And it was concluded that the effect of wine comparable to that of fish may partly explain the protective effects of wine drinking against CHD.[283]

Magnesium

A well performed randomised placebo-controlled trial in a hospital setting using intravenous magnesium sulfate (2.5g over a 20 minute period) in addition to usual care, demonstrated enhanced rate reduction and conversion to sinus rhythm in patients who presented acutely with rapid atrial fibrillation compared with standard rate-reduction therapies, such as digoxin.[284]

Chronic venous insufficiency (CVI)

A Cochrane review of the literature identified a number of RCTs and found horse-chestnut seed extract to be efficacious for the symptomatic relief such as leg pain, oedema and pruritus over a short period of time for patients with CVI.[285] The adverse events reported were mild and infrequent, including gastrointestinal complaints, dizziness, nausea, headache and pruritus.

Congestive heart failure (CHF)

Obesity

Paradoxically, a cohort of outpatients with established CHF, obese patients with higher BMIs, were associated with lower mortality risks compared with those at a healthy weight.[286] All-cause mortality rates increased linearly from 45% in the underweight group to 28.4% in the obese group (P for trend <.001).

Dietary fish consumption

During a 12-year follow-up study of 955 participants, among older adults, consumption of tuna or other broiled or baked fish, but not fried fish, is associated with a significantly lower incidence of CHF.[287]

Fish oils

A placebo-controlled double-blind trial of up to 7000 patients with symptomatic heart failure from any cause, randomised to omega-3 polyunsaturated fatty acid (PUFA) 1g daily or placebo for a median duration of 3.9 years, found a small but significant reduction in risk of all-cause mortality and cardiovascular hospitalisation.[288] The same researchers in a separate study found the statin medication rouvastatin (10mg daily) did not affect the outcome of patients with heart failure.[289] Furthermore, there is now strong evidence available that recommends that fish oils should now join the short list of evidence-based life-prolonging therapies for heart failure.[290]

Fish oil supplementation improved left ventricular function in children with idiopathic dilated cardiomyopathy.[291]

Magnesium

High levels of magnesium orotate (6g for 1 month, then 3g for 11 months) proved to be an effective adjuvant to medical treatment for patients with severe CHF by improving survival rate and improving quality of symptoms and quality of life.[292] Another study demonstrated improved inflammatory marker C-Reactive protein in patients with heart failure after treatment with magnesium 300mg daily compared with standard medical care alone.[293]

Coenzyme Q_{10} (CoQ10)

Good quality trials demonstrate CoQ_{10} improves cardiac function in patients with CHF.

Chinese herb *Shengmai*

A recent Cochrane review identified 19 trials and found that the Chinese herbs *Shengmai* plus usual cardiac treatment showed significant improvement in clinical status, reduced risk of mortality, levels of tumour necrosis factor-alpha and improved hemodynanic tests compared to usual treatment alone for heart failure.[294] The reporters did note most trials were of poor quality and no adverse affects were reported in any of the trials. They concluded that *Shengmai* plus usual treatment may be beneficial compared to usual treatment alone for heart failure, but more long-term, high-quality studies are needed.

Hawthorn berries

A Cochrane review including 14 trials of 855 patients with chronic heart failure found hawthorn extract was more beneficial than placebo for physiological workload capacity, exercise tolerance, and the pressure-heart rate product (an index of cardiac oxygen consumption).[295]

The patients were also less likely to develop the symptoms of shortness of breath and fatigue with treatment. Adverse events were infrequent, mild and transient such, as nausea, dizziness and cardiac and gastrointestinal complaints. The authors concluded there is a significant benefit in symptom control and physiologic outcomes from hawthorn extract as an adjunctive treatment for chronic heart failure. [295]

Venous thromboembolism (VTE)

Natural vitamin E

In the Women's Health Study, intake of 600IU of natural vitamin E on alternate days over a 10-year period reduced the risk of developing VTE by up to 27% compared with placebo. This was especially the case in those with a prior history or genetic predisposition (either factor V Leiden or the prothrombin mutation), where this risk further reduced by 49%.[296]

Peripheral artery disease overweight and/or obese

Paradoxically, a Dutch study of 2392 patients who underwent major vascular surgery at 1 teaching institution, found the overall mortality rates among underweight, normal, overweight, and obese patients were 54%, 50%, 40%, and 31%, respectively. The researchers concluded:

> The excess mortality among underweight patients was largely explained by the overrepresentation of individuals with moderate-to-severe COPD (chronic obstructive pulmonary disease]. COPD may in part explain the 'obesity paradox' in the PAD population.[297]

Arginine

Researchers assessed the effect of 2g or 4g of L-arginine supplementation 3 times daily on nitric oxide (NO) concentration and total antioxidant status (TAS) in patients with atherosclerotic peripheral arterial disease over 28 days.[298] L-arginine increases NO synthesis. Low NO levels can affect vascular endothelium. Supplementation of L-arginine substantially increased NO and TAS levels, which implies L-arginine has an antioxidant effect and may be effective in preventing CVD.

Stroke

Fruit and vegetables

A meta-analysis identified 8 prospective studies that demonstrated 5 servings of fruit and vegetables daily reduces the risk of stroke by 26%, and 3–5 daily by 11%.[299]

Music

A randomised study of 60 patients found listening to music in the early stages following a stroke led to greater improvement in memory and attention than those who listened to audio books, or nothing at all.[300]

Occupational therapy (OT)

According to a Cochrane review of the literature, treatment following a stroke with OT can improve survival length and independence levels compared with no OT.[301]

Intensive nutritional supplement

A randomised, prospective, double-blind, single-centre study comparing intensive nutritional supplementation to standard, routine nutritional supplementation in 116 undernourished patients admitted to a stroke service, demonstrated patients receiving the intensive supplementation improved measures of motor function (estimated by walk tests) and a higher proportion went home compared to those on standard supplementation.[302] However, there were no differences on measures of cognition.

Isoflavone supplements

A study of 102 patients treated over 12 weeks demonstrated daily supplements of isoflavones significantly reduced endothelial dysfunction in patients with a history of ischaemic stroke and reduced serum C-reactive protein levels compared with placbo.[303]

Conclusion

From the foregoing, and emerging aggregate scientific evidence, the prevention and treatment of CV diseases requires a multi-level intervention.

A healthy lifestyle plays an important role in the primary prevention of CHD in middle-aged and older men and women.

The primary objective for health professionals should be to emphasise to the community that CVD can be prevented with lifestyle interventions and within this framework to persuade the community and patients to improve their diets and prudent physical activity and to advise on the safe and cost-effective use of nutritional supplementation when warranted.

One notion that has been advanced is that nutritional supplements cannot be patented, hence the lack of funds for costly clinical trials. This lack of funding most probably explains why it is not conclusively known as to whether reduction of homocysteine can influence CVD, despite the increasing data linking hyper-homocystinemia with CVD. An abstract of a study has demonstrated that multivitamins that contain B group vitamins can significantly reduce blood homocysteine in men at risk for CVD as well as improving depressive symptoms.[304]

The comprehensive cardio-protective lifestyle and supplementation advice suggested by Lewis[17] should be part of routine care of patients by the medical profession.

Many patients need continual reminders, education and support in the importance of lifestyle factors contributing to CVD. Chronic disease self-management education programs are important. The integrative medicine approach must always incorporate the evidence-based use of pharmaceutical therapy. Table 10.3 summarises the level of evidence for some CAM therapies for ASD.

Table 10.3 Levels of evidence for lifestyle and complementary medicines/therapies in the management of cardiovascular conditions

Modality	Level I	Level II	Level IIIa	Level IIIb	Level IIIc	Level IV	Level V
Lifestyle modifications							
Weight reduction / obesity		x					
Cessation of smoking		x					
Sunshine and vitamin D					x		
Mind–body medicine							
Social support				x			
Prevent depression, anxiety and social isolation				x			
Managing life stressors				x			
Cognitive behaviour therapy (CBT), counselling and interpersonal therapy				x			
Music					x		
Sleep					x		
Physical activity		x					
Yoga				x			
Tai chi					x		
Qigong					x		
Diets							
Nutrition generally			x				
Mediterranean and/or Japanese diets	x						
DASH diet			x				
The polymeal diet				x			
Low-fat diet				x			
Vegetarian diet			x				

Continued

Table 10.3 Levels of evidence for lifestyle and complementary medicines/therapies in the management of cardiovascular conditions—cont'd

Modality	Level I	Level II	Level IIIa	Level IIIb	Level IIIc	Level IV	Level V
Nutrition							
Olive oil				x			
High fibre				x			
Fish and Omega-3 PUFAs	x						
Nuts				x			
High vitamin K consumption				x			
Salt and/or sodium reduction				x			
Cocoa and/or chocolate				x			
Tea and/or green tea				x			
Coffee and/or caffeinated beverage restrictions				x			
Pomegranate juice				x			
Vitamin supplements							
Vitamin C and E					x		
B Group vitamins				x			
Vitamin D					x		
Vitamin K					x		
Mineral supplements							
Magnesium and/or IV magnesium			x				
Calcium					x		
Selenium				x			
Chromium					x		
Other supplements							
Omega-3 fatty acids	x						
Coenzyme Q_{10}			x				
Carnitine			x				
Herbal medicines							
Garlic	x						
Panax ginseng	x						
Hawthorn	x						
Flavonoids					x		
Red yeast rice extract					x		
Chinese herb (*Suxiao jiuxin wan*)					x		
Chinese herb (*Shengmai*) for CHF					x		
Physical therapies							
Musculoskeletal therapies				x			
Massage				x			
Acupuncture				x			

Level I — from a systematic review of all relevant randomised controlled trials, meta-analyses.
Level II — from at least 1 properly designed randomised controlled clinical trial.
Level IIIa — from well-designed pseudo-randomised controlled trials (alternate allocation or some other method).
Level IIIb — from comparative studies (including systematic reviews of such studies) with concurrent controls and allocation not randomised, cohort studies, case-control studies, or interrupted time series with a parallel control group.
Level IIIc — from comparative studies with historical control, 2 or more single-arm studies or interrupted time series without a parallel control group.
Level IV — opinions of respected authorities based on clinical experience, descriptive studies or reports of expert committees.
Level V — represents minimal evidence that represents testimonials.

Clinical tips handout for patients with cardiovascular disease

1 Lifestyle advice

Sleep

- Ensure 7–8 hours sleep and regular sleep pattern. A short (20 min) siesta can be protective. (See Chapter 22 for more advice.)

Sunshine

- Amount of exposure varies with local climate.
- At least 15 minutes of sunshine needed daily for vitamin D and melatonin production — especially before 10 a.m. and after 3 p.m. when the sun exposure is safest during summer. Much more exposure required in winter when supplementation needs to be considered.
- Ensure gradual, adequate skin exposure to sun; avoid sunscreen and excess clothing to maximise levels of vitamin D.
- More time in the sun is required for dark skinned people and people with vitamin D deficiency.
- Direct exposure to about 10% of the body (hands, arms, face), without sunscreen and not through glass.
- Vitamin D is obtained in the diet from fatty fish, eggs, liver and fortified foods (some milks and margarines); diet alone is not a sufficient source of vitamin D.

2 Physical activity/exercise

- Exercise 30–60 minutes daily. If exercise is not regular, commence with 5 minutes daily and slowly build up to at least 30 minutes.
- Outdoor exercise in nature, with fresh air and sunshine, is ideal (e.g. brisk walking, light jogging, cycling, swimming, stretching, resistance or weight-bearing exercises).
- Tai chi, qigong and yoga may be particularly helpful.

3 Mind–body medicine (most helpful)

- Stress management program — for example, 6 x 40 minute sessions for patients to understand the nature of their symptoms, the symptom's relationship to stress, and the practice of regular relaxation exercises.
- Regular meditation practice at least 10–20 minutes daily, especially transcendental, mindfulness meditation and autogenic training.
- Anger management may be of help.
- Psychological therapy may help to deal with stressors.

Breathing

- Be aware of breathing from time to time. Notice if tendency to hold breath or over-breathe.
- Snoring and irregular breathing during sleep needs to be reported and further investigated.
- Avoid exposure to polluted air as much as possible.

Rest and stress management

Recurrent stress may cause a return of symptoms. Relaxation is important for a full and lasting recovery.

- Reduce workload and resolve conflicts. Contact family, friends, church or social groups for support.
- Listening to relaxation music helps.
- Relaxation massage therapy is helpful.
- Hypnotherapy, biofeedback, cognitive behavioural therapy, and psychotherapy may be of help.

Fun

- It is important to have fun in life.
- Joy can be found even in the simplest tasks, such as funny movies/videos, comedy, hobbies, dancing, playing with pets and children.

4 Environment

- Avoid smoking, environmental pollutants and chemicals — at work and in the home.

5 Dietary changes

- Do not rush your meals; relax before meals; chew your food thoroughly before swallowing as this aids digestion; have regular relaxed eating patterns.
- Aim to lose weight if you or your medical advisor believe you are overweight. Eating slowly can help with weight loss.
- Eat more fruit and vegetables — a variety of colours and those in season.
- A vegetarian diet high in legumes (e.g. soy), fish (e.g. sardines) vegetables, garlic, nuts and fruit is particularly helpful (Mediterranean diet).
- Increase fibre; for example, add psyllium fibre (husks) to your cereal.

- Eat fresh garlic — 2g daily yields 5–9mg allicin (note: may cause garlic breath and body odour).
- Eat more nuts, seeds, especially flax seeds (best if ground just before use; refrigerate if ground), beans, sprouts (e.g. alfalfa, mung, bean, lentil), soy (best if fermented e.g. miso, soy sauce, natto and tempah).
- Eat more fish (mackerel, sardines, salmon, cod, tuna), especially deep sea fish.
- Reduce red meat intake (preferably use red lean meat e.g. lamb, kangaroo) — no more than twice weekly and not well done — and eat white meat (e.g. free range organic chicken fillets).
- Use cold pressed olive oil (4 teaspoons daily) and avocado oil.
- Use only dark chocolate (25–50g daily) unless not tolerated.
- Eat a variety of wholegrains/cereals (best if not toasted). Cooked traditional rolled oats for breakfast are particularly helpful, as is rice (brown, basmati, Mahatma, Dongara), buckwheat flour, wholegrain organic breads (rye bread, essene, spelt, kamut) — when toasting make hot and crisp, not brown, to avoid acrylamide — brown pasta, couscous, millet, amaranth, etc.
- Use low-fat dairy products, such as low-fat yoghurt, unless there is a dairy intolerance. Soy (organic) milk is an alternative.
- Drink more water 1–2 litres a day and teas, especially green tea, chamomile, peppermint and black teas (best if organic).
- Avoid sea salt.
- Avoid coffee.
- Avoid hydrogenated, saturated fats and trans-fatty acids such as butter, margarines, crispy potato chips, dairy fat (e.g. yellow cheeses and cream), fat in meat and poultry, commercial biscuits, most cakes, pastries and takeaway foods, fast foods, sugar (such as in soft drinks), lollies and processed foods (e.g. white bread, white pasta, pastries).
- Avoid chemical additives — preservatives, colourings and flavourings.
- Minimise alcohol intake — limit to no more than 1–2 glasses daily; red wine may be best.
- Avoid artificial sweeteners — replace with honey (e.g. manuka, yellow box and stringy bark have lowest GI).

6 Physical therapies

- Acupuncture may help.

7 Supplements

Fish oils

- Indication: may reduce blood pressure, help with abnormal heart beat, heart failure and prevent heart disease.
- Dosage: 3–7g daily as tolerated and as indicated for high blood pressure (e.g. EPA 180/DHA 120mg / 1000mg capsule).If consuming fish 2–3 times a week, a 1000mg capsule per day may be sufficient.
- Results: 4–7 days.
- Side-effects: often well tolerated especially if taken with meals. Very mild and rare side-effects; for example, gastrointestinal upset; allergic reactions (e.g. rash, breathing problems if allergic to seafood); blood thinning effects in very high doses > 10g daily (may need to stop fish oil supplements 2 weeks prior to surgery).
- Contraindications: sensitivity reaction to seafood; drug interactions; caution when taking high doses of fish oils >4g per day together with warfarin (your doctor will check your INR test).

Niacin

- Indication: can reduce bad cholesterol and increase good cholesterol; can reduce triglyceride.
- Dosage: the effects are dose dependant — to increase good cholesterol need 1200–1500mg/day. To decrease bad cholesterol need 2000–3000mg/day.
- Results: 2 weeks and beyond.
- Side-effects: flushing is a common side-effect. If using sustained release forms this is less likely to happen; aspirin may also reduce flushing.
- Contraindications: can make gout worse. If high dosage, require liver function test from time to time.

Vitamins and minerals

Vitamins B6, B12, Folate (best given together as a multivitamin + mineral)

- Indication: can reduce homocysteine which may be linked to artery disease.
- Dosage: vitamin B6: best if dosage is no more than 50mg daily. Vitamin B12: 600mcg daily. Folate: 0.5–1mg daily.
- Result: 1 month.

- Side-effects: no toxicity with this group (within dosage); vitamin B6 toxicity with doses above the recommended dose.
- Contraindications: generally safe when used in combination. If anaemia present, cause must be found.

Vitamin D3 (Cholecalciferol)

- Indication: low levels increase CVD. One mechanism could be by increasing risk of hypertension.
- Dosage: safe sunshine exposure of skin is the safest source of vitamin D (cholecalciferol 1000 international units). Doctors should check blood levels and suggest supplementation if levels are low. Adults: 400–1000IU daily for maintenance; 3000–5000 IU daily for 1 month then 1000IU daily if vitamin D level below normal. Ensure repeat blood measurement.
  Children at risk: 200–400IU daily under medical supervision.
  Pregnant and lactating women at risk: under medical supervision.
- Results: 6–9–12 months.
- Side-effects: very high doses can cause vitamin D toxicity; raised calcium levels in the blood. Can increase aluminium and magnesium absorption; prolonged heparin therapy can increase resorption and reduce formation of bone and hence more vitamin D and calcium required.
- Contraindications: thiazide diuretics decrease urinary calcium and hence hypercalcemia possible with vitamin D supplementation; high levels of vitamin D can reduce effectiveness of verapamil.

Vitamin C

- Indication: may reduce risk of artery disease when combined with natural vitamin E and selenium by reducing blood stickiness.
- Dosage: 500–1000mg daily.
- Results: can reduce blood stickiness in 1 week.
- Side-effects: with high doses can cause nausea, heartburn, abdominal cramps and diarrhoea.
- Contraindications: can increase iron absorption. Use with caution if glucose-6-phosphate dehydrogenase deficiency.

Natural vitamin E

- Indication: may reduce artery disease and blood stickiness when combined with vitamin C and selenium. Can help prevent venous thromboembolism.
- Dosage: 200–800 IU daily.
- Results: can reduce blood stickiness in 1 week.
- Side-effects: doses below 1500IU daily are very unlikely to result in haemorrhage. Rarely cause diarrhoea, flatulence, nausea, heart palpitations.
- Contraindications: use with caution if bleeding disorder or if taking with blood thinning medication. If using very high dose, reduce dose before surgery.

Magnesium

- Indication: magnesium can prevent coronary artery spasm. Can help with abnormal heart rhythm, angina, heart failure and hypertension. Intravenous magnesium can be most helpful at time of heart attack. May neutralise side-effects of cholesterol drugs (statins) in the orotate form.
- Dosage: magnesium oral: 400–800mg daily, including pregnant and lactating women.
- Magnesium intravenous: must be given carefully and doses vary depending on disorder being treated. Doses vary from 1–6g given at once and further amounts given progressively.
- Results: 1–2 days.
- Side-effects: oral magnesium can cause gastrointestinal irritation, nausea, vomiting, and diarrhoea. The dosage varies from person to person. Although rare, toxic levels can cause low blood pressure, thirst, heart arrhythmia, drowsiness and weakness.
  Intravenous dose can cause flushing, slow pulse rate, low blood pressure plus other heart disorders.
- Contraindications: patients with kidney disease.

Selenium

- Indication: may protect against artery disease and also decrease sticky blood.
- Dosage: less than 200mcg daily given together with vitamin E and vitamin C.
- Result: 1 month.
- Side-effects: no risk at this dose; toxicity in high doses.
- Contraindications: safe even during pregnancy at this dose.

Chromium Picolinate

- Indication: can reduce blood glucose plus lipid levels.
- Dosage: 50–200mcg/ day.
- Results: unknown.
- Side-effects: doses less than 1000mcg are safe; can reduce hypoglycaemic drug

requirement. Very high doses linked to kidney and liver disease.
- Contradictions: kidney and liver disease, high serum levels.

Coenzyme Q_{10} (CoQ_{10})
- Indication: lowers blood pressure; may also be useful in heart failure. Recommended if on high dose cholesterol drugs (statins); may neutralise side-effects of cholesterol drugs (statins).
- Dosage: adults 100–200mg in divided doses, 2–3 times per day.
- Results: 7–14 days.
- Side-effects: generally well tolerated. May cause gastrointestinal side-effects such as nausea, vomiting, diarrhoea.
- Contraindications: avoid in pregnancy and lactating women and if allergic.

L-carnitine
- Indication: can improve function of heart muscle and could help with heart failure.
- Dosage: 2–4g per day.
- Result: unknown.
- Side-effects: rare, but can cause nausea, vomiting, abdominal pain, heartburn and diarrhoea.
- Contraindications: pregnancy — insufficient evidence. Can reduce effectiveness of thyroid hormone replacement.

Herbal medicines

Garlic (*Allium sativum*)
- Indication: may prevent artery disease, a possible mechanism may be improvement of blood stickiness plus improvement of cholesterol levels.
- Dosage 600–900mg/day (3.6–5.4mg of allicin); avoid aged garlic extract or heat-treated garlic as they are less effective for blood pressure.
- Results: 4–7 days.
- Side-effects: breath and body odour; mouth, stomach and gastrointestinal burning or irritation, heartburn, flatulence, nausea, vomiting and diarrhoea. May increase risk of bleeding as garlic can affect platelet function. Some people are allergic to garlic (by ingestion or even topically) and may cause asthma, runny nose, skin irritation and in rare cases severe allergic reactions.
- Contraindications: avoid if allergic to garlic; beware if taking any blood thinning medication such as warfarin; avoid at least 2 weeks prior to any surgery to minimise risk of bleeding; avoid high doses in pregnancy and lactation.

Hawthorn berries
- Indication: heart failure. Can help with hypertension and abnormal heart rhythm.
- Dosage: adult: 500mg 3 times daily.
- Results: 14–21 days.
- Side-effects: generally well tolerated; may cause dizziness, vertigo, nausea, fatigue, sweating, headache and palpitations.
- Contraindications: pregnancy and lactation.

Red yeast rice
- Indication: helps to normalise blood lipids.
- Dosage: 600mg twice daily or 1200mg once or twice daily.
- Results: more than 2 weeks.
- Side-effects: rare; abdominal discomfort, heartburn, flatulence and dizziness. Liver impairment like cholesterol lowering drugs (statins); muscle aches and pains like statins.
- Contraindications: if hypersensitive to this rice extract; pregnancy and nursing mothers; active liver disease.

Horse chestnut
- Indication: useful for symptoms of venous insufficiency.
- Dosage: start with dose of 50–10mg escin twice daily. After 8 weeks reduce dose to 50mg escin daily.
- Results: about 8 weeks.
- Side-effects: rare; digestive complaints, nausea, dizziness, headaches, pruritis. Extremely high doses can cause toxicity.
- Contraindications: pregnancy. Avoid if you suffer gastric irritation, celiac disease, inflammatory bowel disease. Avoid if hepatic or renal impairment. Avoid Liquorice herb if you suffer hypertension.

References

1 World Health Organization—Cardiovascular disease: prevention and control 2003.
2 Australian Bureau of Statistics 3303.0. Causes of death 2006. Released 14 March 2008 http://www.ausstats.abs.gov.au/ausstats/subscriber.nsf/0/A8CB1F4BD5385085CA2574100010092A/$File/33030_2006.pdf (accessed February 2009)
3 Flegal KM, Carroll MD, Ogden CL, Johnson CL. Prevalence and trends in obesity among US adults, 1999–2000. JAMA 2002;288(14):1723–7.
4 Ascherio A, Rimm EB, Giovannucci EL, et. al. A prospective study of nutritional factors and hypertension among US men. Circulation 1992;86(5):1475–84.

5 Stevens VJ, Obarzanek E, Cook NR, et. al. Trials for the Hypertension Prevention Research Group. Long-term weight loss and changes in blood pressure: results of the Trials of Hypertension Prevention, phase II. Ann Intern Med 2001;134(1):1–11.

6 Sacks FM, Bray GA, Carey VJ, et. al. Comparison of weight-loss diets with different compositions of fat, protein, and carbohydrates. NEJM 2009;360:859–873.

7 Katan MB. Weight-loss diets for the prevention and treatment of obesity. NEJM,2009;360:923–24.

8 Heart Foundation. Information for Health Professionals; Reducing Risk in Heart Disease — Full Guidelines. Online. Available: http://www.heartfoundation.org.au/Professional_Information/Clinical_Practice/CHD/Pages/default.aspx (accessed February 2009)

9 Australian and New Zealand Journal of Public Health 2001;25:24–30.

10 Knowler WC, Barrett-Connor E, Fowler SE, et. al. Reduction in the incidence of type 2 diabetes with lifestyle intervention or metformin. NEJM 2002;346:393–403.

11 Akesson A, Weismayer C, Newby PK, et. al. Combined Effect of Low-Risk Dietary and Lifestyle Behaviours in Primary Prevention of Myocardial Infarction in Women. Arch Intern Med 2007;167(19):2122–27.

12 Ornish D, Scherwitz LW, Billings JH, et. al. Intensive lifestyle changes for reversal of coronary heart disease. JAMA 1998;280(23):2001–7.

13 Ornish D, Brown SE, Scherwitz LW, et. al. Can lifestyle changes reverse coronary heart disease? The Lifestyle Heart Trial. Lancet 1990;336(8708):129–33.

14 Calder PC. n-3 polyunsaturated fatty acids, inflammation, and inflammatory diseases. AJCN 2006;83(6 Suppl):1505S-1519S.

15 Frazao E, Allshouse J. Strategies for intervention: commentary and debate. J Nutr 2003;133(3): 844S–7S.

16 Fairfield KM, Fletcher RH. vitamins for chronic disease prevention in adults: scientific review. JAMA 2002;287(23):3116–26.

17 Lewis GRJ. Should doctors discourage nutritional supplementation?: A cardiovascular perspective. Heart Lung Circ 2004;13(3):245–51.

18 Bibbins-Domingo K, Coxson P, Pletcher MJ, et. al. Adolescent Overweight and Future Adult Coronary Heart Disease. NEJM 357(23):2371–79

19 Summerbell CD, Ashton V, Campbell KJ, Edmunds L, Kelly S, Waters E. Interventions for treating obesity in children. Cochrane Database of Systematic Reviews 2003, Issue 3. Art. No.: CD001872. doi: 10.1002/14651858.CD001872.

20 Stuebe AM, Michels KB, Willett WC, et. al. Duration of lactation and incidence of myocardial infarction in middle to late adulthood. Am J Obstet Gynecol 2009;200(2):138.e1–e8.

21 Laura D. Kubzansky, PhD; Rebecca C. Thurston, PhD. Emotional Vitality and Incident Coronary Heart Disease. Benefits of Healthy Psychological Functioning. Arch Gen Psychiatry 2007;64(12):1393–1401.

22 Nemeroff CB, Musselman DL, Evans DL. Depression and cardiac disease. Depress Anxiety 1998;8(Suppl 1):71–9. Review.

23 Parker GB, Hilton TM, Walsh WF, et. al. Timing is everything: the onset of depression and acute coronary syndrome. outcome. Biol Psychiatry 2008;64(8):660–6.

24 Whooley MA, de Jonge P, Vittinghoff E, et. al. Depressive symptoms, health behaviours, and risk of cardiovascular events in patients with coronary heart disease. JAMA 2008;300(20):2379–88.

25 Kubzansky LD, Kawachi I, Spiro A 3rd, et. al. Is worrying bad for your heart? A prospective study of worry and coronary heart disease in the Normative Ageing Study. Circulation 1997;95: 818–24

26 Mangiafico RA, Malatino LS, Attinà T, et. al. Exaggerated endothelin release in response to acute mental stress in patients with intermittent claudication. Angiology 2002;53:383–87

27 Burg MM, Barefoot J, Berkman L, et. al. Low perceived social support and post-myocardial infarction prognosis in the enhancing recovery in coronary heart disease clinical trial: the effects of treatment. Psychosom Med 2005;67(6):879–88.

28 Dickens CM, McGowan L, Percival C, et. al. Lack of a close confidant, but not depression, predicts further cardiac events after myocardial infarction. Heart 2004;90:518–22

29 Bunker SJ, Colquhoun DM, et. al. Stress' and coronary heart disease: psychological risk factors. National Heart Foundation of Australia position statement update. MJA 2003;178:272–276

30 Friedmann E, Thomas SA, Stein PK, Kleiger RE. Relation between pet ownership and heart rate variability in patients with healed myocardial infarcts. Am J Cardiol 2003;91:718–21

31 James H Fowler, Nicholas A Christakis. Dynamic spread of happiness in a large social network: longitudinal analysis over 20 years in the Framingham Heart Study. BMJ 2008;337:a2338.

32 Orth-Gomér K, Wamala SP, Horsten M, et. al. Marital stress worsens prognosis in women with coronary heart disease: The Stockholm Female Coronary Risk Study. JAMA 2000;284:3008–14.

33 Rohrbaugh MJ, Shoham V, Coyne JC. Effect of marital quality on eight-year survival of patients with heart failure. Am J Card 2006;98:1069–72

34 De Vogli R, Chandola T, Marmot MG. Negative aspects of close relationships and heart disease. Arch Int Med 2007;167:1951–57.

35 Rohrbaugh MJ, Shoham V, Coyne JC. Effect of marital quality on eight-year survival of patients with heart failure. Am J Card 2006;98(8):1069–72.

36 Napadow V, Ahn A, Longhurst J, et. al. The status and future of acupuncture clinical research. J Altern Complement Med 2008;14(7):861–9.

37 Artinian NT, Washington OG, Flack JM, et. al. Depression, stress, and blood pressure in urban African-American women. Prog Cardiovasc Nurs 2006 Spring;21(2):68–75.

38 Wilbert-Lampen U, Leistner D, Greven S et. al. Cardiovascular Events during World Cup Soccer. NEJMe 2008; 358(5):475–83.

39 Wittstein IS, Thiemann DR, Lima JA, et. al. Neurohumoral features of myocardial stunning due to sudden emotional stress.NEJM 2005;352:539–48

40 Connelly KA, MacIsaac AI, Jelinek VM. Stress, myocardial infarction, and the 'tako-tsubo' phenomenon. Heart 2004;90:e52.

41 Vitetta L, Anton B, Cortizo F, Sali A. Mind-body medicine: stress and its impact on overall health and longevity. Ann N Y Acad Sci 2005;1057:492–505.

42 Surtees PG, Wainwright NW, Luben RN, et. al. Psychological distress, major depressive disorder, and risk of stroke. Neurology 2008;70:788–94.

43 Wang HX, Leineweber C, Kirkeeide R, et. al. Psychosocial stress and atherosclerosis: family and work stress accelerate progression of coronary disease in women. The Stockholm Female Coronary Angiography Study. J Intern Med 2007;261:245–54.
44 Brotman DJ, Golden SH, Wittstein IS. The cardiovascular toll of stress. Lancet 2007;370: 1089–100.
45 Aboa-Eboulé C, Brisson C, Maunsell E, et. al. Job strain and risk of acute recurrent coronary heart disease events. JAMA 2007;298:1652–60.
46 Kivimäki M, Ferrie JE, Brunner E, et. al. Justice at work and reduced risk of coronary heart disease among employees: the Whitehall II Study. Arch Int Med 2005;165:2245–51.
47 Marmot MG, Bosma H, Hemingway H, Brunner E, Stansfeld S. Contribution of job control and other risk factors to social variations in coronary heart disease incidence. Lancet 1997;350:235–39.
48 Matthews KA, Gump BB, Harris KF, et. al. Hostile behaviours predict cardiovascular mortality among men enrolled in the Multiple Risk Factor Intervention Trial. Circulation 2004;109:66–70.
49 Williams JE, Nieto FJ, Sanford CP, Tyroler HA. Effects of an angry temperament on coronary heart disease risk: The Atherosclerosis Risk in Communities Study. Am J Epidemiol 2001;154: 230–35.
50 Eaker ED, Sullivan LM, Kelly-Hayes M, et. al. Anger and hostility predict the development of atrial fibrillation in men in the Framingham Offspring Study. Circulation 2004;109:1267–71.
51 Castillo-Richmond A, Schneider RH, Alexander CN, Cook R, Myers H, Nidich S, Haney C, Rainforth M, Salerno J. Effects of stress reduction on carotid atherosclerosis in hypertensive African Americans. Stroke 2000;31(3):568–73.
52 Blumenthal JA, Jiang W, Babyak MA, et. al. Stress management and exercise training in cardiac patients with myocardial ischemia. Effects on prognosis and evaluation of mechanisms. Arch Int Med 1997;157:2213–23.
53 Bernardi L, Porta C, Sleight P. Cardiovascular, cerebrovascular, and respiratory changes induced by different types of music in musicians and non-musicians: the importance of silence.Heart 2006;92(4):445–52.
54 Naska A, Oikonomou E, Trichopoulou A, et. al. Siesta in Healthy Adults and Coronary Mortality in the General Population, Arch Intern Med 2007;167:296–301.
55 Empana JP, Dauvilliers Y, Dartigues JF, et. al. Excessive Daytime Sleepiness Is an Independent Risk Indicator for Cardiovascular Mortality in Community-Dwelling Elderly. The 3 City Study. Stroke 2009 Feb 26. (Epub ahead of print).
56 King CR, Knutson KL, Rathouz PJ, Sidney S, Liu K, Lauderdale DS. Short sleep duration and incident coronary artery calcification. JAMA 2008;300(24):2859–66.
57 Eguchi K, Pickering TG, Schwartz JE,et. al. Short Sleep Duration as an Independent Predictor of Cardiovascular Events in Japanese Patients With Hypertension. Arch Intern Med 2008;168(20): 2225–31.
58 Cohen MC, Rohtla KM, Lavery CE, Muller JE, Mittleman MA. Meta-analysis of the morning excess of acute myocardial infarction and sudden cardiac death. Am J Cardiol 1997;79(11):1512–6.
59 Marin JM, Carrizo SJ, Vicente E, Agusti AG. Long-term cardiovascular outcomes in men with obstructive sleep apnoea-hypopnoea with or without treatment with continuous positive airway pressure: an observational study. Lancet 2005;365:1046–53
60 Gami AS et. al. Day-night pattern of sudden death in obstructive sleep apnea. NEJM 2005;352:1206–1214
61 Lee SA, Amis TC, Byth K, Larcos G, Kairaitis K, Robinson TD, Wheatley JR. Heavy snoring as a cause of carotid artery atherosclerosis. Sleep 2008;31(9):1207–13.
62 Michos ED, Melamed ML. vitamin D and cardiovascular disease risk. Curr Opin Clin Nutr Metab Care 2008;11(1):7–12.
63 Zitterman A, Schleithoff SS, Koerfer R. Putting cardiovascular diseases and vitamin D insufficiency into perspective. Br J Nutr 2005;94:483–92.
64 Rostand SG. Ultraviolet light may contribute to geographic and racial blood pressure differences. Hypertension1997;30(2.1):150–56.
65 Holick MF. Sunlight and vitamin D for bone health and prevention of autoimmune diseases, cancers, and cardiovascular disease. Am J Clin Nutr.2004;80(6):1678S-1688S.
66 Krause R, Buhring M, Hopfenmuller W, Holick MF, Sharma AM. Ultraviolet B and blood pressure (letter). Lancet 1998;352:709–10.
67 Scragg R. Seasonality of cardiovascular disease mortality and the possible protective effect of ultra-violet radiation. Int. J Epidemiol 1981;10(4):337–41.
68 Grant WB, Strange RC, Garland CF. Sunshine is good medicine. The health benefits of ultraviolet-B induced vitamin D production. J Cosmet Dermatol 2003;2(2):86–98.
69 Heaney RP. Nutrition and Chronic Disease. Mayo Clinic Proceedings; March 2006;81(3):297–99.
70 Grant WB, Holick MF. Benefits and requirements of vitamin D for optimal health: a review. Alter Med Rev 2005;10:94–111.
71 Holick MF. The vitamin D Epidemic and its Health Consequences. J Nutr 2005;135:2739S-2748S.
72 Lee JH, O'Keefe JH, Bell D, Hensrud DD, Holick MF. vitamin D deficiency an important, common, and easily treatable cardiovascular risk factor? J Am Coll Cardiol 2008;52(24):1949–56.
73 Autier P, Gandini S. vitamin D Supplementation and Total Mortality.A Meta-analysis of Randomized Controlled Trials. Arch Intern Med 2007;167(16):1730–37.
74 Melamed ML, Muntner P, Michos ED, et. al. Serum 25-Hydroxyvitamin D levels and the prevalence of peripheral arterial disease. Results form NHANES 2001 to 2004. Arterioscler Thromb Vasc Biol 2008 Apr 16; (Epub ahead of print).
75 Holick MF. Sunlight and vitamin D for bone health and prevention of autoimmune diseases, cancers, and cardiovascular disease. AJCN 2004;80(6 Suppl):1678S-88S.
76 Holick MF. vitamin D: important for prevention of osteoporosis, cardiovascular heart disease, type 1 diabetes, autoimmune diseases, and some cancers. South Med J 2005;98(10):1024–7.
77 Dobnig H, Pilz S, Scharnagl H, Renner W, et. al. Independent association of low serum 25-hydroxyvitamin d and 1,25-dihydroxyvitamin d levels with all-cause and cardiovascular mortality. Arch Intern Med 2008;168(12):1340–9.
78 Zittermann A. vitamin D and disease prevention with special reference to cardiovascular disease. Progress of Biophysics and Molecular Biology 2006;82:39–48.

79 Fahrleitner A, Dobnig H, Obernosterer A, et. al. vitamin D deficiency and secondary hyperparathyroidism are common complications inpatients with peripheral arterial disease. J Gen Intern Med 2002;17:663–69.
80 Levin A, Li YC. vitamin D and its analogues: do they protect against cardiovascular disease in patients with kidney disease? Kidney Int 2005;68(5):1973–81.
81 Sepulveda JL, Mehta JL. C-reactive protein and cardiovascular disease: a critical appraisal. Curr Opinion Cardiol 2005;20:407–16.
82 Schmidt-Gayk H, Goossen J, Lendle F, Seidel D. Serum 25-hydroxycholecalciferol in myocardial infarction. Atherosclerosis 1977;26:55–58.
83 Scragg R, Jackson R, Holdaway JM, Lim T, Beaglehole R. Myocardial infarction is inversely associated with plasma 25-hydroxyvitamin D3 levels: a community-based study. Int J Epidemiol 1990;19(3):559–63.
84 Zitterman A, Schleithoff SS, Tenderich G, Berthold HK, Korfer R, Stehle P. Low vitamin D status: a contributing factor in the pathogenesis of congestive heart failure? J Am Coll Cardiol 2003;41:105–12.
85 Dobnig H, Pilz S, Scharnagl H, et. al. Independent association of low serum 25-hydroxyvitamin d and 1,25-dihydroxyvitamin d levels with all-cause and cardiovascular mortality. Arch Internal Medicine 2008;168:1340–49.
86 Pekkanen J, Peters A, Hoek G, et. al. Particulate air pollution and risk of ST-segment depression during repeated submaximal exercise tests among subjects with coronary heart disease: the Exposure and Risk Assessment for Fine and Ultrafine Particles in Ambient Air (ULTRA) study. Circulation 2002;106(8):933–8.
87 Miller KA, Siscovick DS, Sheppard, L et. al. Long-term exposure to air pollution and incidence of cardiovascular events in women. NEJM 2007;356:447–58.
88 Dockery DW, Stone PH. Cardiovascular risks from fine particulate air pollution. NEJM 2007;356: 511–13.
89 Peters A, von Klot S, Heier M, et. al. Exposure to traffic and the onset of myocardial infarction. NEJM 2004;351:1721–30.
90 Stone PH. Triggering myocardial infarction. NEJM 2004;351:1716–18.
91 Brooke RD. Air Pollution: What Is Bad for the Arteries Might Be Bad for the Veins. Arch Int Med 2008; 168:909–11.
92 Mills NL, Törnqvist H, Gonzalez MC, et. al. Ischemic and Thrombotic Effects of Dilute Diesel-Exhaust Inhalation in Men with Coronary Heart Disease. NEJM 2007;357:1075–82.
93 Kenfield SA et. al. Smoking and smoking cessation in relation to mortality in women. JAMA 2008;299:2037–47.
94 Susan F Hurley. Short-term impact of smoking cessation on myocardial infarction and stroke hospitalisations and costs in Australia. MJA 2005;183:13–17.
95 US Department of Health and Human Services: Physical activity and health: A report of the Surgeon General. Atlanta, Centre for Disease Control and Prevention, 1996. Online. Available: www.cdc.gov (accessed 10 March 2009).
96 Gordon-Larsen P, Hou N, Sidney S, et. al.. Fifteen-year longitudinal trends in walking patterns and their impact on weight change. AJCN 200989:19–26.
97 Briffa TG, Maiorana A, Sheerin NJ, et. al. Physical activity for people with cardiovascular disease: recommendations of the National Heart Foundation of Australia. MJA 2006;184(2):71–75.
98 Lett HS, Davidson J, Blumenthal JA. Nonpharmacologic treatments for depression in patients with coronary heart disease. Psychosom Med 2005;67 Suppl 1:S58–62.
99 Jayasinghe SR. Yoga in cardiac health (a review). Eur J Cardiovasc Prev Rehabil 2004;11(5):369–75.
100 Nazzaro P, Triggiani R, Ciancio L, et. al. Insulin resistance in essential hypertension: a psychophysiological approach to the 'chicken and egg' question. Nutr Metab Cardiovasc Dis 2000;10(5):275–86.
101 Schneider RH, Alexander CN, Salerno JW, et. al. Disease prevention and health promotion in the ageing with a traditional system of natural medicine: Maharishi Vedic Medicine. J Ageing Health 2002;14(1):57–78.
102 King MS, Carr T, D'Cruz C. Transcendental meditation, hypertension and heart disease. Aust Fam Phys 2002;31(2):164–8.
103 Fields JZ, Walton KG, Schneider RH, et. al. Effect of a multimodality natural medicine program on carotid atherosclerosis in older subjects: a pilot trial of Maharishi Vedic Medicine. Am J Cardiol 2002;89(8):952–8.
104 Innes KE, Vincent HK, Taylor AG. Chronic stress and insulin resistance-related indices of cardiovascular disease risk, part 2: a potential role for mind-body therapies. Altern Ther Health Med 2007;13(5):44–51.
105 Manchanda SC, Narang R, Reddy KS, et. al. Retardation of coronary atherosclerosis with yoga lifestyle intervention. J Assoc Physicians India 2000;48(7):687–94.
106 Hong Y, Li JX, Robinson PD. Balance control, flexibility, and cardiorespiratory fitness among older Tai Chi practitioners. Br J Sports Med 2000;34:29–34.
107 Rogers CE, Larkey LK, Keller C. A review of clinical trials of tai chi and qigong in older adults. West J Nurs Res 2009;31(2):245–79.
108 Lee MS, Pittler MH, Guo R, Ernst E. Qigong for hypertension: A systematic review of randomized clinical trials. Journal of Hypertension 2007;25(8):1525–32.
109 Yang Y, Verkuilen JV, Rosengren KS, Grubisich, et. al. Effect of combined taiji and qigong training on balance mechanisms: A randomized controlled trial of older adults. Medical Science Monitor 2007;13(8):CR339–CR348.
110 Tsang HWH, Fung KMT, Chan ASM, et. al. Effect of a qigong exercise program on elderly with depression. International J Geriat Psych 2006; 21(9):890–97.
111 Sancier, K. M. (1999). Therapeutic benefits of qigong exercises in combination with drugs. J Alter Complem Med 1999;5(4), 383–89.
112 Arthur HM, Patterson C, Stone JA. The role of complementary and alternative therapies in cardiac rehabilitation: a systematic evaluation. Eur J Cardiovasc Prev Rehab 2006;13(1):3–9.
113 Lee MJ, Kilbreath SL, Singh MF, et. al. Comparison of effect of aerobic cycle training and progressive resistance training on walking ability after stroke: a randomized sham exercise-controlled study. J Am Geriatr Soc 2008;56(6):976–85.

114 Westhoff TH, Schmidt S, Gross V, et. al. The cardiovascular effects of upper-limb aerobic exercise in hypertensive patients. J Hypertens 2008;26(7):1336–42.
115 Smith FW Jr. Acupuncture for cardiovascular disorders. Probl Vet Med 1992;4(1):125–31.
116 VanWormer AM, Lindquist R, Sendelbach SE. The effects of acupuncture on cardiac arrhythmias: a literature review. Heart Lung 2008;37(6):425–31.
117 Ginter E. Vegetarian diets, chronic diseases and longevity. Bratisl Lek Listy 2008;109(10):463–6.
118 Iqbal R, Anand S, Ounpuu S, et. al. on behalf of the INTERHEART Study Investigators. Dietary Patterns and the Risk of Acute Myocardial Infarction in 52 Countries. Results of the INTERHEART Study. Circulation 2008;118:1929–37.
119 Berg CM, Lappas G, Strandhagen E, et. al. Food patterns and cardiovascular disease risk factors: The Swedish INTERGENE research program. AJC N 2008 88;289–97.
120 Brunner EJ, Rees K, Ward K, Burke M, Thorogood M. Dietary advice for reducing cardiovascular risk. Cochrane Database of Systematic Reviews 2007, Issue 4. Art. No.: CD002128. doi: 10.1002/14651858.CD002128.pub3.
121 Keys A. Mediterranean diet and public health: personal reflections. AJCN 1995;61(6 Suppl):1321S-1323S.
122 Costacou T, Edmundowicz D et. al. Progression of coronary artery calcium in type 1 diabetes mellitus 2007;100(10):1543–7.
123 Rosemary Stanton. Australian Doctor 30 January 2009:29–30.
124 Kozue Nakamura, Chisato Nagata, Shino Oba, Naoyoshi Takatsuka and Hiroyuki Shimizu. Fruit and Vegetable Intake and Mortality from Cardiovascular Disease Are Inversely Associated in Japanese Women but Not in Men. J Nutr 2008 138:1129–34.
125 Jarrett PG, Rockwood K, Carver D, et. al. Illness presentation in elderly patients. Arch Intern Med 2007;167:1060–67.
126 Fung TT, Rexrode KM, Mantzoros CS, et. al. Mediterranean diet and incidence of and mortality from coronary heart disease and stroke in women. Circulation 2009;119(8):1093–100.
127 SOLOS (Spanish Olive Oil Study) Study Investigators. Anti-inflammatory effect of virgin olive oil in stable coronary disease patients: a randomized, cross-over, controlled trial. Eur J Clin Nutr 2008; 62, 570–574; doi:10.1038/sj.ejcn.1602724;
128 Franco OH, Bonneux L, de Laet C, et. al. The Polymeal: a more natural, safer, and probably tastier (than the Polypill) strategy to reduce cardiovascular disease by more than 75%. BMJ 2004;329:18–25.
129 Sofi F, et. al. Adherence to Mediterranean diet and health status: a meta-analysis. B MJ 2008;337:a1344.
130 Martínez-González MA, de la Fuente-Arrillaga C, Nunez-Cordoba JM, et. al. Adherence to Mediterranean diet and risk of developing diabetes: prospective cohort study. BMJ 2008;336(7657):1348–51.
131 Appel LJ, Moore TJ, Obarzanek E, et. al. A clinical trial of the effects of dietary patterns on blood pressure. DASH Collaborative Research Group. NEJM 1997;336(16):1117–24.
132 Ascherio A, Rimm EB, Giovannucci EL, et. al. A prospective study of nutritional factors and hypertension among US men. Circulation 1992;86(5):1475–84.
133 Fung TT, Chiuve SE, McCullough ML, et. al. Adherence to a DASH-Style Diet and Risk of Coronary Heart Disease and Stroke in Women Archives of Internal Medicine 2008;168(7):713–20.
134 Pereira MA, O'Reilly E, Augustsson K, et. al. Dietary fibre and risk of coronary heart disease: a pooled analysis of cohort studies. Arch Intern Med 2004;164(4):370–6.
135 Djoussé L, Gaziano MJ. Breakfast Cereals and Risk of Heart Failure in the Physicians' Health Study I. Arch Intern Med 2007;167(19):2080–85.
136 Erkkilä AT, Herrington DM, Mozaffarian D, Lichtenstein AH. Cereal fibre and whole-grain intake are associated with reduced progression of coronary-artery atherosclerosis in post-menopausal women with coronary artery disease. Am Heart J 2005;150:94–101.
137 Andon MB, Anderson JW. State of the Art Reviews: The Oatmeal-Cholesterol Connection: 10 Years Later. Am J Lifestyle Med 2008;2(1): 51–57.
138 Vincent-Baudry S, Defoort D, Gerber M, et. al. The Medi-RIVAGE study: reduction of cardiovascular disease risk factors after a 3-mo intervention with a Mediterranean-type diet or a low-fat diet. AJCN 2005;82:964–71.
139 Segasothy M, Phillips PA. Vegetarian diet: panacea for modern lifestyle diseases? QJM 1999;92(9): 531–44.
140 Howard BV, Van Horn L, Hsia J, et. al. Low-fat dietary pattern and risk of cardiovascular disease: the Women's Health Initiative Randomized Controlled Dietary Modification Trial. JAMA 2006;295(6): 655–66.
141 Mozaffarian D, Rimm EB. Fish intake, contaminants, and human health: evaluating the risks and the benefits. JAMA 2006;296:1885–99.
142 Iso H, M. Kobayashi, et. al. Intake of fish and n3 fatty acids and risk of coronary heart disease among Japanese: the Japan Public Health Center-Based (JPHC) Study Cohort I. Circulation 2006;113(2):195–202.
143 Siscovick DS, Raghunathan TE, King I, et. al. Dietary intake and cell membrane levels of long-chain n-3polyunsaturated fatty acids and the risk of primary cardiac arrest. JAMA 1995;274: 1363–67.
144 Mozaffarian D, Bryson CL, Lemaitre RN, Burke GL, Siscovick DS. Fish intake and risk of heart failure. J Am Coll Cardiol 2005;45:2015–21.
145 Mozaffarian D, Psaty BM, Rimm EB, et. al. Fish intake and risk of incident atrial fibrillation. Circulation 2004;110:368–73.
146 Ros E, Núñez I, Pérez-Heras A, Serra M, et. al. A walnut diet improves endothelial function in hypercholesterolemic subjects: a randomized cross-over trial. Circulation 2004;109:1609–14.
147 Gillen LJ, Tapsell LC, Patch CS, et. al. Structured dietary advice incorporating walnuts achieves optimal fat and energy balance in patients with type 2 diabetes mellitus. J Am Dietet Assoc 2005;105:1087–95.
148 Gebauer SK, West SG, Kay CD, et. al. Effects of pistachios on cardiovascular disease risk factors and potential mechanisms of action: a dose-response study. AJCN 2008;88(3):651–59.
149 Phillips KM, Ruggio DM, Ashraf-Khorassani M. Phytosterol composition of nuts and seeds commonly consumed in the United States. J Agric Food Chem 2005;53:9436–45.

150 Vermeer C, Shearer MJ, Zittermann A, et. al. Beyond deficiency: potential benefits of increased intakes of vitamin K for bone and vascular health. Eur J Nutr 2004;43(6):325–35.
151 Berkner KL, Runge KW. The physiology of vitamin K nutriture and vitamin K-dependent protein function in atherosclerosis. J Thromb Haemost 2004;2(12):2118–32.
152 Geleijnse JM, Vermeer C, Grobbee DE, et. al. Dietary intake of menaquinone is associated with a reduced risk of coronoary heart disease: the Rotterdam Study. J Nutr 2004;134(11):3100–5.
153 Schurgers LJ, Vermeer C. Determination of phylloquinone and menaquinones in food. Effect of food matrix on circulating vitamin K concentrations. Haemostasis 2000;30(6):298–307.
154 Cook NR, Cutler JA, Obarzanek E, et. al. Long term effects of dietary sodium reduction on cardiovascular disease outcomes: observational follow-up of the trials of hypertension prevention (TOHP). BMJ 2007; 334(7599):885.
155 Dickinson KM, Keogh JB, Clifton PM. Effects of a low-salt diet on flow-mediated dilatation in humans. Am J Clin Nutr 2009 Feb;89(2):485–90.
156 Lee R, Balick M. Rx: chocolate. Explore (NY) 2005;1(2):136–9.
157 di Giuseppe R, Di Castelnuovo A, Centritto F, Zito F, De Curtis A, Costanzo S, Vohnout B, Sieri S, Krogh V, Donati MB, de Gaetano G, Iacoviello L. Regular consumption of dark chocolate is associated with low serum concentrations of C-reactive protein in a healthy italian population. J Nutr 2008;138:1939–45.
158 Balzer J, Rassaf T, Heiss C, et. al. Sustained benefits in vascular function through flavanol-containing cocoa in medicated diabetic patients a double-masked, randomized, controlled trial. J Am Coll Cardiol 2008;551:2141–49.
159 Engler MB, Engler MM, Chen CY, et. al. Flavonoid-rich dark chocolate improves endothelial function and increases plasma epicatechin concentrations in healthy adults. J Am Coll Nutr 2004;23:197–204.
160 Britton A, Marmot MG, Shipley M. Who benefits most from the cardio-protective properties of alcohol consumption—health freaks or couch potatoes? Journal of Epidemiology and Community Health 2008;62:905–8.
161 Mukamal KJ, Chiuve SE, Rimm EB. Alcohol consumption and risk for coronary heart disease in men with healthy lifestyles. Arch Intern Med 2006;166:2145–50.
162 de Lorimier AA. Alcohol, wine, and health. Am J Surgg 2000;180(5):357–61.
163 Bertelli AA. Wine, research and cardiovascular disease: instructions for use.Atherosclerosis 2007;195:242–47.
164 Kuriyama S et. al. Green tea consumption and mortality due to cardiovascular disease, cancer, and all causes in Japan: the Ohsaki study. JAMA 2006;296:1255–65.
165 Gardner EJ, Ruxton CH, Leeds AR. Black tea--helpful or harmful? A review of the evidence. Eur J Clin Nutr 2007;61(1):3–18.
166 Adam J Berger, Kevin Alford. Cardiac arrest in a young man following excess consumption of caffeinated 'energy drinks'. MJA 2009;190:41–43.
167 Namdar M, Koepfli P, Grathwohl R, et. al. Caffeine decreases exercise-induced myocardial flow reserve. J Am Coll Cardiol 2006;47:405–10.
168 Lopez-Garcia E, van Dam RM, Willett WC, et. al. Coffee consumption and coronary heart disease in men and women: a prospective cohort study. Circulation 2006;113:2045–53.
169 Silletta MG, Marfisi R, Levantesi G, et. al. Coffee consumption and risk of cardiovascular events after acute myocardial infarction: results from the GISSI (Gruppo Italiano per lo Studio della Sopravvivenza nell'Infarto miocardico)-Prevenzione trial. Circulation 2007;116(25):2944–51.
170 Sumner MD, Elliott-Eller M, Weidner G, et. al. Effects of pomegranate juice consumption on myocardial perfusion in patients with coronary heart disease. Amer J Cardiol 2005;96:810–14.
171 Houston MC, Cooil B, Olafsson BJ, Raggi P. Juice Powder Concentrate and Systemic Blood Pressure, Progression of Coronary Artery Calcium and Antioxidant Status in Hypertensive Subjects: A Pilot Study. Evid Based Complement Alternat Med 2007;4(4):455–62.
172 Gladys Block, Christopher D Jensen, Edward P Norkus, Tapashi B Dalvi, Les G Wong, Jamie F McManus and Mark L Hudes. Usage patterns, health, and nutritional status of long-term multiple dietary supplement users: a cross-sectional study. Nutrition Journal 2007,6:30. doi:10.1186/1475-2891-6-30.
173 Hercberg S, Galan P, Preziosi P, Bertrais S, Mennen L, Malvy D, Roussel AM, Favier A, Briançon S. The SU.VI.MAX Study: a randomized, placebo-controlled trial of the health effects of antioxidant vitamins and minerals. Arch Intern Med 2004;164(21):2335–42.
174 Palinski W, Witztum JL. Immune responses to oxidative neoepitopes on LDL and phospholipids modulate the development of atherosclerosis. J Int Med 2000;247(3):371–80.
175 Engler MM, Engler MB, Malloy MJ, et. al. Antioxidant vitamins C and E improve endothelial function in children with hyperlipidemia: Endothelial Assessment of Risk from Lipids in Youth (EARLY) Trial. Circulation 2003;108(9):1059–63. 272.
176 Blumberg JB. An update: vitamin E supplementation and heart disease. Nutr Clin Care 2002;5(2):50–5. 274.
177 Munteanu A, Zingg JM, Azzi A. Anti-atherosclerotic effects of vitamin E—myth or reality? J Cell Mol Med 2004;8(1):59–76. 277.
178 Colquhoun DM. Nutraceuticals: vitamins and other nutrients in coronary heart disease (Review). Curr Opin Lipidol 2001;12(6):639–46. 280.
179 Celestini A, Pulcinelli FM, Pignatelli P, et. al. vitamin E potentiates the antiplatelet activity of aspirin in collagen-stimulated platelets. Haematologica 2002;87(4):420–6.
180 Hamabe A, Takase B, Uehata A, et. al. Impaired endothelium-dependent vasodilation in the brachial artery in variant angina pectoris and the effect of intravenous administration of vitamin C. Am J Cardiol 2001;87(10):1154–9.
181 Sesso HD, Buring JE, Christen WG, et. al. vitamins E and C in the prevention of cardiovascular disease in men: the Physicians' Health Study II randomized controlled trial. JAMA 2008;300:2123–33.
182 Cook NR, Albert CM, Gaziano MJ, et. al. A Randomized Factorial Trial of vitamins C and E and Beta Carotene in the Secondary Prevention of Cardiovascular Events in Women. Results From the Women's Antioxidant Cardiovascular Study. Arch Intern Med 2007;167(15):1610–1618
183 Sali A, Vitetta L. Nutritional supplements and cardiovascular disease. Heart Lung Circ 2004;13(4):363–6.

184 Goldberg AC. A meta-analysis of randomized controlled studies on the effects of extended-release niacin in women. Am J Cardiol 2004;94(1):121–4.
185 Aleman G, Tovar AR, Torres N. Homocysteine metabolism and risk of cardiovascular diseases: importance of the nutritional status on folic acid, vitamins B6 and B12. Rev Invest Clin 2001;53(2):141–51.
186 Kolling K, Ndrepepa G, Koch W, et. al. Methylenetetrahy-drofolate reductase gene C677T and A1298C polymorphisms, plasma homocysteine, folate, and vitamin B12 levels and the extent of coronary artery disease. Am J Cardiol 2004;93(10):1201–6.
187 Hickling S, Hung J, Knuiman M, et. al. Impact of voluntary folate fortification on plasma homocysteine and serum folate in Australia from 1995 to 2001: a population based cohort study J Epid Comm Health 2005;59:371–76.
188 Quadri P, Fragiacomo C, Pezzati R, et. al. Homocysteine, folate, and vitamin B-12 in mild cognitive impairment, Alzheimer disease, and vascular dementia. AJCN 2004;80(1):114–22.
189 Oakley Jr GP. Global prevention of all folic acid-preventable spina bifida and anencephaly by 2010. Community Genet 2002;5(1):70–7.
190 Bailey LB, Rampersaud GC, Kauwell GP. Folic acid supplements and fortification affect the risk for neural tube defects, vascular disease and cancer: evolving science (Review). J Nutr 2003;133(6):1961S–8S.
191 Ferguson LR, Philpott M, Karunasinghe N. Dietary cancer and prevention using antimutagens. Toxicology 2004;198(1–3):147–59.
192 Martinez ME, Henning SM, Alberts DS. Folate and colorectal neoplasia: relation between plasma and dietary markers of folate and adenoma recurrence. AJCN 2004;79(4):691–7.
193 Zhang SM, Willett WC, Selhub J, et. al. A prospective study 317of plasma total cysteine and risk of breast cancer. Cancer Epidemiol Biomarkers Prev 2003;12(11 Pt 1):1188–93. 319.
194 Albert CM, Cook NR, Gaziano JM, et. al. Effect of folic acid and B vitamins on risk of cardiovascular events and total mortality among women at high risk for cardiovascular disease: a randomized trial. JAMA 2008;299(17):2027–36.
195 Ebbing M, Bleie Ø, Ueland PM, et. al. Mortality and cardiovascular events in patients treated with homocysteine-lowering B vitamins after coronary angiography: a randomized controlled trial. JAMA 2008;300(7):795–804.
196 Li YC. vitamin D regulation of the rennin-angiotensin system. J Cell Biochem 2003;88:327–31.
197 Sepulveda JL, Mehta JL. C-reactive protein and cardiovascular disease: a critical appraisal. Curr Opinion Cardiol 2005;20:407–16.
198 McCarty MF. Secondary hyperparathyroidism promotes the acute phase response-a rationale for supplemental vitamin D in the prevention of vascular events in the elderly. Med Hypotheses 2005;64:1022–26.
199 Vermeer C, Braam L, Knapen M and Schurgers L. vitamin K supplementation: a simple way to improve vascular health. Agr Food Industry Hi Tech Nov 2003.
200 Braam LAJLM. Thesis, Maastricht ISBN 90-5681-145-2, 2002.
201 Spronk HM, Soute BA, Schurgers LJ, et. al. Tissue-specific utilization of menaquinone-4 results in the prevention of arterial calcification in warfarin-treated rats. J Vasc Res 2003;40(6):531–7.
202 Kawashima H, Nakajima Y, Matubara Y, et. al. Effects of vitamin K2 (menatetrenone) on atherosclerosis and blood coagulation in hypercholesterolemic rabbits. Jpn J Pharmacol 1997;75(2):135–43.
203 Sconce E, Khan T, Mason J, et. al. Patients with unstable control have a poor dietary intake of vitamin K compared to patients with stable control of anticoagulation. Thromb Haemost 2005;93(5):872–5.
204 Sconce E, Khan T, Mason J, et. al. Patients with unstable control have a poorer dietary intake of vitamin K compared to patients with stable control of anticoagulation. Thromb Haemost 2005;93(5):872–5.
205 Couris R, Tataronis G, McCloskey W, et. al. Dietary vitamin K variability affects International Normalized Ration (INR) coagulation indices. Int J vitamin Nutr Res 2006;76(2):65–74.
206 Sconce E, Avery P, Wynne H, Kamali F. vitamin K supplementation can improve stability of anticoagulation for patients with unexplained variability in response to warfarin. Blood 2007;109(6):2419–23.
207 Khan T, Wynne H, Wood P et. al. Dietary vitamin K influences intra-individual variability in anticoagulant response to warfarin. Br J Haematol 2004;124(3):348–54.
208 Turlapaty PD, Altura BM. Magnesium deficiency produces spasms of coronary arteries: relationship to etiology of sudden death ischemic heart disease. Science 1980;208(4440):198–200.
209 Altura BM. Ischemic heart disease and magnesium (Review). Magnesium 1988;7(2):57–67.
210 Schecter M, Shahir M, Labrador MJ et. al. Oral magnesium therapy improves endothelial function, in patients with coronary artery disease. Circulation 2000;102(19):2353–8.
211 Schecter M, et. al. Effects of oral magnesium therapy on exercise tolerance, exercise-induced chest pain, and quality of life in patients with coronary artery disease. Am J Cardiol 2003;91(5):517–21.
212 Leone N, Courbon D, Ducimetiere P, Zureik M. Zinc, copper, and magnesium and risks for all-cause, cancer, and cardiovascular mortality. Epidemiology 2006 May;17(3):308–14.
213 Tejada T, Fornoni A, Lenz O, Materson BJ. Nonpharmacologic therapy for hypertension: does it really work? Curr Cardiol Rep 2006;8(6):418–24. Review.
214 Jee SH, Miller ER 3rd, Guallar E, et. al. The effect of magnesium supplementation on blood pressure: a meta-analysis of randomized control trials. Am J Hypertens 2002;15(8):691–6.
215 Teo KK, Yusuf S. Role of magnesium in reducing mortality in acute myocardial infarction. A review of the evidence. Drugs 1993;46(3):347–59.
216 Thogersen AM, Johnson O, Wester PO. Effects of intravenous magnesium sulfate in suspected acute myocardial infarction on acute arrhythmias and long-term outcome. Int J Cardiol 1995;49(2):143–51.
217 Shechter M, Kaplinsky E, Rabinowitz B. The rationale of magnesium supplementation in acute myocardial infarction. A review of the literature. Arch Intern Med 1992;152(11):2189–96.
218 Fourth International Study of Infarct Survival Collaboration Group. ISIS-4: A randomized factorial trial assessing oral captopril, oral mononitrate, and intravenous magnesium sulfate in 58,050 patients with suspected acute myocardial infarction. Lancet 1995;345:669–85.

219 ISIS-4 (Fourth International Study of Infarct Survival) Collaboration Group. ISIS-4: A randomized factorial trial assessing oral captopril, oral mononitrate, and intravenous magnesium sulfate in 58,050 patients with suspected acute myocardial infarction. Lancet 1995;345:669–85.
220 The Magnesium in Coronaries (MAGIC) Trial Investigators. Early administration of intravenous magnesium to high-risk patients with acute myocardial infarction in the Magnesium in Coronaries (MAGIC) Trial: a randomized controlled trial. Lancet 2002;360:1189–96.
221 Bolland MJ, Barber PA, Doughty RN, et. al. Vascular events in healthy older women receiving calcium supplementation: randomised controlled trial. BMJ, doi:10.1136/bmj.39440.525752.BE (15 January 2008).
222 Kardinaal AF, Kok FJ, Kohlmeier L, Martin-Moreno JM, et. al. Association between toenail selenium and risk of acute myocardial infarction in European men. The EURAMIC Study. European Antioxidant Myocardial Infarction and Breast Cancer. Am J Epidemiol 1997;145(4):347 373–9.
223 Rayman MP. The importance of selenium to human health. Lancet 2000;356(9225):233–41.
224 Thomson CD. Selenium and iodine intakes and status in New Zealand and Australia. Br J Nutr 2004;91(5):661–352.
225 Li H, Stampfer MJ, Giovannucci EL, et. al. A prospective study of plasma selenium levels and prostate cancer risk. JNCI 2004;96(9):696–703.
226 Mozaffarian D, Greelen A, Brouwer IA, et. al. Effect of fish oil on heart rate in humans: a meta-analysis of randomized controlled trials. Circulation 2005;112:1945–52.
227 O'Keefe JH Jr, Abuissa H, Sastre A, et. al. Effects of omega-3 fatty acids on resting heart rate, heart rate recovery after exercise, and heart rate variability in men with healed myocardial infarctions and depressed ejection fractions. Am J Cardiol 2006;97:1127–30.
228 Ninio DM, Hill AM, Howe PR, et. al. Docosahexaenoic acid-rich fish oil improves heart rate variability and heart rate responses to exercise in overweight adults. Br J Nutr 2008;100(5):1097–103.
229 Mozaffarian D, Geelen A, Brouwer IA, et. al. Effect of fish oil on heart rate in humans: a meta-analysis of randomized controlled trials Ciculation 2005;112:1945–52.
230 Kris-Etherton PM, Harris WS, Appel LJ, et. al. Omega-3 fatty acids and cardiovascular disease: new recommendations from the American Heart Association (Review). Arterioscler Thromb Vasc Biol 2003;23(2):151–2.
231 Kris-Etherton PM, HarrisWS, Appel LJ, et. al. American Heart Association Nutrition Committee. Fish consumption, fish oil, omega-3 fatty acids, and cardiovascular disease. Circulation 2002;106(21):2747–57.
232 Harris WS, Mozaffarian D, Rimm E, et. al. Omega-6 fatty acids and risk for cardiovascular disease: a science advisory from the American Heart Association Nutrition Subcommittee of the Council on Nutrition, Physical Activity, and Metabolism; Council on Cardiovascular Nursing; and Council on Epidemiology and Prevention. Circulation 2009;119(6):902–7.
233 Colquhoun DFerreira A., Udell T, Eden B. APD, and the Nutrition and Metabolism Committee of the Heart Foundation. Review of evidence: Fish, fish oils, n-3 polyunsaturated fatty acids and cardiovascular health. Position statement on fish, fish oils, n-3 polyunsaturated fatty acids and cardiovascular health (updated November 2008). Heart Foundation. Online. Available: http://www.heartfoundation.org.au/Healthy_Living/Eating_and_Drinking/Fish/Pages/default.aspxhttp,http://www.heartfoundation.org.au/SiteCollectionDocuments/HW_FS_FishOils_PS_FINAL_web.pdfPosition Statement references,Position Statement references: http://www.heartfoundation.org.au/SiteCollectionDocuments/HW_FS_FishOil_PS_References_FINAL.pdf (accessed 01-02-09)
234 Anand RG, Alkadri M, Lavie CJ, Milani RV. The role of fish oil in arrhythmia prevention. J Cardiopul Rehabil Prev 2008;28(2):92–98.
235 GISSI—P trial Authors. Dietary supplementation with n-3 polyunsaturated fatty acids and vitamin E after myocardial infarction: results of the GISSI-Prevenzione trial. Gruppo Italiano per lo Studio della Sopravvivenza nell'Infarto miocardico. Lancet 1999;354(9177):447–55.
236 WoodmanRJ, MoriTA, BurkeV, et. al. Effects of purified eicosapentaenoic acid and docosahexaenoic acid on platelet, fibrinolytic and vascular function in hypertensive type 2 diabetic patients. Atherosclerosis 2003;166(1):85–93.
237 Bhagavan H, Chopra N&R. Potential role of ubiquinone (Co Enzyme Q10) in pediatric cardiomyopathy 2005;Clin Nutr 24(3):331–8.
238 Gaby AR. The role of coenzyme Q10 in clinical medicine:part II. Cardiovascular disease, hypertension, diabetes mellitus and infertility. Alt Med Rev 1996;1:168–75.
239 Thomas SR, Whiting PK, Stocker R: A role of reduced Co Enzyme Q10 in atherosclerosis? Biofactors.1999;9:207–24.
240 Frank Rosenfelt. Editorial. CoEnzyme Q10 therapy for cardiac disease: science of alternative medicine? Asia Pacific Heart J 1998;7(3):160–8.
241 Kuettner A, Pieper A, Koch J, et. al. Influence of coenzyme Q(10) and cerivastatin on the flow-mediated vasodilation of the brachial artery: results of the ENDOTACT study. Int J Cardiol 2005;98(3):413–9.
242 Tiano L, Belardinelli R, Carnevali P, et. al. Effect of coenzyme Q10 administration on endothelial function and extracellular superoxide dismutase in patients with ischaemic heart disease: a double-blind, randomized controlled study. Eur Heart J 2007;28(18):2249–55.
243 Kamikawa T, Kobayashi A, Yamashita T, et. al. Effects of coenzyme Q10 on exercise tolerance in chronic stable angina pertoris. Am J Cardiol 1985;56(4):247–51.
244 Rundek T, Naini A, Sacco R, Coates K, Di Mauro S. Atorvastatin decreases the coenzyme Q10 level in the blood of patients at risk of cardiovascular disease and stroke. Arch Neurol 2004;61(6):889–92.
245 Dyck JR, Hopkins TA, Bonnet S, et. al. Absence of malonyl coenzyme A decarboxylase in mice increases cardiac glucose oxidation and protects the heart from ischemic injury. Circulation 2006;114:1721–28.

246 Arduini A, Bonomini M, Savica V, et. al. Carnitine in metabolic disease: potential for pharmacological intervention. Pharmacol Ther 2008;120(2):149–56.

247 Vescovo G, Ravara B, Gobbo V, et. al. L-Carnitine: a potential treatment for blocking apoptosis and preventing skeletal muscle myopathy in heart failure. Am J Physiol Cell Physiol 2002;283(3):C802–10.

248 Davini P, Bigalli A, Lamanna F, Boem A. Controlled study on L-carnitine therapeutic efficacy in post-infarction. Drugs Exp Clin Res 1992;18:355–65.

249 Iliceto S, Scrutinio D, Bruzzi P, et. al. Effects of L-carnitine administration on left ventricular remodeling after acute anterior myocardial infarction: The L-carnitine Ecocardiografia Digitalizzata Infarto Miocardico (CEDIM) Trial. J Am Coll Cardiol 1995;26:380–87.

250 Tarantini G, Scrutinio D, Bruzzi P, et. al. Metabolic treatment with L-carnitine in acute anterior ST segment elevation myocardial infarction. A randomized controlled trial. Cardiology 2006' 106:215–23.

251 Demeyere, R., Lormans, P., Weidler, B., et. al. Cardio-protective effects of carnitine in extensive aortocoronary bypass grafting: A double-blind, randomized, placebo-controlled clinical trial. Anesth Analg 1990;71:520–28.

252 Malaguarnera M, Cammalleri L, Gargante MP, et. al. L-Carnitine treatment reduces severity of physical and mental fatigue and increases cognitive functions in centenarians: a randomized and controlled clinical trial. Am J Clin Nutr 2007;86(6):1738–44.

253 Yeh GY, Davis RB, Phillips RS. Use of complementary therapies in patients with cardiovascular disease. Am J Cardiol 2006;98(5):673–80.

254 Koscielny J, Klussendorf D, Latza R, et. al. The antiatherosclerotic effect of *Allium sativum*. Atherosclerosis 1999;144(1):237–49.

255 Banerjee SK, Maulik SK. Effect of garlic on cardiovascular disorders: a review. Nutr Jour 2002;1(4):1–14.

256 Bongiorno PB, Fratellone, PM,LoGiudice P. 'Potential Health Benefits of Garlic (*Allium sativum*): A Narrative Review,' Journal of Complementary and Integrative Medicine 2008;5(1) http://www.bepress.com/jcim/vol5/iss1/1/ (accessed February 2009)

257 Breithaupt-Groegler K, Ling M, Boudoulas H, Belz GG. Protective effect of chronic garlic intake on elastic properties of aorta in the elderly. Circulation 1997;96:2649–55.

258 van Doorn MB, Espirito Santo SM, Meijer P, Kamerling IM, Schoemaker RC,Dirsch V, Vollmar A, Haffner T, Gebhardt R, Cohen AF, Princen HM, Burggraaf J. Effect of garlic powder on C-reactive protein and plasma lipids in overweight and smoking subjects. AJ CN 2006;84(6):1324–9.

259 Gardner CD, Lawson LD, Block E, et. al. Effect of raw garlic vs commercial garlic supplements on plasma lipid concentrations in adults with moderate hypercholesterolemia: a randomized clinical trial. Arch Intern Med 2007;167(4):346–53.

260 Allison GL, Lowe GM, Rahman K. Aged garlic extract and its constituents inhibit platelet aggregation through multiple mechanisms. J Nutr 2006;136(3 Suppl):782S-788S.

261 Der Marderosian A, editor. The review of natural products. Facts and comparisons. Philadelphia: Lippincott, Williams and Wilkins; 2001.

262 Patel AK, Rogers JT, Huang X. Flavanols, mild cognitive impairment, and Alzheimer's dementia. Int J Clin Exp Med 2008;1(2):181–91.

263 Joseph JA, Shukitt-Hale B, Denisova NA, et. al. Reversals of age-related declines in neuronal signal transduction, cognitive, and motor behavioural deficits with blueberry, spinach, or strawberry dietary supplementation. J Neurosci 1999;19(18):8114–21.

264 Kendler BS. Recent nutritional approaches to the prevention and therapy of cardiovascular disease (Review). Prog Cardiovasc Nurs 1997 Summer;12(3):3–23.

265 Weng WL, Zhang WQ, Liu FZ, et. al. Therapeutic effect of Crataegus pinnatifida on 46 cases of angina pectoris—a double-blind study. J Tradit Chin Med 1984;4(4):293–4.

266 Pittler MH, Guo R, Ernst E. Hawthorn extract for treating chronic heart failure. Cochrane Database of Systematic Reviews 2008, Issue 1. Art. No.: CD005312. doi: 10.1002/14651858.CD005312. pub2.

267 Liu J, Zhang J, Shi Y, et. al. Chinese red yeast rice (Monascus purpureus) for primary hyperlipidemia: a meta-analysis of randomized controlled trials. Chin Med 2006;1:4.

268 Heber D, Yip I, Ashley JM, et. al. Cholesterol-lowering effects of a proprietary Chinese red-yeast-rice dietary supplement. AJCN 1999;69(2):231–6.

269 Kou W, Lu Z, Guo J. Effect of xuezhikang on the treatment of primary hyperlipidemia. Zhonghua Nei Ke Za Zhi 1997;36(8):529–31.

270 Duan X, Zhou L, Wu T, Liu G, et. al. Chinese herbal medicine suxiao jiuxin wan for angina pectoris. Cochrane Database of Systematic Reviews 2008;(1).

271 Mozaffarian D, Furberg CD, Patsy BM, Siscovick D. Physical activity and incidence of atrial fibrillation in older adults: the cardiovascular health study. Circulation 2008;118(8):800–7.

272 Felty CL, Rooke TW. Compression therapy for chronic venous insufficiency. Semin Vasc Surg 2005 Mar;18(1):36–40.

273 Badger C, Preston N, Seers K, Mortimer P. Physical therapies for reducing and controlling lymphoedema of the limbs. Cochrane Database Syst Rev 2004 Oct 18;(4):CD003141.

274 Anand RG, Alkadri M, Lavie CJ, Milani RV. The role of fish oil in arrhythmia prevention. J Cardiopul Rehabil Prev 2008;28(2):92–8.

275 Mozaffarian D, Psaty BM, Rimm EB, et. al. Fish intake and risk of incident atrial fibrillation. Circulation 2004;110(4):368–73.

276 Boos CJ, Anderson RA, Lip GYH. Is atrial fibrillation an inflammatory disorder? European Heart Journal 2005;27(2):136–49.

277 Korantzopoulos P, Kolettis TM, Galaris D, Goudevenos JA. The role of oxidative stress in the pathogenesis and perpetuation of atrial fibrillation. Intern J Cardiol 2007;115(2):135–43.

278 Ninio DM, Hill AM, Howe PR, et. al. Docosahexaenoic acid-rich fish oil improves heart rate variability and heart rate responses to exercise in overweight adults. Br J Nutr 2008;100(5): 1097–103.

279 Hernando Leo´n, Marcelo C Shibata, Marlene Dorgan, Ross T Tsuyuki. Effect of fish oil on arrhythmias and mortality: systematic review. BMJ 2009;338:a2931. doi:10.1136/bmj.a2931.

280 Mukamal KJ, Psaty BM, Rautaharju PM, et. al. Alcohol consumption and risk and prognosis of atrial fibrillation among older adults: the Cardiovascular Health Study. Am Heart J 2007;153(2):260–6.

281 de Lorgeril M, Salen P, Martin JL, et. al. Interactions of wine drinking with omega-3 fatty acids in patients with coronary heart disease: a fish-like effect of moderate wine drinking. Am Heart J 2008;155(1):175–81.
282 Davey MJ, Teubner D. A randomized controlled trial of magnesium sulfate, in addition to usual care, for rate control in atrial fibrillation. Emerg Med 2005;45:347–53.
283 Pittler MH, Ernst E. Horse chestnut seed extract for chronic venous insufficiency. Cochrane Database of Systematic Reviews 2006, Issue 1. Art. No.: CD003230. doi: 10.1002/14651858.CD003230.pub3.
284 Curtis JP, Selter JG, Wang Y, et. al. The Obesity Paradox. Body Mass Index and Outcomes in Patients With Heart Failure. Arch Intern Med 2005;165: 55–61.
285 Mozaffarian D, Bryson CL, Lemaitre RN, et. al. Fish Intake and Risk of Incident Heart Failure. J Am Coll Cardiol 2005; 45:2015–21.
286 GISSI-HF Investigators. Effect of n-3 polyunsaturated fatty acids in patients with chronic heart failure (the GISSI-HF trial): a randomised, double-blind, placebo-controlled trial. Lancet 2008;372: 1223–30.
287 Mozaffarian D, Fonarow G. Statins and n-3 fatty acid supplementation in heart failure.2008; 372(9645):1195–6.
288 Pauwels EK, Kostkiewicz M. Fatty acid facts, part III: Cardiovascular disease, or, a fish diet is noy fishy. Drug News Persp 2008;21(10):552–61.
289 Olgar, S, Ertugrul T et. al. Fish oil supplementation improves left ventricular function in children with idiopathic dilated cardiomyopathy Congest Heart Fail 2007;13(6):308–12.
290 Stepura OB, Martynow AI. Magnesium orotate in severe congestive heart failutre (MACH). Int J Cardiol 2009;131(2):293–5.
291 Almoznino-Sarafian D et. al. Magnesium and C-reactive protein in heart failure: an anti-inflammatory effect of magnesium administration? Eur J Nutr 2007;46(4):230–7.
292 Chen J, Wu G, Li S, Yu T, Xie Y, Zhou L, Wang L. Shengmai (a traditional Chinese herbal medicine) for heart failure. Cochrane Database of Systematic Reviews 2007, Issue 4. Art. No.: CD005052. doi: 10.1002/14651858.CD005052.pub2.
293 Pittler MH, Guo R, Ernst E. Hawthorn extract for treating chronic heart failure. Cochrane Database of Systematic Reviews 2008, Issue 1. Art. No.: CD005312. doi: 10.1002/14651858.CD005312.pub2.
294 Glynn RJ, Ridker PM, et. al. Effects of Random Allocation to vitamin E Supplementation on the Occurrence of Venous Thromboembolism. Report From the Women's Health Study. Circulation 2007;116:1497–1503.
295 Galal W, van Gestel I, Hoeks SE, at al. The obesity paradox in patients with peripheral arterial disease. Chest 2008;134:925–30.
296 Jablecka A, Checiński P, Krauss H, et. al. The influence of two different doses of L-arginine oral supplementation on nitric oxide (NO) concentration and total antioxidant status (TAS) in atherosclerotic patients. Med Sci Monit 2004;10(1):CR29–CR32.
297 He FJ, Nowson CA, MacGregor GA. Fruit and vegetable consumption and stroke: meta-analysis of cohort studies. Lancet 2006;367:320–26.
298 Särkämö T, Tervaniemi M, Laitinen S, et. al. Music listening enhances cognitive recovery and mood after middle cerebral artery stroke. Brain 2008;131(Pt 3):866–76.
299 Legg LA, Drummond AE, Langhorne P. Occupational therapy for patients with problems in activities of daily living after stroke. Cochrane Database Syst Rev 2006 Oct 18;(4):CD003585.
300 Rabadi MH, Coar PL, Lukin M, et. al. Intensive nutritional supplements can improve outcomes in stroke rehabilitation. Neurology 2008;71(23):1856–61.
301 Chan YH, Lau KK, Yiu KH, et. al. Reduction of C-reactive protein with isoflavone supplement reverses endothelial dysfunction in patients with ischaemic stroke. Eur Heart J 2008;29(22):2800–7.
302 Vitetta L, Harris E, Kirk J, Pipingas A, Sali A. Cognitive Decline in at Risk Adults and the Effect of a Multivitamin/Mineral Supplement. (Abs) Heart Foundation Proceedings 2009;P109.
303 Jordan JE, Osborne RH. Chronic disease self-management education programs: challenges ahead. MJA 2007;186(2):84–7.
304 Mager A, Orvin K, Koren-Morag N, et. al. Impact ofhomocysteine-loweringvitamintherapyonlong-term outcome of patients with coronary artery disease. Am J Cardiol 2009;104(6):745–9.

Chapter 11

Dementia and Alzheimer's disease

With contribution from Dr Andrew Pipingas and Ms Danielle Sestito

Introduction

The dementias are conditions that co-occur with, but are not necessarily caused by, increasing age. They cause marked deterioration of cognitive abilities such as memory, reasoning and judgment abilities and, often as a consequence, physical deterioration (such as severe weight loss in individuals who cannot care for themselves), and poor emotional control and mood problems. The dementias are distinct from normal cognitive impairment due to ageing, with many of the progressive dementias ultimately fatal as the brain deterioration eventually causes physical shutdown. Alzheimer's dementia (AD) is the most common cause of senile dementia, accounting for about 50% of all cases.[1] Other dementias include Lewy Body dementia, frontotemporal dementias, vascular dementia, and sub-cortical degenerative dementias. Dementia can also be caused by exposure to toxins (alcohol or toxic medications), brain trauma, and infections (such as Lyme disease and AIDS). Currently, although there are pharmaceutical therapies which help relieve some of the symptoms of AD, there is still no cure for the disease or definite prevention model. Due to the emotional and financial costs of the disorder to patients and society, as well as the increasing ageing population and limitations of care facilities available, it is important that more is understood about prevention and treatment for the dementias.

Table 11.1 summarises the cognitive, physical and emotional symptoms in dementias.

Incidence and prevalence

A recent (2007) study on an American cohort found that about 13% of those older than 70 years had dementia.[3] The proportion of Americans over 70 years who had AD specifically was 9.7% (comprising almost 75% of all dementia cases within that cohort). They also found that the prevalence of dementia was related to age, with individuals aged between 71–79 years having a 5% prevalence, however, in individuals over 90 years the prevalence increased to 37.4%.

A recent Australian study, published in 2008, reported about 5.6% of males and 6% of females between 70–79 years have dementia. For those aged between 85–89 years, the prevalence in males is 12.8% and females, 20.2%.[4] Similar to the American study, they found prevalence markedly increased again for those aged over 90 years, with dementia seen in 22.1% of males

Table 11.1 The spectrum of symptoms in the dementias[1, 2]

Cognitive symptoms	Physical and emotional symptoms
Memory impairment — including prospective, remote, working, and recent memory	Personality change
	Aggression
Word-finding deficit	Depression and anxiety
Executive dysfunction	Agitation
Visuospatial problems (agnosias)	Paranoia and delusions
Apraxia	Wandering
Delirium	Sleep disturbances
Language impairment	Weight loss

and 30.8% of females.[4] Generally, the risk of developing dementia in middle age is very low (the risk is only about 1% for those who are 65) and then increases rapidly with increasing age.[1] Consistent with many countries with ageing populations, in Australia the prevalence of dementia is expected to increase fourfold by the year 2050, impacting significantly on the community, both financially and socially.[5]

Because the current pharmacological treatments available for the progressive dementias are of limited efficacy, much research effort has also been directed to alternative and natural therapies that the patient can explore for reducing both cognitive and emotional/physical symptoms of dementia. Additionally, due to cross-cultural evidence findings indicating lower dementia prevalence rates among certain cultures in comparison to more Westernised countries, holistic, lifestyle approaches are offered as potential prevention initiatives. While many of the results appear promising, there is need for high-quality research to be conducted. This chapter will explore the evidence for lifestyle and non-pharmaceutical therapies that may benefit dementia and cognitive decline.

Risk factors

Lifestyle — general

Obesity and high body mass index

Previous studies have shown risk factors associated with coronary disease, stroke, or other vascular disease also predict dementia. The research outcomes from a number of studies confirm an association between obesity in middle age and future risk of dementia.

Two longitudinal population-based studies support the link between mid-life obesity and later life dementia. One study analysed health data from 10 276 men and women who were aged between 40–45 when they underwent detailed health evaluations during the period of 1964 to 1973.[6] Upon re-evaluation in later life, it was found that the mid-life weight–dementia risk link appeared to be linear, with obese individuals (those with a Body Mass Index [BMI] calculation >30), having a 74% increased risk of dementia and overweight individuals (with a BMI range of 25–29) having a 35% greater dementia risk in comparison to individuals who were within the normal BMI range. Another study followed a sample of 7402 men who were aged between 47–55 when they attended medical exams during 1970–1973. They underwent a follow-up exam in 1998 and these results displayed a similar pattern to the previous research after controlling for smoking, socioeconomic status, blood pressure, diabetes and serum cholesterol.[7] They found that those individuals with higher BMI (22.50–24.99) had a substantially increased dementia risk than those who had low to normal BMI (20.00–22.49) at mid-life. The results from these studies suggest that obesity in mid-life may pose a substantial risk for developing dementia in later life above and beyond other risk factors (such as smoking and cholesterol).

Interestingly, the results of an American cardiovascular health study yielded different results.[8] While this study also measured the link between mid-life weight and dementia, it also compared obesity in late-life with dementia. While the 2798 participants initially evaluated were found to be free from dementia in mid-life, they observed, in line with other studies, that those who were overweight or obese initially had a higher risk of developing dementia in later life. However, the study prospectively followed participants for a follow-up evaluation and found that in later life, a BMI within the normal range was associated with a higher risk of dementia, while a higher BMI was unrelated to increased dementia risk. The authors concluded that this reverse effect in later life was a reflection of the physical changes that occur in demented individuals as they approach a disabled status. This finding is supported by other studies which show that higher baseline BMI and slower declining BMI during later life is associated with a reduced risk of dementia.[9]

Alcohol intake

A longitudinal study of an elderly community sample free of dementia at baseline looked at cognitive functions and self-reported drinking habits. Drinking habits were assessed every 2 years and were followed for an average of 7 years.[10] Cognitive measures were compared across 3 groups categorised using self-reported drinking habits. The groups compared were: no drinking, minimal drinking and moderate drinking. Interestingly they observed that mild to moderate drinking was associated with lesser declines in learning and memory tests compared with those who abstained from alcohol completely. This relationship was found to be more pronounced when comparing those who had always consumed alcohol or those who no longer drank alcohol to those who had abstained from alcohol consumption over a lifetime.[10]

A recent systematic review and meta-analysis of 23 studies (mainly epidemiological in nature) also concluded that small amounts of alcohol in earlier adult life may be protective against developing dementia (risk ratio [RR] 0.63; 95% CI 0.53–0.75) and Alzheimer's disease (RR 0.57; 0.44–0.74) later in life, and less for vascular dementia (RR 0.82; 0.50–1.35) or cognitive decline (RR 0.89; 0.67–1.17).[11]

Environment

Smoking

Researchers from The Netherlands studied the effect of smoking on cognitive decline over a 5-year period at middle age (43–70 years). They found that among smokers, as numbers of cigarettes smoked and number of years spent smoking increased, functioning in a number of cognitive indices declined.[12] Another study found that having stiff lungs, which impairs an individual's ability to blow out a large volume of air quickly, was associated with increased risk of dementia.[13] Additionally, a recent stratified random sample study of non-smokers found a relationship between exposure to second-hand smoke and cognitive decline.[14]

Sunshine — vitamin D deficiency

Generally, low serum vitamin D levels have been shown to be linked to dementia and poorer performance on cognitive tasks. Vitamin D deficiency is common in the elderly, particularly as they spend more time indoors, especially with hospitalisation and institutionalisation. The majority of cross-sectional research has found a correlation between vitamin D serum levels and cognitive function with low serum 25-hydroxvitamin D concentration being associated with increased probability of cognitive impairment.[15–18] Similarly, low vitamin D status has been linked to higher risk of dementia. Individuals with normal cognitive function had higher levels of serum 25(OH) D than those who were cognitively impaired. Those with lowest serum level concentrations were 4 times more likely to be demented. Interestingly, there has been mixed results with 1 cross-sectional study revealing that between different age ranges, the relationship between levels of vitamin D and cognitive performance is different.[19] They found that for younger age groups there was no relationship between vitamin D status and cognition, however in elderly age groups they found an opposite effect; that those with the *highest* level of serum vitamin D had the largest impairment on the task (4809 participants were in this age group). It must be noted, however, that in this sample while the participants were representative of their age group, none had dementia. Recently, a study found that vitamin D status was a better predictor of dementia than the more commonly evaluated BMI or serum albumin.[20] One very large scale study (the European Male Ageing Study, EMAS) which evaluated 3369 men aged 40–79 found that serum vitamin D was related to cognitive performance.[21] They observed that those with higher serum 25-hydroxyvitamin D levels had better performance in a number of cognitive measures than individuals with lower serum levels, and this effect was observed particularity in older participants.

Generally, large-scale reviews of the relationships between vitamin D and dementia conclude Ethat findings remain unclear, biological plausibility of relationship is supported, and thus there is an argument for the need for long-term, well-designed trials[22].

Heavy metal exposure

Metal exposure is of interest to researchers as a possible risk factor for dementia given that in AD accumulation of metals within the brain form characteristic amyloid plaques, a key pathological trait in the disorder. Additionally, studies have observed that certain metals, such as copper, aluminium and zinc have been implicated in the precipitation and cytotoxicity of amyloid protein.[23] One recent study has found evidence that high exposure to aluminium in drinking water was significantly associated with increased dementia risk,[24] and this finding has been replicated in a number of epidemiological studies.[25]

Mind—body medicine

Education

Research has found that attaining a higher education is an independent protective factor for dementia and cognitive decline, however this has been debated.[26] On the other hand, studies investigating later-life cognitive stimulation practices for individuals who were already demented improved some cognitive domains as well as the individual's quality of life when compared to individuals who received their regular treatment in the absence of cognitive stimulation.[27] This result has been mirrored in prospective studies within non-clinical populations, where older individuals (75 years +) with increased cognitive activity during their leisure activities show reduced risk of developing mild cognitive impairment.[28]

Work complexity

A case-control study, controlling for age, gender, and level of education found that the more complex the work (either with people or with data) was associated with reduced risk of

AD.[29] The study included 10 079 members of the population-based Swedish Twin Registry who were participants in the HARMONY study. They analysed data with case-control and co-twin control designs. The co-twin control design provides control over genetic and familial factors.

Loneliness and socialisation

Social isolation in old age has been associated with the risk of developing dementia, but the risk associated with perceived isolation, or loneliness, is not well understood. A longitudinal clinicopathologic cohort study found that the lonely persons had almost twice the risk of developing dementia compared with those who were not classified as lonely.[30] This effect remained apparent even after controlling for social isolation. This study observed that more lonely people showed lower indices of cognitive function at baseline and increased rapid cognitive decline at follow-up.

Pets

A recent review summarised 9 studies that investigated dog therapy for older people with dementia residing within residential aged care.[31] The most common findings were substantial decreases in agitated episodes and increased socialisation during dog contact. Interestingly, the improvements seen in social behaviour were unrelated to dementia severity. Additionally, improvements on various measures of overall function were also observed in those receiving dog therapy.

Personality

Personality testing found Japanese centenarians have optimistic attitudes, adaptability, and an easy-going approach to life.[32] Strong social integration and a deep spirituality were particularly evident among older women when in their prime of life. They scored low when it came to feelings of 'time urgency' and 'tension' and high in 'self-confidence' and 'unyieldingness.'

In another study, investigators linked high neuroticism, a personality trait, to dementia.[33] They assessed the personality traits among 506 dementia-free individuals participating as part of the Kungsholmen Project (Sweden) and prospectively followed them for 6 years on average. The main trends observed were for participants scoring lowest in trait neuroticism and combined with high trait extraversion were associated with reduced risk of dementia. Additionally, it was also observed that in individuals who were socially isolated, even low neuroticism alone was associated with decreased dementia risk.

Physical activity

The results of a prospective cohort study published in *Annals of Internal Medicine* suggests that regular exercise may assist delaying the onset of dementia and AD.[35] In this study, 1740 individuals aged 65 years and older were tested on cognitive domains, exercise and other health outcomes and re-tested after approximately 6 years. While 158 participants developed dementia during this period (107 developed AD), there was a reduced incidence of dementia and AD in participants who exercised more frequently (greater than 3 times a week).

Recently, researchers investigated whether late life physical activity in elderly men would have an effect on the risk of developing dementia. A key finding they uncovered was that that elderly men who had poor physical functionality and underwent high levels of physical activity, had half the risk of developing dementia than a matched group who underwent minimal physical exercise. This finding remained significant after controlling for other variables. They postulated that general physical activity may protect against or delay the onset of dementia.[36] Outdoor exercise would gain the added benefits of sun exposure for vitamin D and fresh air.

Nutritional influences

Diet

Fruits and vegetables

A study tested whether consumption of fruit and vegetable juices, containing a high concentration of polyphenols, decreases the risk of incident-probable AD. This was a prospective-design study which followed 1836 participants who were dementia-free during baseline testing (between 1992–1994) through to 2001.[37] They found that the hazard ratio for probable AD was much lower in those participants who reported consuming juices at least 3 times per week than those who reported consuming less than 3 serves of juice per week. Interestingly, this effect was more apparent in individuals who both carried an apolipoprotein E ε-4 allele and did not exercise often.

Another study which found a gene–diet relationship evaluated the results from 8085 non-demented participants aged 65 and over as part of the Three-City cohort study. While they also found that frequent consumption of fruits and vegetables was related with a lower dementia risk in all cases, those who consumed a diet high in omega-6 fats and did not carry the ApoE 4 gene had an increased risk of dementia and a diet high in fish and omega-3 rich oils was protective.[38, 39]

Mediterranean diet

There is converging evidence that composite dietary patterns such as the Mediterranean diet are related to lower risk for cardiovascular disease, several forms of cancer, and overall mortality. The Mediterranean diet is generally comprised of a high intake of fruit, vegetables, legumes and grains, preferring fish to red meat, mainly cooking with olive oil and the consumption of a moderate amount of red wine.[40] A recent review concluded that essential components of the Mediterranean diet, including poly-unsaturated fatty acids (PUFA's), cereals and wine, seem to be protective against cognitive decline.[41] A study prospectively evaluated 2258 community-based non-demented individuals in New York every 1.5 years, and found that higher adherence to the Mediterranean diet is associated with a reduction in risk for AD.[42] A multiethnic community study using Cox proportional hazards method found that higher adherence to the Mediterranean diet is associated with a trend for reduced risk of developing MCI and with reduced risk of MCI conversion to AD.[43]

Okinawa diet

Observing inhabitants of the Japanese island, Okinawa, they generally have a long life expectancy and demonstrate low prevalence of dementia. Outside of genetic factors, lifestyle appears to be a main contributor for longevity. Okinawan's consume more nutrient-dense, calorie-starved foods such as soy, fruits, vegetables, wholegrains, sprouts, broth-based soups, seaweed, sweet potatoes, fish, beans, and yogurt, and infrequent consumption of breads, cheese, oil, nuts, meats and sweets. Other features of Okinawan's include eating small frequent meals (till 80% full), drinking water, green and/or black tea, plenty of exercise through physical labour, martial arts, dance and maintaining a strong community bond that uplifts the spirit.[33]

Green tea

In analysis of cross-sectional data from a community-based Comprehensive Geriatric Assessment, Japanese researchers examined the association between green tea consumption and cognitive function in humans.[44] The assessment comprised 1003 individuals aged 70 years or older, who answered self-report questions about the frequency of green tea consumption. The participants had their cognitive function evaluated, scored using the Mini-Mental State Examination (MMSE). The research observed that the higher consumption of green tea, the lower the prevalence of cognitive impairment. Interestingly, the findings for green tea were highly statistically significant whereas a similar analysis for black or oolong tea and coffee was not statistically significant. Currently, however, there is a lack of substantial clinical trials or long-term prospective design studies, which need to be carried out in order to make any definitive claims for green tea.

Caffeine

Caffeine is a drug which is very widely consumed, in the Western world. Previous experimental models have demonstrated some neuroprotective effects of caffeine at low doses when administered chronically.[45] Subsequent research has investigated the association between caffeine consumption in midlife and AD in late life, with mixed results. One study reported mid-life caffeine consumption to be inversely related to AD while controlling for other variables.[46, 47] In a more recent study, the lowest risk of Alzheimer's disease was found in individuals who consumed on average 3–5 cups of coffee per day in midlife.[46] A prospective study into the effects of caffeine consumption over a 2 and 4 year follow-up found that only in women was high daily consumption of caffeine associated with reduced cognitive decline in some measures.[48] The research surrounding caffeine as a possible preventative for later life dementia is lacking and requires larger, long-term studies before any definitive claims can be made.

Nutritional deficiency

Nutrient deficiency is common in the elderly and may impact adversely on cognition and memory.[49, 50, 51] For example, older individuals generally spend less time outdoors and are more likely to be deficient in vitamin D, but those individuals who maintain an outdoor life into older age retain serum vitamin D levels similar to individuals of younger ages.[52] Additionally, research has shown that some essential nutrients are unable to be taken up through food source alone in older individuals, particularly for those in care.[53] The elderly who have a limited range of foods (e.g. tea and toast), those with dentures limiting proper chewing and those on medication and suffering diseases are also more prone to nutrient deficiencies. Given the relationship between nutrient deficiency and cognitive decline it is therefore prudent to maintain adequate nutrient levels in middle to later life and blood screening is advisable to assess nutrient levels such as vitamin B6, B12, folate, vitamin D and magnesium.[51]

Magnesium deficiency

Previous studies have suggested that magnesium may be a useful dietary supplement in the treatment of Alzheimer's disease. A recent study on a clinical sample compared severity of symptoms/clinical stage of the dementia with current magnesium levels.[54] They found a relationship between serum magnesium levels and the degree of severity of dementia symptoms, with lower levels indicating significantly worse scores on measures of cognition.

Table 11.2 summarises the lifestyle risk factors that can contribute to cognitive decline, dementia and AD.

Table 11.2 Summary of lifestyle risk factors for dementia

Obesity
Work complexity
No or high alcohol intake
Low education
Loneliness and social isolation
High neuroticism and stress
High exposure to heavy metals in drinking water
Smoking
Lack of sunshine; vitamin D deficiency
Lack of exercise and/or physical activity
Dietary factors (e.g. high saturated fat intake)
Vitamin and mineral deficiencies (e.g. vitamin D, B6/12, folate and magnesium)

Integrative management of dementia

Mind–body medicine

Meditation

Meditation practices have various health benefits including the possibility of preserving cognition and preventing dementia. While the exact mechanisms remain investigational, there is some evidence from a few cognitive, brain electrical (EEG), and structural neuro-imaging studies. In 1 cross-sectional study, meditation practitioners were found to have a lower age-related decline in the thickness of specific cortical regions.[55] They found that, compared to non-mediators of the same age, the differences in cortical thickness were most pronounced in the older participants, suggesting that meditation may have contributed to offsetting age-related cortical thinning. Additionally, the thickness of 2 cortical regions correlated with meditation experience.

Cognitive behavioural therapy (CBT)

Anxiety is a common symptom in dementia, often contributing to limited independence and a greater need to be placed in nursing home care. One study assessed CBT as a means to treat dementia related anxiety, comparing the results from 2 patients who were treated with a dementia-specific modified version of CBT.[56] The researchers made modifications in the content, structure, and learning strategies of CBT in the treatment process, with the patients receiving education and awareness training and were taught the skills of diaphragmatic breathing, coping self-statements, exposure, and behavioural activation. They found improvements in anxiety as measured by standardised rating scales. CBT has also been shown to be beneficial in treating anxiety in the caregivers and family members of dementia sufferers.[57, 58]

Additionally, positive belief-based CBT has been used for teaching mnemonic strategies to older adults who were still in the early stages of dementia as a means to improve cognitive function. A 7-week group intervention study used CBT to address unhelpful memory-related beliefs in 3 older men with mild/moderate dementia and associated low mood or anxiety.[59] While results were promising, the researchers concluded that further research into the use of CBT is required.

Music and relaxation therapy

Relaxation can help lower the levels of agitation and stress in AD patients and their caregivers. Simple techniques such as massage, therapeutic and physical touching can help keep patients calm by allaying anxiety. A review of the literature of 8 research-based articles, found that demented older individuals who listened to their preferred music during the study intervention period had positive results, one of which was the reduction of some agitated behaviours.[60] The review cautioned that while only the findings in 1 study did not reach statistical significance, the sample numbers were small and further investigation was necessary.

Aromatherapy

Aromatherapy is the use of pure essential oils from fragrant plants to help relieve health problems and improve the quality of life in general. Aggressiveness, restlessness and excitability are experienced by a large proportion of people with severe dementia, and can be distressing for patients and caregivers. Aromatherapy may play a role in helping to alleviate these symptoms.

One study of 72 people living in long-term care facilities in the UK were randomly assigned to aromatherapy (essential lemon balm oil) or placebo (sunflower oil), combined with a base lotion.[61] Caregivers applied the oils onto the patients' faces and arms twice a day. Over 4 weeks of treatment, the aromatherapy treatment group resulted in a 35% improvement in agitation compared to 11% with placebo treatment. Also, scores on quality of life indices also significantly improved. The lemon balm appeared to be well tolerated and safe with no serious adverse side-effects.

A Cochrane review identified 3 randomised control trials (RCTs) of aromatherapy for dementia, however, found several methodological difficulties with 2 of the studies. The review concluded 'a statistically significant treatment effect in favour of the aroma therapy intervention on measures of agitation and neuropsychiatric symptoms' in 1 of the trials.[62] More research is required.

Brain training

A recent Cochrane review investigated whether cognitive training and cognitive rehabilitation improved symptomatology within individuals with dementia.[63] The review concluded that no definite protective effects were observed and the authors argued that more studies of a larger power and of a better methodological design were required before concluding the efficacy of such training.

There have also been a number of studies evaluating the efficacy of brain training on cognitive processes and activities of daily living in older, cognitively healthy participants. Overall, the findings have been positive, with a number of studies investigating large cohorts in controlled clinical trials. In a study of 2832 persons living in 6 US cities, 10 sessions of computerised cognitive training were used that included specific cognitive domains such as episodic memory and reasoning.[64] Each intervention improved the targeted cognitive ability compared with baseline. In addition, booster training improved specific cognitive functions that were sustained at a 2-year follow-up. Improvements due to training were of the same magnitude as the amount of age-associated decline expected over a 7–14 year period in individuals without dementia. In a follow-up study, brain training was shown to improve trained cognitive abilities and this was maintained after 5 years.[65] The intervention included 10 sessions of training and then follow-up booster training at 11 and 35 months. Importantly, brain training also resulted in a reduced functional decline in activities of daily living over this time.

Two other recent studies have also shown benefits associated with cognitive training. In 1 of these studies a cohort of 487 participants used a cognitive training battery and showed improvements in memory and attention after 8 weeks (1 hour per day, 5 days per week).[66] In the other study, improvements were found both in the cognitive domains being trained and also in non-related standardised neuropsychological tasks.[67] The authors concluded that 'intensive plasticity-engaging training can result in an enhancement of cognitive function in normal mature adults'.

There is also evidence of neurobiological changes that occur as a result of brain training suggesting possible neural underpinnings associated with brain training studies outlined above. In a neuro-imaging study, the density of Dopamine D1 receptors were assessed before and after 14 hours (5 weeks) of working memory training.[68] There were significant changes in D1 binding potential in both prefrontal and parietal brain regions 'demonstrating a reciprocal interplay between mental activity and brain biochemistry *in vivo*'.

Sleep

Insomnia

Insomnia is a common problem in AD. In a randomised-control trial of 36 community dwelling patients with AD and suffering sleep problems, 17 were randomised into active treatment with their caregivers receiving specific treatment about setting up a sleep hygiene program and training in behaviour management skills.[69] They were also instructed to walk daily and to increase daytime light exposure with the use of a light box. Control subjects (n = 19) received general dementia education and caregiver support. The active group demonstrated a significant ($p<.05$) reduction in the number of night-time awakenings, total time awake at night, and depression. These benefits persisted at 6-month follow-up.

Sunshine

Sunshine is the main source of vitamin D produced by the body in response to direct skin exposure to UVB. This means that no or minimal exposure to sun can contribute to vitamin D deficiency as seen in community groups with dress codes (e.g. wearing veils), living in geographical prone areas (e.g. in high and low altitudes) especially over winter, working indoors (e.g. office work), institutionalisation, prolonged hospitalisation and bed-bound people, particularly in dark skin people who need longer sun exposure.[70, 71]

There is a growing body of evidence that vitamin D deficiency can contribute to the risk of dementia (see above under risk factors). Vitamin D appears to have a role in neuro-protection and reduce the risk of dementia.[72] Interestingly, an Australian study has found that during heat waves, admissions to hospital for a variety of disorders, including dementias, were significantly increased, as well as increased mortality in individuals with dementia.[73] Heat waves impact upon mental health.

Light therapy

Light therapy may be beneficial in improving some cognitive and non-cognitive symptoms of dementia. A 2008 study showed that light therapy reduced cognitive decline and ameliorated depressive symptoms in individuals with dementia.[74] Moreover, in the same study mood was adversely affected with administration of melatonin, often administered to improve insomnia. The authors recommended that melotonin should only be taken in combination with light therapy. Their results suggested that the bright light therapy did demonstrate an improvement in some cognitive domains, especially in the participants who were in the initial stages of AD. Their results suggested that bright light therapy improved cognitive functions, especially in individuals who were in early stages of AD.[75] However, a 2004 Cochrane review found that there was insufficient evidence to suggest that light therapy is effective in managing sleep, behaviour, cognitive, or mood disturbances associated with dementia.[76] The authors found only 3 studies that fulfilled all inclusion criteria and recommended that more properly constructed studies are necessary to draw solid conclusions.

Physical and mental activity

Exercise

The relationship between physical exercise and cognition in older individuals has been investigated in a number of studies. One study showed that either memory-based cognitive exercises or cardiovascular exercises resulted in older individuals out-performing age-matched participants in tests of memory functioning.[77] Additionally, the implementation of a 24-week physical activity program in adults who believed they had a memory impairment (but were dementia free) found adequate improvements in memory, even after an 18 month follow-up period.[78] Another recent study found that dementia-free elderly individuals significantly improved in fluid intelligence measures after participation in 2 x 1 hour general exercise classes (conducted over a period of 6 months), compared to a no-exercise control group or a group who participated in a flexibility based relaxation class.[79] Recent Cochrane reviews, however, indicated that the bank of research into the effects of exercise and dementia are still inconclusive due to insufficient research methods.[80]

Tai chi

A study compared healthy individuals aged 45–74 years from Fuyang city, 53 of whom practiced tai chi exercise for half a year or more, and 48 were 'no exercise' controls.[81] The participants were compared across 3 age groups: 45–54 years, 55–64 years, and 65–74 years. Additionally, the tai chi group was subdivided into 3 groups according to experience in tai chi: ≤3 years, 4–6 years, and ≥7years. The cognitive function of both tai chi experienced and no exercise control groups declined with age, but this decline was slower in the tai chi group. In addition, people who had practiced tai chi for a longer duration had less cognitive decline than those with less experience. The researchers concluded that long-term tai chi exercise can possibly benefit cognitive function in middle-aged and old people.

A recent study examined performance on cognitive and physical tasks in 20 older adult subjects after participation in a 10-week tai chi program.[82] They found that compared to baseline, 2 measures of executive cognition had improved. Collectively these studies suggest some beneficial effects of tai chi for cognition in older adults; however, more controlled randomised trials are required for conclusive evidence.

Nutritional influences

Diet

A high dietary intake of fruit, vegetables, legumes, wholegrains, fish and olive oil is protective of cognition and towards reducing the risk of dementia (refer to risk factor section above, under diet). Therefore, encouraging a Mediterranean diet may play a role in helping to reduce any further deterioration of cognition and memory in patients with established dementia and Alzheimer's disease.[40–43]

Nutritional supplements

As outlined above (in the risk factor section, under nutrient deficiency), adequate nutrition is essential for maintaining health and cognition in old age. Research has shown that in older persons in particular it can be difficult to obtain optimum nutritional status through food sources alone, and thus additional supplementation may be required.[53] Additionally, as outlined within the following section, research has uncovered evidence of certain vitamins, nutrients and herbs with potential to act as complementary therapeutic agents for dementia.

Vitamins B6, B12 and folate

The majority of conclusions drawn for the importance of substantial B vitamin status, including folic acid, are derived from studies finding that compromised brain functioning is linked to vitamin deficiencies.[83] In the normal elderly population, vitamin deficiency is quite common, leading to the suggestion that B vitamin status is related to cognitive performance or possibly dementia, however, current findings do not paint a clear picture. One study postulates the link between B vitamin deficiency and impairment of methylation reactions leading to the damage of brain tissue.[83] Another theory that relates to B vitamin deficiency postulates that elevated homocysteine levels are responsible for cognitive dysfunction given that elevated homocysteine has been linked to vascular disease, dementia and AD. One recent randomised placebo-controlled trial aimed to determine the effects of folic acid, vitamin B12, riboflavin, and vitamin B6 supplementation on homocysteine levels and cognitive function.[84] The trial was comprised of 185 patients who suffered ischaemic vascular diseases and were aged 65 years or more. After 1 year, homocysteine levels were lower in the group receiving a combination of folic acid and B12 than patients not receiving the treatment. However, this folic acid/vitamin B12 combined treatment did not significantly alter cognitive performance; neither did a riboflavin/vitamin B6 combined treatment. However, a separate more recent cross-sectional study in the Japanese elderly population reported an independent positive association between reduced folate and vitamin B12 levels and cognitive decline.[85]

This prospective 5-year study measured markers of vitamin B12 status and brain volume loss in older individuals (aged 61–87 years). They found that individuals with lower B12 vitamin status displayed greater decreases in brain loss and the relationship remained significant after controlling for 'age, sex, creatinine, education, initial brain volume, cognitive test scores, systolic blood pressure, ApoE 4 status, homocysteine and folate'.[85] Another study revealed that elderly individuals with a pre-existing vitamin B12 deficiency and mild to moderate dementia did show an improvement in cognitive function with B12 supplementation, however those with advanced dementia displayed an improvement in neurological symptoms only.[86]

A cross-sectional and longitudinal analysis published in the *American Journal of Medicine* in 2005 in a cohort of 499, 70–79 year olds, demonstrated those with elevated homocysteine levels or low levels of folate or vitamin B6, demonstrated worse baseline cognitive function.[87] After adjusting for variables, those with bottom quartile folate levels had a 1.6 fold increased risk of being in the worst quartile of 7-year cognitive decline. Reduced folate levels appear to be a greater risk factor for cognitive decline. Chan et. al.[88] examined the efficacy of a vitamin/nutraceutical formulation in a 12-month pilot trial in individuals with early-stage Alzheimer's disease. The formulation contained a mixture of folate, vitamin B6, vitamin E, s-adenosyl methionine, N-acetyl cysteine and acetyl-L-carnitine. Those taking the formulation performed better on neuropsychiatric and daily living measures than the individuals who were taking pharmacological medications or placebo. While a larger clinical trial is required to confirm these preliminary findings, generally previous large cross section studies have found a trend between adequate folate intake (at or above the RDI) and reduced risk of AD.[89, 90] A similar result was found by Wouters-Wesseling et. al. (2005)[90] who administered a vitamin-nutrient enriched drink to elderly individuals in their double-blind, randomised, placebo-controlled study. The 67 participants received either the drink or placebo for 6 months. They found significant differences after 6 months in a word learning test, and a category fluency test compared to the placebo group. Additionally, they observed that vitamin B12 levels significantly increased and homocysteine levels decreased in the supplement group compared to the placebo group.

Generally a large number of studies have observed that increasing folic acid and vitamin B6 and B12 concentrations decrease homocysteine levels.[85, 92–100] Considering the findings of some improved cognition in elderly individuals with supplementation with B vitamins and folate there appears to be merit to the relationship between homocysteine and cognitive decline.

A recent Cochrane review of 8 RCTs found nothing significant or consistent enough to suggest that folic acid, (either with or without vitamin B12), had a beneficial effect on cognitive function in older people, unless possibly when baseline homocysteine levels were high.[101]

A very recent Australian double-blind, placebo-controlled, randomised trial administered 2mg of folate, plus 25mg of B6 and 400 µg of B12, or placebo to 299 men aged 75 years or older, for a period of 2 years.[102] They found that those in the treatment group had significantly lower levels of Aβ protein 1–40 than the placebo group. While the participants in this sample were dementia free, the study demonstrated the possibility of a simple AD prevention strategy given that Aβ protein was lowered significantly with B vitamin supplementation.[102]

Antioxidants

A review of this subject by the *Lancet* in 1997 suggests protective effects of fruit and vegetables against stroke and vascular dementia may be related to their antioxidant content.[103] Recently, research has provided significant findings to link mitochondrial oxidative damage or the 'free radical theory' of ageing and neurodegenerative diseases such as AD. Researchers in the AD field are beginning to recognise the possible involvement of a mutant APP and its derivatives in causing mitochondrial oxidative damage in AD, and are thus looking at the role of dietary antioxidants in older populations. However, there are conflicting reports about the potential role of vitamin antioxidants.

Vitamin antioxidants

Antioxidants such as vitamins C and E may have an important role through scavenging of increased free-radical formation and repair impaired antioxidant defences. Longitudinal data examined from the Canadian Study of Health and Ageing, a population-based, prospective 5-year investigation of the epidemiology of dementia among Canadians aged 65+ years, suggest a possible protective effect for antioxidant vitamins in relation to cognitive decline.[104] The study included 894 subjects with no dementia. Over a 5-year period, subjects who were consuming combined vitamin E and C supplements and/or multivitamin consumption at baseline were significantly less likely to experience significant cognitive decline during the 5-year follow-up period. Subjects reporting any antioxidant vitamin use at baseline also showed a significantly lower risk for vascular cognitive impairment but no evidence for reduced risk of dementia or AD.

A larger scale study of 4740 elderly people, published in *Archives of Neurology*, yielded similar results.[105] This study demonstrated the use of combined vitamin C and E supplements, but not if used alone, was associated with reduced AD prevalence. Additionally, the study revealed that individuals who were taking antioxidant vitamins E and C in combination with non-steroidal anti-inflammatory drugs at baseline declined in Modified-MMSE scores 0.96 points less every 3 years than non-users, and this effect was entirely attributed to individuals who carried the APOE e4 allele (whose scores declined by 2.25 points fewer on the M-MMSE than non-users).

However, in a double-blind study published in the *NEJM* of 769 subjects, 212 who developed AD, compared with placebo, there were no significant differences in the risk of progression to AD in the vitamin E group or the anti-cholinesterase inhibitor donepezil group during 3 years of treatment.[106] On the other hand, Sano et. al. (1997)[107] conducted a double-blind, placebo-controlled, randomised trial including patients with moderately severe AD who received either Selegiline (a selective monoamine oxidase inhibitor), or vitamin E or a combination of both for 2 years. The authors concluded from the study that either treatment appeared to slow the progression of the disease in terms of 'functional deterioration' leading to nursing home placement relative to placebo; however the authors noted that possible problematic methodology may have contributed to the positive findings.[107, 108]

Another study of 2889 elderly residents published in *Archives of Neurology*, found higher vitamin E intake from foods or supplements, is associated with less cognitive decline with age and slowing the progression of AD.[109] After adjusting for other factors that can influence cognitive status, the researchers found a 36% reduction in the rate of cognitive decline among persons consuming the highest amount of total vitamin E (combined food and supplement sources) compared to those getting the least. This finding has been replicated in other previous age-matched cross sectional research.[104]

Subsequent meta analysis of placebo-controlled, randomised trials have yet to find significant cognitive differences with vitamin E supplementation alone despite cross-sectional observations.[110] Vitamin E combined with vitamin C may be the critical factor in demonstrating benefit.[104,105] Additionally, subjects who reported taking antioxidant multivitamins at baseline also displayed a lower risk of vascular cognitive impairment, however no reduced risk for incident dementia or AD was observed.[111]

Other supplements

Melatonin

A small double-blind study that examined the effects of 3mg/day of melatonin in AD patients found that melatonin administration improved sleep time and reduced night activity.[112] Cognitive and non-cognitive functions were also improved.

However, a recent Cochrane review that included 3 studies exploring the effects of melatonin in patients with dementia or cognitive impairment, found currently the available evidence is insufficient to support the effectiveness of melatonin in managing the cognitive and non-cognitive symptoms of dementia.[113]

Herbal supplements

Ginkgo (*Ginkgo biloba*)

Extracts of the leaves of *Ginkgo biloba* tree have been used in traditional Chinese medicine for thousands of years. Studies suggest several mechanisms for its benefits, including vasodilation, reducing blood viscosity, and modifying neurotransmitter systems. In a recent Cochrane review (2009)[35] controlled clinical trials were included that investigated *Ginkgo biloba* in the treatment of cognitive decline and dementia.[114] The authors concluded that *Ginkgo biloba* appears to be safe compared with placebo. Early trials prone to highly variable quality of preparations and use of unsatisfactory methods showed mixed results. The authors commented on 4 recent trials; 1 of these showing positive effects on cognition, activities of daily living, mood, depression and carer burden. The other 3 were negative. Overall the authors conclude: 'The evidence that *Ginkgo biloba* has predictable and clinically significant benefit for people with dementia or cognitive impairment is inconsistent and unreliable'.[114] Examples of findings from a number of these trials will now be discussed.

One 42-month pilot trial found no significant effect of *Ginkgo biloba* to either alter the risk of progression from normal functioning to clinically demented or protect against memory decline, however the authors noted that when participant compliance was taken into account, those with high compliance did show a significant effect although the compliant sample size was too small to be conclusive.[115] A randomised, double-blind placebo-controlled study which was conducted for 26 weeks compared the effects of both 120mg/day and 240mg/day of *Ginkgo biloba* supplementation with placebo. This study also failed to yield any significant results overall, however did report that in a subgroup of patients with neuropsychiatric symptoms there was a significant beneficial effect of the treatment on cognitive and global functioning observed in comparison to no treatment.[116] The researchers suggested that the null findings overall could have been due to the lack of decline in the placebo group, lessening the sensitivity of the results. Another study matched non-demented 60–70 year olds participants on education level and compared 8 months of *Ginkgo biloba* supplementation on both neuropsychological tests as well as tests of blood viscosity and regional cerebral perfusion[117]. The authors reported that those taking *Ginkgo biloba* displayed a reduction in blood viscosity, improved cerebral blood flow in specific areas and improved global cognitive functioning. Very recently, a study compared the effects of 160mg daily dose of a *Ginkgo biloba* special extract, EGb 761; a pharmaceutical used often for the treatment of dementia, Donepezil (5mg/day) and placebo over a period of 24 weeks.[118] The patients (aged between 50–80 years) in the study were all diagnosed as having mild to moderate Alzheimer's dementia. They found that the clinical efficacy of the *Ginkgo biloba* was comparable to the Donepezil, and concluded that it would be an efficient alternative treatment for those in the mild/moderate stages.

It may be that the extract of *Ginkgo biloba* is more effective therapeutically compared with the whole herb used in studies.

Brahmi (*Bacopa monniera*)

Brahmi is an Indian herb and traditional Ayurvedic medicine with reported memory-enhancing, anti-inflammatory, antioxidative, analgesic, sedative, antipyretic and antiepileptic properties. The memory-enhancing properties of the herb however have drawn a greater deal of research attention, with a number of relatively recent randomised placebo-controlled trials finding positive memory effects of the herb in adult and elderly populations. Brahmi contains Bacoside A and Bacoside B which are steroidal saponins believed to be essential for the clinical efficacy of the product and may have several modes of action in the brain all of which may be useful in ameliorating cognitive decline in the elderly which include: (1) direct cholinergic properties; (2) antioxidant (flavonoid) properties; (3) metal chelation; (4) anti-inflammatory; (5) increases blood circulation; (6) adaptogenic activity; and (7) removal of β-amyloid deposits.

One study investigated the effects of 90 days supplementation with 300mg *Bacopa monniera* (BM) compared to placebo.[119] They found that individuals taking the supplement had significantly improved performance on a spatial working memory task. In addition, participants also responded with less false positives in a rapid visual processing task. Another study which utilised the same BM supplement, employing the same dosage but with neuropsychological testing after supplementation of only 5 and 12 weeks also found that, compared to placebo, that those taking the BM supplement performed significantly better on a visual processing inspection time task and demonstrated improved learning rate and memory consolidation.[120] However, previous somewhat conflicting evidence has also been observed in a separate placebo-controlled, randomised independent groups study. Roodenrys et. al. (2002)[121] investigated learning and memory following 3 months of supplementation utilising the same dosage and same BM branded supplement as Stough et. al. (2001)[120] and Stough et. al. (2008),[119] however only found significant differences between experimental and placebo group on 1 measure of delayed recall. They found that less was forgotten in the BM group compared to placebo after about 90 day's supplementation in a paired-word recall task however they found no effects of reduced forgetting in a story reconstruction memory task, or in any other learning indices.

Other studies on elderly individuals and individuals with age-associated memory impairments have found significant improvements following BM supplementation. Calabrese et. al. (2008)[122] tested 48 older men without clinical signs of dementia, with 24 individuals in each experimental and control group. They were supplemented with 300mg/day BM or placebo for 12 weeks. The findings revealed improved performance in BM group relative to placebo after 12 weeks on word recall scores and performance on the Stroop task (filtering of irrelevant information). Another study investigated the effects of only 125mg/day supplementation for 12 weeks on a group of individuals with age-associated memory impairments compared to a matched placebo group. They found that the BM supplement improved performance on mental control, logical memory and paired associated learning tasks.

Overall the results look promising for the use of Brahmi supplementation for improved memory however human clinical trials are required in order to investigate whether the herb is efficacious in dementia patients. While some preliminary animal models of dementia have shown promising results with BM supplementation,[123] whether the same effects can be seen in human patients is not yet known.

Lemon balm (*Melissa officinalis*)

Melissa officinalis or lemon balm is a traditional herbal medicine which can be used as a mild sedative, muscle relaxant and as an antibacterial agent. Due to studies *in vitro* which display the cholinergic binding properties of the herb, it has been postulated that it may be effective in the treatment of AD. One study has investigated the effects of lemon balm extract compared to placebo on 42 patients (aged between 65–80) with mild to moderate AD.[124] The randomised, double-blind trial went over a 4-month period, and at 4 months, those taking the lemon balm extract performed significantly better on cognitive tasks than placebo.

Sage (*Salvia officinalis*)

Sage is a herbal extract which has displayed pharmacological actions in humans which are relevant to AD; for example, antioxidant effects, anti-inflammatory activity, estrogenic activity, and cholinesterase inhibition.[125]

Sage appears to be well tolerated by Alzheimer's patients. An open-label pilot study administered oral *Salvia lavandulaefolia* (part of the *Salvia officinalis* family) to AD patients for 6 weeks and found that generally the herb was well tolerated and improvements in memory were seen.[125] A double-blind, randomised placebo-controlled trial of *Salvia officinalis* has also been conducted in patients with mild to moderate AD.[126] The study lasted 4 months and patients were administered 60 drops/day of the treatment. The researchers observed significantly improved memory measures in the treatment group compared with placebo group and no significant differences were observed in side-effects, with the only exception being that the placebo group did appear to experience agitated episodes more often than the experimental group.

Ginseng (*Panax ginseng*)

Ginseng is a herbal remedy which has been used in eastern Asian cultures for several thousand years. It has been used to treat many different disorders, and recently has been implicated with enhancing mental performance and influencing the ageing process.[127] While there are some clinical trials on cognitive benefits of ginseng within younger populations, to date not much is known about the benefits of chronic ginseng administration and dementia. The limited clinical research indicates that while it is relatively safe to use in small doses, the current evidence for efficacy of the herb for long-term clinical benefit is not well supported.[128] A very recent study investigated the effects of *Panax ginseng* administered 4.5g/day for 12 weeks to Alzheimer's patients. At follow-up, those within the treatment group displayed significant improvements in the ADAS-cog and MMSE scores. However, after discontinuing treatment scores returned to control levels. Overall, the limited recent clinical data appears promising for the use of ginseng in AD as long as the use is continued. There is a need however for larger trials of a longer duration.

Korean Red Ginseng

Clinical data relating ginseng to dementia specifically has found Korean Red Ginseng (KRG) to be beneficial for cognition in patients with AD.[129] They administered either 4.5g/day or 9g/day of KRG or placebo for 12 weeks, and found improvement within the high-dose group compared to control in all cognitive measures. Another study administered a standardised ginseng vitamin complex daily for 9 months and found improvements in memory for the treatment group.[130] All participants within this study had age-associated memory impairment, but an MMSE score no less than 24.

Turmeric (*Curcuma longa*)

Turmeric has been used in India for at least 2500 years, and is known for possessing antiseptic, anti-inflammatory, detoxifying, and carminative properties. Various studies and research results have displayed that the prevalence of AD in India among individuals aged between 70–79 years is 4.4 times less than that US adults of the same age range.[131] Studies have shown that curcumin (polyphenols contained in turmeric) inhibits the formation of beta-amyloid oligomers and fibrils by binding to plaques *in vitro* and *in vivo*.[132] Tze-Ping Ng et.al (2006)[133] conducted an epidemiologic study investigating dietary curry consumption and cognition. They found that in individuals who reported consuming both low and moderate amounts of curry in their diet, better cognitive performance was observed. Additionally, the amount of curry consumed, whether 'low' or 'moderate' was not significantly related to better cognitive performance between groups. This is consistent with biological data which demonstrates that low but not high doses of curcumin reduced beta-amyloid and plaque burden.[134]

Other epidemiologic data shows that among cultures which regularly consume curry (Chinese, Malay, Indian), the difference in MMSE scores are more pronounced in the Indian cultures, who consume curry more frequently than other cultures.[133] Overall however, there is a great need for clinical trials to investigate the causal effects of curcumin in cognition and dementia.

To date, only 1 randomised, placebo-controlled, double-blind clinical trial pilot has been conducted to investigate the effects of curcumin on AD.[135] The study duration was 6 months and included individuals who were 50 years or older and had a diagnosis of either AD or probable AD. Only 27 participants finished the trial, which had 3 arms — 8 subjects on placebo, 8 subjects on 1 gm/day curcumin and 11 subjects taking 8gm of curcumin/day. Overall, the researchers were not able to find a significant decline in the placebo group over the 6 month period, and suggested that this was probably the reason for the nullified results as the curcumin is thought to work by slowing progression of the cognitive decline rather than improving cognitive function. The researchers argue that their findings warrant a larger, longer term study into the effects of curcumin.

Resveratrol (resveratrol-grape skin extract; trans-3,4,5-trihydroxystilbene)

Epidemiological studies have suggested that moderate consumption of red wine, which is enriched in resveratrol, is related to a lower incidence of dementia and Alzheimer's disease.[136] A recent study found that resveratrol significantly lowered levels of amyloid-beta peptides, a finding the authors suggest may have therapeutic potential in AD.[137] Additionally, rodent study findings have suggested theoretical implications for wine in treatment of dementia in humans.[138, 139]

Other supplements

Omega-3 fatty acids/ fish oil

There is a plethora of evidence to support the use of dietary omega-3 polyunsaturated fatty acid (PUFA) for reducing the risk of dementia and cardiovascular disease in the elderly. Postulated mechanisms include its anti-atherogenic, anti-inflammatory, antioxidant, anti-amyloid and neuroprotective properties. A recent Cochrane review (2006) found no randomised trials in the literature, but acknowledged 'a growing body of evidence from biological, observational and epidemiological studies that suggests a protective effect of omega-3 PUFAs against dementia'.[140] This review concluded that until data from randomised trials becomes available that there is no compelling evidence to support the use of omega-3 PUFA for the prevention of cognitive impairment or dementia.

Several systematic review papers suggest an increase of saturated fatty acids could have negative effects on cognitive function, with a clear reduction of risk of cognitive decline found in populations with a high intake of PUFAs, particularly weekly fish consumption.[141, 142]

More recently, several epidemiological studies have demonstrated that regular fish consumption is associated with a decreased risk of dementia and Alzheimer's disease, as well as better cognitive performance overall in the older population.[143, 144] Additionally, total omega-3 PUFAs within the plasma or erythrocyte membranes is related to slower cognitive decline and a reduced dementia risk,[145, 146, 147] and dietary supplementation with PUFAs has been associated with improved cognitive function in individuals with mild cognitive impairment or organic brain impairment.[148]

Recent double-blind, randomised, placebo-controlled trials have yielded some interesting but mixed results. One study supplemented 174 patients diagnosed with AD with 1.7g/day of docosahexaenoic acid and 0.6g/day of eicosapentaenoic acid (ω-3 fatty acid treatment group) or a placebo for 6 months duration.[149] They found that only within a subgroup of patients who had only a mild cognitive dysfunction (an MMSE score >27), compared to the untreated group, a reduction in the MMSE decline rate was observed. In another study 64 mild or moderate AD patients were supplemented with 1.8g/day total omega-3 PUFAs or placebo for a period of 24 weeks.[150] Overall, the treatment group observed better improvement as rated by the Clinician's Interview-Based Impression of Change Scale than the placebo group at 24 weeks, however only the subgroup of individuals with mild cognitive impairment showed improvements on cognitive measures. A third study with a similar study design but employing elderly but cognitively healthy individuals receiving either 1800mg, or 400mg of omega-3 EPA-DHA or placebo for 26 week did not improve on the measures of cognition.[151] Overall, the clinical results show the ω-3 supplementation appears beneficial for patients with quite mild cognitive impairment.

A very recent (2009) systematic review published in *Nature Reviews* found that overall the current findings provide significant evidence that long-chain omega-3 fatty acids slow cognitive decline in elderly individuals without dementia, however does not prevent dementia.[152] They point out however that this may be due to limitations of the current dementia-omega-3 studies.

Coenzyme Q_{10}

The majority of the literature investigating dietary interventions of supplemental CoQ_{10} and dementia is limited to animal models. The beneficial results observed in animal models of neurodegenerative diseases have so far not been observed in human clinical trials.

Bragin et. al. (2005) investigated an integrative treatment approach on cognitive performance.[153] The study sample comprised of 35 individuals (mean age = 71) who were diagnosed with both mild dementia and depression. Patients were given treatment of antidepressants, cholinesterase inhibitors, as well as vitamins and supplements (including CoQ_{10}). The integration of the treatments in conjunction with healthy eating and regular exercise was found to improve cognition, especially executive activity and memory. However, the specific role that CoQ_{10} played in this improvement is unknown.

Physical therapies

Musculoskeletal

One study found that 6 months of a physiotherapeutic intervention improved participants' balance, but overall there were no improvements observed in global cognition with the intervention.[154] However, when the physiotherapeutic intervention was carried out on a multidisciplinary basis, attenuation in the decline of global cognition in specific cognitive domains was observed.

Massage

Agitation in individuals with dementia living in the nursing home environment affects care and quality of life. Relaxation techniques such as music and massage are showing promise to decrease agitation and improve quality of life in individuals with dementia. Massage has been found to significantly decrease agitation in AD patients when combined with the individual's favourite music.[155]

Acupuncture

Acupuncture is often used as a treatment for dementia and is claimed to be effective in improving intelligence. A recent review found that the few studies which have been carried out to date do not demonstrate significant effectiveness of acupuncture for AD.[156] A recent prospective study investigated the effect of electro-acupuncture (EA) in the treatment of vascular dementia compared with a medication group.[157, 158] They found improvements from baseline across measures in the 'acupuncture only' group however far greater improvements were seen in the medication group. Acupuncture could be explored as an adjunctive therapy, however more research is required.

Conclusion

Overall it is evident that there are many options when considering complementary strategies for treatment of the dementias. Currently, while there is good scientific rationale for a complementary medicinal approach using vitamins and herbal extracts, more randomised, double-blind clinical trials are required to confirm safety and efficacy (see Table 11.3). Additionally, it appears that a number of lifestyle and behavioural changes can be considered in middle age for prevention and management of dementia in older age.

Table 11.3 Levels of evidence for lifestyle and complementary medicines/therapies in the management of dementia and Alzheimer's disease

Modality	Level I	Level II	Level IIIa	Level IIIb	Level IIIc	Level IV	Level V
Lifestyle modification							
Obesity				x			
Education (↓risk)			x				
Smoking (↑risk)				x			
Environment							
Heavy metal exposure (↑risk)				x			
Sunshine				x			
Mind–body medicine							
CBT/counselling			x				
Meditation and/or relaxation			x				
Music therapy				x			
Aromatherapy	x						
Light therapy	x (+/-)						
Work complexity (↓risk)				x			
Social isolation/loneliness (↑risk)				x			
Pets (↓risk)				x			
Optimistic attitude/ personality (↓risk)				x			
Brain training	x (+/-)						
Sleep hygiene program		x					
Nutritional influences							
Diets (vegetable, fruit, fish)				x			
Mediterranean diet (see text)				x			
Okinawa diet (see text)							
Alcohol: mild-moderate consumption	x						
Caffeine				x			
Trans fatty acid avoidance					x		
Chemical and toxin avoidance			x				
Green tea (↓risk)				x			
Physical activity							
Exercise	x				x		
Tai chi		x					
Nutritional supplements							
Antioxidant multivitamins	x						
Vitamin Bs (especially B12)	x						
Folate	x						
Vitamin E	x (-)						

Continued

Table 11.3 Levels of evidence for lifestyle and complementary medicines/therapies in the management of dementia and Alzheimer's disease—cont'd

Modality	Level I	Level II	Level IIIa	Level IIIb	Level IIIc	Level IV	Level V
Vitamin D			x				
Coenzyme Q_{10}		x					
PUFA's/Omega-3				x			
Magnesium (↓risk)				x			
Omega-3	x						
Other supplements							
Melatonin	x (+/-)						
Herbal medicines							
Turmeric (*Curcumin longa*)					x		
Ginkgo (*Ginkgo biloba*)	x (+/-)						
Brahmi extract (*Bacopa monniera*)		x					
Green tea extract					x		
Lemon balm extract (*Melissa officionalis*)		x					
Sage (*Salvia officinalis*)		x					
Ginseng (*Panax ginseng*)				x			
Korean red ginseng				x			
Reveratrol (resveratrol-grape skin extract)				x			
Physical therapies							
Massage			x				
Acupuncture	x (-)			x			
Physiotherapy					x		

Caution is advocated in interpreting these results and conclusive, as further evidence is required.

Level I — from a systematic review of all relevant randomised controlled trials — meta-analyses.
Level II — from at least 1 properly designed randomised controlled clinical trial.
Level IIIa — from well-designed pseudo-randomised controlled trials (alternate allocation or some other method).
Level IIIb — from comparative studies (including systematic reviews of such studies) with concurrent controls and allocation not randomised, cohort studies, case-control studies, or interrupted time series with a parallel control group.
Level IIIc — from comparative studies with historical control, 2 or more single-arm studies or interrupted time series without a parallel control group.
Level IV — opinions of respected authorities based on clinical experience, descriptive studies or reports of expert committees.
Level V — represents minimal evidence that represents testimonials.

Clinical tips handout for patients — dementia and Alzheimer's disease

1 Lifestyle advice

Sleep

- Adequate sleep is essential. (See Chapter 22 for more information.)
- Melatonin supplement, exercise, sun exposure and a routine can help improve sleep patterns in patients with dementia.

Sunshine

- Amount of exposure varies with local climate.
- At least 15 minutes of sunshine needed daily for vitamin D and melatonin production — especially before 10 a.m. and after 3 p.m. when the sun exposure is safest during summer. Much more exposure is required in winter, when supplementation needs to be considered.
- Ensure gradual, adequate skin exposure to sun; avoid sunscreen and excess clothing to maximise levels of vitamin D.
- More time in the sun is required for dark skinned people.
- Direct exposure to about 10% of body (hands, arms, face), without sunscreen and not through glass.
- Vitamin D is obtained in the diet from fatty fish, eggs, liver and fortified foods (some milks and margarines). It is unlikely that adequate vitamin D concentrations can be obtained from diet alone.

2 Physical activity/exercise

- Exercise at least 30 minutes per day. Walk daily, in sunshine, especially in parks.
- Yoga and tai chi may be of help.

3 Mind–body medicine

- Stress management program — for example, 6 x 40 minute sessions for patients to understand the nature of their symptoms, the symptoms' relationship to stress, and the practice of regular relaxation exercises.
- Regular meditation practice at least 10–20 minutes daily.
- Support groups can contact family, friends, church, social or other groups for support.
- Avoid loneliness and social isolation.
- Owning a pet such as a dog can help.

Breathing

- Be aware of breathing from time to time. Notice if tendency to hold breath or over-breathe.
- Always aim to relax breath and the muscles around chest wall.

Rest and stress management

- Reduce workload and resolve conflicts.
- Listening to relaxation music helps.
- Massage therapy helps.
- Aromatherapy (e.g. essential lemon balm oil rubbed onto the face daily) may help reduce agitation, and improve relaxation and sleep.

Brain training

- Keep the mind active. Challenge the mind by solving puzzles and problems. There are many brain-training sites on the internet that may be useful.
- Cognitive behavioural therapy and education extremely helpful.
- Read daily and don't stop learning.
- Stimulate the mind by doing crosswords, sudoko, playing cards with friends, Nintendo, using a computer, writing or reading, such as the daily newspaper.

Fun

- It is important to have fun in life. Joy can be found even in the simplest tasks, such as being with friends with a sense of humour funny movies/videos, comedy, hobbies, dancing, playing with pets and children.
- Try to maintain an 'easy-going approach to life'; avoid feeling time-pressured or rushed.

4 Environment

- Avoid changes in environment where possible as this may increase disorientation.
- Maintain a routine and use triggers such as music to assist with memory.
- Working can help prevent memory decline.
- Office or home environment is enhanced with a view overlooking garden or park.
- Don't smoke and avoid smoking environments.
- Avoid environmental pollutants (especially mercury), lead and cadmium exposure, chemicals — at work and in the home.

- Avoid overheating during heatwaves as this can aggravate dementia.

5 Dietary changes

- Do not rush your meals. Chew your food thoroughly as this aids nutrition value of foods and digestion. If it is diffcult to chew, shred raw food, lightly steam and juice, and use gentle cooking methods (e.g. stew fruit, slow bakes or soups).
- If overweight or underweight, aim to normalise weight.
- For sweetener try honey (e.g. yellow box, and stringy bark have lowest GI).
- Add turmeric spice to your cooking.

Eat more:

- fruit (>2 daily) and vegetables (>5 daily)
- nuts (e.g. walnuts, almonds, peanuts) and seeds
- legumes — beans, lentils, soy, chickpeas and beans sprouts (e.g. alfa, mung)
- unprocessed carbohydrate with lower GI (e.g. wholegrain bread, wholemeal pasta and wholegrain rice)
- fish, especially deep sea fish, daily if possible; canned fish is okay (mackerel, salmon, sardines, cod, tuna)
- lean red meat (e.g. lamb, kangaroo) and white meat (e.g. free range organic chicken).

Drink more:

- water, 1–2 litres a day, and teas (especially organic green tea; black tea) plus vegetable juices
- chamomile tea — may help calm behaviour. Drink 1 cup 30–60 minutes before meals.

Avoid:

- excess coffee — only 1 cup of coffee daily at the start of the day
- trans-fats (e.g. French fries, fish burgers, chicken nuggets, corn chips, pies, Danish rolls, donuts)
- hydrogenated fats, salt, fast foods, added sugar (such as in soft drinks, lollies, biscuits, cakes) and processed foods (e.g. white bread, white pasta, pastries)
- high alcohol intake — small amounts such as 1 glass daily may help prevent dementia
- chemical additives — artificial sweeteners, preservatives, colourings and flavourings.

6 Physical therapies

- Acupuncture and physiotherapy can be useful.
- Massage can help reduce agitation.

7 Supplements

Multivitamin especially B-group containing vitamins B6, B12, and folate

- Side-effects: avoid single vitamin B supplementation and high doses of vitamin B6 >50mg daily for prolonged periods of time. Vitamin B6 toxicity may cause neurological problems such as tingling sensation and balance problems that are often reversible but can be permanent.

Folate

- Indication: may improve memory; prevention of dementia.
- Dosage: 0.4–0.5mg/day lowers high homocysteine levels by as much as 30% in individuals with normal renal function. Dosages more than 0.8–1mg/day are not more effective than a lower daily dose.
  - Result: up to 3 months.
- Side-effects: very mild and rare; unsafe in large doses (more than 1000mcg/day).
- Contraindications: avoid in anaemias until assessed by a doctor.

Vitamin B12

- Indication: may improve memory; prevention of dementia.
- Dosage: Between 600–1000mcg daily.
- Result: 3 months.
- Side-effects: does not cause side-effects even in large doses.
- Contraindications: concurrent use with vitamin C may decrease vitamin B12 absorption therefore best if taken at least 2 hours apart. Several drugs can reduce serum vitamin B12 levels. Excess alcohol intake can also decrease vitamin B12 absorption. Likely to be safe during pregnancy although there is insufficient data.

Multivitamins/antioxidants

- Indication: may improve memory; prevention of dementia; useful in elderly (deficiency common).
- Dosage: 1 multivitamin (containing a mixture of multivitamin B, antioxidants, minerals and fish oils) daily.
- Result: 3 months.
- Side-effects: very mild and rare; gastrointestinal irritation can be avoided if taken after meals.
- Contraindications: vitamin A content greater than 2000 IU daily.

Vitamin D (cholecalciferol)

90% of vitamin D sources come from sunshine, however, supplementation may still be required.

Doctors should check blood levels and suggest supplementation if levels are low.

- Indication: may improve memory; prevention of dementia; improves immunity; strengthens bones and muscles; improves balance and prevents falls in elderly.
- Dosage: cholecalciferol 1000 IU.
- Side-effects: well tolerated if not taken in excessive doses. Excessive dosage causes Vitamin D toxicity.
- Contraindications: moderate interactions with aluminum, calcipotriene (Dovonex), digoxin (Lanoxin), diltiazem (Cardisem, Dilacor, Tiazac), thiazised diuretics, and verapamil (Calan, Covera, Isoptin, Verelan).

Vitamin C (best combined with vitamin E)

- Indication: may improve memory; prevention of dementia; improve immunity.
- Dosage: 200mg daily.
- Results: 3 months.
- Side-effects: with high doses can cause nausea, heartburn, abdominal cramps and diarrhoea.
- Contraindications: can increase iron absorption. Use with caution if glucose-6-phosphate dehydrogenase deficiency and hemochromatosis.

Vitamin E

- Indication: memory; cardiovascular disease.
- Dosage: 200mg daily.
- Side-effects: doses below 1500IU daily are very unlikely to result in haemorrhage, diarrhoea, flatulence, nausea, heart palpitations.
- Contraindications: use with caution if bleeding disorder or if taking with blood thinning medication. If using very high dose, reduce dose before surgery.

Minerals

Magnesium and calcium (best provided together)

- Indication: low magnesium blood levels are associated with cognitive decline; may help poor memory; insomnia; may lower blood pressure; may be useful in anxiety, restless sleep and cramps; restless leg.
- Dosage: children up to 65–120mg daily in divided doses; adults 350–400mg daily including pregnant and lactating women.
- Results: 2–3 days.
- Side-effects: oral magnesium can cause gastrointestinal irritation, nausea, vomiting, and diarrhoea. The dosage varies from person to person. Although rare, toxic levels can cause low blood pressure, thirst, heart arrhythmia, drowsiness and weakness.
- Contraindications: patients with kidney disease; if you have high blood calcium or magnesium levels (e.g. in cancer or kidney diseases).

CoEnzyme Q_{10}

- Indication: may improve memory; prevention of dementia; improves cardiac function.
- Dosage: 200 gm daily.
- Result: 6 months.
- Side-effects: no reported significant side-effects, in some cases mild gastrointestinal upset is reported.
- Contraindications: be cautious when using CoQ_{10} alongside chemotherapy, warfarin or other anticoagulants and hypersensitive drugs.

Fish oils

- Indication: may improve memory; prevention of dementia and cardiovascular disease.
- Dosage: take with meals. Adults: 2–4g (1g containing EPA 180/DHA 120mg) 1–2 daily depending on fish consumption. Children: 500mg 1 to 2 x daily (500mg–1g daily EPA and DHA); can be used in pregnancy or lactation as tolerated.
- Results: 2–4 weeks.
- Side-effects: often well tolerated especially if taken with meals. Very mild and rare side-effects — for example, gastrointestinal upset; allergic reactions (e.g. rash); breathing problems if allergic to seafood; blood thinning effects in very high doses > 10g daily (may need to stop fish oil supplements 2 weeks prior to surgery).
- Contraindications: sensitivity reaction to seafood; drug interactions; caution when taking high doses of fish oils >4g per day together with warfarin (your doctor will check your INR test).

Herbal medicines

Ginkgo (*Ginkgo biloba*)

- Indication: may improve memory; prevention of dementia.
- Dosage: 120–200mg/day or 160mg/day Ginkgo extract Egb 761.
- Results: 12–24 weeks.
- Side-effects: can cause mild gastrointestinal (GI) upset, headache, dizziness, palpitations, constipation, and allergic skin reactions in some cases. Large doses can cause restlessness, diarrhoea, nausea, vomiting, lack of muscle tone, and weakness.
- Contraindications: must not take ginkgo if already taking warfarin or other anticoagulant medication or Ibuprofen. Also be cautious if combining with Alprazolam, anticonvulsants, anti-diabetes, buspirone drugs, cytochrome P450 1A2 (CYP1A2), P450 2C9 (CYP2C9), P450 2C19 (CYP2C19), P450 2D6 (CYP2D6), and P450 3A4 (CYP3A4) substrates, Efavirenz, Fluoxetine, seizure threshold lowering drugs or trazodone. Ginkgo may also interfere with seisure lowering herbs.

Brahmi (*Bacopa monniera*)

- Indication: may improve memory; prevention of dementia.
- Dosage: 300mg/day.
- Results: about 12 weeks.
- Side-effects: some cases experience mild nausea, dry mouth and fatigue.
- Contraindications: none known.

Turmeric (*Curcuma longa*)

- Indication: may improve memory; prevention of dementia.
- Dosage: 1+grams/day. Add powder to cooking.
- Side-effects: can cause gastrointestinal (GI) adverse effects such as nausea and diarrhoea in some cases, otherwise generally well tolerated. Can cause allergic dermatitis when used topically.
- Contraindications: moderate interaction with anticoagulant/antiplatelet drugs. Not recommended to be taken after surgery or if suffering from bile duct obstruction or gallstones.

Lemon balm (*Melissa officinalis*)

- Indication: may improve memory; prevention of dementia.
- Dosage: 60 drops per day of liquid containing 500 μg citral/ml Melissa officinalis.
- Results: 4 months.
- Side-effects: mild sedation, muscle relaxant. Additionally it can cause nausea, vomiting, abdominal pain, dizziness, and wheezing in some cases.
- Contraindications: may enhance the effects of sedative herbs and central nervous system depressants.

Sage (*Salvia lavandulaefolia*)

- Indication: may improve memory; prevention of dementia.
- Dosage: 60 drops/day.
- Results: 4 months.
- Side-effects: used in small doses should have no side-effects. May have mild estrogenic effects.
- Contraindicated: is not recommended for long-term use, however more research needed.

Korean Ginseng (*Panax ginseng*)

- Indication: may improve memory; prevention of dementia.
- Dosage: 200mg daily.
- Results: 12 weeks.
- Side-effects: very rarely occurs. Insomnia; even more rarely and with higher doses –breast discomfort, vaginal bleeding, amenorrhea, tachycardia and palpitations. Has mild estrogenic effects.
- Contraindications: avoid stimulants such as excess caffeine and nicotine. There are a number of theoretical interactions with drugs.

Other supplements

Melatonin

- Indication: helps insomnia in elderly by improving circadian rhythm sleep disorders; reduces the time to fall asleep; jet-lag; may help with night-time restlessness / agitation.
- Dosage: 5–10mg at 6pm or closer to bedtime; for short-term use.
- Results: within 1-3 hours.
- Side-effects: usually well tolerated. Avoid long-term use. May cause drowsiness, dizziness, depressive symptoms, reduced alertness, irritability, headaches; all these symptoms can be transient.
- Contraindications: children, pregnant, lactating mothers; epilepsy; taken with alcohol, sedating medication such as benzodiazepines and use with narcotics; depression.

Melatonin is naturally produced by the body from tryptophan and requires various minerals

Proteins

Peptic HCl ↓ Zinc, vit B1, vit B6

L–Tryptophan

Tryptophan hydroxylase ↓ Folate, Fe, Ca, vit B3

5–Hydroxytryptophan

Dopa Decarboxylase ↓ B6, Zn, mg, vit C

5–Hydroxytryptamine (serotonin)

Protein ⟶ Methionine SAMe ↓ vit B5

Melatonin

Figure 11.1 Flow chart demonstrating production of melatonin by the human brain

and vitamins for its production. Deficiency of any of these may lead to reduced production of melatonin.

Vitamin supplement containing low doses of B1, B3, B5, B6, folate and the minerals zinc, iron, calcium and magnesium may be of help in the production of melatonin.

For a diagrammatic representation of how melatonin is produced in the human brain see Figure 11.1

References

1 Kempler D. Dementia. In: J. Brace-Thompson, Neurocogntive Disorders in Aging. Sage Publications: California, USA, 2005:179–201.

2 Kwok J, Schofield. The Molecular basis of Alzheimer's Disease. In:Sachdev. The Ageing Brain; The Neurobiology and neuropsychology of Ageing. Swets & Zeitlinger Publishers, Lisse, The Netherlands, 2003:173–86.

3 Plassman BL, Langa KM, Fisher GG, et. al. Prevalence of Dementia in the United States: The Aging, Demographics, and Memory Study. Neuroepidemiology 2007;29(1-2):125–32.

4 Nepal B, Brown L, Ranmuthugala G. Years of life lived with and without dementia in Australia, 2004-2006: A population health measure. Australian and New Zealand Journal of Public Health 2008;32(6):565–68.

5 Access Economics, Dementia prevalence and incidence among Australians who do not speak English at home. Alzheimer's Australia, 2006:1-27.

6 Whitmer RA, Gunderson EP, Barrett-Connor E, Quesenberry CP, Jr., Yaffe K. Obesity in middle age and future risk of dementia: a 27 year longitudinal population based study. BMJ 2005;330(7504):1360-.

7 Rosengren A, Skoog I, Gustafson D, Wilhelmsen L. Body Mass Index, Other Cardiovascular Risk Factors, and Hospitalization for Dementia. Arch Intern Med 2005;165(3):321–26.

8 Fitzpatrick AL, Kuller LH, Lopez OL, et. al. Midlife and Late-Life Obesity and the Risk of Dementia: Cardiovascular Health Study. Arch Neurol 2009;66(3):336–42.

9 Hughes TF, Borenstein AR, Schofield E, Wu Y, Larson EB. Association between late-life body mass index and dementia: The Kame Project. Neurology 2009;72(20):1741–46.

10 Ganguli M, Bilt JV, Saxton JA, Shen C, Dodge HH. Alcohol consumption and cognitive function in late life: A longitudinal community study. Neurology 2005;65(8):1210–17.

11 Peters R, Peters J, Warner J, Beckett N, Bulpitt C. Alcohol, dementia and cognitive decline in the elderly: a systematic review. Age Ageing 2008;37(5):505–12.

12 Wang HX, Karp A, Herlitz A, et. al. Personality and lifestyle in relation to dementia incidence. Neurology 2009;72(3):253–259.

13 Nooyens ACJ, van Gelder BM, Verschuren WMM. Smoking and Cognitive Decline Among Middle-Aged Men and Women: The Doetinchem Cohort Study. Am J Public Health 2008;98(12):2244–50.

14 Simons LA, Simons J, McCallum J, Friedlander Y. Lifestyle factors and risk of dementia: Dubbo study of the elderly. Medical Journal of Australia 2006;184(2):68–70.

15 Llewellyn DJ, Lang IA, Langa KM, Naughton F, Matthews FE. Exposure to secondhand smoke and cognitive impairment in non-smokers: national cross sectional study with cotinine measurement. BMJ 2009;338(feb12_2):b462-.

16 Przybelski RJ, Binkley NC. Is vitamin D important for preserving cognition? A positive correlation of serum 25-hydroxyvitamin D concentration with cognitive function. Archives of Biochemistry and Biophysics 2007;460(2):202–205.

17 Wilkins CH, Sheline YI, Roe CM, Birge SJ, Morris JC. Vitamin D deficiency is associated with low mood and worse cognitive performance in older adults. American Journal of Geriatric Psychiatry 2006;14(12):1032–1040.

18 Oudshoorn C, Mattace-Raso FUS, Van Der Velde N, Colin EM, Van Der Cammen TJM. Higher serum vitamin D3 levels are associated with better cognitive test performance in patients with Alzheimer's disease. Dementia and Geriatric Cognitive Disorders 2008;25(6):539–43.

19 Jorde R, Waterloo K, Saleh F, Haug E, Svartberg J. Neuropsychological function in relation to serum parathyroid hormone and serum 25-hydroxyvitamin D levels: The Tromsø study. Journal of Neurology 2006;253(4):464–70.

20 McGrath J, Scragg R, Chant D, Eyles D, Burne T, Obradovic D. No association between serum 25-hydroxyvitamin D3 level and performance on psychometric tests in NHANES III. Neuroepidemiology 2007;29(1-2):49–54.

21 Ravaglia G, De Ronchi D, Forti P, et. al. Nutritional status and dementia in oldest-old women. Archives of Gerontology and Geriatrics 1998;26(Suppl1):427–30.

22 Lee DM, Tajar A, Ulubaev A, et. al. Association between 25-hydroxyvitamin D levels and cognitive performance in middle-aged and older European men. J Neurol Neurosurg Psychiatry 2009;80(7):722–29.

23 Barnham KJ, Bush AI. Metals in Alzheimer's and Parkinson's Diseases. Current Opinion in Chemical Biology 2008;12(2):222–28.

24 Domingo JL. Aluminum and other metals in Alzheimer's disease: A review of potential therapy with chelating agents. Journal of Alzheimer's Disease 2006;10(2):331–41.

25 Rondeau V, Jacqmin-Gadda H, Commenges D, Helmer C, Dartigues J-F. Aluminum and Silica in Drinking Water and the Risk of Alzheimer's Disease or Cognitive Decline: Findings From 15-Year Follow-up of the PAQUID Cohort. Am J Epidemiol 2009;169(4):489–96.

26 Shcherbatykh I, Carpenter DO. The Role of Metals in the Etiology of Alzheimer's Disease. Journal of Alzheimer's Disease 2007;11(2):191–205.
27 Ngandu T, von Strauss E, Helkala EL et. al. Education and dementia: What lies behind the association? Neurology 2007;69(14):1442–50.
28 Knapp M, Thorgrimsen L, Patel A, et. al. Cognitive stimulation therapy for people with dementia: cost-effectiveness analysis. The British Journal of Psychiatry 2006;188(6):574–80.
29 Verghese J, LeValley A, Derby C, et. al. Leisure activities and the risk of amnestic mild cognitive impairment in the elderly. Neurology 2006;66(6):821–27.
30 Andel R, Crowe M, Pedersen NL, et. al. Complexity of Work and Risk of Alzheimer's Disease: A Population-Based Study of Swedish Twins. J Gerontol B Psychol Sci Soc Sci 2005;60(5): P251–P258.
31 Wilson RS, Krueger KR, Arnold SE, et. al. Loneliness and risk of Alzheimer disease. Archives of General Psychiatry 2007;64(2):234–40.
32 Jacqueline Perkins, HBCT J.R. Dog-assisted therapy for older people with dementia: A review. Australasian Journal on Ageing 2008;27(4): 177–182.
33 Willcox B, Willcox D, Todoriki H, et. al. Caloric Restriction, the Traditional Okinawan Diet, and Healthy Aging. Annals of the New York Academy of Sciences, 2007. 1114 (Healthy Aging and Longevity Third International Conference):434–455.
34 Buell JS, Dawson-Hughes B. Vitamin D and neurocognitive dysfunction: Preventing "D"ecline? Molecular Aspects of Medicine 2008;29(6):415–22.
35 Larson EB, Wang L, Bowen JD, et. al. Exercise is associated with reduced risk for incident dementia among persons 65 years of age and older. Annals of Internal Medicine 2006;144(2):73–81.
36 Taaffe DR, Irie F, Masaki KH, et. al. Physical Activity, Physical Function, and Incident Dementia in Elderly Men: The Honolulu-Asia Aging Study. J Gerontol A Biol Sci Med Sci 2008;63(5):529–35.
37 Qi D, Amy RB, Yougui W, James CJ, Eric BL. Fruit and Vegetable Juices and Alzheimer's Disease: The Kame Project. The American Journal of Medicine 2006;119(9):751–59.
38 Barberger-Gateau P, Raffaitin C, Letenneur L, et. al. Dietary patterns and risk of dementia: The Three-City cohort study. Neurology 2007;69(20):1921–1930.
39 Yochum L, Kushi LH, Meyer K, Folsom AR. Dietary Flavonoid Intake and Risk of Cardiovascular Disease in Postmenopausal Women. Am J Epidemiol 1999;149(10):943–49.
40 Eckert GP. The Mediterranean diet to prevent Alzheimer's disease. Mediterrane ernährung zur prophylaxe der Alzheimer demenz 2008;55(8):480–85.
41 Panza F, Solfrizzi V, Colacicco AM, et. al. Mediterranean diet and cognitive decline. Public Health Nutrition 2004;7(07):959–63.
42 Nikolaos Scarmeas YSM-XTRMJAL. Mediterranean diet and risk for Alzheimer's disease. Annals of Neurology 2006;59(6):912–21.
43 Scarmeas N, Stern Y, Mayeux R, Manly JJ, Schupf N, Luchsinger JA. Mediterranean Diet and Mild Cognitive Impairment. Arch Neurol 2009;66(2):216–25.
44 Kuriyama S, Hozawa A, Ohmori K, et. al. Green tea consumption and cognitive function: a cross-sectional study from the Tsurugaya Project 1. Am J Clin Nutr 2006;83(2):355–61.
45 de Mendonca A, Sebastiao AM, Ribeiro JA. Adenosine: does it have a neuroprotective role after all? Brain Res Brain Res Rev 2000;33(2-3):258–74.
46 Maia L, De MendoncÌ§a A. Does caffeine intake protect from Alzheimer's disease? European Journal of Neurology 2002;9(4):377–82.
47 Eskelinen MH, Ngandu T, Tuomilehto J, Soininen H, Kivipelto M. Midlife coffee and tea drinking and the risk of late-life dementia: A population-based CAIDE study. Journal of Alzheimer's Disease 2009;16(1): 85–91.
48 Ritchie K, CarriÃ¨re I, De MendonÃ§a A, et. al. The neuroprotective effects of caffeine: A prospective population study (the Three City Study). Neurology 2007;69(6):536–45.
49 Bartali B, Frongillo EA, Guralnik JM, et. al. Serum Micronutrient Concentrations and Decline in Physical Function Among Older Persons. JAMA 2008;299(3):308–15.
50 Loikas S, Koskinen P, Irjala K, et. al. Vitamin B12 deficiency in the aged: a population-based study. Age Ageing 2007;36(2):177–83.
51 Deanne G, Lucinda JB, Elisabeth AI, Stacey H, Fran S, Judith DB. Malnutrition prevalence and nutrition issues in residential aged care facilities. Australasian Journal on Ageing 2008;27(4):189–94.
52 Scragg R, Camargo CA, Jr. Frequency of Leisure-Time Physical Activity and Serum 25-Hydroxyvitamin D Levels in the US Population: Results from the Third National Health and Nutrition Examination Survey. Am J Epidemiol 2008;168(6):577–86.
53 Grieger JA, Nowson CA. Nutrient intake and plate waste from an Australian residential care facility. Eur J Clin Nutr 2006;61(5):655–63.
54 Çilliler AE, Öztürk S, Özbakir S. Serum Magnesium Level and Clinical Deterioration in Alzheimer's Disease. Gerontology 2007;53(6):419–22.
55 Lazar SW, Kerr CE, Wasserman RH, et. al. Meditation experience is associated with increased cortical thickness. NeuroReport 2005;16(17):1893–97.
56 Kraus CA, Seignourel P, Balasubramanyam V, et. al. Cognitive-behavioral treatment for anxiety in patients with dementia: Two case studies. Journal of Psychiatric Practice 2008;14(3):186–92.
57 Akkerman RL, Ostwald SK. Reducing anxiety in Alzheimer's disease family caregivers: The effectiveness of a nine-week cognitive-behavioral intervention. American Journal of Alzheimer's Disease and other Dementias 2004;19(2):117–23.
58 Secker DL, Brown RG. Cognitive behavioural therapy (CBT) for carers of patients with Parkinson's disease: A preliminary randomised controlled trial. Journal of Neurology, Neurosurgery and Psychiatry 2005;76(4):491–97.
59 Kipling T, Bailey M, Charlesworth G. The feasibility of a cognitive behavioural therapy group for men with mild/moderate cognitive impairment. Behavioural and Cognitive Psychotherapy, 1999;27(2):189–93.
60 Sung, HC, Chang AM. Use of preferred music to decrease agitated behaviours in older people with dementia: A review of the literature. Journal of Clinical Nursing 2005;14(9):1133–40.
61 Ballard C, O'Brien J, Reichelt K, Perry E. Aromatherapy as a safe and effective treatment for the management of agitation in severe dementia: the results of a double-blind, placebo-controlled trial with Melissa. Journal of Clinical Psychiatry 2002;63(7):553–8.

62 Thorgrimsen L, Spector A, Wiles A, Orrell M. Aroma therapy for dementia. Cochrane database of systematic reviews (Online) 2003(3).
63 Clare L, Woods RT, Moniz Cook ED, Orrell M, Spector A, et. al. Cognitive rehabilitation and cognitive training for early-stage Alzheimer's disease and vascular dementia. Cochrane Database Syst Rev 2003(4).
64 Ball K, Berch DB, Helmers KF, et. al. Effects of cognitive training interventions with older adults: a randomized controlled trial. JAMA 2002;288(18):2271–81.
65 Willis SL, Tennstedt SL, Marsiske M, et. al. Long-term effects of cognitive training on everyday functional outcomes in older adults. JAMA 2006;296(23):2805–14.
66 Smith GE, Housen P, Yaffe K, et. al. A cognitive training program based on principles of brain plasticity: results from the Improvement in Memory with Plasticity-based Adaptive Cognitive Training (IMPACT) study. J Am Geriatr Soc 2009;57(4):594–603.
67 Mahncke HW, Connor BB, Appelman J, et. al. Memory enhancement in healthy older adults using a brain plasticity-based training program: a randomized, controlled study. Proc Natl Acad Sci U S A 2006;103(33):12523–8.
68 McNab F, Varrone A, Farde L, et. al. Changes in cortical dopamine D1 receptor binding associated with cognitive training. Science 2009;323(5915):800–2.
69 McCurry SM, Gibbons LE, Logsdon RG, Vitiello MV, Teri L et. al. Nighttime Insomnia Treatment and Education for Alzheimer's Disease: A randomized, controlled trial. Journal of the American Geriatrics Society 2005;53(5): 793–802.
70 Caroline AB, Hodan YA, Dianne EC, Angela V, John DW et. al. Vitamin D deficiency: a study of community beliefs among dark skinned and veiled people. International Journal of Rheumatic Diseases 2008;11(1):15–23.
71 Diamond T, Levy S, Smith A, Day P, et. al. High bone turnover in Muslim women with vitamin D deficiency. The Medical Journal of Australia 2002;177:139–141.
72 Grant WB. Does Vitamin D Reduce the Risk of Dementia? Journal of Alzheimer's Disease 2009;17(1):151–159.
73 Hansen A, Bi P, Nitschke M, Ryan P, Pisaniello D, Tucker G. The effect of heat waves on mental health in a temperate Australian City. Environmental Health Perspectives 2008;116(10):1369–1375.
74 Riemersma-van Der Lek RF, Swaab DF, Twisk J, Hol EM, Hoogendijk WJG, Van Someren EJW. Effect of bright light and melatonin on cognitive and noncognitive function in elderly residents of group care facilities: A randomized controlled trial. JAMA - Journal of the American Medical Association 2008;299(22):2642–2655.
75 Ito T, Yamadera H, Ito R, Endo S. Effects of bright light on cognitive disturbances in Alzheimer-type dementia. Nippon Ika Daigaku zasshi 1999;66(4):229–238.
76 Forbes D, Morgan DG, Bangma J, Peacock S, Pelletier N, Adamson J. Light therapy for managing sleep, behaviour, and mood disturbances in dementia. Cochrane database of systematic reviews (Online) 2004(2).
77 Chan AS, Ho YC, Cheung MC, Albert MS, Chiu HFK, Lam LCW. Association between mind-body and cardiovascular exercises and memory in older adults. Journal of the American Geriatrics Society 2005;53(10):1754–1760.
78 Lautenschlager NT, Cox KL, Flicker L, et. al. Effect of Physical Activity on Cognitive Function in Older Adults at Risk for Alzheimer Disease: A Randomized Trial. JAMA 2008;300(9):1027–1037.
79 Brown AK, Liu-Ambrose T, Tate R, Lord S. The Effect of Group-Based Exercise on Cognitive Performance and Mood in Seniors Residing in Intermediate Care and Self-Care Retirement Facilities: A Randomized Controlled Trial. Br J Sports Med 2008:bjsm.2008.049882.
80 Forbes D, Forbes S, Morgan DG, Markle-Reid M, Wood J, Culum I. Physical activity programs for persons with dementia. Cochrane Database of Systematic Reviews 2008(3).
81 Zhang NN, La XB, Ni W, Mao WQ. Effect of long-term Tai Chi exercise on cognitive function of middle-aged and old people. Chinese Journal of Clinical Rehabilitation 2006;10(26):7–9.
82 Matthews M, Williams H. Can Tai chi enhance cognitive vitality? A preliminary study of cognitive executive control in older adults after A Tai chi intervention. Journal of the South Carolina Medical Association 2008;104(8):255–57.
83 Selhub J, Bagley LC, Miller J, Rosenberg IH. B vitamins, homocysteine, and neurocognitive function in the elderly1. Am J Clin Nutr 2000;71(2): 614s-620.
84 Stott DJ, MacIntosh G, Lowe GDO, et. al. Randomized controlled trial of homocysteine-lowering vitamin treatment in elderly patients with vascular disease. Am J Clin Nutr 2005;82(6):1320–26.
85 Vogiatzoglou A, Refsum H, Johnston C, et. al. Vitamin B12 status and rate of brain volume loss in community-dwelling elderly. Neurology 2008;71(11):826–32.
86 Leischker AH, Kolb GF. Vitamin-B12 deficiency in the elderly. Vitamin-B12-mangel im alter 2002;4(3):120–26.
87 Kado DM, Karlamangla AS, Huang M-H, et. al. Homocysteine versus the vitamins folate, B6, and B12 as predictors of cognitive function and decline in older high-functioning adults: MacArthur Studies of Successful Aging. The American Journal of Medicine 2005;118(2):161–67.
88 Chan A, Paskavitz J, Remington R, Rasmussen S, Shea TB. Efficacy of a vitamin/nutriceutical formulation for early-stage Alzheimer's disease: A 1-year, open-label pilot study with an 16-month caregiver extension. American Journal of Alzheimer's Disease and other Dementias 2009;23(6):571–85.
89 Luchsinger JA, Tang MX, Miller J, Green R, Mayeux R. Relation of higher folate intake to lower risk of Alzheimer disease in the elderly. Archives of Neurology 2007;64(1):86–92.
90 Corrada MM, Kawas CH, Hallfrisch J, Muller D, Brookmeyer R et. al. Reduced risk of Alzheimer's disease with high folate intake: The Baltimore Longitudinal Study of Aging. Alzheimer's and Dementia 2005;1(1):11–8.
91 Wouters-Wesseling W, Wagenaar LW, Rozendaal M, et et. al. Effect of an enriched drink on cognitive function in frail elderly persons. Journals of Gerontology - Series A Biological Sciences and Medical Sciences 2005;60(2):265–70.

92 Aisen PS, Schneider LS, Sano M, et. al. High-Dose B Vitamin Supplementation and Cognitive Decline in Alzheimer Disease: A Randomized Controlled Trial. JAMA 2008;300(15):1774–83.
93 Schulz RJ, Homocysteine as a biomarker for cognitive dysfunction in the elderly. Current Opinion in Clinical Nutrition and Metabolic Care 2007;10(6):718–23.
94 Frick B, Gruber B, Schroecksnadel K, Leblhuber F, Fuchs D. Homocysteine but not neopterin declines in demented patients on B vitamins. Journal of Neural Transmission 2006;113(11):1815–19.
95 Troen A, Rosenberg I. Homocysteine and cognitive function. Seminars in Vascular Medicine 2005;5(2):209–14.
96 McMahon JA, Green TJ, Skeaff CM, Knight RG, Mann JI, Williams SM. A controlled trial of homocysteine lowering and cognitive performance. New England Journal of Medicine 2006;354(26):2764–72.
97 Clarke R, Smith AD, Jobst KA, Refsum H, Sutton L, Ueland PM. Folate, vitamin B12, and serum total homocysteine levels in confirmed Alzheimer disease. Archives of Neurology 1998;55(11):1449–55.
98 Zhang CE, Tian Q, Wei W, et. al. Homocysteine induces tau phosphorylation by inactivating protein phosphatase 2A in rat hippocampus. Neurobiology of Aging 2008;29(11):1654–65.
99 Scott TM, Tucker KL, Bhadelia A, et. al. Homocysteine and B vitamins relate to brain volume and white-matter changes in geriatric patients with psychiatric disorders. American Journal of Geriatric Psychiatry 2004;12(6):631–38.
100 Brain shrinkage from homocysteine? Health news (Waltham, Mass.) 2003;9(3):8.
101 Malouf R, Grimley Evans J. Folic acid with or without vitamin B12 for the prevention and treatment of healthy elderly and demented people. Cochrane database of systematic reviews (Online) 2008(4).
102 Flicker L, Martins RN, Thomas J, et. al. B-vitamins reduce plasma levels of beta amyloid. Neurobiology of Aging 2008;29(2):303–05.
103 Rosemary L, Martin O, in The Lancet. 1997;1189–90.
104 Maxwell CJ, Hicks MS, Hogan DB, Basran J, Ebly EM. Supplemental use of antioxidant vitamins and subsequent risk of cognitive decline and dementia. Dementia and Geriatric Cognitive Disorders 2005;20(1):45–51.
105 Zandi PP, Anthony JC, Khachaturian AS, et. al. Reduced Risk of Alzheimer Disease in Users of Antioxidant Vitamin Supplements: The Cache County Study. Arch Neurol 2004;61(1):82–8.
106 Petersen RC, Thomas RG, Grundman M, et. al. Vitamin E and Donepezil for the Treatment of Mild Cognitive Impairment. N Engl J Med 2005;352(23):2379–88.
107 Sano M, Ernesto C, Thomas RG, et. al. A controlled trial of selegiline, alpha-tocopherol, or both as treatment for Alzheimer's disease. New England Journal of Medicine 1997;336(17):1216–22.
108 Grundman M, Vitamin E and Alzheimer disease: The basis for additional clinical trials. American Journal of Clinical Nutrition 2000;71(2).
109 Morris MC, Evans DA, Bienias JL, Tangney CC, Wilson RS. Vitamin E and Cognitive Decline in Older Persons. Arch Neurol 2002;59(7):1125–32.
110 Mgekn I, Quinn R, Tabet N. Vitamin E for Alzheimer's disease and mild cognitive impairment. Cochrane Database of Systematic Reviews 2008(3).
111 Gray SL, Anderson ML, Crane PK, et. al. Antioxidant vitamin supplement use and risk of dementia or Alzheimer's disease in older adults. Journal of the American Geriatrics Society 2008;56(2):291–95.
112 Asayama K, Yamadera H, Ito T, Suzuki H, Kudo Y, Endo S. Double blind study of melatonin effects on the sleep-wake rhythm, cognitive and non-cognitive functions in Alzheimer type dementia. Journal of Nippon Medical School 2003;70(4):334–41.
113 Jansen SL, Forbes DA, Duncan V, Morgan DG. Melatonin for cognitive impairment. Cochrane database of systematic reviews (Online) 2006(1).
114 Birks J, Grimley Evans J. Ginkgo biloba for cognitive impairment and dementia. Cochrane Database Syst Rev 2009(1):CD003120.
115 Dodge HH, Zitzelberger T, Oken BS, Howieson D, Kaye J. A randomized placebo-controlled trial of Ginkgo biloba for the prevention of cognitive decline. Neurology 2008;70(19_Part_2):1809–17.
116 Schneider LS, DeKosky ST, Farlow MR, Tariot PN, Hoerr R, Kieser M. A randomized, double-blind, placebo-controlled trial of two doses of Ginkgo biloba extract in dementia of the Alzheimer's type. Current Alzheimer Research 2005;2(5):541–51.
117 Santos RF, GaldurÃ³z JCF, Barbieri A, Castiglioni MLV, Ytaya LY, Bueno OFA. Cognitive Performance, SPECT, and Blood Viscosity in Elderly Non-demented People Using Ginkgo Biloba. Pharmacopsychiatry 2003;36(4):127–33.
118 Mazzaa M, Capuanob A, Briaa P, Mazza S. Ginkgo biloba and donepezil: a comparison in the treatment of Alzheimer's dementia in a randomized placebo-controlled double-blind study. European Journal of Neurology 2006;13:981–5.
119 Stough C, Downey LA, Lloyd J, et. al. Examining the nootropic effects of a special extract of Bacopa monniera on human cognitive functioning: 90 Day double-blind placebo-controlled randomized trial. Phytotherapy Research 2008;22(12):1629–34.
120 Stough C, Lloyd J, Clarke J, et. al. The chronic effects of an extract of Bacopa monniera (Brahmi) on cognitive function in healthy human subjects. Psychopharmacology 2001;156(4):481–84.
121 Roodenrys S, Booth D, Bulzomi S, Phipps A, Micallef C, Smoker J. Chronic effects of Brahmi (Bacopa monnieri) on human memory. Neuropsychopharmacology 2002;27(2):279–81.
122 Calabrese C, Gregory WL, Leo M, Kraemer D, Bone K, Oken B. Effects of a Standardized Bacopa monnieri Extract on Cognitive Performance, Anxiety, and Depression in the Elderly: A Randomized, Double-Blind, Placebo-Controlled Trial. The Journal of Alternative and Complementary Medicine 2008;14(6):707–13.
123 Bhattacharya SK, Kumar A, Ghosal S. Effect of Bacopa Monniera on animal models of Alzheimer's disease and perturbed central cholinergic markers of cognition in rats. Research Communications in Pharmacology and Toxicology 1999;4(3-4):II1–II12.
124 Akhondzadeh S, Noroozian M, Mohammadi M, Ohadinia S, Jamshidi AH, Khani M. Melissa officinalis extract in the treatment of patients with mild to moderate Alzheimer's disease: A double blind, randomised, placebo controlled trial. Journal of Neurology Neurosurgery and Psychiatry 2003;74(7):863–66.
125 Perry NSL, Bollen C, Perry EK, Ballard C. Salvia for dementia therapy: Review of pharmacological activity and pilot tolerability clinical trial. Pharmacology Biochemistry and Behavior 2003;75(3):651–59.

126 Akhondzadeh S, Noroozian M, Mohammadi M, Ohadinia S, Jamshidi AH, Khani M. Salvia officinalis extract in the treatment of patients with mild to moderate Alzheimer's disease: A double blind, randomized and placebo-controlled trial. Journal of Clinical Pharmacy and Therapeutics 2003;28(1): 53–9.

127 Glenn MB, Lexell J. Ginseng. The Journal of Head Trauma Rehabilitation 2003;18(2):196–200.

128 Vogler B, Pittler MH, Ernst E. The efficacy of ginseng. A systematic review of randomised trials. European Journal of Clinical Pharmacology 1999;55:567–75.

129 Heo J, Lee S, Chu K, et. al. An open-label trial of Korean red ginseng as an adjuvant treatment for cognitive impairment in patients with Alzheimer's disease. European Journal of Neurology 2008;15(8):865–68.

130 Neri M, Andermarcher E, Pradelli JM, Salvioli G. Influence of a double blind pharmacological trial on two domains of well-being in subject's with age associated memory impairment. Archives of Gerontology and Geriatrics 1995;21(3):241–52.

131 Mishra S, Palaniveru K. The effect of curcumin (tumeric) on Alzheimer's disease:an overview. Annals of Indian Academy of Neurology 2008;11:13–9.

132 Yang F, Lim GP, Begum AN, et. al. Curcumin inhibits formation of amyloid Î² oligomers and fibrils, binds plaques, and reduces amyloid in vivo. Journal of Biological Chemistry 2005;280(7):5892–5901.

133 Ng TP, Chiam PC, Lee T, Chua HC, Lim L, Kua EH. Curry consumption and cognitive function in the elderly. American Journal of Epidemiology 2006;164(9):898–906.

134 Lim GP, Chu T, Yang F, Beech W, Frautschy SA, Cole GM. The curry spice curcumin reduces oxidative damage and amyloid pathology in an Alzheimer transgenic mouse. Journal of Neuroscience 2001;21(21):8370–77.

135 Baum L, Lam CWK, Cheung SK-K, et. al. Six-Month Randomized, Placebo-Controlled, Double-Blind, Pilot Clinical Trial of Curcumin in Patients With Alzheimer Disease. Journal of Clinical Psychopharmacology 2008;28(1):110-113 10.1097/jcp.0b013e318160862c.

136 Vingtdeux V, Dreses-Werringloer U, Zhao H, Davies P, Marambaud P. Therapeutic potential of resveratrol in Alzheimer's disease. BMC Neurosci 2008;9(Suppl 2):S6.

137 Marambaud P, Zhao H, Davies. Resveratrol promotes clearance of Alzheimer's disease amyloid-beta peptides. J Biol Chem 2005;280(45):37377–82.

138 Ho L, Chen LH, Wang J, et. al. Heterogeneity in red wine polyphenolic contents differentially influences Alzheimer's disease-type neuropathology and cognitive deterioration. Journal of Alzheimer's Disease 2009;16(1):59–72.

139 Wang J, Ho L, Zhao Z, et. al. Moderate consumption of Cabernet Sauvignon attenuates AÎ² neuropathology in a mouse model of Alzheimer's disease. FASEB Journal 2006;20(13):2313–20.

140 Lim WS, Gammack JK, Van Niekerk J, Dangour AD. Omega 3 fatty acid for the prevention of dementia. Cochrane database of systematic reviews (Online) 2006(1).

141 Issa AM, Mojica WA, Morton SC, et. al. The Efficacy of Omega--3 Fatty Acids on Cognitive Function in Aging and Dementia: A Systematic Review. Dementia and Geriatric Cognitive Disorders 2006;21(2):88–96.

142 Solfrizzi V, D'Introno A, Colacicco AM, et. al. Dietary fatty acids intake: possible role in cognitive decline and dementia. Experimental Gerontology 2005;40(4):257–70.

143 Nurk E, Drevon CA, Refsum H, et. al. Cognitive performance among the elderly and dietary fish intake: the Hordaland Health Study. Am J Clin Nutr 2007;86(5):1470–78.

144 van Gelder BM, Tijhuis M, Kalmijn S, Kromhout D. Fish consumption, n-3 fatty acids, and subsequent 5-y cognitive decline in elderly men: the Zutphen Elderly Study. Am J Clin Nutr 2007;85(4):1142–47.

145 Conquer J, Tierney M, Zecevic J, Bettger W, Fisher R. Fatty acid analysis of blood plasma of patients with alzheimer's disease, other types of dementia, and cognitive impairment. Lipids 2000;35(12):1305–12.

146 Schaefer EJ, Bongard V, Beiser AS, et. al. Plasma Phosphatidylcholine Docosahexaenoic Acid Content and Risk of Dementia and Alzheimer Disease: The Framingham Heart Study. Arch Neurol 2006;63(11):1545–50.

147 Samieri C, Feart C, Letenneur L, et. al. Low plasma eicosapentaenoicacidanddepressivesymptomatologyare independent predictors of dementia risk. Am J Clin Nutr 2008;88(3):714–21.

148 Kotani S, Sakaguchi E, Warashina S, et. al. Dietary supplementation of arachidonic and docosahexaenoic acids improves cognitive dysfunction. Neuroscience Research 2006;56(2):159–64.

149 Freund Levi Y, Eriksdotter-Jonhagen M, Cederholm T, et. al. {omega}-3 Fatty Acid Treatment in 174 Patients With Mild to Moderate Alzheimer Disease: Omega AD Study: A Randomized Double-blind Trial. Arch Neurol 2006;63(10):1402–08.

150 Chiu CC, Su KP, Cheng TC, et. al. The effects of omega-3 fatty acids monotherapy in Alzheimer's disease and mild cognitive impairment: A preliminary randomized double-blind placebo-controlled study. Progress in Neuro-Psychopharmacology and Biological Psychiatry 2008;32(6):1538–44.

151 van de Rest O, Geleijnse JM, Kok FJ, et. al. Effect of fish oil on cognitive performance in older subjects: a randomized, controlled trial. Neurology 2008;71(6): 430–38.

152 Majid F, Payam M, Kristine Y. Fish consumption, long-chainomega-3fattyacidsandriskofcognitivedecline or Alzheimer disease: a complex association. Nature Reviews Neurology 2009;5(3):140–52.

153 Bragin V, Chemodanova M, Dzhafarova N, Bragin I, Czerniawski J, Aliev G. Integrated treatment approach improves cognitive function in demented and clinically depressed patients. American Journal of Alzheimer's disease and Other Dementias 2005;20(1):21–6.

154 Christofoletti G, Oliani MM, Gobbi S, Stella F, Bucken Gobbi LT, Canineu PR. A controlled clinical trial on the effects of motor intervention on balance and cognition in institutionalized elderly patients with dementia. Clinical Rehabilitation 2008;22(7):618–26.

155 Hicks-Moore SL, Robinson BA. Favorite music and hand massage: Two interventions to decrease agitation in residents with dementia. Dementia 2008;7(1):95–108.

156 Lee MS, Shin BC, Ernst E. Acupuncture for Alzheimer's disease: A systematic review. International Journal of Clinical Practice 2009;63(6):874–79.

157 Liu ZB, Niu WM, Yang XH, Niu XM. Clinical investigation on electroacupuncture treatment of vascular dementia with "Xiusanzhen". Zhen ci yan jiu = Acupuncture research/[Zhongguo yi xue ke xue yuan Yi xue qing bao yan jiu suo bian ji] 2008;33(2):131–34.

Chapter 12

Depression

Introduction

Mental health is closely linked to physical health. Depression (e.g. major depression) is highly prevalent and a major cause of disability. The World Health Organization (WHO) expects that by 2020 depression will rank second only to ischemic heart disease in terms of disability, irrespective of gender and age.[1] Currently, depression is ranked as the second cause of disability in terms of disability adjusted life years in the age category 15–44 years for both genders combined.[1] Depression is a common illness affecting at least 1 in 5 people during their lifetime.[2] Depression has no gender, age, or lifestyle background predilection, it can potentially occur in all persons. Depression facts:

- depression affects approximately 121 million people worldwide
- depression is among the leading causes of disability worldwide
- depression can be reliably diagnosed and treated by clinicians in general practice
- less than 25% of patients affected with depression have access to effective treatments.

Patients often present with an overlapping and complex set of symptoms (Table 12.1).

Depression also influences the morbidity and mortality of a number of somatic illnesses. Research strongly documents a significantly higher risk and mortality in depressed patients post acute myocardial infarction.[4] There is also evidence demonstrating that depression is significantly associated with diabetics.[5]

Complementary medicine (CM) encompasses a wide range of therapies that are currently not part of conventional medicine and are often adopted by patients who feel the need to take more control over their illnesses. Unfortunately, this often leads to patients self-medicating to alleviate symptoms, such as emotional distress, to help them cope with serious mental illness problems.[6]

The key to treating the depressed patient is to take an *holistic* approach by addressing both physical and psychological needs. There are many alternative therapies now available for the treatment of mild–moderate depression that a practitioner can easily recommend, especially lifestyle advice, as part of the holistic management of patients with depression. Guarded optimism exists for many of these therapies and further well-designed trials are needed for most alternative therapies. Also, as part of the integrative approach, the medical practitioner needs to take great care not to delay drug treatment in the patient with severe depression.

A recent review[7] has reported that systematic trials are required for promising substances for depression and that meanwhile, those patients wishing to take psychotropic complementary medicines require appropriate medical advice. In this chapter we review the evidence-based research in CM approaches to the treatment of depression, that includes the use of herbal medicines, nutritional and dietary supplements, mind–body medicine approaches such as cognitive behavioural therapy (CBT), meditation, hypnosis, aromatherapy, acupuncture and light therapy.

A recent review of the literature identified a range of possible non-drug treatments for the treatment of depression in the elderly.[8] The review found best evidence for antidepressants, electroconvulsive therapy (ECT), CBT, psychodynamic psychotherapy, reminiscence therapy, problem-solving therapy, bibliotherapy and physical exercise. Limited evidence was identified for transcranial magnetic stimulation, dialectical behaviour therapy, interpersonal therapy, light therapy, St John's wort and folate.

Another review of the literature found the best evidence for the treatment of depression occurred with St John's wort, exercise, bibliotherapy, CBT and light therapy (for winter depression), and promising evidence (but needing more research) for folate vitamin E, vitamin B6, vitamin D, SAMe (s-adenosyl methionine), phenyalanine, *Ginkgo biloba*, acupuncture, light therapy (non-seasonal depression), massage therapy, negative air ionisation (for winter depression), relaxation therapy, yoga, and reducing or avoiding alcohol, sugar and caffeine avoidance and possibly music/dance therapy.[9]

The risk factors for depression are:

- genetic
- disease and chronic illness (e.g. cancer, asthma, diabetes, cardiac disease)

Table 12.1 The spectrum of symptoms in depression[3]

Physical symptoms	Emotional symptoms
Tiredness and fatigue	Sadness and tearfulness
Sleep disturbances	Anxiety and irritability
Headaches	Loss of interest
Gastrointestinal disturbances	Hopelessness
Psychomotor activity changes	Difficulty concentrating
Appetite changes	Guilt
Body aches and pains	Suicidal tendency

- medication (e.g. oral contraceptive pill)
- chronic pain
- stress and/or traumatic experience (e.g. bullying, abuse)
- social isolation, loneliness, unemployment
- lack of spiritual supports (e.g. family, church)
- sleep disturbance
- elderly
- inadequate sunlight exposure and vitamin D deficiency
- smoking
- drug and alcohol abuse
- lack of exercise and/or physical activity
- poor diet and nutritional deficiencies
- food intolerance
- low fish intake.

Healthy lifestyle changes

In the management of depression, emphasis on lifestyle changes is vital, such as stress management, improved diet, sleep, exercise, sunlight exposure and smoking cessation. The treatment of depression requires the health practitioner to spend long consultations exploring all of these areas.[10] A few words of advice can go a long way towards changing patients' health behaviour.[11] A study found that patients were more likely to try to quit smoking, change their diet and perform more exercise when written information leaflets were backed by encouragement and GP advice. The study also concluded that advice on health behaviour may have to be delivered several times before it brought about change.[11]

Mind–body medicine

Cognitive behavioural therapy (CBT), group therapy and support groups

Counselling and CBT carry the greatest weight of scientific evidence for the treatment of depression.[12] The types of psychotherapy that have proven efficacy are mainly CBT and interpersonal psychotherapy (IPT).[13, 14]

A recent study with depressed mothers demonstrated that brief IPT was beneficial in reducing levels of maternal symptoms of depression and improving functioning at the 3– and 9–month follow-ups compared to usual treatment for depression.[12] Moreover, the meta-analysis reported that preventative strategies such as IPT may be more effective than prevention based on CBT.[13]

The health practitioner needs to be alert to stressors the patient is experiencing in the school, home or work environments. Traumatic and stressful experiences in people's lives such as relationship breakdowns, loss, bullying, being excluded by peers, experiencing humiliation, life-threatening events, assault (physical and sexual), and loss of work are potent triggers for depression and feelings of suicidal ideation.[15-19]

The prognosis of depression is worse when the patient has a serious illness such as cancer or heart disease.[20, 21]

CBT is at least as effective as antidepressants in outpatients with severe depression according to a meta-analysis of 4 major randomised trials.[22]

Positive feedback, reassurance, advice and helping to explore stress and dealing with them were essential components reported. If the practitioner is not well trained in this area then referral to a practitioner who is well trained is advised.

Recent reviews[23,24] conclude that psychotherapy and pharmacotherapy generally are of comparable efficacy, and both modalities are superior to usual care in treating depression.

CBT has been investigated in a number of clinical scenarios, and demonstrated better efficacy than medication for post-partum depression.[25] CBT was efficacious in reducing depressive symptoms among HIV-infected individuals,[26] was effective for the treatment of unipolar depression,[27] effective in incurable cancer patients,[28] and a recent meta-analysis suggests that CBT may be of potential benefit in older people with depression.[29] Further, recently it has been reported that CBT may be useful for depressed patients diagnosed with Parkinson's Disease.[30]

Young adolescents with depression and repeated self-harm showed promising results in a Group therapy program.[31] UK child psychiatrists randomised 63 patients aged 12–16 to routine care or to a weekly group therapy program over 6 months. The adolescents in the group therapy program were less likely to harm themselves, less likely to use health care resources, had better school attendance, and a lower rate of behavioural disorders. However, there was no effect on the severity of the depression or its prevalence.

A comprehensive meta-analysis of the literature of 19 randomised controlled trials (RCTs), meeting the inclusion criteria, highlighted that efficacy of preventive psychological interventions can reduce the incidence of depressive disorders by 22% in experimental groups compared with control groups. Therefore, therapies such as counselling and CBT may also play a role in the prevention of depression onset.[14]

Stress management

A 12-week, randomised, clinical trial of 123 outpatients who met the *DSM-IV* criteria for major or minor depression within 1 year after coronary artery bypass surgery significantly improved following 12 weeks of CBT or supportive stress management[32]. The CBT group led to remission of depression at 3 and 9 months in 71% of patients and 57% for those undergoing supportive stress management by 3 months compared with 33% remission in the usual care group. At 9 months remission rates were similar with CBT being far superior to usual care for depression and other secondary psychological outcomes, such as anxiety, hopelessness, stress, and quality of life.[32]

Meditation

Mindfulness meditation-based stress reduction programs have demonstrated effectiveness in decreasing mood disturbance, including depression and stress symptoms in patients with a wide range of types and stages of cancer.[33, 34] A randomised, wait-list controlled design of 90 patients (mean age 51 years, 78% females) was used with the intervention consisting of weekly meditation of 1.5 hours for 7 weeks plus home meditation practice.[33] Patients in the mindfulness meditation intervention group demonstrated significantly lower scores on total mood disturbance by 65% and sub-scales of depression, anxiety, anger and confusion compared with control participants. The treatment group demonstrated less stress symptoms (by 31%), fewer cardiopulmonary and gastrointestinal symptoms, and less emotional irritability and cognitive disturbances. A recent preliminary study investigating mindfulness-based stress reduction reported that participation in the program was associated with enhanced quality of life and decreased stress symptoms, altered cortisol and immune patterns consistent with less stress and mood disturbance, and decreased blood pressure.[34]

Relaxation therapy

A recent Cochrane review and meta-analysis of 15 trials with 11 included in the analysis demonstrated that relaxation was effective for reducing depressive symptoms.[35] Five trials showed relaxation reduced self-reported depression compared to wait-list, no treatment, or minimal treatment post-intervention (SMD –0.59 [95% confidence interval [CI] –0.94 to –0.24]). For clinician-rated depression, 2 trials showed a non-significant difference in the same direction (SMD –1.35 [95% CI –3.06 to 0.37]). A recent assessment of the Cochrane review concluded relaxation techniques were better than either wait-list, no treatment or minimal treatment, but not as effective as psychological therapies such as CBT.[36]

Music therapy

A recent Cochrane review identified 4 studies that reported greater reduction in symptoms of depression among those randomised to music therapy than to those in standard care conditions.[37] A fifth study showed no benefit. Overall there were low dropout rates from music therapy. The Cochrane review reported that music therapy was accepted by people with depression and was associated with improvements in mood.[37] However, the review cited that the trials reviewed were small in number and that they had low methodological quality. Hence, it was not possible to be confident about the effectiveness of music therapy in the treatment of depression. High quality trials evaluating the effects of music therapy on depression are thus required.

Religion and spiritual health

Healthy religious beliefs may assist older patients with depression after a medical illness by providing comfort, support and improved coping strategies to help them manage, according to a US study.[38] In the study, 94 patients aged 60 and older diagnosed with depression during a hospital admission for a physical complaint, were more likely to recover from depression if they had expressed religious beliefs. In a further US study,[39] with data from 2600 male and female twins, has reported a strong association between religious beliefs and a lower intake of alcohol, nicotine and drug dependence or abuse, with less effects on depression. However, in a recent study 503 patients participating in the Enhancing Recovery in Coronary Heart Disease (ENRICHD) trial completed a Daily Spiritual Experiences (DSE) questionnaire within 28 days from the time of their acute myocardial infarction (AMI). The results showed little evidence that self-reported spirituality, frequency of church attendance, or frequency of prayer is associated with cardiac morbidity or all-cause mortality post-AMI in patients with depression and/or low perceived support.[40]

Hence, what is certain is that religiosity has to be viewed as a complex, multidimensional construct with substantial associations with lifetime psychopathology.

Health practitioners require awareness of the potential role of spirituality, religiosity and depression.[41] This field of evidence is important so as to provide a more holistic approach to psychotherapy treatment.[41] Whilst many studies link a lack of religiosity to depression, one important factor is that it may be a lack of meaning and spiritual fulfilment that is part of the increasingly secular and materialistic society contributing to the increased incidence of depression in the Western countries.

A US study[42] of 160 terminally ill cancer patients in a catholic palliative care hospital found that spiritual wellbeing offered some protection against end-of-life despair and depression. The study demonstrated the importance of spiritual wellbeing in reducing psychological distress, in particular in palliative care practice.

Religion plays an important role in the recovery from depression but findings also point to possible benefits of social connection and support people received when they belonged to a church versus the religion alone.

Family support

It is very likely social connection and social rehabilitation due to strong family and social support are beneficial for patients with mental illness such as depression, as compared to the social isolation experienced by many people that may very well be contributing to depression.

An Australian study with terminally ill patients in a catholic hospice reported that family support was correlated with no documented requests for euthanasia, a surrogate marker for possible enhanced depressive dispositions.[43]

Early studies that include a review of the literature have indicated that a healthy marriage is beneficial for both mental (especially depression) and physical health.[44] Also that a healthy marriage is equally protective for both men and women.[45]

Sleep disturbance

Whilst sleep disturbance is common in patients with depression, there is a growing body of evidence to suggest that sleep deprivation may be a contributor to depression.[46, 47]

In an Australian Melbourne study, 86 patients aged 16–88 years (average age = 42 years; female participants = 54%) presented as suffering from chronic insomnia, of which two-thirds were also suffering from depression.[48] Participants were then introduced to a self-help program (a book and 3 audiocassettes), and a manual to assist in non-drug approaches to sleep, which they used at home to improve their sleep. At follow-up, 6–8 weeks later, 70% of the insomnia sufferers who were depressed before treatment and learned to sleep better were no longer depressed, or were significantly less depressed, once their sleep had improved. An additional 13%, while still depressed, had a reduction of at least 40% in their depression scores. By contrast, among people who did not learn to sleep better, none experienced a significant reduction in depression. This study strongly suggests that, for many people who suffer from both depression and insomnia, treating the insomnia successfully without medication may eliminate or significantly reduce their depression. Further, just over half of those participants who were using antidepressant medications at the initial interview had ceased using it by follow-up, were sleeping significantly better, and were no longer depressed. Whilst the findings of this research are quite impressive, more research in this area is required.

Another Australian Melbourne study at the Royal Children's Hospital using a screening questionnaire of 738 mothers with infants 6–12 months of age, also suggested that sleep deprivation was a contributor to post-natal depression (PND).[49] If the mother reported a problem with their child's sleep, they were twice as likely to score the PND threshold than mothers who did not report a problem. Mothers reporting good sleep, despite an infant sleep problem, were not more likely to develop depression. A further study by the same group demonstrated that by treating the mothers' sleep using behavioural interventions, the depression score was reduced significantly as reported in a randomised control trial of 156 mothers with infants aged 6–12 months.[50] This benefit was sustained at 2 months and at 4 months for mothers with high depression scores.

A sample study of 5692 US adults, found those who reported sleeping difficulties such as initiating or maintaining sleep and early morning awakening, was associated with a two-fold increase risk of suicidality than participants without sleep disturbance.[51] Chronic sleep problems were found to be an independent risk factor for depression and suicidality, so it would appear addressing sleep problems could play an important role in prevention of depression and suicidality.

A recent interventional study reported that a sleep intervention program implemented in infancy resulted in sustained positive effects on maternal depression symptoms and found no evidence of longer-term adverse effects on either the mothers' parenting practices or the children's mental health.[52] This intervention demonstrated the capacity of a functioning primary care system to deliver an effective and universally offered secondary prevention program.

Adequate sleep is essential for general health. A study has found that sleep deprivation combined with light therapy was useful in the treatment of drug resistant bipolar depression.[53] The response was effective for acute and long-term remission rates. (See Chapter 22 on insomnia and sleep disorders.)

Sunshine

Vitamin D

Sunshine is the main source of vitamin D produced by the body in response to direct skin exposure to UVB. This means that no or minimal exposure to sun can contribute to vitamin D deficiency as seen in community groups with dress codes (e.g. wearing veils), living in geographical prone areas (e.g. in high and low altitudes) especially over winter, working indoors (e.g. office work), institutionalisation, prolonged hospitalisation and bed-bound people, and particularly in dark skin people who need longer sun exposure.[54, 55] Vitamin D deficiency especially over winter with lower sun exposure is linked with lower moods, depression and seasonal affective disorder. Increasing sun exposure and supplementation with vitamin D3 can improve moods.[56, 57]

Light therapy

Light therapy is a physical intervention that is used to treat depression and depressive disorders such as bipolar.[53] Cognitive decline, mood, behavioural and sleep disturbances, and limitations of activities of daily living commonly burden patients, especially the elderly with cognitive deficits.[58] Circadian rhythm disturbances have been associated with these symptoms.[58] Light therapy exposes patients to a bank of bright lights for a variable number of hours per day, usually 1–3 hours. Patients can engage in activities during the period of exposure, such as reading and computer use or relaxation time. In a recent study that reviewed CM therapies in the treatment of depression in children and adolescents, Jorm and colleagues[59] have described good evidence for the efficacy of light therapy in winter depression. There was, however, no evidence that it would be effective for non-seasonal depression.

Studies suggest that light therapy may be beneficial when used as an adjunct with other treatments.[60, 61] Results from 1 study indicate that there was a positive total sleep deprivation response in major depression patients which can be predicative of beneficial outcome of subsequent light therapy.[60] In a further study, bright light therapy was significantly beneficial compared to placebo for the treatment of depression.[61] It augmented antidepressant effects of medication and wake therapy.[61] Furthermore, in patients with dementia, light therapy was demonstrated to have a modest benefit in improving some cognitive and non-cognitive symptoms of dementia in a randomised control trial with melatonin supplement.[62] To counteract the adverse effect of melatonin on mood, the study recommended its prescriptive use only in combination with light therapy.

However, in a recent study antidepressant response to bright light treatment in older adults was not statistically superior to placebo. Both treatment and placebo groups experienced a clinically significant overall improvement of 16%.[63] There is very limited data which is currently available, suggesting that further research is warranted.

Environment

Smoking and smoking cessation

Whilst it is well recognised that depression is a major risk factor for smoking and there is a strong relationship between mental disorders and smoking,[64, 65] according to a prospective study[66] of more than 15 000 teenagers, smokers were 4 times more likely to develop depressive symptoms over a 1-year period than teenagers who did not smoke. The strong association remained even after accounting for other risk factors (e.g. low socioeconomic status and low self-esteem). The study reports that smoking itself may be a cause for depression via the activity of nicotine on the central noradrenergic receptor systems. Recently it has been reported that there is a relationship between smoking status and continuously distributed depressed mood among a cohort of adolescents.[67] Moreover, the relationship between cigarette smoking and depression may be a factor in the development of subsequent dependence.[67] It would appear that advising against heavy or any cigarette intake may be useful for the management of depression.

Substance abuse and drug intake

Substance abuse and drug intake is common in depression. About one-third of patients with major depressive disorders also have substance use disorders, associated with higher risk of suicide and greater social and personal impairment as well as other psychiatric conditions.[68]

Physical activity

Exercise

There is strong evidence to support the benefits of exercise in the prevention and alleviation of symptoms of depression. Although data from randomised trials are limited, results of studies included in a recent review generally support use of exercise as an alternative or adjunctive treatment for depression.[69]

Early reports highlight the benefits that regular physical activity provides in reducing the risk of developing depression.[70] People who do not participate in physical activity are more likely to develop depression compared with those who regularly exercise.[71] Regular aerobic and strength training activities can lead to 50% reduction in symptoms of acute depression and anxiety, especially in women and older people.[72] Physical activity is equally as effective as some pharmacological treatment (e.g. sertraline) in the management of mild–moderate depression, especially in the elderly. A 10-month study of 156 adult volunteers with major depressive disorders randomly assigned participants to a course of aerobic exercise, sertraline therapy, or a combination of exercise and sertraline. After 4 months all treatment groups exhibited significant therapeutic improvement and after 10 months, the exercise group had significantly lower relapse rates than participants on sertraline therapy alone.[73]

A Scottish study randomised 86 patients older than 53 with depression and not responding to at least 6 weeks of antidepressants, to twice-weekly group exercise classes (45 minutes of predominantly weight-bearing exercise) or health education talks for 10 weeks.[74] Fifty-five percent of the patients in the exercise group compared with 33% in the education talk group experienced a decline of at least 30% in their depressive symptoms. This study suggests that patients with depression should be actively encouraged to attend group exercise activities and regular physical activity, such as aerobic classes, or an early morning walk of greater than 60 minutes daily. This would at least also take advantage of sunshine exposure or *light therapy* even on overcast winter days.[75]

Exercise has been demonstrated to also improve mood in patients with severe affective disorders, according to a small pilot study of 12 participants.[76] The study concluded that exercise produced changes in concentration of several biologically active molecules such as adrenocorticotrophic hormone, cortisol, catecholamines, opioid peptides, and cytokines, which have been reported to affect mood or are involved in the physiopathology of affective disorders.[77] Moreover, endurance exercise may help to achieve substantial improvement in the mood of selected patients with major depression in the short time.[78] Also, there is sufficient evidence to support appropriate physical activity as an intervention to enhance a cancer patient's physical functioning and psychological wellbeing.[79]

A recent Cochrane review evaluated 28 trials which fulfilled the inclusion criteria, and of which 25 provided data for the meta-analyses.[80] Randomisation was adequately concealed in only a few of the studies, and most did not use intention to treat analyses. Also most of the studies used self reported symptoms as outcome measures. For the 23 trials consisting of 907 participants comparing exercise with no treatment or a control intervention, the pooled SMD was –0.82 (95% CI –1.12, –0.51), indicating a large clinical effect. However when trials with robust designs only were included in the analysis namely, adequate allocation concealment and intention to treat analysis and blinded outcome assessment, the pooled SMD was –0.42 (95% CI –0.88, 0.03) that is a moderate, non significant effect was observed.[80] Hence the study concluded that physical activity gives the impression to improve depressive symptoms in people with a diagnosis of depression, but when only methodologically robust trials are included, the effect sizes are only moderate and not statistically significant. Further robust trials are warranted. Further analysis of the Cochrane review confirmed exercise may improve depression but the majority of trials again had weaknesses.[2]

Yoga

An early study[81] has demonstrated that the daily practice of yoga was able to significantly improve symptoms of depression, and in 1 randomised study was statistically as effective as ECT and imipramine.[82] Another study of men and women found yoga significantly improved mood scores for depression and other psychological states such as anxiety, anger and 'neurotic symptoms'.[83]

A review of the evidence reveals that yoga has potentially beneficial effects as an intervention on depressive disorders.[46] Variation in interventions, severity and reporting of trial methodology suggests that the findings must be interpreted with caution. A number of the interventions may not be feasible in those with reduced or impaired mobility and, even so, further investigation of yoga as a therapeutic intervention is warranted.

Nutritional influences

Nutrition and diets

Chocolate

Dark chocolate may play a role in mood enhancement. One study demonstrated that older men who ate chocolate showed statistically significant improvement in feelings of loneliness, happiness, having plans for the future, less depression, better health, optimism and better psychological wellbeing compared with men who ate candy.[84]

Lactose and/or dairy

Diet plays an equally important role in the management of depression. As an example, lactose malabsorption may play a role in the development of depression.[85] Lactose malabsorption is characterised by a deficiency of mucosal lactase (an enzyme) and, as a consequence, lactose that reaches the colon is broken down by bacteria to short-chain fatty acids, CO_2, and H_2. Bloating, cramps, osmotic diarrhoea, and other symptoms of irritable bowel syndrome (IBS) are the consequence and can be seen in about 50% of lactose malabsorbers. Thirty women aged 16–60 were all screened for depression using a questionnaire. The group with lactose malabsorption (n = 6 compared with 24 normal lactose absorbers) had significantly higher scores on the depression questionnaire compared with normal lactose absorbers. The study postulated that lactose malabsorption may cause high intestinal lactose levels that might interfere with L-tryptophan metabolism by binding with L-tryptophan and impeding its absorption, and in turn affect serotonin synthesis and availability.[85] Although more research is warranted, lactose malabsorption in patients with signs of mental depression, particularly in those with digestive problems, should be considered.

Seafood consumption

Seafood consumption has been reported to be associated with a lower prevalence of bipolar disorder, according to a systematic review.[86] A US-based study reviewed population-based epidemiological studies from 17 countries and found greater rates of seafood consumption (n-3 fatty acids) were associated with lower lifetime prevalence for bipolar I, bipolar II, and bipolar spectrum disorders. Greater seafood consumption (deep sea) was also related to lower lifetime prevalence of major depression in 9 countries.[86]

General diet advice

Consequently, the general advice for depressed patients would include eating regular, balanced healthy meals, high in fruit, vegetables and deep sea fish (at least 2–3 times per week). Poor dietary choices have been reported to be associated with the development of depressive symptoms.[87]

Alcohol

Whilst depression can lead to excessive alcohol intake, a cohort study of 1055 individuals followed up from birth to 25 years of age found a clear association of heavy alcohol consumption and alcohol abuse increasing the risk of major depression by 65% after controlling for confounding factors. The authors postulated that alcohol may act as a trigger for genetic markers that increase the risk of mental disorders.[88]

Nutritional supplements

Fish oils and/or omega-3 (n-3) fatty acids

Fish oil supplementation may play a role in the management of depression and bipolar disorder.

Bipolar disorder

In an early preliminary 4-month double-blind, placebo-controlled trial 30 patients with bipolar disorder were randomised to receive either n-3 fatty acids (9.6 g/day) or placebo (olive oil), in addition to their ongoing treatment.[89] The n-3 fatty acids were well tolerated and the group of patients that took n-3 fatty acids had significantly longer periods of remission than the placebo group and a reduction in depressive symptoms over the 4 months of treatment.

A small open label study of bipolar outpatients with depressive symptoms also improved significantly within 1 month of treatment with 1.5–2 g/day of Eicosapentaneoic acid (EPA) with no patients developing hypomania or manic symptoms or side-effects with treatment. The authors concluded that the fatty acids may play a role by regulating neurotransmitter metabolism and larger well-controlled trials are necessary.[90]

Depression

Several trials indicate omega-3 deficiency may contribute to depression and psychiatric diseases, and dietary fish intake and fish oil supplementation may play a useful role in the management of depression.[91, 92]

In a case control study of pregnant women, women with lower omega-3 PUFA levels especially due to low dietary intake and fetal diversion, were 6 times more likely to experience depression antenatally, compared with women with higher levels.[93] The authors conclude there is a role for increased fish intake and fish oil supplementation during the perinatal period.

In 1 study of middle-aged women with moderate-to-severe psychological distress and depression during the menopausal transition (n = 120), participants were randomly assigned to receive 1.05g ethyl-EPA/d plus 0.15g of ethyl-docosahexaenoic acid/d (n = 59) or placebo (n = 61) for 8 weeks.[94]

At baseline, women experiencing psychological distress were mildly to moderately depressed with 24% meeting the major depressive episode (MDE) criteria of the *Diagnostic and Statistical Manual of Mental Disorders* (4th edn). Of interest, compared with baseline, after 8 weeks overall outcomes improved in both groups and no significant differences were noted between them. However, closer analysis of the data revealed that for women without MDE, mood outcome significantly improved with fish oil supplementation compared with the placebo group.

Two recently reported trials with the essential fatty acid eicosapentaenoic acid (EPA) have demonstrated efficacy in depression.[95, 96] One study compared the administration of EPA to fluoxetine in major depression and reported that the combination was significantly more effective than EPA or fluoxetine administered separately.[96]

A review of treatments of depression in children and adolescents identified 1 trial of omega-3 PUFA supplementation was beneficial in depressed children compared with placebo.[97]

A recent meta-analytic review of double-blind, placebo-controlled trials of antidepressant efficacy of n-3 fatty acids has demonstrated efficacy with a cautionary note.[95] Although the meta-analysis showed significant antidepressant efficacy of n-3 PUFAs, it is still premature to validate this finding due to publication bias and heterogeneity of studies available. Large scale, well-controlled trials are needed to find out the favourable target subjects, therapeutic dose of EPA, and the composition of n-3 PUFAs in treating depression.[98]

Recently, Mischoulon reported that the results of n-3 fatty acid supplementation studies, was promising in the treatment of depression.[99] In addition, the n-3 fatty acids have been shown to be safe and might be useful in specific populations, such as the elderly, pregnant or lactating women, and people with medical comorbid conditions. Moreover, patients with mild depression or those who are unresponsive to conventional antidepressants might be the best candidates for alternative treatments such as St John's Wort (SJW) and n-3 fatty acids.[99]

Tryptophan

A shift in tryptophan metabolism elicited by pro-inflammatory cytokines has gained attention as a new concept to explain the aetiological and pathophysiological mechanisms of major depression.[100] Figure 12.1 illustrates how proteins convert to tryptophan which subsequently converts to serotonin and melatonin requiring various co-factors. Within this research paradigm the use of tryptophan for treating depression has gained popularity.

Tryptophan is an essential amino acid precursor of brain serotonin, making it attractive in the use for depression as well as insomnia. 5-Hydroxytryptophan (5-HTP) appears to be the safer form with fewer and milder side-effects and demonstrates equal potency to antidepressants in early clinical trials.[101, 102] However there is much debate about the use of 5-HTP for depression despite its widespread use.

Dietary sources of tryptophan may play a role in mental states. Tryptophan is found in most protein based foods and is particularly rich in red meat, oats, milk, yoghurt, cottage cheese, fish, poultry (chicken and turkey), dried dates, chickpeas, sesame, sunflower and pumpkin seeds. A small group of 15 women who had suffered episodes of recurrent major depression but had recovered were studied.[103] Participants were randomised to drink either a tryptophan-containing or tryptophan-free mixture. The blood tryptophan levels were 75% less in women drinking the tryptophan-free drink and this was associated with a temporary but clinically significant profile of depressive symptoms. The women who drank the tryptophan-rich drinks had no changes in mental state. The study supports the hypothesis that lowering the brain serotonin activity can precipitate depression. More studies are required to test the potential role of tryptophan for the treatment of depression, especially in relation to any adverse risks.

S-Adenosylmethionine (SAMe)

SAMe is a compound that has been used for many years in Europe as an antidepressant. It became available in the USA as a non-FDA regulated compound in 1999. SAMe resembles a naturally occurring compound in the human body, formed by methionine and adenosine triphosphate (Figure 12.1). SAMe is a co-factor to facilitate the conversion of 5-HT to melatonin and appears to increase central turnover of dopamine and serotonin. It increases the main metabolite of central serotonin-5-HIAA (5–hydroxyindoleacetic acid) in the cerebrospinal fluid.[104, 105]

A review of the clinical studies with SAMe demonstrated safety and efficacy in the treatment of mild–moderate depression, although further research is required to clarify its role as a first-line treatment for depression.[106] Although the exact mechanism is not clear, SAMe is able to maintain high concentrations of serotonin and L-dopamine in the central nervous system (CNS) by inhibiting their degradation. An early meta-analysis of 6 RCTs found that 70% of the participants showed some response to SAMe compared with placebo 30%.[107]

In recent clinical trials SAMe has demonstrated further efficacy. Thirty antidepressant-treated adult outpatients with resistant major depressive disorder received 800 to 1600mg of SAMe tosylate over a 6-week trial.[108] Intention-to-treat analyses based on the Hamilton Depression Rating Scale showed a response rate of 50% and a remission rate of 43% following augmentation of SSRIs or venlafaxine with SAMe.

SAMe has also been investigated secondary to the development of chronic diseases such as Parkinson's disease (PD) and HIV/AIDS.[109] In PD patients although uncontrolled and preliminary, the study suggested that SAMe was well tolerated and could be a safe and effective alternative to the antidepressant agents used in patients with PD.[109] In HIV/AIDS patients, SAMe has a rapid effect evident as soon as week 1 with progressive decreases in depression symptom rating scores throughout the 8 week study.[110]

SAMe should be avoided in patients with bipolar disorder because it could result in more frequent switches between depressive and manic products and technically should be avoided in patients taking other antidepressants.

Proteins

Peptic HCl ↓ Zinc, B1, B6

L-Tryptophan

Tryptophan hydroxylase ↓ Folate, Fe, Ca, B3

5-Hydroxytryptophan

Dopa Decarboxylase ↓ B6, Zn, Mg, Vit C

5-Hydroxytryptamine (serotonin)

Protein ⟶ Methionine ⟶ SAMe ↓ B5

Melatonin

Figure 12.1 Production of melatonin and seratonin from tryptophan

Dosage

A dosage of 400–800mg/day of SAMe for patients with mild–moderate depression and up to 1600mg/day for moderate to severe depression is recommended.

Adverse effects

Gastrointestinal symptoms and headaches are the most common side-effects.

Summary

A review conducted by Thachil et. al. on the evidence for CM therapies used in depression by studies on CM as monotherapy reported that 19 studies yielded grade I evidence for the use SJW, tryptophan / 5–hydroxytryptophan, SAMe and folate in depressive disorders.[111] The review also found grade II evidence for the use of saffron in mild to moderate depression, but large-scale trials are warranted to investigate further its potential as an effective treatment.

Vitamins

Folate and B group vitamins

Recent reviews concluded that the available evidence suggests that folate may have a potential role as a supplement for the treatment of depression.[112, 113] This is further supported by a more recent review that concluded that treatment with folate, B12, and B6 can improve cerebral function.[114] It is currently unclear if this is the case both for people with normal folate levels, and for those with folate deficiency.

Folate deficiency and low folate status have been linked in a number of clinical studies to depression and poor antidepressant response.[115, 116] Research has demonstrated that folate concentrations were lower in depressed patients compared with participants who had never been depressed and suggest that supplementation may be indicated following a depressive episode.[116] In a randomised placebo-controlled trial folic acid was observed to be a simple method of greatly improving the antidepressant action of fluoxetine.[117] Folic acid should be given in doses sufficient to decrease plasma homocysteine.[118] In a recent review reporting on the data from several studies it was tabulated that depressive and cognitive function could be rescued with doses of folate ranging from 0.4–1.0mg.[118] Men may require a higher dose of folic acid to achieve this than women, but more work is required to ascertain the optimum dose of folic acid.[113] A recent Cochrane review assessed 3 trials of 247 patients and concluded that folate could have a potential role as a supplement to other treatments for depression.[113]

Vitamin Bs and B6 act as cofactors in the production of CNS serotonin and this may explain its potential role in boosting mental state. Evidence for vitamin B12 supplementation is not as strong, despite a Finnish study of 115 outpatients aged 21–69 years with major depressive disorder demonstrating that higher serum vitamin B12 levels were significantly associated with a better therapeutic outcome for depression.[119] A number of studies have also explored low levels of vitamins B1, B2 and B6 and their association with depression and the possible role in supplementation to augment antidepressants in the treatment of geriatric depression.[120] However, it should be noted that a recent trial reported that treatment with B12, folic acid, and B6 at doses of 400 microgram B12 + 2mg folic acid + 25mg B6 per day was no better than placebo at reducing the severity of depressive symptoms or the incidence of clinically significant depression over a period of 2 years in older men.[121]

Vitamin D

A growing body of evidence suggests merit in screening patients with depression for vitamin D deficiency.[122, 123] Vitamin D deficiency is common in the elderly and is associated with lower mood and worse cognition.[124]

A recent study of 53 inpatients from a private psychiatric hospital demonstrated significantly lower levels of vitamin D of less than or equal to 50mmol/L in 60% of patients compared with 30% of the 691 community-based controls. Vitamin D levels of 25mmol/L or less was detected in 11% of inpatients compared with 7.2% of controls respectively. The researchers concluded that patients with depression may benefit with supplementation of oral vitamin D.[125] In another recent trial, the results appear to strongly suggest that there is a relationship between reduced serum levels of 25(OH)D and symptoms of depression.[126] Moreover, it was concluded that supplementation with high doses of vitamin D ameliorated the symptoms of depression, indicating a possible causal relationship.[125]

Multivitamins

A 1-year randomised, double-blind study in the UK investigated the effects of multivitamin supplementation on mood and mental health status.[127] In the study, 129 healthy adults with a mean age of 20–56 years were randomised to take placebo or vitamin supplements in the form of 2 capsules daily. The vitamin supplement consisted of vitamin A, vitamin E, thiamin, riboflavin, pyridoxine, vitamin B12, vitamin C, folic acid, biotin, nicotinamide at 10 times the recommended daily dose, with the exception of vitamin A. The change of mood was only significant after 1 year. There was reported improvement in sleep, mood parameters and a tendency to feel more agreeable.[127]

Minerals

Magnesium

Magnesium is an important modulator of *N*–methyl *D*–aspartate (NMDA) receptor activity for glutamate.[128] Recent research indicates that disturbances of glutamatergic transmission primarily via the NMDA-receptor are involved in pathogenesis of mood disorders. Magnesium deficiency is related to a variety of psychological symptoms, especially depression.[129, 130] Early reports have documented that psychiatric symptoms of magnesium deficiency are unspecific, ranging from apathy to psychosis, and may be attributed to other disease processes associated with poor intake, defect absorption or excretion of magnesium.[130] In a further study with depressed patients it was reported that there was significant confounding present in this study due to gender differences and clinical subgroup allocation.[131] The erythrocyte magnesium level tended to normalise in parallel with clinical improvement, depending on sex and clinical subgroup, and was hypothesised subsequently to be related to the intensity of the depression.[131] An additional small study by this research group with 53 male and female drug-free major depressed patients further reported that low plasma magnesium in erythrocytes and plasma was shown to be associated with the intensity of the depression.[132]

Calcium

The intracellular calcium concentration has important roles in the triggering of neurotransmitter release and the regulation of short-term plasticity.[133]

A review has reported that clinical trials in women with PMS have found that calcium supplementation effectively alleviates the majority of mood and somatic symptoms.[134] Evidence to date indicates that women with luteal phase symptomatology have an underlying calcium dysregulation with a secondary hyperparathyroidism and vitamin D deficiency.[134] Hence, indeed supplementation with calcium and vitamin D may be warranted.

Zinc

A recent review has concluded that all the data indicates the important role of zinc homeostasis in psychopathology and therapy of depression, and the potential clinical antidepressant activity that zinc may possess.[135] Hence, low blood zinc has been reported to have a role in the development of depression.[135] and has been reported to be a sensitive marker of treatment resistance for depression.[136] Early studies, have reported that serum and plasma zinc levels were significantly lower in major depressed patients than in normal controls, whereas minor depressed patients showed intermediate values.[137, 138] Zinc has been reported to cause toxicity with excess supplementation, hence caution is advised.[139]

Iron

Iron deficiency and iron deficiency anaemia can contribute to fatigue, lack of motivation and lowered moods which can be confused with depression. A blood test can exclude iron and any other suspected nutrient deficiencies.

Herbal medicines

St John's wort (SJW) (*Hypericum perforatum*)

Studies indicate that SJW extracts improve mood, reduce anxiety and somatic symptoms, and assist with sleep in mild to moderate and major depression. Several active constituents have been isolated from the leaves and to a lesser extent the flowers, including melatonin, *hypericin*, *adhyperforin* and *hyperforin*. SJW is thought to act as a serotonergic (5-HT3 and 5-HT4) receptor antagonist and the active constituents, *hyperforin* and *adhyperforin*, may modulate the effect and inhibit reuptake of the neurotransmitters serotonin, dopamine, and noradrenalin. *Hyperforin* may also inhibit synaptic reuptake of gamma-butyric acid (GABA) and L-glutamate.[140, 141]

Recent systematic and Cochrane reviews have reported that SJW is the only herbal remedy found to be effective as a treatment for mild to moderate and major depression.[142–144]

In a meta-analysis, 5 trials were described that involved 2231 patients that compared SJW with conventional antidepressants. Roder et. al. found both approaches to be equally effective.[144] SJW was significantly effective when compared with placebo in 25 trials involving a total of 2129 patients.

An early meta-analysis of 23 randomised trials with a total of 1757 outpatients suffering mild–moderate depression, demonstrated strong evidence for the efficacy of SJW in the treatment of depression.[145] Fifteen trials were tested against a placebo and 8 trials versus antidepressants. The conclusion was that SJW was useful in the treatment of mild–moderate depression, superior to placebo and comparable with conventional drug treatment, with less side-effects and dropouts. A Cochrane review of 37 trials, 26 compared with placebo and 14 compared with an antidepressant concluded that the evidence favoured SJW as being more effective than placebo but results were inconsistent overall for the treatment of mild–moderately severe depression.[146]

Overall it is well tolerated and the reported side-effects were 26% for SJW as compared with 45% for standard antidepressants.

In an RCT of the active extract of SJW ZE 117 (dose of 250mg) it was reported to be comparable with imipramine (75mgs) in the treatment of patients with mild–moderate depression, and better tolerated.[147] Similar findings were found with an RCT of SJW ZE 117 and fluoxetine for the treatment of mild–moderate depression.[148] Moreover recently it was reported that SJW did not differ significantly from SSRIs with respect to efficacy and adverse events in patients with major depressive disorders.[149] This was further supported in a recent extensive Cochrane systematic review where it was concluded that SJW was as effective for treating major depression as standard drugs.[142, 146] This study investigated 29 trials (that included 5489 participants) which consisted of 18 comparisons with a placebo intervention and 17 comparisons with synthetic standard antidepressants and which met the inclusion criteria for the meta-analysis. The results of the placebo-controlled trials showed marked heterogeneity. In 9 larger trials that compared active treatment to placebo demonstrated a combined response rate ratio for *Hypericum* extracts of 1.28 (95% CI, 1.10–1.49) and from 9 smaller trials it was 1.87.95% CI, 1.22–2.87. The results of trials that compared *Hypericum* extracts to standard antidepressants were statistically homogeneous. Compared with tri- or tetracyclic antidepressants and SSRIs, respectively, the relative risks were 1.02 (95% CI, 0.90–1.15) for 5 trials combined and 1.00 (95% CI, 0.90–1.11) for 12 trials combined. It was also noted that the reported findings were more favourable to *Hypericum* and that the studies originated from German-speaking countries in both the placebo-controlled trials and in the trials that compared *Hypericum* to standard antidepressants.[142] Participants given *Hypericum* extracts dropped out of trials due to adverse effects less frequently than those given older antidepressants (odds ration [OR] 0.24 [95% CI, 0.13–0.46] or SSRIs. OR 0.53, 95% CI, 0.34–0.83]). The study suggested that the *Hypericum* extracts tested included in the trials were superior to placebo in patients with major depression, that they had similar effectiveness to standard antidepressants and had fewer side-effects than standard antidepressants.[142]

St John's wort and Sertraline

In a double-blind controlled study of 340 patients with severe major depression (adults with mean age 42 years) 66% women were randomised to receive either SJW 900–1500mg, Sertraline 50–100mgs or placebo for 8 weeks.[150] Of interest both SJW and Sertraline were equally effective but placebo scored better than both in the treatment of depression. The benefit of placebo was 32% improvement in depression symptom score, compared with SJW 24% and Sertraline treated patients 25%. Side-effects were more frequent in the SJW and Sertraline groups than in the placebo group. A recent similar study investigating a *Hypericum perforatum* extract WS 5570 at doses of 600mg/day (once daily) and 1200mg/day (600mg twice daily) were found to be safe and more effective than placebo, with comparable efficacy of the WS 5570 groups for the treatment of moderate to major depression.[151] Extract WS 5570 (dose of 1800mg/day for 6 weeks) was compared to paroxetine 20–40mg/day in patients with moderate to severe depression. At 2 weeks doses were doubled in 57% of SJW group and 48% in paroxetine group, due to slow response.[152] At 6 weeks, 70% and 60% of the SJW and paroxetine group respectively responded to treatment, with a greater mean of improvement in depression scores in the SJW group. Remission occurred in more of the SJW group compared with the paroxetine group. There were fewer adverse events among patients taking *Hypericum* compared with paroxetine. Hence SJW was at least as effective as paroxetine in moderate to severe depression in people with low suicidal risk.[152]

SJW drug interactions

Herb–drug interactions are important aspects associated with SJW.[153] SJW has been reported to induce the action of the hepatic cytochrome P450 enzymes which metabolise a variety of drugs in the liver. By reducing the plasma concentrations of the drugs, SJW has the potential to reduce the effectiveness of at least 50% of all marketed medications.[154] These include the therapeutic effects of drugs such as the Oral Contraceptive Pill, potentially increasing the risk of pregnancy, and reducing blood levels of warfarin, digoxin, protease inhibitors, theophylline, phenytoin, carbamazepine, phenobarbitone, indinavir and cyclosporine as they are all metabolised by the CYTP450 pathway. Further, SJW should be avoided in patients taking any antidepressants including monoamine oxidase inhibitors (MAOI) and selective serotonin reuptake inhibitors (SSRIs), having the potential to cause excess CNS serotonin concentrations, resulting in serotonin syndrome characterised by altered mental status, autonomic dysfunction and neuromuscular abnormalities.

Dosage

Most clinical trials of SJW have used 900mg daily divided into 3 equal doses. Approximately 2–3 weeks of therapy is usually necessary before it has its maximum therapeutic benefit.

Adverse effects

Potential adverse side-effects attributed to SJW can include rash, photosensitivity rash, pruritis, nausea, headache, dry mouth, dizziness and fatigue.[154]

Ginkgo biloba

In a randomised, double-blind, 22-week trial 400 patients with dementia associated with neuropsychiatric features were treated with *Ginkgo biloba* extract EGb 761 (240mg/day) or placebo. The study demonstrated improvements in favour of EGb 761 for apathy/indifference, anxiety, irritability/lability, depression/dysphoria and sleep/night time behaviour.[155]

Ginkgo biloba and SSRIs induced sexual dysfunction

In an open trial, *Ginkgo biloba* was found to be 84% effective in treating antidepressant-induced sexual dysfunction predominately caused by SSRIs.[156] In the trial, 33 women and 30 men participated for 4 weeks. They were prescribed on average 209mg/day ginkgo biloba extract that was well tolerated. Women reported a higher success rate (91%) than men (76%) on all 4 phases of the sexual response cycle. Other noted benefits included improved cognitive functioning, mental clarity and memory, and enhanced energy level, consistent with *Ginkgo biloba's* known cerebral-enhancing effects. Side-effects included GIT disturbances, headache, and general CNS activation. However, a subsequent study did not support these earlier findings.[157]

Dosage

Usually 40–80mg 3 times daily and can take 2–3 weeks or longer to have therapeutic action.

Saffron (*Crocus sativus L.*)

A number of recent preclinical and clinical studies indicate that stigma and petal of *Crocus sativus* may have an antidepressant effect. In a recent double-blind and randomised trial, patients were randomly assigned to receive a capsule of petal of *C. sativus* 15mg bid (morning and evening) (Group 1) and fluoxetine 10mg bid (morning and evening) (Group 2) for an 8-week study. At the end of trial, petal of *C. sativus* was found to be effective similar to fluoxetine in the treatment of mild to moderate depression.[158] In addition, in both treatments, the remission rate was 25%. There were no significant differences in the 2 groups in terms of observed side-effects. Earlier studies have demonstrated a similar trend of efficacy for the treatment of mild to moderate depression.[159–161]

Rhodiola rosea L.

A recent clinical trial with a standardised extract of SHR-5 of rhisomes of *Rhodiola rosea L.* in patients suffering from a current episode of mild to moderate depression demonstrated efficacy.[162] An antidepressive effect when administered in dosages of either 340 or 680mg/day over a 6-week period was reported.

Other herbal therapies

There are other herbs that have been commonly employed for the treatment of depression, but as yet have not been clinically trialled, and these include vervain, oat straw, scullcap and lemon balm.[163]

Aromatherapy

The antidepressant properties of essential oils such as bergamot (*Citrus bergamia*) and geranium (*Pelargonium graveolens*) were summarised in a report offering clinical and neuropharmacological perspectives of aromatherapy in managing psychiatric disorders.[164] Although some studies demonstrated an association between aromatherapy and improvement in mood in healthy adults, there was a notable lack of methodologically useful trials in clinically depressed populations. A study of 56 healthy men and women found essential oil of lemon improved mood, whilst lavender had no sedating effects compared with control odour of distilled water.[165] Hence no conclusions could be drawn regarding the efficacy of aromatherapy in treating depression until controlled trials are conducted.

A recent systematic review of the literature including 18 studies found that 'credible evidence that odours can affect mood, physiology and behaviour exists', however, methodological problems led to inconsistencies in the data.[166]

Hormones

Males and hormones

A recent study of 3987 men found that of the 203 men who suffered depression they had significantly lower total and free testosterone concentrations compared with non-depressed men ($P < .001$ for both). It was concluded that an RCT was required to determine whether the link between low free testosterone level and depression is causal because older men with depression may benefit from systematic screening of free testosterone concentration and testosterone supplementation.

Females and hormones

Accumulating evidence suggests that estrogens may have therapeutic effects in severe mental illnesses, including schizophrenia, via neuromodulatory and neuroprotective activity. Lowered oestrogen, progesterone, DHEA and testosterone hormone levels in women during and after menopause may also contribute to emotional disturbance such as depression and may warrant suitable hormone therapy.[168] In a recent RCT it was demonstrated that estradiol appeared to be a useful treatment for women with schizophrenia and could provide a new adjunctive therapeutic option for patients with severe mental illnesses.[169, 170]

The contraceptive pill

A pilot study has reported that women using the combined oral contraceptive pill were significantly more depressed than a matched group of women who were not prescribed the contraceptive pill.[171] Further studies are warranted to clarify this relationship.

Physical therapies

Acupuncture

A systematic review of RCTs investigating the efficacy of acupuncture in treating depression examined 9 RCTs, 5 of which were considered to be of poor methodological quality, and found that acupuncture tended to be as effective as antidepressants in treating depression.[172] This study concluded that, whilst the overall evidence remained inconclusive because of the varied methodology and study designs used, further research investigating the use of acupuncture in treating depression was warranted. A recent trial investigating the clinical therapeutic effect and safety of combined electro-acupuncture and fluoxetine for treatment of mild or moderate depression with physical symptoms was completed and reported a better therapeutic effect on depression and less adverse reactions.[173]

Massage therapy

A study of 32 depressed adolescent mothers receiving ten 30-minute sessions of massage therapy or relaxation therapy over a 5-week period resulted in both groups reporting lower depression scores but only the massage therapy group demonstrated significant reduction in anxiety, and salivary and urine cortisol levels also.[174]

Another study of 84 depressed 2nd trimester pregnant women were randomly assigned to massage therapy group (twice weekly 20 minutes), or a progressive muscle relaxation group (twice weekly 20 minutes), or a control group that received standard prenatal care alone. Women reported lower levels of anxiety and depressed mood and less leg and back pain in the massage therapy group, and also higher blood dopamine and serotonin levels and lower levels of cortisol and noradrenalin, contributing to better neonatal outcome (lesser incidence of prematurity and low birth weight).[175]

Conclusion

A holistic approach by addressing lifestyle factors and trialling the use of evidence-based CMs would appear to play a role in the management of the patient with depression.[7] There is documented good scientific evidence for the non-drug management of depression (see Table 12.2).

Table 12.2 Levels of evidence for lifestyle and complementary medicines/therapies in the management of mild–moderate–major depression

Modality	Level I	Level II	Level IIIa	Level IIIb	Level IIIc	Level IV	Level V
Lifestyle					x		
Smoking cessation					x		
Contraceptive pill use increases risk						x	
Physical activity	x						
Mind–body medicine							
CBT	x						
Mindfulness meditation		x					
Relaxation	x						
Music therapy	x						
Religion and spiritual health					x		
Family support						x	
Physical therapies							
Yoga		x					
Light therapy/ sunshine				x			

Continued

Table 12.2 Levels of evidence for lifestyle and complementary medicines/therapies in the management of mild–moderate–major depression—cont'd

Modality	Level I	Level II	Level IIIa	Level IIIb	Level IIIc	Level IV	Level V
Acupuncture				x			
Sleep therapy		x					
Aromatherapy						x	
Nutrition and diet					x		
Herbal medicines							
SJW	x						
Ginkgo biloba			x				
Saffron		x					
Rhodiola rosea L.			x				
Supplements							
SAMe		x					
n-3 fatty acids	x*						
tryptophan					x		
Vitamins							
Folate	x						
B Group		x					
Multivitamin		x			x		
Minerals							
Magnesium					x		
Calcium						x	
Zinc					x		
Hormones							
Testosterone Supplementation						x	

* Caution is advocated in interpreting these results as conclusive, as further evidence is required.

Level I — from a systematic review of all relevant randomised controlled trials, meta-analyses.
Level II — from at least 1 properly designed randomised controlled clinical trial.
Level IIIa — from well-designed pseudo-randomised controlled trials (alternate allocation or some other method).
Level IIIb — from comparative studies (including systematic reviews of such studies) with concurrent controls and allocation not randomised, cohort studies, case-control studies, or interrupted time series with a parallel control group.
Level IIIc — from comparative studies with historical control, 2 or more single-arm studies or interrupted time series without a parallel control group.
Level IV — opinions of respected authorities based on clinical experience, descriptive studies or reports of expert committees.
Level V — represents minimal evidence that represents testimonials.

Clinical tips handout for patients — depression

1 Lifestyle advice

Sleep

- Restore normal sleep patterns. Early to bed (about 9–10 p.m.) and awakening upon sunrise.
  (See Chapter 22 for more advice.)

Sunshine

- At least 15 minutes of sunshine needed daily for vitamin D and melatonin production — especially before 10 a.m. and after 3 p.m. when the sun exposure is safest in summer.
- Ensure adequate skin exposure to sun; avoid sunscreen and excess clothing to maximise levels of vitamin D.
- More time in the sun is required for dark skinned people and in winter, when supplementation of vitamin D may be required.

2 Physical activity/exercise

- Yoga may be of help. Other examples: qiqong, tai chi.
- Exercise 30–60 minutes daily. If exercise is not regular, commence with 5 minutes daily and slowly build up to at least 30 minutes a day. Outdoor exercise with nature, fresh air and sunshine is ideal (e.g. brisk walking, light jogging, cycling, swimming, stretching, weight-bearing exercises). The more time you spend outdoors the better.

3 Mind–body medicine

- Stress management program — for example, 6 x 40 minute sessions for patients to understand the nature of their symptoms, the symptoms' relationship to stress, and the practice of regular relaxation exercises.
- Regular meditation practice, at least 10–20 minutes daily.

Breathing

- Be aware of breathing at all times. Notice if tendency to hold breath or over-breathe. Always aim to relax breath and the muscles around the chest wall.

Rest and stress management

Recurrent stress may cause a return of symptoms. Relaxation is important for a full and lasting recovery.

- Reduce workload and resolve conflicts. Contact family, friends, church or social groups for support.
- Listening to relaxation music helps.
- Relaxation massage therapy is helpful.
- Cognitive behavioural therapy and psychotherapy are extremely helpful.
- Hypnotherapy, biofeedback may be of help.
  Focus on wellness, not just the disease.

Fun

- It is important to have fun in life.
- Joy can be found even in the simplest tasks, such as funny movies/videos, comedy, hobbies, dancing, playing with pets and children.

4 Environment

- Avoid smoking, environmental pollutants and chemicals — at work and in the home.

5 Dietary changes

- Eat regular balanced healthy meals, ideally 3 small meals, and 2 snacks, each containing protein in order to avoid fluctuating blood sugar levels and provide amino acids for nerve transmitters such as tryptophan.
- Eat more fruit and vegetables — a variety of colours and those in season.
- For some individuals, raw or steaming food is better; increase dietary fibre if you suffer constipation.
- Bran may be of benefit in some patients; if you are intolerant of wheat you can use alternative bran such as oat bran.
- Eat more nuts, seeds, beans, sprouts (e.g. alfa, mung, bean, lentil).
- Increase fish intake (sardines, tuna, salmon, cod, mackerel) especially deep sea fish >3 servings per week.
- Reduce red meat intake — preferably eat lean red meat (e.g. lamb, kangaroo) and white meat (e.g. free range organic chicken).
- Use cold pressed olive oil and avocado.
- Eat dark chocolate, preferably with 85% or more cocoa.
- Eat wholegrains/cereals (variety): rice (brown, basmati, Mahatmi, Doongara), traditional rolled oats, buckwheat flour, wholegrain organic breads (rye bread, Essene, spelt, Kamut), brown pasta, couscous, millet, amaranth etc.
- Reduce dairy intake; consume low fat dairy products such as yoghurt and cheeses, unless there is a dairy intolerance.
- Drink more water (1–2 litres a day) and teas (especially green tea, black tea).

- Chamomile and peppermint aid digestion. Drink 1 cup of either 30–60 minutes before meals.
- Avoid hydrogenated fats, salt, fast foods, sugar (such as in soft drinks), lollies, biscuits, cakes and processed foods (e.g. white bread, white pasta, pastries).
- Minimise coffee as it can cause restlessness and agitation in high doses and impacts on sleep.
- Minimise alcohol intake to no more than 1–2 glasses daily as it is a brain depressant and can disturb sleep.
- Avoid chemical additives — preservatives, colourings and flavourings.
- For sweetener try honey (e.g. manuka, yellow box and stringy bark have lowest GI).

Exclusion diets — performed under supervision of a dietitian or experienced health practitioner may be helpful to a limited number of patients. Common food intolerances include wheat, milk, cashew nuts, whole egg and yeast. Your doctor will advise you accordingly.

6 Physical therapies

- Acupuncture may help improve general wellbeing.

7 Supplements

St John's wort

- Indication: mild-moderate depression.
- Dosage: 300mg 2-3 x daily.
- Results: 1-3 weeks.
- Side-effects: very mild and rare. Include: photosensitivity skin rash; digestion disturbance; dizziness; fatigue; dry mouth.
- Contraindications: pregnancy, lactation, fertility, drug interaction; avoid use with most pharmaceutical medication, such as the oral contraceptive pill, other antidepressants, epileptic medication — check with your doctor.

SAMe

- Indication: mild–moderate depression.
- Dosage: 400mg 2–3 times daily.
- Results: 1–3 days.
- Side-effects: very mild and rare.
- Contraindicated: pregnancy, lactation, fertility, bipolar disorder, drug interaction; avoid use with other antidepressants.

Fish oils

- Indication: bipolar disorder and depression. Fish oils providing EPA 6.2g and DHA 3.4g daily have been used.
- Dosage: take with meals. Child: 500mg 1–2 times daily. Adults: 1g 1–2 capsules 1–2–3 times daily; can be used in pregnancy or lactation as tolerated.
- Results: 1–4 days.
- Side-effects: often well tolerated especially if taken with meals. Very mild and rare side-effects; for example, gastrointestinal upset; allergic reactions (e.g. rash, breathing problems) if allergic to seafood; blood thinning effects in very high doses > 10g daily (may need to stop fish oil supplements 2 weeks prior to surgery).
- Contraindications: sensitivity reaction to seafood; drug interactions; caution when taking high doses of fish oils >4g per day together with warfarin (your doctor will check your INR test).

Folate

- Indication: mild–moderate depression, high alcohol intake.
- Dosage: 0.5–1.5mgs daily.
- Results: uncertain.
- Side-effects: very mild and rare.
- Contraindicated: avoid in anaemias until assessed by a doctor.

Vitamin B's especially B6 and B12

- Indication: mild-moderate depression, high alcohol intake.
- Dosage: upper level of intake of vitamin B6 should not exceed 50mg/day.
- Results: uncertain.
- Side-effects: overuse of single vitamin products; avoid use of multiple single-vitamin products (e.g. oral and injectable forms of vitamin B6) or concomitant use of multivitamin products could result in some patients routinely exceeding the upper limit for vitamins associated with severe toxicity. Toxicity in high doses of vitamin B6 includes peripheral neuropathy, such as tingling, burning and numbness of limbs.
- Contraindications: avoid in anaemias until assessed by a doctor.

Vitamin D (cholecalciferol 1000 international units)

Doctors should check blood levels and suggest supplementation if levels are low.

Magnesium and calcium (best provided together)

- Indication: may be useful in depression, anxiety, restless sleep, cramps and insomnia.
- Dosage: Children up to 65–120mg daily in divided doses. Adults 350mg daily including pregnant and lactating women.

- Results: 2–3 days.
- Side-effects: Oral magnesium can cause gastrointestinal irritation, nausea, vomiting, and diarrhoea. The dosage varies from person to person. Although rare, toxic levels can cause low blood pressure, thirst, heart arrhythmia, drowsiness and weakness.
- Contraindications: patients with kidney disease; if you have high blood calcium or magnesium levels (e.g. in cancer).

Zinc

- Indication: may help depression, especially if blood levels are low.
- Dosage: zinc sulfate contains 23% elemental zinc; zinc gluconate contains 14.3% elemental zinc. Usual dosage in adult: no more than 5–10mg zinc sulfate daily.
- Side-effects: nausea, vomiting, metallic taste in mouth. Avoid long-term use and high dosage as this may cause copper deficiency, impair the immune system and cause anaemia.
- Contraindications: sideroblastic anaemia, above normal blood levels of zinc, severe kidney disease.

References

1 World Health Organization (WHO). Online Available: http://www.who.int/mental_health/management/depression/definition/en (accessed July 2008).
2 McAvoy BR. Exercise may improve depression PEARLS No. 139, January 2009.
3 Manual of Mental Disorders (4th edn), revised. American OPsychiatric Association, Washington DC, 1999.
4 Alboni P, Favaron E, Paparella N, et. al. Is there an association between depression and cardiovascular mortality or sudden death? J Cardiovasc Med 2008;9(4):356–62.
5 Golden SH. A review of the evidence for a neuroendocrine link between stress, depression and diabetes mellitus. Curr Diabetes Rev 2007;3(4):252–9.
6 van der Watt G, Laugharne J, Janca A. Complementary and alternative medicine in the treatment of anxiety and depression. Curr Opin Psych 2008;21(1):37–42.
7 Werneke U, Turner T, Priebe S. Complementary medicines in psychiatry: review of effectiveness and safety. Br J Psychiatry 2006;188:109–21.
8 Frazer CJ, Christensen H, Griffiths KM. Effectiveness of treatments for depression in older people. Medical Journal of Australia 2005;182(12):627–32.
9 Jorm AF, Christensen H, Griffiths KM, et. al. Effectiveness of complementary and self-help treatments for depression MJA 2002 May 20;176(Sppl):S84–S96.
10 Howie JG, Heaney DJ, Maxwell M, et. al. Quality at general practice consultations: cross sectional survey. BMJ 1999;319(7212):719–20.
11 Kreuter MW, Chheda SG, Bull FC. How does physician advice influence patient behaviour? Evidence for a priming effect. Arch Fam Med 2000;9(5):426–33.
12 Swartz HA, Frank E, Zuckoff A, et. al. Brief interpersonal psychotherapy for depressed mothers whose children are receiving psychiatric treatment. Am J Psychiatry 2008;165(9):1155–62.
13 Driessen E, Van HL, Schoevers RA, et. al. Cognitive Behavioural Therapy versus Short Psychodynamic Supportive Psychotherapy in the outpatient treatment of depression: a randomised controlled trial. BMC Psychiatry 2007;7:58.
14 Cuijpers P, van Straten A, Smit F, et. al. Preventing the onset of depressive disorders: a meta-analytic review of psychological interventions. Am J Psychiatry 2008;165(10):1272–80.
15 Kendler KS, Hettema JM, Butera F, et. al. Life event dimensions of loss, humiliation, entrapment, and danger in the prediction of onsets of major depression and generalised anxiety. Arch Gen Psychiatry 2003 Aug;60(8):789–96.
16 Farmer AE, McGuffin P. Humiliation, loss and other types of life events and difficulties: a comparison of depressed subjects, healthy controls and their siblings. Psychol Med 2003 Oct;33(7):1169–75.
17 van der Wal MF, de Wit CA, Hirasing RA. Psychosocial health among young victims and offenders of direct and indirect bullying. Pediatrics 2003 Jun;111(6 Pt 1):1312–7.
18 Klomek AB, Sourander A, Kumpulainen K, et. al. Childhood bullying as a risk for later depression and suicidal ideation among Finnish males. J Affect Disord 2008 Jul;109(1-2):47–55. Epub 2008 Jan 24.
19 Kumpulainen K. Psychiatric conditions associated with bullying. Int J Adolesc Med Health 2008 Apr-Jun;20(2):121–32.
20 Vitetta L, Anton B, Cortiso F, et. al. Mind-body medicine: stress and its impact on overall health and longevity. Ann NY Acad Sci 2005;1057:492–505.
21 Vlastelica M. Emotional stress as a trigger in sudden cardiac death. Psychiatr Danub 2008;20(3):411–4.
22 DeRubeis RJ, Gelfand LA, Tang TZ, et. al. Medications versus cognitive behaviour therapy for severely depressed outpatients:mega-analysis of four randomised comparisons. Am J Psychiatry 1999;156(7):1007–13.
23 Wolf NJ, Hopko DR. Psychosocial and pharmacological interventions for depressed adults in primary care: a critical review. Clin Psychol Rev 2008;28(1):131–61.
24 Highet N, Drummond P. A comparative evaluation of community treatments for post-partum depression: implications for treatment and management practices. Aust NZJ Psychiatry 2004;38(4):212–8.
25 Bottai T. Non-drug treatment for depression. Presse Med 2008;37(5 Pt 2):877–82.
26 Himelhoch S, Medoff DR, Oyeniyi G. Efficacy of group psychotherapy to reduce depressive symptoms among HIV-infected individuals: a systematic review and meta-analysis. AIDS Patient Care STDS 2007;21(10):732–9.
27 Oei TP, Dingle G. The effectiveness of group cognitive behaviour therapy for unipolar depressive disorders. J Affect Disord 2008;107(1-3):5–21.
28 Akechi T, Okuyama T, Onishi J, et. al. Psychotherapy for depression among incurable cancer patients. Cochrane Database Syst Rev 2008;(2):CD005537.
29 Wilson KC, Mottram PG, Vassilas CA. Psychotherapeutic treatments for older depressed people. Cochrane Database Syst Rev 2008 Jan 23;(1):CD004853.
30 Dobkin RD, Menza M, Bienfait KL. CBT for the treatment of depression in Parkinson's disease: a promising nonpharmacological approach. Expert Rev Neurother 2008;8(1):27–35.

31 Wood A, Trainor G, Rothwell J, et. al. Randomised trial of group therapy for repeated deliberate self-harm in adolescents. J Am Acad Child Adolesc Psychiatry 2001;40(11):1246–53.
32 Freedland KE, Skala JA, Carney RM, et. al. Treatment of Depression After Coronary Artery Bypass Surgery. A Randomised Controlled Trial. Archives of General Psychiatry 2009 Vol 66(4):387–396.
33 Speca M, Carlson LE, Goodey E, et. al. A randomised, wait-list controlled clinical trial: the effect of a mindfulness meditation-based stress reduction program on mood and symptoms of stress in cancer outpatients. Psychosom Med 2000;62(5):613–22.
34 Carlson LE, Speca M, Faris P, et. al. One year pre-post intervention follow-up of psychological, immune, endocrine and blood pressure outcomes of mindfulness-based stress reduction (MBSR) in breast and prostate cancer outpatients. Brain Behav Immun 2007;21(8):1038–49.
35 Jorm AF, Morgan AJ, Hetrick SE. Relaxation for depression. Cochrane Database of Systematic Reviews 2008, Issue 4. Art. No.: CD007142. doi: 10.1002/14651858.CD007142.pub2.
36 McAvoy BR. Relaxation techniques have some benefit in depression PEARLS November 2008;No. 125.
37 Maratos AS, Gold C, Wang X, et. al. Music therapy for depression. Cochrane Database Syst Rev 2008;(1):CD004517.
38 Koenig HG, George LK, Peterson BL. Religiosity and remission of depression in medically ill older patients. Am J Psychiatry 1998;155(4):536–42.
39 Kendler KS, Liu XQ, Gardner CO, et. al. Dimensions of religiosity and their relationship to lifetime psychiatric and substance use disorders. Am J Psychiatry 2003;160(3):496–503.
40 Blumenthal JA, Babyak MA, Ironson G, et. al. For the ENRICHD Investigators. Spirituality, religion, and clinical outcomes in patients recovering from an acute myocardial infarction. Psychosom Med 2007;69(6):501–8.
41 Hassed CS. Depression: dispirited or spiritually deprived? MJA 2000;173(10):545–7.
42 McClain CS, Rosenfeld B, Breitbart W. Effect of spiritual wellbeing on end-of-life despair in terminally-ill cancer patients. Lancet 2003;361(9369):1603–7.
43. Vitetta L, Kenner D, Kissane D, et. al. Clinical outcomes in terminally ill patients admitted to hospice care: diagnostic and therapeutic interventions. J Palliat Care 2001;17(2):69–77.
44 Kiecolt-Glaser J, Newton T. Marriage and health: his and hers.Psychological Bulletin 2001;127(4):472–503.
45 Hibbard JH, Pope CR. The quality of social roles as predictors of morbidity and mortality. Soc Sci Med 1993;36(3):217–25.
46 Pilkington K, Kirkwood G, Rampes H, et. al. Yoga for depression: the research evidence. J Affect Disord 2005;89(1-3):13–24.
47 Riemann D. Insomnia and comorbid psychiatric disorders. Sleep Med 2007;8(Suppl 4):S15–S20.
48 Morawetz D. Insomnia and Depression: Which Comes First? Sleep Research Online 2003;5(2): 77–81.
49 Hiscock H, Wake M. Infant sleep problems and postnatal depression: a community-based study. Pediatrics 2001;107(6):1317–22.
50 Hiscock H, Wake M. Randomised controlled trial of behavioural infant sleep intervention to improve infant sleep and maternal mood. BMJ 2002;324(7345):1062–5.
51 Wojnar M, Ilgen MA, Wojnar J, et. al. Sleep problems and suicidality in the National Comorbidity Survey Replication. J Psychiatr Res 2009 Feb;43(5):526–31. Epub 2008 Sep 7.
52 Hiscock H, Bayer JK, Hampton A, et. al. Long-term mother and child mental health effects of a population-based infant sleep intervention: cluster-randomised, controlled trial. Pediatrics 2008;122(3):e621–7.
53 Benedetti F, Barbini B, Fulgosi MC, et. al. Combined total sleep deprivation and light therapy in the treatment of drug-resistant bipolar depression: acute response and long-term remission rates. J Clin Psychiatry 2005;66(12):1535–40.
54 Brand CA, Abi HY, Cough DE, et. al. Vitamin D deficiency: a study of community beliefs among dark skinned and veiled people. Intern J Rheumatic Dis 2008;11:15–23.
55 Diamond TH, Levy S, Smith A, et. al. High bone turnover in Muslim women with vitamin D deficiency. MJA 2002;177:139–141.
56 Lansdowne AT, Provost SC. Vitamin D3 enhances mood in healthy subjects during winter. Psychopharmacology (Berl) 1998;135(4):319–23.
57 Gloth FM III, Allam W, Hollis B. Vitamin D vs broad spectrum phototherapy in treatment of seasonal affective disorder. J Nutr Health Ageing 1999;3(1):5–7.
58 Kemper KJ, Shannon S. Complementary and alternative medicine therapies to promote healthy moods. Pediatr Clin North Am 2007;54(6): 901–26.
59 Jorm AF, Allen NB, O'Donnell CP, et. al. Effectiveness of complementary and self-help treatments for depression in children and adolescents. MJA 2006;185:368–372.
60 Fritzsche M, Heller R, Hill H, et. al. Sleep deprivation as a predictor of response to light therapy in major depression. J Affect Disord 2001;62(3):207–15.
61 Loving RT, Kripke DF, Shuchter SR. Bright light augments antidepressant effects of medication and wake therapy. Depress Anxiety 2002;16(1):1–3.
62 Riemersma-van der Lek RF, Swaab DF, et. al. Effect of bright light and melatonin on cognitive and noncognitive function in elderly residents of group care facilities: a randomised controlled trial. JAMA 2008;299(22):2642–55.
63 Loving RT, Kripke DF, Elliott JA, et. al. Bright light treatment of depression for older adults. ISRCTN55452501 BMC Psychiatry 2005;5:41.
64 Jorm AF, Rodgers B, Jacomb PA, et. al. Smoking and mental health: results from a community survey. MJA 1999;170:74–77,
65 Jorm AF. Association between smoking and mental disorders: results from an Australian National Prevalence Survey. AN Z J Publ Health 1999;23(3):245–8.
66 Goodman E, Capitman J. Depressive symptoms and cigarette smoking among teens. Pediatrics 2000;106(4):748–55.
67 Munafò MR, Hitsman B, Rende R, et. al. Effects of progression to cigarette smoking on depressed mood in adolescents: evidence from the National Longitudinal Study of Adolescent Health. Addiction 2008;103(1):162–71.
68 Davis L, Uezato A, Newell JM, Frazier E. Major depression and comorbid substance use disorders. Curr Opin Psychiatry 2008 Jan;21(1):14–8.

69 Barbour KA, Edenfield TM, Blumenthal JA. Exercise as a treatment for depression and other psychiatric disorders: a review. J Cardiopulm Rehabil Prev 2007;27(6):359–67.

70 Weyerer S, Kupfer B. Physical exercise and psychological health. Sports Med 1994;17(2):108–16.

71 Weyerer S. Physical inactivity and depression in the community. Evidence from the Upper Bavarian Field Study. Int J Sports Med 1992;13(6):492–6.

72 Dunn AL, Trivedi MH, O'Neal HA. Physical activity dose-response effects on outcomes of depression and anxiety. Med Sci Sports Exerc 2001;33(6 Suppl):S587–97.

73 Babyak M, Blumenthal JA, Herman S, et. al. Exercise treatment for major depression: maintenance of therapeutic benefit at 10 months. Psychosom Med 2000;62(5):633–8.

74 Mather AS, Rodriguez C, Guthrie MF, et. al. Effects of exercise on depressive symptoms in older adults with poorly responsive depressive disorder: randomised controlled trial. Br J Psychiatry 2002;180:411–5.

75 Wirz-Justice A, Graw P, Kräuchi K, et. al. 'Natural' light treatment of seasonal affective disorder. J Affect Dis 1996;37(2-3):109–20.

76 Dimeo F, Bauer M, Varahram I, et. al. Benefits from aerobic exercise in patients with major depression: a pilot study. Br J Sports Med 2001;35(2):114–7.

77 Hyde JS, Mezulis AH, Abramson LY. The ABCs of depression: integrating affective, biological, and cognitive models to explain the emergence of the gender difference in depression. Psychol Rev 2008;115(2):291–313.

78 Knubben K, Reischies FM, Adli M, et. al. A randomised, controlled study on the effects of a short-term endurance training program in patients with major depression. Br J Sports Med 2007;41(1):29–33.

79 Knobf MT, Musanti R, Dorward J. Exercise and quality of life outcomes in patients with cancer. Semin Oncol Nurs 2007;23(4):285–96.

80 Mead GE, Morley W, Campbell P, et. al. Exercise for depression. Cochrane Database of Systematic Reviews 2008, Issue 4. Art. No.: CD004366. DOI: 10.1002/14651858.CD004366.pub3.

81 Naga Venkatesha Murthy PJ, Janakiramaiah N, et. al. P300 amplitude and antidepressant response to Sudarshan Kriya Yoga (SKY). J Affect Disord 1998;50(1):45–8.

82 Janakiramaiah N, Gangadhar BN, Naga Venkatesha Murthy PJ, et. al. Antidepressant efficacy of Sudarshan Kriya Yoga (SKY) in melancholia: a randomised comparison with electroconvulsive therapy (ECT) and imipramine. J Affect Disord 2000;57(1-3):255–9.

83 Shapiro D, Cook IA, Davydov DM, et. al. Yoga as a Complementary Treatment of Depression: Effects of Traits and Moods on Treatment Outcome. Advance Access Publication 28 February 2007 eCAM 2007;4(4)493–502 doi:10.1093/ecam/nel1142007.

84 Strandberg TE, Strandberg AY, Pitkälä K, et. al. Chocolate, wellbeing and health among elderly men. Eur J Clin Nutr 2008 Feb;62(2):247–53. Epub 2007 Feb 28.

85 Ledochowski M, Sperner-Unterweger B, Fuchs D. Lactose malabsorption is associated with early signs of mental depression in females: a preliminary report. Dig Dis Sci 1998;43(11):2513–7.

86 Noaghiul S, Hibbeln JR. Cross-national comparisons of seafood consumption and rates of bipolar disorders. Am J Psychiatry 2003;160(12):2222–7.

87 Avila-Funes JA, Garant MP, Aguilar-Navarro S.Relationship between determining factors for depressive symptoms and for dietary habits in older adults in Mexico Rev Panam Salud Publica 2006;19(5):321–30.

88 Fergusson DM, Boden JM, Horwood LJ. Tests of causal links between alcohol abuse or dependence and major depression. Arch Gen Psychiatry 2009 Mar;66(3):260–6.

89 Stoll AL, Severus WE, Freeman MP, et. al. Omega-3 fatty acids in bipolar disorder: a preliminary double-blind, placebo-controlled trial. Arch Gen Psychiatry 1999;56(5):407–12.

90 Osher Y, et. al. Omega-3 eicosapentaneoic acid in bipolar depression: Report of a small open-label study. J Clin Psychiatry 2005 Jun;66(6):726–9.

91 Mazza M, Pomponi M, Janiri L, et. al. Review article. Omega-3 fatty acids and antioxidants in neurological and psychiatric diseases: An overview. Progress in Neuro-Psychopharmacology and Biological Psychiatry 2007 January 30;31(1):12–26.

92 Frasure-Smith N, Lespérance F and Julien P. Major depression is associated with lower omega-3 fatty acid levels in patients with recent acute coronary syndromes . Biological Psychiatry 2004 May 1;55(9): 891–96.

93 Rees A, Austin M, Owen C, Parker G. Omega-3 deficiency associated with perinatal depression: Case control study. Psychiatry Research 2009 April 30;166(2-3):254–59.

94 Lucas M, Asselin G, Mérette C, et. al. Ethyl-eicosapentaenoic acid for the treatment of psychological distress and depressive symptoms in middle-aged women: a double-blind, placebo-controlled, randomised clinical trial. Am J Clin Nutr 2009 Feb;89(2):641–51. Epub 2008 Dec 30.

95 Jazayeri S, Tehrani-Doost M, Keshavarz SA, et. al. Comparison of therapeutic effects of omega-3 fatty acid eicosapentaenoic acid and fluoxetine, separately and in combination, in major depressive disorder. Aust N Z J Psychiatry 2008;42(3):192–8.

96 Keshavarz S, Jazayeri S, Tehrani-Doost M, et. al. Effects of n-3 fatty acid EPA in the treatment of depression. Proc Nutr Soc 2008;67(OCE):E210.

97 Clayton EH, Hanstock TL, Garg ML, et. al. Long chain omega-3 polyunsaturated fatty acids in the treatment of psychiatric illnesses in children and adolescents. Acta Neuropsychiatrica 2007 19(2): 92–103.

98 Lin PY, Su KP. A meta-analytic review of double-blind, placebo-controlled trials of antidepressant efficacy of omega-3 fatty acids. J Clin Psychiatry 2007;68(7):1056–61.

99 Mischoulon D. Update and critique of natural remedies as antidepressant treatments. Psychiatr Clin North Am 2007; 30:51–68.

100 Miura H, Ozaki N, Sawada M, et. al. A link between stress and depression: shifts in the balance between the kynurenine and serotonin pathways of tryptophan metabolism and the etiology and pathophysiology of depression. Stress 2008;11(3):198–209.

101 Cournoyer G, de Montigny C, Ouellette J, et. al. A comparative double-blind controlled study of trimipramine and amitriptyline in major depression: lack of correlation with 5-hydroxytryptamine reuptake blockade. J Clin Psychopharmacol 1987;7(6):385–93.

102 Kahn RS, Westenberg HG, Verhoeven WM, et. al. Effect of a serotonin precursor and uptake inhibitor in anxiety disorders; a double-blind comparison of 5-hydroxytryptophan, clomipramine and placebo. Int Clin Psychopharmacol 1987;2(1):33–45.

103 Smith KA, Fairburn CG, Cowen PJ. Relapse of depression after rapid depletion of tryptophan. Lancet 1997;349(9056):915–9.

104 Gatto G, Caleri D, Michelacci S, Sicuteri F. Analgesising effect of a methyl donor (S-adenosylmethionine) in migraine: an open clinical trial. Int J Clin Pharmacol Res 1986;6:15–17.

105 Baldessarini RJ: Neuropharmacology of S-aenosyl-L-methionine. Am J Med 1987;83(suppl 5A): 95–103.

106 Nguyen M, Gregan A. S-adenosylmethionine and depression. Aust Fam Physician 2002;31(4): 339–43.

107 Bressa GM. S-adenosyl-l-methionine (SAMe) as antidepressant: meta-analysis of clinical studies. Acta Neurol Scand Suppl 1994;154:7–14.

108 Alpert JE, Papakostas G, Mischoulon D, et. al. S-adenosyl-L-methionine (SAMe) as an adjunct for resistant major depressive disorder: an open trial following partial or nonresponse to selective serotonin reuptake inhibitors or venlafaxine. J Clin Psychopharmacol 2004;24(6):661–4.

109 Di Rocco A, Rogers JD, Brown R, et. al. S-Adenosyl-Methionine improves depression in patients with Parkinson's disease in an open-label clinical trial. Mov Disord 2000;15(6):1225–9.

110 Shippy RA, Mendez D, Jones K, et. al. S-adenosylmethionine (SAM-e) for the treatment of depression in people living with HIV/AIDS. BMC Psychiatry 2004;4:38.

111 Thachil AF, Mohan R, Bhugra D. The evidence base of complementary and alternative therapies in depression. J Affect Dis 2007; 97:23–35.

112 Taylor MJ, Carney SM, Goodwin GM, et. al. Folate for depressive disorders: systematic review and meta-analysis of randomised controlled trials. J Psychopharmacol 2004;18(2):251–6.

113 Taylor MJ, Carney S, Geddes J, et. al. Folate for depressive disorders. Cochrane Database Syst Rev 2003;(2):CD003390.

114 Herrmann W, Lorenzl S, Obeid R. Review of the role of hyperhomocysteinemia and B-vitamin deficiency in neurological and psychiatric disorders--current evidence and preliminary recommendations Fortschr Neurol Psychiatr 2007;75(9):515–27.

115 Bottiglieri T, Laundy M, Crellin R, et. al. Homocysteine, folate, methylation, and monoamine metabolism in depression. J Neurol Neurosurg Psych 2000;69(2):228–32.

116 Morris MS, Fava M, Jacques PF, et. al. Depression and folate status in the US Population. Psychother Psychosom 2003;72(2):80–7.

117 Coppen A, Bailey J. Enhancement of the antidepressant action of fluoxetine by folic acid: a randomised, placebo-controlled trial. J Affect Disord 2000;60(2):121–30.

118 Obeid R, McCaddon A, Herrmann W. The role of hyperhomocysteinemia and B-vitamin deficiency in neurological and psychiatric diseases. Clin Chem Lab Med 2007;45(12):1590–606.

119 Hintikka J, Tolmunen T, Tanskanen A, et. al. High vitamin B12 level and good treatment outcome may be associated in major depressive disorder. BMC Psychiatry 2003;3:17–22.

120 Bell IR, Edman JS, Morrow FD, et. al. Brief communication. Vitamin B1, B2, and B6 augmentation of tricyclic antidepressant treatment in geriatric depression with cognitive dysfunction. J Am Coll Nutr 1992;11(2):159–63.

121 Ford AH, Flicker L, Thomas J, et. al. Vitamins B12, B6, and folic acid for onset of depressive symptoms in older men:results from a 2-year placebo-controlled randomised trial. J Clin Psychiatry 2008;69(8):1203–9.

122 Murphy PK, Wagner CL. Vitamin D and mood disorders among women: an integrative review. J Midwifery Womens Health 2008;53(5):440–6.

123 Hoogendijk WJ, Lips P, Dikmg, et. al. Depression is associated with decreased 25-hydroxyvitamin D and increased parathyroid hormone levels in older adults. Arch Gen Psychiatry 2008;65(5):508–12.

124 Wilkins CH, et. al. Vitamin D deficiency is associated with low mood and worse cognition in older adults. Am J Geriatr Psychiatry 2006;14:1032–40.

125 Berk M, Jacka FN, Williams LJ, et. al. Is this D vitamin to worry about? Vitamin D insufficiency in an inpatient sample. ANZJ Psych 2008;42(10):874–8.

126 Jorde R, Sneve M, Figenschau Y, et. al. Effects of vitamin D supplementation on symptoms of depression in overweight and obese subjects: randomised double-blind trial. J Intern Med 2008 Sep 10. Epub ahead of print.

127 Benton D, Haller J, Fordy J. Vitamin supplementation for 1 year improves mood. Neuropsychobiology 1995;32(2):98–105.

128 Siwek M, Wróbel A, Dudek D, et. al. .The role of copper and magnesium in the pathogenesis and treatment of affective disorders Psych Pol 2005;39(5):911–20.

129 Linder J, Brismar K, Beck-Friis J, et. al. Calcium and magnesium concentrations in affective disorder: difference between plasma and serum in relation to symptoms. Acta Psychiatr Scand 1989;80(6):527–37.

130 Rasmussen HH, Mortensen PB, Jensen IW. Depression and magnesium deficiency. Int J Psychiatry Med 1989;19(1):57–63.

131 Widmer J, Bovier P, Karege F, et. al. Evolution of blood magnesium, sodium and potassium in depressed patients followed for three months. Neuropsychobiology 1992;26(4):173–9.

132 Widmer J, Henrotte JG, Raffin Y, et. al. Relationship between erythrocyte magnesium, plasma electrolytes and cortisol, and intensity of symptoms in major depressed patients. J Affect Disord 1995;34(3):201–9.

133 Neher E, Sakaba T. Multiple roles of calcium ions in the regulation of neurotransmitter release. Neuron 2008;59(6):861–72.

134 Thys-Jacobs S. Micronutrients and the premenstrual syndrome: the case for calcium. J Am Coll Nutr 2000;19(2):220–7.

135 Nowak G, Szewczyk B, Pilc A. Zinc and depression. An update. Pharmacol Rep 2005;57(6):713–8.

136 Maes M, Vandoolaeghe E, Neels H, et. al. Lower serum zinc in major depression is a sensitive marker of treatment resistance and of the immune/inflammatory response in that illness. Biol Psychiatry 1997;42(5):349–58.

137 Maes M, D'Haese PC, Scharpé S, et. al. Hypozincemia in depression. J Affect Disord 1994;31(2):135–40.

138 McLoughlin IJ, Hodge JS. Zinc in depressive disorder. Acta Psychiatr Scand 1990;82(6):451–3.

139 Broun ER, Greist A, Tricot G, et. al. Excessive zinc ingestion. A reversible cause of sideroblastic anemia and bone marrow depression. JAMA 1990;264(11):1441–3.

140 Schule C, Baghai T, Ferrera A, et. al. Neuroendocrine effects of Hypericum extract WS 5570 in 12 healthy male volunteers. Pharmacopsychiatry 2001;34:S127–33.

141 Nautural Database. Online. Available: http://www.naturaldatabase.com (accessed December 2008).
142 Linde K, Berner MM, Kriston L. St John's wort for major depression. Cochrane Database of Systematic Reviews 2008, Issue 4. Art. No.: CD000448. doi: 10.1002/14651858.CD000448.pub3.
143 Ernst E. Herbal remedies for depression and anxiety. Adv Psychiatr Treat 2007;13:312–316.
144 Roder C, Schaefer M, Leucht S. Meta-analysis of effectiveness and tolerability of treatment of mild to moderate depression with St. John's wort. Fortschr Neurol Psychiatr 2004;72:330–343.
145 Linde K, Ramirez G, Mulrow CD, et. al. St John's wort for depression--an overview and meta-analysis of randomised clinical trials. BMJ 1996;313:253–58.
146 Linde K, Mulrow CD. St John's wort for depression. Cochrane Database Systematic Review, 2000;CD 000448.
147 Woelk H. Comparison of St John's wort and imipramine for treating depression: randomised controlled trial. BMJ 2000;321:536–39.
148 Schrader E. Equivalence of St John's wort extract (Ze 117) and fluoxetine: a randomised,controlled study in mild-moderate depression. Int Clin Psychopharmacol 2000;15(2):61–8.
149 Rahimi R, Nikfar S, Abdollahi M. Efficacy and tolerability of Hypericum perforatum in major depressive disorder in comparison with selective serotonin reuptake inhibitors: A meta-analysis. Prog Neuropsychopharmacol Biol Psychiatry 2008 Nov 12.
150 Hypericum Depression Trial Study Group. Effect of Hypericum perforatum (St John's wort) in major depressive disorder: a randomised controlled trial. JAMA 2002;287(14):1807–14.
151 Kasper S, Anghelescu IG, Szegedi A, et. al. Superior efficacy of St John's wort extract WS 5570 compared to placebo in patients with major depression: a randomised, double-blind, placebo-controlled, multi-center trial.ISRCTN77277298 BMC Med 2006;4:14.
152 Szegedi A, Kohnen R, Dienel A, et. al. Acute treatment of moderate to severe depression with Hypericum extract WS 5570(St John's wort): randomised controlled double-blind non-inferiority trial versus paroxetine. BMJ 2005;330(7490):503.
153 Markowitz JS, Donovan JL, DeVane CL, et. al. Effect of St John's wort on drug metabolism by induction of cytochrome P450 3A4 enzyme. JAMA 2003;290(11):1500–4.
154 Schulz V. Incidence and clinical relevance of the interactions and side-effects of Hypericum preparations. Phytomedicine 2001;8:152–60.
155 Scripnikov A, Khomenko A, Napryeyenko O; GINDEM-NP Study Group. Effects of Ginkgo biloba extract EGb 761 on neuropsychiatric symptoms of dementia: findings from a randomised controlled trial. Wien Med Wochenschr 2007;157(13-14):295–300.
156. Cohen AJ, Bartlik B. Ginkgo biloba for antidepressant-induced sexual dysfunction. J Sex Marital Ther 1998;24(2):139–43.
157 Kang BJ, Lee SJ, Kim MD, et. al. A placebo-controlled, double-blind trial of Ginkgo biloba for antidepressant-induced sexual dysfunction. Hum Psychopharmacol 2002;17(6):279–84.
158 Akhondzadeh Basti A, Moshiri E, Noorbala AA, et. al. Comparison of petal of Crocus sativus L. and fluoxetine in the treatment of depressed outpatients: a pilot double-blind randomised trial. Prog Neuropsychopharmacol Biol Psychiatry 2007;31(2):439–42.
159 Moshiri E, Basti AA, Noorbala AA, et. al. Crocus sativus L. (petal) in the treatment of mild-to-moderate depression: a double-blind, randomised and placebo-controlled trial. Phytomedicine 2006;13(9-10):607–11.
160 Akhondzadeh S, Tahmacebi-Pour N, Noorbala AA, et. al. Crocus sativus L. in the treatment of mild to moderate depression: a double-blind, randomised and placebo-controlled trial. Phytoth Res 2005;19(2):148–51.
161 Akhondzadeh S, Fallah-Pour H, Afkham K, et. al. Comparison of Crocus sativus L. and imipramine in the treatment of mild to moderate depression: a pilot double-blind randomised trial.ISRCTN45683816 BMC Complement Altern Med 2004;4:12.
162 Darbinyan V, Aslanyan G, Amroyan E, et. al. Clinical trial of Rhodiola rosea L. extract SHR-5 in the treatment of mild to moderate depression. Nord J Psychiatry 2007;61(5):343–8.
163 Sarris J. Herbal medicines in the treatment of psychiatric disorders: a systematic review. Phytother Res 2007;21(8):703–16.
164 Perry N, Perry E. Aromatherapy in the management of psychiatric disorders:clinical and neuropharmacological perspectives. CNS Drugs 2006; 20:257–280.
165 Kiecolt-Glaser JK, Graham JE, Malarkey WB, et. al. Olfactoryinfluencesonmoodandautonomic,endocrine, andimmunefunction.Psychoneuroendocrinology2008 Apr;33(3):328–39.
166 Herz RS. Aromatherapy facts and fictions: a scientific analysis of olfactory effects on mood, physiology and behaviour. Int J Neurosci 2009;119(2):263–90.
167 Almeida OP, Yeap BB, Hankey GJ, et. al. Low free testosteroneconcentrationasapotentiallytreatablecause ofdepressivesymptomsinoldermen.ArchGenPsychiatry 2008;65(3):283–9.
168 Onalan G, Onalan R, Selam B, et. al. Mood scores in relation to hormone replacement therapies during menopause: a prospective randomised trial. Tohoku J Exp Med 2005;207(3):223–31.
169 Kulkarni J, de Castella A, Fitzgerald PB, et. al. Estrogen in severe mental illness: a potential new treatment approach. Arch Gen Psychiatry 2008;65(8):955–60.
170 Kulkarni J, Gurvich C, Gilbert H, et. al. Hormone modulation: a novel therapeutic approach for women with severe mental illness. Aust N Z J Psychiatry 2008;42(1):83–8.
171 Kulkarni J. Depression as a side-effect of the contraceptive pill. Expert Opin Drug Saf 2007;6(4):371–4.
172 Leo RJ, Ligot A. A systematic review of randomised controlled trials of acupuncture in the treatment of depression. J Affect Dis 2007;97:13–22.
173 Duan DM, Tu Y, Chen LP. Assessment of effectiveness of electroacupuncture and fluoxetine for treatment of depression with physical symptoms Zhongguo Zhen Jiu 2008;28(3):167–70.
174 Field T, Griszle N, Scafidi F, et. al. Massage and relaxation therapies' effects on depressed adolescent mothers. Adolescence 1996 Winter;31(124):903–11.
175 Field T, Diego MA, Hernandez-Reif M, et. al. Massage therapy effects on depressed pregnant women. J Psychosom Obstet Gynaecol 2004 Jun;25(2):115–22.

Chapter 13

Diabetes

Introduction

Type 1 diabetes mellitus (T1DM) — prevalence and incidence

The prevalence of T1DM accounts for about 10% of all cases of diabetes, occurs most commonly in people of European descent and affects more than 2 million people in Europe and North America.[1,2] A recent update reported that in the US the prevalence of diagnosed and undiagnosed diabetes (all forms in all ages as at 2007) totalled 23.6 million people — 7.8% of the population had some form of the disease. That is, those *diagnosed accounted for 17.9 million* people and undiagnosed 5.7 million people.[2]

There is also a wide variation in incidence of T1DM from country to country that is evident globally.[3] For example, the marked geographic variation in incidence is clearly evident from data that show that a child in Finland has approximately 400 times the likelihood than does a child in Venezuela to acquire the disease.[2, 3, 4] Moreover, the incidence of T1DM in children is increasing in Western countries.[2, 5, 6] The global incidence of T1DM in children less than or equal to 14 years of age as calculated per 100 000 population has marked variation within ethnic and racial distribution in the world population, as summarised in Table 13.1. The incidence increases with age, highest at 10–14 years of age.

It is not clear from these worldwide variations the factors contributing to the incidence of T1DM but it appears genetics, environmental, dietary and lifestyle factors all play an important role. The reporting of incidence data for T1DM is further affected by possible under-reporting in some regions due to the quality of the registration system used in poorer countries.

There are also further sub-group variations of T1DM incidence within populations.[2, 3, 4] For instance, in the US, non-Hispanic white youth have a higher risk of T1DM.[2] A multiethnic, population-based study in the United States estimated the incidence of T1DM (per 100 000 person-years) was 24.3 in children (less than 19 years of age) with the highest rate observed in non-Hispanic white youth (18.6, 28.1, and 32.9 for age groups 0–4, 5–9, and 10–14 years, respectively).[7]

Type 2 diabetes mellitus (T2DM) — prevalence and incidence

As with T1DM the prevalence of T2DM also varies extensively for different populations from distinct geographical areas.[8] At the end of the 20th century, it was estimated that 150 million people in the world had diabetes and the World Health Organization (WHO) predicts that, between 1997 and 2025, the number of patients with T2DM will double to reach about 300 million.[9, 10] According to the WHO, T2DM affects up to 7% of Western populations and is increasing in newly industrialised and developing countries.[11]

The ageing of populations and the effects of modernisation of lifestyle have led to a dramatic increase in the prevalence of diabetes globally with very high rates in developing nations, particularly in Asia and the Pacific.

The heightened susceptibility and high prevalence of T2DM of Micronesian and Polynesian Pacific Islanders,[10, 12] Native Americans,[13] Indigenous Australians and Torres Strait Islanders,[10, 14] and Asian Indians[14] has been well documented.

In Australia, the prevalence of T2DM has been reported to have doubled since 1981[6, 10] (Table 13.2).

There are a number of risk factors that have been identified with the development of T1DM and T2DM (Table 13.3).

The number of adolescents with T2DM diagnosed yearly is also increasing globally and has been attributed to factors such as weight gain, poor nutrition and lack of exercise.[16]

Lifestyle — general, education and prevention of T2DM

Intensive lifestyle interventions can reduce the incidence of diabetes in people with impaired glucose tolerance, so encouragement of positive lifestyle strategies is essential where social opportunities arise, such as with school

Table 13.1 Worldwide incidence of T1DM in children less than or equal to 14 years of age

Very low (<1/100 000 per year)	Low (1–4.99/100 000 per year)	Intermediate (5–9.99/100 000 per year)	High (10–19.99/100 000 per year)	Very high (> or = 20/100 000 per year)
China, South America (Venezuela, Paraguay, Peru), Uruguay, Pakistan	Japan, Mauritius, South America (Chile, Colombia)	Africa (Algeria, Tunisia, Sudan) South America (Argentina, Brazil) 18 of 39 European populations: Greece, Hungary, Israel, Russia, Bulgaria, France, Austria, Italy (Lombardia), Latvia, Portugal (Coimbra, Madeira Island), Romania, Slovenia, Slovakia, United States	Australia, Italy (Eastern Sicily), Kuwait, Denmark, Belgium, Estonia, Lithuania, Luxemburg, The Netherlands, New Zealand (Auckland), Portugal (Algarve), Spain (Catalonia), Northern Ireland	Canada, Italy (Sardinia), Finland, Sweden, Norway Portugal, United Kingdom (Aberdeen), Canada, Portugal (Porto Alegre), New Zealand (Canterbury)

(Source: adapted from Karvonen, Viik-Kajander, Moltchanova)[3]

Table 13.2 Australian prevalence of T2DM

	Men	Women
Prevalence	8%	6.8%
Impaired glucose tolerance and/or impaired fasting glucose	17.4%	15.4%

Table 13.3 Risk factors that have been reported to be associated with T1 and T2DM

Risk factors for T1 and T2DM
Genetic predispositions
Life stressors and/or depression
Diet and/or nutrition
Excess weight
Inadequate exercise
Inadequate sunshine and/or vitamin D deficiency
Smoking

(Source: adapted from Adamo, Tesson)[15]

education, religion or in any other social community situations. Lifestyle changes can lead to lifelong changes and reduce the incidence of diabetes or complications associated with diabetes, even after active counselling has ceased.[17] A post-intervention follow-up study of participants found the risk of developing T2DM was reduced by 43% over a 7-year median period for those who received intensive lifestyle counselling compared with standard intervention.[17]

A systematic review and meta-analysis of the literature identified 17 randomised trials of 8084 participants and confirmed the value of intensive lifestyle intervention counselling to prevent and delay T2DM onset in people with impaired glucose tolerance.[18] Healthy diet and exercise is much more effective at preventing T2DM than drug therapy. When comparing lifestyle intervention and metformin, a study of 3234 subjects over 3 years with impaired glucose tolerance were randomly assigned to a group of placebo, metformin, or a lifestyle-modification program involving diet and exercise over a 2.8 year follow-up. Lifestyle intervention reduced the incidence of developing T2DM by 58% compared with metformin by 31%.[19]

The aim of a healthy lifestyle to prevent T2DM:

- waist reduction and weight loss if overweight
- consume less food at meal times
- consume less energy-dense and nutrient-poor foods and beverages
- consume low glycaemic index (GI) foods (e.g. sweet potatoes rather than normal potatoes)
- consume more fish, protein, fibre, complex carbohydrates, legumes, nuts, vegetables and fruit

- reduce sodium/salt intake
- reduce fat intake
- exercise regularly and increase physical activity generally (e.g. walk more)
- reduce stress and improve moods
- maintain regular sleep patterns (e.g. sleep 7–8 hours per night)
- practice prudent sun exposure for vitamin D.

T2DM is associated with a Westernised lifestyle. Lifestyle management is the most effective way of preventing T2DM, especially with dietary measures and exercise. A recent Cochrane review of the literature emphasises the importance that combined diet interventions and exercise significantly reduces the risk of developing T2DM by up to 37% compared with standard recommendations (RR 0.63) with favourable modest effects on reducing blood lipids and blood pressure compared with exercise or dietary changes alone.[20]

A study of 577 Chinese adults with impaired glucose tolerance without T2DM from 33 Chinese medical clinics, were randomised to either a control group, or 1 of 3 lifestyle intervention groups that included diet or exercise alone, or diet with exercise over a 6-year period and an assessment of the lifestyle intervention group again in the 20 year follow-up.[21]

The combined lifestyle intervention group significantly reduced the incidence of developing diabetes by up to 51% over the 6-year period and up to 43% in the 20-year follow-up compared with the control group, and significantly more than the diet and exercise groups alone. This study emphasises the importance of promoting intensive lifestyle changes to prevent diabetes onset, particularly in patients with reported impaired intolerance or at high risk of developing DM.[21]

Dietary factors and T1DM

Cow's milk consumption in early infancy

Children fed cow's milk during the first few days of life are twice as likely to develop T1DM than children who are breast fed.[22] The association between T1DM may be explained by the generation of specific immune response to beta casein from cow's milk exposure, triggering cellular and humoral anti- β casein immune response which may cross-react with beta-cell antigen.[23] Overall high cow's milk consumption (3 or more glasses of cow's milk a day) was associated with a 5.4 fold increased risk of developing T1DM in young children, and this was higher in children who also had HLA genotype for diabetes.[24]

Dietary factors and T2DM

Obesity is the main cause of developing T2DM according to large scale studies. Whilst lack of physical activity also contributes, the risk of T2DM rises progressively with increasing Body Mass Index (BMI), increasing waist circumference, and obesity.[25]

Epidemiologic studies suggest that greater consumption of fruit and vegetables reduces the risk of diabetes mellitus. In a population-based prospective cohort (European Prospective Investigation of Cancer–Norfolk) study, 21 831 individuals aged 40–75 years at baseline were assessed for plasma vitamin C level and habitual intake of fruit and vegetables over a 12-year follow-up period. The researchers found a strong inverse association between plasma vitamin C level and T2DM risk. High plasma vitamin C level and, to a lesser degree, fruit and vegetable intake was associated with a substantially decreased risk of T2DM.[26]

Cultural factors and prevention

Minority ethnic groups found that upper-middle and high-income countries often suffer a higher prevalence of T2DM than the local population, due to cultural and communication barriers, being of lower socioeconomic backgrounds, and having less access to good quality health care.[27]

Education about positive lifestyle and prevention strategies of T1 and T2DM is vital and needs to be tailored to suit cultural differences and racial sub-groups by understanding lay beliefs and attitudes, religious teachings and professional perceptions in relation to diabetes prevention.

For instance, a UK study of a Bangladeshi community found the Islam norms and teachings offers many opportunities for supporting diabetes prevention. The authors noted that interventions designed for the white population needed to be adapted to be meaningful to the Bangladeshi community. So religion may play an important role in supporting health promotion in any sub-community. Working collaboratively between health educators, health professionals and religious leaders should be explored to promote positive lifestyle changes within communities.[28]

Breastfeeding and prevention

Women breastfeeding for over 6 months significantly reduces the woman's risk of developing T2DM later in life. The longer the duration of breastfeeding, the greater the protection against T2DM.

A large scale prospective observational cohort study of 83 585 parous women identified a strong association of duration of breastfeeding and the incidence of T2DM. Whilst controlling for other relevant risk factors such as BMI, the study found that the longer the women breastfed the less likely they would develop T2DM. For each additional year of lactation, women with a birth in the prior 15 years had a decrease in the risk of diabetes of up to 15% amongst participants. Lactation improves glucose homeostasis.[29]

Gender factors and prevention

Studies indicate, in general, women with risk factors and a family history of diabetes were more likely to obtain diabetes education, gain benefits of self-management and reported higher levels of social support from their diabetes health care team than men did. This highlights the special needs for men with respect to diabetes education, understanding risk factors, prevention, self-care and self-management of T2DM.[30]

Genetics

Whilst studies suggest T1DM is associated with a wide spectrum of susceptibility and protective genotypes within the HLA class II system, it is likely that increasing environmental exposure is able to trigger these genes even in subjects who are less genetically susceptible.[31]

T2DM is the most common disease in the Western world today that has a genetic link.[32] It is the phenotype for more than 150 genotypes.[32, 33, 34] Each of these genotypes is characterised by impaired glucose tolerance and impairment of the control of intermediary metabolism.

Mind–body medicine

Meditation, biofeedback, and hypnosis have all been found to improve T2DM.[35]

Life stressors and/or depression

Stress may be a contributor to T1DM onset according to a prospective population-based study of almost 6000 children. The study demonstrated children had a threefold risk of developing autoimmunity T1DM if their parents divorced or experienced violence during the child's infancy within 2.5 years of the event.[36] The authors concluded that 'maternal experiences of serious life events…seem to be involved in the induction or progression of diabetes-related autoimmunity in children'.[36] Bullying, a form of stress for a child, is also known to adversely affect glycaemic control and self-management, and increase feelings of depression in T1DM children.[37]

Research demonstrates that regular use of stress management techniques can significantly reduce blood glucose levels in T2DM. After 1 year, compared with control, stress management reduced HbA1c by up to 1% which is clinically significant. Stress management would be a useful addition to a lifestyle intervention program for diabetics.[38]

Even daily hot baths for relaxation has been shown to lower fasting serum glucose in diabetics.[39] The researchers postulated the benefits could result from increased blood flow to skeletal muscles.

Stress and depression both influence hormonal levels.[40] Stress and depression increase cortisol, growth hormone and adrenaline. Cortisol and growth hormone increase insulin resistance, and adrenaline stimulate the breakdown of glycogen into glucose (glycogenolysis).[41]

Depression is associated with insulin resistance and with diabetes.[35] Low mood, mild and moderate depression is 2 to 3 times more common in diabetics than in non-diabetics, and is frequently not diagnosed or treated.[42] Insulin resistance is positively associated with the development of diabetes.[43] A large prospective scale study of 4847 participants without depression symptoms at baseline, at 3 years, treated T2DM was significantly associated with depression with an odds ratio of 1.52, even after adjusting for BMI, socioeconomic status, lifestyle and diabetes severity, and after excluding T2DM patients on antidepressants possibly for diabetic neuropathy. It was felt that depression contributed to diabetes and diabetes also contributed to depression.[44]

In another large scale study of more than 4600 patients over 65 years or older, depression symptoms over time was associated with a higher incidence of T2DM after adjusting for other diabetic risk factors.[45]

In a study of patients with work-related depression, the authors found the presence of depression or depressive symptoms was associated with subsequent increased risk of developing T2DM. The relative risk was 1.25 (95% confidence interval [CI]:1.02–1.48) compared with workers not experiencing depression.[46]

There is a positive correlation between insulin resistance and severity of depressive symptoms with impaired glucose tolerance before the outbreak of T2DM.[47]

A recent study found that serotonin receptor agonists can improve glucose tolerance, and reduce plasma insulin levels.[48]

Hence, the proper management of depression and stress are key factors in reducing the risk and progression of diabetes (see also Chapter 12).

Sunshine and Vitamin D

Vitamin D deficiency plays an important role with both insulin synthesis and secretion by way of vitamin D receptors and vitamin D binding proteins in pancreatic tissues as demonstrated in both human and animal models. The mechanism of action of vitamin D is also thought to occur as a direct action on pancreatic beta-cell function and mediated through regulation of plasma calcium levels, which may explain why vitamin D deficiency may play a role in the causation in T1 and T2DM.[49]

Lack of sunshine exposure is contributing to vitamin D deficiency as most vitamin D forms in the skin as a result of ultraviolet radiation (UVB wavelength; 290–320 nm) exposure from sunlight.[50]

People living in the southern regions of the southern hemisphere or the northern regions of the northern hemisphere have a higher risk of vitamin D deficiency, particularly during the winter months. Certain ethnic groups are at increased risk of vitamin D deficiency, especially dark skinned people who cover their skin for religious or cultural reasons, the elderly, babies of vitamin D deficient mothers, and people who are housebound or are in institutional care.[51]

Food sources for vitamin D include oily fish, eggs, and meat or fortified foods such as margarine and some milk products. However, food sources make a relatively small contribution to total vitamin D status (less than 10%).

T1DM

There is a significant body of biologically plausible evidence that strongly suggests that vitamin D plays a role in the prevention of T1DM. Giving infants vitamin D supplementation could protect them from T1DM according to a systematic review of 5 observational studies that showed a reduced risk of T1DM by up to 30% compared with infants not supplemented.[52]

T2DM

In a recent meta-analysis of the literature, studies demonstrate a consistent association of low 25-OH vitamin D status, calcium or dairy intake and the prevalence of T2DM.[49, 53]

Sleep

A number of studies have demonstrated a strong link between lack of sleep or over-sleeping with T2DM. The odds of developing T2DM for subjects sleeping 5 hours or less or 9 hours or more was associated with a significant increase risk of developing T2DM or impaired glucose tolerance test. Factors such as more environmental lighting, long working hours, television and personal computers are contributing to shorter sleep durations in Western societies.[54, 55]

Obstructive sleep apnoea may also be a risk factor for T2DM.[56]

Insomnia, anxiety and depression may double the risk of diabetes in men by 2.2 times compared with those with low levels of psychological distress, independent of risk factors such as BMI, family history for diabetes, and smoking, according to a study of 2127 men and 31 000 women followed up over 8–10 years. Of interest, women with psychological distress and insomnia did not have a higher risk of diabetes.[57]

Environment

Smoking

Researchers have combined the best available information from 25 studies in a systematic review which followed the health of 1.2 million people for several years.[58]

There is an increased risk of T2DM of approximately 50% from smoking and the more a person smoked the higher the risk and vice-versa; smoking preceded the development of T2DM.[58] Smoking has an adverse effect on pancreatic function. It may cause internal inflammation and increase abdominal fat, even in thin smokers, which could then lead to an increase in insulin resistance. Smoking becomes even more of a problem when combined with T2DM risk-enhancing behaviours such as obesity and inactivity.[59]

Further studies have confirmed this association. In a study of 906 participants free of DM at baseline and after multivariable adjustment, the researchers found of the current smokers, 25% developed T2DM at 5 years, compared with 14% of those who never smoked.[60]

Arsenic exposure

Environmental exposure to low levels of inorganic arsenic in drinking water has been associated with diabetes development. Millions of people world-wide are exposed to inorganic arsenic in water from natural mineral deposits. A cross-sectional USA study of 788 adults aged 20 years or older based on a 2003–2004 survey, urine arsenic levels, and after adjustment for biomarkers such as seafood intake, total urine arsenic was associated with increased prevalence of T2DM. Participants with T2DM had a 26% higher level of total arsenic in their urine than participants without T2DM. After similar adjustment, the odds of developing T2DM led to a 3.6 fold increase risk associated with exposure of arsenic. The authors speculated that arsenic could induce diabetes through oxidative stress, inflammation or apoptosis.[61]

Physical activity

Physical activity is one of the key modifiable risk factors for hyperglycaemia. Evidence from population-based, cross-sectional studies report that both decreased physical activity and elevated sedentary behaviours, such as television viewing time, are independently associated with raised blood glucose levels in adults without a diagnosis of diabetes.[62, 63] Regular exercise benefits T1DM and T2DM. Children with T1DM showed improved haemoglubin A1c (HbA1c) and glycaemic control with regular exercise of at least 3 times weekly compared with children who did not exercise.[64, 65]

Walking just 30 minutes daily can significantly reduce the incidence of T2DM.[66] Walking 2 hours weekly can reduce mortality from all causes by 39% and by 34% from cardiovascular disease in patients with T2DM.[67] A study of healthy young sedentary men demonstrated a high intensity aerobic exercise protocol comprising a total of 15 minutes of exercise (6 sessions; 4–6 30-second cycle sprints per session) substantially improved insulin action and glucose tolerance test, and supported the important role of exercise in preventing diabetes.[68]

The size of cities can influence the risk of diabetes. When a person migrates from a rural environment or third-world country to the city or a Western country the risk of T2DM is significantly elevated.[69, 70] If that city happens to be of more than 1 million in population, as described in a recent study,[69] then the risk of diabetes increases fourfold. It is thought that the design of cities can influence whether the people walk or not.

The position statements from both the American Diabetes Association and the American College of Sports Medicine, has recommended the use of resistance training as part of a physical activity program to reduce the risk of developing diabetes.[71, 72]

A Cochrane meta-analysis of 14 randomised controlled trials (RCTs) comparing exercise against no exercise in 377 participants with T2DM found that compared with control and independent of weight loss, exercise intervention significantly improved glycaemic control as indicated by a significant decrease in glycated haemoglobin levels of 0.6% (–0.6 % HbA1c, 95%CI –0.9 to –0.3; $P < 0.05$), reduced visceral adipose tissue, plasma triglycerides but not cholesterol levels.[73]

Of interest, studies indicate aerobic and resistance training alone improves glycaemic control in T2DM, but improvements were greatest with a combined exercise training of both aerobic with resistance training.[74]

Tai chi

Tai chi is a Chinese system of slow meditative physical exercise designed for relaxation, balance and health. Tai chi has demonstrated improved balance, gait speed, muscle strength, cardiorespiratory fitness, and quality of life in older adults.[75–80]

However, recent studies including a systematic review have demonstrated that there is some controversy as to its efficacy for patients with T2DM.[81]

Recently reported RCTs have demonstrated a change in fasting blood glucose levels.[79–82] One RCT demonstrated no significant intergroup differences in fasting blood glucose levels compared with a placebo intervention.[83]

One Chinese clinical trial[84] reported superior effects of tai chi on fasting blood glucose levels compared with walking or running, while 2 other Chinese clinical trials[85, 86] reported that there was no difference compared with a self-management program, or no treatment.

Three clinical trials reported assessing the effectiveness of tai chi on HbA1c.[83, 84, 85] Of these only 1 RCT[85] suggested no effectiveness of tai chi on HbA1c compared with a sham exercise regimen whereas 2 Chinese clinical trials[83, 84] failed to report intergroup differences compared with no treatment, self-management, walking or running exercise activities. One recent Chinese clinical trial with women diagnosed with T2DM reported that the tai chi group had significantly improved glycaemic control and serum triglyceride levels.[86]

Qigong

Qigong is another Chinese health practice that is associated with a system of healing and energy medicine. Preliminary studies show positive effects for qigong and reflexology in T2DM.[87, 88]

A recent review has concluded that although qigong has beneficial effects on some of the metabolic risk factors for T2DM, there exist methodologic limitations that hence make it difficult to draw firm conclusions about the purported benefits.[89] Further clinical trials are warranted.

Further, a recent clinical study adds significant strength to the role of tai chi and/or qigong in the management of the metabolic syndrome and glycaemic control in pre-T2DM.[90]

Yoga

There are few studies that have investigated the efficacy of yoga in T2DM.

Three small studies from India have demonstrated and suggested that yoga asanas and pranayama can better manage glycaemic control and stabilise autonomic functions in T2DM cases.[91, 92, 93] Moreover, in 1 of these studies it was reported that yoga improved sub-clinical neuropathy.[93]

A recent community-based study of yoga classes for T2DM aimed to demonstrate benefits of yoga for diabetic patients but unfortunately experienced 'recruitment challenges; practical and motivational barriers to class attendance; physical and motivational barriers to engaging in the exercises; inadequate intensity and/or duration of yoga intervention; and insufficient personalisation of exercises to individual needs' and these factors need to be considered in any future research.[94] It also highlights how research in yoga can be difficult.

A systematic review of the literature identified 25 eligible studies, including 15 uncontrolled trials, 6 non-RCTs and 4 RCTs. Overall, the studies demonstrate yoga showing benefit in several risk indices, including 'glucose tolerance and insulin sensitivity, lipid profiles, anthropometric characteristics, blood pressure, oxidative stress, coagulation profiles, sympathetic activation and pulmonary function, as well as improvement in specific clinical outcomes'.[95] Again, the authors acknowledge the limitations of these studies when drawing firm conclusions and encourage additional high-quality trials to confirm the benefits of yoga in diabetics.[95]

Diet and nutrition

For both Type 1 and Type 2DM, a low-GI diet can 'improve glycaemic control in diabetes without compromising hypoglycaemic events' according to a recent Cochrane review of the literature of 11 relevant RCTs involving 402 participants, although no study reported on mortality, morbidity or costs.[96] Low glycaemic diet led to a significant decrease in the glycated haemoglobin A1c (HbA1c) and less episodes of hypoglycaemia compared to high GI diet.[96]

T1DM

It is clear from the extensive literature, high dietary GI food affects HbA1c and glycaemic control in patients with T1DM. Patients with T1DM should be under the care and supervision of a dietician and diabetes educator to help fine tune their diet.

A study of 1776 young children (less than 11.5 years of age) who were at increased risk of genetic type 1 diabetes demonstrated that high dietary GI (hazard ratio [HR]: 2.20, 95% CI: 1.17–4.15) and high glycaemic load (HR: 1.59, 95% CI: 0.96–2.64) were associated with rapid progression of islet autoimmunity (IA) to T1DM. Furthermore it was reported that this was possible due to an increased demand on pancreas beta-cell release of insulin and that the development of IA was not associated with high GI foods.[97]

High fish consumption in the diet may also play an important role in the prevention of T1DM onset. A 12-year study reported a diet rich in omega-3 oils, primarily from fish and other seafood, can reduce the chances of high-risk children developing pancreatic islet beta cell autoimmunity and T1DM by up to 55%. The researchers speculated that omega-3 fatty acids may accentuate T-helper 1 activity associated with autoimmunity and its anti-inflammatory effects may contribute to its benefits.[98]

A recent study of 532 people over a 5-year period demonstrated that diets high in fat, saturated fat and lower in carbohydrates were associated with worse glycaemic control in T1DM, independent of exercise and BMI.[99]

T2DM

A low GI diet is as effective as medication in improving glycaemic control in diabetics. Patients with T2DM should be under the care of a dietician or diabetic educator to continually monitor their diet. Dietary compliance is fundamental in the management of T2DM.[100]

A recent study has reported that in those individuals that are at risk for developing T2DM a change in lifestyle that includes dietary manipulation with a significant decrease in fat intake and a concomitant increase in vegetable and fruit consumption resulted in marked inhibition of the transition from the pre-diabetic state to manifest T2DM.[40]

It has been documented that a diet rich in wholegrains and seafood will be high in magnesium.[41, 101]

There is a strong inverse relationship to T2DM with magnesium.[102] Also, such diets may be protective against the development of T2DM.[103] Wholegrain intake is inversely associated with homocysteine and markers of glycaemic control, and studies suggest a lower risk of diabetes and heart disease in persons who consume diets high in wholegrains.[104]

Foods rich in soluble fibre such as oats, legumes, guar gum and psyllium are more slowly absorbed and produce lower blood glucose levels.[105] Increasing dietary fibre up to 50g daily (such as raisins and oranges) can improve glycaemic control in patients with T2DM.[106] There is increasing evidence that inflammation plays an important role in the pathogenesis of diabetes, as obesity is associated with a pro-inflammatory state.[107]

A Cochrane review that investigated the potential effects of wholegrain foods for the prevention of T2DM has concluded that studies have consistently demonstrated that a high intake of wholegrain foods or cereal fibre is associated with a lower risk of the development of T2DM.[108] However, the evidence for a protective effect coming from prospective cohort studies only has to be considered as weak as with this design no cause and effect relationship could be recognised. Hence, it was further concluded that well-designed RCTs are warranted that are able to draw definite conclusions about the preventive effects of wholegrain consumption on the development of T2DM.[108]

Fish

Fish is protective towards the development of T2DM apart from having a number of health benefits by preventing cardiovascular disease. In a study of insulin-resistant participants, a high fish diet improved insulin sensitivity compared with participants not eating fish.[109] Greater fish intake was associated with a lower risk of macroalbuminuria in a self-defined diabetic population.[109]

An anti-inflammatory diet can include fish, nuts, flaxseeds, fruits and vegetables, ginger and turmeric.[110, 111] Partially hydrogenated oils, as in vegetable oils and margarines, are pro-inflammatory and can increase the risk of T2DM.[112]

Other protective foods

Garlic, green tea, chilli and onions have all been shown to have beneficial effects in DM. Onion and garlic can decrease blood glucose, cholesterol and blood pressure.[113, 114]

Two RCTs have found that supplementation with soy protein in T2DM improves fasting insulin, insulin resistance, total and low-density lipoprotein (LDL) cholesterol,[115, 116, 117] which also showed soy improved glucose control. They also found that regular consumption of chilli could attenuate postprandial hyperinsulinemia.[118]

Diets with low GI and glycaemic load will modulate swings in blood glucose levels and insulin secretion because of slower absorption and have been shown to improve haemoglobin A1c (HbA1c).[115]

Other food considerations

Rice consumption

There are also cultural dietary differences that may contribute to high prevalence of diabetes in specific population groups. For instance, in a cohort of 64 227 Chinese women with no history of diabetes or other chronic disease over a 4.6 year period the authors noted dietary carbohydrate intake and consumption of rice (high GI and load) was positively associated with increased risk of developing T2DM.[119]

Sugary drinks

Sugary drinks, including artificially sweetened beverages that are energy-dense and nutrient poor, are contributing to obesity and the diabetic epidemic seen in Western societies.

T2DM is a common problem amongst African American women. A prospective follow-up study of 59 000 African American women reported on food and beverage consumption between 1995 and 2001 and found, after adjusting for relevant confounders such as BMI, the incidence of T2DM was associated with higher intake of both sugar-sweetened soft drinks and fruit drinks. Two or more soft drinks per day increased the risk by 1.24 (95% confidence interval, 1.06–1.45) and for fruit drinks, the comparable incidence rate ratio was 1.31 (95% CI, 1.13–1.52).[120]

Artificial flavours

A recent animal study with rats found foods using artificial sweeteners resulted in 'increased caloric intake, increased body weight, and increased adiposity, as well as diminished caloric compensation and blunted thermic responses to sweet-tasting diets'. These results suggest that consumption of foods containing artificial sweeteners may lead to increased body weight and obesity, and so should be avoided.[121]

Meat intake

High intake of red meat significantly increases the risk of fatal coronary heart disease (CHD) in women with T2DM. Women who consumed the highest levels of haeme iron and red meat also had a 50% increased risk of developing CHD compared with women who consumed the lowest intake.[122]

Low fat dairy intake

A large scale prospective women's health study of 37 183 middle-aged non-diabetic women found low fat dairy and yoghurt consumption significantly reduced the risk of developing T2DM.[123]

A diet rich in low fat dairy food in T2DM helps reduce weight in the overweight and the researchers found no association between dairy calcium intake and other diabetes or CVD disease indexes.[124]

Vegetarian, plant-based diet

A review of the literature demonstrates a strong link between vegetarian and plant-based diets in reducing the risk of obesity, T2DM, heart disease and some cancers.[125] A diet high in vegetables and vegetarianism can significantly reduce the risk of diabetes, improve glycaemic and lipid control and reduce cardiovascular complications.[126, 127]

Body weight

Obesity is the main predisposing risk factor for the development of diabetes.[128]

The prevalence of obesity varies among different racial groups and it is associated with approximately 30% of Chinese and Japanese patients with T2DM. Obesity is found in 60–70% of people in Western countries and, although estimates vary, it is thought that the prevalence of T2DM could be as high as 30% of aboriginal people.[129] Pima Indians, Pacific Islanders from Nauru or Samoa will all almost certainly develop T2DM with obesity.[130]

In a study of 1079 participants, intensive lifestyle intervention for overweight patients with impaired glucose tolerance reduced the 3-year incidence of overt T2DM from 35% to 15% by losing 5 kg compared with the control intervention. Every 1 kg of weight loss resulted in a relative risk reduction of developing TSDM by 16%.[131]

A number of dietary regimes have been recently reported as alternatives for macronutrient intake and the prevention of chronic diseases.[132] A comparative study that included the macronutrient contents of 7-day menu plans from the Omni-Heart Study, Dietary Approaches to Stop Hypertension (DASH), Zone, Atkins, Mediterranean, South Beach, and Ornish diets were evaluated for consistency with the US Food and Nutrition Board's Acceptable Macronutrient Distribution Ranges and with the dietary recommendations of several health organisations for the prevention of cardiovascular disease, cancer and metabolic syndrome. The intent of the study/analysis was to evaluate the healthfulness of the 3 Omni-Heart Trial diets high-carbohydrate (Omni-Carb), high-protein (Omni-Protein), and high unsaturated fat (Omni-Unsat) diets — and were compared with that of the DASH diet and 5 other popular diets, namely the Atkins, Ornish, South Beach, Mediterranean, and Zone diets. The resultant analysis reported that all 3 Omni study diets were consistent with US national guidelines to reduce chronic disease risk. Further, that, popular diets vary in their nutritional adequacy and consistency with guidelines for risk reduction.[132]

There is also significantly strong evidence that special diets can substantially reduce the risk of developing T2DM.

The Mediterranean diet

The Mediterranean diet with its emphasis on vegetables, grains, fish and olive oil has been shown to reduce the risk of atherosclerosis in diabetic patients.[133, 134] There is a significant amount of evidence that strongly suggests that the Mediterranean diet could serve as an anti-inflammatory dietary pattern.[135] This could help prevent diseases that are related to chronic inflammations that include visceral obesity, T2DM and the metabolic syndrome.[135] The rationale for this evidence is further supported by a recent study that demonstrates that adherence to the Mediterranean diet is inversely associated with risk of developing diabetes and the clustering of hypertension, diabetes, obesity, and hypercholesterolemia among high-risk patients.[136, 137]

Monounsaturated fatty acids (MUFA) — olive oil and nuts

The MUFA (especially olive oil) in the Mediterranean diet appear to play an important preventative role for T2DM, even in healthy subjects. Insulin sensitivity reduced in healthy subjects on diets high in MUFA compared with diets high in saturated fatty acid. Subjects with the Ala 54 allele of the fatty acid-binding protein 2 gene demonstrated improved insulin sensitivity when the saturated fats were replaced by the MUFA.[137]

High content of MUFA found for instance in the Mediterranean diet may explain the preventative role in reducing insulin resistance leading to T2DM.

A large prospective cohort study involving over 83 000 university graduates without diabetes at baseline demonstrated high adherence to the Mediterranean diet with an 83% reduced risk of developing T2DM.[138]

Consumption of nuts and peanuts is related inversely with diabetes risk.[139] Nuts may also confer cardiovascular benefit and improve lipid profile for patients with T2DM due to their high content of MUFA and nutritional value.[140]

After 6 months of adding 30g of walnut to a low-fat diet of T2DM patients, compared with those on no walnuts, the LDL cholesterol dropped by 10% and HDL cholesterol increased.[141]

(Refer to Table 13.4.)[142]

The Palaeolithic diet

A randomised control study of 29 patients with ischaemic heart disease plus either glucose intolerance or T2DM were randomised to receive (1) a Palaeolithic ('Old Stone Age') diet based on lean meat, fish, fruit, vegetables, root vegetables, eggs and nuts or (2) a Mediterranean-like diet based on wholegrains, low-fat dairy products, vegetables, fruits, fish, oils and margarines. The study demonstrated that the Palaeolithic diet — the basis of diet by humans before the introduction of grains, dairy, salt and refined fats and sugars — improved glucose tolerance with a 26% decrease of GI compared with 7% decrease in patients on the Mediterranean diet and independent of waist circumference.[143]

The Ornish diet

The Ornish diet was originally designed as a therapy to reverse cardiovascular disease and is also applicable to patients with diabetes. The Ornish diet consists of a low fat, high fibre, basically vegetarian diet with 75% of the kilojoules (calories) obtained from carbohydrates.[144–146]

Critical components of the Ornish dietary plan also include physical activity, yoga and relaxation therapy. In a group of T2DM patients requiring insulin who had adhered to the plan, 60% no longer required insulin at the end of the study.[144]

Caffeine

A systematic review of the literature identified coffee consumption as being protective towards the development of T2DM, reducing the risk by up to 35%.[147]

A large-scale longitudinal study demonstrated a significant reduction in incidence of glucose intolerance and T2DM of up to 64% in white middle-class people who drank regular coffee consumption compared with people who never drank coffee.[148] This benefit persisted in those even after ceasing coffee consumption.

Similarly, another large-scale population-based study of approximately 2400 subjects found that coffee consumption was found to be significantly and inversely associated with fasting glucose, 2-hour plasma glucose, and fasting insulin in both men and women compared with non-drinkers of coffee.[149]

A prospective, community-based cohort of 12 204 non-diabetic, middle-aged men and women assessed risk of caffeine consumption as part of the Atherosclerosis Risk in Communities (ARIC) Study. After adjusting for potential confounders, increased coffee consumption was significantly associated with a decreased risk of diagnosed T2DM in community-based US adults.[150]

Cocoa

Based on epidemiological data, diets rich in flavanols are associated with reduced cardiovascular risk and may play a role in reversing vascular dysfunction in diabetics. Cocoa is rich in flavanols. In a study of

Table 13.4 Healthy fats for diabetics' monounsaturated fats

Oils and margarines	Vegetables	Nuts
Canola, olive, macadamia, sunflower oil, peanut	Avocados, olives	Almonds, peanuts, cashews, hazelnuts, macadamias, pecans
Polyunsaturated fats:		
Oils and margarines	**Fish and other seafood**	**Nuts and seeds**
Sunflower, safflower, corn, soybean, sesame, cottonseed, grapeseed, flaxseed oil or linseed	Canned: sardines, salmon, mackerel Fresh: Atlantic salmon, tuna, mullet, gemfish, trevally, snook, flathead, calamari	Walnuts, pine nuts, brazil nuts, sesame seeds, sunflower seeds, flaxseed or linseed

(Source: adapted from Phillips & Carapetis.)[142]

41 medicated diabetic patients over a 30-day period, dietary intervention with flavanol-rich cocoa (321mg flavanols per dose) significantly increased circulating flavanols, vascular function and flow-mediated dilation of the brachial artery compared with a nutrient-matched control (25mg flavanols per dose). The benefits of flavanol-rich cocoa (321mg flavanols per dose) were dose dependent up to 3 times daily.[151]

Alcohol

A large-scale US cross-sectional study of 32 000 people found an inverse relationship between alcohol intake and glycaemic control. On average, T2DM patients who drank alcohol in moderate amounts had HbA1c levels 1.2 less than non-drinkers.[152]

A multicenter trial randomly assigned 109 patients (41–74 years old) with T2DM who abstained from alcohol to receive 150 ml wine (13g alcohol) at dinner or non-alcoholic diet beer (control) each day during a 3-month period. The study found initiation of moderate daily alcohol consumption reduced fasting plasma glucose but not postprandial glucose and improved sleep in T2DM patients. The authors concluded alcohol may have a favourable glycaemic effect on HbA1c. There were no significant changes on liver function tests.[153]

Nutritional supplements

Vitamins

Antioxidant micronutrients may play a role in the prevention of diabetic complications.[154]

Vitamin C

A large population study has reported an inverse relationship between serum vitamin C levels and HbA1c.[155] Vitamin C also improves endothelium-dependent vasodilatation in T2DM.[156] A recently reported trial on the combined use of chromium and vitamins C and E as well as chromium on its own was effective for reducing metabolic dysfunction and improvement of glucose metabolism in T2DM patients.[157]

A study of 84 patients with T2DM were randomly assigned to either 500mgs or 1000mgs of vitamin C for 6 weeks. Whilst the dose of 500mgs daily vitamin C had no impact on blood parameters, the group taking 1000mgs of vitamin C daily demonstrated significant decrease in fasting blood sugars, triglyceride and LDL cholesterol levels, HbA1c and serum insulin. These results suggest 1000mgs vitamin C may be beneficial for patients with T2DM and reducing the risk of complication.[158]

A recent Cochrane review has concluded that there were no relevant clinical trials identified for the effective treatment diabetic eye disease with vitamin C and superoxide dismutase.[159]

Vitamin E

Vitamin E has been reported to be useful in preventing the long-term complications of diabetes through its synergistic antioxidant effect with vitamin C, improvement of insulin sensitivity and reduction of LDL cholesterol oxidation.[160] Vitamin E also has been reported in an early study to reduce platelet aggregation and hence the risk of thrombosis.[161]

Vitamin D and calcium

Our best source of vitamin D is from direct sun exposure.

Vitamin D deficiency is common in T1 and T2DM has been shown to alter insulin synthesis and secretion in animal models of the disease, a result that has also been demonstrated in humans.[53, 162]

There is a significant body of biologically plausible evidence that strongly suggests that vitamin D plays a role in the prevention of T1DM and T2DM development and management.[53, 163]

Furthermore, a recent meta-analysis of the literature has noted an increased association between vitamin D and calcium deficiency and postulate combined supplementation with both nutrients may be beneficial in optimising glucose metabolism in both T1DM and T2DM.[49, 164]

This meta-analysis of data from case-controlled studies demonstrated the risk of T1DM in infants who were supplemented with vitamin D was significantly reduced compared with those who were not. This effect was dose-dependent.

Vitamin D supplementation is increasingly being recognised for its ability to improve glycaemic control.

Vitamin B1 thiamine

A recent randomised placebo-controlled pilot study has demonstrated that high dose thiamine supplementation may be beneficial for patients diagnosed with T2DM.[165] This small pilot study compared a thiamine supplement administered at a dose of 300mg per day for 3 months to placebo. There was a 2-month washout follow-up. The primary endpoint was a change in urinary albumin excretion. Other markers of renal and vascular dysfunction and plasma concentrations of thiamine were also determined. The study concluded that high-dose thiamine therapy produced a regression of urinary albumin excretion in T2DM patients with microalbuminuria. Thiamine supplements at high dose could provide improved therapy for early-stage diabetic nephropathy. There was, however, no effects observed in glycaemic control, dyslipidaemia or blood pressure. There were no reported adverse effects due to thiamine therapy.[165]

Vitamin B3 nicotinic acid

A 16 week trial of 148 patients trialled on low dose extended nicotinic acid of 1000 milligrams and 1500md/day and when compared with placebo led to increases in HDL cholesterol by 19 and 24% and reduction in triglycerides by 13 and 28% respectively, with only a slight reduction of LDL cholesterol with the higher dose.[166] Nicotinic acid may play a role in diabetics for lipid management. Only 1 subject withdrew from the trial due to flushing from nicotinic acid.

Vitamin K

Vitamin K may be potentially beneficial for insulin resistance. A trial assessing the role of vitamin K supplementation (500 μg/d of phylloquinone) on bone loss, also found that Vitamin K supplementation for 36 months at doses attainable in the diet may reduce progression of insulin resistance in older men, but not women.[167]

Vitamin B12

Whilst vegan diets may help in the prevention and management of T2DM, there is a risk of patients developing vitamin B12 deficiency especially those taking metformin which interferes with vitamin B12 absorption.[168]

The risk for vitamin B12 deficiency was accentuated with prolong metformin use or when used in higher doses. Patients on metformin should have their vitamin B12 levels checked annually. The situation is magnified in diabetics on vegan diets, coupled with metformin use needing to have their vitamin B12 levels carefully monitored.[169]

Vitamin E

Vitamin E may reduce the risk of diabetic neuropathy and retinopathy in a small trial of diabetic patients and prevent vascular complications in diabetics. More research is warranted.[170, 171]

Multivitamin/mineral supplements

Elevated C–reactive protein levels have been associated with the risk of cardiovascular disease and T2DM. An analysis of the data from a randomised, double-blind, placebo-controlled study was carried out at the end of the trial and it was reported that multivitamin use was associated with lower C–reactive protein levels.[172] Recently, it was demonstrated in an RCT that the effects of vitamins C and E, and also when in combination with magnesium and zinc, were a significant improvement of glomerular, but not tubular, renal function in T2DM patients.[173] Furthermore, in randomised placebo-control trials after 3 months of using the combined multivitamin and mineral supplements, the treatment group had significant increased HDL cholesterol and apolipoproteins (apo) A1 enzyme levels, and reduced blood pressure in T2DM patients but no change in serum levels of total cholesterol, LDL cholesterol, triglyceride, and apo B levels. This suggests that the multivitamin and mineral supplements may have a favourable cardiovascular benefit by raising HDL levels and reducing blood pressure in T2DM. Supplementation with vitamin C and E and Zn when used alone did not show any benefit.[174, 175]

Other studies have not been able to demonstrate any benefit of antioxidants on fasting blood glucose levels in T2DM.[176]

Middle-aged and elderly patients with T2DM experienced a significant reduction of infections such as flu-like illnesses respiratory, gastrointestinal and urinary tract infections, and days off work (17% of diabetics) in those who took a daily multivitamin supplement compared with those who took placebo (90% of diabetics).[177] Researchers postulated patients with diabetes were more likely to have suboptimal intake of micronutrients which would explain the positive effect.

Diabetics should be educated about the importance of consuming adequate amounts of vitamins and minerals from natural food sources.

Minerals

Chromium

Chromium has been the most widely studied supplement for diabetes as it is essential for the metabolism of glucose and blood lipids by the body. Low levels of chromium are associated with increased risk of T2DM.[178]

Numerous *in vitro* and *in vivo* studies suggest that chromium supplements, particularly niacin-bound chromium or chromium-nicotinate may be effective in attenuating insulin resistance and lowering plasma cholesterol levels.[179] Chromium functions as a co-factor for insulin, regulating the activity of insulin. It has been reported that T2DM patients, who are chromium-deficient, are likely to benefit from chromium supplementation.[180–189]

A recent review has concluded that there was no significant effect of chromium on lipid or glucose metabolism observed in people without diabetes.[190] However, chromium supplementation significantly improved glycaemia among patients with diabetes.[190] A further review reported that there was greater bioavailability of chromium picolinate compared with other forms of chromium, such as niacin-bound or chromium trichloride. This may explain the comparative superior efficacy in glycemic and lipidemic control.[191] The pooled data from the studies that were investigated that used chromium picolinate supplementation for T2DM patients demonstrated substantial reductions in hyperglycaemia and hyperinsulinemia, which then equates to a significant reduced risk for disease complications.[191] Collectively, the data supported the safety and therapeutic value of chromium picolinate for the management of cholesterolemia and hyperglycaemia in those patients diagnosed with T2DM.[191]

Recent studies with selected populations presenting with insulin resistance have also reported significant benefits with chromium picolinate supplementation either alone or in combination with biotin.[192–195] In 1 study it was reported that 1000 μg/day of chromium picolinate therapy improved insulin resistance in some HIV-positive patients, however, highlighting that extra caution was warranted in this population.[192] Chromium in combination with biotin may have a beneficial effect on reducing atherosclerosis in patients with T2DM.[196]

Moreover, clinical trials suggest positive effects of chromium in T2DM patients with hypercholesterolaemia, with hypercholesterolemic patients (prescribed statins), moderately obese to obese T2DM patients (prescribed anti glycemic medications) benefited significantly from the combined use of chromium picolinate and biotin[190, 194, 195, 196] as ascertained by improved blood lipid and glucose profiles.

There have also been negative findings of chromium on T2DM. A double-blind trial of chromium picolinate 800mcg/day showed no difference in impaired glucose tolerance progression compared with placebo[197] and a systematic review of the literature found chromium had no effect on glucose or insulin concentrations in non-diabetics and was inconclusive for diabetics.[198]

Magnesium

Magnesium is the second most abundant intracellular divalent cation and has been established as a cofactor for over 300 metabolic reactions in the body.[199] Magnesium is also essential in glucose metabolism.[199] Magnesium deficiency is common in patients with diabetes[200–204] and a growing body of research suggests a significant inverse association between magnesium intake and diabetes risk.[205–214]

A meta-analysis of prospective cohort studies including more than 286 000 subjects demonstrated that magnesium dietary intake, either dietary or supplemental magnesium (100mg daily), were equally inversely associated with significantly reducing incidence of T2DM and suggest increased consumption of magnesium-rich foods such as wholegrains, beans, nuts, and green leafy vegetables may reduce the risk of T2DM.[202] In another meta-analysis study of the literature, dietary fibre especially high in cereal fibre and magnesium intake is strongly associated with reduced risk of T2DM. The meta-analysis incorporating data from 9 cohort studies on fibre intake and 8 from magnesium intake, showed 33% reduction in diabetes risk with high cereal intake and 23% reduction of diabetes risk with magnesium intake.[215] Another meta-analysis has confirmed this finding.[216]

Magnesium intake is clearly inversely correlated with the risk of developing T2DM.[216–222]

Two large prospective epidemiological studies,[202, 203] demonstrated that magnesium had a significant inverse association between magnesium intake and T2DM. Moreover, 2 RCTs[223, 224] with magnesium supplementation reported that significant reduced homeostasis model analysis for insulin resistance (HOMA-IR) index compared to controls on 1 study (2.5 gm/day for 12 weeks versus placebo)[223] and significantly improved insulin sensitivity and metabolic control (lower HOMA-IR index), lower fasting blood glucose levels, and lower HbA1c compared to controls in the other (50 gm of magnesium chloride/1,000mL of solution for 16 weeks versus placebo).[224]

Zinc

The mineral zinc plays a key role in the synthesis and action of insulin, both physiologically and in T2DM. Zinc seems to stimulate insulin action and insulin receptor tyrosine kinase activity.[225]

Diabetics excrete more zinc in their urine than normal amounts [224] and often serum zinc levels are lower in diabetic patients than in healthy controls.[226] A number of studies indicate oral supplementation of zinc can improve T2DM and metabolic syndromes and reduce cardiovascular and neurological complications.[226–231] A double-blind placebo-controlled study of T2DM patients who received either zinc sulfate (30mg elemental zinc daily) or placebo for 3 months found the treatment group demonstrated elevated zinc levels, improved glycaemic control as evidenced by a decrease in HbA1c levels.[226] Patients diagnosed with T2DM have demonstrated less metabolic dysfunctions when supplemented with 30mg of zinc daily.[231, 232]

A Cochrane review has concluded that there were no significant differences favouring people receiving zinc supplementation compared to placebo. Hence there is no evidence to suggest that the use of zinc supplementation is effective in the prevention of T2DM.[233]

Vanadium

A number of *in vitro* studies demonstrate vanadium salts to mimic the effects of insulin on main target tissues of the hormone, and in animal studies vanadium can induce a sustained fall in blood glucose levels in insulin-deficient diabetic rats, and improve glucose homeostasis in obese, insulin-resistant diabetic rodents suggesting therapeutic potential of vanadium salts in the treatment of T2DM.[234, 235]

References and further reading may be available for these articles by Brichard and Henquin,[234] and by Preet et al.[235]

Other supplements

Alpha lipoic acid

Alpha lipoic acid is a potent antioxidant which enhances glucose uptake, prevents glycosylation and is useful in diabetic neuropathy.[236] A recent meta-analysis has reported that treatment with alpha-lipoic acid (600mg/day IV) over 3 weeks was safe and significantly improved both positive neuropathic symptoms and neuropathic deficits to a clinically meaningful degree in T2DM patients with symptomatic polyneuropathy.[237]

Arginine — amino acid

L-Arginine is an essential amino acid that is used by endothelial cells to produce nitric oxide (NO). Disturbance of the arginine to NO pathway can lead to endothelial dysfunction, resulting in vascular wall damage and directly leading to cardiovascular risk factors such as atherosclerosis and hypertension. Factors that may disturb this pathway include inflammation caused by insulin resistance, hyperglycaemia, elevated visceral fat, smoking and high cholesterol. Studies also indicate that arginine supplementation may benefit patients with cardiovascular risk factors by improving small vessel endothelial function.[238–240]

Research suggests oral supplementation with up to 3g of arginine can help to restore endothelial function and improve insulin sensitivity. For instance, a double-blind trial on T2DM patients demonstrated that a dose of 3g of arginine 3 times daily over 1 month improved cardiovascular risk and insulin sensitivity significantly as evidenced by an increase in baseline forearm blood flow by 36%, increased glucose disposal by 34%, reduced systolic blood pressure by 14% and reduced endogenous glucose production by 29%.[241]

Coenzyme Q_{10} (CoQ_{10})

CoQ_{10} may improve glycaemic control and insulin requirement in patients with T1DM and also blood pressure control in patients with T2DM.[242, 243]

A recent double-blind crossover study of 23 statin-treated T2DM patients with LDL cholesterol <2.5mmol/L and endothelial dysfunction (brachial artery flow-mediated dilatation [FMD] <5.5%) were randomised to oral CoQ_{10} 200mg/day or placebo for 12 weeks. Compared with placebo, CoQ_{10} supplementation increased brachial artery FMD, improving endothelial dysfunction in statin-treated T2DM patients, possibly by altering local vascular oxidative stress.[244]

Fish oils and/or omega-3 fatty acid

A trial of 162 healthy individuals randomly assigned to a 3-month diet rich in monounsaturated fats or saturated fats and a second group randomisation to fish oil (n-3 fatty acids 3.6 g/day or placebo) found fish oil supplements or high dietary intake of n-6 and n-3 fatty acids of did not affect insulin sensitivity, insulin secretion, *beta*-cell function or glucose tolerance.[245]

It is more likely a diet high in fish and fish oil supplements play a more important role in prevention of complications related to diabetes.

Type 1 DM

Supplementing the diets of children who are at increased risk of developing T1DM with omega-3 fatty acid may reduce the risk by up to 37% by helping to prevent the development of autoimmune antibodies towards islet cell within the pancreas.[246]

Type 2 DM

A review of the literature inclusive of 18 randomised trials explored the use of fish oil supplementation in patients with T2DM as they are at increased risk of cardiovascular disease.[247] Whilst blood sugar levels were not affected, the meta-analysis demonstrated a statistically significant effect of fish oil in lowering triglycerides by 0.56mmol/l (95% CI, -0.71 to -0.40mmol/l) and raising LDL cholesterol by 0.21mmol/l (95% CI, 0.02 to 0.41mmol/l). No effect was seen on HbA1c, total or HDL cholesterol. Despite these findings fish oil supplementation may still play a role in patients with T2DM as it has a clear preventative role in patients with cardiovascular disease risk factors according to the National Heart Foundation of Australia.[248] A recent Cochrane review[249] has concluded that although some types of fat in the blood are reduced through omega-3 fatty acid supplementation, others including LDL cholesterol were increased. A concern as it may predispose to CV disease. Moreover, the control of blood sugar levels was not affected by the treatment.

Herbal medicines

A systematic review of the published literature on the efficacy and safety of herbal therapies and vitamin/mineral supplements for glucose control in patients with diabetes identified a total of 108 trials examining 36 herbs (single or in combination) and 9 vitamin/mineral supplements, involving 4565 patients with diabetes or impaired glucose tolerance.[250] There were 58 controlled clinical trials involving individuals with mostly T2DM or impaired glucose tolerance. The direction of the evidence for the 58 trials was for improved glucose control positive in 76% (44 of 58) with very few adverse effects reported. The authors conclude that there is still insufficient evidence to draw definitive conclusions about the efficacy of individual herbs and supplements for diabetes but several supplements warrant further study. The review identified the best evidence for efficacy from adequately designed RCTs is available for *Coccinia indica* (Ivy gourd) and *Panax quinquefolius* (American ginseng). Other herbs with positive preliminary results include *Gymnema sylvestre*, *Aloe vera*, *Momordica charantia* (bitter melon), and nopal (prickly pear cactus).[250]

Metformin

The popular anti-diabetic drug metformin, a biguanide (oral antihyperglycemic), was developed from the French herb lilac or Goat's rue (*Galega officinalis*).

American ginseng (*Panax quinquefolius*)

Doses of 1–3g of American ginseng reduced postprandial glycaemia, fasting glucose and HbA1c in healthy and T2DM subjects in 2 trials.[251, 252]

Korean or Asian Red Ginseng (*Panax ginseng*)

Numerous studies have demonstrated the benefits of *Panax ginseng* as a potential to improve diabetic control. A randomised control trial (RCT) of T2DM who received 2g of ginseng 6 times daily (6g/day) 40 minutes before meals, improved glycaemic control, glucose and insulin levels compared with placebo.[253]

Korean and American ginseng are known to possess sulfonylurea-like activity.

Cinnamon

Cinnamon has been reported to enhance insulin sensitivity.[254] Cinnamon has also been reported to improve blood glucose, triglyceride, HDL cholesterol and LDL cholesterol levels.[255] Chromium and polyphenols from cinnamon may explain its potential benefit for diabetes and improving insulin resistance.[256]

A recent meta-analysis reported on 5 RCTs that had reported data on HbA1c, fasting blood glucose or lipid parameters.[257] The prospective RCTs[258–262] covered 282 participants and it was concluded that the use of cinnamon did not significantly alter on HbA1c, fasting blood glucose or lipid parameters.

Despite these findings a recent small study demonstrated that cinnamon could play an important role as a dietary supplement for poorly controlled diabetics. Ingestion of 3g of cinnamon on 300g of rice pudding daily reduced serum insulin levels after mealtime and increased the concentration of glucagon-like peptide 1 (GLP–1) in 15 healthy Swedish men (n = 9) and women (n = 6) when compared with 1g or no cinnamon after a period of fasting.[263]

Gymnema silvestre

Preliminary studies support the use of *Gymnema silvestre*.[264, 265] *Gymnema silvestre* has been reported to suppress sweet taste in liquid form, which can result in reduced calorie consumption.[264–273]

Fenugreek *(Trigonella foenum)*

This herb is a soluble fibre and hence slows gastric emptying, delaying glucose absorption. Fenugreek also raises the rate of insulin release plus increasing insulin sensitivity.[274] There is an extensive body of *in vitro* and *in vivo* animal evidence for the biological plausible effect of fenugreek in controlling blood glucose levels.[273–306]

Fenugreek seeds has been documented to lower fasting blood glucose in both T1 and T2DM compared to controls.[306, 307] Reduction in triglyceride levels has also been noted.[307]

Bitter melon *(Momordica charantia)*

Bitter melon grows in tropical areas, including parts of the Amazon, east Africa, Asia, and the Caribbean, and is cultivated throughout South America as a food and medicine. It has a long history of traditional use as a hypoglycaemic, antibacterial and as a bitter digestive aid for intestinal gas, bloating, stomach ache and for intestinal parasites. All parts of the plant, including the fruit, taste very bitter. It is a common food in Asian cooking.

Bitter melon has been documented to contain several insulin-like polypeptides with other substances that lower glucose levels and it also has been reported to increase insulin sensitivity.[308] Moreover, it has been in involved regulating glucose uptake in the jejunum and stimulates glucose uptake into skeletal muscle.

A number of clinical and preclinical trials have documented the hypoglycaemic effects of bitter lemon in T2DM.[309] A recent small controlled RCT trial with outpatients who were either newly diagnosed or poorly controlled T2DM with HbA1c levels between 7% and 9% were randomised to either bitter melon capsules or placebo in addition to standard therapy. The study targeted a 1% decline in HbA1c at the outset with an estimated power of 88%. With the observed decline of 0.24%, the study achieved a power of only 11%. Hence no definite conclusions as to the effectiveness of bitter melon were possible.[310] Larger controlled studies though are warranted.

Green tea extract

There have been conflicting studies using green tea extract for T2DM. One study demonstrated favourable effects with a green tea extract demonstrating a significant reduction of haemoglobin A1c levels and borderline reduction in diastolic blood pressure in patients with T2DM.[311]

Another study found green tea extract in obese middle-aged male subjects had no effect on insulin sensitivity, insulin secretion or glucose tolerance, but did reduce diastolic blood pressure and had a positive effect on mood.[312]

Ginkgo *(Ginkgo biloba)*

Whilst it is not clear if ginkgo may help T2DM, and there have been mixed results on insulin sensitivity in animal studies, the herb may have a cardiovascular benefit for patients.[313–331]

Ginkgo is recognised to assist in improving peripheral circulation and intermittent claudication and some studies suggest it may play a role in alleviating early diabetic neuropathic pain.[330, 331]

Other potentially hypoglycaemic herbal medicines

The following herbal medicines may also be useful in the treatment of T2DM. These include bilberry, milk thistle, pycnogenol, *Inolter*, *Ginkgo biloba*, aloe vera, ginseng, mulberry, chamomile, cranberry, Chinese herbal medicines, Tibetan herbal medicine[332] and red clover isoflavone although more studies are required.[319, 331–336]

Chinese herbal medicine

Chinese herbal medicines have been investigated in 2 recent systematic reviews for the treatment of T2DM.[337, 338] A Cochrane review[337] included 66 randomised trials that involved 8302 participants that met the inclusion criteria. Sixty-nine different Chinese herbal medicines were tested in the included trials, which compared herbal medicines with placebo, hypoglycaemic drugs, or herbal medicines plus hypoglycaemic drugs.

In the trials that compared herbs with placebo, *Holy basil leaves*, *Xianzhen Pian*, *Qidan Tongmai*, traditional Chinese formulae, *Huoxue Jiangtang Pingzhi*, and *Inolter* demonstrated a significant hypoglycaemic response. In the trials that compared herbs with hypoglycaemic drugs that included glibenclamide, tolbutamide, or gliclazide, 7 herbal medicines demonstrated a significant better metabolic control, including *Bushen Jiangtang Tang*, *Composite Trichosanthis*, *Jiangtang Kang*, *Ketang Ling*, *Shenqi Jiangtang Yin*, *Xiaoke Tang*, and *Yishen Huoxue Tiaogan*. In 29 trials that assessed herbal medicines combined with hypoglycaemic drugs, 15 different herbal preparations demonstrated additional enhanced effects than hypoglycaemic drugs monotherapy. Two herbal therapies combined with diet and behaviour change showed better hypoglycaemic effects than diet and behaviour change alone. No serious adverse effects from the herbal medicines were reported in these trials.[337] Generally methodological quality was reported to be of a low quality.

In a second review[338] it was reported that the use of Chinese herbal medicines for the treatment of T2DM was promising but there was a strong requisite for further studies.

Ayurvedic herbs

Ayurveda is a traditional healing system which originated in India. Some Ayurvedic herbs have glucose-lowering effects and deserve further study.[339] A systematic review of the literature identified 54 articles reporting the results of 62 studies. The most-studied herbs were *Gymnema sylvestre*, *Coccinia indica*, fenugreek, and *Eugenia jambolana*. A number of herbal formulas were tested, but Ayush-82 and D-400 were most often studied. There were large variations in the quality of the studies. Of the 10 RCTs, case-control trials or natural experiments included in the review, 12 were case series or cohort studies. The study concluded there was evidence to suggest that the following herbs *C. indica*, holy basil, fenugreek, and *G sylvestre*, and the herbal formulas Ayush-82 and D-400 had a glucose-lowering effect and that further studies were warranted.[340]

Other supplements

Psyllium and guar gum both contain soluble fibre, and have been reported to improve glucose levels, as well as lipid levels in T2DM.[341, 342]

Physical therapies

Reflexology

Reflexology (or zone therapy as it is also known) is the practice of massaging, squeezing, or pushing on parts of the feet, or the hands and ears, with the goal of encouraging a beneficial health effect on other parts of the body, thereby improving overall general health.[343] An early study[344] suggested that foot reflexo-therapy was an effective treatment for T2DM. However, a recent review of the scientific literature has concluded that there was no clinical evidence that reflexology had any beneficial effect on T2DM.[345]

T2DM peripheral neuropathy

Diabetic neuropathy is a common late complication of diabetes and is usually associated with neuropathic pain. Its prevalence is estimated at 15% of people with diabetes. There are several different presentations of diabetic neuropathy, the commonest being chronic diabetic peripheral neuropathy characterised by pain in the feet and ankles. The National Prescribing Service recommends non-drug strategies as part of any management plan to include stress reduction, sleep hygiene, physiotherapy, psychological support and transcutaneous electrical nerve stimulation (TENS).[346]

Topical capsaicin

Topical capsaicin (0.075%) may be useful for diabetic neuropathy.[347, 348]

Vitamin D

Vitamin D supplementation may also be an effective treatment of neuropathic pain in T2DM patients. A study of 51 patients with vitamin D deficiency (mean serum 25 hydroxy-vitamin D concentration of 18 ng/mL) and T2DM, and suffering typical neuropathic pain after 3 months, vitamin D supplementation with cholecalciferol (vitamin D3) tablets resulted in a significant reduction in pain scores, with pain severity reducing by up to 50%. The researchers suggest that vitamin D insufficiency may potentiate diabetic nerve damage and impair nociceptor function.[349]

Alpha lipoic acid

In a study of 443 diabetic patients with painful neuropathy, after receiving daily supplementation of 600mg daily alpha–lipoic acid over an average 5-year period, patients were switched onto 600–2400mg daily gabapentin or no treatment. In the no-treatment group 73% developed neuropathic symptoms 2 weeks after cessation of alpha-lipoic acid and 55% of the gabapentin treatment group, did not respond to doses up to 2400mgs daily, requiring other pain relief medication. Moreover, 45% of the gabapenitn group developed intolerable side-effects, requiring outpatient visits up to 7.9 times in 3 months compared with only 3.8 times per 3 months whilst taking alpha-lipoic acid. The authors concluded that alpha–lipoic acid was an effective, safer and more cost-effective method of treating diabetic neuropathy.[350]

Studies also suggest alpha-lipoic acid supplementation in T2DM may assist in accelerating chronic wound healing in patients undergoing hyperbaric oxygen therapy.[351]

Acetyl–L–Carnitine (ALC)

Research supports the role of carnitine for the treatment of diabetic peripheral neuropathic pain.[352] Carnitine is produced from the amino acids lysine and methionine and is essential for the breakdown of fat into energy. Carnitine may improve the utilisation of fats for energy and may be beneficial in heart disease, enhancing physical performance and diabetes. ALC is often deficient in diabetes.

Two randomised placebo-controlled clinical diabetic neuropathy trials over a 52-week period tested 2 doses of ALC: 500 or 1000mg/day given 3 times daily demonstrated that supplementation with ALC, especially at 1000mgs, is efficacious in alleviating symptoms, particularly pain, and improving nerve fibre regeneration and vibration perception in patients with established diabetic neuropathy. Nerve conduction velocities and amplitudes did not improve.[353, 354]

In another review of the literature that identified 2 large clinical trials involving 1679 subjects, those who received at least 2g daily of ALC showed significant reduction in pain scores in patients with diabetic neuropathic pain. One study showed improvements in electrophysiologic factors, such as nerve conduction velocities, and nerve regeneration was documented in 1 trial. ALC was well tolerated and the authors suggested it should be recommended to patients early in the disease process to provide maximal benefit.[355]

Magnetic insoles

Magnetic insoles may reduce the pain, burning, numbness and tingling of diabetic neuropathy according to a study of 375 patients compared with those who wore placebo soles.[356]

Conclusion

Often it is difficult for patients to take on the responsibility for their illnesses. Taking responsibility is essential for the best outcome in patients diagnosed with T1DM and T2DM, particularly as lifestyle plays an important role in the prevention and management of diabetes. T2DM is the leading cause of death from cardiovascular disease associated complications such as macrovascular and microvascular disease. An integrative approach to management is essential (see Table 13.5). (For management of gestational diabetes, see Chapter 32.)

The integrative approach to caring and managing a patient with T1DM and T2DM is to essentially first determine why the illness has developed and, most importantly henceforth, to prevent the further decline in health by abrogating the risk factors.

The most important risk factors in this patient population are stressors, depression, poor diet, obesity and lack of exercise. An integrative approach which highlights patient participation as a key factor in their care is most applicable and would be most beneficial. A diet which is high in unrefined carbohydrates and restricts fats, except for fish fats plus monounsaturated fats, would be ideal. Foods with a GI less than 55 are desirable, combined with exercise, preferably outdoors to maximise sun exposure for vitamin D and stress management.

Table 13.5 Levels of evidence for lifestyle and complementary medicines/therapies in the management of type 2 diabetes mellitus

Modality	Level I	Level II	Level IIIa	Level IIIb	Level IIIc	Level IV	Level V
Lifestyle modification		x					
Sleep restoration					x		
Smoking cessation	x						
Mind–body medicine							
Meditation / Relaxation			x				
Diets — weight management							
Palaeolithic diet			x				
Mediterranean diet			x				
Ornish diet			x				
Alcohol			x				

Continued

Table 13.5 Levels of evidence for lifestyle and complementary medicines/therapies in the management of type 2 diabetes mellitus—cont'd

Modality	Level I	Level II	Level IIIa	Level IIIb	Level IIIc	Level IV	Level V
Physical activity	x						
Exercise	x						
Tai chi	x						
Qigong			x				
Yoga	x						
Nutritional influences							
Low GI diet	x						
High fibre diet (see text)	x						
Fish intake					x		
Coffee consumption	x			x			
Cocoa			x				
Nutritional supplements							
Chromium	x(-)	x(+/-)					
Magnesium		x					
Zinc	x(-)	x					
Vitamin C	x(-)	x					
Vitamin E			x				
Vitamin D	x						
Alpha Lipoic Acid	x						
Multivitamins/ minerals supplements		x					
Coenzyme Q_{10}			x				
L-anginine				x			
Acetyl-L-Carnitine		x					
Herbal medicines							
American ginseng					x		
Coccinia indica				x			
Cinnamon					x		
Gymnema Silvestre				x			
Fenugreek seeds				x			
Bitter melon					x		
Green tea extract					x		
Chinese herbal medicine	x						
Panax ginseng		x					
Ginkgo biloba		x					
Physical therapies							
Reflexology	x(-)			x			

Level I — from a systematic review of all relevant randomised controlled trials, meta–analyses.
Level II — from at least 1 properly designed randomised controlled clinical trial.
Level IIIa — from well-designed pseudo-randomised controlled trials (alternate allocation or some other method).
Level IIIb — from comparative studies (including systematic reviews of such studies) with concurrent controls and allocation not randomised, cohort studies, case-control studies, or interrupted time series with a parallel control group.
Level IIIc — from comparative studies with historical control, 2 or more single-arm studies or interrupted time series without a parallel control group.
Level IV — opinions of respected authorities based on clinical experience, descriptive studies or reports of expert committees.
Level V — represents minimal evidence that represents testimonials.

Clinical tips handout for patients with cardiovascular disease

1 Lifestyle advice

Sleep

- Restore normal sleep patterns. Most adults require about 7 hours sleep a night. (See Chapter 22 for more advice.)

Sunshine

- Amount of exposure varies with local climate.
- At least 15 minutes of sunshine needed daily for vitamin D and melatonin production — especially before 10 a.m. and after 3 p.m. when the sun exposure is safest during summer. Much more exposure is required in winter, when supplementation needs to be considered.
- Ensure gradual adequate skin exposure to sun; avoid sunscreen and excess clothing to maximise levels of vitamin D.
- More time in the sun is required for dark skinned people.
- Direct exposure to about 10% of body (hands, arms, face), without sunscreen and not through glass.
- Vitamin D is obtained in the diet from fatty fish, eggs, liver and fortified foods (some milks and margarines); it is unlikely that adequate vitamin D concentrations can be obtained from diet alone.

2 Physical activity/exercise

- Exercise 30 minutes or more daily. If exercise is not regular, commence with 5 minutes daily and slowly build up to at least 30 minutes. Outdoor exercise in nature, fresh air and sunshine is ideal (e.g. brisk walking, light jogging, cycling, swimming, stretching). The more time you spend outdoors the better.
- Weight-bearing exercises or resistance exercise are beneficial.
- Yoga may be of help; other examples include qiqong, tai chi.

3 Mind–body medicine

- Stress management program — for example, 6 x 40 minute sessions for patients to understand the nature of their symptoms, the symptoms' relationship to stress, and the practice of regular relaxation exercises.
- Regular meditation practice, at least 10–20 minutes daily.

Breathing

- Be aware of breathing at all times. Notice if tendency to hold breath or over-breathe. Always aim to relax breath and the muscles around the chest wall.

Rest and stress management

Recurrent stress may cause a return of symptoms. Relaxation is important for a full and lasting recovery.

- Reduce workload and resolve conflicts. Contact family, friends, church, social or other groups for support.
- Listening to relaxation music and daily baths help.
- Massage therapy is helpful.
- Hypnotherapy, biofeedback may be of help.
- Cognitive behavioural therapy and psychotherapy are extremely helpful.

Fun

- It is important to have fun in life. Joy can be found even in the simplest tasks, such as being with friends with a sense of humour, funny movies/videos, comedy, hobbies, dancing, playing with pets and children.

4 Environment

- Don't smoke and avoid smoking environments.
- Avoid environmental pollutants and chemicals — at work and in the home.
- Ensure office or home has a view overlooking garden or park.

5 Dietary changes

- Eat regular healthy low GI meals, ideally 3 small meals, and 2 snacks per day; each containing protein in order to avoid fluctuating blood sugar levels and provide amino acids for nerve transmitters, such as tryptophan.
- Eat more fruit (>2/day) and vegetables (>5/day) — variety of colours and those in season.
- Include bitter melon vegetable and cinnamon as part of your diet. Add 1 tsp of bitter melon and cinnamon powder to food or cooking (e.g. sprinkle on meals or add to stews and soups).
- Increase dietary fibre. Psyllium and guar gum can improve glucose control.
- Eat more nuts; for example, walnuts, peanuts; seeds, beans (e.g. soy), sprouts (e.g. alfa, mung bean, lentils).
- Increase fish intake — canned is okay (mackerel, salmon, sardines, cod, tuna, salmon), and especially deep sea fish — daily if possible.

- Reduce red meat intake — preferably eat lean red meat (e.g. lamb, kangaroo) and white meat (e.g. free range organic chicken).
- Use cold pressed olive oil and avocado.
- Use only dark chocolate — preferably 85% or more of cocoa.
- Eat low GI wholegrains/cereals (variety): rice (brown, basmati, Mahatmi, Doongara), traditional rolled oats, buckwheat flour, wholegrain organic breads (rye bread, Essene, spelt, Kamut), brown pasta, millet, amaranth etc.
- Reduce dairy intake: low-fat dairy products such as yoghurt and occasionally cheeses, unless there is a dairy intolerance.
- Drink more water 1–2 litres a day.
- Drink more teas (e.g. especially organic green tea, black tea) plus vegetable juices.
- Chamomile tea may help diabetes. Drink 1 cup of 30–60 minutes before meals.
- Moderate levels of caffeine can help diabetes control. Avoid high dosage as it can cause restlessness and agitation.
- Avoid hydrogenated fats, salt, fast foods, sugar (such as in soft drinks), lollies, biscuits, cakes and processed foods (e.g. white bread, white pasta, pastries).
- Minimise alcohol intake to no more than 1–2 glasses daily (non-sweet) as it is a brain depressant and can disturb sleep.
- Avoid chemical additives — preservatives, colourings and flavourings.
- Avoid artificial sweeteners. For sweetener try honey (e.g. manuka, yellow box and stringy bark have lowest GI).

6 Physical therapies

- Reflexology may improve blood glucose.
- Magnetic insoles may help reduce pain, burning, numbness and tingling of neuropathy.

7 Supplements

Fish oils

- Indication: reduces triglycerides; cardio protection prevents heart disease; fish oils 2–4g (1g containing EPA 180/ DHA 120mg) daily depending on fish consumption.
- Dosage: take with meals. Adult: 1g 1–2 capsules twice daily. Child 500mg 1 to 2 x daily (500mg–1g daily EPA and DHA); can be used in pregnancy or lactation as tolerated.
- Results: 1–4 days.
- Side-effects: Often well tolerated especially if taken with meals. Very mild and rare side-effects; for example, gastrointestinal upset; allergic reactions (e.g. rash, breathing problems) if allergic to seafood; blood thinning effects in very high doses > 10g daily (may need to stop fish oil supplements 2 weeks prior to surgery).
- Contraindications: sensitivity reaction to seafood; drug interactions; caution when taking high doses of fish oils >4g per day together with warfarin (your doctor will check your INR test).

Folate

- Indication: elevated homocysteine.
- Dosage: 0.5–1mg daily as in a multivitamin and mineral supplement.
- Results: uncertain.
- Side-effects: very mild and rare.
- Contraindications: avoid in anaemias until assessed by a doctor.

Vitamin B's especially B6 and B12

- Indication: Elevated homocysteine; metformin can reduce vitamin B12.
- Dosage: upper level of intake of vitamin B6 should not exceed 50mg/day.
- Results: uncertain.
- Side-effects: avoid overuse of single vitamin products (e.g. oral and injectable forms of vitamin B6) or concomitant use of multivitamin products could result in some patients routinely exceeding the upper limit for vitamins associated with severe toxicity. Toxicity in high doses of vitamin B6 includes: peripheral neuropathy, such as tingling, burning and numbness of limbs.
- Contraindications: avoid in anaemias until assessed by a doctor.

Vitamin D3 (cholecalciferol 1000 international units)

Doctors should check blood levels and suggest supplementation if levels are low.

Can help diabetes and neuropathic pain.

Vitamin C and vitamin E (best given together)

Vitamin C

- Indication: can reactivate vitamin E. May help to prevent vascular disease.
- Dosage: 500–1000mg daily or as tolerated.
- Results: unknown.

- Side-effects: with high doses can cause nausea, heartburn, abdominal cramps and diarrhoea.
- Contraindications: can increase iron absorption. Use with caution if glucose-6-phosphate dehydrogenase deficiency.

Vitamin E (natural)

- Indication: can help reduce platelet aggregation.
- Dosage: 200–500–1000IU daily (D-alpha-tocopherol or mixed isomers).
- Side-effects: doses below 1500IU daily are very unlikely to result in haemorrhage, diarrhoea, flatulence, nausea, heart palpitations.
- Contraindications: use with caution if bleeding disorder or if taking with blood thinning medication. If using very high dose, reduce dose before surgery.

Magnesium and calcium (best provided together)

- Indication: improves insulin sensitivity and hence glucose level.
- Dosage: children: up to 65–120mg daily in divided doses. Adults: 350mg daily including pregnant and lactating women.
- Results: 2–3 days.
- Side-effects: oral magnesium, especially at a dose greater than 400mg daily, can cause gastrointestinal irritation, nausea, vomiting and diarrhoea. The dosage varies from person to person. Although rare, toxic levels can cause low blood pressure, thirst, heart arrhythmia, drowsiness and weakness.
- Contraindications: patients with kidney disease and heart block.

Zinc

- Indication: can improve insulin sensitivity and hence decrease glucose level.
- Dosage: usual dosage in adult no more than 5–10mgs zinc sulfate daily. Zinc amino avid chelate 50mg.
- Side-effects: nausea, vomiting, metallic taste in mouth. Avoid long term use and high dosage as this may cause copper deficiency, impair the immune system and cause anaemia.
- Contraindications: sideroblastic anaemia, above normal blood levels of zinc, severe kidney disease.

Chromium picolinate

- Indication: an reduce blood glucose plus lipid levels.
- Dosage: 50–200mcg per day.
- Results: unknown.
- Side-effects: doses less than 1000mcg are safe.
- Contradictions: can reduce hypoglycaemic drug requirement. Very high doses linked to kidney and liver disease.

Acetyl-L-carnitine (amino acid)

- Indications: diabetic peripheral neuropathy; Alzheimer's disease.
- Dosage: 500–1000mg 3 x daily.
- Results: can reduce blood glucose in 2–4 hours.
- Side-effects: well tolerated; gastrointestinal upset.
- Contraindications: avoid with blood thinners; hypothyroidism; seizures.

Alpha-lipoic acid

- Indication: may prevent nerve damage and can repair existing damage; diabetic neuropathy.
- Dosage: 600–1200mg daily (oral).
- Side-effects: nausea and skin rashes have been reported.
- Contraindications: must not be taken if thiamine deficient (e.g. alcoholic) unless thiamine supplementation is given.

Herbs

Bitter melon

- Indications: lowers blood glucose.
- Dosage: juice 50–100ml per day containing 45–60g bitter melon.
- Results: can reduce blood glucose in 2–4 hours.
- Side-effects: can reduce hypoglycaemic drug requirement. Diarrhoea, epigastric pain and head aches can occur.
- Contraindications: during pregnancy. Has been documented to reduce fertility in males and females. Do not use if glucose-6-phosphate dehydrogenase deficient. Contraindicated while breastfeeding.

Capsaicin cream

Topical capsaicin cream (0.075%) may help diabetic neuropathy.

Fenugreek

- Indication: can help reduce blood glucose. May help to improve blood lipids.
- Dosage: 10–15g per day as a single dose or divided doses. Lower doses can normalise lipids.
- Results: within 2–4 hours.

- Side-effects: diarrhoea, abdominal discomfort and bloating. May need to decrease hypoglycaemic medications.
- Contraindications: monitor blood glucose as may have to reduce hypoglycaemic medication. May be unsafe in children. Do not use if allergic to legumes (e.g. peas, beans, peanuts).

Gymnema sylvestre

- Indication: a decrease blood glucose by several mechanisms.
- Dosage: 200mg twice daily.
- Results: within 2–4 hours.
- Side-effects: none reported. May need to decrease hypoglycaemic medication.
- Contraindications: none reported but necessary to monitor blood glucose levels.

Panax ginseng (Korean)

- Indication: lowers blood glucose.
- Dosage: 200mg daily.
- Results: 2–4 hours.
- Side-effects: very rarely occur, but include insomnia. Even more rarely, and with higher doses, breast discomfort, vaginal bleeding, amenorrhea, tachycardia and palpitations.
- Contraindications: avoid stimulants such as excess caffeine and nicotine.

American ginseng

- Indication: can reduce blood glucose levels.
- Dosage: 3g up to 2 hours before meals.
- Results: 3–4 hours.
- Side-effects: may cause gastrointestinal, nervous and hormonal effects (e.g. breast discomfort or vaginal bleeding).
- Contraindications: avoid stimulants such as excess caffeine and nicotine.

Cinnamon

- Indication: decreases blood glucose by increasing insulin and increasing glucose uptake through increased insulin sensitivity.
- Dosage: can vary from 1–6g per day; sprinkle 1–2 tsps onto cereal or porridge.
- Side-effects: generally very safe. May need to decrease hypoglycaemic medication.
- Contraindications: very high doses of cinnamon must not be used in those with liver disease who may have increased bleeding tendency.

References

1. EURODIAB ACE Study Group. Variation and trends in incidence of childhood diabetes in Europe. Lancet 2000;355:873–6.
2. http://diabetes.niddk.nih.gov/dm/pubs/statistics/#allages Accessed December 2008.
3. Karvonen M, Viik-Kajander M, Moltchanova E, et. al. Incidence of childhood type 1 diabetes worldwide. Diabetes Mondiale (DiaMond) Project Group. Diabetes Care 2000;23:1516–26.
4. Gillespie KM. Type 1 diabetes: pathogenesis and prevention. CMAJ 2006;175(2):165–70.
5. Taplin CE, Craig ME, Lloyd M, et. al. The rising incidence of childhood type 1 diabetes in New South Wales, 1990-2002. MJA 2005;183:243–46.
6. Australian Institute of Health and Welfare (AIHW). Online. Available: www.aihw.gov.au/publications/cvd/daf08/daf08pdf (accessed December 2008).
7. The SEARCH for Diabetes in Youth Study Writing Group. Incidence of Diabetes in Youth in the United States. JAMA 2007;297:2716–24.
8. Amos A, McCarty D, Zimmet P. The rising global burden of diabetes and its complications: estimates and projections to the year 2010. Diabet Med 1997;14:S1–S85.
9. King H, Aubert R, Herman W. Global burden of diabetes, 1995–2025: prevalence, numerical estimates and projections. Diab Care 1998;21: 1414–31.
10. Dunstan DW, Zimmet P, Welborne TA, et. al. The rising prevalence of diabetes and impaired glucose tolerance. Diab Care 2002;25;829–34.
11. World Health Organization. http://www.who.int/mediacentre/factsheets/fs312/en/(accessed May 2009).
12. Serjeantson SW, Owerbach D, Zimmet P et. al. Genetics of diabetes in Nauru: effects of foreign admixture, HLA antigens and the insulin-gene-linked polymorphism. Diabetologia 1983;25:13–17.
13. Knowler WC, Williams RC, Pettitt DJ, et. al. Gm3;5,13,14 and type 2 diabetes mellitus: an association in American Indians with genetic admixture. Am J Hum Genet 1988;43 520–26.
14. Simmons D, Williams DR, Powell MJ. The Coventry Diabetes Study: prevalence of diabetes and impaired glucose tolerance in Europids and Asians. Q J Med 1991;81:1021–30.
15. Adamo KB, Tesson F. Gene-environment interaction and the metabolic syndrome. Novartis Found Symp 2008;293:103–19.
16. Pinhas-Hamiel, O and Zeitler P. The global spread of type 2 diabetes mellitus in children and adolescents. J Pediatr 2005;146(5):693–700.
17. Lindström J, Ilanne-Parikka P, Peltonen M, et. al.Finnish Diabetes Prevention Study Group. Sustained reduction in the incidence of type 2 diabetes by lifestyle intervention: follow-up of the Finnish Diabetes Prevention Study. Lancet 2006;368(9548):1673–9.
18. Gillies CI, Abrams KR, Lambert PC, et. al. Pharmacological and lifestyle interventions to prevent or delay type 2 diabetes in people with impaired glucose tolerance: systematic review and meat-analysis. BMJ 2007;334:299.
19. Knowler WC, Barrett-Connor E, Fowler SE, et. al. and Diabetes Prevention Program Research Group. Reduction in the incidence of type 2 diabetes with lifestyle intervention or metformin. NEJM 2002;346:393–403.

20 Orozco LJ, Buchleitner AM, Gimenez-Perez G, et. al. Exercise or exercise and diet for preventing type 2 diabetes mellitus. Cochrane Database of Systematic Reviews 2008, Issue 3. Art. No.: CD003054. doi: 10.1002/14651858.CD003054.pub3.
21 Li G, Zhang P, Wang J, et. al. The long-term effect of lifestyle interventions to preventdiabetes in the China Da Qing Diabetes Prevention Study: a 20-year follow-up study. Lifestyle intervention, diabetes, and cardiovascular disease. Lancet 2008;371:1731–33.
22 Gimeno SG, de Souza JM. IDDM and milk consumption. A case-control study in São Paulo, Brazil. Diabetes Care 1997;20(8):1256–60.
23 Cavallomg, Fava D, Monetini L, et. al. Cell-mediated immune response to β casein in recent-onset insulin-dependent diabetes: implications for disease pathogenesis. Lancet 1996;348:926–28.
24 Virtanen SM, Läärä E, Hyppönen E, et. al. Cow's milk consumption, HLA-DQB1 genotype, and type 1 diabetes: a nested case-control study of siblings of children with diabetes. Childhood diabetes in Finland study group. Diabetes 2000;49(6):912–7.
25 Rana JS, Li TY, Manson JE, et. al. Adiposity compared with physical inactivity and risk of type 2 diabetes in women. Diabetes Care 2007;30(1):53–8.
26 Harding AH, Wareham NJ, Bingham SA, et. al. Plasma Vitamin C Level, Fruit and Vegetable Consumption, and the Risk of New-Onset Type 2 Diabetes Mellitus. The European Prospective Investigation of Cancer–Norfolk Prospective Study. Arch Intern Med 2008;168(14):1493–99.
27 Cochrane PEARLS. http://www.cochraneprimarycare.org/en/newPage1.html Practical Evidence About Real Life Situations. No. 95, September 2008.
28 Grace C, Begum R, Subhani S, et. al. Prevention of type 2 diabetes in British Bangladeshis: qualitative study of community, religious, and professional perspectives BMJ 2008 November 4;337:a1931.
29 Alison M. Stuebe, Janet W. Rich-Edwards, et. al. Duration of Lactation and Incidence of Type 2 Diabetes. JAMA 2005;294:2601–10.
30 Gucciardi E, Chi-Tyan Wang S, De Melo M, et. al. Characteristics of men and women with diabetes. Observations during patients' initial visit to a diabetes education centre. Can Fam Phys 2008;54:219–27.
31 Vehik K, Hamman RF, Lezotte D, et. al. Trends in High-Risk HLA Susceptibility Genes Among Colorado Youth With Type 1 Diabetes. Diabetes Care 2008;31:1392–1396; doi: 10.2337/dc07-2210.
32 Barroso I. Genetics of Type 2 diabetes. Diabet Med 2005;22(5):517–35.
33 Lammert E. The vascular trigger of type II diabetes mellitus. Exp Clin Endocrinol Diabetes 2008;116(Suppl 1):S21–S5.
34 Moore AF, Florez JC. Genetic susceptibility to type 2 diabetes and implications for antidiabetic therapy. Annu Rev Med 2008;59:95–111.
35 McGrady AV, et. al. In: Spencer JW, Jacobs JJ. Complementary and Alternative Medicine: an evidence-based approach. St. Louis, Mosby, 2003.
36 Sepa A, Frodi A, Ludvigsson J. Mothers' experiences of serious life events increase the risk of diabetes-related autoimmunity in their children. Diabetes Care 2005;28(10):2394–9.
37 Storch EA, Heidgerken AD, Geffken GR, et. al. Bullying, regimen self-management, and metabolic control in youth with type I diabetes. J Pediatr 2006;148(6):784–7.
38 Surwit RS, van Tilburg MAL, Zucker N, et. al. Stress Management Improves Long-Term Glycemic Control in Type 2 Diabetes. Diab Care 2002;25:30–4.
39 Hooper PL. Hot-tub therapy for type 2 diabetes mellitus. NEJM 1999;341(12):924–5.
40 Haslam D. Understanding obesity in the older person: prevalence and risk factors. Br J Community Nurs 2008;13(3):115–22.
41 Keller U. From obesity to diabetes. Int J Vitam Nutr Res 2006;76(4):172–7.
42 Anderson RJ, Freedland KE, et. al. The prevalence of comorbid depression in adults with diabetes: a meta-analysis. Diabetes Care 2001;24(6):1069–78.
43 Lawlor DA, Ebrahim S, Smith GD. Association of insulin resistance with depression: cross-sectional findings from the British Women's Heart and Health Study. BMJ 2003;327:383–4.
44 Golden SH, Lazo M, Carnethon M, et. al. Examining a bidirectional association between depressive symptoms and diabetes. JAMA 2008;299:2751–59.
45 Carnethon MR, Biggs ML, Barzilay JI, et. al. Longitudinal association between depressive symptoms and incident type 2 diabetes mellitus in older adults: the cardiovascular health study. Arch Intern Med 2007;167(8):802–7.
46 Martin P. Cosgrove, Lincoln A, et. al. Does depression increase the risk of developing type 2 diabetes? Occupational Medicine 2008;58(1):7–14.
47 Timonen M, Laakso M, Jokelainen J, et. al. Insulin resistance and depression: cross-sectional study. BMJ 2005;330:17–18.
48 Zhou L, Sutton GM, Rochford JJ, et. al. Serotonin 2C receptor agonists improve Type 2 diabetes via melanocortin-4 receptor signaling pathways. Cell Metab 2007;6:398–405.
49 Pittas AG, Lau J, Hu F, et. al. The role of vitamin D and calcium in type 2 diabetes. A systematic review and meta-analysis. J Clin Endocrinol Metab 2007;92:2017–29.
50 Vitamin D and adult bone health in Australia and New Zealand: a position statement. Working Group of the Australian and New Zealand Bone and Mineral Society, Endocrine Society of Australia and Osteoporosis Australia MJA 2005;182:281–285.
51 National Prescribing Service, Australia. Published 1 December 2008. http://www.nps.org.au/health_professionals/publications/nps_radar/issues/current/december_2008/alendronate_with_cholecalciferol?SQ_BACKEND_PAGE=main&backend_section=am&am_section=edit_asset&assetid=65713&sq_asset_path=1,43,72,360,686,24894,25055,65656,65712&asset_ei_screen=contents&sq_link_path=,0,43,93,526,1081,33528,33753,128772,128852#revhistory] (accessed December 2008)
52 Zipitis CS, Akobeng AK. Vitamin D Supplementation in Early Childhood and Risk of Type 1 Diabetes: a Systematic Review and Meta-analysis. Archives of Disease in Childhood. 2008 doi:10.1136/adc.2007.128579.
53 Palomer X, Gonzalez-Clemente J.M. Role of vitamin D in the pathogenesis of type 2 diabetes mellitus. Diabetes Obes Metab 2008;10(3):185–97.
54 Chaput JP, Després JP, Bouchard C, et. al. Association of sleep duration with type 2 diabetes and impaired glucose tolerance. Diabetol 2007;50:2298–304.
55 Gottlieb DJ, Naresh Punjabi NM, Newman AB, et. al. Association of Sleep Time With Diabetes Mellitus and Impaired Glucose Tolerance. Arch Intern Med 2005;165:863–67.

56 West SD, Nicoll DJ, Stradling JR. Prevalence of obstructive sleep apnoea in men with type 2 diabetes. Thorax 2006;61(11):945–50.
57 Eriksson AK, Ekbom A, Granath F, et. al. Psychological distress and risk of pre-diabetes and Type 2 diabetes in a prospective study of Swedish middle-aged men and women. Diabetic Medicine 2008;25:834–42.
58 Willi C, et. al. Active smoking and the risk of Type 2 diabetes. A systematic review and meta-analysis. JAMA 2007;289:2654–64.
59 Kruger J, Ham SA, Prohaska TR. Behavioural risk factors associated with overweight and obesity among older adults: the 2005 National Health Interview Survey. Prev Chronic Dis 2009;6(1):A14. Epub 2008 Dec 15.
60 Foy CG, Bell RA, Farmer DF, et. al. Smoking and incidence of diabetes among U.S. adults: findings from the Insulin Resistance Atherosclerosis Study. Diabetes Care 2005;28(10):2501–7.
61 Navas-Acien A, Silbergeld EK, Pastor-Barriuso R, et. al. Arsenic Exposure and Prevalence of Type 2 Diabetes in US Adults. JAMA 2008;300(7):814–22.
62 Healy GN, Dunstan DW, Shaw JE, et. al. Beneficial associations of physical activity with 2-h but not fasting blood glucose in Australian adults: Aus Diab Study. Diabetes Care 2006;29:2598–2604.
63 Dunstan DW, Salmon J, Healy GN, et. al. Association of television viewing with fasting and 2-hr post-challenge plasma glucose levels in adults without diagnosed diabetes. Diabetes Care 2007;30:516–22.
64 Herbst A, Bachran R, Kapellen T, et. al. Physical activity, also, has a major influence on obesity control and is a significant predictor of mortality in T2DM. Arch Pediatr Adolesc Med 2006;160:573–77.
65 Jeon CY, Lokken RP, Hu FB, et. al. Physical activity of moderate intensity and risk of type 2 diabetes: a systematic review. Diabetes Care 2007;30(3):744–52.
66 Kriska AM, Saremi A, Hanson RL, et. al. Physical activity, obesity, and the incidence of type 2 diabetes in a high-risk population. Am J Epidemiol 2003;158(7):669–75.
67 Gregg EW, Gerzoff RB, Caspersen CJ, et. al. Relationship of Walking to Mortality Among US Adults With Diabetes. Arch Intern Med 2003;163:1440–47.
68 Babraj JA, Vollaard NBJ, Keast C, et. al. Extremely short duration high intensity interval training substantially improves insulin action in young healthy males. BMC Endocrine Disorders 2009;9:3 doi:10.1186/1472-6823-9-3.
69 Silink M. http://www.abc.net.au/am/content/2006/s17869.
70 Hosper K, Deutekom M, Stronks K. The effectiveness of 'Exercise on Prescription' in stimulating physical activity among women from ethnic minority groups in the Netherlands: protocol for a randomised controlled trial. BMC Public Health 2008;8(1):406.
71 American Diabetes Association: Diabetes mellitus and exercise (position statement). Diabetes Care 2000;23(Suppl. 1):S50-S54.
72 Albright A, et. al. American College of Sports Medicine position stand: exercise and Type 2 diabetes. Med Sci Sports Exerc.2000;32:1345–60.
73 Thomas DE, Elliott EJ, Naughton GA. Exercise for type 2 diabetes mellitus. The Cochrane Database of Systematic Reviews 2006(3).
74 Sigal RJ, Kenny GP, Boulé NG, et. al. Effects of Aerobic Training, Resistance Training, or Both on Glycemic Control in Type 2 Diabetes. A Randomised Trial. Ann Intern Med 2007;147:357–69.
75 Christou EA, Yang Y, Rosengren KS. Taiji training improves knee extensor strength and force control in older adults. J Gerontol A Biol Sci Med Sci 2003;58:763–66.
76 Lan C, Lai JS, Chen SY, et. al. Tai Chi Chuan to improve muscular strength and endurance in elderly individuals: a pilot study. Arch Phys Med Rehabil 2000;81:604–07.
77 Tsang WW, Hui-Chan CW. Effect of 4-and 8-wk intensive Tai Chi training on balance control in the elderly. Med Sci Sports Exerc 2004;36:648–57.
78 Hong Y, Li JX, Robinson PD. Balance control, flexibility, and cardiorespiratory fitness among older Tai Chi practitioners. Br J Sports Med 2000;34: 29–34.
79 Richerson S, Rosendale K. Does Tai Chi improve plantar sensory ability? A pilot study. Diabetes Technol Ther 2007;9(3):276–86.
80 Taylor-Piliae RE, Haskell WL, et. al. Improvement in balance, strength, and flexibility after 12 weeks of Tai chi exercise in ethnic Chinese adults with cardiovascular disease risk factors. Altern Ther Health Med 2006;12(2):50–8.
81 Lee MS, Pittler MH, Kim MS, et. al. Tai chi for Type 2 diabetes: a systematic review. Diabet Med 2008;25(2):240–1.
82 Orr R, Tsang T, Lam P, et. al. Mobility impairment in type 2 diabetes: association with muscle power and effect of Tai Chi intervention. Diabetes Care.2006;29(9):2120–2.
83 Song R, Lee EO, Bae SC, et. al. Effects of tai chi self-help program on glucose control, cardiovascular risks and quality of life in type II diabetic patients (in Korean). J Muscle Joint Health 2007;14:13–25.
84 Wang J, Cao Y. Effects of tai chi exercise on plasma neuropeptide Y of type 2 diabetes mellitus with geriatric obesity (in Chinese). J Sports Sci 2003;24:67–8.
85 Tsang T, Orr R, Lam P, et. al. Effects of Tai Chi on glucose homeostasis and insulin sensitivity in older adults with type 2 diabetes: a randomised double-blind sham-exercise-controlled trial. Age Ageing 2008;37(1):64–71. Epub 2007 Oct 25.
86 Zhang Y, Fu FH. Effects of 14-week Tai Ji Quan exercise on metabolic control in women with type 2 diabetes. Am J Chin Med 2008;36(4):647–54.
87 Jeong IS, Lee HJ, Kim MH. The effect of the Taeguk Gi-gong exercise on insulin resistance and blood glucose in patients with type II diabetes mellitus (in Korean). J Korean Acad Fundam Nurs 2007;14: 44–52.
88 Tsujiuchi T, Kumano H, Yoshiuchi K, et. al. The effect of Qi-gong relaxation exercise on the control of Type 2 diabetes mellitus: a randomised controlled trial. Diab Care 2002;25:241–42.
89 Xin L, Miller YD, Brown WJ. A qualitative review of the role of qigong in the management of diabetes. J Altern Complement Med 2007;13(4):427–33.
90 Liu X., Brown W, Miller Y. Effects of Chinese medical exercise on indicators of metabolic syndrome in Australian adults with elevated blood glucose level: A randomised controlled trial. J of Sci and Med in Sport 2007;10(6):54.
91 Singh S, Malhotra V, Singh KP, et. al. Role of yoga in modifying certain cardiovascular functions in type 2 diabetic patients. J Assoc Phys India 2004;52:203–6.
92 Malhotra V, Singh S, Singh KP, et. al. Study of yoga asanas in assessment of pulmonary function in NIDDM patients. Indian J Phys Pharm 2002;46(3):313–20.

93 Malhotra V, Singh S, Tandon OP, et. al. Effect of Yoga asanas on nerve conduction in type 2 diabetes. Indian J Physiol Pharmacol 2002;46:298–306.
94 Skoro-Kondza L, Tai SS, Gadelrab R, et. al. Community based yoga classes for type 2 diabetes: an exploratory randomised controlled trial. BMC Health Services Research 2009,9:33 doi:10.1186/1472-6963-9-33.
95 Innes KE, Vincent HK. Review: The Influence of Yoga-Based Programs on Risk Profiles in Adults with Type 2 Diabetes Mellitus: A Systematic Review. Advance Access Publication 11 December 2006. eCAM 2007;4(4)469–86.
96 Thomas D, Elliott EJ. Low glycaemic index, low glycaemic load diets for diabetes mellitus. Cochrane Database of Systematic Reviews 2009, issue 1. Art. No: CD006296. Do1: 10.1002/14651858 CD 006296. pub2.
97 Lamb MM, Yin X, Barriga K, et. al. Dietary Glycemic Index, Development of Islet Autoimmunity, and Subsequent Progression to Type 1 Diabetes in Young Children. J Clin Endocrin Metabol Accepted July 24, 2008.
98 Norris JM, Yin X, Lamb MM, et. al. Omega-3 polyunsaturated fatty acid intake and islet autoimmunity in children at increased risk for type 1 diabetes. JAMA 2007;298(12):1420–8.
99 Delahanty LM, Nathan DM, Lachin JM, et. al. Association of diet with glycated hemoglobin during intensive treatment of type 1 diabetes in the Diabetes Control and Complications Trial. America Journal of Clinical Nutrition 2009;89:518–24.
100 Brand-Miller J, Hayne S, Petocz P, et. al. Low–Glycemic Index Diets in the Management of Diabetes: A meta-analysis of randomised controlled trials Diabetes Care 2003;26:2261–67.
101 Schulze MB, Schulz M, Heidemann C, et. al. Fiber and Magnesium Intake and Incidence of Type 2 Diabetes A Prospective Study and Meta-analysis. Arch Intern Med 2007;167:956–65.
102 Meyer KA, et. al. Carbohydrates, dietary fiber, and incident Type 2 diabetes in older women. Am J Clin Nutr 2000;71:921–30.
103 Feldeisen SE, Tucker KL. Nutritional strategies in the prevention and treatment of metabolic syndrome. Appl Physiol Nutr Metab 2007; 32(1):46–60.
104 Jensen MK, Koh-Banerjee P, Franz M, et. al. Wholegrains, bran, and germ in relation to homocysteine and markers of glycemic control, lipids, and inflammation. AJCN 2006;83:275–83.
105 McKeown NM. Wholegrain intake and insulin sensitivity: evidence from observational studies. Nutr Rev 2004;62(7 Pt 1):286–91.
106 Chandalia M, Garg A, Lutjohann D. Beneficial effects of high dietary fiber intake in patients with type 2 diabetes mellitus. NEJM 2000;342(19): 1392–8.
107 Wellen KL et. al. Inflammation, stress and diabetes. J Clin Invest 2005;115:1111–19.
108 Priebemg, van Binsbergen JJ, de Vos R, et. al. Whole grain foods for the prevention of type 2 diabetes mellitus. Cochrane Database of Systematic Reviews 2008, Issue 1. Art. No.: CD006061. doi: 10.1002/14651858.CD006061.pub2.
109 Lee CT, Adler AI, Forouhi NG, et. al. Cross-sectional association between fish consumption and albuminuria: the European Prospective Investigation of Cancer-Norfolk Study. Am J Kidney Dis 2008;52(5):876–86.
110 Santangelo C, Varì R, Scazzocchio B, et. al. Polyphenols, intracellular signalling and inflammation. Ann Ist Super Sanita 2007;43(4): 394–405.
111 Ordovas J. Diet/genetic interactions and their effects on inflammatory markers. Nutr Rev 2007;65(12 Pt 2):S203–7.
112 Salmeron J, et. al. Dietary fat intake and risk of Type 2 diabetes in women. Am Clin Nutr 2001;73: 1019–26.
113 Sharma KK, et. al. Anti-hyperglycemic effect of onion: effect on fasting blood sugar and induced hyperglycemia in man. Ind J Med Res 1977;65: 422–29.
114 Sheela CG, et. al. Anti-diabetic effects of S-allylcysteine sulphoxide isolated from garlic (Allium sativum). Ind J Exp Biol 1992;192: 523–26.
115 Jaimenez-Cruz A, Bacardi-Gascon M, Turnbull WH, et. al. A flexible low glycemic index Mexican-style diet in overweight and obese subjects with Type 2 diabetes improves metabolic parameters during a 6-week treatment period. Diabetes Care 2003;26:1967–70.
116 Teixeira SR, Tappenden KA, Carson L, et. al. Isolated soy protein consumption reduces urinary albumin excretion and improves the serum lipid profile in men with type 2 diabetes mellitus and nephropathy. J Nutr 2004;134(8):1874–80.
117 Jayagopal V, Albertazzi P, Kilpatrick ES, et. al. Beneficial Effects of Soy Phytoestrogen Intake in Postmenopausal Women With Type 2 Diabetes. Diabetes Care 25:1709–14.
118 Ahuja KD, Robertson IK, Geraghty DP, et. al. Effects of chili consumption on postprandial glucose, insulin, and energy metabolism. AJCN 2006;84: 63–9.
119 Villegas R, Liu S, Gao YT, et. al. Prospective Study of Dietary Carbohydrates, Glycemic Index, Glycemic Load, and Incidence of Type 2 Diabetes Mellitus in Middle-aged Chinese Women. Arch Intern Med 2007;167:2310–16.
120 Palmer JR, Boggs DA, Krishnan S, et. al. Sugar-Sweetened Beverages and Incidence of Type 2 Diabetes Mellitus in African American Women. Arch Intern Med 2008;168:1487–92.
121 Swithers SE, Davidson TL. A Role for Sweet Taste: Calorie Predictive Relations in Energy Regulation by Rats. Behavioural Neuroscience 2008;122: 161–73.
122 Lu Qi, Rob M. van Dam, Kathryn Rexrode, et. al. Hu Heme Iron From Diet as a Risk Factor for Coronary Heart Disease in Women With Type 2 Diabetes Diabetes Care 2007;30:101–6.
123 Liu S, Choi HK, Ford E, et. al. A prospective study of dairy intake and risk of type 2 diabetes in women. Diabetes Care 2006;29:1579–84.
124 Shahar DR, Abel R, Elhayany A, et. al. Does Dairy Calcium Intake Enhance Weight Loss Among Overweight Diabetic Patients? Diabetes Care 2007;30:485–89.
125 Teixeira Rde C, Molina Mdel C, et. al. Cardiovascular risk in vegetarians and omnivores: a comparative study. Arq Bras Cardiol 2007;89(4):237–44.
126 Barnard ND, Cohen J, Jenkins DJA, et. al. A Low-Fat Vegan Diet Improves Glycemic Control and Cardiovascular Risk Factors in a Randomised Clinical Trial in Individuals With Type 2 Diabetes. Diabetes Care 2006;29:1777–83.

127 Turner-McGrievy GM, Barnard ND, Cohen J, et. al. Changes in nutrient intake and dietary quality among participants with type 2 diabetes following a low-fat vegan diet or a conventional diabetes diet for 22 weeks. J Am Diet Assoc 2008;108(10): 1636–45.

128 Wing SS. The UPS in diabetes and obesity. BMC Biochem 2008;9(Suppl 1):S6.

129 Rowley K, et. al. Diabetes in Australian aborigines and Torres Strait islander peoples. PNG Med J 2001;44:164–70.

130 Wild S, et. al. Global prevalence of diabetes: estimates for the year 2000, and projections for 2030. Diabetes Care 2004;27:1047–53.

131 Knowler WC, Barrett-Connor E, Fowler SE, et. al. Diabetes Prevention Program Research Group. Reduction in the incidence of type 2 diabetes with lifestyle intervention or metformin. N Eng J Med 2002;346:393–403.

132 Dansinger ML, Tatsioni A, Wong JB, et. al. Meta-analysis: the effect of dietary counseling for weight loss. Ann Intern Med 2007;147(1):41–50.

133 Jossa F. A Mediterranean diet in the prevention of arteriosclerosis. Recent Prog Med 1996;87: 175–81.

134 Martinez-Gonzalez MA, Estruch R, Bulló M, et. al. Adherence to a Mediterranean diet and risk of developing diabetes: prospective cohort study. BMJ 2008;336:1348–51.

135 Giugliano D, Esposito K. Mediterranean diet and metabolic diseases. Curr Opin Lipidol 2008;19(1):63–8.

136 Martínez-González MA, de la Fuente-Arrillaga C, Nunez-Cordoba JM, et. al. Adherence to Mediterranean diet and risk of developing diabetes: prospective cohort study. BMJ 2008;336(7657):1348–51.

137 Sánchez-Taínta A, Estruch R, Bulló M, et. al. Adherence to a Mediterranean-type diet and reduced prevalence of clusteredcardiovascular risk factors in a cohort of 3,204 high-risk patients. Eur J Cardiovasc Prev Rehabil 2008;15(5):589–93.

138 Marin C, Perez-Jimenez F, et. al. The Ala54Thr polymorphism of the fatty acid-binding protein 2 gene is associated with a change in insulin sensitivity after a change in the type of dietary fat. AJCN 2005;82(1):196–200.

139 Jiang R, Manson JE, Stampfer MJ, et. al. Nut and peanut butter consumption and risk of type 2 diabetes in women. JAMA 2002;288:2554–60.

140 Jenkins DJA, Hu FB, Tapsell LC, et. al. Possible Benefit of Nuts in Type 2 Diabetes. J Nutr 2008;138:1752S-56S.

141 Tapsell LC, Gillen LJ, Patch CS, et. al. Including Walnuts in a Low-Fat/Modified-Fat Diet Improves HDL Cholesterol-to-Total Cholesterol Ratios in Patients With Type 2 Diabetes. Diabetes Care 2004;27:2777–83.

142 Phillips M, Carapetis M. Six steps to a healthy lifestyle- the keystone in managing type 2 diabetes. Medicine Today 2008;8:51–58.

143 Lindeberg S, Jönsson T, Granfeldt Y, et. al. A Palaeolithic diet improves glucose tolerance more than a Mediterranean-like diet in individuals with ischaemic heart disease. Diabetologia 2007;50:1795–807.

144 Ornish DM. Can lifestyle changes reverse coronary heart disease? Lancet 1990;336:129–33.

145 Pischke CR, Scherwitz L, Weidner G, et. al. Long-term effects of lifestyle changes on well-being and cardiac variables among coronary heart disease patients. Health Psychol 2008;27(5):584–92.

146 Pischke CR, Weidner G, Elliott-Eller M, et. al. Lifestyle changes and clinical profile in coronary heart disease patients with an ejection fraction of <or=40% or >40% in the Multicenter Lifestyle Demonstration Project. Eur J Heart Fail 2007;9(9):928–34.

147 van Dam RM, Hu FB. Coffee consumption and risk of type 2 diabetes: a systematic review. JAMA 2005;294(1):97–104.

148 Smith B, Wingard DL, Smith TC, et. al. Does coffee consumption reduce the risk of type 2 diabetes in individuals with impaired glucose? Diabetes Care 2006;29:2385–90.

149 Bidel S, Hu G, et. al. Effects of coffee consumption on glucose tolerance, serum glucose and insulin levels-a cross-sectional analysis. Horm Metabol Res 2006;38:38–43.

150 Paynter NP, Yeh HC, Voutilainen S, et. al. Coffee and sweetened beverage consumption and the risk of type 2 diabetes mellitus: the atherosclerosis risk in communities study. Am J Epidemiol 2006;164:1075–84.

151 Balzer J, Rassaf T, Heiss C, et. al. Sustained Benefits in Vascular Function Through Flavanol-Containing Cocoa in Medicated Diabetic Patients. A Double-Masked, Randomised, Controlled Trial. J Am Coll Cardiol 2008;51:2141–49.

152 Mackenzie T, Brooks B, O'Connor G. Beverage intake, diabetes, and glucose control of adults in America. Ann Epidemiol 2006;16:688–91.

153 Shai I, Wainstein J, Harman-Boehm I, et. al. Glycemic Effects of Moderate Alcohol Intake Among Patients With Type 2 Diabetes. A multicenter, randomised, clinical intervention trial. Diabetes Care 2007;30:3011–16.

154 Bonnefont-Rousselot D. The role of antioxidant micronutrients in the prevention of diabetic complications. Treat Endocrinol 2004;3(1): 41–52.

155 Sargeant LA, Wareham NJ, Bingham S, et. al. Vitamin C and hyperglycemia in the European Prospective Investigation into Cancer--Norfolk (EPIC- Norfolk) study: a population-based study. Diabetes Care 2000;23:726–32.

156 Ting HH, Timimi FK, Boles KS, et. al. Vitamin C improves endothelium-dependent vasodilatation in patients with non-insulin dependent diabetes mellitus. J Clin Invt 1996;97:22–8.

157 Lai MH. Antioxidant effects and insulin resistance improvement of chromium combined with vitamin C and e supplementation for type 2 diabetes mellitus. J Clin Biochem Nutr 2008;43(3):191–8.

158 Afkhami-Ardekani M, Shojaoddiny-Ardekani A. Effect of vitamin C on blood glucose, serum lipids and serum insulin in type 2 diabetes payients. Indian J Med Res 2007;126(5):471–4.

159 Lopes de Jesus CC, Atallah AN, Valente O, et. al. Vitamin C and superoxide dismutase (SOD) for diabetic retinopathy. Cochrane Database of Systematic Reviews 2008, Issue 1. Art. No.: CD006695. doi: 10.1002/14651858.CD006695.pub2.

160 Paolisso G, D'Amore A, Galzerano D, et. al. Daily vitamin E supplements improve metabolic control but not insulin secretion in elderly Type 2 diabetic patients. Diabetes Care 1993;16:1433–37.

161 Huijgens PC, van den Berg CA, Imandt LM, et. al. Vitamin E and platelet aggregation. ACTA Haematol 1981;65:217–8.

162 Luong K, Nguyen LTH, Nguyen DNP. The role of vitamin D in protecting type 1 diabetes mellitus. Diabetes Metab Res Rev 2005;21:338–46.

163 Mathieu C, Gysemans C, Guilietti A, et. al. Vitamin D and diabetes. Diabetologia 2005; 48:1247–57.
164 Zipitis CS, Akobeng AK. Vitamin D Supplementation in Early Childhood and Risk of Type 1 Diabetes: a Systematic Review and Meta-analysis. Archives of Disease in Childhood 2008;93:512–17.
165 Rabbani N, Alam SS, Riaz S, et. al. High-dose thiamine therapy for patients with type 2 diabetes and microalbuminuria: a randomised, double-blind placebo-controlled pilot study. Diabetologia 2008 Dec 5. Epub ahead of print.
166 Janssen I, Powell LH, Crawford S, et. al. Menopause and the metabolic syndrome: the Study of Women's Health Across the Nation. Arch Intern Med 2002;162:1568–75.
167 Yoshida M, Jacques PF, Meigs JB, et. al. Effect of vitamin K supplementation on insulin resistance in older men and women. Diabetes Care 2008;31:2092–96.
168 Sahin M, Tutuncu NB, Ertugrul D, et. al. Effects of metformin or rosiglitazone on serum concentrations of homocysteine, folate, and vitamin B12 in patients with type 2 diabetes mellitus. J Diabetes Complications 2007;21(2):118–23.
169 Ting RZ, Szeto CC, Chan MH, et. al. Risk factors of vitamin B12 deficiency inpatients receiving metformin. Archives of Internal Medicine 2006; 166:1075–79.
170 Bursell SE, Clermont AC, Aiello LP, et. al. High-dose vitamin E supplementation normalises retinal blood flow and creatinine clearance in patients with type 1 diabetes. Diabetes Care 1999;22:1245–51.
171 Skyrme-Jones RA, O'Brien RC, et. al. Vitamin E supplementation improves endothelial function in type I diabetes mellitus: a randomised, placebo-controlled study. J Am Coll Cardiol 2000;36(1):94–102.
172 Church TS, Earnest CP, Wood KA, et. al. Reduction of C-reactive protein levels through use of a multivitamin. Am J Med 2003;115(9):702–7.
173 Farvid MS, Jalali M, Siassi F, et. al. Comparison of the effects of vitamins and/or mineral supplementation on glomerular and tubular dysfunction in type 2 diabetes. Diabetes Care 2005;28(10):2458–64.
174 Farvid MS, Siassi F, Jalali M, et. al. The impact of vitamin and/or mineral supplementation on lipid profiles in type 2 diabetes. Diabetes Res Clin Pract 2004;65(1):21–8.
175 Farvid MS, Jalali M, Siassi F, et. al. The impact of vitamins and/or mineral supplementation on blood pressure in type 2 diabetes. J Am Coll Nut 2004;23(3):272–9.
176 Czernichow S, Couthouis A, Bertrais S, et. al. Antioxidant supplementation does not affect fasting plasma glucose in the SU.VI.MAX study in France: association with dietary intake and plasma concentrations. AJCN 2006;84(2):395–9.
177 Barringer TA, Kirk JK, Santaniello AC, et. al. Effect of a multivitamin and mineral supplement on infection and quality of life. A randomised, double-blind, placebo-controlled trial. Ann Intern Med 2003;138(5):365–71.
178 Anderson RA. Chromium in the prevention and control of diabetes. Diabetes Metab 2000;26(1):22–7.
179 Lau FC, Bagchi M, Sen CK, et. al. Nutrigenomic basis of beneficial effects of chromium(III) on obesity and diabetes. Mol Cell Biochem 2008;317(1-2):1–10.
180 Finney LS, et. al. Dietary chromium and diabetes: is there a relationship? Clin Diabetes 1997;15:6–10.
181 Roussel AM, Andriollo-Sanchez M, Ferry M, et. al. Food chromium content, dietary chromium intake and related biological variables in French free-living elderly. Br J Nutr 2007;98(2):326–31.
182 Vladeva SV, Terzieva DD, Arabadjiiska DT. The effect of chromium on the insulin resistance in patients with type II DM. Folia Med 2005;47(3-4):59–62.
183 Aguilar MV, Saavedra P, Arrieta FJ, et. al. Plasma mineral content in Type II diabetic patients and their association with the metabolic syndrome. Ann Nutr Metab 2007;51:402–6.
184 Vladeva SV, Terzieva DD, Arabadjiiska DT. The effect of chromium on the insulin resistance in patients with type II DM. Folia Med 2005;47(3-4):59–62.
185 Mark DA. Chromium picolinate supplementation attenuates body weight gain and increases insulin sensitivity in subjects with type II DM. Diab Care 2006;29:2764.
186 Sreekanth R, Pattabhi V, Rajan SS. Molecular basis of chromium insulin interactions. Biochem Biophys Res Commun 2008;369(2):725–9.
187 Singer GM, Geohas J. The effect of chromium picolinate and biotin supplementation on glycaemic control in poorly controlled patients with type II DM: A placebo-controlled, double-blinded, randomised trial. Diabetes Technol Ther 2006;8:636–43.
188 Martin J, Wang ZQ, Zhang XH, et. al. Chromium picolinate supplementation attenuates Body weight gain and increases insulin sensitivity in subjects with type II DM. Diabetes Care 2006;29:1826–32.
189 Yang X, Li SY, Dong F, et. al. Insulin-sensitising and cholesterol-lowering effects of chromium (D-phenylalanine). J Inorg Biochem 2006;100(7):1187–93.
190 Balk EM, Tatsioni A, Lichtenstein AH, et. al. Effect of chromium supplementation on glucose metabolism and lipids: a systematic review of randomised controlled trials. Diabetes Care 2007;30(8):2154–63.
191 Broadhurst CL, Domenico P. Clinical studies on chromium picolinate supplementation in diabetes mellitus—a review. Diabetes Technol Ther 2006;8(6):677–87.
192 Feiner JJ, McNurlan MA, Ferris RE, et. al. Chromium picolinate for insulin resistance in subjects with HIV disease: a pilot study. Diabetes Obes Metab 2008;10(2):151–8.
193 Komorowski JR, Greenberg D, Juturu V. Chromium picolinate does not produce chromosomal damage. Toxicol in Vitro 2008;22(3):819–26.
194 Albarracin C, Fuqua B, Geohas J, et. al. Combination of chromium and biotin improves coronary risk factors in hypercholesterolemic type 2 diabetes mellitus: a placebo-controlled, double-blind randomised clinical trial. J Cardiometab Syndr 2007;2(2):91–7.
195 Albarracin CA, Fuqua BC, Evans JL, et. al. Chromium picolinate and biotin combination improves glucose metabolism in treated, uncontrolled overweight to obese patients with type 2 diabetes. Diab Metab Res Rev 2008;24(1):41–51.
196 Geohas J, Daly A, Juturu V, et. al. Chromium picolinate and biotin combination reduces atherogenic index of plasma in patients with type 2 diabetes mellitus: a placebo-controlled, double-blinded, randomised clinical trial. Am J Med Sci 2007;333(3):145–53.
197 Gunton JE, Cheung WN, Hitchman R, et. al. Chromium Supplementation Does Not Improve Glucose Tolerance, Insulin Sensitivity, or Lipid Profile: A randomised, placebo-controlled, double-blind trial of supplementation in subjects with impaired glucose tolerance. Diabetes Care 2005;28:712–13.

198 Althius MD, Jordan NE, Ludington EA, et. al. Glucose and insulin responses to dietary chromium supplements: a meta-analysis. AJCN 2002;76:148–55.
199 Takaya J, Higashino H, Kobayashi Y. Intracellular magnesium and insulin resistance. Magnes Res 2004;17(2):126–36.
200 Wells IC. Evidence that the etiology of the syndrome containing type 2 diabetes mellitus results from abnormal magnesium metabolism. Can J Physiol Pharmacol 2008;86(1-2):16–24.
201 Volpe SL. Magnesium, the metabolic syndrome, insulin resistance, and type 2 diabetes mellitus. Crit Rev Food Sci Nutr 2008;48(3):293–300.
202 Larsson SC, Wolk A. Magnesium intake and risk of type 2 diabetes: a meta-analysis. J Intern Med 2007;262(2):208–14.
203 Lopez-Ridaura, Willett WC, Rimm EB, et. al. Magnesium intake and risk of Type 2 diabetes in men and women. Diabetes Care 2004;27:134–40.
204 Song Y, Ridker PM, Manson JE, et. al. Magnesium intake, C-reactive protein, and the prevalence of metabolic syndrome in middle-aged and older U.S. women. Diabetes Care 2005;28(6):1438–44.
205 Huertamg, Rascón-Pacheco RA, Rodríguez-Morán M, et. al. Magnesium deficiency is associated with insulin resistance in obese children. Diabetes Care 2005;28(5):1175–81.
206 Chambers EC, Heshka S, Gallagher D, et. al. Serum magnesium and Type II DM in African-Americans and Hispanics: A New York cohort. J Am Coll Nutr 2006;25(6):509–13.
207 Van Dam RM, Hu FB, Rosenberg L, et. al. Dietary calcium and magnesium major food sources, and risk of Type II DM in US black women. Diab Care 2006;29(10):2238–43.
208 Sharma A, Dabla S, Agrawal RP, et. al. Serum magnesium: An early predictor of course and complications of DM. J Indian Med Assoc 2007;105(1):16–20.
209 Mayer-Davis EJ, Nichols M, Liese AD, et. al. Dietary intake among youth with DM: the SEARCH for DM in youth study. J Am Diet Assoc 2006;106(5): 689–97.
210 He K, Liu K, Daviglus ML, et. al. Magnesium intake and incidence of metabolic syndrome among young adults. Circulation 2006;113(13): 1675–82.
211 Pham PC, Pham PM, Pham SV. Hypomagnesemia in patients with type 2 diabetes mellitus. Clin J Am Soc Nephrol 2007;2(2):366–73.
212 Brabagallo M, Dominguez LJ. Magnesium metabolism in Type II DM, metabolic syndrome and insulin resistance. Arch Biochem Biophys 2007;458(1):40–7.
213 Volpe SL. Magnesium, the metabolic syndrome, insulin resistance and type II DM. Crit Rev Food Sci Nutr 2008;48(93):293–300.
214 Longstreet DA, Heath DL, Panaretto KS, et. al. Correlations suggest low magnesium may lead to higher rates of type II DM in indigenous Australians. Rural Remote Health 2007;7:843.
215 Schulze MB, Schulz M, Heidemann C, et. al. Fiber and Magnesium Intake and Incidence of Type 2 Diabetes A Prospective Study and Meta-analysis. Arch Intern Med 2007;167:956–65.
216 Larsson SC, Wolk A. Magnesium intake and risk of Type II DM: A meta-analysis. J Intern Med 2007;262(2):208–14.
217 Sales CH, Pedrosa Lde F. Magnesium and DM: Their relation. Clin Nutr 2006;25(4):554–62.
218 Corica F, Corsonello A, Ientile R, et. al. Serum ionised magnesium levels in relation to metabolic syndrome in Type II DM patients. J Am Coll Nutr 2006;25(3):210–5.
219 Rumawas ME, McKeown NM, Rogers G, et. al. Magnesium intake is related to improved insulin homeostasis in the Framingham Offspring cohort. J Am Coll Nutr 2006;25(6):486–92.
220 Bo S, Durazzo M, Guidi S, et. al. Dietary magnesium and fibre intakes and inflammatory and metabolic indicators in middle-aged subjects from a population-based cohort. Am J Clin Nutr 2006;84(5):1062–9.
221 Ma B, Lawson AB, Liese AD, et. al. Dairy, magnesium and calcium intake in relation to insulin sensitivity: Approaches to modeling a dose-dependent association. Am J Epidemiol 2006;164(5):449–58.
222 Song Y, Buring J, Manson AE, et. al. Dietary magnesium intake in relation to plasma insulin levels and risk of Type 2 Diabetes in women. Diabetes Care 2004;27:59–65.
223 Guerrero-Romero F, Tamez-Perez HE, Gonzalez-Gonzalez G, et. al. Oral magnesium supplementation improves insulin sensitivity in non-diabetic subjects with insulin resistance. A double-blind placebo-controlled randomised trial. Diabetes Metab 2004;30(3):253–58.
224 Rodrıguez-Moran M, Guerrero-Romero F. Oral Magnesium supplementation improves insulin sensitivity and metabolic control in Type 2 diabetic subjects. A randomised, double-blind controlled trial. Diabetes Care 2003;26:1147–52.
225 Beletate V, El Dib RP, Atallah AN. Zinc supplementation for the prevention of type 2 diabetes mellitus. Cochrane Database Syst Rev 2007;(1):CD005525.
226 Al-Maroof RA, Al-Shaarbatti SS. Serum zinc levels in diabetic patients and effect of zinc supplementation on glycemic control of type 2 diabetics. Saudi Med J 2006;27(3):344–50.
227 Adachi Y, Yoshida j, kodera Y, et. al. Oral administration of a zinc complex improves type II DM and metabolic syndromes. Biochem Biophys Res Commun 2006;8351(1):165–70.
228 Yoshikawa Y, Adachi Y, Sakurai H. A new type of orally active anti-diabetic Zn(II)-dithiocarbamate complex. Life Sci 2007;80(8):759–66.
229 Soinio M, Marniemi J, Laakso M, et. al. Serum zinc level and coronary heart disease events in patients with type II DM. Diabetes Care 2007;30(3):523–8.
230 Hayee MA, Mohammed QD, Haque A. Diabetic neuropathy and zinc therapy. Bangladesh Med Res Counc Bull 2005;31(2):62–7.
231 Blostein-Fujii A, DiSilvestro RA, Frid D, et. al. Short-term zinc supplementation in women with non-insulin-dependent diabetes mellitus: effects on plasma 5′-nucleotidase activities, insulin-like growth factor I concentrations, and lipoprotein oxidation rates in vitro. Am J Clin Nutr 1997;66:639–42.
232 Anderson RA, Roussel AM, Zouari N, et. al. Potential antioxidant effects of zinc and chromium supplementation in people with Type 2 diabetes mellitus. J Am Col Nutr 2001;20:212–18.
233 Beletate V, El Dib RP, Atallah AN. Zinc supplementation for the prevention of type 2 diabetes mellitus. Cochrane Database of Systematic Reviews 2007, Issue 1. Art. No.: CD005525. doi: 10.1002/14651858.CD005525.pub2.
234 Brichard SM, Henquin JC. The role of vanadium in the management of diabetes. Trends in Pharmacological Sciences 1995;16:265–70.

235 Preet A, Gupta BL, Yadava PK, et. al. efficacy of lower doses of vanadium in restoring altered glucose metabolism and anti-oxidant status in diabetic rat lenses. J Biosci 2005;30(2):221–30.

236 Bartlett HE, Eperjesi F. Nutritional supplementation for type 2 diabetes: a systematic review. Ophthalmic Physiol Opt 2008;28(6):503–23.

237 Ziegler D, Hanefeld M, Ruhnau KJ, et. al. Treatment of symptomatic diabetic neuropathy with the antioxidant alpha-lipoic acid: a meta-analysis. Diab Med 2004; 21:114–12.

238 Boger RH, Ron ES. L–Arginine improves vascular function by overcoming deleterious effects of ADMA, a novel CV risk factor. Altern Med Rev 2005;10(1):14–23.

239 Piatti PM, et. al. Long term oral L–arginine administration improves peripheral and hepatic insulin sensitivity in Type 2 diabetic patients. Diabetes Care 2001;24(5):875–80.

240 Lerman A, et. al. Long term L-arginine supplementation improves small-vessel coronary endothelial function in humans. Circulation 1998;97(21):2123–8.

241 Piatti PM, Monti LD, Valsecchi G, et. al. Long term oral L-arginine administration improves peripheral and hepatic insulin sensitivity in Type 2 diabetic patients. Diabetes Care 2001;24(5):875–80.

242 Hodgson JM, Watts GF, Playford Da, et. al. Coenzyme Q10 improves blood pressure and glycemic control: a controlled trial of subjects with type 2 diabetes. Eur J Clin Nutr 2002;56(11):1137–42.

243 Henriksen JE, et. al. Impact of ubiquinone (coenzyme Q10) treatment on glycemic control, insulin requirement and well-being in patients with Type 1 diabetes mellitus. Diabet Med 1999;16(4):312–8.

244 Hamilton SJ, Chew GT, Watts GF. Co Enzyme Q_{10} improves endothelial dysfunction in statin-treated type 2 diabetic patients. Diabetes Care 2009 February 19. doi: 10.2337/dc08-1736.

245 Giacco R, Cuomo V, Vessby B, et. al. Fish oil, insulin sensitivity, insulin secretion and glucose tolerance in healthy people: Is there any effect of fish oil supplementation in relation to the type of background diet and habitual dietary intake of n-6 and n-3 fatty acids? Nutr Metabol Cardiovasc Dis 2007;17:572:e580.

246 Norris JM, Yin X, Lamb MM, et. al. Omega-3 polyunsaturated fatty acid intake and islet autoimmunity in children at increased risk for type 1 diabetes. JAMA 2007;298:1420–8.

247 Farmer A, Montori V, Dinneen S, et. al. Fish oil in people with type 2 diabetes mellitus. The Cochrane Database of Systematic Reviews 2006(3).

248 Heart Foundation Australia. Online. Available: www.heartfoundation.org.au/http://www.heartfoundation.org.au/SiteCollectionDocuments/HW_FS_Fish Oils_PS_FINAL_web.pdf (accessed December 2008)

249 Hartweg J, Perera R, Montori V, et. al. Omega-3 polyunsaturated fatty acids (PUFA) for type 2 diabetes mellitus. Cochrane Database of Systematic Reviews 2008, Issue 1. Art. No.: CD003205. doi: 10.1002/14651858.CD003205.pub2.

250 Yeh GY, Eisenberg DM, Kaptchuk TJ, et. al. Systematic Review of Herbs and Dietary Supplements for Glycemic Control in Diabetes. Diab Care 2003;26:1277–94.

251 Vuksan V, Sievenpiper JL, Wong J, et. al. American ginseng (Panax quinquefolius L) attenuates postprandial glycemia in a time-dependent but not dose-dependent manner in healthy individuals. AJCN 2001;73(4):753–58.

252 Vuksan V, Sievenpiper JL, Koo VY, et. al. American ginseng (Panax quinquefolius L) reduces postprandial glycemia in nondiabetic subjects and subjects wit type 2 diabetes mellitus. Arch Int Med 2000;160:1009–13.

253 Vuksan V, Sung MK, Sievenpiper JL, et. al. Korean red ginseng (*Panax ginseng*) improves glucose and insulin regulation in well-controlled, type 2 diabetes: results of a randomised, double-blind, placebo-controlled study of efficacy and safety. Nutr Metab Cardiovasc Dis 2008;18(1):46–56.

254 Khan A, Bryden N, Polansky M, et. al. Cinnamon improves glucose and lipids of people with Type 2 diabetes. Diabetes Care 2003;26:3215–18.

255 Yeh GY, Eisenberg DM, Kaptchuk TJ, et. al. Systematic review of herbs and dietary supplements for glycaemic control in diabetes. Diabetes Care 2003;26:1277–94.

256 Anderson RA. Chromium and polyphenols from cinnamon improve insulin sensitivity. Proc Nutr Soc 2008;67(1):48–53.

257 Baker WL, Gutierrez-Williams G, White CM, et. al. Effect of cinnamon on glucose control and lipid parameters. Diabetes Care 2008;31(1):41–3.

258 Altschuler JA, Casella SJ, MacKenzie TA.The effect of cinnamon on A1C among adolescents with type 1 diabetes. Diabetes Care 2007;30(4):813–6.

259 Blevins SM, Leyva MJ, Brown J, et. al. Effect of cinnamon on glucose and lipid levels in non insulin-dependent type 2 diabetes. Diab Care 2007;30(9):2236–7.

260 Khan A, Safdar M, Ali Khan MM, et. al. Cinnamon improves glucose and lipids of people with type 2 diabetes. Diabetes Care 2003;26(12):3215–8.

261 Mang B, Wolters M, Schmitt B, et. al. Effects of a cinnamon extract on plasma glucose, HbA, and serum lipids in diabetes mellitus type 2. Eur J Clin Invest 2006;36(5):340–4.

262 Vanschoonbeek K, Thomassen BJ, Senden JM, et. al. Cinnamon supplementation does not improve glycemic control in postmenopausal type 2 diabetes patients. J Nutr 2006;136(4):977–80.

263 Hlebowicz J, Hlebowicz A, Lindstedt S, et. al. Effects of 1 and 3 g cinnamon on gastric emptying, satiety,and postprandial blood glucose, insulin, glucose-dependent insulinotropic polypeptide, glucagon-like peptide 1, and ghrelin concentrations in healthy subjects. AJCN 2009;89:815–21.

264 Porchezhian E, Dobriyal RM. An overview on the advances of Gymnema sylvestre: chemistry, pharmacology and patents. Pharmazie 2003;58(1):5–12.

265 Persaud SJ, Al-Majed H, Raman A, et. al. Gymnema silvestre stimulates insulin release in vitro by increasing membrane permeability. J Endocrinol 1999;163:207–13.

266 Brala PM, Hagen RL. Effects of sweetness perception and calorie value of a preload on short-term intake. Physiol Behav 1983;30:1–9.

267 Kanetkar P, Singhal R, Kamat M. Gymnema sylvestre: A Memoir. J Clin Biochem Nutr 2007;41(2):77–81.

268 Chattopadhyay RR. A comparative evaluation of some blood sugar lowering agents of plant origin. J Ethnoopharmacol 1999;30;67(3):367–72.

269 Leach MJ. Gymnema sylvestre for DM: a systematic review. J Alt Comp Med 2007;13(9):977–83.

270 Kanetkar PV, Singhal RS, Laddha KS, et. al. Extraction and quantification of gymnemic acids through gymnemagenin from callus cultures of Gymnema sylvestre. Phytochem Anal 2006;17(6):409–13.

271 Kimura I. Medical benefits of using natural compounds and their derivatives having multiple pharmacological actions. Yakugaku Zasshi 2006;126(3):133–43.

272 Baskaran K, Kisar Ahamath B, Radha Shanmugasundarum K, et. al. Anti-diabetic effects of a leaf extract from gymnema sylvestre in NIDDM patients. J Ethnopharmacol 1990;30(3):295–300.

273 Al Habori M, Raman A, Lawrence MJ, et. al. In vitro effect of fenugreek extracts on intestinal sodium-dependent glucose uptake and hepatic glycogen phosphorylase A. Int J Exp Diabetes Res 2001;2: 91–9.

274 Raju J, Patiolla JM, Swamy MV, et. al. Diosgenin, a steroid saponin of Trigonella foenum graecum inhibits azoxymethane-induce aberrant crypt foci formation in F344 rats and induces apoptosis in HT-29 human colon cancer cells. Cancer Epidemiol biomarkers Prev 2004 Aug;13(8):1392–8.

275 Broca C, Breil V, Cruciani-Guglielmacci C, et. al. Insulinotropic agent ID-1101 (4-hydroxyleucine) activates insulin signaling in rat. Am J Physiol Endocrinol Metab 2004 Sept;287(3):E463–71.

276 Flammang AM, Cifone MA, Erexson GL, et. al. Genotoxicity testing of a fenugreek extract. Food Chem Toxicol 2004 Nov;42(11):1769–75.

277 Vijayakumar MV, Singh S, Chhipa RR, et. al. The hypoglycaemic activity of fenugreek seed extract is mediated through the stimulation of an insulin signaling pathway. Br J Pharmacol 2005;146(1): 41–8.

278 Puri D, Prabhu KM, Murthy PS. Mechanism of action of a hypoglycaemic principle isolated from fenugreek seeds. Indian J Physiol Pharmacol, 2002;46(4):457–62.

279 Vijayakumar MV, Bhat MK. Hypoglycaemic effect of a novel dialysed fenugreek seeds extract is sustainable and is mediated, in part, by the activation of hepatic enzymes. Phytother Res 2008;22(4):500–5.

280 Hannan JM, Ali L, Rokeya B, et. al. Soluble dietary fibre fraction of trigonella foenum graecum seed improves glucose homeostasis in animal models of Type I and II DM by delaying carbohydrate carbohydrate digestion and absorption, and enhancing insulin action. Br J Nutr 2007;97(3):514–21.

281 Kumar GS, Shetty AK, Salimath PV. Modulatory effect of fenugreek seed mucilage and spent turmeric on intestinal and renal disaccharidases in STZ induced diabetic rats. Plant Foods Hum Nutr 2005;60(2):87–91.

282 Mohammed S, Taha A, Akhtar K, et. al. In vivo effect of trigonella on the expression of pyruvate kinase, phosphoenolpyruvate carboxykinase, and distribution of glucose transporter (GLUT4) in alloxan-diabetic rats. Can J Physiol Pharmacol 2006;84(6):647–54.

283 Raju J, Gupta D, Rao AR, et. al. Trigonella seed powder improves glucose homeostasis in alloxan diabetic rat tissues by reversing the altered glycolytic, gluconeogenic and lipogenic enzymes. Mol Cell Biochem 2001;224(1-2):45–51.

284 Vats V, Yadav SP, Grover JK. Effect of Trigonella on glycogen contant of tissues of tissues and the key enzymes of carbohydrate metabolism. J Ethnopharmacol 2003;85(2-3):237–42.

285 Pathak P, Srivastava S, Grover S. Development of food products based on millets, legumes and fenugreek seeds and their suitability in the diabetic diet. Int J Food Sci Nutr 2000 Sept;51(5):409–14.

286 Mohamed S, Taha A, Bamezai RN, et. al. Lower doses of vanadate in combination with trigonella restore altered carbohydrate metabolism and anti-oxidant status in alloxan-diabetic rats. Clin Chem Acta 2004;342(1-2):105–14.

287 Siddiqui MR, Taha A, Moorthy K, et. al. Amelioration of altered antioxidant status and membrane linked functions by vanadium and Trigonella in alloxan diabetic rat brains. J Biosci 2005 Sept;30(4):483–90.

288 Mohamed S, Taha A, Bamezai RN, et. al. Modulation of glucose transporter (GLUT4) by vanadate and Trigonella in alloxan diabetic rats. Life Sci 2006;78(8):820–4.

289 Siddiqui MR, Taha A, Moorthy K, et. al. Low doses of vanadate and Trigonella synergistically regulate Na/K and ATPase activity and GLUT4 translocation in alloxan diabetic rats. Mol cell Biochem 2006;285(1-2):17–27.

290 Xue WL, li XS, Zhang J, et. al. effect of Trigonella extract on blood glucose, blood lipids and haemorrheological properties in STZ-induced diabetic rats. Asia Pac J Clin Nutr 2007;16(Suppl 1): 422–6.

291 Kaviarasan S, Vijayalakshmi K, anuradha CV. Polyphenol rich extract of fenugreek seeds protect erythrocytes from oxidative damage. Plant Foods Hum Nutr 2004 Fall;59(4):143–7.

292 Petit PR, Sauvaire YD, Hillaire-buys DM, et. al. Steroid saponins from fenugreek seeds: extraction, purification and pharmacological investigation on feeding behaviour and plasma cholesterol. Steroids 1995;60(10):674–80.

293 Valette G, Sauvaire Y, Baccou JC, et. al. Hypocholesterolaemic effect of fenugreek seeds in dogs. Atherosclerosis 1984;50(1):105–11.

294 Sauvaire Y, Ribes G, Baccou JC, et. al. Implication of steroid saponins and sapogenins in the hypocholesterolaemic effect of fenugreek. Lipids 1991;26(3):191–7.

295 Ravikumar P, Anuradha CV. Effect of fenugreek seeds on blood lipid peroxidation and antioxidants in diabetic rats. Phytother Res 1999;13(3):197–201.

296 Annida B, Stanely Mainzen Prince P. Supplementation of fenugreek leaves lower lipid profile in STZ-induced diabatic rats. J Med Food 2004 Summer;7(2):152–6.

297 Narender T, Puri A, Shweta A, et. al. 4-Hydroxyleucine an unusual amino acid as antidyslipidaemic and antihyperglycaemic agent. Bioorg Med Chem Lett 2006;16(2):293–6.

298 Hannan JM, Rokeya B, Faruque O, et. al. Effect of soluble dietary fibre fraction of Trigonella on glycaemic, insulinaemic, lipidaemic and platelet aggregation status of type II diabetic model rats. J Ethnopharmacol 2003;88(1):73–7.

299 Gupta A, Gupta R, Lai B. Effect of Trigonella seeds on glycaemic control and insulin resistance in Type II DM: A double-blind placebo-controlled study. J Assoc Physicians India 2001;49:1057–61.

300 Bordia A, Verma SK, Srivastava KC. Effect of ginger and fenugreek on blood lipids, blood sugar and platelet aggregation in patients with coronary artery disease. Prostaglandins Leukot Fatty Acids 1997;56(5):379–84.

301 Genet S, Kale RK, Baquer NZ. Alterations in antioxidant enzymes and oxidative damage in experimental diabetic rat tissues: effect of vanadate and fenugreek. Mol Cell biochem 2002;236(1-2): 7–12.

302 Anuradha CV, Ravikumar P. restoration on tissue antioxidants by fenugreek seeds in alloxan diabetic rats. Indian J Physiol Pharmacol 2001;45(4):408–20.
303 Preet A, Siddiqui MR, taha A, et. al. Long-term effect of trigonella and its combination with sodium orthovanadate in preventing histopathological and biochemical abnormalities in diabetic rat ocular tissues. Mol Cell Biochem 2006;289(1-2):137–47.
304 Vats V, yadav SP, Biswas NR, et. al. Anti-cataract activity of Pterocarpus marsupium bark and Trigonella seed extract in alloxan diabetic rats. J Ethnopharmacol 2004;93(2-3):289–94.
305 Preet A, Gupta BL, Siddiqui MR, et. al. Restoration of ultrastructural and biochemical changes in alloxan-induced diabetic rat sciatic nerve on treatment with Na3VO4 and Trigonella- a promising anti-diabetic agent. Mol Cell Biochem 2005;27891-2:21–31.
306 Sharma RD, Raghuram TC, Rao NS. Effect of fenugreek seeds on blood glucose and serum lipids in Type 1 diabetes. Eur J Clin Nutr 1990;44:301–8.
307 Gupta A, Gupta R, Lal B. Effect of Trigonella foenum-graecum (fenugreek) seeds on glycaemic control and insulin resistance in Type 2 diabetes mellitus: a double-blind placebo-controlled study. J Assoc Phys India 2001;49:1057–61.
308 Grover JK, Yadav SP. Pharmacological actions and potential uses of Momordica charantia: a review. J Ethnopharmacol 2004;93:123–32.
309 Basch E. Bitter lemon (Momordica charantia): a review of the efficacy and safety. Am J Health Syst Pharm 2003;60:356–59.
310 Dans AM, Villarruz MV, Jimeno CA, et. al. The effect of Momordica charantia capsule preparation on glycemic control in type 2 diabetes mellitus needs further studies. J Clin Epidemiol 2007;60(6):554–9.
311 Fukino Y, Ikeda A, Maruyama K, et. al. Randomised controlled trial for an effect of green tea-extract powder supplementation on glucose abnormalities. European Journal of Clinical Nutrition 2008;62:953–60.
312 Brown AL, Lane J, Coverly J, et. al. Effects of dietary supplementation with the green tea polyphenol epigallocatechin-3-gallate on insulin resistance and associated metabolic risk factors: randomised controlled trial. Br J Nutr 2008;19:1–9.
313 Kudulo GB. The effect of 3 month ingestion of Ginkgo biloba extract (EGb761) on pancreatic beta-cell function in response to glucose loading in individuals with NIDDM. J Clin Phrmacol 2001;41(6):600–11.
314 Kudulo GB, Delaney D, Blodgett J. Short-term ingestion of Ginkgo biloba extract (EGb761) reduces malondialdehyde levels in washed platelets of Type II DM subjects. Diabetes res Clin Pract 2005;68(1):29–38.
315 Kudolo GB, Wang W, Javors M et. al. The effect of the ingestion of EGb761 on the pharmacokinetics of metformin in non-diabetic and Type II DM subjects – a double-blind, placebo-controlled, crossover study. Clin Nutr 2006;25(4):606–16.
316 Kudulo GB, Dorsey S, Blodgett J. Effect of the ingestion of Ginkgo biloba extract on platelet aggregation and urinary prostanoid excretion in healthy and Type II DM subjects. Thromb Res.2002;108(2-3):151–60.
317 Kudulo GB, Wang W, Elrod R, et. al. Short-term ingestion of Ginkgo biloba extract does not alter whole body insulin sensitivity in non-diabetic, pre-diabetic or type II diabetic subjects –a randomised double-blind placebo-controlled crossover study. Clin Nutr 2006;25(1):123–34.
318 Tanaka S, Han LK, Zheng YN, et. al. Effects of the flavonoid fraction from Ginkgo biloba extraction on the postprandiol blood glucose elevation in rats. Yakugaku Zasshi 2004;124(9):605–11.
319 Fodor JI, Keve T. New phytotherapical opportunity in the prevention and treatment of Type II DM. Acta Pharm Hung 2006;76(4):200–7.
320 Welt K, Fitzl G, Schepper A. Experimental hypoxia of STZ-diabetic rat myocardium and protective effects of Ginkgo biloba extract. Ultrastructural investigation of microvascular endothelium. Exp Toxic Pathol 2001;52(6):503–12.
321 Fitzl G, Welt K, Martin R, et. al. The influence of hypoxia on the myocardium of experimentally diabetic rats with and without protection by ginkgo biloba extract. Ultrastructural and biochemical investigations on cardiomyocytes. Exp toxicol pathol 2000;52(5):419–30.
322 Welt K, Weiss J, Martin R, et. al. Ultrastructural, immunohistochemicalandbiochemicalinvestigationsofthe ratliverexposedtoexperimentaldiabetesandacutehypoxia with and without application of Ginkgo extract. Exp Toxicol Pathol 2004;55(5):331–45.
323 Witte S, Anadere I, Walitza E. Improvement of haemorrheology with ginkgo biloba extract. Decreasing a cardiovascular risk factor. Fortschr Med 1992;110(13):247–50.
324 Huang SY, Jeng C, Kao SC, et. al. Improved haemorrheological properties by Ginkgo biloba extract (EGb761) in Type II DM complicated by retinopathy. Clin Nutr 2004;23(4):615–21.
325 Bernardczyk-Meller J, Siwiec-Proscinska J, Stankiewicz W, et. al. Influence of EGb761 on the function of the retina in children and adolescent with long-lasting DM-preliminary report. Klin Oczna 2004;106(4-5):569–71.
326 Welt K, Weiss J, Martin R, et. al. Ginkgo biloba extracts protect rat kidney from diabetic and hypoxic damage. Phytomedicine 2007;14(2-3): 196–203.
327 Punkt K, Psinia I, Welt K, et. al. Effects on skeletal muscle fibres of diabetes and ginkgo biloba extract treatment. Acta Histochem 1999;101(1):53–69.
328 Wang GX, Cao FL, Chen J. Progress in researches on the pharmaceutical mechanism and clinical application of Ginkgo biloba extract on various kinds of diseases. Chin J Integr Med 2006;12(3): 324–9.
329 Lu J, He H. Clinical observation of Ginkgo biloba extract injection in treating early diabetic nephropathy. Chin J Integr Med 2005;11(3):226–8.
330 Zhu HW, Shi ZF, Chen YY. Effect of ginkgo biloba onearlydiabeticnephropathy.ZhongguoZhongXiYiJie He Za Zhi, 2005;25(10):889–91.
331 Ernst E, et. al. The Desktop Guide to Complementary and Alternative Medicine: an evidence-based approach. Mosby, Philadelphia, 2006.
332 Namdul T, Sood A, Ramakrishnan L, et. al. Efficacy ofTibetanmedicineasanadjunctinthetreatmentoftype 2 diabetes. Diabetes Care 2001;24:176–77.
333 Campbell MJ, Woodside JV, Honour JW, et. al. Effect of red clover-derived isoflavone supplementation on insulin-like growth factor, lipid and antioxidant status in healthy female volunteers: a pilot study. EJCN 2004;58:173–79.
334 Kato A, Minoshima Y, Yamamoto J, et. al. Protective effects of dietary chamomile tea on diabetic complications. J Agric Food Chem 2008;56(17):8206–11.

335 McKay DL, Blumberg JB. A review of the bioactivity and potential health benefits of chamomile tea (Matricaria recutita L.). Phytother Res 2006;20(7):519–30.

336 Apostolidis E, Kwon YI, Kalidas Shetty K. Potential of cranberry-based herbal synergies for diabetes and hypertension management. Asia Pac J Clin Nutr 2006;15:433–41.

337 Liu JP, Zhang M, Wang WY, et. al. Chinese herbal medicines for type 2 diabetes mellitus. Cochrane Database Syst Rev 2004;(3):CD003642.

338 Wang E, Wylie-Rosett J. Review of selected Chinese herbal medicines in the treatment of type 2 diabetes. Diabetes Educ 2008;34(4):645–54.

339 Grover JK, Yadav S, Vats V. Medicinal plants of India with anti-diabetic potential. J Ethnopharmacol 2002;81(1):81–100.

340 Moghaddam MS, Kumar PA, Reddy GB, et. al. Effect of Diabecon on sugar-induced lens opacity in organ culture: mechanism of action. J Ethnopharmacol 2005;97(2):397–403.

341 Brown L, Rosner B, Willett WW, et. al. Cholesterol-lowering effects of dietary fibre: a meta-analysis. Am J Clin Nutr 1999;69:30–42.

342 Anderson JW, Allgood LD, Turner J, et. al. Effects of psyllium on glucose and serum lipid responses in men with Type 2 diabetes and hypercholesterolaemia. AJCN 1999;70:466–73.

343 Hodgson DM, Nakamura T, Walker AK. Prophylactic role for complementary and alternative medicine in perinatal programming of adult health. Forsch Komplementmed 2007;14(2):92–101.

344 Wang XM. Treating Type 2 diabetes mellitus with foot reflexotherapy. Zhongguo Zhong Zxi Yi Jie He Za Zhi 1993;13:536–38.

345 Wang MY, Tsai PS, Lee PH, et. al. The efficacy of reflexology: systematic review. J Adv Nurs 2008;62(5):512–20.

346 National Prescribing Service NPS Newsletter 60, October 2008 ISSN 1441-7421.

347 Sowerby Centre for Health Informatics at Newcastle (SCHIN). Diabetes Type 1 and 2- foot disease. Clinical Knowledge Summaries. Newcastle upon Tyne, UK: National Library for Health, 2007.

348 Neal JM. Diabetic neuropathic cachexia: a rare manifestation of diabetic neuropathy. South Med J 2009;102(3):327–9.

349 Lee P, Chen R. Vitamin D as an analgesic for patients with type 2 diabetes and neuropathic pain. Arch Int Med 2008;168:771–72.

350 Reussmann HJ. On behalf of the German Society of outpatient diabetes centres AND. Switching from pathogenetic treatment with alpha-lipoic acid to gabapentin and other analgesics in painful diabetic neuropathy: a real world study in outpatients. J Diabetes Complications 2008 April 8.

351 Alleva, R, Nasole, et. al. Alpha-lipoic acid supplementation inhibits oxidative damage, accelerating chronic wound healing in patients undergoing hyperbaric oxygen therapy. Biochem Res Commun 2005;333(2):404–10.

352 Cha YS. Effects of L-carnitine on obesity, diabetes, and as an ergogenic aid Asia Pac J Clin Nutr 2008;17(Suppl 1):306–8.

353 Sima AA, Calvani M, Mehra M, et. al. Acetyl-L-Carnitine Study Group. Acetyl-L-carnitine improves pain, nerve regeneration, and vibratory perception in patients with chronic diabetic neuropathy: an analysis of two randomised placebo-controlled trials. Diabetes Care 2005;28(1):89–94.

354 De Grandis D, Minardi C. Acetyl-L-carnitine (levacecarnine) in the treatment of diabetic neuropathy. A long-term, randomised, double-blind, placebo-controlled study. Drugs R D 2002;3(4): 223–31.

355 Evans JD, Jacobs TF, Evans EW. Role of acetyl-L-carnitine in the treatment of diabetic peripheral neuropathy. Ann Pharmacother 2008;42(11): 1686–91.

356 Weintraub MI, Wolfe GI, Barohn RA, et. al. Static magnetic field therapy for symptomatic diabetic neuropathy: a randomised, double-blind, placebo-controlledtrial.ArchPhysMedRehabil2003;84:736–46.

Chapter 14

Eczema, psoriasis, skin cancers and other skin disorders

Introduction

The integument (the skin) is the largest and heaviest organ in the human body consisting of approximately 16% of body weight and is the primary interface between the internal environment and the outside surroundings.[1] Given that the thickness of skin has an extremely thin foundation, the epidermis protects animals against major environmental stresses, such as water loss and microorganism infection. Hence, the skin's primary function is to act as a barrier to protect the body from damage caused by outside forces, contaminants, microorganisms and radiation exposure.

The skin epidermis and its appendages undergo ongoing renewal by a process called *homeostasis*. Stem cells in the epidermis have a crucial role in maintaining tissue homeostasis by providing replacement cells to those that are constantly lost during tissue turnover or following traumatic injury. A number of different skin stem cell pools contribute to the maintenance and repair of the various epidermal tissues of the skin. These include the inter-follicular epidermis, hair follicles and sebaceous glands. It is interesting to note that the basic mechanisms and signalling pathways that orchestrate epithelial morphogenesis in the skin are reused during adult life to regulate skin homeostasis.[2]

In clinical practice, dermatology includes about 3000 diseases that affect the skin and its accessory tissues (e.g. hair and nails).[3] While many infamous epidemics with prominent skin manifestations such as small pox, plague, leprosy, and anthrax, have been largely controlled,[4] other dermatologic diseases such as warts, acne, and dermatitis remain especially common.

In 2004, more than 50% (165 million) of the US population suffered from herpes simplex virus (HSV) and herpes zoster virus (HZV) infections, and 83.3 million cases of human papilloma virus (HPV) infection were noted.[2] Indeed, at any given time, it has been reported that at least 25% of the population of the US suffer from at least 1 skin disease[5,6] — a state that constitutes a significant global burden of disease.[2, 7–10] A recent study from the US on the burden of skin diseases demonstrated that skin disease was 1 of the top 15 groups of medical conditions for which prevalence and health care spending increased the most between 1987 and 2000, with approximately 1 in 3 persons diagnosed with a skin disease at any given time (see Table 14.1).

Exposure of the skin to UV light has the potential to induce the formation of high concentrations of reactive oxygen species (ROS) which can destabilise ROS signalling functions and damage organelles and modify the structures of important molecules such as proteins, lipids and genetic material.[12] Sunlight, particularly ultraviolet B (UVB) (wavelength 290–320 nm), is responsible for sunburn, but also causes cellular damage. UVA light (wavelength 320–400 nm) burns less than UVB (wavelength 290–320 nm) and penetrates deep into the dermis (as far as the boundary with the epidermis). UVA light makes up the majority of sunlight, and is absorbed by a wide range of molecules, which can become photosensitisers, and can do more damage to the skin due to its greater ability to penetrate. Environmental pollutants such as ozone and oxides of nitrogen and sulphur are also able to produce free radicals in the skin, thereby also risking skin damage.[13] Although formed in the outer layers of the epidermis, these radicals induce damage in deeper layers in a manner similar to UV light.

A number of nutraceuticals have been claimed to exhibit useful activities in the area of skin health, including proanthocyanidins and the pine bark extract Pycnogenol, carotenoids, polyunsaturated fatty acids (PUFAs), tea, soy, glucosamine and melatonin.[14]

Table 14.1 Prevalence of selected skin diseases in the US

Skin disease	Prevalence in millions as at 2004
Acne (cystic and vulgaris)	50.2
Actinic keratosis	39.5
Atopic dermatitis	15.2
Benign neoplasms/keloid	29.4
Bullous diseases	0.14
Contact dermatitis	72.3
Cutaneous fungal infections	29.4
Cutaneous lymphoma	0.02
Drug eruptions	2.6
Hair and nail disorders	70.5
Herpes simplex and zoster	165.0
Human papillomavirus/warts	58.5
Lupus erythematosus	0.36
Psoriasis	3.1
Rosacea	14.7
Seborrheic dermatitis	5.9
Seborrheic keratosis	83.8
Skin cancer— melanoma	0.72
Skin cancer— non-melanocytic	1.2
Skin ulcers and wounds	4.8
Solar-radiation damage	123.1
Vitiligo	1.5

(Source: adapted and modified from Bickers et. al. 2006)[11]

Lifestyle factors

Smoking

The adverse health risks associated with smoking are well documented and this is also important for overall skin health. Smoking has been associated with the positive and negative prevalence of numerous diseases and conditions of the skin (see Table 14.2).[15, 16]

Epidemiological studies have demonstrated that tobacco smoking is one of many factors that significantly contributes to premature skin ageing in addition to other factors such as age, sex, skin pigmentation, sun exposure history, and alcohol consumption.[17–20] Moreover, smoking is the causal factor of smoker's wrinkles. Similarly, as with chronic exposure of the skin to ultraviolet radiation, tobacco also promotes manifested alterations in the structure and composition of the epidermis and dermis, similarly to that observed with photoageing. [21, 22, 23] In a recent study, tobacco smoking, but not ultraviolet exposure, was determined to be a strong predictor of skin ageing.[24]

Although smoking may have certain beneficial effects on some skin diseases (as described in Table 14.2), it is exceptionally difficult to favour this habit which is highly damaging to overall health. Tobacco smoking is currently the leading preventable cause of disease and death in Western countries, and some of its beneficial effects on the skin are significantly dwarfed when compared to the hazard risks to health encountered with habitual tobacco use for both smokers and those who are exposed to secondary tobacco smoke, therefore it cannot be recommended.

Alcohol

The long-term consumption of alcohol in excessive quantities can damage every organ system in the body. A recent report has documented that chronic excessive alcohol consumption in alcoholics was associated with a wide range of skin disorders that included urticaria, porphyria cutanea tarda, flushing, cutaneous stigmata of cirrhosis, psoriasis, pruritus, seborrheic dermatitis and rosacea.[25]

Life stressors

Psycho-emotional stressors have long been expected to exacerbate or even trigger allergic diseases such as atopic dermatitis (see Figure 14.1).[26, 27]

Psychodermatological or psychocutaneous disorders are conditions resulting from the interaction between the mind and the skin. There are 3 major groups of psychodermatological disorders recognised; psychophysiologic disorders, psychiatric disorders with dermatologic symptoms, and dermatologic disorders with psychiatric symptoms.[28]

A number of human studies have reported associations between personality traits and psychic disturbances such as stress perception, anxiety, or depression and atopic dermatitis severity or even onset.[29–32]

Table 14.2 Skin diseases and the effect of smoking

Diseases/conditions increased frequency and/or exacerbation	Diseases/conditions decreased frequency and/or improvement	Association contentious	No association
Psoriasis	Rosacea	Melanoma	Atopic dermatitis
Palmoplantar pustulosis	Oral aphthous ulcers	SCC of the skin	Mucosal pemphigoid
Scar formation	Herpes simplex labialis	BCC	Oral lichen planus
SCC of the lip SCC of the oral cavity SCC Anus and genitalia	Pemphigus vulgaris Dermatitis herpetiformis	Acne	
Hidradenitis Allergic contact dermatitis Favre-Racouchot syndrome Systemic lupus erythematosus Discoid lupus erythematosus Poor wound healing Premature skin ageing Hair loss			

*SCC = squamous cell carcinoma
**BCC = basal cell carcinoma
(Source: adapted from Just-Sarobé M, 2008)[15,16]

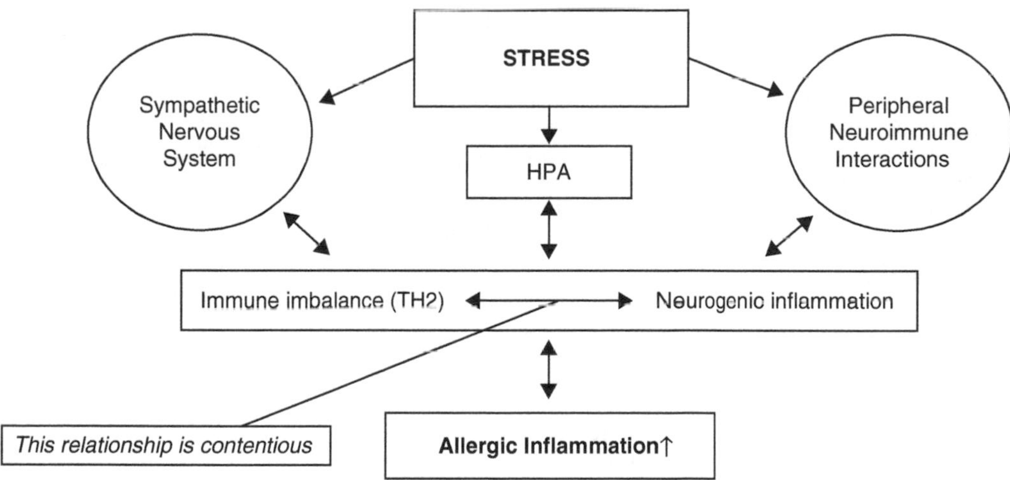

Figure 14.1 Stress axes exacerbating inflammatory skin diseases/conditions

Depression in dermatology patients often is multi-factorial in its cause. Genetic factors, psychosocial stressors, age of patients at onset of skin disease, body areas involved, physical discomfort (i.e. pruritus, pain, or burning), and clinical severity all are potential contributors.

The nature of the mechanisms that link stress and exacerbation of skin inflammation remain largely unknown. Recent studies suggest psycho–neuro–immunologic factors and emotional stressors are important in its evolution (Figure 14.1).[33]

The established explanation is that immune balance is altered by activation of 2 stress axes; namely, activation of the hypothalamic–pituitary–adrenal (HPA) axis that raises cortisol levels, and activation of the sympathetic nervous systems which raises adrenaline levels (Figure 14.1).[34] This mechanism of activity has been further investigated in wound-healing experiments. For more than a decade it has been extant that stress/stressors (which can range in magnitude and duration) can significantly slow wound healing.[35, 36]

Itch is a major feature of many skin diseases, which adversely affects patient's quality of life. Recently it was shown that cognitive factors, such as helplessness and worrying, and the behavioural response of scratching were indicated as possible worsening factors. This is consistent with overall findings that implicate a biopsychosocial model for the itch sensation.[37]

Environmental insults

There is increasing evidence that over-exposure of the skin to damaging environmental influences such as ultraviolet radiation, climatic determinants, chemicals and infections can significantly disrupt skin homeostasis.

Sunlight/ultraviolet (UV) exposure

Sunlight exposure produces a variety of adverse cutaneous effects, such as erythema, photosensitivity, and immunologic alterations, that represent acute events.

Among harmful environmental factors that contribute to extrinsic ageing, are the long-term effects of repeated exposure to UV that leads to carcinogenesis and photo-ageing as long-term consequences.

Acute adverse effects of sun exposure

Acute overexposure to sunlight causes sunburn, primarily because of ultraviolet B (UVB) (290–320 nm) radiation. This is characterised by erythema, oedema, and tenderness. Sunburn represents injury to both epidermal and dermal layers.[38]

Lentigo maligna

Repeated acute exposure over time may enhance the risk of skin disease as reported in a recent epidemiological study. The study reported that although chronically sun-exposed skin was recognised as a prerequisite for *lentigo maligna*, the risk of *lentigo maligna* did not increase with the cumulative dose of sun exposure; however, that *lentigo maligna* was associated with sunburn history, like all other types of melanomas. The main epidemiological characteristic of *lentigo maligna* reported in this study was the absence of an apparent relation with the genetic propensity to develop nevi.[39]

Skin cancers

The influence of painful sunburns and lifetime sun exposure to the skin has also been studied in other skin diseases.[40] Lifetime sun exposure was predominantly associated with an increased risk of squamous cell carcinoma (SCC) and actinic keratoses and to a lesser degree with basal cell carcinoma (BCC). By contrast, lifetime sun exposure appeared to be associated with a lower risk of malignant melanoma, despite the fact that lifetime sun exposure did not diminish the number of melanocytic nevi or atypical nevi. Neither painful sunburns nor lifetime sun exposure were associated with an increased risk of seborrheic warts.

Chronic adverse effects of sun exposure

Carcinogenesis

Over 100 years ago, Paul Gerson Unna correctly identified chronic solar exposure as the cause of SCC.[41] The vast majority of the non-melanoma forms of skin cancer (SCC and BCC) result from chronic or intense intermittent solar exposure, and perhaps two-thirds of melanoma worldwide have solar UV radiation (UVR) as an aetiological causal factor.[42]

The 3 types of skin cancer are: basal cell carcinoma (BCC), squamous cell carcinoma (SCC); and melanoma.[43] (See also Chapter 9.)

BCC is the most common type of skin cancer accounting for approximately 75% of all skin cancers. It grows slowly and rarely occurs in children. SCC accounts for 20% of skin cancers and is more aggressive than BCC, but less aggressive than melanoma. It also rarely occurs in children. Melanoma is the most aggressive form of skin cancer. It arises from pigment-producing cells called melanocytes. Therefore, most melanoma begins as a mole. It accounts for 4% of all skin cancer, but causes 79% of all deaths from skin cancer. In the US approximately 300 cases of melanoma arise in children per year.

Photo-ageing

Photo-ageing is a multisystem degenerative process that involves the skin and its support system. Photo-ageing results from repeated sun exposure rather than to those changes resulting from the passage of time alone.[44]

Avoiding over-exposure of the skin to the sun can beneficially promote smooth, unblemished skin even in the ninth decade of life, showing only laxity and deepening of the expression lines. Photo-aged skin displays a telangiectatic, leathery, dry, coarse, nodular yellowish surface, with deep wrinkles, accentuated skin furrows, mottled pigmentation, and purpura, as well as a variety of benign, premalignant, and malignant neoplasms. Lifetime sun exposure is also positively associated with xerosis, spider angioma, and superficial varicose veins.[45]

Contact allergy and the skin

Contact allergy caused by ingredients in cosmetic products is a well-known problem (see Table 14.3). In the US it has been reported that

Table 14.3 Important allergens for consideration in cosmetics

Allergen	Function
Amerchol™ L101	Emulsifier
p-Aminobenzoic acid	Sunscreens
Balsam of Peru (*Myroxylon pereirae*)	Fragrance
Benzophenone 3	Sunscreens
2–Bromo–2–nitropropane–1,3–diol (Bronopol)	Preservative
Butylated hydroxyanisole	Antioxidant
Butylated hydroxytoluene	Antioxidant
Cetyl/stearyl alcohol	Emulsifier
Cocamidopropyl betaine	Surfactant
DMDM hydantoin	Antimicrobial Formaldehyde releaser preservative
Fragrance mix	Fragrance
Formaldehyde	Preservative
Glyceryl thioglycolate	Hair permanent wave (perming) compound
Hydroxy–isohexyl–3–cyclohexane carboxaldehyde (HMPPC Lyral®)	Fragrance
Imidazolidinyl urea	Preservative
Iodopropynyl butylcarbamate	Preservative
Kathon CG	Preservative
Lanolin alcohol (wool alcohol)	Binder Emulsion stabiliser Viscosity increasing agent
Methyl methacrylate	Nail Industry
Methylisothiazolinone/methylchloroisothiazolinone	Preservative
Methyldibromo glutaronitrile	Preservative
p-Phenylenediamine	Hair dye
Oxybenzone	Sunscreens
Parabens	Preservative
Quaternium–15	Preservative
Toluene sulphonamide (formaldehyde resin)	Nail polish cosmetic
Tosylamide/formaldehyde resin	Nail cosmetic
Tea tree oil	Essential oil
Thimerosal	Preservative

(Source: data adapted and modified from Ortis, Yiannias[49] and Orton, Wilkinson)[50]

approximately 6% of the general population has a cosmetic-related contact allergy, mainly caused by constituent compounds such as preservatives or fragrances in the cosmetic product.[46–49]

Mind–body medicine

The endocrine system serves as a central gateway for psychologic influences on health. Stress and depression can cause the release of pituitary and adrenal hormones that have multiple effects on immune function that can subsequently influence skin physiology. Furthermore, skin problems associated with depression and or anxiety can be classified accurately as psychophysiologic disorders. They can be elicited and worsened by psychologic factors and, in turn, living with them can be associated with a higher prevalence of emotional disorders, such as depression and anxiety.[51] Hence, there is a brain–skin connection via psychoneuroimmunological–endocrine mechanisms that, through human behaviours, can strongly influence the initiation and exacerbation of skin disorders.

Cognitive behavioural therapy (CBT)

It has been reported that CBTs deal with dysfunctional thought patterns (cognitive) or actions (behavioural) that can damage the skin or can interfere with dermatologic therapies.[52] CBT-responsive skin disorders include:

- acne excoriee
- atopic dermatitis
- factitious cheilitis
- hyperhidrosis
- lichen simplex chronicus
- needle phobia
- neurodermatitis
- onychotillomania
- prurigo nodularis
- trichotillomania
- urticaria.

Moreover, it has also been reported that addition of hypnosis to CBT can facilitate aversive therapy and enhance desensitisation and other CBTs.

Hypnosis

Dermatologic conditions that responded to hypnosis are presented in Table 14.4.

The mechanism by which hypnosis produces improvement in symptoms and in skin lesions is not completely understood. Hypnosis may help regulate blood flow and other autonomic functions not usually under conscious control. The relaxation response that accompanies hypnosis may alter neurohormonal systems that in turn regulate many body functions.[53]

Table 14.4 Skin conditions responsive to hypnosis[54, 55]

Randomised controlled trials
Verruca vulgaris Psoriasis
Non-randomised controlled trials
Atopic dermatitis
Case series
Urticaria Single or few case reports (weak evidence of effectiveness) Acne excoriee Alopecia areata Congenital ichthyosiform erythroderma Dyshidrotic dermatitis Erythromelalgia Furuncles Glossodynia Herpes simplex Hyperhidrosis Ichthyosis vulgaris Lichen planus Neurodermatitis Nummular dermatitis Postherpetic neuralgia Pruritus Rosacea Trichotillomania Vitiligo

Hypnosis may be used to help control harmful habits, such as scratching. It also can be used to provide immediate and long-term analgesia, reduce symptoms such as pruritus, improve recovery from surgery, and facilitate the mind–body connection to promote healing of the skin.

Biofeedback

Biofeedback can be a training program in which a person is given information about physiological processes (e.g. heart rate or blood pressure) that is not normally available with the goal of gaining conscious control of them.

Instrumentation that can measure galvanic skin resistance, skin temperature, or other manifestations of autonomic nervous system activity in the skin and then display it in a visual, auditory, or kinesthetic mode gives the individual sensory biofeedback. With training, individuals may learn consciously how to alter autonomic nervous system associated responses for skin problems, and with enough repetition may establish new habit patterns.[56]

Early reports show that biofeedback of galvanic skin resistance for hyperhidrosis and biofeedback of skin temperature for dyshidrosis and Raynaud's syndrome can be effective.[57, 58] When biofeedback was combined with hypnosis the efficacy was reported to be enhanced.

Psychological/educational interventions

Atopic eczema

Psychological and educational interventions have been incorporated as adjuncts to conventional therapies for children with atopic eczema. These interventions enhance the effectiveness of topical therapy. A recent systematic review has reported that there is a lack of rigorously designed trials (that excluded a recent German study) that provided only a limited amount of evidence of the effectiveness of psychological and educational interventions in assisting to manage atopic eczema in children.[59]

There is low-level evidence for the use of affirmations, prayer and meditation in ameliorating skin disorders and further studies are required because it has been long recognised that there is a significant link between stress and the development of skin disorders.[60]

Physical activity

There are no studies investigating the benefits of regular physical activity on skin health. However, given that there is a plethora of scientific evidence for the benefits of physical activity for overall health (see other chapters) it is strongly recommended that physical activity be adopted for overall health maintenance and disease prevention. Exercise combined with fresh air and prudent sun exposure benefit skin health.

Furthermore, there are numerous studies that have investigated the beneficial effects of physical activity, tai chi and yoga for the management of stress[61–65] and it is biologically plausible to conclude that providing advice to patients about the benefits of physical activity, tai chi and yoga may also be favourable options for the management of stress that could indirectly also assist with skin conditions.

Nutrition and the skin

Nutritional dermatology is the use of elimination diets, nutritional regimens and supplements to augment treatment and prevention of dermatologic disorders.

Treatment regimens have their origins from numerous areas that are diversely derived from complementary medicine techniques, historical use and traditional healing systems such as Ayurveda, and the systems fashioned by various empirical nutritional therapists.[66]

As is well known, diet has been recognised to be important in the treatment of several disorders. For example, stimulants and hot foods have been related to acne rosacea,[67] wheat gluten to dermatitis herpetiformis,[68] and zinc deficiency to acrodermatitis enteropathica.[69] Other nutritional deficiencies have historically been recognised to play a role in dermatitis, such as in vitamin B1 deficiency that leads to pellagra.[70]

Food sensitivities

Population-based assessments of food allergy are scarce.[71] Despite the difficulties in obtaining firm population-based data on the prevalence of food allergies, there has been evidence for a general increase in food allergies, documented best for peanut, sesame, and kiwi, that could be attributed to environmental and dietary factors including reduced immune stimulation from infection; that is, the hygiene hypothesis. There have been changes in the components of the diet, including antioxidants, fats, and nutrients such as vitamin D, as well as the use of medications.[72, 73, 74]

Addressing *food allergies* (food sensitivities), is an important nutritional elimination procedure. These are reactions to foods that are far broader than the classical reactions such as urticaria, itchy eyes, and rhinitis. They include any inflammatory manifestation as well as a variety of neurological and other non-inflammatory conditions.[75]

Food hypersensitivity can be the first stage in the development of allergic diseases, such as atopic eczema.[76] It has been reported that clinicians have found that elimination of specific foods found by food challenge to elicit symptoms can lead to significant improvement in eczematous symptoms.[77] There is a vast amount of scientific literature claiming that dietary elimination causes improvement of atopic eczema in some cases. However, a recent systematic review portrays the evidence available as weak and the issue of exclusion diets in atopic eczema remains contentious.[78]

Diets

The eradication from the diet of chemicals is an effective way to eliminate potential skin diseases that are aggravated by chemicals. The Palaeolithic diet has addressed such issues in the scientific/medical literature.[79] The essential of this diet involves the consumption of those foods that have a low glycemic index (GI) and consists of meat, fish, vegetable, fruit, roots, and nut consumption and excludes grains, legumes, dairy products, salt, refined sugar, and processed oils. Adherence to this diet in turn minimises the consumption of pesticides, petroleum-based fertilisers, preservatives, artificial flavourings, and artificial food colours.

Acne vulgaris

Studies have reported that excessive intake of refined carbohydrates might contribute to the high rates of acne seen in Western countries through a mechanism involving insulin-stimulated androgen production and that hence nutrition-related lifestyle factors play a role in the pathogenesis of acne and that adhering to a diet with low GI foods improves skin health.[80, 81, 82] A recent Cochrane review has reported that improving lifestyle eating profiles such as adhering to a low-GI dietary regimen can improve health outcomes,[83] which could in turn improve skin health. The systematic review reported that overweight or obese people on a low-GI diet lost more weight and had more improvement in lipid profiles than those receiving carbohydrate diets. Body mass, total fat mass, body mass index (BMI), total cholesterol and LDL cholesterol all decreased significantly more in the low GI group. In studies that compared *ad libitum* low-GI diets to conventional restricted energy low-fat diets, participants fared as well or better on the low-GI diet, even though they could eat as much as desired. Therefore, this review concluded that lowering the glycaemic load of the diet appears to be an effective method of promoting weight loss and improving lipid profiles and can be simply incorporated into a person's everyday lifestyle. This improvement may well extend to include better skin health. A recent study further emphasises that there could be a possible role of desaturase enzymes in sebaceous lipogenesis and the clinical manifestation of acne.[84]

Atopic eczema

Systematic reviews of the literature demonstrate mixed results for dietary exclusion in patients with atopic eczema.

Given that many studies were of a low statistical power indicates that study design was not appropriate and that the lack of benefit was hence not proven.[85, 86]

Nutritional supplements

Different data support the notion that dietary bioactive molecules such as vitamins, carotenoids, polyphenols and trace elements such as zinc and selenium contribute to the maintenance and improvement of skin integrity and physiology, as well as preventing deleterious effects induced by ageing and environmental stressors.

Beneficial effects have been demonstrated in various experimental model systems including topical application of these ingredients. Recently, oral supplements containing various dietary bioactive molecules have also been reported to be beneficial for skin.[87]

Vitamins

Vitamin A and analogues

Vitamin A includes all naturally occurring, nutritionally active forms of vitamin A (i.e. retinol, retinyl esters) and the carotenoids. Retinoids include natural metabolic products and synthetic analogues of vitamin A. Vitamin A is physiologically essential for the reproductive system, bone formation, vision, and epithelial tissues. Cutaneous signs of its deficiency include xerosis and phrynoderma. Beta-carotene is a precursor to vitamin A, and is a putative antioxidant, that can protect cell membranes from lipid peroxidation and plants from UV light-induced damage. Retinoids have long historical therapeutic uses since the first introduction of topical tretinoin (retinoid) for the treatment of acne vulgaris.[88] An early study demonstrated that orally administered vitamin A to benefit acne when used in high doses (300,000 units per day for women, 400,000 to 500,000 units daily for men) with adverse events reported limited to xerosis and cheilitis.[89]

High doses of vitamin A should be avoided (for used cautiously with contraception) in women who may wish to conceive due to potential teratogenicity effects on the fetus.

There have been approximately 2500 new retinoid compounds synthesized.[90] Vitamin A stimulates various aspects of wound repair. It affects fibroplasia, collagen synthesis, epithelialisation, and angiogenesis and is involved in inflammatory processes with specific effects on macrophages, which play a dominant role in wound healing.[91]

Retinoids already approved for the treatment of dermatological conditions include:

- natural all-*trans*-retinoic acid (tretinoin; approved for the treatment of acne and photo-ageing)
- 13-*cis* retinoic acid (isotretinoin; approved for the treatment of severe nodular acne)

- synthetic compounds:
  - etretinate (approved for severe psoriasis)
  - acitretin (approved for severe psoriasis)
  - adapalene (approved for acne)
  - tazarotene (approved for psoriasis and acne).

The treatment of disorders of abnormal keratinisation, such as Darier's disease and Kyrle's disease, has been ascribed to etretinate and acitretin which are established in Europe for the treatment of Darier's disease and ichthyosis, especially the nonbullous congenital type.[92] In the US, however, these compounds have only been approved by the FDA for psoriasis. Palmoplantar keratoderma also responds well to these drugs, but treatment is justified only in severe cases.[93] *Pityriasis rubra pilaris* has been treated successfully with isotretinoin in the past,[94] but now acitretin seems to be the drug of choice in Europe.

It has been reported that retinoids possess certain properties that make them good candidates for cancer prevention and therapy. They are metabolically active compounds that can induce changes in cellular function and appearance, and that can modify the expression of a variety of genes involved in cell growth and differentiation.[95]

Topical tretinoin, at concentrations of 0.05% and 0.1%, have been used in combination with hydroquinone and corticosteroids for the treatment of melasma.[96] Isotretinoin, etretinate, and acitretin have all been used in recalcitrant cases of lichen planus and cutaneous lupus erythematosus with good results.[97] Erythropoietic protoporphyria responds to treatment with beta-carotene.

The use of retinoids has been significantly more successful in skin cancer prevention in high-risk patients. Treatment of patients suffering from *xeroderma pigmentosum* with 2mg/kg/day isotretinoin for 2 years resulted in an average reduction of 63% in the number of skin cancers compared with the 2-year interval before intervention.[98]

Furthermore, patients with nevoid basal cell carcinoma (BCC) syndrome have been reported to benefit from the same dose of isotretinoin treatment, as there was a rapid decrease in the number of new BCCs.[99] Also transplant recipients are also a high-risk group for the development of skin cancer. It has been reported that etretinate at a dose of 50mg/day and acitretin at 30mg/day reduced the incidence of skin cancer in renal transplant recipients.[100] An additional group that is appropriate for skin cancer chemo-prevention includes patients with premalignant lesions and a history of 1 or a few skin cancers. Vitamin A (25 000IU per day) appears to benefit patients with many actinic keratoses and a history of fewer than 3 skin cancers[101] but not those with 4 or more cancers.[102] Albeit retinoids have shown promise as skin cancer chemo-prevention agents, their benefits do not persist after discontinuation of treatments. It should be also noted that long-term use is associated with possible severe side-effects and therefore careful patient monitoring is required.

Researchers have reported favourable responses to isotretinoin and etretinate in patients with multiple keratoacanthomas.[103,104] Other studies with patients with SCC were also reported to be successfully treated with oral isotretinoin.[105] However, in most cases responses of advanced skin cancers to retinoids have been largely disappointing.

Vitamin C (Ascorbate)

Ascorbate has a known catalytic role and hence is a co-factor for a number of enzymes. Most cutaneous manifestations of ascorbate deficiency (scurvy) can be attributed to its role as a cofactor for prolyl and lysyl hydroxylase. Ascorbate plays a critical role in wound healing.[106]

Moreover, ascorbate has the potential to act as a photo-protectant. Skin damage caused by UV radiation includes acute events like sunburn and photosensitivity reactions as well as long-term exposure events that can lead to photo-ageing and skin cancer. It is important to note that ascorbate levels of the skin can be severely depleted after UV irradiation.[107]

Vitamin C has been reported to protect the skin from UVA-mediated and UVB-mediated phototoxic reactions,[108, 109] and when it is combined with a UVA sunscreen, a greater than additive protection is noted. Reduced sunburn reaction, measured by minimal erythema dose and cutaneous blood flow, has also been reported in human studies after systemic administration of 2g vitamin C and 1000IU of vitamin E for 8 days.[110] Orally administered vitamin C has been shown to protect mice from UV induced dermal neoplasms. These studies have reported that increases in dietary vitamin C decreased the incidence and delayed the onset of malignant lesions.[111, 112]

Numerous reviews have consistently reported on studies that have demonstrated that ascorbate can be photo-protective and aid skin repair.[113–118]

Vitamin E

Vitamin E includes tocopherols and tocotrienols and is a putative antioxidant with no known catalytic roles. However, given that it is a fat soluble (lipophilic) vitamin, it may have important intracellular metabolism modifying functions.[118]

Skin damage, UV radiation

Research has demonstrated that topically applied alpha-tocopherol can inhibit thymine dimer formation after UVB irradiation in a dose-dependent manner, providing a mechanism through which vitamin E can prevent gene mutations and thus development of skin cancer.[119] Vitamin E hence, can be topically applied to skin protecting it from UV-induced damage.

Topical application to the skin of laboratory animals (mice), with vitamin E, has demonstrated a significant benefit immediately after UVB exposure to reduce sunburn-associated erythema, oedema, and skin sensitivity.[120] Also chronic photo-damage, assessed by skin wrinkling and tumour development, has also been shown to be delayed by topical application of 5% tocopherol before UVB exposure.[121] The efficacy in humans is contentious.

In contrast, a study by Werninghaus and colleagues[122] has reported that daily supplementation of healthy individuals with 400IU of natural-source vitamin E for up to 6 months did not significantly alter UV-induced skin damage, as assessed by minimal erythema dose and sunburn cell formation.

A recent review[123] has cited numerous topical studies (laboratory animal and human studies) that have demonstrated that vitamin E application prior to UV exposure significantly reduced:

- lipid peroxidation
- immunosuppression
- chemiluminescence
- DNA adduct formation
- UVA-induced binding of photosensitisers
- gacute skin responses, such as erythema and edema, sun burn cell formation
- chronic skin reactions owing to prolonged UVB or UVA exposure, such as skin wrinkling and skin tumour incidence.

Herpetic cold sores

Early uncontrolled trials, using topical application of vitamin E have demonstrated relief of pain and aided in the healing of oral herpetic lesions (gingivostomatitis or herpetic cold sores). In 2 studies, the affected area was dried and cotton saturated with vitamin E oil (20 000–28 000IU per ounce) was spread over the lesions for 15 minutes.[124, 125] Pain relief was noted within 15 minutes to 8 hours, and the lesions regressed more rapidly than normal. In some cases, a single application was beneficial, but large or multiple lesions responded better when treated 3 times daily for 3 days. In a further study of 50 patients with herpetic cold sores, the content of a vitamin E capsule was applied to the lesions every 4 hours. The results of this study[126] demonstrated prompt and sustained relief of pain and the lesions healed more rapidly than was otherwise expected.

When assessing studies on the use of vitamin E, the natural versus the synthetic form of the vitamin needs to be taken into consideration. There are numerous studies that have reported on negative effects and these studies have utilised the synthetic form of the vitamin.

Vitamin D

The essential biochemistry of vitamin D3 begins with it being one of the major regulators of calcium homeostasis. It is absorbed from the gut but is also synthesized in the skin following exposure to UV light. It is activated by hydroxylation first in the liver to form 25-hydroxyvitamin D3 (25OHD3) and then in the kidneys to form a variety of metabolites, the most potent of which is 1,25(OH)2D3.

Psoriasis

Chronic plaque psoriasis is the most common type of psoriasis and is characterised by redness, thickness and scaling. A recent systematic review that investigated the efficacy of cortecosteroid medication and vitamin D on chronic plaque psoriasis has concluded that dithranol and tazarotene performed better than placebo and that comparisons of vitamin D against potent or very potent corticosteroids found no significant differences. However, combined treatment with vitamin D/corticosteroid performed significantly better than either vitamin D alone or corticosteroid alone.[127]

Calcipotriol, a vitamin D analogue (and a synthetic derivative of calcitriol), has been reported in a randomised controlled trial (RCT) of supervised treatment of psoriasis in a day-care setting can be considered as a first-line approach in clinical practice.[128] Patients who participated in this multi-centre clinical trial were treated at the day-care centre, using the care instruction principle of daily visits during the first week and twice-weekly visits subsequently for up to 12 weeks. The study concluded that topical treatment in combination with interventions explicitly focusing on improvement of coping behaviour and psychosocial functioning may further increase the degree of improvement in the psychosocial domains of quality of life in this patient group.

Recently a clinical trial reported that calcitriol ointment at a concentration of 3μ /g was a safe, effective, and well-tolerated option for the long-term treatment of chronic plaque psoriasis. Clinical improvement was maintained for up to 52 weeks, with no clinical effect on calcium homeostasis or other relevant laboratory test parameters observed.[129]

Atopic dermatitis

In a recent double-blinded randomly assigned pilot study participants took ergocalciferol 1000IU or an identical-looking placebo once daily for 1 month for winter-related atopic dermatitis in children.[130] Four out of the 5 child participants who received vitamin D compared with 1 out of the 5 who received placebo had a documented improvement but the difference was not statistically significant when the differences between baselines for the 2 groups were calculated. A study with larger participant numbers is required. The role of vitamin D in inflammatory skin diseases such as atopic dermatitis in children remains to be elucidated. Recently the American Academy of Paediatrics in the US recommended an *increase to the daily dose of vitamin D in children from* 200 to 400IU per day.[131] Noticeable effects, on the incidence of atopic dermatitis hence remain to be reported.

Skin cancers and malignant melanomas

New scientific findings convincingly demonstrate that Vitamin D deficiency is associated with a variety of severe diseases including various types of cancer.[132] Hence sun exposure has been reported from various locations [133–136] to be associated with a relatively favourable prognosis and increased survival rate in various malignancies, including malignant melanoma. A recent meta-analysis concluded that there is a growing body of evidence that Vitamin D may be of significant importance for the pathogenesis of cutaneous malignant melanoma.[137]

B Group Vitamins

The vitamin B complex consists mainly of thiamine (vitamin B1), riboflavin (vitamin B2), niacin (vitamin B3), pyridoxine (vitamin B6), cyanocobalamin (vitamin B12) and folate (vitamin B9). Also vitamins of the B complex are not widely used for the treatment of dermatological disorders.

Sporadic studies have been reported in the scientific literature which investigated the topical application of specific B group vitamins to the skin. Topical nicotinamide, the physiologically active form of niacin, was reported to have efficacy comparable to that of topical clindamycin in the treatment of acne vulgaris[138] and has produced good results in patients with necrobiosis lipoidica.[139] In combination with tetracycline, nicotinamide was successful in 1 patient with dermatitis herpetiformis.[140] The combination of nicotinamide and tetracycline has also been proposed as an alternative to systemic steroids in the treatment of bullous pemphigoid.[141] The success of nicotinamide in the treatment of these skin disorders perhaps is attributable to a re-regulation of the inflammatory state of the skin.

Other B-complex vitamins that have been used in the treatment of skin disorders include pyridoxine, for the management of erythropoietic protoporphyria,[142] and vitamin B12, in combination with folic acid, for the treatment of vitiligo.[143]

Minerals

Zinc

Zinc is an essential component of many metallo-enzymes involved in cell activities such as protein synthesis DNA and RNA replication, and cell division and it is crucial for the normal development of the skin.[144]

Acne vulgaris

Studies detecting low serum zinc levels in patients with acne have a long history.[145,146] The finding that zinc was bacteriostatic against Propionibacterium *acnes*, inhibited chemotaxis, and could decrease tumour necrosis factor-alpha production provided evidence of its usefulness. Subsequently numerous studies have demonstrated that oral zinc was effective in the treatment of severe and inflammatory acne,[147–153] more so than it was for mild or moderate acne.[154, 155]

Despite the hopeful results, oral doses used in these studies (i.e. 200mg of zinc gluconate/day, 400 or 600mg of zinc sulfate/day) were associated with nausea, vomiting, and diarrhoea.

Gastrointestinal side-effects can be ameliorated somewhat by ingesting zinc directly after meals. One to 2 milligrams of copper supplementation may be recommended with long-term zinc therapy to prevent copper deficiency as zinc decreases the absorption of copper. Oral zinc salt supplementation has been shown to be equally or less effective than oral tetracyclines.[156–159]

One study, however, showed that oral zinc sulfate had no effect on male patients with moderate acne after 8 weeks of therapy, despite evidence of systemic absorption.[160] Limited efficacy and poor patient compliance caused by gastrointestinal side-effects have limited the use of oral zinc for the treatment of acne. Further trials need to be conducted to assess the efficacy and side-effects of lower doses of orally administered zinc.

Seborrheic dermatitis and dandruff

Topical zinc pyrithione (1%) has been approved for the treatment of seborrheic dermatitis and dandruff of the scalp.[161]

Selenium

Selenium has a catalytic role, as a component of glutathione peroxidase, in the regulation of oxygen metabolism, particularly in catalysing the breakdown of H_2O_2. Studies with laboratory animals have implicated selenium deficits in skin cancer tumorigenesis.[162] Human studies however have proven controversial.

Cancer studies

Early clinical studies have demonstrated that skin cancer patients in good general health had a significantly lower mean plasma selenium concentration than did controls, and have reported that serum selenium is predictive of future skin cancer risk in humans.[163, 164] A multicenter RCT from the Nutritional Prevention of Cancer Study Group, demonstrated that selenium treatment (200mg) of skin cancer patients for 4.5 years reduced significantly total cancer incidence and mortality and incidences of lung, colorectal, and prostate cancer, but it did not protect against development of another basal or squamous cell carcinoma.

Investigators emphasised the need for confirmation of their results before new public health recommendations regarding selenium supplementation could be made.[165]

A recent Cochrane review has confirmed this notion.[166]

In a recent study on the effect of selenium intake on the prevention of cutaneous epithelial lesions in organ transplant recipients it was reported that selenium (at a dose of 200 µg/day) did not prevent the occurrence of skin lesions linked to HPV.[167]

Recent zinc/selenium trace element supplementation studies have demonstrated significant associations with higher circulating plasma and skin tissue contents of zinc/selenium and improved antioxidant status. These physiological changes were associated with improved clinical outcome, including fewer pulmonary infections and better wound healing.[168, 169]

Other nutritional supplements

Alpha-hydroxy acids (AHAs)

AHAs are weak organic acids that can be found in fruits, milk sugars, and plants. Glycolic acid (from sugar cane) and lactic acid (from milk) are 2 types of AHAs found in over the counter acne products, but these AHAs are often chemically synthesized rather than isolated from natural sources. Moreover, fruit acids are a special group of organic acids found in many natural foods and consist of citric, gluconic, gluconolactone, glycolic, malic and tartaric acids.

Acne vulgaris

Studies have demonstrated that AHAs are safe and efficacious, in combination, such as in glycolic acid/retinaldehyde preparations,[170, 171, 172] as well as its ability to accompany common topical anti-acne therapies. Also, this combination has been reported to prevent and repair post-inflammatory hyper-pigmented skin that was associated with acne.[173] Retinaldehyde, a precursor of retinoic acid, has shown de-pigmenting activity whereas glycolic acid decreases excessive pigmentation by a wounding and re-epithelization process. There appears to be a synergistic effect when these 2 compounds are used in combination.

An early double-blind clinical trial on 150 patients to evaluate the efficacy and skin tolerance of the alpha hydroxy acid gluconolactone 14% in solution (Nuvoderm lotion) in the treatment of mild to moderate acne was compared to its vehicle (placebo) and 5% benzoyl peroxide lotion. The results of the study demonstrated that both gluconolactone and benzoyl peroxide had a significant effect in improving patients' acne by reducing the number of lesions (i.e. inflamed and non-inflamed). Furthermore, fewer side-effects were reported by patients treated with gluconolactone when compared with benzoyl peroxide.[174] Irritation was the main adverse effect when gluconolactone was in high concentrations.

Salicylic acid

Salicylic acid is a phytohormone, a plant product that acts like a hormone by regulating cell growth and differentiation. It is a beta hydroxy acid that is chemically similar to the active component of aspirin. It functions as a topical desquamating agent, dissolving the intercellular cement holding the cells of the stratum corneum together. It is used as a topical keratolytic agent.

Hyperpigmentation

A recent small study of 10 participants with Fitzpatrick skin phototypes IV to VI were randomised to receive two 20% salicylic acid peels followed by three 30% salicylic acid peels to half of the face. The contralateral half of the face remained untreated.[175] The results of this study demonstrated that salicylic acid peels were safe in this population of adults. Measured quality of life improved nominally.

Acne vulgaris

In an RCT study, 80 participants with mild to moderate facial acne were randomised to receive either a *lipophillic derivative of salicylic acid* formulation twice a day or 5% benzoyl peroxide once a day for 12 weeks. The study compared efficacy and tolerance between the treatments for facial *acne vulgaris* and reported that the lipophillic derivative of salicylic acid formulation could be a treatment option to consider in mild to moderate acne vulgaris patients that are intolerant to benzoyl peroxide.[176]

Human Papilloma Virus

Salicylic acid is commonly used in over-the-counter products for the treatment of warts.

Coenzyme Q_{10} (CoQ_{10})

CoQ_{10} is ubiquitous in human tissues, although its level is variable. The level of CoQ_{10} is highest in organs with high rates of metabolism such as the heart, kidney and liver.[177] Compounds such as coenzyme Q_{10} have been reported to play an increasing beneficial role in skin care. The benefits range from skin conditions such as acne and psoriasis to protection against environmental insults.[178]

Psoriasis

A recent study that evaluated the clinical effects of supplementation with antioxidants to patients with severe erythrodermic and arthropathic forms of psoriasis reported that co-supplementation with antioxidants such as vitamin E, and selenium plus CoQ_{10} could be feasible for the management of patients with severe forms of psoriasis.[179]

The use of CoQ_{10} has also been heavily promoted for use in cosmeceutical products as a beneficial agent for ageing skin.[180, 181]

Lipoic acid

Low molecular weight compounds such as lipoic acid have also been reported to be protective low molecular weight antioxidants through a diet rich in fruits and vegetables or by direct topical application for photo-damaged skin.[182] However, studies investigating the efficacy of lipoic acid in treating photo-damaged skin are lacking.

Functional foods

Probiotics

A recent review has documented the numerous experimental studies that have found that probiotics exert specific effects in the intestinal lumen and on epithelial cells and immune cells with anti-allergic potential.[183] The review also documented that the barrier function and the innate immune system of the skin indicates that the skin's microbiota have a beneficial role, much like that observed with the gut microflora.[184]

Atopic dermatitis

Studies worldwide have shown that an environment rich in microbes in early life reduces the subsequent risk of developing allergic diseases such as atopic dermatitis.[185] Continuous stimulation of the immune system by environmental saprophytes via the skin, respiratory tract and gut appears to be necessary for activation of the regulatory network including regulatory T-cells and dendritic cells. Substantial evidence now shows that the balance between allergy and tolerance is dependent on regulatory T-cells. Tolerance induced by allergen-specific regulatory T-cells appears to be the normal immunological response to allergens in non-atopic healthy individuals. Healthy subjects have an intact functional allergen-specific regulatory T-cells response, which in allergic subjects is impaired. Evidence on this exists with respect to atopic dermatitis, contact dermatitis, allergic rhinitis and asthma.

In a large meta-analysis of the current literature regarding the use of prenatal and postnatal probiotics for the prevention and treatment or either of atopic dermatitis, Lee and colleagues have reviewed and analysed the data from 10 studies.[186] Six of the 10 studies showed evidence to support the use of probiotics both prenatally and postnatally for the prevention of atopic dermatitis. A risk reduction as high as 61% was seen that was attributed mainly to the prenatal use of probiotics. For the treatment of atopic dermatitis there was no significant difference detected between those that used probiotics and those that did not. Patient education may further increase the likelihood of successful preventative measures.[187]

Eczema

Probiotic bacteria have been proposed as an effective treatment for eczema, and recently a number of clinical trials have been undertaken and recent systematic reviews have analysed the published data. Two reviews by the same research group have found that there was significant heterogeneity between the results of individual studies, which could be explained by the use of different probiotic strains.[188,189] A subgroup analysis by age of participant, severity of eczema, presence of atopy or presence of food allergy did not identify a population with different treatment outcomes to the population as a whole. The adverse events reported identified some case reports of infections and bowel ischaemia caused by probiotics. The overall conclusions from the reviewed was that probiotics were not an effective treatment for eczema, and probiotic treatment carried a small risk of adverse events.

A significant caveat is that there was a strong heterogeneity in probiotic formulations used and this may well be the most important explanation as to probiotic efficacy failure thereby significantly weakening the conclusions of the systematic reviews.

Essential fatty acids (omega-3 and -6)

Atopic dermatitis

There has been conflicting evidence on the use of omega-3 and omega-6 supplementation for the prevention of allergic diseases. A recent systematic review has investigated RCTs and contrary to the evidence from basic science and epidemiological studies, the review suggested that supplementation with omega-3 and omega-6 oils was unlikely to play an important role as a strategy for the primary prevention of sensitisation or allergic disease.[190] The evidence hence remains highly contentious as it is out of line with the plethora of additional data that is available.[191–194]

Herbal medicines

Herbal medicines that are used as medicines comprise plants/plant part(s) that contain specific active ingredients that enable it to be used for healing purposes or symptom relief. There are a number of herbs that have been reported to have traditional uses for skin problems and these include examples such as chamomile, fennel, lavender, lemon balm, pot marigold, red clover, rose, sage and thyme.[195] The following discussion follows the use of herbal medicines by treatment type.

Herbal medicines for acne

The topical application and oral ingestion of herbal medicines and plants that have been indicated for acne problems and with anti infective properties such as that produced by *P acnes* are presented in Tables 14.5 and 14.6.[196, 197]

It has been reported that *tannins* (substances present in the seeds and stems of grapes, the bark of some trees, and tea leaves) have been employed topically to treat acne because of their natural astringent properties.[198] A herb that is known for its astringent and anti-viral properties is witch-hazel (*Hamamelis virginiana*). This herb is from a genus of flowering plants in the family *Hamamelidaceae*, with 2 species in North America (*H virginiana* and *H vernalis*), and 1 each in Japan (*H. japonica*) and China (*H mollis*).[199, 200] There are no studies that have reported the efficacy of witch-hazel in the treatment of acne.

Tea tree oil (*Melaleuca alternifolia*)

Tea tree oil was studied in an early Australian study[201] by comparing the efficacy of 5% tea tree oil to that of 5% benzoyl peroxide. A single-blinded, RCT on 124 patients was performed to evaluate the efficacy and skin tolerance of 5% tea tree oil gel in the treatment of mild to moderate acne. The study concluded that both preparations, namely 5% tea tree oil and 5% benzoyl peroxide, had a significant effect in ameliorating the patients' acne by reducing the number of inflamed and non-inflamed lesions (i.e. open and closed comedones), although the onset of action in the case of tea tree oil was slower. Also fewer side-effects were reported by patients treated with tea tree oil. A further study supported the use of tea tree oil in the treatment of acne, and demonstrated that the terpinene-4-ol was not the sole active constituent of the oil that may have antimicrobial activity.[202] A subsequent systematic review, although not finding conclusive evidence that tea tree oil was useful in the treatment of acne, did specify that the emerging evidence was promising.[203, 204]

Tea tree oil has been recently studied in a double-blind RCT of 60 patients with mild to moderate acne vulgaris.[205] Participants were randomly divided into 2 groups and were treated with tea tree oil gel (n = 30) or placebo (n = 30) and were followed every 15 days for a period of 45 days. The study concluded that topically applied 5% tea tree oil is an effective treatment for mild to moderate acne vulgaris.

Tea tree oil may also have additional effects on the skin as reported recently with the first study to show experimentally that tea tree oil reduced histamine-induced skin inflammation.[206]

Vitex (*Vitex agnus castus L*)

The traditional use of this herb has been reported to be for the efficacious treatment

Table 14.5 Topically applied herbal medicines and plants/plant parts for the treatment of acne, condyloma and verruca vulgaris

Aloe vera/Aloe Barbadensis	Ironweed/*Veronia antihelminitica*
American may apple/*Podophyllum peltatum*$^{\Phi}$	*Kramiria triandra* Ruis plus escin–beta–sitosterol plus lauric acid
Bittersweet nightshade/*Solanum dulcamara*$^{\Phi}$	Lilac/*Azadirachta indica*$^{\Omega}$
Black walnut/*Juglans regia*	Oak bark/*Quercus robur*
Borage/*Borago officinalis*	Oat straw/*Avena sativa*$^{\Phi}$
Compositae/Artemesia vulgaris and A. Absinthum	Onion/*Allium cepa*
Calotropis/Calotropis procera$^{\Phi}$ (used in India to treat warts)	Oregon grape root/*Mahonia aquifolia/berberine*
Crinum/*Crinum macowanii*	Pea/*Pisum sativum*
Cucumber	Pomegranate/*Punica granitum*
Duckweed/*Lemma minor*	Pumpkin/*Cucurbita pepo*
English walnut/*Juglans regia*	Rue/*Ruta graveolens*
Fresh lemon	East Indian globe thistle/*Sphaeranthus indicus L*$^{\Omega}$
Fruit acids (citric/gluconic/gluconolactone/glycolic/malic/tartric)	White Marudah/*Ternialia arjuna*
Garlic/*Allium sativum*	Tea Tree Oil/*Melaleuca alternifolia*$^{\Omega}$
Grapefruit seeds	Turmeric/*Curcuma longa*$^{\Omega}$
Greater celandine/*Chelidonium majus*$^{\Phi}$ (used in China to treat warts)	Vinegar
Indian Madder/*Rubia cordifolia*$^{\Omega}$	Vitex/*Vitex agnus–castus L*
Indian Sarsaparilla/*Hemidesmus indicus*$^{\Omega}$	Witch-hazel/*Hamamelis virginiana sp*

Note: These herbal medicines and plants/plant parts are effective in inhibiting the pathogenesis of *P acnes*$^{\Omega}$ *in vitro, in vivo* and for condyloma$^{\Phi}$ and verruca vulgaris$^{\Phi}$

Table 14.6 Orally administered herbal medicines and plants/plant parts and other$^{\Delta}$ for the treatment of acne

Burdock root/*Arctium lappa*
$^{\Delta}$Brewer's yeast/*Saccharomyces cerevisiae*
Ku shen/*Sophora flavescens*
Indian ginseng/*Withania somnifera*
Mukul myrrh tree/Commiphora mukul

(Source: modified from Magin et. al. 2006)[196]

of premenstrual acne.[207, 208] The whole fruit extract is thought to act to rebalance follicle stimulating hormone and luteinising hormone levels in the pituitary gland therby increasing progesterone and simultaneously decreasing oestrogen levels.[207] The German Commission E Monographs (hereafter referred to as the German Commission) have recommended an oral dose of 40mg/day.[209] The main adverse effects reported were gastrointestinal upset and rash. From the published scientific data, Vitex has been recently reported to be a safe medicinal herb.[208] There is though a requisite for more controlled studies to demonstrate the efficacy of this herb.

For an extensive review that has recently documented the extensive literature on herbal medicines for the treatment of acne refer further to the review by Magin and colleagues.[196]

Herbal medicines for wounds, burns and radiation dermatitis

Aloe vera

Several case reports have documented that *Aloe vera* reduced itching, burning and scarring associated with radiation dermatitis.[210] An early study demonstrated that *Aloe vera* was effective in skin wound caused by burns.[211] This study showed the effectiveness of *Aloe vera* gel on a partial thickness burn wound, concluding that additional studies were warranted. Also, that only some minor adverse effects, such as discomfort and pain were encountered in the 27 cases.

A recent systematic review while accepting that *Aloe vera* has been traditionally used for burn healing the clinical evidence for its efficacy remains unclear.[212] The study concluded that due to the differences of products and outcome measures employed by different study designs, there was paucity of information and hence to draw specific conclusions regarding the effect of *Aloe vera* for burn wound healing was difficult. However, the authors did also comment that given the cumulative scientific evidence that exists, this would tend to support that *Aloe vera* might be an effective intervention used in burn wound healing for first to second degree burns. Moreover it was also concluded that well-designed trials with sufficient details of the contents of the *Aloe vera* products used (percent content of the gel and liquid extracts) should be carried out to determine the efficacy of the herb.

Honey

For centuries the use of honey has provided a therapeutic ointment option for wounds.[213] There is a growing body of scientific literature promoting the use of sterilised honey-based products in wound care, demonstrating their efficacy, cost-effectiveness and exceptional record of safety.[214, 215]

A recent Cochrane review concluded that honey may improve healing times in mild to moderate superficial and partial thickness burns compared with some conventional dressings.[216]

Marigold (*Calendula officinalis*)

Marigold has been used topically for skin wounds for centuries. The German Commission has approved its use as an antiseptic for wound healing.[209]

A number of studies have reported that *Calendula officinalis* was effective in treating radiation induced wounds in cancer patients.[217, 218, 219]

A recent systematic review has demonstrated preliminary data in support of the efficacy of topical calendula for prophylaxis of acute dermatitis during radiotherapy.[220]

Tannins in herbs

Common tannin-containing herbs that may be useful for treating skin wounds when topically applied include English walnut leaf (*Juglans regia*), goldenrod, Labrador tea, lavender, mullein, oak bark, rhatany, Chinese rhubarb and yellow dock.[207] The efficacy for these herbal medicines is largely anecdotal and good quality trials are required.

Herbal medicines for skin wounds due to herpes simplex

Lemon balm (*Melissa Oficinalis* L)

Extracts of the leaves of lemon balm (*Melissa officinalis*) have been investigated as a topical treatment for herpes simplex. Randomised trials have demonstrated that Lemon balm was effective for herpes simplex. In 1 study with 116 patients with an acute herpes simplex outbreak applied a lemon balm preparation or a placebo cream. Treatment was begun within 72 hours of the onset of symptoms and administered 2–4 times daily for 5–10 days. Healing was assessed as very good by 41% of patients in the lemon balm group and by 19% in the placebo group.[221] A further study which was a DBRCT was carried out with the same balm preparation with the aim of proving efficacy of the standardised balm mint cream (active ingredient: 1% Lo–701 dried extract from *Melissa officinalis* L leaves [70:1]).[222] The lemon balm cream or placebo cream was applied to the affected area 4 times daily for 5 days. On the second day of therapy, the symptom score was significantly lower in the active-treatment group than in the placebo group, with a non significant trend in favour of the lemon balm treatment at the end of the study.

Liquorice (Glycyrrhiza glabra and Glycyrrhiza uralensis)

The topical application of *Glycyrrhiza sp* has been associated with historical sources from ancient manuscripts from China, India and Greece.[223] Laboratory studies have demonstrated inhibition of the varicella zoster virus. Human clinical trials have yet to be conducted, although the topical application of liquorice is reported to be safe.[207]

Herbal medicines for bacterial and fungal infections

As previously outlined a number of herbal medicines can inhibit the growth of *P acnes in vitro* (Table 14.5).[197] Similarly tea tree oil has demonstrated significant antibacterial activity *in vitro* against a variety of micro-organisms that include, *Propionibaterium acnes*, *Staphylococcus aureus*, *Escherichia coli*, *Candida albicans*, *Tricophyton mentagrophytes* and *Trichophyton rubrum*.[198]

Tea tree oil has also been used as a topical antiseptic agent since the early part of the 20th century for a wide variety of skin infections, including bacterial and fungal.[224] In a study with a fungal infection tea tree oil cream (10% w/w) appeared to reduce the symptomatology of tinea pedis as effectively as tolnaftate 1% but was no more effective than placebo in achieving a mycological cure.[225] In a further study which assessed the efficacy and tolerability of topical application of 1% clotrimazole solution compared with that of 100% tea tree oil for the treatment of toenail onychomycosis, the study concluded that the topical therapy, provided improvement in nail appearance and symptomatology by both treatments.[226] However it was concluded by another study that it should not be employed in burn wounds to the skin because of tea tree oil's cytolytic effect on epithelial cells and fibrolasts.[227]

Garlic (*Allium sativum*)

Reports document that ajoene, an organic trisulphur originally isolated from garlic, has an antimycotic activity which has been widely demonstrated both *in vitro* and *in vivo*.[228] A study of short duration demonstrated that the use of ajoene as a 0.4% (w/w) cream resulted in complete clinical and mycological cure in 27 of 34 patients (79%) after 7 days of treatment. The remaining 7 patients (21%) achieved complete cure after 7 additional days of treatment.[229] At a 3-month follow up all participants remained free of fungus.

Herbal medicines for condyloma and verruca vulgaris

A number of herbal medicines have been reported to treat skin warts (see Table 14.5).[198] However, rigorous clinical trials are warranted to test efficacy and safety.

Herbal medicines for scabies

Herbal preparations from essential oils such as anise (*Pimpinella anisum*) seeds that has displayed antibacterial and insecticidal activity *in vitro* has been employed topically to treat scabies.[198] Neem (*Azadirachta indica*) is an Indian plant that has been used medicinally in that country.[198] In a report of more than 800 villagers in India the paste of neem and turmeric was used topically to treat chronic ulcers and scabies.[198] Rigorous data is lacking and further studies are warranted.

Herbal medicines for psoriasis and dermatitis

TCM herbs

Traditional Chinese medicine (TCM) for the treatment of psoriasis and atopic dermatitis has gained significant attention in the last decade.[198] TCM deals with the whole-body medicine system whereby the role of the therapy is to regain metabolic balance for the individual. This requires a mixture of herbs.[230]

Two recent cross-over RCTs investigated the use of TCM in the treatment of atopic dermatitis in which conventional medicine had failed to respond adequately to currently available therapies.[231, 232]

A Chinese practitioner aided the investigators to formulate a mixture of herbal medicines for the RCTs. The Chinese herbal medicines included *Potentilla chinensis*, *Tribulus terrestris*, *Rehmannia glutinosa*, *Lophatherum gracile*, *Clematis armandi*, *Ledebouriella sacleoides*, *Dictamnus dasycarpus*, *Paeonia lactiflora*, *Schisonepeta tenuifolia* and *G glabra*. This mixture of herbs was placed in sachets and boiled and then provided to participants as a tea to be consumed daily.[231] The 2 (8-week) studies investigated children (atopic eczema) and adults (atopic dermatitis) and the mixed herbal tea was significantly more effective than the placebo tea preparation. The efficacy was associated with significant decreases in erythema and surface damage to the skin. The only serious adverse event reported was elevation of aspartate aminotransferase levels in 2 children which decreased to normal on treatment discontinuation.

Psoriasis is a common, chronic, recurrent inflammatory skin disorder whose aetiology is still unknown. Traditional Chinese herbal medicines have demonstrated efficacy in treating psoriasis, with TCM characterised by a variety of methods of treatment, flexible use of drugs, high efficacy, low recurrence, and few side-effects.[233, 234] A recent study with 80 patients randomly assigned to 2 groups, 39 in Group A and 41 in Group B, investigating blood-heat syndrome type psoriasis has demonstrated that the effect of Chinese herbal medicines combined with acitretin capsule was superior to

Chinese herbal medicines alone in treating this skin problem.[235] This result, though, requires replication by conducting larger trials.

Aloe vera

As discussed previously, *Aloe vera* has a historical use for treating skin wounds. In an early double-blind RCT study 60 patients were treated with a topical *Aloe vera* extract 0.5% in a hydrophilic cream to cure patients with psoriasis vulgaris.[236]

The results from this study suggest that topically applied *Aloe vera* extract 0.5% in a hydrophilic cream is more effective than placebo. No toxic or any other objective side-effects were demonstrated hence the regimen was deemed as safe and as an alternative treatment to cure patients suffering from psoriasis. A systematic review that followed this study concluded that even though there were some promising results, clinical effectiveness of oral or topical *Aloe vera* was reported not to be sufficiently defined.[237]

A recent double-blind RCT reported the effect of the commercial *Aloe vera* gel on stable plaque psoriasis to be modest and not better than placebo. However, the high response rate of placebo indicated a possible effect of this in its own right, which would make the *Aloe vera* gel treatment appear less effective.[238]

Capsaicin (*Capsicum frutescens*)

Capsaicin is the active component of cayenne peppers (chilli peppers). Two early trials have demonstrated that 0.025% capsaicin cream was effective in treating psoriasis.[239, 240] One study showed significant reductions in scaling and erythema during a 6-week treatment of 44 participants presenting with moderate to severe psoriasis.[237] The second study was a double-blind study in patients with pruritic psoriasis randomised to receive either the capsaicin cream or vehicle 4 times a day for 6 weeks.[220] Topically applied capsaicin effectively treated pruritic psoriasis.

A review that followed these studies concluded that capsaicin was effective for psoriasis.[241]

Reported side-effects include a short-lived burning sensation. The German Commission suggest that capsaicin not be used for more than 2 consecutive days with a 2 week lapse between consecutive treatments.[198]

St Johns wort (*Hypericum perforatum L*)

A recent double-blind RCT study with a cream containing *Hypericum* extract standardised to 1.5% *hyperforin* (verum) in comparison to the corresponding vehicle (placebo) for the treatment of subacute atopic dermatitis.[242] The study concluded that the *Hypericum* cream showed a significant superiority compared to the vehicle in the topical treatment of mild to moderate atopic dermatitis. However, the therapeutic efficacy has to be evaluated in further studies with larger patient cohorts, in comparison to therapeutic standards such as glucocorticoids.

Other herbal medicines

A number of herbs have been approved by the German Commission for the use in atopic dermatitis and psoriasis. These include: *Arnica montana*, German chamomile (*Matricaria recutita*), bittersweet nightshade (*S. dulcamara*), *as* we all as Breyer's yeast (*S. cereviceae*) which are thought to possess anti-inflammatory activity and anti-bacterial effects. Heartseases (*Viola tricolor*), English plantain (*Plantago lanceolata*), fenugreek (*Trigonella foenum-gaecum*), and flax (*Linum usitatissium*) contain mucilages which can act as emollients that can soothe the skin.[198] Furthermore, agrimony (*Agrimonia eupatoria*), oak (*Quercus robur*), walnut (*Juglans regia*), and St John's wort (*Hypericum perforatum*) contain tannins and can act as astringents. Oak straw (*A. sativa*) was also approved for its soothing and antipruritic qualities.[198]

Aromatherapy

Aromatherapy is the therapeutic use of volatile, aromatic essential oils which are extracted from plants. Aromatherapy may also be regarded as having a close and overlapping relationship to herbal medicine. Aromatic compounds have been used throughout history for spiritual, medicinal, social, and beauty purposes.[243]

The aromatic oils depicted in Table 14.7 have been reported to be useful in a variety of dermatological conditions especially acne.[242] Further, there are only a few clinical trials that have been published on the topical treatment of atopic dermatitis with herbal ointments and the quality of these trials was largely poor. Whereas a review of clinical trials with *Mahonia aquifolium* reported that taken together, these clinical studies indicated that *Mahonia aquifolium* was a safe and effective treatment for patients with mild to moderate psoriasis.[244]

A reported RCT of a Toto ointment/soap combination (containing Shea butter/ *Butyrospermum paradoxicum* oils with multiple constituents) reported efficacy after an average of approximately 4 weeks of treatment.[245] The RCT was of a poor quality.

A further low-quality, open, non-comparative study was of the efficacy and safety of *Acalypha wilkesiana* ointment in superficial fungal skin diseases. Thirty-two Nigerian patients with

Table 14.7 Aromatherapy — essential oils useful in dermatology

Australian eucalyptus/*Eucalyptus radiata*	Lavender (French)/*Lavandula latifolia*
Basil/*Ocimum sactum, O basilicum and O gratissimum*	Lemon grass/*Cymbopogon citratus*
Bay essential oil/*Pimenta racemosa*	Lemon/*Citrus limon*
Benzoin/*Styrax benzoe*	Nialouli/*Melaleuca quinquenervia/Viridifolia*
Black cumin/*Nigella sativa*	Orange/*Citrus aurantium*
Black pepper/*Piper nigrum*	Orange (sweet)/*Citrus senesis*
Benzoin/*Styrax benzoe*	Patchouli/*Pogostemon cablin*
Bergamot/*Citrus bergamia*	Petitgrain/*Citrus aurantium* var *amara* fol
Cajeput/*Melaleuca leucodendron*	Peppermint/*Mentha x piperita*
Chamomile/*Chamaemelum nobile*	Moroccan chamomile/*Ormensis mixta flos*
Dandelion/*Taraxacum officinale*	Ravensara/*Ravensara aromatica*
Frankincense/*Boswellia carterii*	Rose water/*Rosa damascena*
Fijian fire plant/*Acalypha wilkesiana*	Rosemary (verbenone)/*Rosmarinus officinalis*
German chamomile/*Matricaria recutita*	Safflower oil, Linoleic acid
Geranium/*Pelargonium asperum*	Sandalwood/*Santalum album and S. spicatum*
Heartsease/*Viola tricolor*	Scotch pine/*Pinus sylvestrus*
Holly-leaved barberry/*Mahonia aquifolium*	Sunflower oil, linoleic acid
Jasmine/*Jasminum officinalis*	Tea tree oil/*Malaleuca alternifolia*
Juniper berry/*Juniperus communis*	Thick-leaved pennywort/*Centella asiatica*
Juniper twig/*Juniperus communis ram*	Thyme linalool/*Thymus vulgaris* L.
Knight's milfoil/*Achillea millefolium*	Verbenone/*Rosemarinus officinulis* verbenone
Lavender (true)/*Lavandula angustifolia and L. spicula*	Winter Savory/*Satureja montana*

clinical and mycological evidence of superficial mycoses were recruited. The study concluded that *Acalypha* ointment may be used for the treatment of superficial mycoses.[246]

A recent study with a combination herbal ointment containing *Mahonia aquifolium*, *Viola tricolor* and *Centella asiatica* was reported for the treatment of mild–moderate atopic dermatitis.[247] Patients were treated for 4 weeks with the ointment. The primary endpoint was a summary score for erythema, edema/papulation, oozing/crust, excoriation and lichenification according to a 4-point scale. The study concluded that the ointment was not proven to be superior to a base cream. However, a sub-analysis of the data indicated that the cream could be effective under conditions of cold and dry weather.

Low level quality studies investigating *Ocimum gratissimum* oil products tested were reported to produce a significantly greater reduction in acne lesion count compared with 10% benzoyl peroxide.[248, 249, 250]

A recent review has investigated the literature and the evidence that exists on the influence that essential oils have on wound healing and their potential application in clinical practice.[251] The review concludes that although there is some evidence for efficacy for such essential oils as further larger studies are required.

Herbal medicines for alopecia

Garlic gel/betamethasone valerate

A recent double-blind RCT study investigated a combination of topical garlic gel and betamethasone valerate cream in the treatment of localised alopecia areata.[252]

Patients were randomly divided into 2 groups of garlic gel and placebo. The 2 groups were advised to follow the treatments twice daily, for 3 months. Both groups received topical application of corticosteroid (betamethasone cream 0.1% in isopropyl alcohol) twice daily. The study concluded that the use of garlic gel significantly added to the therapeutic efficacy of topical betamethasone valerate in alopecia areata and that it can be an effective adjunctive topical therapy for alopecia areata.

Aromatherapy oils

The efficacy of aromatherapy in the treatment of patients with alopecia areata was investigated in an RCT.[253] Eighty-six patients diagnosed as having alopecia areata were randomised into 2 groups. The active group massaged essential oils (thyme/rosemary/lavender/cedarwood) in a mixture of carrier oils (jojoba/grapeseed) into their scalp daily whereas the control group used only carrier oils for their daily massages for 7 months. The results demonstrated aromatherapy safety and efficacy of treatment for alopecia areata. Treatment with these essential oils was significantly more effective than treatment with the carrier oil alone.

Other herbal medicines for skin cancer

Laboratory animal data demonstrate that a number of other herbal medicines may have a protective role in skin carcinogenesis and these include rosemary, propolis, red ginseng and silymarin.[198]

Tea

Tea has been reported in the scientific literature as nature's defence against malignancies (see also Chapter 9).[253] Descriptive and observational epidemiological studies have reported that tea consumption is associated with an inverse risk of skin malignancies.[255–259]

Physical therapies

Electrical impulses

A recent review of the literature concludes that electrical stimulation of chronic wounds may be efficacious in some instances and that the evidence suggests it is a potentially useful, accessible and cheap therapy, which could play a valuable role in everyday clinical practices.[260] A systematic review, however, has concluded that there was no evidence of benefit in using electromagnetic therapy to treat pressure ulcers.[261]

Acupuncture

Acupuncture has been demonstrated to influence neurologic, endocrine, immune, and psychologic systems. In dermatology numerous acupuncture methods are recognised (Table 14.8).[262]

Acupuncture includes original acupuncture (acus-puncture) and many related methods such as the use of moxibustion, cupping, acupressure and can be divided according to the use or absence of needles.[262]

- Needle acupuncture:
  - filiform needle
  - lancet or blood-letting needle
  - cutaneous needle
  - ear needle.
- Non-needle acupuncture:
  - moxibustion
  - cupping
  - acupressure.

Acne

Acupuncture for acne has been reported in a review of TCM applications.[263] A recent small study with He–Ne laser auricular irradiation plus body acupuncture for acne vulgaris reported a significant benefit.[264] The results showed that the cure rate was approximately 80% in the treatment group and 47% in the control group indicating that He–Ne laser auricular irradiation plus body acupuncture may exhibit better effects for acne vulgaris.

A recent RCT from China that investigated 26 patients with acne conglobata treated by encircling acupuncture combined with ventouse and cupping demonstrated efficacy.[265] The study concluded that both acupuncture and medication effectively promoted the recovery of the affected skin, and lowered serum IL-6 levels in acne conglobata patients. The effect of acupuncture was stronger than that of isotretinoin in lowering serum IL-6 content and was associated with fewer adverse effects.

A review article also from China has concluded that acupuncture–moxibustion was safe and effective for treatment of acne, and that it was possibly better than routine Western medicine. Moreover, that the comprehensive acupuncture–moxibustion therapy was better than single acupuncture–moxibustion therapy.[266] These data need to be further evaluated.[267]

Table 14.8 Different forms of acupuncture used in dermatology

Type of acupuncture	Methodology employed
Corporal acupuncture	Involves needling with metal needles on 365 known points, located on the so-called meridians (Chinese *Jing Luo*)
Auricle acupuncture	Richly innervated area consisting of 130 points on the auricle that can evoke various changes in the physiological functions of the body
Electro-acupuncture	Consists of electric stimulation using a light electric current with different frequencies. This is applied to the needles influencing the skin and underlying tissues in the region of the acupuncture point
Electro-puncture	Effect is rendered directly with electric current by means of electrodes inserted into the acupuncture point. The effect with this method is more superficial compared to electro-acupuncture
Moxibustion	Cones are placed on the acupuncture point — wormwood or the wormwood cigar is held at a distance (pecking method), which results in burning or warming of the skin up to 45°C
Acupressure	Massage of the acupuncture points is the oldest of all possible techniques for the external treatment in TCM Unlike ordinary massage this method uses rounded movements of the fingers over the acupuncture point
Cryopuncture	Cooling and slight freezing of the skin in the region of the acupuncture point thereby influencing thermo-receptors and a non-specific cryodestructive effect is obtained
Medicamentous acupuncture	This method injects pharmaceuticals, vitamins, phytoproducts, procaine and other materials, most often in the given acu-point
Auto-hemopuncture	The patient's own blood is injected subcutaneously into the region of the acu-point
Apitherapy	Bee honey is inserted in the region of the acupuncture point on the skin
Cupping	Bars of different sizes are applied to the specific zone or on the acu-point of the skin. One of the purposes, among others, is blood-letting, which is very widely used in the practice of TCM
Magnito-puncture	Acupuncture point that is influenced by magnetic fields
Laser acupuncture	By contact or at distance of acupuncture points that are irradiated with low-density laser from sources with different characteristics. Most often: • Helium–Neon (He–Ne) lasers are used with wavelength 632.8 n • Diode lasers with wavelength from 780 to 904 n
Other methods	Acupuncture points treated with: • ultraviolet (UV) rays, using microphoto–electrophoresis • different drugs can be applied etc

(Source: adapted from Iliev)[262]

The effectiveness of pharmaceutical therapies for acne has discouraged the use of acupuncture, however, in those individuals who have a history of drug allergy or intolerance, needle acupuncture may still be useful.

Herpes zoster

An early study that investigated a total of 62 cases diagnosed with herpes zoster were enrolled in a single-blinded RCT that evaluated the effect of auricular and body acupuncture compared with placebo. The results showed that 7 patients in the placebo group and 7 patients in the acupuncture group experienced pain relief at the end of treatment. There was no difference in the pain relief between these 2 groups.[268]

A recent review from China indicates that correct randomisation, concealment, blinding and placebo-control, and the RCTs with generally accepted criteria for assessment of diagnosis and therapeutic effects, safety evaluation and rational design of follow-up are needed. Also, that preliminary studies identified in the scientific literature indicate that blood-letting acupuncture and cupping at *Ashi* points are the predominant methods for the treatment of herpes zoster.[269]

Psoriasis

An early study progressed the use of acupuncture as a treatment option for psoriasis.[270] Using filiform needle acupuncture to stimulate a number of key points and related acu-points, this study investigated 61 patients with psoriasis who had poor response to Western medical management. Subsequent to an average of 9 sessions of acupuncture treatment, approximately 50% of the 61 patients had complete or near-complete clearance of their skin lesions, approximately one-third had partial improvement, and 15% did not improve. This study's results are weakened by the lack of a control group however, the results were considered important at the time.

A subsequent Swedish study reported that classical needle acupuncture was not superior to sham therapy in the treatment of psoriasis.[271] Though methodologically more robust, the primary weakness of this study was its lack of description in terms of acupuncture points and techniques employed. In addition, the sample size was small with 35 participants receiving acupuncture, and 19 receiving sham acupuncture.

A recent multi-centre study from China and review of the literature has reported that the meridian three-combined therapy was effective and safe for treatment of ordinary psoriasis.[272] Hence, this multi-centre, randomised and positive drug controlled trial consisted of 233 cases that were divided into an observation group of 116 cases and a control group of 117 cases. The observation group was treated with thread embedding at points, blood-letting puncture on the back of the ear and auricular point pressing (i.e. meridian three-combined therapy).

Atopic dermatitis

Small early studies have demonstrated some efficacy for atopic dermatitis, however more robust research is warranted.[273, 274]

Urticaria

Acupuncture has been reported to be effective for both acute and chronic urticaria.[275]

A recent study from China has reported that acupuncture had a benign regulatory effect on IgE, showing a favourable regulation on the immune functions in patients with chronic urticaria.[276]

A subsequent study also from China investigated the therapeutic effects of acupuncture plus point-injection for obstinate urticaria.[277] Sixty-four cases of obstinate urticaria were randomly divided into 2 groups. The results demonstrated that the therapeutic effect in the treatment group was significantly better than that in the control group, with a much lower relapse rate in the test group than in the control group.

Vitiligo

Briefly vitiligo is a chronic disorder that causes de-pigmentation in patches of skin. A recent study utilising low-energy He–Ne laser therapy induced re-pigmentation and improved the appearance of the skin in segmental vitiligo.[278] After an average of 17 treatment sessions, initial re-pigmentation was noticed in the majority of patients. Marked re-pigmentation (> 50%) was observed in 60% of the patients with successive treatments. Furthermore cutaneous blood flow was significantly higher at segmental vitiligo lesions compared with contralateral skin, but this was normalised after He–Ne laser treatment. The study concluded that He–Ne laser therapy was an effective treatment for segmental vitiligo by normalising dysfunctions of cutaneous blood flow and adrenoceptor responses in these patients. It was hypothesized that the beneficial effects of He–Ne laser therapy could be mediated in part by a reparative effect on sympathetic nerve dysfunction.

Other therapies[279, 280]

Balneotherapy is a natural therapy which makes use of natural elements, such as hot springs, climatic factors, chrono-biological and circadian rhythmic phases and natural herbal substances for treatment of disease. Dermatology perhaps is one of the oldest users of this form of therapy. Wet to dry soaks, salt water baths, tar baths, the use of the Dead Sea for the treatment of many papulosquamous and eczematous disorders — all have been mainstream dermatologic therapy for many decades.[281]

Phototherapy or light therapy is a form of treatment for skin conditions using artificial light wavelengths from the ultraviolet wavelength range (blue light). A recent study has demonstrated that photo-modulation with a 590 nm wavelength LED array decreased the intensity and duration of post-fractional laser treatment erythema.[282]

Massage therapy has also been reported to be useful for all skin diseases offering a mode of relaxation, particularly if combined with suitable aromatherapy oils.

Photopheresis, originally developed in dermatology, has become a treatment method accepted across various disciplines.[283]

Conclusion

General practice dermatology refers to the assessment, treatment and referral of disorders affecting the skin, nail, hair or mucous membranes. Skin topography and microvasculature undergo characteristic changes with ageing as well as with environmental exposures. Hence there are important implications for clinical practice and research of skin diseases. There are a number of studies that are appropriate for the integrative management of the patient with skin diseases given that there is a significant amount of evidence of extensive CAM use among patients with skin diseases.

Common sense suggests that studies of food allergy exclusions should be carried out on people with a history of suggested food allergy, confirmed by appropriate allergy testing or challenge tests. A distinction should be made between young children, grown-up children and adults, because food allergy in children tends to improve over time. Disease severity should be measured using valid instruments and include quality of life assessments such as adherence to prudent physical activity regimens, nutritional practices and life stressors so that patient-centred outcomes can be interpreted clinically.

Also, it should be noted that CAM products are also extensively used by people to improve skin appearance as a form of anti-ageing therapy. A large number of complementary medicine therapies have been advocated for skin as cosmeceuticals. Commercial anti-ageing creams can contain 1 or more of the following:

- antioxidants (vitamin A [retinol]), retinoic acid, tretinoin (all-trans retinoic acid), retinyl palmitate, retinyl acetate; vitamin C (L-ascorbic acid), more acidic forms penetrate better but are more irritant, ascorbate tetrapalmitate; vitamin E (α-tocopherol); α-lipoic acid and Green tea, with gamma glutamyl cysteine under development
- α-β-hydroxy acids (AHAs naturally occurring glycolic, lactic, citric, malic, tartaric acids exfoliation, stimulate collagen, elastin; BHAs e.g. salicylic acid)
- other compounds (biotin, ceramides, CoQ_{10}; collagen and elastin (moisturising or lubricating properties only, no penetration); glycerin (humectant); hyaluronic acid; liposomes; pro-vitamin B5; vita-niacin (complex of vitamin E, pro-vitamin B5 and vitamin B3
- sunscreens (physical blocking agents [zinc oxide, titanium dioxide] — may be nanosized; octyl methoxycinnamate).

Hence clinicians need to be aware of the plethora of compounds that may find their way into skin products that may be effective or alternatively that may cause irritability to the skin or perhaps may have the potential to be toxic (e.g. idebenone).

Table 14.9 summarises the level of evidence for some CAM therapies for eczema, psoriasis and other skin disorders.

Table 14.9 Levels of evidence for lifestyle and complementary medicines/therapies in the management of eczema, psoriasis and other skin disorders

Modality	Level I	Level II	Level IIIa	Level IIIb	Level IIIc	Level IV	Level V
Lifestyle modification							
Smoking				x			
Alcohol				x			
Life stressors				x			
Environmental factors							
Sunlight exposure/UV				x			
Contact allergy				x			

Continued

Table 14.9 Levels of evidence for lifestyle and complementary medicines/therapies in the management of eczema, psoriasis and other skin disorders—cont'd

Modality	Level I	Level II	Level IIIa	Level IIIb	Level IIIc	Level IV	Level V
Mind–body medicine							
Cognitive behavioural therapy		x					
Hypnosis		x					
Biofeedback					x		
Psychosocial education	x(-)				x		
Physical activity							
Indirect effects				x			
Nutrition							
Diets							
Exclusion diets	x(-)			x			
Food sensitivities				x			
Low GI diet		x					
Nutritional supplements							
Vitamins							
Vitamin A	x						
Vitamin A Analogs (topically applied)	x						
Vitamin C (oral ingestion* and topically applied†)	x†			x*			
Vitamin E (oral ingestion and topically applied)			x				
Vitamin D (oral ingestion* and topically applied†)	x†	x*					
B group vitamins			x				
Minerals							
Zinc		x					
Selenium		x(+/-)					
Other nutrients							
Alpha hydroxy acids (oral ingestion and topically applied)		x					
Salicylic acid				x			
Coenzyme Q_{10} (oral ingestion and topically applied)					x		
Lipoic acid (oral ingestion and topically applied)					x		
Essential fatty acids (omega-3 and omega-6)	x(+/-)						
Functional foods							
Probiotics	x						
Herbal medicines							
Tea tree oil (topical)		x					
Vitex agnus castus (oral)				x			
Aloe vera (topical)	x(+/-)	x					

Continued

Table 14.9 Levels of evidence for lifestyle and complementary medicines/therapies in the management of eczema, psoriasis and other skin disorders—cont'd

Modality	Level I	Level II	Level IIIa	Level IIIb	Level IIIc	Level IV	Level V
Honey (topical)	x						
Marigold (topical)		x					
Tannins in herbs						x	
Lemon balm (topical)				x			
Licorice (topical)						x	
Garlic (topical)				x			
Capsaicin (topical)			x				
St John's wort (topical)				x			
Other medicines/treatments							
Traditional Chinese medicines (oral)				x			
Aromatherapy (topical)		x					
Physical therapies							
Electrical impulses	x(-)			x			
Acupuncture (see detailed discussion in text for different types of acupuncture)				x x			
Balneotherapy					x		
Phototherapy					x		
Massage therapy					x		
Photopheresis					x		

Level I — from a systematic review of all relevant randomised controlled trials — meta-analyses.
Level II — from at least 1 properly designed randomised controlled clinical trial.
Level IIIa — from well-designed pseudo-randomised controlled trials (alternate allocation or some other method).
Level IIIb — from comparative studies (including systematic reviews of such studies) with concurrent controls and allocation not randomised, cohort studies, case-control studies, or interrupted time series with a parallel control group.
Level IIIc — from comparative studies with historical control, 2 or more single-arm studies or interrupted time series without a parallel control group.
Level IV — opinions of respected authorities based on clinical experience, descriptive studies or reports of expert committees.
Level V — represents minimal evidence that represents testimonials.

Clinical tips handout for patients–skin diseases

1 Lifestyle advice

Sleep

- Restore normal sleep patterns. Most adults require about 7 hours sleep a day. (See Chapter 22 for more advice.)

Sunshine

- Eye protection should be worn in the form of sunglasses at all times when exposed to the sun for prolonged periods of time.
- Amount of exposure varies with local climate.
- At least 15 minutes of sunshine needed daily for vitamin D and melatonin production — especially before 10 a.m. and after 3 p.m. when the sun exposure is safest during summer. Much more exposure is required in winter when supplementation needs to be considered.
- Ensure gradual adequate skin exposure to sun; avoid sunscreen and excess clothing to maximise levels of vitamin D.
- More time in the sun is required for dark skinned people.
- Aim for direct exposure to about 10% of body (hands, arms, face), without sunscreen and not through glass.
- Vitamin D is obtained in the diet from fatty fish, eggs, liver and fortified foods (some milks and margarines), but it is unlikely that adequate vitamin D concentrations can be obtained from diet alone.

2 Physical activity/exercise

- Exercise 30 minutes or more daily. If exercise is not regular, commence with 5 minutes daily and slowly build up to at least 30 minutes. Outdoor exercise in nature, fresh air and sunshine is ideal (e.g. brisk walking, light jogging, cycling, swimming, stretching.) The more time you spend outdoors the better.
- Yoga may be of help; other examples include qiqong, tai chi.

3 Mind–body medicine

Stress

- Stress management program — for example, 6 x 40 minute sessions for patients to understand the nature of their symptoms, the symptoms' relationship to stress, and the practice of regular relaxation exercises.
- Regular meditation practice at least 10–20 minutes daily.

Breathing

- Be aware of breathing from time to time. Notice if tendency to hold breath or over-breathe.
- Always aim to relax breath and the muscles around chest wall.

Rest and stress management

Recurrent stress may cause a return of symptoms. Relaxation is important for a full and lasting recovery.

- Reduce workload and resolve conflicts.
- Listening to relaxation music helps.
- Massage therapy helps.
- Aromatherapy (e.g. essential lemon balm oil rubbed onto the face daily) may help reduce agitation, and improve relaxation and sleep.
- Exercise, hypnotherapy, and biofeedback may be of help.
- Cognitive behavioural therapy and psychotherapy are extremely helpful.

Fun

- It is important to have fun in life. Joy can be found even in the simplest tasks, such as being with friends with a sense of humour funny movies/videos, comedy, hobbies, dancing, playing with pets and children.
- Try to maintain an 'easy-going approach to life'; avoid feeling time-pressured or rushed.

4 Environment

- Don't smoke and avoid smoking environments.
- Avoid environmental pollutants (especially mercury), lead and cadmium exposure, chemicals — at work and in the home.

5 Dietary changes

- Eat regular healthy low GI meals, ideally 3 small meals, and 2 snacks a day, each containing protein in order to avoid fluctuating blood sugar levels and provide amino acids for nerve transmitters such as tryptophan.
- Eat more fruit and vegetables — variety of colours and those in season.

- Increase dietary fibre — nuts (e.g. walnuts, peanuts); seeds, beans (e.g. soy); sprouts (e.g. alfa, mung bean); lentils.
- Increase fish intake, especially deep sea fish, and eat fish daily if possible. Canned is okay (mackerel, salmon, sardines, cod, tuna, salmon).
- Reduce red meat intake (preferably use red lean meat e.g. lamb, kangaroo) and white meat (e.g. free range organic chicken is okay).
- Use cold pressed olive oil and avocado.
- Use dark chocolate, preferably 85% or more of cocoa.
- Consume low-GI wholegrains/cereals (variety); rice (brown, basmati, Mahatmi, Doongara); traditional rolled oats; buckwheat flour; wholegrain organic breads (rye bread, Essene, spelt, Kamut), brown pasta; millet; amaranth etc.
- Reduce dairy intake; low-fat dairy products such as yoghurt and occasionally cheeses, unless there is a dairy intolerance.
- Drink more water 1–2 litres a day and teas, especially organic green tea and black tea, plus vegetable juices.
- Avoid hydrogenated fats, salt, fast foods, added sugar such as in soft drinks, lollies, biscuits, cakes and processed foods (e.g. white bread, white pasta, pastries).
- Minimise alcohol intake to no more than 1–2 glasses daily (non-sweet) as it is a brain depressant and can disturb sleep.
- Avoid chemical additives — preservatives, colourings and flavourings.
- For sweetener try honey (e.g. yellow box and stringy bark have the lowest GI).
- A trial elimination diet under the supervision of a nutritionist may help relieve symptoms of some skin diseases such as dermatitis and eczema. See www.integrative-medicine.com.au for more information.

6 Physical therapies

- Various forms of acupuncture and other physical therapies may be very useful for the treatment of a number of skin conditions.

7 Supplements

Fish oils

- Indication: anti-inflammatory; allergic dermatitis fish oils 2–4g (1g containing EPA 180/DHA 120mg) daily depending on fish consumption.
- Dosage: take with meals. Adult: 1g 1-2 capsules twice daily. Child: 500mg 1 to 2 x daily (500mg–1g daily EPA and DHA); can be used in pregnancy or lactation as tolerated.
- Side-effects: often well tolerated especially if taken with meals. Very mild and rare side-effects; for example, gastrointestinal upset; allergic reactions (e.g. rash, breathing problems if allergic to seafood); blood thinning effects in very high doses > 10g daily (may need to stop fish oil supplements 2 weeks prior to surgery).
- Contraindications: sensitivity reaction to seafood; drug interactions; caution when taking high doses of fish oils >4g per day together with warfarin (your doctor will check your INR test).

Multivitamin especially B-group containing B6, B12 and folate

- Indication: for atopic dermatitis; pellagra.
- Dosage: 1 tablet daily.
- Side-effects: usually well tolerated in this dosage; avoid single vitamin B >50md/day for prolonged periods of time. Vitamin B6 toxicity may cause neurological problems such as tingling sensation and balance problems that are often reversible, but can be permanent.
- Contraindications: vitamin A content greater than 2000IU/day.

Vitamin D3 (cholecalciferol 1000IU)

Doctors should check blood levels and suggest oral supplementation if levels are low.

Various forms of vitamin D products are available for the treatment of psoriasis and atopic dermatitis. Check with your doctor.

Vitamin C and Vitamin E (best given together)

Vitamin C

- Indication: can reactivate vitamin E. May help repair skin lesions; anti-bacterial; protects against UV damage.
- Dosage: 500–1000mg daily or as tolerated.
- Side-effects: with high doses can cause nausea, heartburn, abdominal cramps and diarrhoea.
- Contraindications: can increase iron absorption. Use with caution if glucose-6-phosphate dehydrogenase deficiency.

Vitamin E (natural form)

- Indication: can promote growth and hence help repair skin; topical to herpetic coldsores; protects against harmful UV radiation effects.

- Dosage: 200–500–1000IU daily (D-alpha-tocopherol or mixed isomers).
- Side-effects: doses below 1500IU daily are very unlikely to result in haemorrhage diarrhoea, flatulence, nausea, heart palpitations.
- Contraindications: use with caution if bleeding disorder or if taking with blood thinning medication. If using very high dose, reduce dose before surgery.

Zinc

- Indication: can improve innate immune function and aid in skin repair; acne; seborrheic dermatitis; dandruff.
- Dosage: usual dosage in adult no more than 5–10mcg zinc sulfate daily. Zinc amino acid chelate 50mg topical (1%).
- Side-effects: nausea, vomiting, metallic taste in mouth. Avoid long-term use and high dosage as this may cause copper deficiency, impair the immune system and cause anaemia.
- Contraindications: sideroblastic anaemia, above normal blood levels of zinc, severe kidney disease.

Selenium (sodium selenite, organic selenium found in yeast)

- Indication: may help with reducing metabolic dysfunction of the skin; prevention of some cancers but not skin cancers.
- Dosage: 50–100mcg daily; do not exceed >600 microgram daily (health professional supervision required to avoid toxicity).
- Results: uncertain.
- Side-effects: very mild and rare; nausea, vomiting, rash, sensitivity reactions, toxicity in high doses; nail changes, irritability, fatigue.
- Contraindications: pregnancy, lactation, children <12 years of age; avoid yeast derived selenium if allergic to yeast.

Coenzyme Q_{10} (CoQ_{10})

- Indication: may be useful for skin repair mechanism; psoriasis.
- Dosage: Adults 100–200mg in divided doses, 2–3 times per day with meals.
- Side-effects: generally well tolerated. May cause gastrointestinal side-effects such as nausea, vomiting, diarrhoea.
- Contraindicated: avoid in pregnancy and lactating women and if allergic.

Alpha-lipoic acid

- Indication: may prevent nerve damage and can repair existing damage of the skin.
- Dosage: 600–1200mg daily (oral).
- Side-effects: nausea and skin rashes have been reported.
- Contraindications: must not be taken if thiamine deficient (e.g. alcoholic) unless thiamine supplementation is given.

Probiotics

- Indications: to enhance Gut Associated Lymphoid Tissue (GALT), thereby providing balance between Th1 and Th2 cytokines in order to prevent and treat auto-immune and infectious diseases; eczema; atopic dermatits.
- Dosage: depending upon condition, different probiotics may be required. Generalised treatment dose before breakfast (multi-strain formula is best).
  - *Lactobacillus rhamnosus* 12 billion CFU
  - *Lactobacillus acidophilus* 4 billion CFU
  - *Lactobacillus casei* 2 billion CFU
  - *Bifidobacterium bifidum* 1 billion CFU
  - *Bifidobacterium longum* 1 billion CFU
- Results: few days to few weeks depending on condition.
- Side-effects: gastrointestinal disturbance if wrong probiotic.
- Contraindications: true cow's milk allergy if contained in product.

Herbal medicines (all for external/topical use only)

Word of caution: always patch-test a small area of skin to check sensitivity before wider application. Take great care with babies and infants — apply to smaller areas after a test dose (patch-test). Immediately cease using a product if it causes pain, redness, itchiness, burning, or any irritation of the skin. Avoid contact with eyes. Not for oral ingestion.

A number of herbal medicines have been researched and promoted for topical use and these include the following.

Tea tree oil

- Indications: For adults, this oil has been used in gels, creams shampoo, body washes and in tinctures or extracts. Most doses used in studies are applied topically (on the skin). These doses have not necessarily been proven conclusively to be effective or safe. While 100% tea tree oil is sometimes used (e.g. for fungal nail infections), it is often diluted with inactive ingredients (e.g. oils).

Typically, preparations contain about 4–5% tea tree oil and are used daily for 4 weeks to 6 months depending on condition.

- Dosage: Tea tree oil 5% gel has been applied to acne-prone areas of the skin daily.
  For athlete's foot (tinea pedis), 10% tea tree oil cream, applied twice daily to the feet after they have been thoroughly washed and dried or 25–50% tea tree oil solution applied twice daily to the affected area for 4 weeks has been studied.[284]
  For genital herpes, a 6% tea tree oil gel has been used.
  For head or pubic lice add a few drops of tea tree oil and lavender oil to hair conditioner and slowly comb through the hair, using a fine-toothed steel comb, on a daily basis for up to 1–2 weeks, then weekly as required.
- Side-effects: Reports of severe side-effects after tea tree oil ingestion it is strongly recommended that tea tree oil not be taken by mouth. Although tea tree oil solution has been used as a mouthwash, it should not be swallowed.
- Contraindications: Use cautiously if allergic to eucalyptol as many tea tree preparations contain eucalyptol.
  Skin reactions range from mild contact dermatitis to severe blistering rashes.
  NOT recommended for children under 18 years — insufficient research available.

Aloe vera

Used externally to treat different skin conditions, such as psoriasis, and reduces inflammation.

Used for the treatment of burns and bruises.

Speeds the healing of insect bites, and relieves itching and dandruff.

Manuka honey

- Indications: partial thickness burns, ulcerations, wound healing; throat infections. Use under medical supervision.
- Dosage: topical application as directed; 1tsp of honey for sore throats.
- Results: within a week; may have immediate soothing effect on throat.
- Side-effects: none.
- Contraindications: allergy to honey.

Note: numerous other herbs are available for topical use. Request manufacturer information on products.

Evening primrose oil

- Indications: atopic eczema; psoriasis; mastalgia; breast discomfort.
- Dosage: 2–4g/day.
- Side-effects: usually well tolerated; may increase bleeding time so take care with other anticoagulants.
- Contraindications: avoid if you suffer seizures or epilepsy.

References

1 Mukhtar H, Mercurio MG, Agarwal R. Murine skin carcinogenesis: Relevance to humans. In: Mukhtar H. Skin Cancer: Mechanism and Human Relevance. CRC Press, Boca Raton, 1995:3–8.

2 Blanpain C, Fuchs E. Epidermal homeostasis: a balancing act of stem cells in the skin. Nat Rev Mol Cell Biol 2009;10(3):207–17.

3 Bickers DR, Lim HW, Margolis D, et. al. The burden of skin diseases: 2004 a joint project of the American Academy of Dermatology Association and the Society for Investigative Dermatology. J Am Acad Dermatol 2006;55:490–500.

4 Khatami, M. San Sebastian Skin Disease: A Neglected Public Health Problem. Dermatologic Clinics 2007;27(2):99–101.

5 Wolkenstein P, Grob JJ, Bastuji-Garin S, et. al. Societe Francaise de Dermotologie. French people and skin diseases: results of a survey using a representative sample. Arch Dermat 2003;139:1614–9.

6 Figueroa JI, Fuller LC, Abraha A, et al. Dermatology in the south western Ethiopia: rational for a community approach. Int J Dermatol 1998;37:752–8.

7 Chen SC, Bayoumi AM, Soon SL, et. al. A catalogue of dermatology utilities: a measure of the burden of skin diseases. J Investig Dermatol Symp Proc 2004;9:160–8.

8 Insinga RP, Dasbach EJ, Elbasha EH, et. al. Assessing the annual economical burden of preventing and treating anogenital human papillomavirus-related disease in the US: analytic framework and review of the literature. Pharmacoeconomics 2005;23: 1107–22.

9 Walker N, Lewis-Jones MS. Quality of life and acne in Scottish adolescent schoolchildren: use of the Children's Dermatology Life Quality Index (CDLQI) and the Cardiff Acne Disability Index (CADI). J Eur Acad Dermatol Venereol 2006;20:45–50.

10 Carroll CL, Balkrishnan R, Feldman SR, et. al. The burden of atopic dermatitis: impact on the patient, family, and society. Pediatr Dermatol 2005;22:192–9.

11 Bickers DR, Lim HW, Margolis D, et al. The burden of skin diseases: 2004 a joint project of the American Academy of Dermatology Association and the Society for Investigative Dermatology. J Am Acad Dermatol 2006;55(3):490–500.

12 Linnane AW, Kios M, Vitetta L. Healthy ageing: regulation of the metabolome by cellular redox modulation and prooxidant signaling systems: the essential roles of superoxide anion and hydrogen peroxide. Biogerontology 2007;8(5):445–67.

13 Verhoeven EW, Kraaimaat FW, van Weel C, et. al. Skin diseases in family medicine: prevalence and health care use. Ann Fam Med 2008;6(4):349–54.

14 Morganti P. The photoprotective activity of nutraceuticals. Clin Dermatol 2009;27(2):166–74.

15 Just-Sarobé M. Smoking and the Skin. Actas Dermosifiliogr 2008;99:173–84.

16 Morita A. Tobacco smoke causes premature skin ageing. J Dermatol Sci 2007;48(3):169–75.

17 Frances C. Smoker's wrinkles: epidemiological and pathogenic considerations. Clin Dermatol 1998;16:565–70.

18 Ernster VL, Grady D, Miike R, et. al. Facial wrinkling in men and women, by smoking status. Am J Public Health 1995;85:78–82.

19 Grady D, Ernster V. Does cigarette smoking make you ugly and old? Am J Epid 1992;135:839–42.

20 Kadunce DP, Burr R, Gress R, et. al. Cigarette smoking: risk factor for premature facial wrinkling. Ann Intern Med 1991;114:840–4.

21 Wenk J, Brenneisen P, Meewes C, et. al. UV-induced oxidative stress and photo-ageing. Curr Probl Dermatol 2001;29:83–94.

22 Fisher GJ, Talwar HS, Lin J, et. al. Molecular mechanisms of photo-ageing in human skin in vivo and their prevention by all-trans retinoic acid. Photochem Photobiol 1999;69:154–7.

23 Grether-Beck S, Buettner R, Krutmann J. Ultraviolet A radiation-induced expression of human genes: molecular and photobiological mechanisms. Biol Chem 1997;378:1231–6.

24 Leung W-C, Harvey I. Is skin ageing in the elderly caused by sun exposure or smoking? Br J Dermatol 2002;147:1187–91.

25 Kostović K, Lipozencić J. Skin diseases in alcoholics. Acta Dermatoven Croat 2004;12(3):181–90.

26 Peters EM, Kuhlmei A, Tobin DJ, et. al. Stress exposure modulates peptidergic innervation and degranulates mast cells in murine skin. Brain Behav Immun 2005;19:252–62.

27 Joachim RA, Sagach V, Quarcoo D, et al. Neurokinin-1 receptor mediates stress-exacerbated allergic airway inflammation and airway hyperresponsiveness in mice. Psych Med 2004;66:564–71.

28 Buljan D, Buljan M, Zivkovic MV, et. al. Basic aspects of psychodermatology. Psychiatr Danub 2008;20(3):415–8.

29 Hashisume H, Horibe T, Ohshima A, et. al. Anxiety accelerates T-helper 2-tilted immune responses in patients with atopic dermatitis. Br J Dermatol 2005;152:1161–4.

30 Kilpelainen M, Koskenvuo M, Helenius H, Terho EO. Stressful life events promote the manifestation of asthma and atopic diseases. Clin Exp Allergy 2002;32:256–63.

31 Kodama A, Horikawa T, Suzuki T, et. al. Effect of stress on atopic dermatitis: investigation in patients after the great hanshin earthquake. J Allergy Clin Immunol 1999;104:173–6.

32 Buske-Kirschbaum A, Geiben A, Hellhammer D. Psychobiological aspects of atopic dermatitis: an overview. Psychother Psychosom 2001;70:6–16

33 Arndt J, Smith N, Tausk F. Stress and atopic dermatitis. Curr Allergy Asthma Rep 2008;8(4): 312–7.

34 Hendrix S. Neuroimmune Communication in Skin: Far from Peripheral. J Invest Dermatol 2008;128:260–261.

35 Christian LM, Graham JE, Padgett DA, et. al. Stress and wound healing. Neuroimmunomodulation. 2006;13(5-6):337–46.

36 Godbout JP, Glaser R. Stress-induced immune dysregulation: implications for wound healing, infectious disease and cancer. J Neuroimmune Pharmacol 2006;1(4):421–7.

37 Verhoeven EW, de Klerk S, Kraaimaat FW, et. al. Biopsychosocial mechanisms of chronic itch in patients with skin diseases: a review. Acta Derm Venereol 2008;88(3):211–8.

38 Nolan BV, Feldman SR. Ultraviolet tanning addiction. Dermatol Clin 2009;27:109–12.

39 Gaudy-Marqueste C, Madjlessi N, Guillot B, et. al. Risk factors in elderly people for lentigo maligna compared with other melanomas: a double case-control study. Arch Dermatol 2009;145(4):418–23.

40 Kennedy C, Bajdik CD, Willemze R, et. al. The influence of painful sunburns and lifetime sun exposure on the risk of actinic keratoses, seborrheic warts, melanocytic nevi, atypical nevi, and skin cancer. J Invest Dermatol 2003;120(6):1087–93.

41 Armstrong BK, Kricker A. How much melanoma is caused by sun exposure? Melanoma Res 1993;3:395–401.

42 Taylor CR, Sober AJ. Sun exposure and skin disease. Annu Rev Med 1996;47:181–91.

43 Skin Cancer Fact Sheet – from American Academy of Dermatology. Online. Available: http://www.aad.org/media/background/factsheets/fact_skincancer.html (accessed June 2009).

44 Young AR. 1990. Cumulative effects of ultraviolet radiation in the skin: cancer and photo-ageing. Semin Dermatol 1990;9:25–31.

45 Engel A, Johnson ML, Haynes SG. Health effects of sunlight exposure in the United States. Arch Dermatol 1988;124:72–79.

46 de Groot AC, Bruynzeel DP, Bos JD, et. al. The allergens in cosmetics. Arch Dermatol 1988;124:1525–29.

47 Goossens A, Beck MH,Haneke E, McFadden JP, et. al. Adverse cutaneous reactions to cosmetic allergens. Contact Dermatitis 1999;40:112–13.

48 Nielsen NH, Linneberg A, Menne T, et. al. Allergic contact sensitisation in an adult Danish population: two cross-sectional surveys eight years apart (the Copenhagen Allergy Study). Acta Derm Venereol, 2001;81:31–34.

49 Ortis KJ, Yiannias JA. Contact dermatitis to cosmetics, fragrances, and botanicals. Dermatol Ther 2004;17(3):264–71.

50 Orton DI, Wilkinson JD. Cosmetic allergy: incidence, diagnosis, and management. Am J Clin Dermatol 2004;5(5):327–37.

51 Fried RG, Gupta MA, Gupta AK. Depression and skin disease. Dermatol Clin 2005;23(4):657–64.

52 Shenefelt PD. Therapeutic management of psychodermatological disorders. Expert Opin Pharmacother 2008;9(6):973-85.

53 Tausk FA. Alternative medicine: is it all in your mind? Arch Dermatol 1998;134:1422–5.

54 Shenefelt PD. Hypnosis in dermatology. Arch Dermatol 2000;136:393–9.

55 Spiegel H, Spiegel D. Trance and treatment: clinical uses of hypnosis (2nd edn). DC7 American Psychiatric Publishing, Washington, 2004:51–92.

56 Shenefelt PD. Therapeutic management of psychodermatological disorders. Expert Opin Pharmacother 2008;9(6):973–85.

57 Sarti MG. Biofeedback in dermatology. Clin Dermatol 1998;16(6):711–4.

58 Freedman RR. Quantitative measurements of finger blood flow during behavioural treatments for Raynaud's disease. Psychophysiology 1989;26(4):437–41.

59 Ersser SJ, Latter S, Sibley A, et. al. Psychological and educational interventions for atopic eczema in children. Cochrane Database Syst Rev 2007 Jul 18;(3):CD004054.

60 Bilkis MR, Mark KA. Mind-body medicine. Practical applications in dermatology. Arch Dermatol 1998;134(11):1437–41.
61 Ospina MB, Bond K, Karkhaneh M, et. al. Meditation practices for health: state of the research. Evid Rep Technol Assess (Full Rep) 2007;(155):1–263.
62 Javnbakht M, Hejazi Kenari R, Ghasemi M. Effects of yoga on depression and anxiety of women. Complement Ther Clin Pract 2009;15(2):102–4.
63 Grodin MA, Piwowarczyk L, Fulker D, et. al. Treating survivors of torture and refugee trauma: a preliminary case series using qigong and t'ai chi. J Altern Complement Med 2008;14(7):801–6.
64 Kuramoto AM. Therapeutic benefits of Tai Chi exercise: research review. WMJ 2006;105(7):42–6.
65 Wall RB. Teaching Tai Chi with mindfulness-based stress reduction to middle school children in the inner city: a review of the literature and approaches. Med Sport Sci 2008;52:166–72.
66 Dattner AM. Nutritional dermatology. Clin Dermatol 1999;17(1):57–64.
67 Guin JD, Hoskyn J. Aggravation of rosacea by protein contact dermatitis to soy. Contact Dermatitis 2005;53(4):235–6.
68 Humbert P, Pelletier F, Dreno B, et. al. Gluten intolerance and skin diseases. Eur J Dermatol 2006;16(1):4–11.
69 Ackland ML, Michalczyk A. Zinc deficiency and its inherited disorders –a review. Genes Nutr 2006;1(1):41–9.
70 Lee BY, Thurmon TF. Nutritional disorders among workers in North China during national turmoil. Ann Nutr Metab 2001;45(4):175–80.
71 Sicherer SH, Leung DY. Advances in allergic skin disease, anaphylaxis, and hypersensitivity reactions to foods, drugs, and insects in 2008. J Allergy Clin Immunol 2009;123(2):319–27.
72 Lack G. Epidemiologic risks for food allergy. J Allergy Clin Immunol 2008;121:1331–6.
73 Untersmayr E, Jensen-Jarolim E. The role of protein digestibility and antacids on food allergy outcomes. J Allergy Clin Immunol 2008;121:1301–8.
74 Pistiner M, Gold DR, Abdulkerim H, et. al. Birth by caesarean section, allergic rhinitis, and allergic sensitisation among children with a parental history of atopy. J Allergy Clin Immunol 2008;122:274–9.
75 Hare ND, Fasano MB. Clinical manifestations of food allergy: differentiating true allergy from food intolerance. Postgrad Med 2008;120(2):E01-5.
76 Chandra RK. Food hypersensitivity and allergic diseases. Eur J Clin Invest 2002;56:S54–S56.
77 Sampson HA. The evaluation and management of food allergy in atopic dermatitis. Clin Dermatol 2003;21:183–192.
78 Bath-Hextall F, Delamere FM, Williams HC. Dietary exclusions for improving established atopic eczema in adults and children: systematic review. Allergy 2009;64(2):258–64.
79 Eaton SB, Konner M. Paleolithic nutrition; A consideration of its nature and current implications. NEJM 1985;312:283–9.
80 Smith RN, Mann NJ, Braue A, et. al. The effect of a high-protein, low glycemic-load diet versus a conventional, high glycemic-load diet on biochemical parameters associated with acne vulgaris: a randomised, investigator-masked, controlled trial. J Am Acad Dermatol 2007;57(2):247–56.
81 Smith RN, Mann NJ, Braue A, et. al. A low-glycemic-load diet improves symptoms in acne vulgaris patients: a randomised controlled trial. Am J Clin Nutr 2007;86(1):107–15.
82 Berra B, Riszo AM. Glycemic index, glycemic load, wellness and beauty: the state of the art. Clin Dermatol 2009;27(2):230–5.
83 Thomas DE, Elliott EJ, Baur L. Low glycaemic index or low glycaemic load diets for overweight and obesity. Cochrane Database Syst Rev 2007;(3):CD005105.
84 Smith RN, Braue A, Varigos GA, Mann NJ. The effect of a low glycemic load diet on acne vulgaris and the fatty acid composition of skin surface triglycerides. J Dermatol Sci 2008;50(1):41–52.
85 Bath-Hextall F, Delamere FM, Williams HC. Dietary exclusions for established atopic eczema. Cochrane Database Syst Rev 2008 Jan 23;(1):CD005203.
86 Bath-Hextall F, Delamere FM, Williams HC. Dietary exclusions for improving established atopic eczema in adults and children: systematic review. Allergy 2009;64(2):258–64.
87 Richelle M, Sabatier M, Steiling H, et. al. Skin bioavailability of dietary vitamin E, carotenoids, polyphenols, vitamin C, zinc and selenium. Br J Nutr 2006;96(2):227–38.
88 Kligman AM, Fulton JE, Plewig G. Topical vitamin A acid in acne vulgaris. Arch Dermatol 1969;99:469–76.
89 Kligman AM, Mills OH Jr, Leyden JJ, et. al. Oral vitamin A in acne vulgaris. Preliminary report. Int J Dermatol 1981;20:278–285.
90 Kligman AM. The growing importance of topical retinoids in clinical dermatology: A retrospective and prospective analysis. J Am Acad Dermatol 1998;39:S2–7.
91 Hunt TK. Vitamin A and wound healing. J Am Acad Dermatol 1986;15:817–21.
92 Saurat JH. Retinoids. In: Katsambas AD, Lotti TM. European handbook of dermatologic treatments. Berlin, Heidelberg: Springer-Verlag, 1999:812–18.
93 Fritsch PO. Retinoids in psoriasis and disorders of keratinisation. J Am Acad Derm 1992;27:S8–14.
94 Goldsmith LA, Weinrich AE, Shupack J. Pityriasis rubra pilaris response to 13-*cis*-retinoic acid (isotretinoin). J Am Acad Dermatol 1982;6(Suppl):710 –5.
95 Levine N. Role of retinoids in skin cancer treatment and prevention. J Am Acad Dermatol 1998;39:S62–6.
96 Katsambas AD, Lotti TM. Melasma. In: Katsambas AD, Lotti TM. European handbook of dermatologic treatments. Springer-Verlag, Berlin, Heidelberg, 1999:368–73.
97 Laszlo Keller K, Fenske NA. Uses of vitamins A, C, and E and related compounds in dermatology: A review. J Am Acad Dermatol 1998;39:611–25.
98 Kraemer KH, DiGiovanna JJ, Moshell AN, et. al. Prevention of skin cancer in xeroderma pigmentosum with the use of oral isotretinoin. NEJM 1998;318:1633–7.
99 Goldberg LH, Hsu SH, Alcalay J. Effectiveness of isotretinoin in preventing the appearance of basal cell carcinomas in basal cell nevus syndrome. J Am Acad Dermatol 1989;21:144–5.
100 DiGiovanna JJ. Retinoid chemoprevention in the high-risk patient. J Am Acad Dermatol 1998;39:S82–5.
101 Moon TE, Levine N, Cartmel B, et. al. Effect of retinol to prevent squamous cell skin cancer in moderate-risk subjects. Cancer Epidemiol Biomarkers Prev 1997;6:949–56.
102 Levine N, Moon TE, Cartmel B, et. al. Trial of retinol and isotretinoin in skin cancer prevention. Cancer Epidemiol Biomarkers Prev 1997;6:957–61.
103 Haydey RP, Reed ML, Dzubow LM, et. al. Treatment of keratoacanthomas with oral 13-*cis*-retinoic acid. NEJM 1980;303:560–2.

104 Benoldi D, Alinovi A. Multiple persistent keratoacanthomas: Treatment with oral etretinate. J Am Acad Dermatol 1984;10:1035–8.
105 Lippman SM, Meyskens FL Jr. Treatment of advanced squamous cell carcinoma of the skin with isotretinoin. Ann Intern Med 1987;107:499–502.
106 Sies H, Stahl W. Nutritional protection against skin damage from sunlight. Annu Rev Nutr 2004;24: 173–200.
107 Dreher F, Maibach H. Protective effects of topical antioxidants in humans. Curr Probl Dermatol 2001;29:157–64.
108 Oresajo C, Stephens T, Hino PD, et. al. Protective effects of a topical antioxidant mixture containing vitamin C, ferulic acid, and phloretin against ultraviolet-induced photodamage in human skin. J Cosmet Dermatol 2008;7(4):290–7.
109 Darr D, Dunston S, Faust H, et. al. Effectiveness of antioxidants (vitamin C and E) with and without sunscreens as topical photoprotectants. Acta Derm Venereol (Stockh) 1996;76:264–8.
110 Eberlein-Konig B, Placzek M, Przybilla B. Protective effect against sunburn of combined systemic ascorbic acid (vitamin C) and *d*-alpha-tocopherol (vitamin E). J Am Acad Dermatol 1998;38:45–8.
111 Dunham WB, Zuckerkandl E, Reynolds R, et al. Effects of intake of l-ascorbic acid on the incidence of dermal neoplasms induced in mice by ultraviolet light. PNAS 1982;79:7532–6.
112 Pauling L. Effect of ascorbic acid on incidence of spontaneous mammary tumors and UV-light-induced skin tumors in mice. Am J Clin Nutr 1991;54(6 Suppl):S1252–5.
113 Oresajo C, Stephens T, Hino PD, et. al. Protective effects of a topical antioxidant mixture containing vitamin C, ferulic acid, and phloretin against ultraviolet-induced photodamage in human skin. J Cosmet Dermatol 2008;7(4):290–7.
114 Samuel M, Brooke RC, Hollis S, et. al. Interventions for photodamaged skin. Cochrane Database Syst Rev 2005;25:CD001782. Review.
115 Farris PK. Topical vitamin C: a useful agent for treating photo-ageing and other dermatologic conditions. Dermatol Surg 2005;31(7 Pt 2):814–7.
116 Catani MV, Savini I, Rossi A, et. al. Biological role of vitamin C in keratinocytes. Nutr Rev 2005 Mar;63(3):81–90.
117 Lévêque N, Mac-Mary S, Muret P, et. al. Evaluation of a sunscreen photoprotective effect by ascorbic acid assessment in human dermis using microdialysis and gas chromatography mass spectrometry. Exp Dermatol 2005;14(3):176–81.
118 Placzek M, Gaube S, Kerkmann U, et. al. Ultraviolet B-induced DNA damage in human epidermis is modified by the antioxidants ascorbic acid and D-alpha-tocopherol. J Invest Dermatol 2005;124(2):304–7.
119 McVean M, Liebler DC. Inhibition of UVB-induced DNA photodamage in mouse epidermis by topically applied alpha-tocopherol. Carcinogenesis 1997;18:1617–22.
120 Trevithick JR, Xiong H, Lee S, et. al. Topical tocopherol acetate reduces post-UVB sunburn-associated erythema, edema, and skin sensitivity in hairless mice. Arch Biochem Biophys 1992;296:575–82.
121 Bissett DL, Chatterjee R, Hannon DP. Photoprotective effect of superoxide-scavenging antioxidants against ultraviolet radiation-induced chronic skin damage in the hairless mouse. Photodermatol Photoimmunol Photomed 1990;7:56–62.
122 Werninghaus K, Meydani M, Bhawan J, et. al. Evaluation of the photoprotective effect of oral vitamin E supplementation. Arch Dermatol 1994;130:1257–61.
123 Thiele JJ, Hsieh SN, Ekanayake-Mudiyanselage S. Vitamin E: critical review of its current use in cosmetic and clinical dermatology. Dermatol Surg 2005;31(7 Pt 2):805–13.
124 Starasoler S, Haber GS. Use of vitamin E oil in primary herpes gingivostomatitis in an adult. N Y State Dent J 1978;44:382–83.
125 Nead DE. Effective vitamin E treatment for ulcerative herpetic lesions. Dent Surv 1976;52:50–51.
126 Fink M, Fink J. Treatment of Herpes simplex by alpha-tocopherol (vitamin E). Br Dent J 1980;148:246.
127 Mason AR, Mason J, Cork M, et. al. Topical treatments for chronic plaque psoriasis. Cochrane Database Syst Rev 2009 Apr 15;(2):CD005028.
128 de Korte J, van der Valk PG, Sprangers MA, et. al. A comparison of twice-daily calcipotriol ointment with once-daily short-contact dithranol cream therapy: quality-of-life outcomes of a randomised controlled trial of supervised treatment of psoriasis in a day-care setting. Br J Dermatol 2008;158(2):375–81.
129 Lebwohl M, Ortonne JP, Andres P, et. al. Calcitriol ointment 3 microg/g is safe and effective over 52 weeks for the treatment of mild to moderate plaque psoriasis. Cutis 2009;83(4):205–12.
130 Sidbury R, Sullivan AF, Thadhani RI, et. al. Randomised controlled trial of vitamin D supplementation for winter-related atopic dermatitis in Boston: a pilot study. Br J Dermatol 2008;159:245–247.
131 Anderson PC, Dinulos JG. Atopic dermatitis and alternative management strategies. Curr Opin Pediatr 2009;21(1):131–8.
132 Holick MF. High prevalence of vitamin D inadequacy and implications for health. Mayo Clin Proc 2006;81:353–73.
133 Berwick M, Armstrong BK, Ben-Porat L, et. al. Sun exposure and mortality from melanoma. JNCI 2005;97:195–9.
134 Boniol M, Armstrong BK, Dore JF. Variation in incidence and fatality of melanoma by season of diagnosis in New South Wales, Australia. Cancer Epidemiol Biomarkers Prev 2006;15:524–6.
135 Porojnicu AC, Dahlback A, Moan J. Sun exposure and cancer survival in Norway: changes in the risk of death with season of diagnosis and latitude. Adv Exp Med Biol 2008;624:43–54.
136 Rosso S, Sera F, Segnan N, et. al. Sun exposure prior to diagnosis is associated with improved survival in melanoma patients: results from a long-term follow-up study of Italian patients. Eur J Cancer 2008;44:1275–81.
137 Gandini S, Raimondi S, Gnagnarella P, et. al. Vitamin D and skin cancer: A meta-analysis. Eur J Can 2009;45;634–641.
138 Parish LC, Sofman MS, Chalker DK. Topical nicotinamide compared with clindamycin gel in the treatment of inflammatory acne vulgaris. Int J Dermatol 1995;34:434–7.
139 Handfield-Jones S, Jones S, Peachey R. High-dose nicotinamide in the treatment of necrobiosis lipoidica. Br J Dermatol 1988;118:693–6.
140 Zemtsov A, Neldner KH. Successful treatment of dermatitis herpetiformis with tetracycline and nicotinamide in a patient unable to tolerate dapsone. J Am Acad Dermatol 1993;28:505–6.

141 Fivenson DP, Breneman DL, Rosen GB, et. al. Nicotinamide and tetracycline therapy of bullous pemphigoid. Arch Dermatol 1994;130:753–8.
142 Ross JB, Moss MA. Relief of the photosensitivity of erythropoietic protoporphyria by pyridoxine. J Am Acad Dermatol 1990;22:340–2.
143 Juhlin L, Olsson MJ. Improvement of vitiligo after oral treatment with vitamin B12 and folic acid and the importance of sun exposure. Acta Derm Venereol (Stockh) 1997;77:460–2.
144 Prasad AS: Zinc deficiency. BMJ 2003;326:409–10.
145 Michaelsson G, Vahlquist A, Juhlin L. Serum zinc and retinol-binding protein in acne. Br J Dermatol 1977;96:283–86.
146 Amer M, Bahgat MR, Tosson Z, et. al. Serum zinc in acne vulgaris. Int J Dermatol 1982;21:481–84.
147 Hillstrom L, Pettersson L, Hellbe L, et. al: Comparison of oral treatment with zinc sulphate and placebo in acne vulgaris. Br J Dermatol 1977;97:681–84.
148 Michaelsson G, Juhlin L, Vahlquist A. Effects of oral zinc and vitamin A in acne. Arch Dermatol 1977;113:31–6.
149 Goransson K, Liden S, Odsell L. Oral zinc in acne vulgaris: A clinical and methodological study. Acta Derm Venereol 1978;58:443–48.
150 Verma KC, Saini AS, Dhamija SK. Oral zinc sulphate therapy in acne vulgaris: A double-blind trial. Acta Derm Venereol 1980;60:337–40.
151 Liden S, Goransson K, Odsell L. Clinical evaluation in acne. Acta Derm Venereol Suppl (Stockh) 19890;89:47–52.
152 Dreno B, Amblard P, Agache P, et. al. Low doses of zinc gluconate for inflammatory acne. Acta Derm Venereol 1989;69:541–43.
153 Dreno B, Moyse D, Alirezai M, et. al. Multicenter randomised comparative double-blind controlled clinical trial of the safety and efficacy of zinc gluconate versus minocycline hydrochloride in the treatment of inflammatory acne vulgaris. Dermatology 2001;203:135–40.
154 Orris L, Shalita AR, Sibulkin D, et. al. Oral zinc therapy of acne. Absorption and clinical effect. Arch Dermatol 1978;114:1018–20.
155 Weimar VM, Puhl SC, Smith WH, et. al. Zinc sulfate in acne vulgaris. Arch Derm 1978;114:1776–78.
156 Cochran RJ, Tucker SB, Flannigan SA. Topical zinc therapy for acne vulgaris. Int J Dermatol 1985;24:188–90.
157 Schachner L, Eaglstein W, Kittles C, et. al. Topical erythromycin and zinc therapy for acne. J Am Acad Dermatol 1990;22:253–60.
158 Schachner L, Pestana A, Kittles C. A clinical trial comparing the safety and efficacy of a topical erythromycin-zinc formulation with a topical clindamycin formulation. J Am Acad Dermatol 1990;22:489–95.
159 Van Hoogdalem EJ, Terpstra IJ, Baven AL. Evaluation of the effect of zinc acetate on the stratum corneum penetration kinetics of erythromycin in healthy male volunteers. Skin Pharm 1996;9: 104–10.
160 Orris L, Shalita AR, Sibulkin D, et. al. Oral zinc therapy of acne. Absorption and clinical effect. Arch Dermatol 1978;114:1018–20.
161 Guthery E, Seal LA, Anderson EL. Zinc pyrithione in alcohol-based products for skin antisepsis: persistence of antimicrobial effects. Am J Infect Control 2005;33(1):15–22.
162 Pence BC, Delver E, Dunn DM. Effects of dietary selenium of UVB-induced skin carcinogenesis and epidermal antioxidant status. J Invest Dermatol 1994;102:759–61.
163 Clark LC, Graham GF, Crounse RG, et. al. Plasma selenium and skin neoplasms: A case control study. Nutr Cancer 1984;6:13–21.
164 Combs GF Jr, Clark LC, Turnbull BW, et. al. Low plasma selenium predicts the 24-month incidence of squamous cell carcinoma of the skin in a cancer prevention trial. FASEB J 1993;7:A278.
165 Clark LC, Combs GF Jr, Turnbull BW, et. al. Effects of selenium supplementation for cancer prevention in patients with carcinoma of the skin: A randomised controlled trial. Nutritional Prevention of Cancer Study Group. JAMA 1996;276:1957–63.
166 Bath-Hextall F, Leonardi-Bee J, Somchand N, et. al. Interventions for preventing non-melanoma skin cancers in high-risk groups. Cochrane Database Syst Rev 2007 Oct 17;(4):CD005414.
167 Dreno B, Euvrard S, Frances C, et. al. Effect of selenium intake on the prevention of cutaneous epithelial lesions in organ transplant recipients. Eur J Dermatol 2007;17(2):140–5.
168 Berger MM, Binnert C, Chiolero RL, et. al. Trace element supplementation after major burns increases burned skin trace element concentrations and modulates local protein metabolism but not whole-body substrate metabolism. AJCN 2007;85(5):1301–6.
169 Berger MM, Baines M, Raffoul W, et. al. Trace element supplementation after major burns modulates antioxidant status and clinical course by way of increased tissue trace element concentrations. AJCN 2007;85(5):1293–300.
170 Dreno B, Nocera T, Verriere F, et. al. Topical retinaldehyde with glycolic acid: Study of tolerance and acceptability in association with anti-acne treatments in 1,709 patients. Dermatology 2005;210:22–29.
171 Poli F, Ribet V, Lauze C, et. al. Efficacy and safety of 0.1% retinaldehyde/6% glycolic acid (diacneal) for mild to moderate acne vulgaris. A multicentre, double-blind, randomised, vehicle-controlled trial. Dermatology 2005;210:14–21.
172 Tran C, Kasraee B, Grand D, et. al. Pharmacology of RALGA, a mixture of retinaldehyde and glycolic acid. Dermatology 2005;210:6–13.
173 Katsambas AD. RALGA (Diacneal), a retinaldehyde and glycolic acid association and postinflammatory hyperpigmentation in acne—a review. Dermatology 2005;210:39–45.
174 Hunt MJ, Barnetson RS. A comparative study of gluconolactone versus benzoyl peroxide in the treatment of acne. Australas J Dermatol 1992;33(3):131–4.
175 Joshi SS, Boone SL, Alam M, et. al. Effectiveness, safety, and effect on quality of life of topical salicylic acid peels for treatment of postinflammatory hyperpigmentation in dark skin. Dermatol Surg 2009;35(4):638–44.
176 Bissonnette R, Bolduc C, Seite S, et. al. Randomised study comparing the efficacy and tolerance of a lipophillic hydroxyl acid derivative of salicylic acid and 5% benzoyl peroxide in the treatment of facial acne vulgaris. J Cosmet Dermatol 2009;8(1):19–23.
177 Hoppe U, Bergemann J, Diembeck W, et. al. Coenzyme Q10, a cutaneous antioxidant and energiser. Biofactors 1999;9(2-4):371–8.

178 Shapiro SS, Saliou C. Role of vitamins in skin care. Nutrition 2001;17(10):839–44.
179 Kharaeva Z, Gostova E, De Luca C, et. al. Clinical and biochemical effects of coenzyme Q(10), vitamin E, and selenium supplementation to psoriasis patients. Nutrition 2009;25(3):295–302.
180 Blatt T, Lenz H, Koop U, et. al. Stimulation of skin's energy metabolism provides multiple benefits for mature human skin. Biofactors 2005;25(1-4):179–85.
181 Puisina-Ivic N. Skin ageing. Acta Dermatovenerol Alp Panonica Adriat 2008;17(2):47–54.
182 Podda M, Grundmann-Kollmann M. Low molecular weight antioxidants and their role in skin ageing. Clin Exp Dermatol 2001;26(7):578–82.
183 Caramia G, Atzei A, Fanos V. Probiotics and the skin. Clin Dermatol 2008;26(1):4–11.
184 Krutmann J. Pre- and probiotics for human skin. J Dermatol Sci 2009;54(1):1–5.
185 von Hertzen LC, Savolainen J, Hannuksela M, et. al. Scientific rationale for the Finnish Allergy Program 2008-2018: emphasis on prevention and endorsing tolerance. Allergy 2009;64:678–701.
186 Lee J, Seto D, Bielory L. Meta-analysis of clinical trials of probiotics for prevention and treatment of pediatric atopic dermatitis. J Allergy Clin Immunol 2008;121:116.e11–121.e11
187 Nicol NH, Boguniewicz M. Successful strategies in atopic dermatitis management. Dermatol Nurs 2008;(Suppl):3–18.
188 Boyle RJ, Bath-Hextall FJ, Leonardi-Bee J, et. al. Probiotics for treating eczema. Cochrane Database Syst Rev 2008 Oct 8;(4):CD006135.
189 Boyle RJ, Bath-Hextall FJ, Leonardi-Bee J, et. al. Probiotics for the treatment of eczema: a systematic review. Clin Exp Allergy. 2009 Jul 1. (Epub ahead of print).
190 Anandan C, Nurmatov U, Sheikh A. Omega 3 and 6 oils for primary prevention of allergic disease: systematic review and meta-analysis. Allergy 2009;64(6):840–8.
191 Schnappinger M, Sausenthaler S, Linseisen J, et. al. Fish consumption, allergic sensitisation and allergic diseases in adults. Ann Nutr Metab 2009;54(1): 67–74.
192 Olsen SF, Osterdal ML, Salvig JD, et. al. Fish oil intake compared with olive oil intake in late pregnancy and asthma in the offspring: 16 y of registry-based follow-up from a randomised controlled trial. AJCN 2008;88(1):167–75.
193 Sala-Vila A, Miles EA, Calder PC. Fatty acid composition abnormalities in atopic disease: evidence explored and role in the disease process examined. Clin Exp Allergy 2008;38(9):1432–50.
194 Blumer N, Renz H. Consumption of omega3-fatty acids during perinatal life: role in immuno-modulation and allergy prevention. J Perinat Med 2007;35(Suppl 1):S12–8.
195 Jones CLA. Introduction. In: Herbs for Healthy Skin. Mushroom eBooks 2002. ISBN 1843190672.
196 Magin PJ, Adams J, Pond CD, et. al. Topical and oral CAM in acne: A review of the empirical evidence and a consideration of its context. Complem Ther Med 2006;14:62–76.
197 Jain A, Basal E. Inhibition of Propionibacterium acnes-induced mediators of inflammation by Indian herbs. Phytomedicine 2003;10(1):34–8.
198 Bedi MK, Shenefelt PD. Herbal therapy in dermatology. Arch Dermatol 2002;138(2):232–42.
199 Gabler H. (100 years of Hamamelis ointment). Dtsch Apoth 1978;30:202–204.
200 Erdelmeier CA, Cinatl J Jr, Rabenau H, et. al. Antiviral and antiphlogistic activities of Hamamelis virginiana bark. Planta Med 1996;62:241–245.
201 Bassett IB, Pannowitz DL, Barnetson RS. A comparative study of tea-tree oil versus benzoylperoxide in the treatment of acne. MJA 1990;153(8):455–8.
202 Raman A, Weir U, Bloomfield SF. Antimicrobial effects of tea-tree oil and its major components on Staphylococcus aureus, Staph. epidermidis and Propionibacterium acnes. Lett Appl Microbiol 1995;21(4):242–5.
203 Ernst E, Huntley A. Tea tree oil: a systematic review of randomised clinical trials. Forsch Komplementarmed Klass Naturheilkd 2000;7(1):17–20.
204 Martin KW, Ernst E. Herbal medicines for treatment of bacterial infections: a review of controlled clinical trials. J Antimicrob Chemother 2003;51(2):241–6.
205 Enshaieh S, Jooya A, Siadat AH, et. al. The efficacy of 5% topical tea tree oil gel in mild to moderate acne vulgaris: a randomised, double-blind placebo-controlled study. Indian J Dermatol Venereol Leprol 2007;73(1):22–5.
206 Koh KJ, Pearce AL, Marshman G, et. al. Tea tree oil reduces histamine-induced skin inflammation. Br J Dermatol 2002;147(6):1212–7.
207 Bedi MK, Shenefelt PD. Herbal therapy in dermatology. Arch Dermatol 2002;138:232–242.
208 Daniele C, Thompson Coon J, Pittler MH, et. al. Vitex agnus castus: a systematic review of adverse events. Drug Saf 2005;28:319–32.
209 PDR for Herbal Medicines (4th edn). Thompson Healthcare Inc, Montvael NJ, 2007. ISBN 1-56363-678-6.
210 Klein AD, Penneys NS. Aloe vera. J Am Acad Dermatol 1988;118:714–20.
211 Visuthikosol V, Chowchuen B, Sukwanarat Y, et. al. Effect of aloe vera gel to healing of burn wound a clinical and histologic study. J Med Assoc Thai 1995;78(8):403–9.
212 Maenthaisong R, Chaiyakunapruk N, Niruntraporn S, et. al. The efficacy of aloe vera used for burn wound healing: a systematic review. Burns 2007;33(6):713–8.
213 Vitetta L, Sali A. Treatments for damaged skin. AFP 2006;37:501–502.
214 Langemo DK, Hanson D, Anderson J, et. al. Use of honey for wound healing. Adv Skin Wound Care 2009;22(3):113–8.
215 Evans J, Flavin S. Honey: a guide for healthcare professionals. Br J Nurs 2008;17(15):S24, S26, S28–30.
216 Jull AB, Rodgers A, Walker N. Honey as a topical treatment for wounds. Cochrane Database Syst Rev 2008 Oct 8;(4):CD005083.
217 McQuestion M. Evidence-based skin care management in radiation therapy. Semin Oncol Nurs 2006;22(3):163–73.
218 Bolderston A, Lloyd NS, Wong RK, et. al. Supportive Care Guidelines Group of Cancer Care Ontario Program in Evidence-Based Care. The prevention and management of acute skin reactions related to radiation therapy: a systematic review and practice guideline. Support Care Canc 2006;14(8): 802–17.
219 Pommier P, Gomez F, Sunyach MP, et. al. Phase III randomised trial of Calendula officinalis compared with trolamine for the prevention of acute dermatitis during irradiation for breast cancer. J Clin Oncol 2004;22(8):1447–53.

220 Kassab S, Cummings M, Berkovitz S, et. al. Homeopathic medicines for adverse effects of cancer treatments. Cochrane Database Syst Rev 2009 Apr 15;(2):CD004845.

221 Wolbling RH, Leonhardt K. Local therapy of Herpes simplex with dried extract from Melissa officinalis. Phytomedicine 1994;1:25–31.

222 Koytchev R, Alken RG, Dundarov S. Balm mint extract (Lo-701) for topical treatment of recurring herpes labialis. Phytomedicine 1999;6(4):225–30.

223 Fiore C, Eisenhut M, Krausse R, et. al. Antiviral effects of Glycyrrhiza species. Phytother Res 2008;22(2):141–8.

224 Satchell AC, Saurajen A, Bell C, et. al. Treatment of interdigital tinea pedis with 25% and 50% tea tree oil solution: a randomized, placebo-controlled, blinded study. Australas J Dermatol 2002;43:175–8.

225 Tong MM, Altman PM, Barnetson RS. Tea tree oil in the treatment of tinea pedis. Australas J Dermatol 1992;33(3):145–9.

226 Buck DS, Nidorf DM, Addino JG. Comparison of two topical preparations for the treatment of onychomycosis: Melaleuca alternifolia (tea tree) oil and clotrimazole. J Fam Pract 1994;38(6):601–5.

227 Faoagali J, George N, Leditschke JF. Does tea tree oil have a place in the topical treatment of burns? Burns 1997;23(4):349–51.

228 Ledezma E, López JC, Marin P, et. al. Ajoene in the topical short-term treatment of tinea cruris and tinea corporis in humans. Randomised comparative study with terbinafine. Arzneimittelforschung 1999;49(6):544–7.

229 Ledezma E, DeSousa L, Jorquera A, et. al. Efficacy of ajoene, an organosulphur derived from garlic, in the short-term therapy of tinea pedis. Mycoses 1996;39(9-10):393–5.

230 Atherton DJ, Sheehan MP, Rustin MH, et. al. Treatment of atopic eczema with traditional Chinese medicinal plants. Pediatr Dermatol 1992;9(4):373–5.

231 Sheehan MP, Atherton DJ. A controlled trial of traditional Chinese medicinal plants in widespread non-exudative atopic eczema. Br J Dermatol 1992;126(2):179–84.

232 Sheehan MP, Rustin MH, Atherton DJ, et. al. Efficacy of traditional Chinese herbal therapy in adult atopic dermatitis. Lancet 1992;340(8810): 13–7.

233 Zhang H, Qu X. Advances in experimental studies on treatment of psoriasis by traditional Chinese medicine. J Tradit Chin Med 2002;22(1):61–6.

234 Tse TW. Use of common Chinese herbs in the treatment of psoriasis. Clin Exp Dermatol 2003;28(5):469–75.

235 Zhang LX, Bai YP, Song PH, et. al. Effect of Chinese herbal medicine combined with acitretin capsule in treating psoriasis of blood-heat syndrome type. Chin J Integr Med 2009;15(2):141–4.

236 Syed TA, Ahmad SA, Holt AH, et. al. Management of psoriasis with Aloe vera extract in a hydrophilic cream: a placebo-controlled, double-blind study.Trop Med Int Health 1996;1(4):505–9.

237 Vogler BK, Ernst E. Aloe vera: a systematic review of its clinical effectiveness. Br J Gen Pract 1999;49(447):823–8.

238 Paulsen E, Korsholm L, Brandrup F. A double-blind, placebo-controlled study of a commercial Aloe vera gel in the treatment of slight to moderate psoriasis vulgaris. J Eur Acad Dermatol Venereol 2005;19(3):326–31.

239 Bernstein JE, Parish LC, Rapaport M, et. al. Effects of topically applied capsaicin on moderate and severe psoriasis vulgaris. J Am Acad Dermatol 1986;15(3):504–7.

240 Ellis CN, Berberian B, Sulica VI, et. al. A double-blind evaluation of topical capsaicin in pruritic psoriasis. J Am Acad Dermatol 1993;29(3):438–42.

241 Hautkappe M, Roisen MF, Toledano A, et. al. Review of the effectiveness of capsaicin for painful cutaneous disorders and neural dysfunction. Clin J Pain 1998;14(2):97–106.

242 Schempp CM, Windeck T, Hezel S, et. al. Topical treatment of atopic dermatitis with St. John's wort cream--a randomised, placebo controlled, double-blind half-side comparison. Phytomedicine 2003;10(Suppl 4):31–37.

243 Stevensen CJ. Aromatherapy in dermatology. Clin Dermatol 1998;16(6):689–94.

244 Gulliver WP, Donsky HJ. A report on three recent clinical trials using Mahonia aquifolium 10% topical cream and a review of the worldwide clinical experience with Mahonia aquifolium for the treatment of plaque psoriasis. Am J Ther 2005;12(5):398–406.

245 Alebiosu CO, Ogunledun A, Ogunleye DS. A report of clinical trial conducted on Toto ointment and soap products. JNMA 2003;95:95–105.

246 Oyelami OA, Onayemi O, Oladimeji FA, et. al. Clinical evaluation of Acalypha ointment in the treatment of superficial fungal skin diseases. Phytother Res 2003;17(5):555–7.

247 Klovekorn W, Tepe A, Danesch U. A randomised, double-blind, vehicle-controlled, half-side comparison with a herbal ointment containing Mahonia aquifolium, Viola tricolor and Centella asiatica for the treatment of mild-to-moderate atopic dermatitis. Int J Clin Pharm Ther 2007;45(11): 583–91.

248 Orafidiya LO, et. al. Preliminary clinical tests on topical preparations of *Ocimum gratissimum* Linn Leaf essential oil for the treatment of acne vulgaris. Clin Drugs Under Invest 2002;22(5):313–9.

249 Orafidiya LO, et. al. The effect of *aloe vera* gel on the antiacne properties of the essential oil of *Ocimum gratissimum* Linn leaf—a preliminary clinical investigation. Int J Aromather 2004;14:15–21.

250 Balambal R, et. al. *Ocimum basilicum* in acne vulgaris—a controlled comparison with a standard regime. J Assoc Physicians India 1985;33(8):507–8.

251 Woollard AC, Tatham KC, Barker S. The influence of essential oils on the process of wound healing: a review of the current evidence. Wound Care 2007;16(6):255–7.

252 Hajheydari Z, Jamshidi M, Akbari J, et. al. Combination of topical garlic gel and betamethasone valerate cream in the treatment of localised alopecia areata: a double-blind randomised controlled study. Indian J Dermatol Venereol Leprol 2007;73(1): 29–32.

253 Hay IC, Jamieson M, Ormerod AD. Randomised trial of aromatherapy. Successful treatment for alopecia areata. Arch Dermatol 1998;134(11): 1349–52.

254 Butt MS, Sultan MT. Green tea: nature's defense against malignancies. Crit Rev Food Sci Nutr 2009;49(5):463–73.

255 Rees JR, Stukel TA, Perry AE, et. al. Tea consumption and basal cell and squamous cell skin cancer: results of a case-control study. Am Acad Dermatol 2007;56(5):781–5.

256 Hakim IA, Harris RB, Weisgerber UM. Tea intake and squamous cell carcinoma of the skin: influence of type of tea beverages. Cancer Epidemiol Biomarkers Prev 2000;9(7):727–31.
257 McNaughton SA, Marks GC, Green AC. Role of dietary factors in the development of basal cell cancer and squamous cell cancer of the skin. Can Epidemiol Biomarkers Prev 2005;14(7):1596–607.
258 van Dam RM, Huang Z, Giovannucci E, et. al. Diet and basal cell carcinoma of the skin in a prospective cohort of men. AJCN 2000;71(1):135–41.
259 Hsu S. Green tea and the skin. J Am Acad Dermatol 2005;52(6):1049–59.
260 Ramadan A, Elsaidy M, Zyada R. Effect of low-intensity direct current on the healing of chronic wounds: a literature review. J Wound Care 2008;17(7):292–6.
261 Olyaee Manesh A, Flemming K, et. al. Electromagnetic therapy for treating pressure ulcers. Cochrane Database Syst Rev 2006 Apr 19;(2):CD002930.
262 Chen CJ, Yu HS. Acupuncture, electrostimulation, and reflex therapy in dermatology. Dermatol Ther. 2003;16(2):87–92.
263 Iliev E. Acupuncture in Dermatology. Clinics in Dermatology 1998;16:659–688.
264 Nie Y, Wang C. A survey of treatment of acne by acupuncture. J Tradit Chin Med 2008;28(1):71–4.
265 Lihong S. He-Ne laser auricular irradiation plus body acupuncture for treatment of acne vulgaris in 36 cases. J Tradit Chin Med 2006;26(3):193–4.
266 Liu CZ, Lei B, Zheng JF. Randomised control study on the treatment of 26 cases of acne conglobata with encircling acupuncture combined with venesection and cupping. Zhen Ci Yan Jiu 2008;33(6):406–8.
267 Li B, Chai H, Du YH, et. al. Evaluation of therapeutic effect and safety for clinical randomised and controlled trials of treatment of acne with acupuncture and moxibustion. Zhongguo Zhen Jiu 2009;29(3):247–51.
268 Chen CJ, Yu HS. Acupuncture, electrostimulation, and reflex therapy in dermatology. Dermatol Ther 2003;16(2):87–92.
269 Lewith GT, Field J, Machin D. Acupuncture compared with placebo in post-herpetic pain. Pain 1983:17:361-368.
270 Peng WN, Liu ZS, Deng YH, et. al. Evaluation of literature quality of acupuncture for treatment of herpes zoster and approach to the laws of treatment. Zhongguo Zhen Jiu 2008;28(2):147–50.
271 Liao SJ, Liao TA. Acupuncture treatment for psoriasis: a retrospective case report. Acupunct Electrother Res 1992;17:195–208.
272 Jerner B, Skogh M, Vahlquist A. A controlled trial of acupuncture in psoriasis: no convincing effect. Acta Derm Venereol 1997;77:154–156.
273 Qing H, Tian YS, Fan JM, et. al. Meridian three-combined therapy for treatment of ordinary psoriasis: a multi-center randomised controlled study. Zhongguo Zhen Jiu 2009;29(3):181–4.
274 Wang DZ. Indirect moxibustion with herb cake for treatment of atopic dermatitis: dermatitis: 20 cases (in Chinese). China Acupunct 2000;20:612.
275 Adaskevich VP. Clinical efficacy and immunoregulatory and neurohumoral effects of MM therapyinpatientswithatopicdermatitis.CritRevBiomed Eng 2000;28:11–21.
276 Chen CJ, Yu HS. Acupuncture treatment of urticaria. Arch Dermatol 1998;134:1397–1399.
277 Jianli C. The effect of acupuncture on serum IgE level in patients with chronic urticaria. J Tradit Chin Med 2006;26(3):189–90.
278 Zhao Y. Acupuncture plus point-injection for 32 cases of obstinate urticaria. J Tradit Chin Med 2006;26(1):22–3.
279 Wu CS, Hu SC, Lan CC, et. al. Low-energy helium-neon laser therapy induces repigmentation and improves the abnormalities of cutaneous microcirculation in segmental-type vitiligo lesions. Kaohsiung J Med Sci 2008;24(4):180–9.
280 Millikan LE. Unapproved Treatments or Indications in Dermatology: Physical Therapy Including Balneotherapy Clinics in Dermatology 2000;18: 125–129.
281 Millikan LE. Complementary Medicine. Clinics in Dermatology 2002;20:602–605.
282 Benedetto AV, Millikan L. Mineral water and spas in the United States. Clin Derm 1996;14:583–600.
283 Alster TS, Wanitphakdeedecha R. Improvement of postfractional laser erythema with light-emitting diode photomodulation. Dermatol Surg 2009;35(5):813–5.
284 Mathur K, Morris S, Deighan C, et. al. Extracorporeal photopheresis improves nephrogenic fibrosing dermopathy/nephrogenic systemic fibrosis: three case reports and review of literature. J Clin Apher 2008;23(4):144–50.

Chapter 15

Epilepsy

With contribution from Dr Lily Tomas

Introduction

Epilepsy is a chronic neurological disorder that is characterised by recurrent and unprovoked seizures. The lifetime risk of developing epilepsy is 3.2% with more than of 90% of these cases having partial or localisation-related epilepsy. Despite the introduction of newer anti-epileptic drugs (AEDs), nearly 50% of patients with partial epilepsy will not attain a seizure remission with the use of medication.[1, 2, 3] In fact, a recent UK study indicated that although 30 000 people develop epilepsy annually, only 6000 have medically refractory seizures.[1] Adverse effects of antiepileptic drugs are a further major impediment to optimal dosing for seizure control.[4] In the North American continent more than 3 million people have epilepsy.[5]

It is therefore easy to understand why at least 25–50% individuals with epilepsy have trialled some form of complementary and alternative medicine (CAM) therapy. Commonly used therapies include mind–body, dietary modification, nutritional and/or herbal supplementation, massage, homeopathy and acupuncture.[6–9] It is important to note that many patients use CAM therapies without notifying their physician. Thus, it becomes the responsibility of the physician to actively inquire and then monitor therapies to ensure safety and effectiveness of combined CAM and traditional treatment.[6, 10]

In many instances, CAM therapies are not substitutes for traditional medications, however, depending on the effectiveness of the intervention(s), dosage reductions or cessation of medications under professional supervision may be possible.[11]

Lifestyle — general

Weight gain or loss is not an integral part of epilepsy although a sedentary lifestyle can contribute to weight gain. This is an important consideration because pharmacological treatment for epilepsy may be associated with substantial weight changes that may increase morbidity and impair adherence to the treatment regimen.[12]

Sleep

The close relationship between the physiological state of sleep and the pathological process underlying epileptic seizures has been known for centuries, however, it is still not well understood secondary to its complexity.[13] Individuals with epilepsy demonstrate multiple sleep abnormalities including increased sleep latency, fragmented sleep, increased awakenings and stage shifts and an increase in stages 1 and 2 of non-REM sleep.[14]

Indeed, sleep is one of the best documented factors influencing the expression of seizures and interictal discharges. Many seizures are potently activated by sleep or arousal from sleep.[14, 15] In fact, seizures occur during sleep in nearly one-third of patients. It has also been demonstrated that non-REM sleep components generally promote, and REM sleep components generally suppress, seizure discharge propagation.[16, 17] Sleep deprivation can also increase the frequency of epileptiform discharges and seizures.[18, 19, 20] The effective treatment of sleep disorders can improve seizure control. Indeed, AEDs, use of ketogenic dietary principles and vagus nerve stimulation can all improve sleep quality, daytime alertness and neurocognitive function.[18]

Poor sleep can also be an adverse effect of some AEDs. This should be identified and rectified where possible as sleep disturbance exerts greater effect than short-term seizure control on quality of life scores of patients with epilepsy.[4, 21]

Mind–body medicine

The historical relationship between the study of epilepsy and religious experience suggests particular potential associations between CAM therapies (especially spiritual healing and care for those with epilepsy).[22] Traditional healers still use spiritual healing, often in combination with special magical concoctions, in order to exorcise evil spirits in their treatment of epilepsy.[23, 24]

Meditation practices

A recent systematic review of various meditative practices (meditation, meditative prayer, yoga, relaxation) has demonstrated strong evidence for the efficacy of meditation in the treatment of epilepsy.[25] Clinical studies have shown that transcendental meditation (TM), derived from ancient yogic teachings, may be a potential anti-epileptic treatment. However, TM may possibly also be a double-edged sword as many of the EEG recordings during TM (increased alpha, theta, gamma frequencies with increased coherence and synchrony) are similar to seizure activity, with neuronal hypersynchrony being a cardinal feature of epilepsy. More rigorous trials are needed to determine this.[26]

Cognitive behaviour therapy

Overall, the current evidence for cognitive behavioural therapy remains contentious as reported by a recent Cochrane review.[27] The review reports that 2 trials found CBT to be effective in reducing depression, among people with epilepsy with a depressed affect, whilst another did not. Two trials of CBT found improvement in quality of life scores. One trial of group cognitive therapy found no significant effect on seizure frequency while another trial found statistically significant reduction in seizure frequency as well as in seizure index (product of seizure frequency and seizure duration in seconds) among participants treated with CBT.[27]

Relaxation therapy and biofeedback

Two trials of combined relaxation and behaviour therapy and 1 of EEG biofeedback and 4 of educational interventions did not provide sufficient information to assess their effect on seizure frequency.[27] One small study of galvanic skin response biofeedback reported significant reduction in seizure frequency. Combined use of relaxation and behaviour modification was found beneficial for anxiety and adjustment in 1 study. In 1 study EEG biofeedback was found to improve the cognitive and motor functions in individuals with greatest seizure reduction.[27]

Educational interventions

Educational interventions were found to be beneficial in improving the knowledge and understanding of epilepsy, coping with epilepsy, compliance to medication and social competencies.[27]

Sunshine

The long-term treatment with various anticonvulsants may result in hypocalcaemia, osteomalacia and osteopaenia independent from Vitamin D metabolism. Regional variances in the incidences of drug-induced bone disease has been attributed to differences in sunlight exposure, with most reports from areas of little sunshine or from institutionalised patients.[28, 29]

Environment

Toxins

Toxic causes of seizures are numerous and include alcohol and other substances of abuse, drugs, and industrial and household products. Epileptic seizures have been induced by occupational nickel and other heavy metal exposure.[30] There is also a reduction in the threshold for seizures in animals whose blood contents of lead are similar to those of humans from some urban areas with high levels of air pollution.[31]

Diurnal and seasonal variations

Research on hospital admissions with status epilepticus reveals an important association with several environmental protective and precipitating factors. There is a significant diurnal pattern, with most admissions between 4–5 p.m. and least admissions in early morning hours. Admissions also vary significantly across the lunar cycle, peaking at day 3 after the new moon and being minimal 3 days before new moon. Admissions are greatest on bright, sunny days whereas dark days, high humidity and high temperature appear to be significantly protective factors.[32]

Physical activity

Exercise

Many people with epilepsy, especially those with uncontrolled seizures, live a sedentary life and have poor physical fitness.[33] Despite a shift in medical recommendations towards encouraging rather than restricting exercise, epileptics often fear they may suffer with exercise-induced seizures.[34] Although there are rare cases of exercise induced seizures, clinical and experimental data has shown that physical activity can decrease seizure frequency, as well as lead to improved cardiovascular and psychological health in patients with epilepsy.[35, 36, 37] Indeed, regular physical exercise may have a moderate seizure-preventative effect in 30–40% of this population.[33]

Animal studies are currently investigating whether physical activity is beneficial for preventing or treating chronic temporal lobe epilepsy.[38]

The majority of sports, including contact sports, are safe to participate in. Water sports and swimming are also considered to be safe if seizures are well controlled and supervision is present. Sports such as hang-gliding and scuba diving are not recommended given the risk of severe injury or death if a seizure was to occur.[36]

However, as this patient group is highly heterogeneous, counselling regarding exercise should be individualised and take into account both seizure type and frequency.[33]

Yoga

Recent studies have shown that yoga can significantly reduce seizure index and increase quality of life in people with epilepsy.[39] Yoga also significantly improves parasympathetic parameters, indicating that yoga may have a role as an adjuvant therapy in the treatment of autonomic dysfunction in patients with refractory epilepsy.[40]

Nutritional influences

Diets

Potentially beneficial dietary interventions should always include the identification and treatment of blood glucose dysregulation, the identification and elimination of allergenic foods and the avoidance of suspected triggers such as alcohol, artificial sweeteners, diet soft-drinks, energy drinks and MSG.[11, 41, 42]

Growth retardation is common amongst children with epilepsy and this appears to be primarily due to poor dietary intake. Approximately 30% of children with intractable epilepsy have been noted to have intakes below the recommended daily allowance (RDA) for Vitamins D, E and K, folate, calcium, linoleic acid and alpha-linolenic acid. It is the physician's responsibility to be aware of this pattern of low nutrient intake and to educate families to provide an adequate diet or consider vitamin and mineral supplementation.[43]

Dietary treatments for epilepsy (ketogenic, modified Atkins, low glycaemic index diets) have been in continuous use since 1921. These dietary interventions have been well studied, with approximately 50% children having a 50% reduction in seizures after 6 months. Approximately one-third will attain >90% reduction in their seizures. It is important to note that the diet maintains its efficacy when provided continuously for several years. Furthermore, long-term benefits may be seen even when the diet is ceased after only a few months, indicating neuroprotective effects.[44]

Ketogenic diet (KD)

The KD is a high-fat, low-carbohydrate, high-protein diet used to treat medically refractory epilepsy.[45] A recent RCT in children with refractory epilepsies showed that the KD was superior to continuation of medical treatment in reducing seizure frequency in this population. The KD has also been used successfully in a variety of epilepsy syndromes, such as Lennox-Gastaut syndrome.[46] Despite nearly a century of use, however, the mechanisms underlying its clinical efficacy remain unknown.[47] As the KD is effective in syndromes of various aetiologies, this suggests there are multiple mechanisms of action.[45,46–53] It is beyond the scope of this chapter to discuss these in detail, however, 4 such hypotheses include the pH, metabolic, amino acid and the ketone hypotheses.[54] The KD is principally high in fat, has adequate protein and is low in carbohydrates (no more than 4:1 ratio weight of fat: combined protein/ carbohydrate).

Chronic ketosis is thought to modify the TCA cycle to increase GABA synthesis in the brain, limit ROS generation and boost energy production in brain tissue.[47, 55] Acetone is the principal ketone body elevated in the KD with demonstrated robust anticonvulsant properties. Recent research has shown that acetone enhances the anticonvulsant effects of valproate, carbamazepine, lamotrigine and phenobarbital without affecting their pharmokinetic or side-effect profiles.[56] Indeed, therapeutic indices in animal models are comparable to or better than those of valproate, a standard broad-spectrum anticonvulsant.[57]

At least 15–20% patients using the KD experience a >50% reduction in seizure frequency. For this reason, the KD should be considered as an early treatment for drug-resistant epilepsy, not only as a 'last resort'.[58, 59, 60] Unfortunately, 10–40% discontinue this strict diet secondary to a lack of response or adverse side-effects. Available data indicates that genetic factors are likely to affect the efficacy of this diet.[61]

A recent blinded cross-over trial involved children with Lennox-Gastaut syndrome placed on the KD with an addition of 60g glucose daily to negate the ketosis. This additional glucose did not significantly alter the frequency of EEG-assessed seizures, however, it did decrease the frequency of parent-reported 'drop' seizures during the follow-up period of 12 months. Fasting had significant effects on both seizures and EEG-assessed events.[62]

The efficacy of the KD develops over 1–3 weeks, suggesting that adaptive changes in gene expression are involved in its anticonvulsant effects.[63] It has proven to be a valuable therapeutic option for children with drug-resistant focal epilepsy, particularly those with a recent deterioration of seizure control. Because of its rapid effects, the KD may also be a useful support to IV emergency drugs in such a situation.[64]

Modified Atkins diet

The modified Atkins diet is a less restrictive ketogenic diet which does not involve fasting and has no restrictions on calories, fluids or protein. The consumption of 10g/day of carbohydrates in children and 15g/day carbohydrates in adults is allowed whilst high fat foods are encouraged. Approximately 45% patients have 50–90% seizure reduction with 28% having >90% seizure reduction, results that are very similar to those produced by the KD.[65] The KD appears to exert its seizure-reducing effects quicker than the modified Atkins diet, however, by 6 months the difference is no longer considered significant.[59]

Low glycaemic index diet (LGIT)

Children on the KD may exhibit poor weight gain and have lower blood glucose levels compared with children on standard balanced diets. One recent study reported on the efficacy, safety and tolerability of the LGIT in paediatric intractable epilepsy. Greater than 50% reduction from baseline seizure frequency was seen respectively in 42%, 50%, 54%, 64% and 66% of children at 1, 3, 6, 9 and 12 months. No significant changes were seen in BMI. Of the participants, 24% discontinued the LGIT secondary to its restrictiveness.[66]

Nutritional supplementation

Vitamins and minerals

Antioxidants

Neuronal hyperexcitability and excessive production of free radicals have been strongly implicated in the pathogenesis of idiopathic epilepsy. As such, there is a possible role of antioxidants as an adjunct to AEDs for better seizure control.[67, 68, 69]

The pro-oxidant/antioxidant balance is modulated by both seizure activity and by AEDs.[67] Gingival hyperplasia is a side-effect of some of these drugs and appears secondary to increased oxidative stress. Studies reveal reduced levels of superoxide dismutase, glutathione peroxidase, glutathione reductase, ascorbic acid and alpha-tocopherol with elevated lipid peroxides in these patients.[70] Oxidative stress after long-term treatment with valproate has only been found to occur in overweight children. This is important as it may contribute to endothelial dysfunction and atherosclerosis that is of increased incidence in the adult life of many people with epilepsy.[71] Antioxidant markers are again increased when valproate is ceased.[72, 73]

Plasma and RBC levels of the antioxidants Vitamins A, C and E, superoxide dismutase, glutathione reductase and selenium are markedly lower in epileptic patients compared with controls. These levels improve with supplementation.[74, 75]

Anti-epileptic medications may also deplete total body selenium stores and failure to give appropriate Se supplementation, especially to pregnant women taking valproate, may increase the risk of neural tube defects or other free radical mediated damage.[76]

Alpha-tocopherol is the antioxidant most studied with respect to reducing frequency of epileptic activity in both animal models and humans. Results have thus far been mixed and more studies are required before definitive recommendations can be made.[77–86]

Selenium deficiency has also been implicated in the pathogenesis of epilepsy.[87] Recent studies have shown that topiramate and Vitamin E have protective effects on pentylenetetrazol-induced (PTZ-induced) nephrotoxicity by inhibition of free radicals and support of the antioxidant redox system.[88] Similarly, topiramate and selenium exert protective effects on PTZ-induced brain injury and blood toxicity by inhibiting free radical production, regulating calcium-dependent processes and supporting the antioxidant redox system.[89, 87]

Better regulation of the lipid peroxidation and antioxidants and fewer disturbances in mineral metabolism have been observed with patients on monotherapy vs polytherapy and with carbemazepine vs valproate therapy.[90]

Zinc

Zinc is a fundamental trace element present in high levels in many structures of the limbic circuitry. Altered zinc homeostasis appears to be associated with epilepsy, however, the definitive role of zinc as a neuromodulator in synapses is still uncertain.[91–96] Intracellular zinc homeostasis is sensitive to pathophysiological environmental changes such as acidosis, inflammation and oxidative stress.[97] Zinc itself can also induce oxidative stress by promoting mitochondrial and extra-mitochondrial production of reactive oxygen species.[98] Studies have revealed that zinc chelation decreases the duration of behavioural seizures and electrical after-discharges and the duration of EEG spikes frequency.[99]

Animal studies reveal that zinc deficiency is associated with an increase in epileptic seizures and hippocampal cell death. This appears to happen through abnormal calcium metabolism.[100, 101, 102]

Other vitamins and minerals

Most AEDs reduce folic acid levels, thereby raising homocysteine (Hcy) levels. Hcy, however, is a convulsing agent resulting in heightened seizure recurrence and intractability to AEDs. Furthermore, AEDs can disturb lipid metabolism with subsequent hypercholesterolaemia and dyslipidaemia, with additional altered uric acid metabolism. As such, routine supplementation with folic acid, Vitamin B12, B6, C, E and beta-carotene for all those on AEDs becomes increasingly important.[103]

A recent Cochrane review has found that thiamine improves neuropsychological and cognitive functions in patients with epilepsy. In the same review, Vitamin D was found to improve bone mineral density in those taking AEDs. However, more trials are obviously needed.[11, 77]

A recent systematic review has demonstrated that manganese deficiency can also be accompanied by seizures in both animals and humans. As yet, it is unclear as to whether this is a cause or effect of the convulsions, justifying the need for more intensive research.[104]

Individuals with seizures may also have lower levels of vitamin A, B1, B12, C, folate, magnesium, selenium, zinc, carnitine, carnosine, choline and possibly serine. Furthermore, disorders of metabolism involving vitamin B6, D, calcium and tryptophan may play important roles.[105] Seizure type and number of stimuli seem to be the determinant factors for changes in zinc, copper and magnesium levels.[106, 107, 108] There has also been found a statistically significant increase in serum copper levels in patients with epilepsy compared with controls.[109]

Other supplements

Polyunsaturated fatty acids (PUFAs)

A higher dietary intake of PUFAs may be partially responsible for the potent anticonvulsant effects of the KD as concentrations of both ketone bodies and PUFAs have been found to be increased in the CSF and plasma of patients.[2, 110] Animal studies have shown that increased intake of PUFAs may reduce the risk of epileptic seizures through various biochemical mechanisms, including PUFA-induced openings of voltage-gated potassium channels.[2, 110] Omega-3 supplementation has also been shown to prevent status epilepticus-associated neuropathological changes in the hippocampus in animals.[111]

Some AEDs, such as carbemazepine, are known to decrease levels of long-chain omega-3 PUFAs, particularly DHA, and thereby increase the risk of cardiovascular events (arrhythmias, sudden unexplained death in epilepsy) in this population. Following 3 months of omega-3 supplementation (1g EPA/0.7g DHA daily), plasma and RBC levels increased significantly and patients taking carbemazepine (or not) exhibited a more favourable cardiovascular profile.[112, 113, 114] Furthermore, omega-3 supplementation may be associated with reduced membrane phospholipid breakdown in the brain with an improvement in brain energy metabolism.[115]

Recent animal studies with Evening Primrose Oil (EPO) have conflicted previous thoughts that EPO could potentiate seizures. Rather, prolonged supplementation of linoleic acid and gamma-linolenic acid appears to exert anticonvulsant activity through various biochemical pathways.[116] Nevertheless, more research is warranted to ensure the safety of EPO in epileptic patients.

Although PUFAs reduce seizures in several animal models, available data regarding the effects of supplementation with PUFAs (1–3g EPA/DHA daily) in epileptic patients reveal mixed results with respect to seizure frequency.[114, 117, 118, 119, 120] Therefore, more research is required before PUFAs can be presented as a treatment option for epilepsy.[2]

Amino acids

Because of the high proportion of patients with drug-resistant epilepsy, new hypotheses about the mechanisms of pharmacoresistance are actively being researched. In particular, the role of brain serotonin in epilepsy has been turned upside down in recent years with current thoughts being that serotonin has an anti-epileptic effect. Serotonin receptors are expressed in almost all networks involved in epilepsies. Some SSRIs, such as Fluoxetine, have indeed improved seizure control and some AEDs have recently been found to increase endogenous serotonin levels.[121, 122, 123]

Tryptophan

Tryptophan, an essential amino acid, is the only brain precursor of serotonin. It has been estimated that patients with epilepsy have approximately 30% lower brain intake of tryptophan compared with controls. Increasing plasma tryptophan results in increased brain synthesis of serotonin. However, there is competition between tryptophan and other large neutral amino acids (LNAAs) for entry across the blood brain barrier. Whey proteins that are high in tryptophan but lower in other LNAAs are currently being tested as a combination with anti-epileptic medications.[121]

Taurine

Taurine is one of the most abundant free amino acids which is found mainly in excitable tissues. Taurine is required for the synthesis of GABA, one of the major inhibitory neurotransmitters in the limbic system.[124] For this reason, drugs that target GABA receptors are the mainstay of treatment of seizures with the recent transplantation of GABA-producing cells effectively reducing seizures in several well-established models.[125, 126] Humans are mostly dependent on dietary sources of taurine and previous studies have shown that supplementation can protect against oxidative stress, neurodegenerative diseases and atherosclerosis.[127, 128]

There have been multiple animal studies demonstrating that taurine-fed animals have increased expression of glutamic acid decarboxylase, the enzyme responsible for GABA synthesis, with increased levels of GABA. They also have a higher threshold for seizure onset compared to controls.[124] Furthermore, increased taurine levels in the hippocampus improve membrane stabilisation, significantly reducing neuronal cell death and favouring recovery after neuronal hyperactivity.[129, 130, 131] Acute injections of taurine also result in a reduction or total absence of tonic/clonic seizures with reduced duration and mortality rate in animal models.[130]

Carnosine

Carnosine is a naturally occurring compound that is made from beta-alanine and l-histidine. It has many features of a neurotransmitter and can act as both a neuromodulator and neuroprotective agent. It may indirectly influence neuronal excitability by modulating the effects of zinc and copper.[132, 133, 134] Recent findings indicate that carnosine has a significant anticonvulsant effect on penicillin-induced epilepsy in animals. Thus it may be a potential anticonvulsant treatment for clinical therapy of epilepsy in the future.[135]

Indeed, the concentrations of many amino acids, including alanine, arginine, glutamate, aspartate, carnitine as well as taurine, impact upon seizure activity in animal models. Although not yet well understood, there appears to be a specific role of these amino acids in the shaping of a new equilibrium between excitatory and inhibitory processes in the hippocampus.[11, 136]

Homeopathy

A case series of the clinical management of idiopathic epilepsy in dogs has demonstrated that the homeopathic Belladonna 200C is very effective in preventing or reducing seizure frequency.[137, 138] There are no studies in the literature of the use of homeopathy in patients with epilepsy.

Herbal medicines

Herbal medicine has been used for centuries in many cultures around the world for the treatment of epilepsy. Today, many people try herbal therapies for better control of seizures or to counteract adverse effects from AEDs. Indeed, herbs are considered by many to be safe and effective and use them without the knowledge of their physician.[139] However, many herbs can increase the risk for seizures through intrinsic anticonvulsant properties, contamination by heavy metals or by affecting cytochrome P450 enzymes and P-glycoproteins, altering AED disposition. Health care professionals should therefore always inquire as to the use of herbal preparations in order to prevent complications with the combined regime.[140]

Well-designed clinical trials of herbal therapies for epilepsy are scarce. However, based on animal studies and numerous anecdotal observations of clinical benefits in humans, further research is certainly warranted.[139, 140]

Some traditional medicinal herbs have been found to exert anticonvulsant effects by exhibiting significant affinity for the GABA (A) receptor benzodiazepine binding site. These include flavonoid derivatives from *Scutellaria baicalensis Georgi*, *Artemesia herba-alba*, *Melissa officinalis* and *Salvia triloba*.[141, 142] *Gingko biloba* possesses the capacity to both induce and inhibit seizures.[143]

Some Chinese herbs, including *Chaihu-longu-muli-tang*, have both anti-epileptic and antioxidant potential. It is thought that the reduction in seizure frequency may be related to the antioxidant effects of the herbs.[144] *Shitei-To* is another TCM formulation that may have therapeutic effects in the prevention of secondarily generalised seizures. It is made from 3 medicinal herbs: *Shitei* (calyx of *Diospyros kaki L.f*), *Shokyu* (rhizome of *Zingiber officinale Roscoe*) and *Choji* (flowerbud of *Sysygium aromaticum*).[145]

Curcumin has also been recently shown to significantly prevent generalisation of electro-clinical seizure activity as well as the pathogenesis of iron-induced epileptogenesis.[146, 147]

Physical therapies

Acupuncture

A recent Cochrane review has investigated the use of acupuncture in epilepsy. Compared to phenytoin, patients who received needle acupuncture appeared more likely to achieve 75% or greater reduction in seizure frequency. Compared to valproate, catgut implantation at acu-points appeared more likely to result in 75% or greater reduction in seizure frequency. However, the studies were of poor methodological quality and it was concluded that current evidence does not support acupuncture as a treatment for epilepsy.[148] Results are generally mixed and as such, more rigorous trials are warranted to establish the role of acupuncture in epilepsy.[149–152]

There have been multiple animal studies demonstrating the anticonvulsant effects of electro-acupuncture.[153, 154] It has been shown that stimulation of acupuncture points on the extremities results in stimulation of the vagus nerve and this may partially explain its neuroprotective effects.[155]

As stated previously, taurine may play an inhibitory role against epilepsy by its action as an inhibitory amino acid in the central nervous system. Recent animal studies have shown that electro-acupuncture may partially inhibit epilepsy by up-regulating the concentration of taurine transporter to increase the release of taurine.[156, 157, 158] Exogenous taurine further enhances the anti-convulsive effect of electro-acupuncture.[159]

Electro-acupuncture may also exert its anti-seizure effects by elevating melatonin levels in the pineal gland and hippocampus and reducing nitric oxide synthases.[11, 160, 161,]

Chiropractic

A systematic review from 1970–2000 has concluded that chiropractic care may represent a valid non-pharmaceutical health care approach for paediatric epileptic patients. Case reports and anecdotal evidence suggest that correction of potential upper cervical vertebral subluxation complexes might be most beneficial. Further investigation into upper cervical trauma as a contributing factor to epilepsy should be pursued.[162, 163, 164]

Reiki

There has been only 1 published study of inferior quality on epilepsy and reiki.[165] In a randomly selected sample population with refractory epilepsy from a single neurology department, data were collected on 15 patients before treatment and 3 months after treatment. The participants were aged 20–30 years and had no comorbidities. Seizure frequency at the end of treatment was reduced and there was also a significant increase in serum magnesium.

Conclusion

Epilepsy is the most common neurological disorder in the world, with important and serious physical, psychological, social and economic costs. Epilepsy is widespread across the globe, with the World Health Organization estimating that approximately 85% of the people afflicted with this disorder live in developing countries.[166]

Epilepsy is a difficult illness to control — up to 35% of patients do not respond fully to traditional medical treatments.[167] This is a primary reason as to why many sufferers choose to rely on or incorporate CAM into their treatment regimens. Epileptics can employ diverse modalities to prevent and treat seizures, such as: mind–body medicines, such as relaxation therapy, hypnosis and CBT; biologic-based medicine, such as herbal remedies, dietary supplements, and manipulative-based medicine such as chiropractic, acupuncture, massage, cranio-sacral therapies, homeopathy, ketogenic diets and aromatherapy.[168] CAM therapies should be embraced as having a potentially important role in the integrated holistic management of patients with epilepsy.

Table 15.1 summarises the level of evidence for some CAM therapies for epilepsy.

Table 15.1 Levels of evidence for lifestyle and complementary medicines/therapies in the management of epilepsy

Modality	Level I	Level II	Level IIIa	Level IIIb	Level IIIc	Level IV	Level V
Lifestyle – general							
Weight gain				x			
Sleep					x		
Mind–body medicine							
Cognitive behavioral therapy	x						
Meditation	x						
Meditative prayer	x						
Relaxation	x						
Biofeedback	x						
Behaviour modification through education	x						
Environmental							
Nickel and heavy metal exposures					x		
Sunshine and vitamin D						x	
Physical activity							
Yoga	x						
Nutrition							
Diets					x		
Ketogenic diet				x			
Modified Atkins diet						x	
Low glycemic index diet						x	
Nutritional supplements							
Vitamin E		x					
Antioxidants (C, E, carotenoids, selenium)					x		
Zinc					x		
Multivitamin/minerals						x	
Other supplements							
PUFAs/omega-3FA		x					
Evening primrose oil					x		
Amino acids							
Tryptophan						x	
Taurine						x	
Carnosine							x
Homeopathy							x
Herbal medicines							
Scutellaria baicalensis Georgi					x		
Artemesia herba-alba					x		
Melissa officinalis					x		
Salvia triloba					x		
Gingko biloba					x		

Continued

Table 15.1 Levels of evidence for lifestyle and complementary medicines/therapies in the management of epilepsy—cont'd

Modality	Level I	Level II	Level IIIa	Level IIIb	Level IIIc	Level IV	Level V
Traditional Chinese medicines							
Chaihu-longu-muli-tang					x		
Shitei-To					x		
Physical therapies							
Acupuncture	x(+/–)						
Chiropractic	x						
Reiki					x		

Level I — from a systematic review of all relevant randomised controlled trials, meta–analyses.
Level II — from at least 1 properly designed randomised controlled clinical trial.
Level IIIa — from well-designed pseudo-randomised controlled trials (alternate allocation or some other method).
Level IIIb — from comparative studies (including systematic reviews of such studies) with concurrent controls and allocation not randomised, cohort studies, case-control studies, or interrupted time series with a parallel control group.
Level IIIc — from comparative studies with historical control, 2 or more single-arm studies or interrupted time series without a parallel control group.
Level IV — opinions of respected authorities based on clinical experience, descriptive studies or reports of expert committees.
Level V — represents minimal evidence that represents testimonials.

Clinical tips handout for patients — epilepsy

1 Lifestyle advice

Sleep

- Individuals with epilepsy demonstrate multiple sleep abnormalities with both sleep and sleep deprivation being triggers for seizures. Eliminating and treating underlying sleep disorders can improve seizure control. (See Chapter 22 for more advice)
- Ketogenic diet principles can improve sleep quality.
- It is important to identify and rectify where possible if medications are contributing to sleep disturbances.
- Magnesium (up to 350mg elemental twice daily) can be used to assist sleep and reduce restless legs at night (3 month trial).
- L-Tryptophan (200mg bd) may be trialled for 1 month in the morning and 1 hour before bedtime (not with antidepressant medications).
- Melatonin (3–6mg at bedtime) may be trialled for 1 month (not with L-tryptophan, antidepressant medications).
- Herbal supplements, including chamomile, passionflower and valerian, may be helpful in some cases.
- Herbal teas such as chamomile can be helpful in some cases.

Sunshine

- Long-term treatment with various anticonvulsants can result in poor bone health. This is greater in areas with reduced sunlight or for institutionalised patients. Therefore, increase outdoor activities whenever possible.
- At least 15 minutes sunshine is needed daily for Vitamin D production. More sun exposure is required in winter and for dark-skinned people.
- Sunscreen can block the conversion to Vitamin D so this should be avoided during this specified time period.

2 Physical activity/exercise

- Many patients with epilepsy do not exercise for fear of inducing seizures. Although there are rare cases of this, physical activity can decrease the frequency of seizures.
- Contact sports do not increase the risk of seizures.
- Water sports and swimming are safe if supervised and if seizures are well-controlled.
- The only exercises that are not recommended include activities such as hang-gliding and scuba-diving, given the risk of severe injury or death if a seizure was to occur.
- Counselling regarding exercise should always be individualised and take into account both seizure type and frequency.
- Yoga can significantly reduce seizure frequency and improve quality of life.

3 Mind-body medicine

- CBT and psychotherapy can be of help.
- Meditation, meditative prayer and relaxation training can all be very effective in the treatment of epilepsy.
- More trials are needed before transcendental meditation can be recommended as it may be potentially seizure-provoking.

4 Environment

- Any known environmental triggers for seizures should be avoided. These include substances of abuse, drugs, industrial chemicals and some household products.
- Exposure to heavy metals such as lead and nickel can provoke seizures. Testing for heavy metals is therefore important in suspicious cases. This can be done by blood, hair mineral analysis or comprehensive urinary element profiling.
- People suffering with epilepsy should be aware that episodes of status epilepticus are generally more frequent on bright, sunny days and tend to peak at day 3 after the new moon.

5 Dietary modification

- Possible blood glucose dysregulations need to be identified and treated as they may provoke seizures. Eating small meals more often with regular snacks (on foods such as seeds, nuts and protein sources) is the easiest way to avoid hypoglycaemia (low blood sugar).
- Magnesium (up to 350mg elemental Mg twice daily) in adults can also help to regulate blood sugar.
- Identify and eliminate any allergenic foods in the diet.

- Avoid suspect seizure triggers such as alcohol, artificial sweeteners, diet soft drinks, energy drinks and MSG.
- 30% of children with intractable epilepsy are deficient in nutrients, hence detailed dietary histories and referral to nutritionists/dietitians are important.
- The ketogenic diet (high fat, high protein, low carbohydrate) is the diet most studied in epilepsy. At least 20–50% patients experience a >50% reduction in seizure frequency. For this reason, dietary modifications should be one of the first line therapies for people with epilepsy. The Ketogenic diet is very restrictive, however, therefore long-term counselling with nutritionists and dietitians is recommended.
- The modified Atkins diet is a less restrictive ketogenic diet which allows 10g/day carbohydrates in children and 15g/day carbohydrates in adults. It has shown similar results in reducing seizure frequency as the ketogenic diet, however, its effects are slower.

6 Physical therapies

- Although controversial, acupuncture and electro-acupuncture are generally safe and well-tolerated. Consider a trial period.
- An assessment by a chiropractor or cranial osteopath appears worthwhile to exclude potential upper cervical vertebral subluxation complexes as a contributing factor to seizures.

7 Supplementation

Polyunsaturated fatty acids-EPA/DHA

- Indication: to reduce seizures and neuronal damage and to improve cardiovascular health.
- Dosage: 1–3g EPA/DHA.
- Results: 3 month trial.
- Side-effects: fishy burps, diarrhoea, gastrointestinal discomfort.
- Contraindications: caution with anticoagulants at very high doses; >10g/day can cause bleeding tendencies, stop 1–2 weeks before surgery.

L-Tryptophan

- Indication: to increase serotonin levels and possibly reduce seizures.
- Dosage: up to 200mg twice daily in adult.
- Results: 1–3 months trial.
- Side-effects: may aggravate aggressive behaviour.
- Contraindications: not to be used with antidepressant drugs, MAOIs, adrenal insufficiency, scleroderma.

Taurine

- Indication: to increase GABA and possibly reduce seizures.
- Dosage: 500mg bd.
- Results: 3 month trial.
- Side-effects: may aggravate individuals with gastrointestinal upset, ulcers.
- Contraindications: caution to be taken with anti-epileptic drugs.

Folate

- Indication: to counteract reduced folate levels by some anti-epileptic drugs (phenytoin). To reduce homocysteine and improve cardiovascular health. To lower seizure frequency and intractability to medications.
- Dosage: depending on red cell levels, 500mg–5g/day.
- Results: supplementation needs to be ongoing whilst anti-epileptic medications are used.
- Side-effects: urticaria with allergy, nausea, flatulence, bitter taste in mouth, irritability, excitability.
- Contraindications: close supervision required as folate may reduce efficacy of some anti-epileptic medications.

Thiamine

- Indication: to improve neuropsychological and cognitive functions in epilepsy.
- Dosage: 50mg/day.
- Results: 3 month trial.
- Side-effects: mild and rare.
- Contraindications: caution with cancer patients.

Vitamin D3 (cholecalaferol)

- Indication: to improve bone health in patients taking anti-epileptic medications.
- Dosage: depending upon blood 25(OH) D3 levels, may need 1000–6000IU vitamin D3/day.
- Results: 3 month trial.
- Side-effects: mild and rare when used appropriately.
- Contraindications: hypersensitivity to vitamin D, SLE, hypercalcaemia. Caution in sarcoidosis and hyperparathyroidism. Possible interaction with calcium channel blockers and digitalis.

Selenium

- Indication: to reduce the risk of neural tube defects in pregnant women taking valproate.
- Dosage: up to 150mcg/day.
- Results: to continue throughout pregnancy and lactation.
- Side-effects: nausea, vomiting, irritability, fatigue, nail changes at doses > 1mg/day.
- Contraindications: sensitivity to selenium or yeast if selenium is yeast-derived.

References

1 Cascino GD. When drugs and surgery don't work. Epilepsia 2008;49(Suppl 9):79–84.
2 Farman AH, Lossius MI, Nakken KO. PUFAs and Epilepsy. Tidsskr Nor Laegeforen 2009;129(1):26–8.
3 Vicente-Hernandez M, Garcia-garcia P, Gil-Nagel A, et. al. Therapeutic approach to epilepsy from the nutritional view: current status of dietary treatment. Neurologia 2007;2298:517–25.
4 Perucca P, Carter J, Vahle V, et. al. Adverse antiepileptic drug effects: towards a clinically and neurobiologically relevant taxonomy. Neurology 2009;72(14):1223–9.
5 Theodore WH, Spencer SS, Wiebe S, et. al. Epilepsy in North America: a report prepared under the auspices of the global campaign against epilepsy, the International Bureau for Epilepsy, the International League Against Epilepsy, and the World Health Organization. Epilepsia 2006;47(10):1700–22.
6 Schachter SC. CAM Therapies. Curr Opin Neurol 2008;21(2):184–9.
7 Ricotti V, Delanty N. Use of CAM in epilepsy. Curr Neurol Neurosci Rep 2006;6(4):347–53.
8 Gross-Tsur V, Lahad A, Shalev RS. Use of complementary medicine in children with ADHD and epilepsy. Paediatr Neurol 2003;29(1):53–5.
9 Peebles CT, McAuley JW, Roach J. Alternative medicine use by patients with epilepsy. Epilepsy Behav 2000;1(1):74–77.
10 Tandon M, Prabhaker S, Pandhi P. Pattern of use of CAM in epileptic patients in a tertiary care hospital in India. Pharmacoepidemiol Dug Saf 2002;11(6):457–63.
11 Gaby AR. Natural approaches to epilepsy. Altern Med Rev 2007;12(1):9–24.
12 Ben-Menachem E. Weight issues for people with epilepsy–a review. Epilepsia. 2007;48(Suppl 9):42–5.
13 Rocamora R, Sanchez-Alvarez JC, Salas-Puig J. The relationship between sleep and epilepsy. Neurologist 2008;14(6 Suppl 1):S35–S43.
14 Mendez M, Radtke RA. Interactions between sleep and epilepsy. J Clin Neurophysiol 2001;18(2):106–27.
15 Dinner DS. Effect of sleep on epilepsy. J Clin Neurophysiol 2002;19(6):504–13.
16 Shouse MN, Farber PR, Staba RJ. Physiological basis: how NREM sleep components can promote and REM sleep components can suppress seizure discharge propagation. Clin Neurophysiol 2000;111(Suppl 2):S9–S18.
17 Shouse MN, Scordato JC, Farber PR. Sleep and arousal mechanisms in experimental epilepsy: epileptic components of NREM and antiepileptic components of REM sleep. Ment retard Dev Disabil Res Rev 2004;10(2):117–21.
18 Kotagal P, Yardi N. The relationship between sleep and epilepsy. Semin Pediatr Neurol 2008;15(2): 42–9.
19 DeRoos ST, Chillag KL, Keeler M, et. al. Effects of sleep deprivation on the paediatric EEG. Pediatrics 2009;123(2):703–8.
20 Sebit MB, Mielke J. Epilepsy in sub-Saharan Africa: its socio-demography, aetilogy, diagnosis and EEG characteristics in Harare, Zimbabwe. East afr Med J 2005;82(3):128–37.
21 Kwan P, Yu E, Leung H, et. al. Association of subjective anxiety, depression and sleep disturbance with QOL ratings in adults with epilepsy. Epilepsia 2008 Dec 15. Epub ahead of print.
22 Cohen MH. Regulation, religious experience and epilepsy: a lens on comp therapies. Epilepsy Behav 2003;4(6):602–6.
23 Gross RA. A brief history of epilepsy and its therapy in the Western Hemisphere. Epilepsy Res 1992;12(2):65–74.
24 Millogo A, Ratsimbazafy V, Nubukpo P, et. al. Epilepsy and traditional medicine in Bobo-Dioulasso. Acta Neurol Scand 2004;109(4):250–4.
25 Arias AJ, Steinberg K, Banga A, et. al. illness, Systematic review of the efficacy of meditation techniques as treatments for mental. J Altern Complement Med 2006;12(8):817–32.
26 Lansky EP, St Louis EK. TM: a doubl-edged wsord in epilepsy? Epilepsy Behav 2006;9(3):394–400.
27 Ramaratnam S, Baker GA, Goldstein LH. Psychological treatments for epilepsy. Cochrane Database Syst Rev. 2008 Jul 16;(3):CD002029.
28 Weinstein RS, Bryce GF, Sappington LJ, et. al. Decreased serum ionised calcium and normal Vitamin D metabolite levels with anticonvulsant drug treatment. J Clin endocrin Metab 1984;58(6):1003–9.
29 Williams C, Netzloff M, folkerts L, et. al. Vit D metabolism and anticonvulsant therapy: effect of sunshine on incidence of osteomalacia. Soth Med J 1984;77(7):834–6, 842.
30 Denays R, Kumba C, Lison D, et. al. First epileptic seizure induced by occupational nickel poisoning. Epilepsia 2005;46(6):961–2.
31 Arrieta O, Palencia G, Garcia-Arenas G, et. al. Prolonged exposure to lead lowers the threshold of pentylenetetrazole-induced seizures in rats. Epilepsia 2005;46(10):1599–602.
32 Ruegg S, Hunziker P, Marsch S, et. al. Association of environmental factors with the onset of status epilepticus. Epilepsy Behav 2008;12(1):66–73.
33 Nakken KO. Should people with epilepsy exercise? Tidsskr Nor Laegeforen 2000;120(25):3051–3.
34 Ablah E, Haug A, Konda K, et. al. Exercise and epilepsy: a survey of Midwest epilepsy patients. Epilepsy Behav 2009;14(1):162–6.
35 Arida RM, Scorza CA, Schmidt B, et. al. Physical activity in SUDEP: much more than a simple sport. Neurosci Bull 2008;24(6):374–80.
36 Howard GM, Radloff M, Sevier TL. Epilepsy and sports participation. Curr Sports Med Rep 2004;3(1):15–9.
37 Arida RM, Cavalheiro EA, da Silva AC, et. al. Physical activity and epilepsy: proven and predicted benefits. Sports Med 2008;38(7):607–15.
38 Arida RM, Scorza FA, Scorza CA, et. al. Is physical activity beneficial for recovery in TLE? Evidences from animal studies. Neurosci Biobehav Rev 2009;33(3):422–31.

39 Lundgren T, Dahl J, Yardi N, et. al. Acceptance and Commitment Therapy and yoga for drug-refractory epilepsy: a RCT. Epilepsy Behav 2008;13(1): 102–8.
40 Sathyaprabha TN, Satishchandra P, Pradhan C, et. al. Modulation of cardiac autonomic balance with adjuvant yoga therapy in pts with refractory epilepsy. Epilepsy Behav 2008;12(2):245–52.
41 Mortelmans LJ, Van Loo M, De Cauwer HG, et. al. Seizures and hyponatremia after excessive intake of diet coke. Eur J Emerg Med 2008;15(1):51.
42 Iyadurai SJ, Chung SS. Nutrient intake of children with intractable epilepsy compared with healthy children. New onset seizures in adults: possible association with consumption of popular energy drinks. Epilepsy Behav 2007;10(3):504–8.
43 Volpe SL, Schall JI, Gallagher PR, et. al. J Am Diet Assoc 2007;107(6):1014–8.
44 Kossoff EH, Rho JM. KD: Evidence for short and long term efficacy. Neurotherapeutics 2009;6(2):406–14.
45 Weinshenker D. The contribution of NorAd and orexigenic neuropeptides to the anticonvulsant effect of the KD. Epilepsia 2008;49(Suppl 8):104–7.
46 Hartman AL. Does the effectiveness of the KD in different epilepsies yield insights into its mechanisms? Epilepsia 2008;49(Suppl 8):53–6.
47 Bough KJ, Rho JM. Anticonvulsant mechanisms of the KD. Epilepsia 2007;48(1):43–58.
48 Rho JM, Sankar R. The KD in a pill: is this possible? Epilepsia 2008;49(Suppl 8):127–33.
49 Nikanorova M, Miranda MJ, Atkins M, et. al. KD in the treatment of refractory continuous spikes and waves during slow sleep. Epilepsia 2009 Feb 12. Epub ahead of print.
50 Masino SA, Geiger JD. The KD and epilepsy: Is adenosine the missing link? Epilepsia 2009;50(2):332–3.
51 Noh HS, Kim YS, Choi WS. Neuroprotective effects of the KD. Epilepsia 2008;49(Suppl 8):120–3.
52 Allen CN. Circadian rhythms, diet and neuronal excitability. Epilepsia 2008;49(Suppl 8):124–6.
53 Yamada KA. Calorie restriction and glucose regulation. Epilepsia 2008;49(Suppl 8):94–6.
54 Nylen K, Likhodii S, Burnham WM. The KD: proposed mechanisms of action. Neurotherapeutics 2009;6(2):402–5.
55 Bough K. Energy metabolism as part of the anticonvulsant mechanism of the KD. Epilepsia 2008; 49(Suppl 8):91–3.
56 Zarnowska I, Luszczki JJ, Zarnowski T, et. al. Pharmacodynamic and pharmacokinetic interactions between common AED and acetone, the chief anticonvulsant ketone body elevated in the KD in mice. Epilepsia 2008 Oct 24. Epub ahead of print.
57 Likhodii S, Nylen K, Burnham WM. Acetone as an anticonvulsant. Epilepsia 2008;49(Suppl 8):83–6.
58 Nordli DR, Jr. The KD, four score and seven years later. Nat Clin Pract Neurol 2009;5(1): 12–3.
59 Porta N, Vallee L, Boutry E, et. al. Comparison of seizure reduction and serum FA levels after receiving the ketogenic and modified Atkins diet. Seizure 2009 Feb 2 [Epub ahead of print].
60 Kozak N, Csiba L. Dietary aspects of epilepsy. Ideggyogy Sz 2007;60(5–6):234–8.
61 Dutton SB, Escayg A. Genetic influences on KD efficacy. Epilepsia 2008;49(Suppl 8):67–9.
62 Freeman JM. The KD: additional information from a crossover study. J Child Neurol 2009;24(4): 509–12.
63 Bough K. Energy metabolism as part of the anticonvulsant mechanism of the KD. Epilepsia 2008;49(Suppl 8):91–3.
64 Villeneuve N, Pinton F, Bahi-Buisson N, et. al. The KD improves recently worsened focal epilepsy. Dev Med Child Neurol 2009;51(4):276–81.
65 Kossoff EH, Dorward JL. The Modified Atkins Diet. Epilepsia 2008;49(Suppl 8):37–41.
66 Muzykewicz DA, Lyczkowski DA, Memon N, et. al. Efficacy, safety and tolerability of the LGIT in paediatric epilepsy. Epilepsia 2009 Feb 12. Epub ahead of print.
67 Devi PU, Manocha A, Vohora D. Seizures, antiepileptics, antioxidants and ox stress: an insight for researchers. Expert Opin Pharmacother 2008;9(18):3169–77.
68 Hayashi M. Ox stress in developmental brain disorders. Neuropathology 2009;29(1):1–8.
69 Gupta RC, Milatovic D, Dettbarn WD. Depletion of energy metabolites following acetlycholinesterase inhibitor-induced status epilepticus: protection by anti-oxidants. Neurotoxicogy 2001;22(2):271–82.
70 Sobaniec H, Sobaniec W, Sendrowski K, et. al. Antiox activity of blood serum and saliva in patients with periodontal disease treated due to epilepsy. Adv Med Sci 2007;52(Suppl 1):204–6.
71 Hamed SA, Nabeshima T. The high atherosclerotic risk among epileptics: the atheroprotective role of multivitamins . J Pharmacol Sci 2005;98(4):340–53.
72 Verrotti A, Scardapane A, Franzoni E, et. al. Increased ox stress in epileptic children treated with valproic acid. Epilepsy Res 2008;78(2–3):171–7.
73 Verrotti A, Greco R, Latini G, et. al. Obesity and plasma concentrations of alpha-tocopherol and beta-carotene in epileptic girls treated with valproate. Neuroendocrinology 2004;79(3):157–62.
74 Liao KH, Mei QY, Zhou YC. Determination of anti-ox in plasma and RBC in pts with epilepsy. Zhong Nan Da Xue Xue Bao Yi Xue ban 2004;29(1):72–4.
75 Sudha K, Rao AV, Rao A. Ox stress and antioxidants in epilepsy. Clin Chim Acta 2001;303(1–2):19–24.
76 Gutierrez-Alvarez AM, Moreno CB, Gonzalez-Reyes RE. Changes in Se levels in epilepsy. Rev Neurol 2005;40(2):111–6.
77 Ranganathan LN, Ramaratnam S. Vitamins for epilepsy. Cochrane Database Syst rev 2005;(2):CD004304.
78 Ayyildiz M, Yildirim M, Agar E. The effects of Vit E on penicillin-induced epileptiform activity in rats. Exp brain Res 2006;174(1):109–13.
79 Ribeiro MC, de Avila DS, Schnider CY, et. al. Alpha-tocopherol protects against pentylenetetrazol and methylmalonite induce convulsions. Epilepsy Res 2005;66(1–3):185–94.
80 Komatsu M, Hiramatsu M. The efficacy of an antioxidant cocktail on lipid peroxide level and SOD activity in aged rat brain and DNA damage in iron-induced epileptogenic foci. Toxicology 2000; 148(2–3):143–8.
81 Rauca C, Wiswedel I, Zerbe R, et. al. The role of SOD and alpha-tocopherol in the devt of seizures and kindling induced by pentylenetetrazol-influence of the radical scavenger alpha-phenyl-N-tert-butyl nitrone. Brain Res 2004;1009(1–2):203–12.
82 Cao L, Xu J, Lin Y, et. al. Autophagy is upregulated in rats with status epilepticus and partly inhibited

by Vitamin E. Biochem Biophys Res Commun 2009;379(4):949–53.
83 Oztas B, Kilic S, Dural E, et. al. Influence of antioxidants on the BBB permeability during epileptic seizures. J Neurosci res 2001;66(4):674–8.
84 Frantseva MV, Perez Velazquez JL, Tsoraklidis G, et. al. Ox stress is involved in seizure-induced neurodegeneration in the kindling model of epilepsy. Neuroscience 2000;97(3):431–5.
85 Ogunmekan AO, Hwang PA. A randomised double-blind, placebo-controlled trial of D-alpha-tocopheryl actate (vitamin E) as add-on therapy, for epilepsy in children. Epilepsia 1989;30(1):84–9.
86 Raju GB, Behari M, Prasad K, et. al. Randomised double-blind placebo-controlled clinical trial of D-alpha-tocopherol (vitamin E) as add-on therapy in uncontrolled epilepsy. Epilepsia 1994;35(2):368–72.
87 Kutluhan S, Naziroglu M, Celik O, et. al. Effects of Se and TPM on lipid peroxidation and anti-oxidant vitamin levels in blood of PTZ-induced epileptic rats. Biol Trace Elem res 2009 Jan 6. Epub ahead of print.
88 Armagan A, Kutluhan S, Yilmaz M, et. al. Topiramate and Vitamin E modulate antiox enzyme activities, nitric oxide and lipid peroxidation levels in pentylenetetrazol-induced nephrotoxicity in rats. Basic Clin Pharmacol Toxic 2008;103(2):166–70.
89 Naziroglu M, Kutuhan S, Yilmaz M. Se and TPM modulates brain microsomal ox stress values, Ca2+-ATPase activity and EEG records in PTZ-induced seizures in rats. J MZembr Biol 2008;22591–3): 39–49.
90 Hamed SA, Abdellah MM, El-Melagy N. Blood levels of tace elements, electrolytes and ox stress/anti-ox systems in epileptic pts. J Pharmacol Sci 2004;96(4):465–73.
91 Moreno CB, Gutierrez-Alvarez AM, Gonzalez-Reyes RE. Zn and epilepsy: Is there a causal relation between them? Rev Neurol 2008;42(12):754–9.
92 Domingeuz MI, Blasco-Ibanez JM, Crespo C, et. al. Neural overexcitation and implication of NMDA and AMPA receptors in a mouse model of temporal lobe epilepsy implying zinc chelation. Epilepsia 2006;4795):887–99.
93 Takeda A, Itoh H, Hirate, et. al. Region-specific loss of zinc in the brain in PTZ-induced seizures and seizure susceptibility in Zn deficiency. Epilepsy Res 2006;70(1):41–8.
94 Mathie A, Sutton GL, Clarke CE, et. al. Zn and Cu: pharmacological probes and endogenous modulators of neuronal excitability. Pharmacol Ther 2006;111(3):567–83.
95 Horning MS, Trombley PQ. Zn and Cu influence excitability of rat olfactory bulb neurons by multiple mechanisms. J Neurophysiol 2001;86(4):1652–60.
96 Levenson CW. Zn supplementation: neuroprotective or neurotoxic? Nutr Rev 2005;63(4):122–5.
97 Capasso M, Jeng JM, Malavolta M, et. al. Zn dyshomeostasis: a key modulator of neuronal injury. J alzheimers Dis 2005;8(2):93–108.
98 Frazzini V, Rockabrand E, Mocchegiani E, et. al. Ox stress and brain aging: is zinc the link? Biogerontology 2006;7(5–6):307–14.
99 Foresti ML, Arisi GM, Fernandaz A, et. al. Chelatable Zn modulatesx excitability and seizure duration in the amygdala rapid kinding model. Epilepsy Res 2008;79(2–3):166–72.
100 Takeda A, Tamano H, Nagayoshi A, et. al. Increase in hippocampal death after treatment with kainate in zinc deficiency. Neurochem Int 2005;47(8):539–44.
101 Takeda A, Itoh H, Nagayoshi A, et. al. Abnormal calcium mobilisation in hippocampal slices of epileptic animals fed a zinc deficient diet. Epilepsy Res 2009;83(1):73–80.
102 Chwiej J, Winiarski W, Ciarach M, et. al. The role of trace elements in the pathogenesis and progress pf pilocarpine-induced epileptic seizures. J Biol Inorg chem 2008;13(8):1267–74.
103 Hamed SA, Nabeshima T. The high atherosclerotic risk among epileptics: the atheroprotective role of MV. J pharmacol sci 2005;98(4):340–53.
104 Gonzalez-reyes RE, Gutierrez-Alvarez AM, Moreno CB. Mn and epilepsy: a SR of the literature. Brain Res Rev 2007;53(2):332–6.
105 Thiel RJ, Fowkes SW. Downs Syndrome and Epilepsy-a nutritional connection? Med Hypotheses 2004;62(1):35–44.
106 Doretto MC, Simoes S, Paiva AM, et. al. Zn, Mg and Cu profiles in 3 experimental models of epilepsy. Brain Res 2002;956(1):166–72.
107 Ilhan A, Uz E, Kali S, et. al. Serum and hair trace element levels in patients with epilepsy and healthy subjects: does the AEDs affect the element concentrations of hair? Eur J Neurol 1999;6(6):705–9.
108 Motta E, Miller K, Ostrowska Z. Conc of copper and ceruloplasmin in serum of patients treated for epilepsy. Wiad Lek 1998;51(3–4):156–61.
109 Ilhan A, Ozerol E, Gulec M, et. al. The comparison of nail and serum trace elements in patients with epilepsy and healthy subjects. Prog Neuropsychopharmacol Biol Psychiatry 2004;28(1):99–104.
110 Xu XP, Erichsen D, Borjesson SI, et. al. PUFAs and CSF from children on the KD open a voltage-gated K channel: a putative mechanism of antiseizure action. Epilepsy Res 2008;80(1):57–66.
111 Ferrari D, Cysneiros RM, Scorza CA, et. al. Neuroprotective activity of n-3 FAs against epilepsy-induced hippocampal damage: Quantification with immunohistochemical for Ca-binding proteins. Epilepsy Behav 2008;13(1):36–42.
112 Yuen AW, Sander JW, Flugel D, et. al. RBC and plasma FA profiles in patients with epilepsy: does carbemazepine affect Omega-3 FA concentrations? Epilepsy Behaviour 2008;12(2):317–23.
113 Dahlin M, Hjelte L, Nilsson S, et. al. Plasma PUFAs are influenced by a KD enriched with n-3 FAs in children with epilepsy. Epilepsy Res 2007;73(2):199–207.
114 DeGeorgio CM, Miller P, Meymandi S, et. al. Omega-3 FAs for epilepsy, cardiac risk factors and risk of SUDEP: clues from a pilot, double-blind exploratory study. Epilepsy Behav 2008;13(4):681–4.
115 Puri BK, Koepp MJ, Holmes J, et. al. A 31 P neurospectoscopy study of n-3 LCPUFA intervention with EPA and DHA in patients with chronic refractory epilepsy. Prostaglandins Leukot Essent Fatty Acids 2007;77(2):105–7.
116 Puri BK. The safety of EPO in epilepsy. Prostaglandins Leukot Essent fatty Acids 2007;77(2):101–3.
117 Taha AY, Huot PS, Reza-Lopez S, et. al. Seizure resistance in fat-1 transgenic mice endogenously synthesising high levels of n-3 PUFAs. J Neurochem 2008;105(2):380–8.
118 Pifferi F, Tremblay S, Plourde M, et. al. Ketones and brain function: possible link to PUFAs and availability of a new brain PET tracer, 11C-acetoacetate. Epilepsia 2008;49(Suppl 8):76–9.

119 Borges K. Mouse models: the KD and PUFAS. Epilepsia 2008;49(Suppl 8):64–6.
120 Bromfield E, Dworetsky B, Hurwitz S, et. al. A randomised trial of PUFAs for refractory epilepsy. Epilepsy Behav 2008;12(1):187–90.
121 Mainardi P, Leonardi A, Albano C. Potentiation of brain serotonin activity may exhibit seizures, especially in drug-resistant epilepsy. Med Hypotheses 2008;70(4):876–9.
122 Bagdy G, Kecskemeti V, Riba P, et. al. Serotonin and epilepsy. J Neurochem 2007;100(4):857–73.
123 Isaac M. Serotonergic 5-HT2C receptors as a potential therapeutic target for the design of antiepileptic drugs. Curr Top Med Chem 2005;5(1):59–67.
124 El idrissi A, L'Amoreaux WJ. Selective resistance of taurine-fed mice to isoniazid-potentiated seizures: in vivo functional test for the activity of glutamic acid decarboxylase. Neuroscience 2008;156(3):693–9.
125 Galanopoulou AS. GABA(A) Receptors in normal development and seizures: friends or foe? Curr Neuropharmacol 2008;6(1):1–20.
126 Thompson K. Transplantation of GABA-Producing cells for seizure control in models of temporal lobe epilepsy. Neurotherapeutics 2009;6(2):284–94.
127 Bouckenooghe T, Remacle C, Reusens B. Is taurine a functional nutrient? Curr Opin Clin Nutr Metab Care 2006;9(6):728–33.
128 Gupta RC, Win T, Bittner S. Taurine analogues; a new class of therapeutics: retrospect and prospects. Curr Med Chem 2005;12(17):2021–39.
129 Baran H. Alterations of taurine in the brain of chronic kainic acid epilepsy model. Amino Acids 2006;31(3):303–7.
130 El Idrissi A, messing J, Scalia J, et. al. Prevention of epileptic seizures by taurine. Adv Exp Med Biol 2003;526:515–25.
131 Junyent F, Utrera J, Romera R, et. al. Prevention of epilepsy by taurine treatments in mice experimental model. J Neurosci Res 2009;87(6):1500–8.
132 Trombley PQ, Horning MS, Blakemore LJ. Carnosine modulates zinc and copper effects on amino acid receptors and synaptic transmission. Neuroreport 1998;9(15):3503–7.
133 Trombley PQ, Horning MS, Blakemore LJ. Interactions between carnosine and zinc and copper: implications for neuromodulation and neuroprotection. Biochemistry (Mosc 2000;65(7):807–16.
134 Horning MS, Blakemore LJ, Trombley PQ. Endogenous mechanisms of neuroprotection: role of zinc, copper and carnosine. Brain Res 2000;852(1):56–61.
135 Kozan R, sefil F, Bagirici F. Anticonvulsant effect of carnosine on penicillin-induced epileptiform activity in rats. Brain Res 2008 Aug 16. Epub ahead of print.
136 Szyndler J, Maciejak P, Turzynska D, et. al. Changes in the concentration of amino acids in the hippocampus of pentylenetetrazole-kindled rats. Neurosci lett 2008;439(3):245–9.
137 Varshney JP. Clinical management of idiopathic epilepsy in dogs with homeopathic Belladonna 200C: a case series. Homeopathy 2007;96(1):46–8.
138 Mathie RT, Hansen L, Elliott MF, et. al. Outcomes from homeopathic prescribing in vet practice: a prospective research-targeted, pilot study. Homeopathy 2007;96(1):27–34.
139 Schacter SC. Botanics and herbs: a traditional approach to treating epilepsy. Neurotherapeutics 2009;6(2):415–20.
140 Samuels N, Finkelstein Y, Singer SR, et. al. Herbal medicine and epilepsy: proconvulsive effects and interactions with AEDs. Epilepsia 2008;49(3): 373–80.
141 Huen MS, Leung JW, ng W, et. al. 5,7-dihydroxy-6-methoxyflavone, a benzodiazepine site ligand isolated grom Scutellaria baicalensis Georgi, with selective antagonistic properties. Biochem Pharmacol 2003;66(1):125–32.
142 Salah SM, Jager AK. Screening of traditionally used Lebanese herbs for neurological activities. J Ethnopharmacol 2005;97(1):145–9.
143 Harms SL, Garrard J, Schwinghammer P, et. al. *Gingko biloba* use in nursing home elderly with epilepsy or seizure disorder. Epilepsia 2006;47(2):323–9.
144 Hung-Ming W, Liu CS, Tsai JJ, et. al. Antiox and anti-convulsant effect of a modified formula of chaihu-longu-muli-tang. Am J Chin Med 2002; 30(2–3):339–46.
145 Minami E, Shibata H, Nomoto M, et. al. Effect of shitei-to, a TCM formulation, on PZT-induced kindling in mice. Phytomedicine 2000;7(1):69–72.
146 Jyoti A, Sethi P, Sharma D. Curcumin protects against electrobehavioural progression of seizures in the iron-induced experimental model of epileptogenesis. Epilepsy Behav 2009;14(2):300–8.
147 Sumanont Y, Murakami Y, Tohda M. Effects of Mn complexes of curcumin and diacetylcurcumin on kainic acid-induced neurotoxic responses in the rat hippocampus. Biol Pharm Bull 2007;30(9):1732–9.
148 Cheuk DK, Wong V. Acupuncture for epilepsy. Cochrane Database Syst Rev 2008;(4):CD005062.
149 Lee H, Park HJ, Park J. Acupuncture application for neurological disorders. Neurol Res 2007;29(Suppl 1):S49–S54.
150 Chen XH, Yang HT. effects of acupuncture under guidance of qi street theory on endocrine function in the patient of epilepsy. Zhongguo Zhen jiu 2008;28(7):481–4.
151 Yongxia R. Acupuncture treatment of Jacksonian epilepsy-a report of 98 cases. J Tradit Chin Med 2006;26(3):177–8.
152 Zhao HY, Li J. Clinical application of '8 acupoints at the head' by Professer QIN Liang-fu. Zhongguo Zhen Jiu 2007;27(10):745–8.
153 Shu J, Liu RY, Huang XF. Efficacy of ear-point stimulation on experimentally induced seizure. Acupunct Electrother Res 2005;30(1–2):43–52.
154 Guo J, Liu J, Fu W, et. al. The effect of EA on spontaneous recurrent seizure and expression of GAD(67 mRNA in dentate gyrus in a rat model of epilepsy. Brain Res 2008;1188:165–72.
155 Cakmak YO. Epilepsy, EA and the nucleus of the solitary tract. Acupunct Med 2006;24(4):164–8.
156 Jin HB, Li B, Gu J, et. al. EA improves epileptic seizures induced by kainic acid in taurine-depletion rats. Acupunct Electrother Res 2005;30(3–4):207–17.
157 Shu J, Liu RY, Huang XF. The effects of ear-point stimulation on the contents of somatostatin and amino acid neurotransmitters in brain of rat with experimental seizure. Acupunct Electrother Res 2004;29(1–2):43–51.
158 Yang R, Li Q, Guo JC, et. al. Taurine participates in the anticonvulsant effect of EA. Adv Exp Med Biol 2006;583:389–94.

159 Li Q, Guo JC, Jin HB, et. al. Involvement of taurine in penicillin-induced epilepsy and anti-convulsion of acupuncture: a preliminary report. Acupunct Electrother Res 2005;30(1–2):1–14.

160 Chao DM, Chen G, Cheng JS. Melatonin might be one possible medium of EA anti-seizures. Acupunct Electrother Res 2001;26(1–2):39–48.

161 Yang R, Huang ZN, Cheng JS. Anticonvulsion effect of acupuncture might be related to the decrease of neuronal and inducible nitric oxide synthases. Acupunct Electrother Res 2000;25(3–4):137–43.

162 Pistolese RA. Epilepsy and seizure disorders: a review of the literature relative to chiropractic care of children. J Manipulative Physiol Ther 2001;24(3):199–205.

163 Alcantara J, Heschong R, Plaugher G, et. al. Chiropractic management of a patient with subluxations, low back pain and epileptic seizures. J Manipulative Physiol Ther 1998;21(6):410–8.

164 Elster EL. Treatment of bipolar, seizure and sleep disorders and migraine headaches utilizing a chiropractic technique. J Manipulative Physiol Ther 2004;27(3):E5.

165 Kumar AR, Kurup PA. Changes in the isoprenoid pathway with transcendental meditation and Reiki healing practices in seizure disorder. Neurol India 2003;51:211–214.

166 Carpio A, Bharucha NE, Jallon P, et. al. Mortality of epilepsy in developing countries. Epilepsia 2005;46(Suppl 11):28–32.

167 Epilepsy. Control, Centre for Disease. Online. Available: http://www.cdc.gov/epilepsy/basics/faqs.htm (accessed May 2009).

168 Ricotti V, Delanty N. Use of complementary and alternative medicine in epilepsy. Curr Neurol Neurosci Rep 2006;6(4):347–53.

Chapter 16

Fibromyalgia

With contribution from Dr Lily Tomas and Greg de Jong

Introduction

Fibromyalgia is a functional condition typified by widespread muscle and joint pain affecting at least 2% of the general population[1] and as high as 15%.[2] While the American College of Rheumatology classification criteria consists of the identification of at least 11 of 18 standardised tender points, a range of symptoms also exists including fatigue, insomnia and mood disorders (anxiety and depression).[3] Furthermore, demonstrated affects on cognitive function ('fibrofog') have been confirmed with demonstrated influences on memory and attention.[4, 5] Indeed, fibromyalgia is considered a functional somatic syndrome[2] rather than a disease, in that it is a diagnosis of exclusion concluded only after other musculoskeletal disorders have been ruled out.[6]

Significantly, fibromyalgia is frequently found to exist contemporaneously with other functional somatic syndromes.[7] Two studies of the relationship between fibromyalgia and irritable bowel syndrome (IBS) identified that IBS existed in 77%[8] and 70%[9] of fibromyalgia patients (compared to controls in which 18% and 10% had IBS). Of patients with fibromyalgia, 70% were also found to meet the criteria of chronic fatigue syndrome (CFS); [10] 33 of 60 (55%) with fibromyalgia were considered to meet the criteria of multiple chemical sensitivity.[11] As a result it has been suggested that these conditions may represent different symptoms and expressions of common pathogenetic mechanisms due to their substantial overlap,[8] such that specific diagnosis between functional somatic syndromes may depend considerably upon the pragmatics of the assessment rather than definitive pathology.[7]

Due to the debilitating nature of fibromyalgia, long-term consequences and only partial effectiveness of pharmaceutical medicines to alleviate the symptoms, let alone affect a 'cure', many patients explore complementary and alternative medicines (CAM). In fact a study of patients presenting to a tertiary clinic identified that 96% of patients with a diagnosis of fibromyalgia had used CAM in the prior 6 months.[12] Of the most frequently used CAM therapies, 48% used exercise, 45% spiritual healing, 44% massage, 37% chiropractic, and 20% weight loss programmes.[12]

Organic factors

As fibromyalgia is considered a functional syndrome and, subsequently, a condition diagnosed by exclusion, there is the danger that it is assumed to be solely psychosomatic in origin. However, as shall be outlined, numerous organic changes are noted in patients with fibromyalgia suggesting that it is instead a complex condition in which identifying individual factors may be significant in maximising patient outcomes.

Genetic factors

Family studies of fibromyalgia patients demonstrate that the condition aggregates in families. Furthermore it is possible that mood disorders and fibromyalgia may share inherited factors.[13] Inheritability appears to be of a polymorphic nature with evidence of influence amongst serotoninergic, dopaminergic and catecholaminergic systems.[14, 15, 16] Furthermore it has been postulated that subgroups of fibromyalgia patients exist with genetic factors likened to the differentiation of immune cells.[17] Thus emerging evidence suggests that the individual existence, variance and degree of fibromyalgia may be influenced by heterogenous genetic influences.

Muscle changes

Fibromyalgia patients demonstrate definitive muscle changes according to pathology testing. DNA fragmentation has been noted, with disorganisation of actin and myofibre filaments and accumulation of glycogen and lipids within tissues. Muscles appear 'moth eaten', however inflammatory changes are not noted.[18] One possible explanation for such changes is vasomotor dysregulation and vasoconstriction in muscles with a resulting low level ischemia leading to metabolic consequences.[19] Muscle performance and electromyography has demonstrated an inability to relax during work activity as significant in fibromyalgia patients.[20] Muscle strength has also been found to be 35% less per unit.[21]

Results regarding muscle energy metabolism are mixed. In some instances no difference has been found between fibromyalgia patients and controls during rest, exercise or recovery according to measures of phosphocreatine, inorganic phosphate and intracellular pH.[22] However, measures of pyruvate, lactate, adenosine triphosphate and muscular isoenzymes of lacticodeshydrogenase have been found to be altered suggesting biochemical abnormalities during glycolysis may exist.[23] Histological studies may also indicate abnormalities of the mitochondria, reduced capillary circulation and endothelial thickness may lead to oxygen debt, impaired oxidative phosphorylation and reduced ATP synthesis.[24] Mitochondrial numbers have also been found to be significantly lowered,[25] however in other instances a slight increase in type 1 muscle fibres have been noted, with type II muscle fibre atrophy.[26]

Oxidative stress and nutrient deficiencies

Fibromyalgia patients also appear to be under oxidative stress as identified by a comparison of oxidative stress parameters with myalgic scores and associated depression.[27] Total antioxidant capacity has been observed to be significantly lower and total peroxide levels higher in fibromyalgia patients when compared to normals. A significant negative correlation between total antioxidant capacity and visual analogue scale for pain was also noted.[28] These findings are consistent with investigations of female fibromyalgia patients that identified increased free radical parameters and decreased antioxidant parameters (Superoxide Dismutase) leading to oxidant/antioxidant imbalances as compared to normals.[28] Hence it has been hypothesised that oxidative stress and nitric oxide balance may play an important role in fibromyalgia.[30]

Coenzyme Q_{10} is both an important aspect of the mitochondrial respiratory chain and anti-oxidant and has also been found to be abnormally distributed in patients with fibromyalgia, increased reactive oxygen species being identified in mononuclear cells of fibromyalgia patients, but decreased in the presence of CoQ_{10}.[31] Vitamin A and E have been found to be significantly reduced but not Vitamin C and beta–carotene in a study that also identified raised lipid perioxidation in patients with fibromyalgia.[32]

Vitamin D

In a small study of 40 female fibromyalgia patients, 17 demonstrated 25-hydroxyvitamin D concentrations less than 20nmol/l as compared to 7 normals.[33] In a cross-sectional study of 150 patients with non-specific musculoskeletal pain, ages ranging between 10 and 65, 28% demonstrated severe Vitamin D deficiency (<20nmol), 55% of whom were younger than 30 years. Young women and immigrants had the highest levels of deficiency, however the authors emphasised that risks extended beyond patients traditionally suspected of Vitamin D deficiency (aged, housebound, immigrant).[34] Low Vitamin D levels have also been noted amongst rheumatology patients in general[35] and associated with fibromyalgia patients presenting with associated anxiety and depression.[36]

Calcium/magnesium

Preliminary studies comparing ATP, calcium and magnesium platelet levels in fibromyalgia patients were indicative of a trend towards higher calcium concentrations and significant elevations in magnesium simultaneous with lower ATP platelet levels suggesting that abnormal calcium–magnesium flow regulation may be of relevance in fibromyalgia.[37] Intracellular evaluations demonstrate similar calcium–magnesium flow abnormalities exist with a possible influence on muscle contractility in fibromyalgia patients.

Amino acid/neurotransmitter balance

It has been hypothesised that an altered tryptophan metabolism may be responsible for fibromyalgia, however investigations suggest this may only be present in a subgroup of patients.[38] A study of plasma levels of amino acids indicated that patients with fibromyalgia have significantly decreased levels of the branch chain amino acids; valine, leucine and isoleucine, and phenylalanine than normals, but no difference in measures related to tryptophan uptake or serotonergic markers.[39] However, in contrast a second study indicated multiple individual amino acids (taurine, alanine, tyrosine, valine, methionine, phenylalanine and threonine) and the sum total of amino acids competing with tryptophan for brain uptake were found to be lower in fibromyalgia patients, suggesting gut protein malabsorption may be indicated with subsequent potential influences on neurotransmitter balance.[40]

Cerebrospinal fluid analysis indicated that in patients with fibromyalgia with other overlapping conditions (as compared to normals and primary fibromyalgia), pain intensity and tender point index co-varied with concentrations of metabolites of the excitatory neurotransmitters, glutamate and asparagines, with glycine and taurine also showing covariance with tender point index measures.[41] Arginine, a precursor to nitric oxide, co-varied with tender point index scores for both primary and fibromyalgia associated with other conditions. The authors concluded that an increase in excitatory amino acid release may be associated with increased nitric oxide synthesis eventually leading to increase pain in fibromyalgia patients.[41]

Central nervous system (CNS)

A 2008 review of literature concluded that recent studies of fibromyalgia highlight abnormalities in the CNS processing of pain leading to increased sensitivity and a lowered threshold for pain. Persistent nociceptive input may lead to plastic changes provoking central sensitisation and chronic pain states. The authors suggested that these central changes were indicative of many of the syndromes that overlap with fibromyalgia, such as IBS, low back pain, migraine and temporomandibular disorders.[42]

It has also been suggested that autonomic nervous system dysregulation may exist in some patients as exemplified by the common finding of postural orthostatic tachycardia.[43] However, the autonomic response in fibromyalgia patients to stress tasks appears to differ within subgroups. Although patients with fibromyalgia consistently demonstrated reduced surface electromyographic (EMG) readings at baseline, subsets of fibromyalgia patients present with increased sympathetic vasomotor reactivity and reduced muscular response with or without increased sudomotor reactivity during stress tasks, while others demonstrated parasympathetic vasomotor reactivity, reduced sudomotor activity and reduced muscular response. These variant autonomous system responses to stress subsequently imply that heterogenous groups of fibromyalgia exist.[44] Abnormal responses of the sympathetic nervous system may be related to exaggerated norepinephrine (noradrenaline release) that have been observed amongst female patients with fibromyalgia.[45]

Neuroendocrine systems

Emerging evidence suggests that the neuroendocrine system is subtly involved in fibromyalgic presentation in an overlapping relationship with disturbances in neurotransmitters. Again, changes may be relevant in a subgroup of patients only rather than the entire spectrum of fibromyalgia patients.

Cortisol

A review of papers in 2001 found that in one-third of studies, cortisol at baseline was significantly low in one-third of patients while 24-hour urinary cortisol levels are frequently within the lower part of normal.[46, 47] Cortisol responses to increased ACTH in stress, exercise and during hypoglycaemic events are often blunted[48, 49, 50] suggestive of an impaired ability to activate the hypothalamic pituitary portion of the hypothalamic–pituitary–adrenal (HPA) axis with subsequent adrenal hyporesponsiveness leading to a relative adrenal insufficiency.[47–52] A lower expression of corticosteroid receptors has also been observed which may be compounded by lower levels of anti-inflammatory mediators.[53]

Consistent with this clinical studies have revealed that cortisol levels at waking and 1 hour after waking have a relationship to morning pain scores in women with fibromyalgia, although this relationship does not appear relevant later in the day.[54] In the late evening an elevation of cortisol levels was evident in half of all fibromyalgia patients compared to normals and tending towards being statistically lower overnight, again suggesting a loss of resilience in the basal circadian function of the HPA axis.[55]

Thyroid hormone

Autoimmune thyroid disease (ATD) has been identified in a subgroup of patients presenting with fibromyalgia. An examination of 56 patients with a diagnosis of ATD identified 31% could be classified as having fibromyalgia.[56] A study of thyroid antibodies in 128 fibromyalgia patients demonstrated that thyroid autoimmunity existed in 34% of fibromyalgia patients as compared to 18.8% of normals, with the highest frequencies in those patients with previous psychiatric treatment, postmenopausal women and patients presenting with a frequent history of dry mouth.[57] In a further study, 41% of fibromyalgia patients had thyroid antibodies despite normal basal ranges, however age and depression were not found to be significant. Frequent symptoms reported in this study included dry eyes, burning/pain with urination, allodynia, blurred vision and a sore throat.[58] There is a 4.5 times calculated likelihood of detecting thyroid antibodies associated with fibromyalgia.[59]

Growth hormone

A physiological dysregulation of the HPA also appears to be a factor in impaired growth hormone secretion (rather than production) frequently reported in patients with fibromyalgia.[60, 61] Growth hormone stimulation tests often demonstrate blunted responses suggesting the possibility of hypothalamic origin for growth hormone dysfunction.[62]

Sleep, melatonin and the immune system

Fibromyalgia patients commonly report early morning awakenings, feeling tired, lack of sleep, cognitive disturbances and on occasion, sleep apnoea. Poor sleep quality has been noted to parallel pain intensity. Fibromyalgia patients often demonstrate sleep abnormalities consistent with normals during sleep deprivation (alpha-delta sleep anomaly), increased stage 1, decreased delta sleep and an increase in the number of sleep arousals.[63] Dysfunctional beliefs regarding sleep may also play a role in fibromyalgia.[64]

Melatonin is important in regulating wake–sleep cycles. Fibromyalgia sufferers appear to have significantly lower levels of melatonin than normal controls. In a study comparing total melatonin secreted between 1800hr and 0800hr and hours of darkness (2300hr to 700hr) fibromyalgia patients were observed to be 31% lower in the latter measure and peak serum levels of melatonin were also considerably lower. It was concluded that these variations in melatonin may lead to the impaired night sleep, day fatigue and altered perceptions of pain associated with fibromyalgia pain.[65]

Elevations in cytokine levels have also been implicated in sleep–wake dysregulation in fibromyalgia patients. These immune mediators form a link between the periphery and the neuroendocrine, autonomic, limbic and cortical areas of the CNS and have hence been found to mediate sleep, sleepiness and fatigue.[66, 67] However, views and evidence appear varied on the input of the immune system and whether it is in an excited or inhibited state. While some papers suggest there is no evidence that fibromyalgia is associated with a heightened immune system response, indeed immunosuppression may be a significant factor, trials with immunotherapies risk inducing fibromyalgia like symptoms.[67] Results of C-reactive protein (CRP) studies, however, have indicated raised CRP levels are often present in patients with fibromyalgia.[69]

Infections

Consistent with findings of immune system involvement is the preliminary evidence that viral and other infections may be present in patients with fibromyalgia. Indeed a review of tender points during acute viral infection indicates that tender points are common and transient features during acute illness.[70] Patients with acute episodes of fibromyalgia have been demonstrated to have an increase in IgM antibodies to enterovirus as compared to both chronic fibromyalgia and normal controls, suggesting a variance in their immune response.[71] Of fibromyalgia patients, 13% who had muscle biopsies were found to have enterovirus present within their muscle tissue. Persistence of infection was suspected as an influence on fibromyalgia by the reporters due to these associated biopsy findings.[72]

A study of the presence of mycoplasmal infections in patients with chronic fatigue and/or fibromyalgia indicated that single or multiple mycoplasma organism infections (fermentans, pneumonia, hominis, penetrans) were present in over 50% of these individuals. Infections with mycoplasmal species were consistent with longer symptoms of fibromyalgia.[73] Furthermore, it has been hypothesised that mycoplasmal infection may be a significant factor in thyroid abnormalities noted to occur in some fibromyalgia patients.[74]

A statistical association also appears to exist between Human T Cell Lymphotropic Virus Type 1 infections and patients with fibromyalgia — 38% of patients with this infection experiencing fibromyalgia as compared to 3% of normals.[75] There does not appear to be a relationship between fibromyalgia and either hepatitis C (HCV) or human parvovirus B19.[76, 77]

Gastrointestinal system

As noted 30–70% of patients with fibromyalgia have concurrent IBS. It has been suggested that altered microbial balance in the gastrointestinal system may be responsible for some aspects of fibromyalgia.[78, 79]

Lifestyle factors

Psychological

Studies of psychological and psychosocial influences on, and comorbidities with, fibromyalgia also suggest that it is not a homogenous syndrome, with mixed elements individual to each patient being significant dependent upon their psychosocial background.[80] For example, a degree of somatization appears to be a significant predictive factor in the development of fibromyalgia. A prospective study of 1658 adult patients demonstrated that patients who developed widespread pain often had a prior tendency towards somatisation.[81]

A comparison of psychological factors of fibromyalgia when compared to rheumatoid arthritis amongst patients attending a tertiary clinic indicated a high percentage of fibromyalgia patients. Ninety percent (N = 36) had a prior psychiatric diagnosis as compared to less than 50% for rheumatoid arthritis.[82] However, while the presence of anxiety and depression are common and may exist in definable subgroups, it has been shown that the degree of the psychological comorbidities of anxiety and depression varies between patients with a subgroup of patients ('adaptive copers') demonstrating very few comorbidities at all.[80]

Psychosocial

A cross-sectional study of the community observed that people with fibromyalgia and chronic widespread pain reported more health impairments than people with no pain, or regionalised pain. There was also an increased incidence of fibromyalgia amongst people of low socioeconomic status, low educational levels, low social support and a family history of chronic pain,[83] and amongst employed women and housewives.

Stress

Stress-related issues also appear to be pertinent. Indeed, fibromyalgia patients commonly demonstrate clinically significant levels of post traumatic stress disorder (PTSD)-like syndromes,[84] while registering greater levels of significant disability (85% vs 50%). Those fibromyalgia patients with PTSD-like symptoms reported significantly greater levels of pain, emotional distress, life interference and disability as compared to fibromyalgia patients without PTSD symptoms. Only 15% of fibromyalgia patients with PTSD syndromes were considered adaptive copers as compared to 48% without symptoms.

Consistent with this, fibromyalgia patients appear to be associated with higher levels of victimisation than other patients (control group consisted of rheumatoid arthritis patients and other rheumatology patients).[85, 86] Forms of victimisation included abuse of a sexual, physical or emotional basis (neglect);[87] in particular, adult physical abuse, although childhood abuse was also significant. A further study suggested this relationship (without reaching clinical significance), however, did determine with significance that frequency of abuse was a correlate with fibromyalgia,[88] even if this relationship has not always been demonstrated for all forms of abuse.[89] Links have also been determined with frequency of drug abuse.[88] Work stress, including workplace bullying (almost 4 times as likely), high workload (twice as likely) and low decision latitude also appear pertinent associated related/causal factors.[90]

Tobacco

People who smoke appear to have higher pain intensities, numbness, severity and functional difficulties than non-smokers with fibromyalgia, however, no significant difference has been associated with number of tender points or fatigue levels.[91, 92] Psychiatric therapy use and alcohol consumption were higher in fibromyalgia patients who smoked as was the level of un-restorative sleepiness and anxiety-depression.[93] Smokers experienced fewer good days and more days of work missed per week.[92]

Obesity

Fibromyalgia patients who are overweight or obese generally have poorer quality of life, lower pain thresholds, reduced function and increased tender point counts than patients with lower Body Mass Indexes (BMIs).[94, 95] A trend towards significance was identified between BMI and fatigue.[95]

Overview of treatment evidence for fibromyalgia

A review of the multi-factorial causation and associations with fibromyalgia identifies why it is a difficult condition to treat. As a heterogenetic syndrome with multiple overlaps with other functional syndromes and conditions (IBS, chronic fatigue, mood disorders etc.) it is essential that both a multi-disciplinary yet individualised approach is undertaken for each patient with fibromyalgia. This may also explain why many treatment approaches have only a low level of evidence, given that evidential support for treatment methods that might only be successful in particular subsets of patients would be statistically blunted if applied to undifferentiated groups of fibromyalgia patients. This further infers that comprehensive assessment is essential when addressing the patient with fibromyalgia in order to establish which therapy amongst the many advocated for the condition is both pertinent and a priority to the individual.

Multidisciplinary treatment approaches

Given the multi-factorial nature of fibromyalgia, it is unsurprising that multidisciplinary programmes are often applied to fibromyalgia patients. However, while some individual studies have demonstrated improvements from multidisciplinary approaches (group behavioural therapies, stress management, relaxation plus exercise),[96–99] a Cochrane review (2000) found there was little evidence that such programmes were of benefit, given the poor quality of existing studies.[100] However, subsequent clinical trials continue to indicate the potential of multidisciplinary programmes[101] with growing evidence to their efficacy when combinations of behavioural therapies, exercise, relaxation and other such sessions are included.[102, 103]

Mind–body medicine

Like most treatments for fibromyalgia, only low-level evidence exists for the efficacy of independent mind–body therapies due predominantly to low numbers in studies and methodological flaws.

A study of 28 fibromyalgia patients showed that cognitive behaviour therapy (CBT) was superior to pharmacological intervention (cyclobenzaprine) during treatment and follow-up.[103] Small studies of electromypgraphy and electro–encephalography biofeedback also suggests that it has the potential of being effective.[105, 106] Pilot and small studies of hypnosis also advocate continued investigation.[107–110]

Small-scale evaluation of mindfulness meditation indicated that 8 by 2.5 sessions of mindfulness-based stress reduction may reduce the depressive symptoms in women with fibromyalgia.[111] A trial of meditation-based stress management during a 10-week outpatient group programme indicated effectiveness, however, identified a specific subgroup (51%) of responders who gained through better sleep, reduced fatigue and increased feelings of rejuvenation in the morning.[112] A 7-week trial of qigong indicated potential benefits amongst 29 female fibromyalgia patients,[113] however a combined meditation–qigong intervention was found to be only equivalent to education and support.[114] The use of guided imagery focusing on pleasant imagery as a distraction from the pain of fibromyalgia was found to be effective, however the use of attention imagery was not.[115] Relaxation and guided imagery was also found to be of benefit in a small trial of Hispanic patients.[116]

In summary, while various mind–body therapies have been recommended for fibromyalgia and pooled evidence is suggestive of benefit,[117] further evidence is required before we can conclude definitive benefits for specific treatment approaches.

Physical activity

A Cochrane review (2007) identified exercise as being moderately beneficial in certain aspects of fibromyalgia management depending on the type of exercise. Aerobic exercise (a moderate intensity 12-week programme) may increase feelings of wellbeing and function, although may not effect pain or tender point number. Strength training has been noted to reduce pain, tender points, depression and wellbeing, although not physical function. Exercise programmes should be initiated in a graded manner and balanced with symptoms. Compliance is often difficult for fibromyalgia patients.[118] A 2008 systematic review supported many of these conclusions, however advocated further studies are required.[119]

In particular, aquatic therapy has been demonstrated to be effective in fibromyalgia.[120] Aquatic therapy has been suggested as an introduction for patients who may fear that pain will exacerbate their symptoms.[121] While both patients on a home-based exercise programme and undertaking aquatic therapy may benefit from exercise, aquatic therapy appears to have long-term effects on pain reduction.[122]

Small studies have shown statistically significant benefits for fibromyalgia patients participating in tai chi[123] and yoga.[124]

Nutritional influences

Diet

Evidence is weak regarding the benefits of diet on fibromyalgia. A pilot study on the effects of weight loss on fibromyalgia suggests that a behavioural weight loss programme leading to an average 4.4% weight reduction in overweight/obese patients predicted reduced fibromyalgia symptoms, body satisfaction and quality of life.[125] While it has been noted by some studies that vegan and predominantly raw vegetable diets may have short-term benefits on fibromyalgia symptoms,[126, 127] these results are questionable as other studies indicate vegetarian diets as being of little benefit as compared to medication with amitrytilline.[128] A trial of 4 patients demonstrated the possibility that excitotoxin removal (e.g. MSG and aspartamine) may assist in a subgroup of fibromyalgia patients.[129] Soy and casein (protein) shakes may also decrease fibromyalgia symptoms.[130] In summary, as with many areas of fibromyalgia intervention, evidence is inconclusive due to the low evidential value of current studies.

Nutritional supplements

Most forms of supplementation are only supported by single low-level studies such that evidence remains inconclusive.

Intravenous vitamin therapy may assist to decrease symptoms and increase function in long-term fibromyalgia patients.[131]

An open pilot study of 200mg Coenzyme Q_{10} and 200mg *Gingko biloba* extract given to fibromyalgia patients for 84 days, resulted in many reporting quality of life improvements; 64% recording that they felt better as compared to 9% stating they felt worse.[132] In a second trial, 2 capsules of 500mg acetyl L-carnitine per day over 10 weeks led to an improvement in pain scores and depression as compared to control groups.[133]

A double-blind placebo cross-over trial of intravenous S-adenosyl-l-methionine (SAMe) reported a tendency towards significance in response to pain at rest, pain on movement and wellbeing and only slight improvements in fatigue, quality of sleep and morning stiffness, with no effect on muscle strength.[134] A further SAMe injection trial indicated an improvement in tender point scores and associated depression.[135] An oral supplementation investigation of SAMe using 800mg daily for 6 weeks demonstrated improvements in clinical disease activity, pain experienced over a week, morning stiffness, mood (as measured by Face Scale) and fatigue, although tender point scores, muscle strength and mood (as evaluated by Beck Depression Inventory) did not differ as compared to a control.[136]

It has been suggested that the use of 5-Hydroxytryptophan (5-HTH) as a serontonin precursor is effective in treating fibromyalgia, particularly since, unlike tryptophan, it cannot be shunted into niacin or protein production.[137] A 90-day open study of 50 patients with 5-HTH demonstrated it was effective in providing good or fair clinical improvement in 50% of patients.[138]

Vitamin D deficient (25 [OH]D 10-25ng/mL) fibromyalgia patients treated with 50 000 units cholecalciferol (vitamin D3) showed significant improvement in fibromyalgia assessment when treated over an 8-week period. However, those patients considered severely deficient (<10ng/mL) showed no benefit.[139] However, these results differ to trials in which ergocalciferol (vitamin D2) 50000IU once weekly for 3 months did not significantly change fibromyalgia symptoms amongst patients with low vitamin D levels (<20ng/ml).[140]

Trials of combination treatment with malic acid (1200 to 2400mg) and magnesium (300 to 600mg) over 8 weeks indicated decreases in tender-point measures as early as 48 hours, with resumption of symptoms on cessation.[141] A further study at the lowest dosage levels identified that the half dose did not appear significant enough to lead to symptoms reduction, and that the higher double dosage could take up to 2 months to be effective.[142]

Physical therapies

A 2003 systematic review of chiropractic manipulation for non-spinal conditions including fibromyalgia indicates that there is not enough evidence to suggest that they are effective.[143] A further review in 2009 suggested that there was only limited evidence that chiropractic manipulation was effective in treating fibromyalgia.[144]

In comparison moderate evidence appears to exist for the use of massage therapies (twice per week, 5 weeks) during the course of treatment.[145] The sleep of fibromyalgia patients also appears to improve after massage.[146] A trial of reiki therapy in fibromyalgia patients indicates that there is little evidence of effectiveness.[147]

A systematic review (2007) of acupuncture suggests only short-term limited effects such that acupuncture could not be recommended for fibromyalgia.[148] However, a subsequent small trial (2008) differs in stating acupuncture may provide quality of life improvements up to 3 months post-treatment.[149] It should be noted that the use of sham needling in evaluating acupuncture has been challenged by acupuncturists as being inappropriate to this form of modality.[150]

The use of static magnetic therapies has been demonstrated to only be as effective as sham or usual treatment.[151]

Conclusion

Growing knowledge as to the multi-factorial causes, dysfunctions and associations of fibromyalgia indicates that this is a heterogenetic syndrome requiring an essential individualisation of therapy. At present, non–pharmacological treatment evidence remains scant, other than for aerobic and strengthening exercise, yet it is likely that multidisciplinary programmes that provide a combination of mind–body, exercise and supplementation approaches are necessary if maximum achievable gains are to be made by the patient. (See Table 16.1.)

Table 16.1 Levels of evidence for lifestyle and complementary medicines/therapies in the management of fibromyalgia

Modality	Level I	Level II	Level IIIa	Level IIIb	Level IIIc	Level IV	Level V
Organic factors							
Genetics			x				
Muscle changes					x		
Oxidative stress and nutritional deficits					x		
Vitamin D				x			
Magnesium					x		
Amino acid/ neurotransmitter balance					x		
CNS					x		
Neuroendocrine							
Cortisol					x		
Thyroid hormone					x		
Growth hormone					x		
Sleep/melatonin					x		
Infections					x		
Gastrointestinal					x		
Lifestyle factors							
Psychological					x		
Psychosocial					x		
Multidisiciplinary (behavioural therapies/ exercise/ relaxation)		x					
Tobacco					x		
Obesity					x		
Mind–body medicine							
Cognitive behavioural therapy				x			
Electromyography					x		
Electro-encephalography biofeedback					x		
Mindfulness-based stress reduction		x					
Hypnosis					x		
Guided imagery					x		
Physical activity	x						
Qigong		x					
Hydrotherapy/ aquatherapy	x						
Nutrition							
Diet and weight loss					x		
Vegetarian diet				x			

Continued

Table 16.1 Levels of evidence for lifestyle and complementary medicines/therapies in the management of fibromyalgia—cont'd

Modality	Level I	Level II	Level IIIa	Level IIIb	Level IIIc	Level IV	Level V
Nutritional supplements							
IV multivitamin therapy				x			
Vitamin D (cholecalciferol)		x					
Coenzyme Q_{10} + *Gingko biloba*					x		
L-Carnitine		x					
S-adenosyl-l-methionine			x				
5-Hydroxytryptophan					x		
Malic acid + magnesium		x					
Physical therapies							
Chiropractic manipulation		x(–)					
Acupuncture		x					
Masage therapy			x				
Static magnetic therapies					x(–)		
Reiki			x(–)		x		

Level I — from a systematic review of all relevant randomised controlled trials — meta-analyses.
Level II — from at least 1 properly designed randomised controlled clinical trial.
Level IIIa — from well-designed pseudo-randomised controlled trials (alternate allocation or some other method).
Level IIIb — from comparative studies (including systematic reviews of such studies) with concurrent controls and allocation not randomised, cohort studies, case-control studies, or interrupted time series with a parallel control group.
Level IIIc — from comparative studies with historical control, 2 or more single-arm studies or interrupted time series without a parallel control group.
Level IV — opinions of respected authorities based on clinical experience, descriptive studies or reports of expert committees.
Level V — represents minimal evidence that represents testimonials.

Clinical tips handout for patients — fibromyalgia

1 Lifestyle advice

Sunshine

- Amount of exposure varies with local climate.
- At least 15 minutes of sunshine needed daily for vitamin D and melatonin production — especially before 10 a.m. and after 3 p.m. when the sun exposure is safest during summer. Much more exposure required in winter when supplementation needs to be considered.
- Ensure gradual, adequate skin exposure to sun; avoid sunscreen and excess clothing to maximise levels of vitamin D.
- More time in the sun is required for dark-skinned people and people with vitamin D deficiency.
- Direct exposure to about 10% of the body (hands, arms, face), without sunscreen and not through glass.
- Vitamin D is obtained in the diet from fatty fish, eggs, liver and fortified foods (some milks and margarines); diet alone is not a sufficient source of vitamin D.

2 Physical activity/exercise

- Aerobic exercise — 30–60 minutes daily within the limits of functional disability. If exercise is not regular, commence with 5 minutes at a time and slowly build up increment length towards 30 minutes over several weeks. Exercising several short manageable sessions per day that total 30 minutes while increasing increment time is also beneficial. Outdoor exercise with nature, fresh air and sunshine is ideal.
- Stretching and muscle strengthening programs may be beneficial; perform 2–3 sessions per week involving all major muscle groups.
- Yoga and tai chi may also be considered for balance and flexibility.
- Start slowly and recognise and respect fatigue.

3 Mind–body medicine

- Cognitive behavioural techniques, hypnosis, biofeedback and other psychological interventions may be of benefit for some people. You should assess the benefits on an individual basis.
- Stress management programmes may be helpful, including journaling/verbal disclosure of emotions. The use of a counsellor does not appear to provide additional benefit.
- Meditation and/or relaxation, at least 10-20 minutes per day, can be helpful.

Fun

- Enjoy life! Find ways to make life as pleasurable as possible. Seek joy in the simple aspects of life.

4 Environment

- Avoid environmental pollutants and chemicals — at work and in the home.
- Quit smoking through whatever means are available. Support is often essential as smoking cessation over the long-term is a challenge.

Education

- Participate in a self-management program to increase your knowledge of the disease and available coping strategies.

Community

- Actively engage in your community in order to increase your support networks.

5 Dietary changes

- Consider undertaking a food elimination and re-introduction regime to establish if you have any food intolerances/allergies (grain, milk, beef, eggs etc) that affect fibromyalgia. This is preferable to strict long-term elemental, vegan or vegetarian diets as it may not be as limiting once food reintroduction is complete.
- Eat regular balanced healthy meals; ideally 3 main meals and 2 snacks per day, each containing protein.
- The use of a high-quality protein powder may be considered to increase amino acid intake, particularly of the branch chain amino acids. Consume separate to any tryptophan/5-Hydroxytryptopgan supplementation.
- Increase fish intake (sardines, tuna, salmon, cod, mackerel), especially deep sea fish. Eat 3 or more fish meals per week.

- Two small serves of red meat per week should be consumed to ensure adequate iron levels.
- Trial a vegetarian diet as this may help.
- Consume high quantities of fruit (>2/day) and vegetables (>5/day) (in particular red fruit and vegetables).
- Use extra virgin cold-pressed olive oil and avocado in dressings.
- Eat more nuts, seeds and bean sprouts (e.g. alfalfa, mung, bean, lentil).
- Enjoy dark chocolate.
- Reduce dairy intake but consume full-fat varieties to increase vitamin D intake from fat-soluble sources.
- Add wholegrains (e.g. rice, buckwheat flours, wholegrain organic breads, millet etc.)
- Drink 1–2 litres of water per day.
- Short-term fasting may be of benefit during symptom exacerbation.
- Avoid hydrogenated fats, salt, fast foods, sugar such as soft drinks, lollies, biscuits, cakes and other processed foods (e.g. white breads, white pasta, pastries).
- Moderate coffee and alcohol consumption only; 1–2 serves per day. Assess whether either affect your symptoms.
- Avoid chemical additives — preservatives, colourings, flavourings.
- For sweeteners try honey (e.g. manuka, yellow box and stringy bark).

6 Physical therapies

- Hydrotherapy/aquatherapy can help.
- Regular massages may provide both short and long-term benefits.

7 Supplements

- Your choice of supplementation may depend upon the nature of overlapping conditions (e.g. irritable bowel syndrome, chronic fatigue syndrome, depression).

Protein supplementation (e.g. rice whey, soy, casein)

- A broad-based protein powder may be of benefit in providing quality amino acid supply as a meal replacement or snack.
- Consider use with pancreatic enzymes to improve digestion.

Probiotics

- Probiotics and other appropriate supplementation is recommended when fibromyalgia coexists with gastrointestinal conditions and irritable bowel syndrome.

Carnitine

- Additional indications: low energy (co-existing chronic fatigue syndrome).
- Dosage: 2 x 500mg acetyl-L-carnitine over 8–12 weeks to determine benefits.
- Contraindications: use with caution in case of liver disease, epilepsy or if you are using anti-coagulant therapy (monitor bleeding time).

Coenzyme Q_{10}

- Additional indications: low energy (co-existing chronic fatigue syndrome).
- Dosage: 200mg coenzyme Q_{10} daily; 8–12 weeks.
- Contraindications: review INR levels if taking warfarin.

S-adenosyl-l-methionine (SAMe)

- Additional indications: fibromyalgia; pre-existing mild-moderate depression.
- Dosage: supplementation trials have used 800mg/day.
- Contraindications: not to be used during pregnancy, lactation, fertility, or by people with bipolar disorder. Should not be used with anti-depressants.

Tryptophan/5-Hydroxytryptophan

- Additional indications: pre-existing mild–moderate depression.
- Dosage: 100–200mg/day for 1–3 months to assess results.
- Contraindications: should not be taken by patients on anti-depressives (monoamine oxidase inhibitors or selective serotonin uptake inhibitors).

Melatonin

Melatonin is derived from tryptophan and requires various minerals and vitamins for its production. Deficiency of any of these may lead to reduced production of melatonin.

- Indication: helps insomnia by improving circadian rhythm sleep disorders; reduces the time to fall asleep; jet lag.
- Dosage: adult: 0.3–6 mg at 6 p.m. or closer to bedtime; for short-term use. Requires a prescription from your doctor. Children — smaller doses required, up to 3mg.
- Results: within 1–3 hours.
- Side-effects: usually well tolerated. Avoid long-term use. May cause drowsiness, dizziness, depressive symptoms, reduced alertness, irritability, headaches; all these symptoms can be transient.

- Contraindications: children, pregnant, lactating mothers; epilepsy sufferers; with alcohol, sedating medication such as benzodiazepines and use with narcotics; depression.

Vitamins and minerals

Vitamin D3 (Cholecalciferol)

- Additional indications: recommendation based on clinical tests performed by a doctor.
- Dosage: may begin with supplementation up to 50 000IU per week (7500IU/ day) until levels normalised, after which 1000IU is the maintenance dosage.
- Contraindications: some people may be sensitive to vitamin D supplementation.
  - Potentially, vitamin D may reduce the effectiveness of calcium channel blockers and therefore need to be used under medical supervision (e.g. for patients with cardiac conditions).
  - Patients with systemic lupus erythematosus, hypercalcemia, sarcoidosis, hyperparathyroidism and patients taking digitalis should take care with high doses and, therefore, require medical supervision.

Magnesium + malic acid

- Indications: fibromyalgia; myofascial trigger points, muscle twitches, heart palpitations in absence of cardiac conditions.
- Dosage: 300–600mg magnesium with 1200–2400mg malic acid/day.
- Contraindications: some people have gastrointestinal side-effects from high dosages. Not to be used in patients with severe kidney disease or heart blocks.

References

1 Mease P. Fibromyalgia syndrome: a review of clinical presentation, pathogenesis, outcome measures and treatment. J Rheumatol Supp 2005 Aug;75:6–21.

2 Neumann L, Buskila D. Epidemiology of fibromyalgia. Curr Pain Headache Rep 2003 Oct;7(5):362–8.

3 Wolfe F, Smythe HA, Yunus MB, et. al. The American College of Rheumatology Criteria for the Classification of Fibromyalgia. Report of the Multicenter. Criteria Committee Arthritis and Rheumatism 1990;33:160–172.

4 Glass JM. Fibromyalgia and cognition. J Curr Clin Psychiatry 2008;69(Suppl 2):20–4.

5 Sephton SE, Studts JL, Hoover K, et. al. Biological and psychological factors associated with memory function in fibromyalgia syndrome. Health Psychol 2003 Nov:22(6):592–7.

6 Nampiaparampil DF, Shmerling RH. A review of fibromyalgia. Am J Manag Care 2004;10(11 Pt1):794–800.

7 Kanaan RA, Lepine JP, Wessely SC. The association or otherwise of the functional somatic syndrome. Psychosom Med 2007 Dec;69(9):855–9.

8 Veale D, Kavanagh G, Fielding JF, et. al. Primary fibromyalgia and the irritable bowel syndrome: different expressions of a common pathogenetic process. Br J Rheum 1991 Jun 30;(3):220–2.

9 Overlapping conditions among patients with chronic fatigue syndrome, fibromyalgia and temporomandibular disorder. Arch Intern Med 2000 Jan 25;160(2):221–7.

10 Buchwald D, Garrity D. Comparison of patients with chronic fatigue syndrome, fibromyalgia, and multiple chemical sensitivities. Arch Int Med 1994 Sep 26;154(18):2049–53.

11 Slotkoff AT, Radulovic DA, Clauw DJ. The relationship between fibromyalgia and the multiple chemical sensitivity syndrome Scand. J Rheumatol 1997;26(5):364–7.

12 Wahner-Roedler DL, Elkin PL, Vincent A. Use of complementary and alternative medical therapies by patients referred to a fibromyalgia treatment program at a tertiary care center. Mayo Clinic Proc 2005 Jan;80(1):55–60.

13 Arnold LM, Hudson JI, Hess EV. Family study of fibromyalgia. Arthritis Rheum 2004 Mar;50(3): 944–52.

14 Buskila D. Genetics of chronic pain states. Best Pract Clin Rheumatol 2007 Jun;21(3):553–47.

15 Buskila D, Neumann L. Genetics of fibromyalgia. Curr Pain Headache Rep 2005 Oct;9(5):313–315.

16 Ablin JN, Cohen H, Buskila D. Mechanisms of Disease; genetics of fibromyalgia. Nat Clin Pract Rheum 2006 Dec;2(12):671–8.

17 Carvalho LS, Correa H, Silva GC, et. al. May genetic factors in fibromyalgia help to identify patients with differentially altered frequencies of immune cells? Clin Exp Immunol 2008 Dec;154(3):346–52.

18 Yunas MB, Kanyan-Raman UP, Kalyan-Raman K. Primary fibromyalgia and myofascial pain syndrome: clinical features and muscle pathology. Arch Phys Med Rehabil 1988 Jun;69(6):451–4.

19 Katz DL, Greene L, Ali A, et. al. The pain of fibromyalgia is due to muscle hypoperfusion induced by regional vasomotor dysregulation. Med Hypotheses 2007;69(3):517–25. Epub 2007 Mar 21.

20 Elert JE, Rantapaa-Dahiqvist SB, Henriksson-Larsen K, et. al. Muscle performance electromyography and fibre type composition in fibromyalgia and work related myalgia. Scand J Rheumatol 1992;21(1):28–34.

21 Norregaard J, Bulow PM, Danneskiold-Samson B. Muscle strength, voluntary activation, twitch properties, and endurance in patients with fibromyalgia. J Neurol Neurosurg Psychiatry 1994 Sep;57(9):1106–11.

22 Simms RW, Roy SH, Hrovat M, et. al. Lack of association between fibromyalgia syndrome and abnormalities in muscle energy metabolism. Arthritis Rheum 1994 Jun;37(6):794–800.

23 Elsinger J, Plantamura A, Ayavou T. Glycolysis abnormalities in fibromyalgia. J Am Coll Nutr 1994 Apr;13(2):144–8.

24 Le Goff. Is fibromyalgia a muscle disorder? Joint Bone Spine 2006 May;73(3):239–42.

25 Sprot H, Salemi S, Gay RE, et. al. Increased DNA fragmentation and ultrastructural changes in fibromyalgic muscle fibres. Ann Rheum Dis 2004 Mar;63(3):245–51.

26 Pongratz DE, Spath M. Morphologic aspects of fibromyalgia. Z Rheumatol 1998;57(Suppl 2):47–51.

27 Ozgoenmens S, Ozyurt H, Sogut S, et. al. Antioxidant status, lipid peroxidation and nitric oxide in fibromalgia: etiologic and therapeutic concerns. Rheumatol Int 2006 May;26(7):598–603.
28 Altindag O, Celik H. Total antioxidant capacity and the severity of the pain in patients with fibromyalgia. Redox Rep 2006;11(3):131–5.
29 Bagia S, Tamer L, Sahin G. Free radicals and antioxidants in primary fibromyalgia: an oxidative stress disorder?
30 Ozgocmens S, Ozyurt H, Sodut S. Current concepts in the pathophysiology of fibromyalgia: the potential role of oxidative stress and nitric oxide. Rheumatol Int 2006 May;26(7):585–97.
31 Cordero MD, Moreno-Fernandez AM, deMiguel M, et. al. Coenzyme Q10 distribution in blood is altered in patients with fibromyalgia. Clin Biochem 2009 May;42(7-8):732–5.
32 Akkus S, Naziroglu M, Eris S, et. al. Levels of lipid perioxidation and antioxidant vitamins in plasma of patients with fibromyalgia. Cell Bioch Funct 2009 Mar 14.
33 Al-Allaf AW, Mole PA, Paterson CR. Bone health in patients with fibromyalgia. Rheumatology 2003 Oct;42(10):1202–6.
34 Plotnikoff GA, Quigley JM. Prevalence of severe hypovitaminosis in patients with persistent, nonspecific musculoskeletal pain. Mayo Clin Prac 2003 Dec;78(12):1463–70.
35 Mouyis M, Ostor AJ, Crisp AJ. Hypovitaminosis D among rheumatology outpatients in clinical practice. Rheumatology 2008 Sep;47(9):1348–51.
36 Armstrong DJ, Meenagh GK, Bickle I. Vitamin D deficiency is associated with anxiety and depression in fibromyalgia. Clin Rheumatol 2007;26(4):551–4.
37 Bazzichi L, Giannaccini G, Betti L, et. al. ATP, calcium and magnesium levels in platelets of patients with primary fibromyalgia. Clin Biochem 2008;41(13):1084–90.
38 Schwarz MJ, Offenbaecher M, Neumeister, et. al. Experimental evaluation of an altered tryptophan metabolism in fibromyalgia. Adv Exp Med Biol 2003;532:265–75.
39 Maes M, Verkerk R, Delmeire L, et. al. Serotonergic markers and lowered plasma branch chain amino acid concentrations in fibromyalgia. Psychiatry Res 2000 Dec 4;97(1):11–20.
40 Bazzichi L, Palego L, Giannaccini G, et. al. Altered amino acid homeostasis in subjects affected by fibromyalgia. Clin Biochem 2009 Mar 9.
41 Larson AA, Giovengo SL, Michalek JE. Changes in the concentration of amino acids in cerebrospinal fluid that correlate with pain in patients with fibromyalgia: implications for nitric oxide pathways. Pain 2000;87(2):201–11.
42 Staud R, Spaeth M. Psychophysical and neurochemical abnormalities of pain processing in fibromyalgia. CNS Spectr 2008 Mar;13(3 Suppl 5):12–7.
43 Staud R. Autonomic dysfunction in the fibromyalgia syndrome: postural orthostatic tachycardia. Curr Rheumatol Rep 2008 Dec;10(6):463–6.
44 Thieme K, Turk DC. Heterogeneity of psychophysiological stress responses in fibromyalgia syndrome patients. Arthritis Res Ther 2006;8(1):R9.
45 Torpy DJ, Papanicolaou DA, Lotsikas AJ, et. al. Responses of the sympathetic nervous system and the hypoithalamic-pituatary-adrenal axis to interleukin-6: a pilot study in fibromyalgia. Arthritis Rheum 2000 Apr;43(4):872–80.
46 Geenen R, Jacob JW, Bijisma JW. Evaluation and management of endocrine dysfunction in fibromyalgia. Rheum Dis Clin North Am 2002;28(2):389–404.
47 Izquierdo-Alvarez S, Bocos-Terraz JP, Bancalero-Floes JL, et. al. BMC Res Notes 2008 Dec 22;1:134.
48 Adler GK, Kinsley BT, Hurwitz S, et. al. Reduced hypothalamic-pituatary and sympathoadrenal responses to hypoglycaemia in women with fibromyalgia. Am J Med 1999 May;106(5):534–43.
49 Crofford LJ, Engleberg NC, Demitrack MA. Neurohormonal pertunation in fibromyalgia. Baillieres Clin Rmeumatol 1996 May;10:365–78.
50 Riedel W, Schlapp U, Leck, et. al. Blunted ACTH and cortisol responses to systemic injection of corticotrophin releasing hormone (CRH) in fibromyalgia: role of somatostatin and CRH-binding protein. Ann N Y Acad Sci 2002;966:483–90.
51 Griep EN, Boersma JW, de Kloet ER. Altered reactivity of the hypothalamic-pituitary-adrenal axis in the primary fibromyalgic syndrome. J Rheumatol 1993 Mar;20(3):469–74.
52 Calis M, Gokce C, Ates F. Investigation of the hypothalamo-pituitary-adrenal axis (HPA) by 1microg ACTH test and mtyrapone test in patients with primary fibromyalgia syndrome. J Endocrinol Invest 2004 Jan;27(1):42–6.
53 Macedo JA, Hesse J, Turner JD. Glucocorticoid sensitivity in fibromyalgia patients: decreased expression of corticosteroid receptors and glucocorticoid-induced leucine zipper. Psychoneuroendicrinology 2008 Jul;33(6):799–809.
54 McClean SA, Willias DA, Harris RE, et. al. Momentary relationships between cortisol secretion and symptoms in patients with fibromyalgia. Arthritis Rheum 2005 Nov;52(11):3600–9.
55 Crofford LJ, Young EA, Engleberg NC, et. al. Basal circadian and pulsatile ACTH and cortisol secretion in patients with fibromyalgia and/or chronic fatigue syndrome. Bran Behav Immun 2004 Jul;18(4):314–25.
56 Soy M, Guidikin S, Arikan E, et. al. Frequency of rheumatic diseases in patients with autoimmune thyroid disease. Rheumatol Int 2007 Apr;27(6):575–7.
57 Pamuk ON, Cakir N. The frequency of thyroid antibodies in fibromyalgia patients and their relationship with symptoms. Clin Rheum 2007;26(1):55–9.
58 Bazzichi L, Rossi A, Giuliano T, et. al. Association between thyroid autoimmunity and fibromyalgic disease severity. Clin Rheumatol 2007 Dec;26(12):2115–20.
59 Ribiero LS, Proietti FA. Interrelations between fibromyalgia, thyroid autoantibodies and depression. J Rheumatol 2004 Oct;31(10):2036–40.
60 Bennett RM. Adult growth hormone deficiency in patients with fibromyalgia. Curr Rheumatol Rep 2002 Aug;4(4):306–12.
61 Bennet RM. Growth hormone in musculoskeletal pain states. Curr Pain Headache Rep 2005 Oct;9(5):331–8.
62 Jones RD, Deodhar P, Lorentzen A, et. al. Growth hormone perturbations in fibromyalgia: a review. Semim Arthritis Rheum 2007 Jun;36(6):357–79.
63 Harding SM. Sleep in fibromyalgia patients: subjective and objective findings. Am J Med Sci 1998 Jun;315(6):367–76.
64 Theadon A, Cropley M. Dysfunctional beliefs, stress and sleep disturbances in fibromyalgia. Sleep Med 2008 May;9(4):376–81.

65 Wilkner J, Hirsch U, Wetterberg L, et. al. Fibromyalgia – a syndrome associated with decreased nocturnal melatonin secretion. Clin Endocrinol 1998 Aug;49(2):179–183.

66 Mullington JM, Hinze-Selch D, Polimacher T. Mediators of inflammation and their interaction with sleep: relevance for chronic fatigue syndrome and related conditions. Ann N Y Acad Sci 2001 Mar;993:201–10.

67 Lorton D, Lubahn CL, Estus, et. al. Bidirectional communication between the brain and the immune system: implications for physiological sleep and disrupted sleep. Neuroimmunomodulation 2006;13(5-6):357–74.

68 Van West D, Maes M. Neuroendocrine and immune aspects of fibromyalgia. Biodrugs 2001;15(8):521–31.

69 Haheim LL, Nafstad P, Olsen I, et. al. C-reactive protein variations for different chronic somatic disorders. Scand J Public Health 2009 Apr 16.

70 Rea T, Russo J, Katon W, et. al. A prospective study of tender points and fibromyalgia during and after an acute viral infection. Arch Intern Med 1999 Apr 26;159(8):865–70.

71 Wittrup IH, Jensen B, Biddal H, et. al. Comparison of viral antibodies in 2 groups of patients with fibromyalgia. J Rheumatol 2001 Mar;28(3):601–3.

72 Douche-Aourik F, Serleir F, Ferasson L, et. al. Detection of enterovirus in human skeletal muscle from patients with chronic inflammatory muscle disease or fibromyalgia and healthy subjects. J Med Virol 2003;71(4):540–7.

73 Nasralia M, Naier J, Nicolson GL. Multiple mycoplasmal infections in blood of patients with chronic fatigue syndrome and/or fibromyalgia syndrome. Eur J Clin Microbiol Infect Dis 1999 Dec;18(12):859–65.

74 Garrison RL, Breeding PC. A metabolic basis for fibromyalgia and its related disorders: the possible role of resistance to thyroid hormone. Med Hypotheses 2003 Aug;61(2):182–9.

75 Cruz BA, Catalan-Soares B, Proietta F. Higher prevalence of fibromyalgia in patients infected with human T cell lymphotropic virus type 1. J Rheumatol 2006 Nov;33(11):2300–3.

76 Narvaez J, Nolla JM, Valverde-Garcia J. Lack of association of fibromyalgia with hepatitis C virus infection. J Rheumatol 2005 Jun;32(6):1118–21.

77 Narvaez J, Nolla JM, Valverde J. Joint Bone Spine 2005 Dec;73(6):592–4.

78 Othman M, Aguero R, Lin HC. Alterations in intestinal microbial flora and human disease. Curr Opin Gastroenterol 2008 Jan;24(1):11–6.

79 Wallace DJ, Hallequa DS. Fibromyalgia: the gastrointestinal system. Curr Pain Headache Resp 2004 Oct;8(5):364–8.

80 Thieme K, Turk DC, Flor H. Comorbid depression and anxiety in fibromyalgia syndrome: relationship to somatic and psychosocial variable. Psychosom Med 2004 Nov-Dec;66(6):837–44.

81 McBeth J, Macfarlane GJ, Benjamin S, et. al. Features of somatisation predict the onset of chronic widespread pain: results of a large population based study. Arthritis Rheum 2001 Apr;44(4):940–6.

82 Walker EA, Keegan D, Gardner G. Psychosocial factors in fibromyalgia compared with rheumatoid arthritis: I. Psychiatric diagnoses and functional disability. Psychosom Med 1997 Nov-Dec;59(6):565–71.

83 Bergman S. Psychosocial aspects of chronic widespread pain and fibromyalgia. Disabil Rehabil 2005 Jun 17;27(12):675–83.

84 Sherman JJ, Turk Dc, Okifuji Prevalence and impact of posttraumatic stress disorder-like symptoms on patients with fibromyalgic syndrome. Clin J Pain 2000 Jun;16(2):127–34.

85 Boisset-Piero MH, Esdalle JM, Fitzcharles MA. Sexual and physical abuse in women with fibromyalgia syndrome. Arthritis Rheum 1995 Feb;38(2):235–44.

86 Walker EA, Keenan D, Gardner G, et. al. Psychosocial factors in fibromyalgia compared with rheumatoid arthritis: II Sexual, physical and emotional abuse and neglect. Psychosom Med 1997 Nov-Dec;59(6):572–7.

87 Van Houdenhove B, Neerinchx E, Lysens R, et. al. Victimisation in chronic fatigue syndrome and fibromyalgia in tertiary care: a controlled study on prevalence and characteristics. Psychosomatics 2001 Jan Feb;42(1):21–8.

88 Ruiz- Perez I, Plazaola-Castano J, Caliz-Caliz R, et. al. Risk factors for fibromyalgia the role of violence against women. Clin Rheum 2009 Mar 10.

89 Ciccone DS, Elliot DK, Chandler HK, et. al. Sexual and physical abuse with fibromyalgia syndrome: a test of the trauma hypothesis. Clin J Pain 2005 Sep Oct;21(5):378–86.

90 Kivimaki M, Leiros-Arjas P, Virtanen M, et. al. Work stress and incidence of newly diagnosed fibromyalgia: prospective cohort study. J Psychosom Res 2004 Nov;57(5):417–22.

91 Yunus MB, Arsian S, Aldag JC, et. al. Relationship between fibromyalgia and smoking. Scand J Rheumatol 2002;31(5):301–5.

92 Weingarten TN, Podduturu VR, Hooten WM, et. al. Impact of tobacco use in patients presenting to multidisciplinary outpatient treatment programme in fibromyalgia. Clin J Pain 2009 Jan;25(1):39–43.

93 Pamuk ON, Donmez S, Cakir N. The frequency of smoking in fibromyalgia patients and its association with symptoms. Rheumatol Int 2009 Jan 20.

94 Neumann L, Lerner E, Glazer Y, et. al. A cross-sectional study of the relationship between body mass index and clinical characteristics, tenderness measures, quality of life and physical function in fibromyalgia patients. Clin Rheumatol 2008 Dec;27(15):1543–7.

95 Yunus MB, Arsian S, Aldag JC. Relationship between body mass index and fibromyalgia features. Scand J Rheumatol 2002;31(1):27–31.

96 Burckhardt CS, Mannerkorpi K, Hedenberg L, et. al. A randomized controlled clinical trial of education and physical training with fibromyalgia. J Rheumatol 1994 Apr;21(4):714–20.

97 Havermark Am, Languis Ekiof. A Long term follow up of a physical therapy programme for patients with fibromyalgia syndrome. Scand J Caring Sc 2006 Sep;20(3):315–22.

98 Keel PJ, Bodoki C, Gerhard U, et. al. Comparison of integrated group therapy and relaxation training for fibromyalgia. Clin J Pain 1998 Sep;14(3):232–8.

99 Creamer P, Singh BB, Hochberg BM. Sustained improvement produced by nonpharmacological intervention in fibromyalgia: results of a pilot study. Arthritis Care Research 2000 Aug;13(4):198–204.

100 Karjalainen K, Malmivaara A, van Tulder M, et. al. Multidisciplinary rehabilitation for fibromyalgia and musculoskeletal pain in working age adults. Cochrane Date Base Systematic Review 2000(2):CD001984.

101 Goldenberg DL. Multidisciplinary modalities in the treatment of fibromyalgia. J Clin Psychiatry 2008;69(Suppl 2):30–4.

102 Lemstra M, Olsznski WP. The effectiveness of multidisciplinary rehabilitation in the treatment of fibromyalgia: a randomised controlled trial. Clin J Pain Mar-Apr;21(2):166–174.
103 Angst F, Brioschi R, Main CJ. Interdisciplinary rehabilitation in fibromyalgia and chronic back pain: a prospective outcome study. J Pain 2006;7:807–15.
104 Garcia J, Simon Ma, Duran M. Differential efficacy of a cognitive behavioural intervention versus pharmacological treatment in the management of fibromyalgic syndrome. Psychol Health Med 2006 Nov;11(4):498–506.
105 Babu As, Matthew E, Danda D. Management of patients with fibromyalgia using biofeedback: a randomised control trial Indian. J Med Sci 2007 Aug;61(8):455–61.
106 Kayiran S, Dursan E, Ermutiu N. Neurofeedback in fibromyalgia. Agri 2007 Jul;19(3):47–53.
107 Castel A, Perez M, Sala J, et. al. Effect of hypnotic suggestion on fibromyalgic pain: comparison between hypnosis and relaxation. Eur J Pain 2007 May;11(4):463–8.
108 Martinez-Valero C, Castel A, Capafons A, et. al. Hypnotic treatment synergizes the psychological treatment of fibromyalgia: a pilot study. Am J Clin Hyn 2008 Apr;50(4):311–21.
109 Alvarez-Nemegyei J, Negreros-Castillo A, Nuno-Gutierrez BL, et. al. Eriksonian hypnosis in women with fibromyalgia syndrome. Rev Med Inst Mex Seguro Soc 2007 Jul-Aug;45(4):395–401.
110 Derbyshire SW, Whalleymg, Oakley DA. Fibromyalgia pain and its modulation by hypnotic and non-hypnotic suggestion: an MRI analysis.
111 Sephton SE, Salmon P, Weissbecker I, et. al. Mindfulness meditation alleviates symptoms in women with fibromyalgia: results of a randomized clinical trial. Arthritis Rheum 2007 Feb 15;57(1): 77–85.
112 Kaplan KH, Goldenberg DL, Galvin Nadeau M. The impact of a meditation-based stress reduction program on fibromyalgia. Gen Hosp Psychiatry 1993 Sep;15(5):284–9.
113 Haak T, Scott The effect of Qigong on fibromyalgia (FMS): a controlled randomized study Disabil Rehabil 30(8):625–33.
114 Astin JA, Berman BM, Bausell B, et. al. The efficacy of mindfulness meditation plus Qigong movement therapy in the treatment of fibromyalgia: a randomized controlled trial. J Rheumatol 2003 Oct;30(10):2257–62.
115 The effect of guided imagery and amitriptyline on daily fibromyalgia pain: a prospective, randomized, controlled trial. J Psychiatr Res 2002 May-Jun;36(3):179–87.
116 Menzies V, Kim S. Relaxation and guided imagery in Hispanic persons diagnosed with fibromyalgia: a pilot study. Fam Community Health 2008 Jul-Sep;31(3):204–12.
117 Hadhazy VA, Ezzo J, Creamer P, et. al. Mind-body therapies for the treatment of fibromyalgia. A systematic review. J Rheumatol 2000 Dec;27(12):2911–8.
118 Busch AJ, Barber KA, Peloso PMJ, et. al. Exercise for treating fibromyalgia syndrome. Cochrane Database of Systematic Reviews 2007(4). Art No.: CD0003786.
119 Busch AJ, Schachter CL, Overend TJ, et. al. Exercise for fibromyalgia: a systematic review. J Rheumatol 2008 Jun;35(6):1130–44.
120 McVeigh JG, McGaughey H, Hall M, et. al. The effectiveness of hydrotherapy in the management of fibromyalgia syndrome: a systematic review. Rheumatol Int 2008 Dec;29(2):119–30.
121 Gowan SE, deHueck A. Pool exercise for individuals with fibromyalgia. Curr Opin Rheumatol 2007 Mar;19(2):168–73.
122 Ecvik D, Yigit I, Pusak H. Rheumatol Int 2008 Jul;28(9):885–90.
123 Taggart HM, Arsianian Cl, Baea, et. al. Effects of Tai Chi exercise in fibromyalgia symptoms and health relates quality of life. Orthop Nurs 2003 Sep-Oct;22(5):353–60.
124 Da Silva GD, Lorenzi-Filho G, Lage LV. Effects of yoga and the addition of Tui Na in patients with fibromyalgia. J Altern Complement Med 2007 Dec;13(10):1107–13.
125 Shapiro JR, Anderson DA, Danoff-Burg S. A pilot study of the effects of behavioural weight loss treatment on fibromyalgia symptoms. J Psychosom Res 2005 Nov;59(5):275–82.
126 Kaartinen K, Lammi K, Hypen M, et. al. Vegan diet alleviates fibromyalgia symptoms. Scand J Rheumatol 2000;29(5):308–13.
127 Donaldson MS, Speight N, Loomis S. Fibromyalgia syndrome improved using a mostly raw vegetarian diet: an observational study. BMC Complement Altern Med 2001;1:7.
128 Azad KA, Alam MN, Haq SA, et. al. Vegetarian diet in the treatment of fibromyalgia. Bangladesh Med Res Counc Bull 2000 Aug;26(2):41–7.
129 Smith JD, Terpening CM, Schmidt SO, et. al. Relief of fibromyalgia symptoms following discontinuation of dietary excitotoxins. Ann Pharmacother 2001 Jun;25(6):702–6.
130 Wahner-Roedler DL, Thompson JM, Luedtke CA. Dietary Soy Supplement on Fibromyalgia Symptoms: A randomised, double-blind, placebo-controlled, early phase trial. Evid Based Complement Alternat Med 2008 Nov 6.
131 Massey PB. Reduction of fibromyalgic symptoms through intravenous nutrient therapy: results of a pilot study. Altern Ther Health Med 2007;13(3):32–4.
132 Lister RE. An open, pilot study to evaluate the potential benefits of coenzyme Q10 combined with Gingko biloba extract in fibromyalgia syndrome. J Int Med Res 2002;30(2):195–9.
133 Rossine M, Di Munno O, Valentini G, et. al. Double-blind, multicentre trial compating acetyl l carnitine with placebo in the treatment of fibromyalgia patients. Clin Exp Rheumatol 2007 Mar-Apr;25(2):182–8.
134 Volkmann H, Norregard S, Danneskoid-Samsoe B, et. al. Double-blind placebo controlled cross-over study of intravenous S-adenyl-L-methionine in patients with fibromyalgia. Scand J Rheum 1997;26(3):206–211.
135 Tavoni A, Vitali C, Bombardieri S, et. al. Evaluation of S-adenosylmethionine in primary fibromyalgia. A double-blind crossover study. Am J Med 1987 Nov 20;83(5A):107–10.
136 Jacobsen S, Danneskioid-Samsoe B, Andersen RB. Oral S-adenosylmethionine in primary fibromyalgia. Double-blind clinical evaluation. Scand J Rheum 1991;20(4):294–302.
137 Birdsall TC. 5-Hydroxytryptophan: a clinically effective serotonin precursor. Altern Med Rev 1998 Aug;3(4):271–80.

138 Sarzi Puttini P, Caruso I. Primary fibromyalgia syndrome and 5-Hydroxy-L-tryptophan: a 90 day open trial. J Int Med Res 1992 Apr;20(2):182–9.
139 Arvold DS, Odean MJ, Dornfeld MJ, et. al. Correlation of symptoms with vitamin D deficiency and symptoms responses to cholecalciferol treatment: a randomised controlled trial. Endocr Prac 2009 May-Jun;15(3):203–12.
140 Diffuse musculoskeletal pain is not associated with low vitamin D levels or improved by treatment with Vitamin D. J Clin Rheumatol 2008 Feb;14:12–6.
141 Abraham GE, Flechens JD. Management of fibromyalgia: rational for use of magnesium and malic acid. J Nutr Med 1992:349–59.
142 Russell IJ, Michalek JE, Flechas JD, et. al. Treatment of fibromyalgia syndrome with Supper Malic: a randomised double-blind. Placebo controlled, cross over study. J Rheumol 1995:22(5):953–8.
143 Ernst E. Chiropractic manipulation for non-spinal pain-a systematic review. NZ Med 2003 Aug 8;116(1179):U539.
144 Schneider M, Vernon H, Ko G, et. al. Chiropractic management of fibromyalgia syndrome: a systematic review of the literature. J Manipulative Physiol Ther 2009 Jan;32(1):25–40.
145 Sunshine W, Field TM, Quintino O, et. al. Fibromyalgia benefits from massage therapy and transcutaneous electrical stimulation. L Clin Rheumatol 1996 Feb;2(1):18–22.
146 Field T, Diego M, Cullen C, et. al. Fibromyalgia pain and substance P decreases and sleep improves after massage therapy. J Clin Rheumatol 2002 Apr;8(2):72–6.
147 Assefi N, Bogart A, Goldberg J, et. al. Reiki for the treatment of fibromyalgia: a randomised controlled trial. J Altern Complement Med 2008 Nov;14(9).
148 Mayhew E, Ernst E. Acupuncture for fibromyalgia – a systematic review of randomized clinical trials. J Rheumatology 2007 May;46(5):801–4.
149 Targino RA, Imamura M, Kaziyama HH, et. al. A randomised controlled trial of acupuncture added to usual treatment for fibromyalgia. J Rehabil Med 2008 Jul;40(7):582–8.
150 Lundeberg T, Lund I. Are reviews based on sham acupuncture procedures in fibromyalgia syndrome (FMS) valid? Acupunct Med 2007 Sep;25(3):100–6.
151 Alfano AP, Taylor AG, Foresman PA, et. al. Statics magnets fields for treatments of fibromyalgia: a randomised controlled trial. J Altern Complement Med 2001 Feb;7(1):53–64.

Chapter 17

Headaches and migraines

Introduction

Headache is the most prevalent neurological symptom encountered in medical practice.[1] It is experienced by almost everyone at some stage of their lives. Headache can be a symptom of a serious life-threatening disease, such as a brain tumour, although in most cases it is a benign disorder that can comprise a primary headache, such as a migraine, or a tension-type headache.[2] Nevertheless, migraines and tension-type headaches can cause considerable levels of disability, not only to patients and their families but also to society as a whole owing to its high prevalence in the general population.

There is a significant burden associated with headache and it is a major public health problem.[2] The most common types of headaches are migraines and tension headaches. Globally, the percentage of the adult population with an active headache disorder is 47% for headaches in general, 10% for migraine, 38% for tension-type headaches, and 3% for chronic headaches that last for more than 15 days per month.[2, 3]

General lifestyle and behavioural interventions

Numerous lifestyle factors can trigger headaches. These can be caused by lifestyle stressors, particular foods and beverages, sleep problems, sinus and allergy problems, muscle tension, and mood disorders.[4] People who report having relatives who get migraine headaches are more likely to get them as well.[4]

Health practitioners are ideally placed to treat most patients with chronic headaches and migraines. Once organic causes are excluded, management needs to focus on lifestyle and dietary changes to help prevent and promote self-management of headaches and migraines. A multi-disciplinary approach may be required till the exact causes are identified. This was demonstrated in a recent study where 80 men and women with migraine were randomly assigned to 1 of 2 groups. The intervention group consisted of supervised exercise therapy, stress management and relaxation therapy lectures, dietary lecture, and massage therapy sessions.[5] The control group consisted of standard care with the patient's family clinician. There were no significant differences between the 2 groups before intervention. At the end of the 6-week intervention and at a 3-month follow-up, the intervention group experienced statistically significant improvement in pain frequency, pain intensity and duration, described better quality of life and health status and reduced symptoms of depression. Healthy behaviour patterns involving relaxation practice and lifestyle modifications of diet, regular meals, exercise, and correcting sleep deprivation consistently demonstrate significant improvement in reducing headaches and migraines and improved mood levels.[5]

Mind–body therapies

Stress management, biofeedback, cognitive behaviour therapy (CBT)

Chronic tension and mixed type headaches appear to benefit from mind–body interventions, especially where the evidence for mind–body therapies is quite strong such as migraine headaches.[6] Several clinical trials for chronic tension-type headaches and chronic migraines have found that relaxation training significantly reduced headache activity compared to talk therapy, self-monitoring, muscle relaxant (chlormezanone), information/education, and no treatment.[7–14] Penzien and colleagues estimate that behavioural interventions yielded approximately 35–50% reduction in migraine and tension-type headaches.[13]

Relaxation therapies have been described to be as effective, or more effective, in reducing the frequency of migraine headaches comparable to pharmacologic medication.[14] This review investigated the evidence for mind–body therapies for chronic pain disorders including chronic headaches and migraines. Based on evidence from randomised controlled trials (RCTs) and systematic reviews of the literature, relaxation and thermal biofeedback were deemed effective treatments for recurrent migraine while relaxation and muscle biofeedback was an effective adjunct or stand alone therapy for recurrent tension headaches.[14] The physiological basis for their effectiveness is unclear, but data from 1 trial suggest that levels of plasma beta-endorphin can be altered by relaxation and biofeedback therapies.[15]

Children appear to be very responsive to mind–body related therapies. An early systematic review of 7 relaxation trials and 5 biofeedback-assisted relaxation trials examined a total of 252 children with headaches.[16] Overall *relaxation training* was better than an information-giving intervention, a discussion group, or treatment with propranolol 3mg/kg/day, including at 5–6 month follow-up. *Relaxation training together with biofeedback* experienced greater reduction in headache frequency, intensity and duration than the control group, post-treatment and at 6-month follow-up. A more recent Cochrane review identified 28 RCTs and concluded that:

> there was very good evidence that psychological treatments, principally relaxation and cognitive behavioural therapy, were effective in reducing the severity and frequency of chronic headache in children and adolescents.[17]

In summary, mind–body therapies may be more effective in treating headaches compared to no treatment or in combination with standard care. However, when compared to each other, there may not be a significant difference. A systematic review of autogenic relaxation training reported equivalency among several different relaxation techniques in the treatment of headaches.[18] Mind–body interventions for migraine have been better studied than those for tension headache. The US Headache Consortium treatment guidelines for migraines now include cognitive and behavioural treatment recommendations based on evidence from 39 controlled trials.[19, 20] It suggests that relaxation training, thermal biofeedback combined with relaxation training, electromyographic biofeedback, and cognitive behavioural therapy (CBT) may be considered as treatment options for prevention of migraine and combined with preventive drug therapy to achieve additional clinical improvement for migraine relief based on the highest level I evidence rating. Furthermore, a recent Cochrane meta-analysis of the literature assessed 29 randomised control studies (1432 patients) and found children and adolescents who suffer chronic headaches significantly benefit from psychological therapies — namely relaxation, hypnosis, coping skills, biofeedback and CBT — and concluded there is a strong case to include these therapies as routine care.[17]

Sleep

Sleep disturbance is implicated with specific headache patterns and severity.[21, 22] In a recent study it was reported that a short sleep group, who routinely slept 6 hours per night, exhibited the more severe headache patterns and more sleep-related headache compared with those who slept longer.[23] Also sleep complaints occurred with greater frequency among chronic than episodic migraine sufferers.[24] A study of 49 men and women from headache clinics with onset of headache during the night or early morning, were investigated.[25] Fifty-five percent were found to have specific sleep disorders. Also participants were found to have excessive daytime somnolence. After treatment for defined sleep disorders, all participants reported improvement or absence of their headache (65%). All patients who reported sleep apnoea found that their headaches disappeared with appropriate treatment.[25] Assessing patients for sleep disorders may be important in the management of patients with chronic headaches.

Environmental factors

In a recent study it was reported that from a cohort of 120 participants the most common trigger factors that were associated with precipitating a migraine or tension-type headache were the weather (82.5%), stress (66.7%) and menstruation (51.4%).[23] There have been numerous factors that have been implicated with triggering migraines and tension-type headaches not related to diet (Table 17.1).[24] In a further study it was reported that there are precipitating and aggravating factors differentiating migraine from tension-type headache but not vice versa.[25] Three of the migraine-specific precipitating factors were the weather, smell, and smoke which involved the nose and sinus system, suggesting a greater significance of this system in headache causation than is generally considered.[25]

A recent US study of over 7000 people diagnosed with headache identified frequency and severity of headaches and hospital admission increased with climacteric changes namely, higher ambient temperatures and to a lesser extent lower barometric air pressure, but not air pollution.[26]

In addition, people who tend to spend a lot of time indoors may suffer chronic headaches due to environmental toxins, such as volatile organic compounds released from new furniture and renovations, and poor air quality.[27, 28] Airing the house or workplace frequently and spending more time outdoors is helpful. Other known environmental factors which have

Table 17.1 Non-alimentary trigger factors for migraines and tension-type headaches (4 frequency ranges)*

	Migraines				Tension-type headaches			
Trigger factors	[<10%]	[10–25%]	[<26–50%]	[>50%]	[<10%]	[<10–25%]	[26–50%]	[>50%]
Light — bright	2	1	6 (iv)	-	3 (ii)(v)	3 (vi)	2 (iii)	-
Light — sunshine	-	2	2	-	-	1 (ii)	-	-
Light — neon	-	1	-	-	-	-	-	-
Computer screen	-	1	-	-	-	-	-	-
Cinema	-	-	-	-	-	1 (iii)	-	-
Reading	-	1	-	-	-	1	1 (iii)	-
Depression and/or disappointment	-	-	2	-	-	-	-	-
Worries	-	-	1	-	-	-	-	-
Fear	-	-	-	1	-	-	-	-
Anger	1	-	1	-	1 (ii)	-	-	-
Noise (light noise)	-	-	1	-	-	-	1	-
Noise	2	-	-	1	(ii)	-	2 (iii)	-
Driving trips	1	-	1	1 (ii)	1	1 (iii)	1	1
Holidays	-	1	-	-	-	-	-	-
Shopping	-	-	-	-	-	1 (iii)	-	-
Inconvenience	1	-	-	-	1 (ii)	-	-	-
Psychological stress	-	-	1 (i)	-	-	-	-	-
Stress and/or strains	-	-	7 (i)	4	-	1 (ii)	2	3 (iii)
Following stress–relaxation	-	2	-	-	-	-	-	-
Smell	2	-	3	2	2 (ii)(iii)	1	-	1
Smoking	5 (i)	1	2	1	4 (ii)(v)(vi)	-	2	-
Overworked — strain	-	-	1	-	-	2	-	-
Sleeping patterns altered	-	-	-	1	-	-	-	1
Sleep	-	-	1	-	--	-	-	-
Sleep — lack of	-	-	1	2	-	-	-	2 (iii)

Continued

Table 17.1 Non-alimentary trigger factors for migraines and tension-type headaches (4 frequency ranges)*—cont'd

	Migraines				Tension-type headaches			
Trigger factors	[<10%]	[10–25%]	[<26–50%]	[>50%]	[<10%]	[<10–25%]	[26–50%]	[>50%]
Sleep problems — tiredness	-	-	1	1	-	-	1	1(ii)
Late nights	-	2	-	-	-	-	1 (iii)	-
Tiredness, exhaustion	1	1	2	2	-	1 (v)	2 (vi)	2
Physical or sexual activity	3 (i)	4 (iv)	3	-	3 (v)(vi)	1 (iii)	2	-
Altered posture	1	2	-	-	1 (iii)	-	-	-
Cough, sneeze	1	-	-	-	-	1	-	-
Neck problems	1	-	-	-	2 (ii)(iii)	-	-	-
Head trauma	1 (i)	-	-	-	-	-	-	-
Infections	-	1	-	-	-	1 (ii)	-	-
Menstruation	-	2 (i)	7 (i)	4 (i)	-	1 (ii)	4 (iii)	1
Ovulation	1	-	-	-	-	-	-	-
Contraceptive pill	-	-	3	-	-	-	2	-
Weather	2 (i)	4	4 (i)	2	1 (i)	1 (ii)	4	-
Wind	1	-	1	-	1c	-	-	-
Heat	1	-	1	-	-	-	1 (iii)	-
No triggers	-	1	2 (vii)	-	-	-	-	-

* The numerals indicate how many studies were included.
(i) A study on migraine with aura.
(ii) A study without migraine but on headache.
(iii) A study without differentiating between migraine/headache, and other headache.
(iv) Three studies of migraine with aura.
(v) A study of tension and migraine without aura.
(vi) A study of tension and migraine without aura.
(vii) In 2 studies of migraine with aura.
(Source: adapted and modified from Holzhammer, Wöber)[24]

been implicated as possible causes of migraines and headaches include: cigarette smoking; perfumes; watching excessive television; bright lights; loud noises; working in front of TV/VCR/computer screens; and medications, such as the oral contraceptive pill.[23, 24, 29]

Physical activity

Excercise, especially outdoors in a natural setting for fresh air and sunshine, is *highly* recommended for people who suffer headaches and migraines.

An 8-month RCT evaluated the effectiveness of a workplace educational and physical program in reducing headache, neck and shoulder pain.[30] In the study, 192 employees participated, using diaries for the daily recording of pain episodes. Compared with baseline, those randomised to education and physical exercise program, there was significant reduction in headache frequency, frequency of neck and shoulder pain and reduced analgesic drug consumption compared with the control group. The study suggests that an educational and physical program reduces headache and neck and shoulder pain in a working community.

Nutritional influences

Diet

Over a quarter of patients with migraines recognise hypoglycaemia, caffeine withdrawal and certain foods as migraine triggers.[31–34] Such triggers can include monosodium glutamate (also labelled as hydrolysed yeast extract, natural flavouring, hydrolysed vegetable protein), that is often found in soups and Chinese food. Nitrites (a preservative found in numerous meats and hot dog products), tyramines (found in wines and aged foods such as cheeses), and phenylethylamine (found in chocolate, garlic, nuts, raw onions, and seeds) comprise other potential migraine triggers. Any type of alcohol, artificial sweeteners, citrus fruits, pickled products, and vinegars are additional possible triggers. It should be noted that not everyone will have all of these foods as triggers, so a diet totally eliminating these items may not be warranted in all those suffering from migraines or headaches.

A study emphasised the need to explore diet in the precipitation of headaches in children and adolescents with migraine.[33]

The risk-associated foods that have been listed include cheeses, chocolate, citrus fruits, hot dogs, monosodium glutamate, aspartame, fatty foods, ice cream, caffeine withdrawal, and alcoholic drinks, especially red wine and beer, as potential precipitants.[34] A large-scale study of 577 patients with migraines found a definite statistical association between sensitivity to cheese/chocolate, red wine, beer but not to alcohol in general.[35] Tyramine, phenylethylamine, histamine, nitrites and sulphites are involved in the mechanism of food intolerance headache, by influencing the release of serotonin and noradrenalin, causing vasoconstriction or vasodilatation, or by direct stimulation of trigeminal ganglia, brainstem, and cortical neuronal pathways.[36] This study found 93% of 88 children with severe frequent migraine recovered on oligo-antigenic diets, with recurrence of migraines after reintroduction of the suspected foods, suggesting an allergenic, not idiosyncratic, response. Associated symptoms which improved in addition to headache included abdominal pain, behaviour disorder, fits, asthma, and eczema. Patients who developed migraines by non-specific factors, such as blows to the head, exercise, and flashing lights, no longer experienced migraines while they were on the diet.

A later study by the same group demonstrated similar findings on 45 children with migraines and epilepsy.[37] The oligo-antigenic diet alleviated most symptoms of migraines, abdominal pains, hyperkinetic behaviour and epilepsy.

However, an evaluation of the scientific evidence of 13 oral challenge tests to dietary biogenic amines in susceptible patients[38] found no relation with migraines, some of the studies were poorly designed and more research is required to support this association.

Patients with headaches, abdominal symptoms and/or obscure neurologic dysfunction such as ataxia may warrant testing for anti-gliadin antibodies.[39]

Missing a meal can cause hypoglycaemia (low blood sugar) which in turn can precipitate a migraine, so it is important to eat regularly and not miss any meals.

Caffeine consumption and withdrawal are also known causes of headaches and migraines and, thus, caffeine is best minimised or avoided.[40] If consuming caffeine, increasing water intake helps as dehydration from caffeine may also contribute to headaches and migraines.[41]

Fluids

Dehydration is commonly believed to result in headache.[42] A recent pilot study has demonstrated a significant reduction in the total number of hours and intensity of headache episodes after increased water intake.[43] Further studies are required though.

Nutritional supplements

Riboflavin (vitamin B2)

For many migraine sufferers, taking riboflavin regularly may help decrease the frequency and shorten the duration of migraine headaches. Several studies have demonstrated benefits of riboflavin supplement as a prophylactic in reducing migraine frequency. A pilot trial followed up with a randomised placebo-controlled trial by the same group found patients taking a daily dose of 400mgs riboflavin were significantly better for migraine prophylaxis over placebo.[44, 45] The number of days with migraine was halved in approximately 60% of the participants taking riboflavin compared with 15% in placebo group.[45] A more recent study of 23 patients also demonstrated a reduction of headache frequency by 50% from an average of 4 days a month to 2 days following 3–6 months of treatment with 400mgs of riboflavin daily.[46]

The use of medications by headache sufferers reduced by one-third, but there was no change in headache intensity duration. Adverse events reported from the studies investigating riboflavin have been limited to diarrhoea and polyuria, both occurring in extremely low numbers and is generally well tolerated. Although it appears to have low toxicity no long-term safety data exist for vitamin B2. Further research is warranted to assess the role of lower doses of riboflavin.

Magnesium (Mg^{++})

Magnesium deficiency

It has been reported that studies of low-brain magnesium have been associated with migraine sufferers.[47] Hence magnesium supplementation may play a role in the prophylaxis and treatment of migraines. Magnesium deficiency is reported in some studies of migraine sufferers and is suspected in promoting muscle irritability and sensitivity during migraine attacks.[48, 49] Reduced intracellular free magnesium in the brain and body tissues of migraine sufferers may cause instability of neuronal function and thus increasing the risk of developing an attack.[50]

Recent review of the literature suggest deficiencies in magnesium play a role in the pathogenesis of migraine headaches that the use of intravenous and oral magnesium could provide a simple, inexpensive, safe option for acute and preventative treatment.[51]

Oral magnesium

The first RCT of Mg^{++} for migraine prevention involved only 20 participants and was positive. The active therapy was 360mg Mg^{++} pyrrolidone carboxylic acid divided TDS.[52] A further, earlier, RCT of 81 migraine patients, who were randomised to receive either 600mg/day of magnesium or placebo for 12 weeks, demonstrated that by 9–12 weeks there was significant reduction in frequency and duration of migraine attacks, and reduction in medication use.[53] Magnesium daily intake demonstrated a 41.6% improvement versus 15.8% for placebo. In a further double-blind placebo-controlled trial designed for migraine prophylaxis involving 69 participants taking 486mg Mg^{++} there was no benefit for Mg^{++} observed at the end of the 3-month treatment phase.[54] The positive responser rate was 28.6% in the magnesium group and 29.4% in placebo subjects with respect to the primary efficacy endpoint. Diarrhoea was reported in significant numbers of both patients receiving placebo (23.5%) and double the risk in patients receiving magnesium (45.7%). The high rate in the active arms suggests that a poorly absorbed magnesium preparation added to the negative outcome.[54, 55]

In a placebo-controlled RCT with children and adolescents aged 3 to 17 years, magnesium oxide was administered at a dose of 9mg/kg divided TID.[56] Approximately three-quarters of the eligible participants completed the study, with a significant decrease in trend in headache days in the active treatment group versus placebo. However, given the small participant numbers this study did not unequivocally determine whether oral magnesium oxide was or was not superior to placebo in preventing frequent migrainous headache in children.

Reports that debate the conflicting data from migraine treatments of patients as either being likely to respond (low levels) or unlikely to respond (normal levels) allude to the notion that low levels of intracellular Mg^{++} ion and serum ionised Mg^{++} may correlate with the element's efficacy.[57, 58, 59]

In a study designed to determine Mg^{++} effects on sumatriptan non-responders (83% of who had low ionised Mg^{++} levels), Cady and colleagues found that although ionised Mg^{++} levels could be normalised intravenously; a daily dose of 250mg of oral magnesium taurate for 5.5 months failed to maintain normal levels.[60] It was recommended that a daily dose of 600mg of chelated or slow-release oral Mg^{++} be employed for sustained supplementation.[61]

IV magnesium

A number of trials indicate IV magnesium may play a valid role in the acute treatment of severe migraine, especially in a hospital setting. The use of IV magnesium sulfate has been explored for treatment of acute severe migraine attacks but caution and further research is required with its potential use.[61]

A recent single-blind, placebo-controlled trial of 30 patients, with acute moderate or severe migraine attacks, were randomised to receive 1g intravenous magnesium sulfate (given over 15 minutes) or 10 mL of 0.9% saline intravenously.[62] Those in the placebo group with persisting complaints of pain or nausea and vomiting after 30 minutes also received 1g magnesium sulfate intravenously. All patients in the treatment group responded to treatment with magnesium sulfate with significant reduction in pain in up to 87% of patients and all patients (100%), accompanying symptoms disappeared. Symptoms persisted in the placebo group, such as nausea, irritability or photophobia, who then responded to the

IV magnesium treatment causing symptoms to completely disappear. The authors concluded that 1g intravenous magnesium sulfate is an efficient, safe, and well-tolerated drug in the treatment of migraine attacks.[62]

Coenzyme Q_{10} (CoQ_{10})

CoQ_{10} has been used in neurologic and non-neurologic conditions and is considered to have an acceptable safety, tolerance and non-adverse effects profile.

A recent, not dose-ranging, RCT study reported the use of CoQ_{10} involving 42 participants given either a non-commercially available liquid formulation of water-dispersed nano-particles comprising a super-cooled melt of CoQ_{10} with modified physicochemical properties taken 300mg/day divided TID or placebo.[63] Migraine attack frequency in month 4 was reduced ≥50% in 47.6% of patients in the active arm (i.e. those taking CoQ_{10}) as compared to 14.4% for placebo. Adverse events were not statistically different between the 2 treatment groups. One participant who was in the treatment group withdrew and was not considered in the analysis due to a cutaneous allergy to CoQ_{10}.

In a recent study of CoQ_{10} deficiency and response to supplementation in paediatric and adolescent migraine it was suggested that determination of deficiency and subsequent supplementation may result in clinical improvement.[64] However further analysis involving more scientifically rigorous methodology is required.

Fish oils

A well-performed double-blind, cross-over study consisting of a 2-month period on fish oil supplementation, 1 month wash-out period, and 2 months of placebo (olive oil), demonstrated significant reduction in duration and severity of headaches in adolescents with recurrent migraines in both the treatment and placebo group.[65] The authors concluded that the marked benefit in both groups compared with baseline was beyond a placebo effect and suggested that olive oil may also demonstrate benefit for recurrent migraines.[65]

Herbal medicines

Feverfew (*Tanacetum parthenium*)

Feverfew is a popular herbal remedy recommended for the prevention of migraine.

There have been some positive trials, such as a positive trial showing efficacy for feverfew in migraine sufferers[66] and a positive trial using feverfew CO_2 extract (MIG-99, 6.25mg TID).[67] A reduction in headache attacks per month was reported during the second and third recording periods (from 4.8 attacks to 2.9 with MIG-99 versus 3.5 attacks with placebo [a reduction in attacks per month of 1.9 versus 1.3]) (P = 046, and OR 3.4).[67] Greater than 50% reduction in headache attacks per 28 days occurred in 30.3% of the feverfew treatment group and 17.3% of the placebo arm, a therapeutic gain of 13% (P = 047). Adverse events occurred in 8.4% of the participants receiving feverfew and 10.2% of placebo controls.

However, the totality of evidence, including systematic reviews, does not support feverfew as representing an unequivocally effective therapy for migraine, nor has its safety with long-term use been established. One systematic review[68] of feverfew showed potential for prophylaxis against migraine attacks, however a more recent Cochrane review[69] of all the literature found most trials lacked methodological quality and its efficacy was concluded not to have been established. Adequate long-term studies, including extension safety trials, are warranted.

A RCT study to determine the efficacy for migraine prophylaxis of a compound containing a combination of riboflavin, magnesium, and feverfew was recently completed.[70] The combination compound provided a daily dose of riboflavin 400mg, magnesium 300mg, and feverfew 100mg. The placebo contained 25mg riboflavin alone. The study documented that 49 participants completed the 3-month trial. For the primary outcome measure, a 50% or greater reduction in migraines was observed, however, there was no difference between active and placebo (riboflavin) group, achieved by 10 (42%) and 11 (44%) participants respectively. Similarly, there was no significant difference in secondary outcome measures, for active versus placebo groups, respectively. Also, no change in mean number of migraines, migraine days, migraine index, or triptan doses was observed. Compared to baseline, however, both groups showed a significant reduction in number of migraines, migraine days, and migraine index.[70] It was concluded that riboflavin (25mg) showed an effect comparable to a combination of riboflavin (400mg), magnesium (300mg), and feverfew (100mg).

Physical therapies

Musculoskeletal manipulation

Non-invasive physical treatments are often used to treat common types of chronic/recurrent headache. Cervicogenic headaches are well documented and respond well to daily walking to develop better postural alignment, stretching, and physical therapies, such as manipulation.[71] Spinal manipulative therapy (SMT) appears to have a better effect than massage for cervicogenic headache. It also appears that SMT has an effect comparable to commonly used first-line prophylactic prescription medication for tension-type headache and migraine headache. This conclusion emerged from several trials of adequate methodological quality.[71]

A recent Cochrane review of 22 studies with a total of 2628 patients (age 12 to 78 years) met the inclusion criteria.[72] Five types of headache were studied namely — migraine, tension-type, cervicogenic, a mix of migraine and tension-type, and post-traumatic headache. It was reported that a few non-invasive physical treatments may be effective as prophylactic treatments for chronic/recurrent headaches. Based on trial results, these treatments appear to be associated with little risk of serious adverse effects.[72] The authors concluded the clinical effectiveness and cost-effectiveness of non-invasive physical treatments require further research using scientifically rigorous methods as there was significant heterogeneity of the studies included in the review.

Despite these positive findings, a more recent systematic review looked at the role for cervical musculoskeletal dysfunction in migraine and based on the evidence the review found that there is currently no convincing evidence to confirm this phenomenon in humans.[73]

Acupuncture

A recent general practice study that investigated 400 patients with chronic headache and migraine found acupuncture to be significantly effective.[74] Patients were randomised to 12 sessions of acupuncture treatment or standard medical care. Acupuncture treatment led to 34% reduction in headache severity, 15% less medication use, 25% fewer visits to GPs and 22 fewer days of headache a year compared with 16% reduction in headache severity in patients given standard care at 1-year follow-up. The acupuncture treatment appeared long-lasting.[74]

A critical review reported its findings from 13 clinical trials and agreed with previous literature reviews that the majority of studies of acupuncture for migraine research were of a poor quality, with conflicting results,[75] noting that large high-quality trials were required.

Recently a number of additional conflicting studies have been conducted on the use of acupuncture to treat and prevent headaches.[76–80] Nevertheless acupuncture has been increasingly advocated and used in Western countries for migraine treatment, but the evidence of its effectiveness remains weak. A large variability of treatments is present in published studies and no acu-point selection according to Traditional Chinese Medicine (TCM) has ever been investigated so far. Therefore, the low level of evidence of acupuncture effectiveness might partly have depended on the inappropriate treatments that have been investigated in the most recent past.[76, 77] In 1 trial, acupuncture was reported to be no more effective than sham acupuncture in reducing migraine headaches although both interventions were more effective than a waiting list control.[76] The effectiveness of a true acupuncture treatment according to TCM in migraine without aura, comparing it to a standard mock acupuncture protocol, an accurate mock acupuncture healing ritual, and untreated controls, has demonstrated significant efficacy.[78, 79, 80]

Idiopathic headache

A Cochrane review[81] of 26 trials including a total of 1151 patients concluded that the existing evidence supported the value of acupuncture for the treatment of idiopathic headaches. However, the quality and amount of evidence was not fully convincing.

Chronic-tension headache

A recent Cochrane review of the literature including 11 trials of 2317 participants (mean age 62 years) found overall statistically significant benefits over control for chronic-tension headache (reduction in number of days and pain intensity) in 2 large major trials, but only small benefits when compared with sham acupuncture in 5 smaller trials.[82]

Migraine prophylaxis

A recent Cochrane meta-analysis of the literature identified 22 trials inclusive of 4419 participants and found overall 14 trials comparing 'true' acupuncture with sham acupuncture, and there were no statistically significant differences, but in 4 trials acupuncture was superior to proven prophylactic drug treatment, associated with slightly better outcomes and fewer adverse effects in the acupuncture group. The authors concluded the 'evidence in support of acupuncture for migraine prophylaxis was considered promising but insufficient …' and '… should be considered a treatment option for patients willing to undergo this treatment'.[83]

Conclusion

What CAM modalities can be stated to be evidence-based and hence efficacious for the treatment of migraine and headache?

There is solid evidence that mind–body modalities have significant efficacy in the treatment of migraines and headaches. Health practitioners have access to a wide range of well-evidenced behavioural and mind–body therapies for the treatment of headache in children and adults. Combined with knowledge on documented alimentary and non-alimentary trigger factors, practitioners can effectively treat and prevent migraines and headaches with alternative treatment options.

The overall evidence for integrative and complementary therapies is summarised in Table 17.2. Lifestyle, exercise, relaxation and psychological therapies, as well as dietary factors, play an important role in the management of headache and migraine. With respect to supplements, there currently is at best level II evidence for most of the supplement compounds discussed in this chapter. Level II evidence represents limited evidence from a single randomised trial, or non-randomised trials or multiple trials with inconsistent outcomes. No firm consensus yet exists as to the relative treatment efficacy of these multiple agents, but given the number of patients, data consistency, or lack thereof, we tentatively suggest that the rank order may be of the order of — Mg^{++} > feverfew > riboflavin > CoQ_{10}. At present, TCM-based acupuncture may offer the best modality of its kind for the treatment of migraines and headaches.

Table 17.2 Levels of evidence for lifestyle and complementary medicines/therapies in the management of migraines and/or headaches

Modality	Level I	Level II	Level IIIa	Level IIIb	Level IIIc	Level IV	Level V
Lifestyle modifications							
[diet, exercise, smoking cessation, stress management]		x					
Behavioural interventions		x					
Sleep restoration			x				
Environmental factors							
Visual stimulus (trigger)			x				
Mind–body medicine		x					
Psychological support (e.g. CBT]	x						
Relaxation therapies	x						
Biofeedback		x					
Autogenic training	x						
Physical activity/ exercise							
Exercise program at work		x					
Nutrition							
Amine free diet		x					
Oligoantigenic diet		x					
Gluten sensitivity			x				
Food, wine, beer triggers			x				

Continued

Table 17.2 Levels of evidence for lifestyle and complementary medicines/therapies in the management of migraines and/or headaches—cont'd

Modality	Level I	Level II	Level IIIa	Level IIIb	Level IIIc	Level IV	Level V
Caffeine withdrawal				x			
Food colourings				x			
Fluid/water intake				x			
Herbal medicines							
Feverfew	x (+/–)	x					
Fish oil/Olive oil		x					
Supplements							
B2 Riboflavin		x					
Coenzyme Q_{10}		x					
Magnesium (oral)	x						
Physical therapies							
Acupuncture	x						
Spinal manipulative therapy	x (+/-)	x					

Level I — from a systematic review of all relevant randomised controlled trials — meta-analyses.
Level II — from at least 1 properly designed randomised controlled clinical trial.
Level IIIa — from well-designed pseudo-randomised controlled trials (alternate allocation or some other method).
Level IIIb — from comparative studies (including systematic reviews of such studies) with concurrent controls and allocation not randomised, cohort studies, case-control studies, or interrupted time series with a parallel control group.
Level IIIc — from comparative studies with historical control, 2 or more single-arm studies or interrupted time series without a parallel control group.
Level IV — opinions of respected authorities based on clinical experience, descriptive studies or reports of expert committees.
Level V — represents minimal evidence that represents testimonials.

Clinical tips handout for patients — migraines and headaches

1 Lifestyle advice

Sleep

- Restore normal sleep patterns. Most adults require about 7 hours sleep; early to bed, about 9–10 p.m., and awake with sunrise. (See Chapter 22 for more advice.)

Sunshine

- Amount of exposure varies with local climate.
- At least 15 minutes of sunshine needed daily for vitamin D and melatonin production, especially before 10 a.m. and after 3 p.m. when the sun exposure is safest during summer. More exposure in winter is required when supplementation may need to be considered.
- Ensure gradual adequate skin exposure to sun; avoid sunscreen and excess clothing to maximise levels of vitamin D.
- More time in the sun is required for dark skinned people.
- Ensure direct exposure to about 10% of the body (hands, arms, face), without sunscreen and not through glass.
- Vitamin D is obtained in the diet from fatty fish, eggs, liver and fortified foods (some milks and margarines). It is unlikely that adequate vitamin D concentrations can be obtained from diet alone.

2 Physical activity/exercise

- Exercise at least 30–60 minutes daily. If exercise is not regular, commence with 5 minutes daily and slowly build up to at least 30 minutes. Outdoor exercise with nature, fresh air and sunshine is ideal (e.g. brisk walking, light jogging, cycling, swimming, stretching, weight bearing exercises), especially in outdoor parkland.
- A regular exercise program and stretching at work can be particularly helpful.
- Yoga may be of help; other examples include qiqong and tai chi.
- Pilates and Alexander technique can improve posture, which may help reduce cervicogenic headaches.

3 Mind–body medicine (most helpful)

- Stress management program; for example, 6 x 40 minute sessions for patients to understand the nature of their symptoms, the symptoms' relationship to stress and the practice of regular relaxation exercises.
- Regular meditation practice at least 10-20 minutes daily.
- Biofeedback and autogenic training can be helpful.

Breathing

- Be aware of breathing from time to time. Notice if tendency to hold breath or over-breathe.
- Always aim to relax breath and the muscles around chest wall.

Rest and stress management

Recurrent stress may cause a return of symptoms. Relaxation is important for a full and lasting recovery.

- Reduce workload and resolve conflicts.
- Contact family, friends, church or social groups for support.
- Listening to relaxation music helps.
- Regular relaxation massage therapy helps.
- Cognitive behavioural therapy and psychotherapy are particularly helpful.
- Hypnotherapy and biofeedback may be helpful.

Fun

- It is important to have fun in life. Joy can be found even in the simplest tasks, such as being with friends with a sense of humour funny movies/videos, comedy, hobbies, dancing, playing with pets and children.
- Try to maintain an 'easy-going approach to life'; avoid feeling time-pressured or rushed.

4 Dietary changes

- Low amine and salicylate diet (see Chapter 2 for a list of amine and salicylate-free foods).
- In some individuals food intolerances (e.g. gluten) may cause headaches. Discuss with your practitioner.
- Consume frequent, small healthy snacks and avoid missing meals. This can help reduce onset of migraine attacks.
- Eat fruit (>2/day) and vegetables (>5/day) — variety of colours and those in season.
- Eat legumes (e.g. beans, lentils, chickpeas).
- Eat nuts, seeds, sprouts (e.g. alfalfa, mung beans).

- Increase fish intake (sardines, tuna, salmon, cod, mackerel), especially deep sea fish. Canned fish is quite acceptable.
- Consume lean red meat intake (preferably lamb, kangaroo) and white meat (e.g. free range organic chicken fillets).
- Use only cold-pressed olive oil and avocado instead of butter or margarine.
- Enjoy dark chocolate, but avoid excessive quantities due to amine content.
- Consume low-GI wholegrains/cereals (variety); rice (brown, basmati, Mahatma, Doongara); traditional rolled oats; buckwheat flour; wholegrain organic breads (rye bread, Essene, spelt, Kamut), brown pasta; millet; amaranth etc.
- Avoid any food intolerances.
- Consume low-fat dairy products such as yoghurt and cheeses, unless there is a dairy intolerance.
- Drink more filtered water, 1–2 litres a day, and teas, especially green tea, black tea, and herbal teas (e.g. chamomile, peppermint).

Avoid

- Hydrogenated fats, salt, fast foods, sugar such as soft drinks, lollies, biscuits, cakes and processed foods (e.g. white bread, white pasta, pastries).
- More than 1 cup of coffee daily; reduce intake slowly as caffeine withdrawal can cause onset of headaches.
- Excess alcohol — minimise intake to no more than 1 glass daily (avoid red wine).
- Food and chemical additives — preservatives, colourings and flavourings (e.g. monosodium glutamate, sulfites, sulphur dioxide, preservative 220 in wines).
- Artificial sweeteners. For sweetener try honey (e.g. manuka, yellow box and stringy bark have the lowest GI).

5 Environment

- Do not smoke and avoid smoking environments.
- Avoid environmental pollutants, chemicals, at work and in the home.
- Instigate measures to cool down during hot weather.
- Have a regular daily exercise regime, and get plenty of fresh air and sunshine.
- Some people are sensitive to indoor pollutants, such as renovations that can cause 'Sick Building Syndrome'. Headaches are a feature of this.
- Avoid excessive computer work, bright lights and television use.

6 Physical therapies

- Acupuncture may help — improves general wellbeing and can alleviate headaches.
- Spinal manipulative therapy may be of help.

7 Supplements

Vitamins

Riboflavin, vitamin B2

- Indication: for prevention of headaches.
- Dosage: children: up to 100mg daily in divided doses. Adults 400mg daily; probably safe in pregnancy and lactation.
- Results: may take 2–4 weeks.
- Side-effects: not common. Diarrhoea, gastrointestinal irritation, nausea, vomiting; excessive urination. Vitamin Bs can cause dark yellow discolouration of urine.
- Contraindications: avoid in known vitamin B toxicity.
- **Hint:** Do not take vitamin B2 alone. Use with 1 multi-B vitamin.

Pro-vitamin

Coenzyme Q_{10}

- Indication: migraines, headaches. May also assist cardiac muscle, heart failure, hypertension, Parkinson's disease and immune system.
- Dosage: 100mgs 1–3 times daily in adults. Children: up to 50mg daily. Avoid in pregnant and lactating women.
- Results: 7–14 days.
- Side-effects: rare. Gastrointestinal irritation, nausea, vomiting, and diarrhoea in very high doses.
- Contraindications: avoid prior to surgery; care with concomitant use of anti-hypertensive medication as it lowers blood pressure.

Minerals

Magnesium oxide and calcium (best provided together)

- Indication: headaches; insomnia; may lower blood pressure; be useful in anxiety; restless sleep; restless legs and cramps.
- Dosage: children: up to 65–120mg daily in divided doses. Adults: 350–400mg daily to twice daily as tolerated, including pregnant and lactating women.
- Results: immediately or 1–3 days.
- Side-effects: oral magnesium can cause gastrointestinal irritation, nausea,

vomiting, and diarrhea. The dosage varies from person to person. Although rare, toxic levels can cause low blood pressure, thirst, heart arrhythmia, drowsiness and weakness.
- Contraindications: patients with kidney disease; if you have high blood calcium or magnesium levels (e.g. in cancer or kidney diseases).

Fish oils

- Indication: may help inflammation, bronchospasm, asthma.
- Dosage: 3–7g daily as tolerated. If consuming fish 2–3 times a week, a 1000mg capsule per day may be sufficient.
- Results: 4–7 days.
- Side-effects: often well tolerated especially if taken with meals. Very mild and rare side-effects; for example, gastrointestinal upset; fishy burps; allergic reactions (e.g. rash, breathing problems if allergic to seafood); blood thinning effects in very high doses > 10g daily (may need to stop fish oil supplements 2 weeks prior to surgery).
- Contraindications: sensitivity reaction to seafood; drug interactions; caution when taking high doses of fish oils >4g per day together with warfarin (your doctor will check your INR test).

Herbs

Feverfew

- Indication: may prevent headaches and migraines.
- Dosage: adults 50–150mg/day, up to 3 months use. Avoid in children, pregnant and lactating women.
- Results: 14–28 days.
- Side-effects: uncommon. Mouth ulcers, allergic reactions, rashes, gastrointestinal irritation, nausea, vomiting, and diarrhoea.
- Contraindications: avoid 2 weeks prior to surgery and concomitant use with blood thinners.

References

1 Andlin-Sobocki P, Jönsson B, Wittchen HU, et. al. Cost of disorders of the brain in Europe. Eur J Neurol 2005;12:1–27.

2 Jensen R, Stovner LJ. Epidemiology and comorbidity of headache. Lancet Neurol 2008;7(4):354–61.

3 Speciali JG, Eckeli AL, Dach F. Tension-type headache. Expert Rev Neurother 2008;8(5):839–53.

4 Sierpina V, Astin J, Giordano J. Mind–body therapies for headache. Am Fam Physician 2007;76(10):1518–22.

5 Hoodin F, Brines BJ, Lake AE III, et. al. Behavioural self-management in an inpatient headache treatment unit: increasing adherence and relationship to changes in affective distress. Headache 2000;40(5):377–83.

6 Wahbeh H, Elsas SM, Oken BS. Mind–body interventions: applications in neurology. Neurology 2008;70(24):2321–8.

7 Fumal A, Schoenen J. Tension-type headache: current research and clinical management. Lancet Neurol 2008;7(1):70–83.

8 Holroyd KA, Penzien DB. Client variables and behavioural treatment of recurrent tension headaches: a meta-analytic review. J Behav Med 1986;9:515–36.

9 Holroyd KA, Martin PR. Psychological treatments for tension-type headache. In: Olesen J, Tfelt-Hansen P, Welch KMA. The Headaches (2nd edn). Lippincott Williams & Wilkins, Philadelphia, 2000:643–49.

10 Blanchard EB, Appelbaum KA, Guarnieri P, et. al. Two studies of the long-term follow-up of minimal-therapist contact treatments of vascular and tension headache. J Consult Clin Psychol 1988;56:427–32.

11 Schoenen J, Pholien P, Maertens de Noordhout A. EMG biofeedback in tension-type headache: is the 4th session predictive of outcome? Cephalalgia 1985;5:132–33.

12 Holroyd KA. Tension-type headache, cluster headache, and miscellaneous headaches: Psychological and behavioural techniques. In: Olesen J, Tfelt-Hansen P, Welch KMA. The Headaches. Raven Press, New York, 1993:515–20.

13 Penzien DB, Rains JC, Andrasik F. Behavioural management of recurrent headache: three decades of experience and empiricism. Appl Psychophysiol Biofeedback 2002;27(2):163–81.

14 Astin JA. Mind body therapies for the management of pain. Clin J Pain 2004;20:27–32.

15 Helm-Hylkema H, Orlebeke JF, Enting LA, et. al. Effects of behaviour therapy on migraine and plasma beta-endorphin in young migraine patients. Psychoneuroendocrinology 1990;15(1):39–45.

16 Duckro PN, Cantwell-Simmonds E. A review of studies evaluating biofeedback and relaxation training in the management of pediatric headache. Headache 1989;29:428–33.

17 Eccleston C, Yorke L, Morley S, et. al. Psychological therapies for the management of chronic and recurrent pain in children and adolescents. Cochrane Database Syst Rev 2003;(1):CD003968.

18 Kanji N, White AR, Ernst E. Autogenic training for tension type headaches: a systematic review of controlled trials. Complement Ther Med 2006;14(2):144–50.

19 http://www.aan.com/professionals/practice/pdfs/gl0089.pdf (accessed July 2008).

20 Goslin RE, Gray RN, McCrory DC, et. al. Behavioural and Physical Treatments for Migraine Headache. Technical Review 2.2, February 1999. (Prepared for the Agency for Health Care Policy and Research under Contract No. 290-94-2025. Available from the National Technical Information Service; NTIS Accession No. 127946).

21 Kelman L, Rains JC. Headache and sleep: examination of sleep patterns and complaints in a large clinical sample of migraineurs. Headache 2005;45:904–10.

22 Paiva T, Farinha A, Martins A, et. al. Chronic headaches and sleep disorders. Arch Intern Med 1997;157(15):1701–5.

23 Wöber C, Holzhammer J, Zeitlhofer J, et. al. Trigger factors of migraine and tension-type headache: experience and knowledge of the patients. J Headache Pain 2006;7(4):188–95.

24 Holzhammer J, Wöber C. Non-alimentary trigger factors of migraine and tension-type headache. Schmerz 2006;20(3):226–37.
25 Spierings EL, Ranke AH, Honkoop PC. Precipitating and aggravating factors of migraine versus tension-type headache. Headache 2001;41(6):554–8.
26 Phipps RA. A comparison of two studies reporting the prevalence of the sick building syndrome in New Zealand and England. NZ Med J 1999;112:228–30.
27 Ando M. Indoor air and human health--sick house syndrome and multiple chemical sensitivity. Kokuritsu Iyakuhin Shokuhin Eisei Kenkyusho Hokoku 2002;(120):6–38.
28 Mukamal KJ, Wellenius GA, Suh HH, et. al. Weather and air pollution as triggers of severe headaches. Neurology 2009;72(10):922–7.
29 Harle DE, Shepherd AJ, Evans BJ. Visual stimuli are common triggers of migraine and are associated with pattern glare. Headache 2006;46(9):1431–40.
30 Mongini F, Ciccone G, Rota E, et. al. Effectiveness of an educational and physical programme in reducing headache, neck and shoulder pain: a workplace controlled trial. Cephalalgia 2008;28:541–52.
31 Kelman L. The triggers or precipitants of the acute migraine attack. Cephalalgia 2007;27(5):394–402.
32 Patel RM, Sarma R, Grimsley E. Popular sweetener sucralose as a migraine trigger. Headache 2006;46(8):1303–4.
33 Torelli P, Manzoni GC. Fasting headache. Correct Pain Headache Rep 2010;14(4):284–91.
34 Millichap JG, Yee MM. The diet factor in pediatric and adolescent migraine. Pediatr Neurol 2003;28(1):9–15.
35 Peatfield RC. Relationships between food, wine and beer-precipitated migrainous headaches. Headache 1995;35(6):355–7.
36 Egger J, Carter CM, Wilson J, et. al. Is migraine food allergy? A double-blind controlled trial of oligoantigenic diet treatment. Lancet 1983;2(8355):865–9.
37 Egger J, Carter CM, Soothill JF, et. al. Oligoantigenic diet treatment of children with epilepsy and migraine. J Pediatr 1989;114(1):51–8.
38 Jansen SC, van Dusseldorp M, Bottema KC, et. al. Intolerance to dietary biogenic amines: a review. Ann Allergy Asthma Immunol 2003;91(3):233–40.
39 Hadjivassiliou M, Grunewald RA, Lawden M, et. al. Headache in CNS white matter abnormalities associated with gluten sensitivity. Neurol 2001;56:385–8.
40 Mueller LL. Diagnosing and managing migraine headache. J Am Osteopath Assoc 2007;107(10 Suppl 6):ES10–6.
41 Silverman K, Evans SM, Strain EC, et. al. Withdrawal syndrome after the double-blind cessation of caffeine consumption. NEJM 1992;327(16):1109–14.
42 Maughan RJ. Impact of mild dehydration on wellness and on exercise performance. Eur J Clin Nutr 2003;57(Suppl 2):S19-S23.
43 Spigt MG, Kuijper EC, Schayck CP, et. al. Increasing the daily water intake for the prophylactic treatment of headache: a pilot trial. Eur J Neurol 2005;12(9):715–18.
44 Schoenen J, Lenaerts M, Bastings E. High-dose riboflavin as a prophylactic treatment of migraine: results of an open pilot study. Cephalalgia 1994;14:328–9.
45 Schoenen J, Jacquy J, Lenaerts M. Effectiveness of high-dose riboflavin in migraine prophylaxis. A randomised controlled trial. Neurology 1998;50:466–70.
46 Boehnke C, Reuter U, Flach U, et. al. High-dose riboflavin treatment is efficacious in migraine prophylaxis: an open study in a tertiary care centre. Eur J Neurol 2004;11(7):475–7.
47 Evans RW, Taylor FR. 'Natural' or alternative medications for migraine prevention. Headache 2006;46(6):1012–8.
48 Thomas J, Tomb E, Thomas E, et. al. Migraine treatment by oral magnesium intake and correction of the irritation of buccofacial and cervical muscles as a side effect of mandibular imbalance. Magnes Res 1994;7(2):123–7.
49 Thomas J, Thomas E, Tomb E. Serum erythrocyte magnesium concentrations and migraine. Magnes Res 1992;5(2):127–30.
50 Welch KM, Ramadan NM. Mitochondria, magnesium and migraine. J Neurol.Sci 1995;134(1-2):9–14.
51 Sun-Edelstein C, Mauskop A. Role of magnesium in the pathogenesis and treatment of migraine. Expert Rev Neurother 2009 Mar;9(3):369–79.
52 Facchinetti F, Sances G, Borella P, et. al. Magnesium prophylaxis of menstrual migraine: Effects on intracellular magnesium. Headache 1991;31:298–301.
53 Peikert A, Wilimzig C, Köhne-Volland R. Prophylaxis of migraine with oral magnesium- results from a prospective multi-center, placebo-controlled and double-blind, randomised study. Cephalagia 1996;16(4):257–63.
54 Pfafferath V, Wessely P, Meyer C, et. al. Magnesium in the prophylaxis of migraine—A double-blind, placebo-controlled study. Cephalalgia 1996;16: 436–40.
55 Mauskop A. Editorial: Evidence linking magnesium deficiency to migraines. Cephalalgia 1999;19: 766–67.
56 Wang F, Van Den Eeden SK, Ackerson LM, et. al. Oral magnesium oxide prophylaxis of frequent migrainous headache in children: A randomised, double-blind, placebo-controlled trial. Headache 2003;43:601–10.
57 Mazzotta G, Sarchielli P, Alberti A, et. al. Intracellular Mg++ concentration and electromyographical ischemic test in juvenile headache. Cephalalgia 1999;19:802–9.
58 Mauskop A, Altura BT, Cracco RQ, et. al. Deficiency in serum ionised magnesium but not total magnesium in patients with migraines. Possible role of ICa2+/IMg2+ ratio. Headache 1993;33:135–38.
59 Mauskop A, Altura BT, Altura BM. Serum ionised magnesium in serum ionised calcium/ionised magnesium ratios in women with menstrual migraine. Headache 2002;42:242–8.
60 Cady RK, Farmer K, Altura BT, et. al. The effect of magnesium on the responsiveness of migraineurs to a 5-HT1 agonist. Neurology 1998;50(Suppl 4):A340. Abstract.
61 Mauskop A, Altura BM. Role of magnesium in the pathogenesis and treatment of migraines. Clin Neurosci 1998;5:24–7.
62 Demirkaya S, Vural O, Dora B, et. al. Efficacy of intravenous magnesium sulfate in the treatment of acute migraine attacks. Headache 2001;41(2): 171–7.
63 Sandor PS, Di Clemente L, Coppola G, et. al. Efficacy of coenzyme Q10 in migraine prophylaxis: A randomised controlled trial. Neurology 2005;64:713.
64 Hershey AD, Powers SW, Vockell AL, et. al. Coenzyme Q10 deficiency and response to supplementation in pediatric and adolescent migraine. Headache 2007;47(1):73–80.

65 Harel Z, Gascon G, Riggs S, et. al. Supplementation with omega-3 polyunsaturated fatty acids in the management of recurrent migraines in adolescents. Journal of Adolescent Health 2002;31:154–61.

66 Pfaffenrath V, Diener HC, Fischer M, et. al. The efficacy and safety of Tanacetum parthenium (feverfew) in migraine prophylaxis--a double-blind, multicentre, randomised placebo-controlled dose-response study. Cephalalgia 2002;22(7):523–32.

67 Diener HC, Pfaffenrath V, Schnitker J, et. al. Efficacy and safety of 6.25mg t.i.d. feverfew CO2-extract (MIG-99) in migraine prevention--a randomised, double-blind, multicentre, placebo-controlled study. Cephalalgia 2005;25(11):1031–41.

68 BK Vogler, MH Pittler, E Ernst. Feverfew as a preventive treatment for migraine: a systematic review. Cephalalgia 1998 18:704–8.

69 Pittler MH, Vogler BK, Ernst E. Feverfew for preventing migraine. The Cochrane Database of Systematic Reviews 2001;(4).

70 Maisels M, Blumenfeld A, Burchette R. A combination of riboflavin, magnesium, and feverfew for migraine prophylaxis: a randomised trial. Headache 2004;44(9):885–90.

71 Bronfort G, Assendelft WJ, Evans R, et. al. Efficacy of spinal manipulation for chronic headache: a systematic review. J Manipulative Physiol Ther 2001;24:457–66.

72 Bronfort G, Nilsson N, Haas M, et. al. Non-invasive physical treatments for chronic/recurrent headache. Cochrane Database Syst Rev 2004;(3):CD001878.

73 Robertson BA, Morris ME. The role of cervical dysfunction in migraine: a systematic review Cephalalgia 2008;28:474–83.

74 Vickers AJ, Rees RW, Zollman CE, et. al. Acupuncture for chronic headache in primary care: large, pragmatic, randomised trial. BMJ 2004;328(7442):744–7.

75 Griggs C, Jensen J. Effectiveness of acupuncture for migraine: critical literature review. J Adv Nurs 2006;54(4):491–501.

76 Linde K, Streng A, Jürgens S, et. al. Acupuncture for patients with migraine: a randomised controlled trial. JAMA 2005;293(17):2118–25.

77 Diener HC, Kronfeld K, Boewing G, et. al. Efficacy of acupuncture for the prophylaxis of migraine: a multicentre randomised controlled clinical trial. Lancet Neurol 2006;5(4):310–6.

78 Linde K, Streng A, Hoppe A, et. al. Treatment in a randomised multicenter trial of acupuncture for migraine (ART migraine). Forsch Komplementmed 2006;13(2):101–8.

79 Alecrim-Andrade J, Maciel-Júnior JA, Cladellas XC, et. al. Acupuncture in migraine prophylaxis: a randomised sham-controlled trial. Cephalalgia 2006;26(5):520–9.

80 Facco E, Liguori A, Petti F, et. al. Traditional acupuncture in migraine: a controlled, randomised study. Headache 2008;48(3):398–407.

81 Melchart D, Linde K, Fischer P, et. al. Acupuncture for idiopathic headache. Cochrane Database Syst Rev 2001;(1):CD001218.

82 Linde K, Allais G, Brinkhaus B, et. al. Acupuncture for tension-type headache. Cochrane Database of Systematic Reviews 2009, Issue 1. Art. No.: CD007587. doi: 10.1002/14651858.CD007587.

83 Linde K, Allais G, Brinkhaus B, et. al. Acupuncture for migraine prophylaxis. Cochrane Database of Systematic Reviews 2009, Issue 1. Art. No.: CD001218. doi: 10.1002/14651858.CD001218.pub2.

Chapter 18

Hyperlipidemia

With contribution from Professor Manohar Garg

Introduction

Hyperlipidemia is a heterogeneous disorder characterised by increased circulating levels of plasma cholesterol, low-density lipoprotein (LDL)-cholesterol, triglycerides and apolipoprotein-B (apoB) as well as reduced high-density lipoprotein (HDL)-cholesterol concentration.[1] The primary lipid abnormality involved in the development of hyperlipidemia is an increase in circulating free (non-esterified) fatty acids originating from adipose tissue, caused by a down-regulation of signalling pathways, as well as inadequate esterification and metabolism.[2] Reduced retention of fatty acids by adipose tissue results in an increased flux of non-esterified or free fatty acids (FFA) returning to the liver, stimulating hepatic triglyceride synthesis, promoting production of apoB and assembly/secretion of very low-density lipoprotein (VLDL).[3] Presence of increased plasma triglyceride concentration results in the increased production of triglyceride rich HDL particles that are more likely to be catabolized resulting in reduced HDL-cholesterol. Elevated VLDL particles are lipolyses, converted into small dense (highly atherogenic) LDL particles with reduced receptor-mediated clearance, prolonged retention in circulation and an increased susceptibility to peroxidation.[4] A strong independent association between elevated levels of LDL-cholesterol and increased incidence of coronary heart disease (CHD) has been established.[5, 6]

Prevalence and economy of burden

The World Health Organization (WHO) estimated that hyperlipidemia is associated with more than 50% of global cases of ischemic heart disease and >4 million deaths/year.[7] Most (80%) lipid disorders are related to diet and lifestyle, although familial disorders (20%) are important as well. The basic categories of hyperlipidemia include: increased LDL-cholesterol, reduced HDL-cholesterol, excess lipoprotein(a) (LPa), hypertriglyceridemia, atherogenic dyslipidemia, and mixed lipid disorders.[8] Most patients with CHD have mixed hyperlipidemia (e.g. elevated LDL-cholesterol and low HDL-cholesterol), which is also commonly seen in patients with diabetes mellitus.

The American Heart Association estimates that more than 98 million Americans have total cholesterol levels >5.18mmol/L (200mg/dL), which is considered a moderately high level, and more than 34 million adult Americans have levels >6.2mmol/L (240mg/dL), which is considered a high level necessitating treatment.[9] A recent Australian study set out to estimate the prevalence of selected diagnosed chronic diseases among patients (n = 9156) attending general practice reported prevalence of hyperlipidemia to be 15.9%.[10] Prevalence of dyslipidemia in a professional population in Beijing, China has been reported to be 52.7% for males and 42.9% for females with at least 1 abnormality in the blood lipid profile.[11]

Increasing evidence supports triglyceride (TG) concentration as a risk factor for cardiovascular disease,[12] however, the exact role of hypertriglyceridemia in the development of CVD is not known. A recent study examined the prevalence of hyperlipidemia in 5610 adults aged 20 years or older enrolled in the National Health and Nutrition Examination Surveys (NHANES) from 1999 to 2004.[13] Unadjusted prevalence rates (percentages) of TG concentration of 1.695mmol/L (150mg/dL) or higher occurred in 33.1% of participants, a concentration of 2.26mmol/L (200mg/dL) or higher occurred in 17.9% of participants, a concentration of 5.65mmol/L (500mg/dL) or higher occurred in 1.7% of participants, and a concentration of 11.3mmol/L (1000mg/dL) or higher occurred in 0.4% of participants.

The total cost associated with cardiovascular diseases and stroke in the United States, many of which are related to dyslipidemia, was estimated to exceed $400 billion in 2006.[14] Total costs include medical services (direct costs) as well as lost wages (indirect costs). While the health care system is only associated with the direct costs, these are nearly two-thirds of total costs. Costs of cardiovascular disease and stroke vary widely around the world, but in every instance, costs are substantial.[15]

Closely related to dyslipidemia is diabetes mellitus. Persons with diabetes mellitus have average LDL-cholesterol levels in excess of 140mg/dL, and most require drug therapy.[16]

In light of the increasing prevalence and health consequences associated with CHD, there is an emerging need to identify lifestyle factors and treatments which alleviate risk factors associated with its development and progression. Hyperlipidemia contributes to the underlying mechanisms of atherosclerotic disease, promoting endothelial dysfunction, oxidative stress and pro-inflammatory pathways.

The National Heart Foundation (NHF) of Australia recommends lifestyle advice supplemented by pharmacological measures for the appropriate management of hyperlipidemia.[17] Management should be based on both the individual's measured serum cholesterol levels and estimated absolute cardiovascular risk. The management aims to lower the plasma lipid levels as part of the absolute risk profile of the individual, which is particularly relevant in high-risk groups such as diabetics, people with familial hypercholesterolemia, vascular disease, chronic kidney disease and those with a family history of coronary heart disease.[17]

Table 18.1 summarises the NHF recommendation of lifestyle factors for reducing cholesterol levels and risk of developing cardiovascular disease.

Table 18.2 summarises the NHF recommendations for drug and nutrient therapy in patients with hyperlipidemia.

The NHF goals and targets for therapy, especially in people with existing coronary heart disease or other high-risk groups, are summarised as:[17]

- an emphasis on lowering LDL-C (target LDL-C of <2.0mmol/L)
- raising HDL-C levels (>1.0mmol/L)
- lowering triglyceride levels (<2.0mmol/L).

Lipid management recommendations, if adopted, have immense potential for significant health gain; however conventional lipid-modifying treatments such as statins and fibrates are underused, due to both under-prescription and non-adherence to treatment in Australia and overseas.[18, 19] The Adult Treatment Panel III (ATP III) guidelines of the US National Cholesterol Education Program (NCEP) emphasise the importance on lowering cholesterol but also place greater emphasis on lowering triglyceride levels.[20] Therefore statin monotherapy may not be sufficient to achieve the recommended non-LDL goals, especially given their modest effects on triglyceride concentration.

Table 18.1 NHF recommendation of lifestyle factors[17]

Dietary advice
• Variety of fruit, vegetables, wholegrains • Low saturated fat • Moderate amounts of polyunsaturated and monounsaturated fats and oils • Marine omega-3s (2–3 fish meals per week) • At least 2g of plant omega-3s (alpha-linolenic acid) per day • Plant sterols and stanols
Exercise — be physically active; at least 30 minutes of moderate-intensity daily
Maintain a healthy weight
Avoidance of smoking; being smoke-free

Table 18.2 NHF recommendations of drug/nutrient therapy[17]

Statins (HMG-CoA Reductase Inhibitors)	Reduces the level of LDL-C; modest triglyceride-lowering; HDL-C-raising effects
Fibrates	Reduces coronary risk, especially in people with type 2 diabetes or with features of the metabolic syndrome (particularly high triglycerides, low HDL-C or overweight) Less effective than statins in lowering LDLC May be combined with a statin
Fish oils	
Bile acid binding resins in selected patients	

Pharmacological therapies including bile acid sequestrant resins, statins, fibrates, niacin and cholesterol absorption inhibitors are common treatment options for hyperlipidemia, however the use of alternative therapies is also becoming increasingly popular. Controlled trials using a range of dietary supplements, herbal extracts and functional foods (e.g. policosanols, flaxseed, red yeast rice, guggulipid, garlic, viscous fibre, tree nuts and soy proteins) have been examined as potential complementary treatments in the management of hyperlipidemia.[21] A recent survey found that as many as 50% of respondents with elevated cholesterol levels would prefer non-prescription drugs such as garlic, yeast, or soy products as an alternative to pharmaceutical drugs.[22]

This chapter reviews the data from human clinical trials that have studied the efficacy of lifestyle changes, pharmaceutical and complementary medicines (CMs) to treat lipid aberrations. The discussion on CMs is limited to hyperlipidemias and will not encompass relationship with cardiovascular disease. Evidence for the complementary and synergistic efficacy of the combined pharmaceutical and alternative therapies is also presented.

Risk factors for hyperlipidemia

Risk factors for hyperlipidemia include:

- age (men over 45 years of age; women over 55 years)
- genetic predisposition; familial hypercholesterolemia
- disease — vascular disease (e.g. coronary heart disease, stroke, peripheral arterial disease, diabetes, hypothyroidism, chronic kidney disease)
- Aboriginal and Torres Strait Islander peoples
- menopause
- stress
- diet (e.g. high saturated fat intake)
- obesity
- lack of exercise.

Familial hypercholesterolemia

Familial hypercholesterolemia (FH) is caused by a defect on the short arm of chromosome 19 via an autosomal dominant gene.[23] FH is a result of mutations that influence the binding of LDL particles to the cell-surface receptor (LDL-receptor). Five classes of mutations in the LDL-receptor have been identified with each class having multiple alleles.[24] Class 1 mutations are null mutations as these result in a complete failure to express any LDL-receptor protein. Most common are the class 2 mutations resulting in intracellular transport defects so that the LDL-receptor does not move between the intracellular membranes (endoplasmic reticulum and the golgi membranes). Class 3 mutations involve LDL-receptors that are expressed and transported to the cell surface but fail to bind with LDL particles. Class 4 mutations are the rarest that result in failure of the LDL-receptor/LDL particle complexes be internalised. Class 5 mutations cause failure of the LDL-receptor recycling back to the cell surface. Regardless of the class of mutation, the body's ability to remove LDL-cholesterol from the bloodstream is impaired and that results in raised blood levels of LDL-cholesterol, contributing to increased risk of atherosclerosis, cardiovascular and coronary heart disease.

Symptoms of hyperlipidemia

There are no specific symptoms related to hyperlipidemia, the mainstay of diagnosis being a blood test for fasting serum cholesterol, triglyceride, HDL- and LDL-cholesterol levels. Fasting glucose and thyroid function tests are also advisable as both diabetes and hypothyroidism may contribute to raise lipids. The main signs on examination include fatty, cholesterol-rich skin deposits (xanthomas) and cholesterol deposits in the eyelids (xanthelasmas). Body mass index, waist circumference and early detection of signs of cardiovascular disease (including CVD risk factors such as hypertension) are also important hallmarks of the medical consultation in a patient with hyperlipidemia.

Pharmaceutical treatment of hyperlipidemia: key factors to consider

Compliance

Despite all of the positive research and trial data about statins and other pharmacologic interventions for treating elevated cholesterol, many patients do not take these drugs. Drug companies have reported that over 30% of patients initiated on statins do not continue their prescriptions. These reasons warrant a review of the efficacy of dietary and non-pharmacologic measures to lower cholesterol compared with pharmacologic therapy.[25]

Efficacy of treatment

Several treatment or preventive strategies may significantly reduce lipid levels; however, the reduction may not be large enough to be of clinical significance. Strategies that demonstrate sustainable efficacy over a long period of time would be of greater value than the ones to which the body develops resistance/adaptation over time. Most non-pharmaceutical treatments reduce total and LDL-cholesterol with no or little effects on triglyceride or HDL-cholesterol levels. Modalities that have multiple effects for optimising the circulating lipid profile are preferred over those that only modify 1 of the lipid risk factors.

Cost of treatment

In Australia, a Pharmaceutical Benefits Scheme (PBS) non-concessional prescription for statins, which would lower LDL-cholesterol by 30–40%, costs about $1 per day (the cost to the PBS is about $1.50–$3.00 per day). In comparison, a daily serving of phytosterol enriched spread sufficient to lower LDL-cholesterol by 10% costs the Australian consumer about 17 cents per day.[26] Cost of the treatment must be taken into consideration when looking at long-term management of hyperlipidemia.

Adverse health effects

Although statins are generally well tolerated, many clinicians believe that, in practice, statin-related side-effects occur more commonly than reported in randomised trials. Recently, researchers identified a common variant of a gene on chromosome 12 that predisposes patients to statin myopathy.[27] Another point of controversy is whether statins cause cognitive problems in some people. Yet another concern about statins and cognition was raised in a recently published Canadian study in which the researchers used a national database to conduct a retrospective analysis of nearly 300 000 patients who had undergone elective surgery. Patients who had been prescribed statins during the previous 90 days had a significantly higher risk for developing post-operative delirium than did statin non-users. Intriguingly, no other class of cardiovascular drugs was associated with postoperative delirium. The authors speculated that altered cerebral blood flow, resulting from the effects of statins on vascular smooth muscle, could be 1 mechanism for statin-induced post-operative delirium. The beneficial effects of statins in high-risk patient populations are indisputable. However, these drugs increasingly are being prescribed to asymptomatic people on the basis of somewhat arbitrary serum lipid thresholds, without regard to overall cardiovascular risk.

The most common adverse reactions associated with the use of statins are myopathy, muscle pain and weakness, which are reversible upon cessation of the statins. However, if severe, statins can cause rhabdomyolysis, severe myopathy and hepatitis in sensitive individuals.

Lifestyle factors

Diet and exercise, apart from genetic predisposition, are the most important factors contributing to the development of hyperlipidemia, and should be considered as the primary management of hyperlipidemia.

Stress management

A number of studies have demonstrated the possible link between stress and hyperlipidaemia. With prolonged stress, the pituitary-adrenal cortical system is activated to secrete cortisol. This is lipogenic and the plasma cholesterol levels can rise up to 60% above baseline.[28, 29] An American study including a survey of 187 394 respondents from the Behavioural Risk Factor Surveillance System (BRFSS), aged 35 years or older from 37 states and territories, confirmed the linear relationship between psychological distress and blood cholesterol.[30] However, whether stress is the cause or consequence of increased blood cholesterol or whether it is a casual relationship remains unclear. A recent study, in which participants were asked to increase dietary fibre intake to >30g/day; reduce saturated fat intake to <16g/day; trained to reach 70-85% of their maximum heart rate; perform strength training for 3 days/week and engage in 10-20 minutes of stress management activities daily, demonstrated a reduction in the ratio of total to HDL-cholesterol by 8.9% and plasma cholesterol lowering by 7.3%.[31]

Randomised controlled trials (RCTs) involving specific intervention with stress management alone are required to delineate further the relationship between blood lipids and stress.

Yoga

Yoga has become increasingly popular in Western cultures as a means of exercise and training fitness. It has been used clinically as a therapeutic intervention and its practice includes muscle stretching, breathing exercises, behavioural modification, and dietary control through mental discipline. An Indian RCT examined the effects of yoga and meditation on biochemical parameters of metabolic syndrome.[32] In this study, 101 participants were randomised to receive either the usual care (n = 46) or yogic intervention in addition to usual care for 3 months (n = 55). At the end of the intervention period, plasma triglyceride levels decreased from 210 to 152mg/dL and HDL-cholesterol increased from 33.4 to 44.5mg/dL in the group receiving yogic intervention.

Physical activity and exercise

A 5-year follow-up study of more than 7000 men with average age of 66, demonstrated that physical activity was associated with positive changes to lipid profile.[33] Cross-sectional and longitudinal exercise training studies indicate that 15 to 20 miles/week of brisk walking or jogging, which elicit between 5000 to 9000 kilojoules of energy expenditure per week, is associated with triglyceride lowering from 5 up to 38mg/dL and HDL-cholesterol increases of 2 to 8mg/dL. Halverstadt et. al.[34] showed that endurance exercise training induced favourable changes in plasma lipoprotein and lipid profiles independent of diet and baseline or change in body fat. Another small study involving 12 healthy unfit men and women, subjected to 6 weeks of exercise, demonstrated that endurance training results in a decrease of LDL-cholesterol by 21%, apoB levels by 19% and an increase in HDL-cholesterol by 10%.[35] Exercise training rarely alters serum cholesterol or LDL-cholesterol unless dietary fat intake is reduced and body weight loss is associated with the exercise training program, or both. The decrease in plasma triglyceride concentrations is related to baseline concentrations[36, 37, 38] with greater reductions in people, previously inactive and higher baseline concentrations.[37, 39, 40, 41] Resistance training, however, appears to have no effects on blood lipids, even when initial blood lipid levels are elevated.[42–46] A recent Portuguese study compared the effects of 2 exercise programs of 8 months duration on lipid profiles in older women.[47] Women (n = 77) aged 60-79 years were randomly assigned to either a multi-component exercise program or resistance exercise program. Significant decreases in plasma triglyceride (–5.1%), and significant increases in HDL-cholesterol (9.3%) were observed in the multi-component exercise group while no significant changes in lipid profile were observed in the resistance exercise group.[47]

Only a small number of studies have investigated the effects of physical activity on blood lipids and lipoproteins in a race- and sex-specific manner. African American and white participants of the Atherosclerosis Risk in Communities (ARIC) study were investigated for the longitudinal effects of physical activity on plasma lipids and lipoproteins.[48] Nine years of follow up data on 8764 individuals aged 45-64 years at baseline demonstrated that increases in the level of activity were associated with increases in HDL and decreases in triglycerides among white participants. Physical activity was associated with reduced LDL in all women, while the association with total cholesterol was limited to African American women.

Nutritional influences

Diet

Diet plays the most important role in the management of hyperlipidemia.

Low (saturated) fat — epidemiological studies

A wealth of epidemiological and interventional studies over the last 60 years has established a link between saturated fat intake and serum cholesterol levels. Perhaps the most quoted of these is the Seven Countries Study,[49] in which the dietary habits of 12 763 middle-aged men comprising 16 cohorts from 7 countries were studied, and the relationship to serum cholesterol and coronary disease mortality analysed over subsequent years. This study was carried out between 1958 and 1964, with the information on dietary intake collected by the dietary record method. It allowed inter-cohort comparisons to be made, but analysis on an individual level was not possible. Large variations were seen in the average intake of different saturated fats, and correlations were found between the intake of lauric and myrisitic acids and serum cholesterol increases. In the Western Electric Study,[50] 1900 middle-aged men randomly chosen from the Western Electric Company's Hawthorne Works in the Chicago area were analysed for their dietary intake, and serum cholesterol concentrations were measured. The information was collected through interviews and questionnaires by nutritionists. Again, a positive correlation was apparent between serum cholesterol and saturated fat intake. In Belgium, an epidemiological analysis was performed on the differences between the dietary intakes of Belgians living in the north and south of the country.[51] Food intake was gathered through 3 independent sources: an investigation of 451 families in the north and 752 in the south, a survey by the Ministry of Agriculture, and through the Ministry of Economic Affairs by way of the National Institute of Statistics. This information revealed a much higher intake of saturated fat in the south compared to the north, and also a lower intake of total polyunsaturated fats in the south. Evidence gathered over 10 years revealed decreasing average serum cholesterol in the north of the country, and a higher serum cholesterol in the south, allowing the authors to conclude a positive relationship between saturated fat intake and serum cholesterol. Kato et. al.[52] undertook a large scale study of men of Japanese ancestry living in 3 different environments, which was a useful approach as it limited the effects of genetic influences on serum cholesterol changes. Information was collected by 24-hour recall dietary interviews. Dietary intake patterns varied markedly between the men in Japan, Hawaii and California, with serum cholesterol levels showing an apparent positive regression with saturated fat intake.

Low (saturated) fat — interventional studies

Along with epidemiological evidence, there have been a number of interventional studies attempting to establish the link between saturated fat intake and serum cholesterol. Keys et. al.[53] in 1957 used 66 middle-aged schizophrenic men for a dietary experiment to establish a link between fat intake and serum cholesterol. On a fixed calorie diet, the type of fat fed to the subjects was varied, with 2–9 weeks spent on each experimental diet. The fats used were butter fat, hydrogenated coconut oil, olive oil, cotton-seed oil, corn oil, sunflower-seed oil, safflower oil and fish oil. The percentage of the caloric intake from saturated, monoethenoid and polyethenoid fats were estimated, and serum cholesterol was measured in duplicate at the end of each dietary period. The authors came to the conclusion from their results that saturated fatty acids (especially fats containing 10 or more carbons) such as butter fat and coconut oil have about twice the effect in raising total serum cholesterol as the cholesterol depressing effect of equal amounts of polyethenoid fats. Another major study often used as apparent evidence is that of Hegsted et. al.[54] Two groups of 10 normocholesterolaemic male subjects were tested whilst being fed diets with fixed fat (38% caloric intake) and protein proportions, with carbohydrates varied to make caloric intake appropriate for each subject. Each test period lasted for 4 weeks, with the type of fat varied (coconut, olive, safflower). Samples taken were measured for total serum cholesterol, beta-lipoprotein cholesterol, total fatty acids, and lipid phosphorus. It was concluded that myristic acid is most hypercholesterolemic. Another highly referenced article on the saturated fat theory is that of Ahrens et. al.,[55] who examined 40 patients who were either hyperlipidaemic, hypercholesterolaemic or normocholesterolaemic with arteriosclerotic heart disease. The subjects were observed for 4–6 months under controlled dietary conditions, with fixed calories, total fat (40% of total calories), carbohydrates and proteins. The type of fat fed to the subjects varied between corn oil and coconut oil. Serum cholesterol levels were found to be higher on the coconut oil diet (high in saturated fat) and lower on the corn oil diet (high in polyunsaturated fat). Shepherd et. al.[56] studied the effect of dietary fatty acids on low density lipoprotein (LDL) in 8 young normocholesterolaemic adult males. During study 1, the subjects received a diet rich in saturated fat, derived mainly from dairy products. In study 2, the fat intake from the dairy products was replaced by safflower oil, lower in saturated fat and higher in polyunsaturated fats. Both diets were controlled for total caloric intake and dietary cholesterol. Serum samples were measured for triglyceride, plasma cholesterol, and lipoprotein cholesterol concentrations. It was concluded that compared to the saturated fat diet, the polyunsaturated diet lowered both plasma cholesterol and triglyceride, with 67% of the cholesterol reduction due to a fall in LDL-cholesterol. Similar results were seen by Turner et. al.,[57] where 15 subjects (7 normal and 8 with type II hyperlipoproteinaemia) were fed diets with 40% calories as either safflower oil or lard. The diets were chosen to maximise the difference in the degree of saturation of the dietary fat whilst maintaining constant cholesterol and total fat intake.

A strict, very low saturated fat, low cholesterol American Heart Association Step 2 diet only minimally lowers serum cholesterol. A 5% reduction in LDL-cholesterol in patients following this program was reported and, discouragingly, an equivalent 6% fall in HDL cholesterol, so that ratios were unchanged.[58] Low-fat diets as commonly prescribed rarely produce significant LDL declines. Studies performed on controlled metabolic units where intakes are rigidly enforced can demonstrate cholesterol reductions of 15% with diet alone; however, in the real world, people can rarely replicate these results.[59] One exception to this, however, is the Dean Ornish-style diet, which was studied in the Lifestyle Heart Trial.[60] This vegetarian diet consists of fruits, vegetables, soybean products, non-fat milk, and yoghurt with no oils or animal fats. Roughly 7% of calories are from fat, 15% to 20% from protein, and the remainder from complex carbohydrates. Only 12mg of cholesterol per day is allowed. On average, Ornish's patients had a 37% reduction in LDL-cholesterol levels (HDL-cholesterol levels were unchanged).

What is most provocative about this diet/lifestyle program is that there was a 91% reduction in angina frequency and a significant degree of angiographically measured coronary stenosis regression. It is unclear to what degree other lifestyle modifications, such as exercise and stress reduction, which are integral parts of the Ornish program, play in these results. The problem with the Ornish diet is that it is so stringent that most Americans find adhering to it nearly impossible. In addition, critics of this study note that it had only 48 subjects; thus, the outcome should be viewed sceptically until larger trials are completed. The greatest scientific objection to the Ornish-style diet is that it is now known that high-carbohydrate, low-fat diets raise triglyceride levels, lower HDL levels, and may convert LDL lipoproteins into smaller, denser, and more atherogenic particles.[61] Nevertheless, the Ornish diet provides the greatest absolute LDL reduction available by diet alone and is of a magnitude similar to that of high-dose statin therapy, which can reduce cholesterol by 25% to 60% depending upon the drug dose.[62] A recent meta-analysis of 60 controlled trials revealed that as the chain length of the saturated fatty acids increase, their cholesterol-raising effects tapers off. Accordingly, lauric acid (C12:0) is most hypercholesterolemic and the longer chain stearic acid (C18:0) in fact is cholesterol neutral or even slightly hypocholesterolemic.[63] Based on the above evidence, most international dietary guidelines recommend that total fat intake should be limited to 30% of daily energy intake with saturated fat contributing no more than 10% of daily energy intake to control blood lipid levels. Families with high cardiovascular risk factors such as familial hypercholesterolemia may also warrant for children to be on a diet low in saturated fats and cholesterol. Researchers demonstrated a diet low in saturated fats (30–35% of daily energy) and cholesterol (less than 200mg/day) in early children, aged 7 months to 5 years, reduced cholesterol levels by 3–5% compared with controls without affecting development which may reduce the risk of cardiovascular disease in adulthood.[64] The authors warned against over-restricting dietary fat intake in young children.

Monounsaturated fats

A large majority of the published literature suggests that consumption of monounsaturated fatty acids (MUFA), primarily oleic acid rich sources including olive oil, high oleic safflower oil, canola oil, sunola (genetically modified sunflower) oil, macadamia oil and avocado oil, are cholesterol neutral; that is, they do not significantly affect plasma cholesterol. Therefore, not surprisingly, MUFA consumption is not factored in any of the equations used to predict the change in blood cholesterol levels such as those put forward by Hegsted et. al.[54] and Keys.[65] Intervention studies involving 24–28% of daily energy in the form of MUFA conducted in the 1980s reported reduction in LDL-cholesterol to the same extent to that of a low fat, high-carbohydrate diet.[66]

Monounsaturated fats and the Mediterranean diet

More widely studied and perhaps more practical for the treatment of patients with coronary artery disease is the Mediterranean diet rich in MUFA. In the 1950s, Ancel Keys began studying the dietary habits of 1770 inhabitants of various countries and correlating them with subsequent mortality.[67] His landmark study found that the mortality rates from heart disease were 2–3 times lower in the countries bordering the Mediterranean Sea compared with Northern Europe and the USA. Notably, studies conducted in North America, where MUFA source was not olive oil but other plant or animal oils, failed to demonstrate benefits of MUFA-rich diets, raising possibilities of benefits of Mediterranean diet components other than MUFA. Another potential mechanism is that a diet rich in fruits and legumes provides folic acid, which may reduce cardiac risk by lowering plasma homocysteine.[68] Also, moderate alcohol consumption is associated with decreased cardiovascular risk, in part by increasing HDL levels,[69] and both red wine and some Mediterranean plant foods contain large amounts of flavonoids, which are natural antioxidants and antithrombotic substances.[70] But the most provocative explanation is that the Mediterranean diet contains α-linolenic acid which is an omega-3 fatty acid and has been shown to possess antithrombotic properties and may also be antiarrhythmic.[71,72] This α-linolenic acid is a precursor of other omega-3 fatty acids found in fish and fish oil, such as eicosapentaenoic acid (EPA) and docosahexaenoic acid (DHA), which may have independent beneficial effects that are discussed later in this review.

Nevertheless, based on the reported studies, Adult Treatment Panel III (ATP-III) recommended that human diets should contain at least 15% energy from MUFA for optimisation of blood cholesterol levels.

Polyunsaturated fats

Most polyunsaturated fatty acids in the diet belong to the omega-6 (mainly linoleic acid) family, present in large amounts in seed oils such as corn, sunflower, soybean and cottonseed. Consumption of these has been shown to lower serum cholesterol, LDL-cholesterol and, in clinical trials, the risk of heart disease. Every 1 gram increase in linoleic acid consumption resulted in plasma cholesterol lowering by 1mg/dL.[73] Increased consumption of linoleic acid may induce increased expression of hepatic LDL-receptors, thereby enhancing increased LDL uptake in the liver for further metabolism.[74]

Controversy surrounds omega-6 polyunsaturated fatty acids, because even though they lower LDL-cholesterol levels, excessive intakes do not appear to be correlated with cardiovascular benefit.[75] Recently, Jakobsen et. al.[76] pooled data on diet and the incidence of heart disease in 340 000 people from the United States, Scandinavia, and Israel. Metabolic trials of diet and blood lipids show that replacing 5% of energy from saturated fatty acids with polyunsaturated fatty acids reduces the serum total/HDL-cholesterol ratio by 0.17.[77] In prospective observational studies, such a reduction in the total-to-HDL-cholesterol ratio is associated with a reduction in heart disease risk of 9%.[78] The effect of omega-6 fatty acids on blood lipids, combined with prospective data on blood lipids and heart disease, predicts a 9% risk reduction. The randomised clinical trials predict an 8% reduction, and the observational studies pooled by Jakobsen et. al.[76] predicted a 13% reduction for people who eat 5% of calories as polyunsaturated instead of saturated fatty acids.

Based on the information in the literature, The American Adult Treatment Panel III (ATP-III) recommended that 10% of daily energy will make an optimal intake of polyunsaturated fatty acids, of which at least 1% of total energy should originate from omega-3 fatty acids for control of blood lipid profiles.

Tree nuts

Nuts are energy-rich foods and are an excellent source of unsaturated fatty acids. The favourable fatty acid profile perhaps contributes to the health benefits of nuts observed in epidemiologic studies and cholesterol-lowering potential in feeding trials.[79, 80] Besides, the nuts contain many bioactive compounds such as vegetable protein, fibre, minerals, vitamin E, and polyphenols.[81] RCTs involving dietary supplementation with peanuts, walnuts, pistachio nuts, almonds, hazelnuts and macadamia nuts have demonstrated a reduction in serum total cholesterol and LDL-cholesterol.

A systematic review of studies investigating independent effects of nuts show reduction in total cholesterol between 2–16% and LDL-cholesterol between 2–19% in subjects consuming almonds or walnuts or pecan nuts or peanuts or macadamia nuts compared with those consuming control diets.[79] Another review of clinical studies concluded that tree nuts lower LDL-cholesterol by 3–19% compared with Western and lower-fat diets.[80] In summary, nuts as part of a healthy diet can play an important role in maintenance of blood cholesterol levels. Of all the nuts, walnut is the most extensively studied tree nut and appears to possess hypocholesterolemic properties. A recent crossover randomised control trial in which 25 normal or mildly hypercholesterolemic subjects were supplemented with 42.5g of walnuts daily for 4 weeks, confirmed serum cholesterol reduction of 9.5% and LDL-cholesterol reduction of 5.2%.[82]

High-protein diets

One of the initial concerns with the high-protein diets for weight loss, such as the Atkins diet, was that it allows unrestricted fat consumption, including saturated fats known to increase total and LDL-cholesterol. When the Atkins diet was studied by Samaha[83] in comparison to a low-fat diet (16% fat) in severely obese subjects, they found that the high-protein diet significantly lowered triacylglycerol (TGL) by 20% versus 4% in the low-fat group ($p = 0.001$). The Atkins diet was also tested in a study by Foster,[84] where at 3 months a significant reduction in LDL-cholesterol and triglyceride and a significant increase in HDL-cholesterol were found, compared to a low-fat diet group. Changes in LDL-cholesterol were not maintained at 1 year, therefore significant differences between the groups was lost. In view of the fact that adherence to the diet was very poor, the relevance of this is not yet clear.

Other studies[85, 86] demonstrated significant reductions in triglyceride and oxidised LDL-cholesterol, with high-protein diets. By contrast, Parkers study[87] in 54 type-2 diabetics on a high-protein diet (30% protein) compared to a high-carbohydrate group (15% protein), did not find any significant changes in triglyceride. Findings in regards to both LDL-cholesterol and HDL-cholesterol are even more varied. In a systematic review on low-carbohydrate diets, Bravata[88] found that no change was detected overall in any serum lipids. They note that the studies were few in number and there was a wide variety in the design. However, from limited evidence, it does appear that higher protein diets do not have any adverse effects on total and LDL-cholesterol, though their effect on HDL-cholesterol is less clear. While more research is needed in these areas, it appears that moderately high-protein diets are not harmful to cardiovascular health and may indeed be beneficial.

Low carbohydrate, high vegetable protein and vegetable oil diet ('Eco-Atkins')

A 4-week trial of 47 overweight hyperlipidemic men and women randomised to consume either a low-carbohydrate (26% of total calories), high vegetable protein (31% from gluten, soy, nuts, fruit, vegetables, and cereals), and vegetable oil

(43%) plant-based diet — termed the 'Eco-Atkin diet' — was compared to a high-carbohydrate lacto-ovo vegetarian diet (58% carbohydrate, 16% protein, and 25% fat), with both diets providing 60% of calorie requirements.[89]

The study found that whilst weight loss was similar in both diets, there were significant reductions in LDL-cholesterol concentration and total cholesterol to HDL-C and apolipoprotein-B apolipoprotein-AI ratios, and also for systolic and diastolic blood pressures, for the low-carbohydrate compared with the high-carbohydrate diet.

A dietary portfolio for hyperlipidemia

Efforts to lower cholesterol through dietary manipulations have had only modest effects. In an attempt to increase the efficacy of diet in the prevention of cardiovascular disease, the Adult Treatment Panel of the National Cholesterol Education Program has recommended adding plant sterols and viscous fibres to the diet.[20] Soy proteins and tree nuts may have additional health benefits. Jenkins and colleagues examined the cholesterol-lowering potential of a diet low in saturated-fat that included these ingredients.[90] Forty-six hyperlipidemic, otherwise healthy subjects completed the 4-week study. After 4 weeks of following their own diet that was low in saturated fat, participants were randomised into 1 of the following groups: a very-low-saturated-fat diet without a statin control group; the same diet with a statin; or a similar diet with added viscous fibres, plant sterols, soy foods, and almonds (portfolio diet).

After 4 weeks, the control group lowered their LDL-cholesterol by 8% and increased the LDL-cholesterol to HDL-cholesterol ratio by 3%. The group receiving a statin lowered their LDL-cholesterol by 30.9% and decreased the LDL-cholesterol to HDL-cholesterol ratio by 28.4%. The portfolio diet group lowered their LDL-cholesterol by 28.6% and decreased the LDL-cholesterol to HDL-cholesterol ratio by 23.5%. Clearly the reductions in blood lipid levels in the statin and portfolio diet groups were considerably greater than the changes in the control group; however, no significant differences were apparent in the statin versus the portfolio diet groups. The authors concluded that diet alone, if selecting for foods with a combination of cholesterol-lowering properties, can lower cholesterol to the same extent as statins.[90] Compliance in all the 3 groups was reported to be 93%. These results were subsequently confirmed by another similar study.[91] The long-term sustainability of clinically meaningful reduction in LDL-cholesterol of >20% by dietary means in motivated individuals has also been reported.[92]

Additional benefits of a portfolio diet include weight loss,[92, 93] reduced blood pressure,[93] and reduced inflammation as indicated by a reduction in CRP levels.[90, 94] It has also been shown that the reduction in serum cholesterol following the consumption of the portfolio diet is attributable to decrease in the level of the highly atherogenic, smallest subclass of LDL.[95] More importantly, these health benefits can be achieved without side-effects. Notably the portfolio diet had no effect on the HDL-cholesterol or triglyceride levels. Long-chain omega-3 fatty acids, particularly docosahexanoic acid (DHA), is known to decrease triglyceride and increase HDL-cholesterol levels, therefore, addition of DHA may enhance the lipid-lowering potential of the portfolio diet.

Alcohol

Moderate alcohol consumption is associated with decreased cardiovascular risk in part by increasing HDL levels.[69] Red wine, rich in flavonoids, a natural antioxidant with antithrombotic properties, is particularly more beneficial.[70]

Grapefruit juice

Israeli grapefruit juice, with a high level of bioactive compounds, has been shown to possess cholesterol-lowering properties. An RCT of 72 hypercholesterolemic patients were divided into either a control group or experimental groups supplemented daily with 100 or 200 mL of fresh grapefruit juice for 30 days.[96] Following the intervention period, total cholesterol decreased by 9.5%, and 16.1%; LDL-cholesterol by 11.6% and 21.0%; and triglycerides by 11.5%, and 24.7% in the groups supplemented with 100mL and 200 mL of grapefruit juice respectively. In a follow-up study by the same authors,[97] the lipid-lowering potential of red versus blonde grapefruit was compared. Fifty-seven hypercholesterolemic patients, after coronary bypass surgery, were divided into either a control group or experimental groups supplemented daily with 1 equal weight of red or blond grapefruit. Following the 30-day intervention period, total cholesterol decreased by 15.5%, and 7.6%; LDL-cholesterol by 20.3% and 10.7%; and triglycerides by 17.2%, and 5.6% in the red and blond grapefruit fed groups respectively.[97] It is conceivable that addition of grapefruit (especially red variety) juice may be beneficial for hypercholesterolemic individuals in a dose-dependent manner. The magnitude of the lipid-lowering following red grapefruit consumption should prompt further interest in this food as part of a healthy diet.

However, care is required as grapefruit juice is known to interact and augment the drug bioavailability with many pharmaceutical drugs. (See chapter on Herb-drug interactions). The mechanism for this interaction is via the inhibition of cytochrome P-450 3A4 in the small intestine, reducing the metabolism of the drug, and also the inhibition of P-glycoprotein resulting in further increases in absorption of the drug, potentially leading toxic levels.[98] Drugs metabolised by the pathways that are most affected by grapefruit juice include some calcium channel antagonists (e.g. nifedipine, verapamil), blood thinning medications such as warfarin (increasing risk of bleeding), benzodiazepines (e.g. midazolam and diazepam increasing risk of sedation), HMG-CoA reductase inhibitors /statins (increasing risk of side-effects such as myopathies) and cyclosporine. Even a single glass of juice can produce a significant interaction.[99]

Soybean products

Soybean-derived protein has been shown to possess considerable cholesterol-lowering potential in clinical studies involving hypercholesterolemic subjects. In 1995, a meta-analysis concluded that partial or full replacement of dietary animal proteins by soy protein resulted in an average reduction of 23mg/dL in plasma total and 22mg/dL in LDL-cholesterol concentrations.[100] The observed effects of soybeans on plasma lipids were not extended to triglycerides or HDL-cholesterol. Moreover, reductions in plasma cholesterol were dependent on baseline levels with greater reductions noted in subjects with established hypercholesterolemia.[100] Another recent meta-analysis confirmed these effects of soy proteins.[101] It has been shown that the cholesterol-lowering ability of soy proteins may be attributed to its ability to up-regulate apo-B receptor gene expression.[102, 103]

Another component of soybeans, isoflavones, structurally similar to oestrogen, have been examined for their cholesterol-lowering potential. Isolated soy isoflavones introduced in amounts from 28–150mg have achieved statistically insignificant reductions in LDL-cholesterol in the range of 1–6.5%.[104] These minor declines in non-HDL/LDL-cholesterol concentrations would be of little clinical significance in terms of a reduction in the risk of developing coronary artery disease, but when combined with dietary changes may have an additive beneficial effect.

Based on the published scientific evidence, the United States Food & Drug Administration issued a health claim that 25g/day of soy protein, when supplemented in the diet may significantly reduce the risk of cardiovascular disease via an average fall of up to 10% in plasma cholesterol levels, depending on initial values.[105]

Nutritional supplements

Phytosterols

Phytosterols, also referred to as plant sterols are structurally similar to cholesterol, with the same basic functions in plants as cholesterol in animals; that is, to regulate membrane fluidity and other physiological functions associated with plant biology.[106] The only difference between phytostanols and phytosterols is the saturation of the double bond, consequently the former are less abundant in nature.[107]

Phytosterols are effective in reducing the absorption of both dietary and biliary cholesterol from the gastrointestinal tract, by displacing cholesterol from micelles.[107–110] The inhibition of cholesterol absorption by this mechanism produces a state of relative cholesterol deficiency, which is followed by an up-regulation of cholesterol biosynthesis and LDL-receptor activity.[110] Chronic phytosterol feeding studies, show whole body cholesterol biosynthesis increases by 38–53%, LDL-receptor expression increases by 25–45%, VLDL-cholesterol production by the liver was reduced by 20% and plasma concentration of dense LDL-cholesterol was reduced by 22%.[111, 112] Cholesterol-lowering potential of phytosterols were first documented more than 50 years ago,[113] however a fortified functional food (fat spread) was developed in 1995 and since then a number of studies have investigated the safety/efficacy of the spread to modify blood lipids.[114, 115] Research has demonstrated that plant sterol and stanol ester-enriched margarine spreads lower LDL-cholesterol by 9–14%.[116] Maximal LDL reduction is achieved at plant sterol or stanol ester doses of 1.6–2.0g/day.[117, 118] Plant sterols also provide additional LDL-lowering when used in conjunction with statins.[117, 119] It should be noted that neither phytosterols nor statin drugs have any significant effect on plasma triglycerides. Recent studies have shown that combined plant sterols and long-chain omega-3 fatty acid supplementation have complementary and synergistic lipid-lowering effects.[120, 121] Therefore, for optimisation of blood lipid profile in order to maximise cardio-protection, it may be advisable to develop functional foods with the 2 supplements together.

In the 21st century, plant sterols have been added to other food matrices, including juices, non-fat beverages, milk and yoghurt, cheese, croissants, muffins, cereal bars and chocolates.[122] Plant sterol-enriched fermented milk can significantly reduce LDL-Cholesterol and also triglyceride levels in moderately hypercholesterolemic patients. A multi-centre, randomised, double-blind, placebo-controlled, parallel clinical trial of 83 hypercholesterolemic patients who received a 100 ml serving of either plain (control) low-fat or phytosterol enriched (1.6g of free sterol equivalents) drinkable yoghurt per day along with their main meal for 42 days[123] demonstrated a significant reduction in LDL-cholesterol without affecting the HDL-cholesterol.

Efficacy of phytosterols in low-fat or non-fat products may be a concern, however, fortified low-fat dairy products have been shown to be as effective as fortified fat spreads for lipid-lowering.[115, 122] The beneficial physiologic effects of plant sterols could be further enhanced by combining them with other beneficial foods and substances, such as olive and fish oils, fibres, and soy proteins, enhanced by the additive effects of exercise. In 2006 Food Standards Australia New Zealand (FSANZ) granted permission to market plant sterols in low-fat milks, yoghurts and breakfast cereals. A meta-analysis of 6 randomised controlled intervention trials investigated the effects of phytosterols/stanols on lipid concentrations in familial hypercholesterolemic subjects that used fat spreads (dosages ranging from 1.6–2.8g/day) over a 4–12 week period, and found fat spreads enriched with 2.3 +/– 0.5 gram phytosterols/stanols per day significantly reduced total cholesterol by 7–11% and LDL-cholesterol from 10–15% compared with control. There were no changes in triglyceride and HDL-cholesterol concentrations.[124]

Vitamin B3 — niacin or nicotinic acid

Niacin or nicotinic acid appears to lower LDL-cholesterol and increase HDL-cholesterol. Vitamin B3 includes niacin (nicotinic acid) and niacinamide (nicotinamide), although niacinamide has no effect on lipid levels in patients with hyperlipidemia. Well-designed studies have found that niacin/nicotinic acid lowers LDL-cholesterol by approximately 10%, lowers triglycerides by 25%, and raises 'good' HDL-cholesterol by 15% to 30%. When compared with statins, niacin can raise HDL levels up to 5 times although statins are more effective in lowering total and LDL-cholesterol.[125–128] In a randomised open-label controlled (n = 30) study of 6 months duration, extended release niacin (1000mg/day) significantly reduced LDL-cholesterol by 24% and triglycerides by 12% in patients with impaired glucose tolerance.[129]

Combined extended release niacin and statin therapy

Niacin combined with statins may provide additional benefit for achieving LDL-cholesterol, non-HDL-cholesterol, HDL-cholesterol and triglyceride target goals for cardiovascular prevention. A number of trials demonstrated that combined niacin and statins have significant additional benefits of lowering total cholesterol, LDL-cholesterol, triglyceride and raising HDL-cholesterol levels compared with statins alone, and for prevention of coronary artery disease.[130–134] Extended-release niacin (1000mg/day) combined with simvastatin (20mg) reduced LDL-cholesterol by 6%, non-HDL-cholesterol by 7% and triglycerides by 13%, and raised HDL-cholesterol by 11% compared to simvastatin alone, over a 52-week period. The higher niacin dose of 2000mg combined with simvastatin 20–40mg reduced LDL-cholesterol by up to 24%, non-HDL-cholesterol by up to 28%, and triglycerides by up to 34%, and increased HDL-cholesterol by up to 22% compared to similar dose simvastatin monotherapy.[135] A randomised study of 520 patients with mixed dyslipidemia over a 52-week period compared niacin extended release combined with simvastatin therapy (dosage of 2000/40mg/day) to simvastatin monotherapy[136] and examined their safety and efficacy.[136] Combined niacin/simvastatin therapy was well tolerated with about 70% of patients experiencing mostly mild–moderate flushing that subsided over time and 20% of participants withdrew from the treatment group due to side-effects (7% due to flushing). Overall, when compared with simvastatin monotherapy, combined niacin/simvastatin therapy significantly reduced non-HDL-cholesterol and LDL-cholesterol levels, increased HDL-cholesterol and reduced triglyceride levels.

Niacin may also play a role in metabolic syndrome. A recent study compared the effects of aerobic exercise and extended-release niacin on post-prandial triglyceride levels in 15 men with the metabolic syndrome over a 16-week period.[137] This study reported that aerobic exercise lowers the postprandial triglyceride response to a high-fat meal, whereas niacin lowered fasting but not postprandial triglycerides. When the 2 were combined, niacin attenuated the triglyceride-lowering effect of exercise and decreased postprandial insulin concentrations after niacin administration.[137]

Mechanism of action

There are several possible mechanisms of action for niacin. These include inhibiting free fatty acid release from adipose tissue, inhibiting hepatic diacylglycerol acyltransferase (DGAT), resulting in inhibition of triglyceride synthesis and reducing apolipoprotein B-containing lipoproteins and reducing the rate of synthesis of LDL-cholesterol and VLDL-cholesterol.[138, 139, 140]

Adverse effects

Niacin's therapeutic benefit to lower cholesterol and triglyceride levels is dose related. However, at the level required to produce significant results (500–1500mg), niacin is a powerful vasodilator, especially of cutaneous blood vessels of the face, neck and chest, mediated by prostaglandins, and can create an adverse effect of 'flushing' for 30 minutes. Tolerance to these effects occurs within 2 weeks in most people with continued use. Also, there have been reports of hepatotoxicity, especially in the extended release forms, although a number of studies using these forms, including with statins, have reported low rates of adverse effects.

Over-the-counter complementary medicines such as multivitamins in Australia cannot contain over 100mg of nicotinic acid per dosage unit. For therapeutic purposes, nicotinic acid containing 250mg or less of nicotinic acid is included in Schedule 3 of the *Standards for the Uniform Scheduling of Drugs and Poisons* (SUSDP; Pharmacist only) or in Schedule 4 of the SUSDP (Prescription only) for the indication of treatment of both hypercholesterolemia and hypertriglyceridemia. Because of side-effects, niacin should not be used to lower cholesterol unless under the supervision of a qualified medical practitioner.

Viscous (soluble) fibre

Soluble fibre appears to reduce LDL-cholesterol by reducing cholesterol absorption in the intestines. Soluble fibre binds with cholesterol so that it is excreted. Soluble fibre can be found as a dietary supplement, such as psyllium powder, or in foods such as oats, barley, rye, legumes (peas, beans), some fruits such as apples, prunes, and berries and some vegetables, such as carrots, brussel sprouts, broccoli, and yams. Five to 10g a day of soluble fibre has been found to decrease LDL-cholesterol by approximately 5%. Well-controlled intervention studies have now shown that 4 major water-soluble fibre types — β-glucan, psyllium, pectin and guar gum — effectively lower serum LDL-cholesterol concentrations, without affecting HDL-cholesterol or triglyceride concentrations. It is estimated that for each additional gram of water-soluble fibre in the diet, serum total and LDL-cholesterol concentrations decrease by -0.028mmol/L and -0.029mmol/L, respectively.[141]

Oats and barley

Several studies have been carried out on the cholesterol-lowering effects of oats, which were later found to be due to their β-glucan content.[142] Results of several uncontrolled metabolic ward trials have been summarised by Anderson et. al. and reductions in serum total cholesterol (mainly LDL-cholesterol) from 13% to 26% were reported,[143] however a few studies demonstrated virtually no benefit.[144, 145, 146] Although a few individual studies showed virtually no effects, a number of meta-analyses concluded that water-soluble fibre from oat products effectively lowered serum total and LDL-cholesterol concentrations.[147, 148, 149] Brown et. al. estimated that 1g of water-soluble fibre from oats lowered total and LDL-cholesterol concentrations with −0.037mmol/L and −0.032mmol/L, respectively.[149] Obviously, more research is needed to confirm the cholesterol-lowering effects of this source of β-glucan and its potential beneficial effects on HDL-cholesterol concentrations. A recent systematic review of 8 RCTs (n = 391 patients) of 4–12 weeks' duration evaluated the lipid-lowering effects of barley, another source of β-glucan.[150] The use of barley significantly lowered total cholesterol (−13.38mg/dL), LDL-cholesterol (−10.02mg/dL) and triglycerides (−11.83mg/dL) but did not appear to significantly alter HDL-cholesterol.

Psyllium

Psyllium has been shown to reduce total cholesterol and LDL-cholesterol levels in animals and humans. One study demonstrated a 3.5% reduction in total cholesterol and a 5.1% reduction in LDL-cholesterol levels after consuming 5.1g of psyllium husk twice daily for 8 weeks.[151]

Another study began with individuals on the American Heart Association Step-1 diet, then with the addition of 8 weeks of psyllium supplements, resulted in decreased total cholesterol (4.8%) and LDL (8.8%).[152] An analysis of all double-blind studies concluded that psyllium-enriched cereals lowered cholesterol levels by 5% and LDL by 9%.[153] In a study examining age and gender differences in the effect of psyllium on blood lipids, men and pre- and post-menopausal women were given psyllium or placebo. Psyllium lowered plasma LDL-cholesterol levels by 7–9% in all groups. Triglyceride levels were lowered by 17% in men, but increased by 16% in post-menopausal women. Pre-menopausal women displayed no significant shift in triglycerides.[154]

Pectin

Keys et. al.[155] published the first human study involving 24 healthy subjects that suggested that pectin supplementation lowered serum total cholesterol concentrations. Consumption of biscuits with pectin (15g/day) reduced total cholesterol by 5%. Since then, many studies have confirmed that pectin lowers serum cholesterol levels in hypercholesterolemic as well as normocholesterolemic subjects. All sources of pectin, including guava fruit, prunes, grapefruit gelatin capsules, and citrus pectin desserts were all effective. Despite some controversy,[156, 157] meta-analysis by Brown et. al.[149] concluded that pectin effectively lowered total and LDL-cholesterol concentrations. The range of effects on total cholesterol varied from –16% to –5%. On average, each gram of pectin decreased total and LDL-cholesterol concentrations by –0.070mmol/L and –0.055mmol/L respectively. Pectin did not significantly alter serum HDL-cholesterol and triglyceride levels.

Guar gum (*Cyamopsis tetragonoloba*)

Guar gum, a bulk laxative, is not only used to relieve constipation but also to decrease serum cholesterol concentrations. Fahrenbach et. al. were the first to report that guar gum effectively reduced serum cholesterol levels in normocholesterolemic subjects.[158] Since then, this serum lipid-lowering effect of guar gum has been investigated in a large number of human trials. The results of these studies were consistent in that total and LDL-cholesterol were effectively decreased by guar gum supplementation, whereas HDL-cholesterol and triglyceride remained unchanged. From their meta-analysis, Brown et. al. estimated that 1g of water-soluble fibre from guar gum lowered serum total and LDL-cholesterol by –0.026mmol/L and –0.033mmol/L respectively.[149] Guar gum lowered total cholesterol concentrations in healthy and hyperlipidemia subjects, and in subjects with diabetes mellitus. Guar gum exhibited additional cholesterol-lowering effects in subjects already receiving lipid-lowering drugs.

Glucomannan

Glucomannan, another soluble fibre derived from *Amorphophallus konjac,* available in numerous over-the-counter products, such as Lipozene®, has been the subject of several intervention trials evaluating its influence on blood lipids.[159–162] A meta-analysis of 14 RCTs, including patients receiving glucomannan, had statistically significantly lower total cholesterol, LDL-cholesterol, and triglycerides; however, the use of glucomannan did not appear to alter HDL-cholesterol.[163]

Fish oil

Omega-3 fatty acids are pleiotropic molecules with the potential to play a key role in the management of hyperlipidemia for the prevention of coronary heart disease. Supplementation with omega-3 fatty acids favourably modifies serum lipids; the most consistent finding being a drastic reduction in fasting and postprandial triglycerides levels.[164] This has been observed with EPA and DHA alone[165] and with their combination in fish oil.

Grimsgaard et. al.[166] reported on the effects of supplementation with highly purified eicosapentanoic acid (EPA) (3.8 g/d) or docasahexanoic acid (DHA) (3.6 g/d) for 7 weeks in healthy, non-smoking male volunteers. They found a reduction in plasma triglycerides that was at least as marked in the DHA group (26%) as in the EPA group (21%). In addition, HDL-cholesterol increased only in the DHA group.[166] These results provide convincing evidence that EPA and DHA are equally effective at reducing serum triglycerides, but that DHA may raise HDL-cholesterol as well as LDL particle size (i.e. both anti atherogenic outcomes). Omega-3 fatty acids have contrasting effects on LDL-cholesterol, with a general tendency toward slightly increased LDL-cholesterol concentrations, however the size of the LDL molecule is also increased, which is thought to be less atherogenic.[167]

A recent meta-analysis quantitatively evaluated RCTs of fish oils in hyperlipidemic subjects.[168] The final analysis comprising of 47 trials showed that consuming fish oils (average intake of 3.25g/day of EPA/DHA) produced a clinically significant reduction of triglyceride (–0.34mmol/L), no change in serum cholesterol (–0.01mmol/L) and slight increase in HDL (0.01mmol/L) and LDL-cholesterol (0.06mmol/L). The reduction in triglyceride concentration correlated with both EPA/DHA intake and initial triglyceride levels. A recent trial supports the observations that dietary supplementation with a DHA rich oil, reduces plasma triglyceride by 22.3% and increases HDL-cholesterol by 7.1% with no significant change in total or LDL-cholesterol.[120]

A systematic review comparing the effects of lipid-lowering interventions for the prevention and treatment of hyperlipidemias concluded that statins and omega-3 fatty acids are by far the most favourite agents to reduce the risk of cardiovascular disease.[169] Another recent study demonstrated that fish oil supplements may work slightly better than a popular cholesterol-reducing drug to help patients with chronic heart failure.[170] Indeed, combined therapy with cholesterol-lowering agents (statin drugs or phytosterols) and omega-3 fatty acid may offer complementary or even synergistic effects on blood lipid levels.[120, 121, 171] Monotherapy with statins or phytosterols may not be sufficient to treat target goals for hyperlipidemia, especially given their modest effects on triglyceride concentration, and co-supplementation with omega-3 fatty acids may optimise plasma lipid profile in people with mixed hyperlipidemia.

Herbal therapies

Extract from *Commiphora mukul* (guggul), artichoke leaf extract, and garlic extract have all been marketed to the general public as treatment options for hyperlipidemia. This section reviews interventional studies involving herbal remedies for lipid-lowering and provides evidence as to how these remedies stand up to vigorous scientific scrutiny.

Guggulipid

Guggulipid, a petroleum extract from the plant *Commiphora mukul* (guggul), is an approved treatment for elevated cholesterol in India and has been the mainstay of the Ayurvedic approach to preventing atherosclerosis since its discovery in 1987.

One trial studying the effects of guggul reported that serum cholesterol dropped by 17.5%.[172] In another report comparing guggul to the drug clofibrate, average fall in serum cholesterol was slightly greater in the guggul group; moreover, HDL-cholesterol rose in 60% of people responding to guggul, while clofibrate did not elevate HDL.[173] In another Indian placebo-controlled study from 1994, guggulipid lowered the average level of total cholesterol by 11.7%, LDL-cholesterol by 12.5%, triglycerides by 12% and total cholesterol/HDL ratio by 11.1%.[174] In the first clinical trial of guggul extract outside of India, neither the commonly used dose, nor a high dose of standardised guggul improved any of the measured levels of lipoproteins in a sample of 103 healthy patients with hypercholesterolemia (moderate) and eating a Western diet.[175] Guggul also appeared to cause a dermatologic hypersensitivity reaction in some patients

A recent Norwegian double-blind, randomised, placebo-controlled trial including 43 women and men, age 27–70 years, with moderately increased cholesterol, randomised to use 2160mg guggul daily, or a placebo for 12 weeks, showed a significant decrease in serum cholesterol and HDL-cholesterol with no change in LDL-cholesterol, triglycerides, and total cholesterol/HDL-C ratio between the 2 groups.[176] Further larger studies are needed to establish effects and safety of guggul-based formulations in the treatment for hypercholesterolemia.

Artichoke leaf extract

Artichoke (*Cynara scolymus*) leaf extract (ALE) is a herbal remedy marketed as an aid to lowering cholesterol. ALE may work by limiting the synthesis of cholesterol in the body. Artichokes also contain a compound called cynarin, believed to increase bile production in the liver and speed the flow of bile from the gallbladder, both of which may increase cholesterol excretion. A review of 11 clinical studies conducted between 1936–1994 on the lipid-lowering effects of ALE showed an average decrease in either total cholesterol or triglycerides of between 5% and 45%,[177] although the robustness of some of the trial designs is unclear.

In a recent UK study, 75 hypercholesterolemic volunteers were randomised to examine the effects of feeding 1280mg of a standardised ALE, or a matched placebo, daily for 12 weeks.[178] Plasma total cholesterol decreased in the treatment group by an average of 4.2%. No significant differences between groups were observed for LDL-cholesterol, HDL-cholesterol or triglyceride levels. An Indian study including 30 volunteers with type II diabetes reported that 6g of globe artichoke powder per day for 90 days significantly lowered total cholesterol by 11mg/dL, LDL-cholesterol by 17mg/dL (9%), triglyceride by 18mg/dL (9.5%) and surprisingly increased HDL-cholesterol by a massive 38% or 9mg/dL, compared to the baseline values.[179] A meta-analysis looked at RCTs for artichoke extract for high cholesterol.[180] Two trials involving a total of 167 people met the quality criteria. One trial found artichoke significantly reduced total cholesterol after 42 days of treatment.[181] The other study found artichoke significantly reduced total cholesterol in a subgroup of patients with total cholesterol levels of more than 230mg/dl.[182] Adverse events were mild, transient and infrequent. Larger clinical trials over longer periods are needed.

Garlic extract

There have been numerous studies with conflicting results regarding garlic's ability to lower lipids. Positive findings in 3 trials exhibited a lowering of cholesterol from 6.1 to 11.5%, primarily due to the lowering of LDL levels over a 1–4 month period.[183, 184, 185] More recent studies have yielded conflicting results.[186, 187] A 12-week study using garlic powder in ambulatory patients resulted in a

14% reduction of serum cholesterol. An earlier meta-analysis of the controlled trials of garlic to reduce hypercholesterolemia suggested a significant reduction in total cholesterol levels.[188] The best available evidence suggests that garlic, in an amount approximating one-half to 1 clove per day, decreased total serum cholesterol levels by about 9% in the groups of patients studied. It should be noted that only 5 of 28 studies were selected for review while the rest did not meet the criteria for homogeneity with respect to study design, patient characteristics, interventions, duration of therapy, and cholesterol measurements. Another meta-analysis of randomised double-blind, placebo-controlled clinical trials published in 2001 suggested that garlic is superior to placebo in reducing serum cholesterol levels, however, the effect size is modest, and the robustness of the effect is debatable, raising doubts about the treatment of hypercholesterolemia by garlic use.[189] A recent systematic review evaluated the effects of garlic on cholesterol levels in both healthy and hypercholesterolaemic subjects. RCTs with garlic ranging from 11–24 weeks in duration concluded that garlic therapy did not produce any statistically significant reduction in serum total cholesterol levels.[190] As moderate to high heterogeneity exists among pooled studies, the available evidence from RCTs does not demonstrate beneficial effects of garlic on serum cholesterol.

Other supplements

Policosanols

Policosanol is a natural product derived from sugar cane wax, which may inhibit cholesterol synthesis although studies have demonstrated conflicting results. A single daily dose of 5–10mg policosanol reduced cholesterol by 8–18% and LDL-cholesterol by 11–28% (equivalent to low dose statin) within 2 months of therapy. It also increased HDL-cholesterol from 10–29%.[191–194] More than 80 placebo-controlled or comparative trials suggest that policosanol at doses of 5–40mg/d has lipoprotein-lowering effects comparable with statins.

Hypocholesterolemic effects of policosanol have been compared with lipid-lowering drugs, bezafibrate[195] and statins.[196] A multi-centre controlled double-blind randomised trial in 113 hypercholesterolemic subjects demonstrated that a daily dose of 10mg of policosanol possessed superior lipid-lowering effects compared to 400mg/day dose of bezafibrate.[195] Another double-blind randomised study conducted in Chile showed greater lipid-lowering effects of policosanol compared with statins.[197] In this trial, Frencini-Presenti et. al.[197] failed to demonstrate cholesterol-lowering potential of policosanol at a dose of 20mg/day for 8 weeks. Another randomised, double-blind, placebo-controlled, parallel-group trial conducted in Germany using a daily dose of up to 80mg of policosanol for 12 weeks showed no significant effects on blood lipids.[198] Yet another randomised, parallel, double-blind, double-dummy, placebo-controlled trial[199] with policosanol with or without statin therapy failed to show cholesterol-lowering effects and the authors suggested that policosanol should be added to the list of nutritional supplements lacking scientific validity to support their use. A recent study demonstrated that dietary supplementation with 30mg/day of octacosanol (policosanol) for 4 weeks did not alter blood lipid profile; however, neutral sterol and bile excretion in the faeces decreased following the intervention suggesting a systemic effect of policosanol on cholesterol metabolism.[200] A meta-analysis of 4596 patients from 52 eligible studies that compared the benefits of policosanol and plant sterols and stanols with placebo, found that policosanol affected total cholesterol, HDL-cholesterol, triglyceride levels more favourably than plant sterols and stanols.[201] Both groups had favourable safety profile. The net reduction of LDL-cholesterol were –24% for policosanol versus –10% for plant sterols ($p<0.0001$) after accounting for the placebo groups, and a clinically significant decrease in the LDL:HDL ratio with the policosanol group.

However, a number of recent RCTs for policosanol suggest it has no benefit for the treatment of hypercholesterolemia demonstrating no significant change in LDL-cholesterol levels or reduced LDL oxidation compared to control in hypercholesterolaemic individuals.[202–205] Therefore, the overall weight of current evidence at present suggests policosanol may not play a role in the treatment of hypercholesterolemia.

Chinese red yeast rice extract (RYRE) *(Monascus purpureus)*

The benefit of Chinese RYRE, a fungus, has been known for over a decade to have cholesterol-lowering effects.[206–211] It contains a natural source of lovastatin, possessing statin properties, and many other substances such as flavonoids, polyunsaturated fats, pyrrolinic compounds.[212] Like statin cholesterol-lowering agents, Chinese RYRE is an inhibitor of HMG-CoA reductase and can potentially have similar side-effects such as liver impairment and hepatitis with elevation of alanine-amino transferase (ALT) and aspartate-amino transferase (AST), and myopathy or rhabdomyolysis with elevation of creatinine kinase (CK).[213, 214, 215] The biosynthesis of ubiquinone (CoQ_{10}) is well recognised to be affected by the inhibition of HMG-CoA reductase with significant reduction in plasma levels with statin treatment. CoQ_{10} is essential for the production of energy, has antioxidative properties and reduced levels are thought to be responsible for membrane alteration and consequent cellular damage leading to myopathy. Anaphylaxis to the yeast extract is also reported in a case report.[216]

A number of short-term, placebo-controlled trials of *Monascus purpureus* Went rice (dosage 600mg daily for 8 weeks), demonstrated significant reduction in LDL-cholesterol levels, total cholesterol/HDL-lipoprotein cholesterol ratio, LDL-cholesterol/HDL-cholesterol ratio and apolipoprotein B/apolipoprotein A-I ratios in hypercholesterolemic patients (aged 23–65 years) when compared with placebo.[217, 218] *Monascus purpureus* Went rice therapy was able to reduce LDL-cholesterol by up to 27.7%, total cholesterol by 21.5%, triglycerides by 15.8% and apolipoprotein B by 26.0% with 8 weeks therapy.[218] There was a non-significant rise in HDL-cholesterol and apolipoprotein A-I levels by 0.9% and 3.4% respectively.

A longer trial of *Monascus purpureus* Went rice (600mg twice daily 1st month, then daily) for a total of 6–12 months in subjects with secondary nephrotic hyperlipidemia demonstrated it was equally as effective as fluvastatin (20mgs/day) in reducing cholesterol levels and well-tolerated with no significant side-effects, including myopathy.[219] A recent meta-analysis of trials of Chinese RYRE for primary hyperlipidemia identified 93 randomised trials (9625 participants) of namely 3 RYRE preparations (Cholestin, Xuezhikang and Zhibituo), and found from the combined results significant reduction of serum total cholesterol levels, triglycerides levels and LDL-cholesterol levels, and increase of HDL-cholesterol levels compared with placebo and on par to statins such as pravastatin, simvastatin, lovastatin, atorvastatin, or fluvastatin.[220] Another recent RCT involving 62 patients with dyslipidemia and history of discontinuation of statin therapy due to myalgias have demonstrated that those receiving 1800mg/day of RYRE for 24 weeks had a significant reduction in LDL-cholesterol of 0.9mmol/L without adverse effects on HDL-cholesterol, triglyceride, liver enzyme, CPK, weight loss, and pain severity scores.[221] More long-term research is warranted.

Conclusion

Lipid management guidelines from the National Heart Foundation (NHF) of Australia emphasise the importance of advising lifestyle factors, especially in high-risk groups, with the aim to reduce absolute cardiovascular risk and also of lowering plasma lipid levels LDL-cholesterol and raising HDL-cholesterol, as atherogenic and antiatherogenic components, respectively, and lowering triglyceride levels. The NHF recommendations for lifestyle advice and pharmacological measures for the appropriate management of hyperlipidemia and targets for therapy are summarised at the beginning of the chapter. The Adult Treatment Panel III (ATP III) guidelines of the US National Cholesterol Education Program (NCEP) emphasise the importance of lowering cholesterol and place greater emphasis on lowering triglyceride levels.

Taken together, for maximum defence against the risk of developing cardiovascular disease the following targets have been set:[17, 20]

1. total blood cholesterol <4.0mmol/L
2. LDL-cholesterol <2.5mmol/L
3. HDL-cholesterol >1.0mmol/L
4. triglyceride levels <1.5mmol/L.

It is evident that hyperlipidemia, being a heterogenous condition, cannot be managed optimally by any of the monotherapies described in this chapter, may they be pharmaceutical or complementary. A majority of the treatment strategies for hyperlipidemia (including statins, phytosterols, RYRE etc.) influence total and LDL-cholesterol while only a few (fibrates, niacin, fish oil, exercise) have the potential to influence HDL-cholesterol and triglyceride levels also. The following combinations might achieve the best results, particularly for people with mixed hyperlipidemia:

1. diet, exercise, statins and fibrates/niacin (lifestyle and pharmaceutical)
2. diet, exercise, statins, niacin, phytosterols and fish oil (lifestyle, pharmaceutical and dietary supplements)
3. diet, exercise, niacin, phytosterol and fish oil (lifestyle and dietary supplements).

In summary, non-pharmaceutical management of hyperlipidemia should include a combination of lifestyle changes such as diet, exercise, stress management and consideration for co-supplementation such as with phytosterols, niacin, Chinese RYRE, and omega-3 fatty acids to optimise plasma

Table 18.3 Levels of evidence for lifestyle and complementary medicine/therapies in the management of hyperlipidemia

Modality	Level I	Level II	Level IIa	Level IIIb	Level IIIc	Level IV	Level V
Lifestyle — diet							
Fat intake	x						
Saturated fat intake (↑risk)	x						
Monounsaturated fat intake			x				
Polyunsaturated fat intake		x					
High-protein diet		x					
Portfolio diet	x						
Tree nuts	x						
Grapefruit juice		x					
Soybean products		x					
Exercise and physical activity	x						
Mind–body therapy							
Stress management		x					
Nutritional supplements							
Phytosterols	x						
Fish oil	x						
Niacin		x					
Viscous fibre	x						
Glucomannan	x						
Other supplements							
Policosanols	x (+/-)	x (+/-)					
Herbal therapies							
Garlic	x						
Guggulipid		x					
Artichokes	x						
Red yeast rice extract	x						

*Caution is advocated in interpreting these results as conclusive — further evidence is required.
Level I— from a systematic review of all relevant randomised controlled trials, meta-analyses.
Level II— from at least 1 properly designed randomised controlled clinical trial.
Level IIIa— from well-designed pseudo-randomised controlled trials (alternate allocation or some other method).
Level IIIb— from comparative studies (including systematic reviews of such studies) with concurrent controls and allocation not randomised, cohort studies, case-control studies, or interrupted time series with a parallel control group.
Level IIIc— from comparative studies with historical control, 2 or more single-arm studies or interrupted time series without a parallel control group.
Level IV— opinions of respected authorities based on clinical experience, descriptive studies or reports of expert committees.
Level V— represents minimal evidence that represents testimonials.

lipid profile, particularly in people with mixed hyperlipidemia. Where stronger therapy is necessary, pharmaceutical medication may be warranted.

Table 18.3 summarises the level of scientific evidence for the treatment of hyperlipidemia for lifestyle factors and CAM (complementary and alternative medicine) therapies.

Clinical tips handout for patients — hyperlipidemia

1 Lifestyle advice

Sleep

- Restore normal sleep patterns. Most adults require about 7 hours sleep a day. (See Chapter 22 for more advice.)

Sunshine

- Amount of exposure varies with local climate.
- At least 15 minutes of sunshine needed daily for vitamin D and melatonin production — especially before 10 a.m. and after 3 p.m. when the sun exposure is safest during summer. Much more exposure required in winter when supplementation needs to be considered.
- Ensure gradual, adequate skin exposure to sun; avoid sunscreen and excess clothing to maximise levels of vitamin D.
- More time in the sun is required for dark skinned people and people with vitamin D deficiency.
- Direct exposure to about 10% of the body (hands, arms, face), without sunscreen and not through glass.
- Vitamin D is obtained in the diet from fatty fish, eggs, liver and fortified foods (some milks and margarines); diet alone is not a sufficient source of vitamin D.

2 Physical activity/exercise

- Exercise 30–60 minutes daily. If exercise is not regular, commence with 5 minutes daily and slowly build up to at least 30 minutes.
- Outdoor exercise in nature, with fresh air and sunshine, is ideal (e.g. brisk walking, light jogging, cycling, swimming, stretching, resistance or weight-bearing exercises). The more time you spend outdoors the better.

3 Mind–body medicine

- Stress management program — for example, 6 x 40 minute sessions for patients to understand the nature of their symptoms, the symptoms' relationship to stress, and the practice of regular relaxation exercises.
- Regular meditation practice at least 10–20 minutes daily, especially transcendental mindfulness meditation and autogenic training.

Breathing

- Be aware of breathing from time to time. Notice if tendency to hold breath or over-breathe.
- Snoring and irregular breathing during sleep needs to be reported and further investigated.
- Avoid exposure to polluted air as much as possible.

Rest and stress management

Relaxation is important for a full and lasting recovery.

- Reduce workload and resolve conflicts. Contact family, friends, church or social groups for support.
- Listening to relaxation music and daily baths may help.
- Relaxation massage therapy is helpful.
- Exercise is a stress reliever.
- Cognitive behavioural therapy and psychotherapy are extremely helpful for resolving issues and reducing stress levels (only if needed).

Fun

- It is important to have fun in life.
- Joy can be found even in the simplest tasks, such as funny movies/videos, comedy, hobbies, dancing, playing with pets and children.

4 Environment

- Avoid smoking, environmental pollutants and chemicals — at work and in the home.
- Walks in parks, office areas or around the home, with a view overlooking the garden or a park can help with daily relaxation.

5 Dietary changes

- Eat regular healthy low-GI meals; ideally 3 small meals a day.
- A low-carbohydrate, high-protein diet (fish, legumes, nuts, seeds, cereals) and high vegetable oil plant-based diet is best.
- Eat more fruit (>2/day), such as apples, prunes, guava fruit, avocado, olives and berries.
- Eat more vegetables (>5/day) with skin (for fibre), and use a variety of colours (e.g. carrots, brussel sprouts, broccoli, artichoke, okra, eggplant, yams) and preferably vegetables in season.
- Increase dietary fibre — oats, oat bran, barley, psyllium husks (1 tsp of psyllium husk twice daily). Pectin is a soluble fibre (polysaccharide) found in fruits.
- Add 20–30g of lecithin to meals.

- Eat more nuts (30–100g/day), especially walnuts and macadamia, and seeds (e.g. sunflower seeds, flaxseed).
- Eat more legumes (e.g. peas, beans, soy, chickpeas) — 25–50g/day of soy protein can help reduce cholesterol.
- Increase fish intake to 2–3–4 times weekly (daily if possible), especially deep sea fish. Canned fish is okay (mackerel, salmon, sardines, cod, tuna, salmon).
- Reduce red meat intake (preferably use red lean meat e.g. lamb, kangaroo) and white meat (e.g. free range organic chicken).
- Use cold-pressed olive oil, avocado or tahini (in place of butter).
- Eat more low-GI wholegrains/cereals (variety): traditional rolled oats and barley are particularly helpful for lowering lipids; rice (brown, basmati, Mahatmi, Dongara), buckwheat flour, wholegrain organic breads (rye bread, Essene, spelt, Kamut), brown pasta, millet, amaranth etc.
- Reduce dairy intake; consume only low-fat dairy products such as yoghurt and occasionally cheeses, unless there is a dairy intolerance.
- Drink more water, 1–2 litres a day, and teas, especially organic green tea and black tea.
- Minimise alcohol intake. Red wine is best; no more than 1–2 glasses daily.
- Drink grapefruit juice (especially red variety); 100–200mls/day may be beneficial (beware if taking other medication e.g. warfarin; check with your doctor).
- Plant sterols or phytosterols (2-3g/day phytosterols or stanols/day) are effective in reducing the absorption of both dietary and biliary cholesterol from the gastrointestinal tract. It is now added to some foods such as margarine (1 tbs/day), juices, non-fat beverages, fermented milk or yoghurt (containing average 1.6g of free sterol,100 ml/day).
- Reduce intake of eggs and shellfish.

Avoid:

- high-fat animal products (e.g. high-fat cheeses and butter)
- hydrogenated fats, salt, fast foods, and added sugar such as in soft drinks, lollies, biscuits, cakes and processed foods (e.g. white bread, white pasta, pastries)
- coconut and palm oil
- chemical additives — preservatives, colourings and flavourings
- sugars — for sweetener try honey (e.g. yellow box and stringy bark have lowest GI).

6 Supplements

Fish oils (EPA/DHA)

- Indication: lowering lipids, particularly triglycerides.
- Dosage: take with meals. Adult: 2–4g (1g containing EPA 180/DHA 120mg) once or twice daily depending on fish consumption. Child 500mg once or twice daily (500mg–1g daily EPA and DHA); can be used in pregnancy or lactation as tolerated.
- Results: 2–4 weeks.
- Side-effects: often well tolerated especially if taken with meals. Very mild and rare side-effects (e.g. gastrointestinal upset); allergic reactions (e.g. rash, breathing problems if allergic to seafood); blood thinning effects in very high doses > 10g/day (may need to stop fish oil supplements 2 weeks prior to surgery).
- Contraindications: sensitivity reaction to seafood; drug interactions; caution when taking high doses of fish oils >4g per day together with warfarin (your doctor will check your INR test).

Vitamin B3 — niacin (nicotinic acid)

- Indication: vitamin B3 as nicotinic acid appears to lower LDL-cholesterol and triglycerides and increase HDL-cholesterol.
- Dosage: nicotinic acid 250mg, 3 times a day; up to 3–4.5g/day.
- Results: 3–6 months; start with lowest dose to minimise flushing; aspirin 30 minutes before taking niacin can reduce flushes.
- Side-effects: hot flushing and perfused sweating to face, chest and neck usually within 30 minutes of tablet (tolerance to these effects occurs within 2 weeks in most people); avoid taking niacin with hot drinks; headache; dizziness; burning, tingling, itching, rashes, redness of face, arms and chest; liver impairment with high doses of niacin; change in glucose levels (beware in diabetics); gastrointestinal upset (e.g. vomiting, heartburn, anorexia, abdominal pain and diarrhoea); raised uric acid and gout.
- Contraindications: slow release niacin due to its association with liver toxicity. Liver impairment/disease.

Guar gum

Guar gum is high in fibre.

- Indications: relieves constipation, reduces serum cholesterol concentrations.

- Dosage: adult: 1g of water-soluble fibre from guar gum combined with pectin. Start with smallest dose and build up slowly; up to 10–15g/day as tolerated. Possibly safe in pregnancy.
- Results: 2–4 weeks.
- Side-effects: often well tolerated, especially if taken with meals. Very mild and rare side-effects (e.g. gastrointestinal upset; diarrhoea, gas, and loose stools; may reduce glucose levels requiring reduction of diabetes medication).
- Contraindications: concurrent use with some medication may reduce absorption of drugs.

Glucomannan

Glucomannan is high in fibre, derived from *Amorphophallus konjac.*

- Indications: reduce serum cholesterol concentrations, relieve constipation, may assist diabetes and irritable bowel syndrome.
- Dosage: 1g 1–3 times daily.
- Results: 2–4 weeks.
- Side-effects: often well tolerated, especially if taken with meals. Very mild and rare side-effects (e.g. gastrointestinal upset, dry throat). May interfere with absorption of fat soluble vitamins A, D, E, K. May need to reduce diabetic medication.
- Contraindications: pregnancy, lactation, elderly.

Soybean products

- Dosage: 25g soy protein per day.
- Side-effects: a component of soybeans, isoflavones, structurally similar to oestrogen.
- Results: 2–4 weeks.
- Side-effects: often well tolerated. Very mild and rare side-effects; transient abdominal discomfort; theoretically may stimulate estrogenic receptors causing breast discomfort, heavy menstrual bleeding and endometrial hyperplasia.
- Contraindications: more evidence is required to determine effect of soy on patients with existing hormone sensitive cancers, such as breast and uterine cancer.

Herbs

Guggulipid

Guggulipid is a gum resin extract from the plant *Commiphora mukul* (guggul).

- Indication: lowering total cholesterol; may assist with acne.
- Dosage: 1–2g guggul daily.
- Results: 10–12 weeks.
- Side-effects: usually well tolerated; digestive problems, allergic reaction, estrogenic activity.
- Contraindications: avoid with anticoagulants and estrogenic medication (e.g. oral contraceptive pill); estrogenic-sensitive diseases.

Artichoke (*Cynara scolymus*) leaf extract (ALE)

- Indication: lowering total cholesterol; nausea, dyspepsia, irritable bowel syndrome.
- Dosage: 1280mg of a standardised ALE.
- Results: 6–12 weeks.
- Side-effects: usually well tolerated; digestive problems, flatulence; allergic reaction (topical or systemic) especially in patients sensitive to the *Asteraceae/Compositae* family (e.g. chrysanthemums, marigolds, daisies and ragweed).
- Contraindications: allergy or sensitivity to the *Asteraceae/Compositae* family (e.g. chrysanthemums, marigolds, daisies and ragweed); pregnancy, lactation.

Red rice yeast extract (*Monascus purpureus*)

These products contain low dose of the enzyme HMG-CoA reductase inhibitor and work similar to 'statin' drugs, such as lovastatin. Consider co-supplementing with coenzyme Q_{10}.

- Indication: lowering total and LDL-cholesterol and triglycerides.
- Dosage: 600mg/day.
- Results: 8–12 weeks.
- Side-effects: usually well tolerated; similar side-effects to statins such as hepatitis, muscle aches and pains; rhabdomyolysis; digestive problems, flatulence; allergic reaction; anaphylaxis in rare cases.
- Contraindications: liver or renal impairment; allergy to fungi or yeast; avoid taking with statin medication as they have an additive effect.

References

1 Kolovou GD, Anagnostopoulou KK, Cokkinos DV. Pathophysiology of dyslipidaemia in the metabolic syndrome. Postgrad Med J 2005;81:358–66.

2 Bernard J. Free fatty acid receptor family: novel targets for the treatment of diabetes and dyslipidemia. Curr Opin Investig Drugs 2008;9:1078–83.

3 Funatsu T, Suzuki K, Goto M, et. al. Prolonged inhibition of cholesterol synthesis by atorvastatin inhibits apo B-100 and triglyceride secretion from HepG2 cells. Atherosclerosis 2001;157:107–15.

4 Holvoet P, Jenny NS, Schreiner PJ, et. al. The relationship between oxidised LDL and other cardiovascular risk factors and subclinical CVD in different ethnic groups: The Multi-Ethnic Study of Atherosclerosis (MESA). Atherosclerosis 2007;194:245–52.

5 Gordon T, Kannel WB. Premature mortality from coronary heart disease. The Framingham study. JAMA 1971;215:1617–25.

6 Iso H, Jacobs DRJ, Wentworth D, et. al. Serum cholesterol levels and six-year mortality from stroke in 350,977 men screened for the multiple risk factor intervention trial. N Engl J Med 1989;320:904–10.

7 World Health Organization. Quantifying selected major risks to health. In: The World Health Report 2002 - Reducing Risks, Promoting Healthy Life. Chapter 4. World Health Organization, Geneva, 2002:47–97.

8 Eaton CB. Hyperlipidemia. Prim Care Clin Office Pract 2005;32:1027–55.

9 American Heart Association. High Blood Cholesterol and Other Lipids – Statistics (2009 Update). Available at: http://www.americanheart.org/downloadable/heart/1236205246237CHOL.pdf (accessed 18 June 2009).

10 Knox SA, Harrison CM, Britt HC, et. al. Estimating prevalence of common chronic morbidities in Australia. Medical Journal of Australia 2008;189:66–70.

11 Li Z, Yang R, Xu G, et. al. Serum lipid concentrations and prevalence of dyslipidemia in a large professional population in Beijing. Clinical Chemistry 2005;51:144–50.

12 Rana JS, Visser ME, Arsenault BJ, et. al. Metabolic dyslipidemia and risk of future coronary heart disease in apparently healthy men and women: The EPIC-Norfolk prospective population study. Int J Cardiol Epub ahead of print, doi:10.1016/j.ijcard.2009.03.123.

13 Ford ES, Li C, Zhao G, Pearson WS, et. al. Hypertriglyceridemia and its pharmacologic treatment among US adults. Arch Intern Med 2009;169:572–8.

14 Thom T, Haase N, Rosamond W, et. al. Heart disease and stroke statistics - 2006 update: a report from the American Heart Association Statistics Committee and Stroke Statistics Subcommittee. Circulation 2006;113:e85–e151.

15 Palmer AJ, Valentine WJ, Roze S, et. al. Overview of costs of stroke from published, incidence-based studies spanning 16 industrialised countries. Curr Med Res Opin 2005;21:19–26.

16 Erdman DM, Cook CB, Greenlund KJ, et. al. The impact of outpatient diabetes management on serum lipids in urban African-Americans with type 2 diabetes. Diabetes Care 2002;25:9–15.

17 National Heart Foundation of Australia and The Cardiac Society of Australia & New Zealand. Position Statement on Lipid Management – 2005. Heart and Lung Circulation 2005;14:275–291. Online. Available: http://www.heartfoundation.org.au/SiteCollectionDocuments/Lipids%20HLC%20Pos%20Statement.pdf (accessed 18 June 2009).

18 Euroaspire. A European Society of Cardiology survey of secondary prevention of coronary heart disease. Euroaspire Study Group. European action on secondary prevention through intervention to reduce events. Principal results. Eur Heart J 1997;18: 1569–82.

19 Simons LA, Levis G, Simons J. Apparent discontinuation rates in patients prescribed lipid-lowering drugs. Med J Aust 1996;164:208–11.

20 NCEP. Executive summary of the Third Report of The National Cholesterol Education Program (NCEP) Expert Panel on Detection, Evaluation, And Treatment of High Blood Cholesterol in Adults (Adult Treatment Panel III). JAMA 2001;285:2486–97.

21 Nies LK, Cymbala AA, Kasten SL, et. al. Complementary and alternative therapies for the management of dyslipidemia. Ann Pharmacother 2006;40:1984–92.

22 Caron MF, White CM. Evaluation of the anti-hyperlipidemic properties of dietary supplements. Pharmacotherapy 2001;21:451–7.

23 Beekman M, Heijmans BT, Martin Nicholas G, et. al. Evidence for a QTL on chromosome 19 influencing LDL-cholesterol levels in the general population. European Journal of Human Genetics 2003;11:845–50.

24 Jensen HK. The molecular genetic basis and diagnosis of familial hypercholesterolemia in Denmark. Dan Med Bull 2002;49:318–45.

25 Rosenthal RL. Effectiveness of altering serum cholesterol levels without drugs. BUMC Proceedings 2000;13:351–5.

26 Clifton P. Lowering cholesterol: A review on the role of plant sterols. Australian Family Physician 2009;38:218–21.

27 SEARCH Collaborative Group, Link E, Parish S, et. al. SLCO1B1 variants and statin-induced myopathy - A genomewide study. N Engl J Med 2008;359:789–99.

28 Dimsdale JE, Herd JA. Variability of plasma lipids in response to emotional arousal. Psychosomatic Medicine 1982;44:413–30.

29 Brindley DN, Rolland Y. Possible connections between stress, diabetes, hypertension and altered lipoprotein metabolism that mey result in athersclerosis. Clinical Science 1989;77:453–61.

30 Fan AZ, Strine TW, Muppidi SR, et. al. Psychological distress associated with self-reported high blood pressure and high blood cholesterol in U.S. adults, 2007. Int J Public Health 2009 April 14, Epub ahead of print.

31 Masley SC, Weaver W, Peri G, et. al. Efficacy of lifestyle changes in modifying practical markers of wellness and ageing. Altern Ther Health Med 2008;14:24–9.

32 Khatri D, Mathur KC, Gahlot S, et. al. Effects of yoga and meditation on clinical and biochemical parameters of metabolic syndrome. Diabetes Research and Clinical Practice, Epub ahead of print 2008; doi:10.1016/j.diabres.2007.05.002.

33 Lee IM, Sesso HD, Paffenbarger RS Jr. Physical activity and coronary heart disease risk in men: does the duration of exercise episodes predict risk? Circulation 2000;102:981–6.

34 Halverstadt A, Phares DA, Wilund KR, et. al. Endurance exercise training raises high-density lipoprotein cholesterol and lowers small low-density lipoprotein and very low-density lipoprotein independent of body fat phenotypes in older men and women. Metabolism Clinical and Experimental 2007;56:444–50.

35 Vislocky LM, Pikosky MA, Rubin KH, et. al. Habitual consumption of eggs does not alter the beneficial effects of endurance training on plasma lipids and lipoprotein metabolism in untrained men and women. Journal of Nutritional Biochemistry 2009;20:26–34.

36 Grandjean PW, Crouse SF, O'Brian BC, et. al. The effects of menopausal status and exercise training on serum lipids and the activities of intravascular enzymes related to lipid transport. Metabolism 1998;47:377–83.

37 Kokkinos PF, Holland JC, Narayan P, et. al. Miles run per week and high-density lipoprotein cholesterol levels in healthy, middleaged men. Arch Intern Med 1995;155:415–20.

38 Kokkinos PF, Narayan P, Colleran J. Effects of moderate intensity exercise on serum lipids in African-American men with sever systemic hypertension. Am J Cardiol 1998;81:732–5.

39 Seip RL, Moulin P, Cocke T, et. al. Exercise training decreases plasma cholesteryl ester transfer protein. Arterioscler Thromb 1993;13:1359–67.

40 Thompson PD, Yurgalevitch SM, Flynn MM, et. al. Effect of prolonged exercise training without weight loss on high-density lipoprotein metabolism in overweight men. Metabolism 1997;46:217–23.

41 Wilson PW, D'Agostino RB, Levy D, et. al. Prediction of coronary heart disease using risk factor categories. Circulation 1998;97:1837–47.

42 Ullrich IH, Reid CM, Yeater RA, et. al. Increased HDL-cholesterol levels with a weight lifting program. South Med J 1987;80:328–31.

43 Boyden TW, Pamenter RW, Going SB, et. al. Resistance exercise training is associated with decreases in serum low-density lipoprotein cholesterol levels in premenopausal women. Arch Intern Med 1993;153:97–100.

44 Kokkinos PF, Hurley BF, Smutok MA, et. al. Strength training does not improve lipoprotein-lipid profiles in men at risk for CHD. Med Sci Sports Exerc 1993;32:1134–9.

45 Smutok MA, Reece C, Kokkinos PF, et. al. Aerobic versus strength training for risk factor intervention in middle-aged men at high risk for coronary artery disease. Metabolism 1993;42:177–84.

46 Durstine JL, Grandjean PW, Cox CA, et. al. Lipids, Lipoproteins, and Exercise. Journal of Cardiopulmonary Rehabilitation 2002;22: 385–98.

47 Marques E, Carvalho J, Soares JMC, et. al. Effects of resistance and multi-component exercise on lipid profiles of older women. Maturitas Epub ahead of print, doi:10.1016/j.maturitas.2009.03.003.

48 Monda KL, Ballantyne CM, North KE. Longitudinal impact of physical activity on lipid profiles in middle-aged adults: the Atherosclerosis Risk in Communities (ARIC) Study. J Lipid Res 2009; Epub ahead of print, doi:10.1194/jlr.P900029-JLR200.

49 Keys A. Coronary heart disease in seven countries. Circulation 1970;41(Suppl. 1):1–211.

50 Skekelle RB, Shryock AM, Paul O, et. al. Diet, serum cholesterol, and death from coronary heart disease: the Western Electric study. New England Journal of Medicine 1981;304:65–70.

51 Joossens JV, Vuylsteek K, Brems-Heyns E, et. al. The pattern of food and mortality in Belgium. Lancet 1977;1:1069–72.

52 Kato H, Tillotson J, Nichaman MZ, et. al. Epidemiologic studies of coronary heart disease and stroke in Japanese men living in Japan, Hawaii and California: serum lipids and diet. American Journal of Epidemiology 1993;97:372–85.

53 Keys A, Anderson JT, Grande F. Prediction of serum-cholesterol responses of man to changes in fats in the diet. Lancet 1957;2:959–66.

54 Hegsted DM, McGandy RB, Myers ML, et. al. Quantitative effects of dietary fat on serum cholesterol in man. American Journal of Clinical Nutrition 1965;17:281–95.

55 Ahrens EH, Insull W, Blomstrand R, et. al. The influence of dietary fats on serum-lipid levels in man. Lancet 1957;1:943–53.

56 Shepherd J, Packard CJ, Grundy SM, et. al. Effects of saturated and polyunsaturated fat diets on the chemical composition and metabolism of low density lipoproteins in man. Journal of Lipid Research 1980;21:91–9.

57 Turner JD, Le NA, Brown WV. Effect of changing dietary fat saturation on low density lipoprotein metabolism in man. American Journal of Physiology 1981;241:E57-E63.

58 Hunninghake DB, Stein EA, Dujovne CA, et. al. The efficacy of intensive dietary therapy alone or combined with lovastatin in outpatients with hypercholesterolemia. N Engl J Med 1993;328:1213–19.

59 Schaefer EJ, Brosseau ME. Diet, lipoproteins, and coronary heart disease. Endocrinol Metab Clin North Am 1998;27:711–27.

60 Ornish D, Brown SE, Scherwitz LW, et. al. Can lifestyle changes reverse coronary heart disease? The Lifestyle Heart Trial. Lancet 1990;336:129–33.

61 Grundy SM. What is the desirable ratio of saturated, polyunsaturated, and monounsaturated fatty acids in the diet? Am J Clin Nutr 1997;66(Suppl):988S-990S.

62 Knopp RH. Drug treatment of lipid disorders. N Engl J Med 1999;341:498–511.

63 Mensink RP, Zock PL, Kester ADM, et. al. Effects of dietary fatty acids and carbohydrates on the ratio of serum total to HDL-cholesterol and on serum lipids and lipoproteins: a meta-analysis of 60 controlled trials. Amer J Clin Nutr 2003;77:1146–55.

64 Rask-Nissilä L, Jokinen E, Terho P, et. al. Neurological development of 5-year-old children receiving a low-saturated fat, low-cholesterol diet since infancy: A randomised controlled trial. Journal of the American Medical Association 2000;284: 993–1000.

65 Keys A. Serum cholesterol response to dietary cholesterol. Amer J Clin Nutr 1984;40:351–9.

66 Grundy SM, Florentin L, Nixand D, et. al. Comparison of monounsaturated fatty acids and carbohydrates for reducing raised levels of plasma cholesterol in man. Am J Clin Nutr 1988;47: 965–9.

67 Keys A, Anderson JT, Grande F. Serum cholesterol response to changes in the diet, IV: particular saturated fatty acids in the diet. Metabolism 1965;14:776–87.

68 Nygard O, Nordrehaug JE, Refsum H, et. al. Plasma homocysteine levels and mortality in patients with coronary artery disease. N Engl J Med 1997;337:230–6.

69 Gaziano JM, Buring JE, Breslow JL, et. al. Moderate alcohol intake, increased levels of high density lipoprotein and its subfractions, and decreased risk of myocardial infarction. N Engl J Med 1993;329:1829–34.

70 Trichopoulou A, Vasilopoulou E, Liagiou A. Mediterranean diet and coronary heart disease: are antioxidants critical? Nutr Rev 1999;57:253–5.

71 de Lorgeril M, Renaud S, Mamelle N, et. al. Mediterranean alpha-linolenic acid-rich diet in secondary prevention of coronary heart disease. Lancet 1994;343:1454–9.

72 de Lorgeril M, Salen P, Martin J-L, et. al. Mediterranean diet, traditional risk factors, and the rate of cardiovascular complications after myocardial infarction: final report of the Lyon Diet Heart Study. Circulation 1999;99:779–85.
73 Denke MA. Dietary fats, fatty acids, and their effects on lipoproteins. Curr Atheroscler Rep 2006;8:466–71.
74 Fernandez ML, West KL. Mechanisms by which dietary fatty acids modulate plasma lipids. J Nutr 2005;135:2075–8.
75 Lecerf JM. Fatty acids and cardiovascular disease. Nutr Rev 2009;67:273–83.
76 Jakobsen MU, O'Reilly EJ, Heitmann BL, et. al. Major types of dietary fat and risk of coronary heart disease: a pooled analysis of 11 cohort studies. Am J Clin Nutr 2009;89:1425–1432.
77 Mensink RP, Zock PL, Kester ADM, et. al. Effects of dietary fatty acids and carbohydrates on the ratio of serum total to HDL-cholesterol and on serum lipids and apolipoproteins: a meta-analysis of 60 controlled trials. Am J Clin Nutr 2003;77:1146–55.
78 Stampfer MJ, Sacks FM, Salvini S, et. al. A prospective study of cholesterol, apolipoproteins, and the risk of myocardial infarction. N Engl J Med 1991;325:373–81.
79 Mukuddem-Petersen J, OosthuisenW, Jerling J. A systematic review of the effects of nuts on blood lipid profiles in humans. J Nutr 2005;135:2082–9.
80 Griel AE, Kris-Etherton PM. Tree nuts and the lipid profile: a review of clinical studies. Br J Nutr 2006;96(Suppl 2):S68–S78.
81 Ros E. Nuts and novel biomarkers of cardiovascular disease. Am J Clin Nutr 2009;89(suppl):1649S–1656S.
82 Rajaram S, Haddad EH, Mejia A, et. al. Walnuts and fatty fish influence different serum lipid fractions in normal to mildly hyperlipidemic individuals: a randomised controlled study. Am J Clin Nutr 2009;89 (suppl):1657S–1663S.
83 Samaha FF, Iqbal N, Seshadri P, et. al. A low-carbohydrate as compared with a low-fat diet in severe obesity. N Engl J Med 2003;348:2074–81.
84 Foster GD, Wyatt HR, Hill JO, et. al. A randomised trial of a low-carbohydrate diet for obesity. N Engl J Med 2003;348:2082–90.
85 Skov AR, Toubro S, Rønn B, et. al. Randomised trial on protein vs carbohydrate in ad libitum fat reduced diet for the treatment of obesity. Int J Obes Relat Metab Disord 2003;23:528–36.
86 Jenkins DJ, Kendall CWC, Vidgen E, et. al. High-protein diets in hyperlipidemia: effect of wheat gluten on serum lipids, uric acid, and renal function. Am J Clin Nutr 2001;74:57–63.
87 Parker B, Noakes M, Luscombe N, et. al. Effect of a high-protein, high-monounsaturated fat weight loss diet on glycemic control and lipid levels in type 2 diabetes. Diabetes Care 2002;25:425–30.
88 Bravata DM, Sanders L, Huang J, et. al. Efficacy and safety of low-carbohydrate diets: a systematic review. JAMA 2003;289:1837–50.
89 Jenkins DJA, Julia MW, Wong RD et. al. The Effect of a Plant-Based Low-Carbohydrate ('Eco-Atkins') Diet on Body Weight and Blood Lipid Concentrations in Hyperlipidemic Subjects. Arch Intern Med 2009;169(11):1046–1054.
90 Jenkins DJ, Kendall CWC, Marchie A, et. al. Effects of a dietary portfolio of cholesterol-lowering foods vs lovastatin on serum lipids and C-reactive protein. JAMA 2003;290:502–10.
91 Jenkins DJA, Kendall CWC, Faulkner DA, et. al. The Effect of Combining Plant Sterols, Soy Protein, Viscous Fibres, and Almonds in Treating Hypercholesterolemia. Metabolism 2003;52:1478–83.
92 Jenkins DJ, Kendall CW, Faulkner DA, et. al. Assessment of the longer-term effects of a dietary portfolio of cholesterol-lowering foods in hypercholesterolemia. Am J Clin Nutr 2006;83:582–91.
93 Jenkins DJA, Kendall CWC, Faulkner DA, et. al. Long-term effects of a plant-based dietary portfolio of cholesterol-lowering foods on blood pressure. European Journal of Clinical Nutrition 2008;62:781–8.
94 Jenkins DJ, Kendall CW, Marchie A, et. al. Direct comparison of dietary portfolio vs statin on C-reactive protein. European Journal of Clinical Nutrition 2005;59:851–60.
95 Gigleux I, Jenkins DJA, Kendall CWC, et. al. Comparison of a dietary portfolio diet of cholesterol-lowering foods and a statin on LDL particle size phenotype in hypercholesterolaemic participants. British Journal of Nutrition 2007;98:1229–36.
96 Gorinstein S, Caspi A, Libman I, et. al. Fresh israeli jaffa sweetie juice consumption improves lipid metabolism and increases antioxidant capacity in hypercholesterolemic patients suffering from coronary artery disease: studies in vitro and in humans and positive changes in albumin and fibrinogen fractions. J Agric Food Chem 2004;52:5215–22.
97 Gorinstein S, Caspi A, Libman I, et. al. Red grapefruit positively influences serum triglyceride level in patients suffering from coronary atherosclerosis: studies in vitro and in humans. J Agric Food Chem 2006;54:1887–92.
98 Dahan A, Altman H. Food-drug interaction: grapefruit juice augments drug bioavailability--mechanism, extent and relevance. Eur J Clin Nutr 2004;58:1–9.
99 Gateway IM, Braun L. Drug-Food Supplement Interactions. Journal of Complementary Medicine 2004;3:80–84.
100 Anderson JW, Johnstone BM, Cook-Newell ME. Meta-analysis of the effects of soy protein intake on serum lipids. New Engl J Med 1995;333:276–82.
101 Sirtori CR, Eberini I, Arnoldi A. Hypocholesterolaemic effects of soya proteins: results of recent studies are predictable from the Anderson meta-analysis data. Br J Nutr 2007;97:816–22.
102 Descovich GC, Ceredi C, Gaddi A, et. al. Multicentre study of soybean protein diet for outpatient hyper-cholesterolaemic patients. Lancet 1980;ii:709–12.
103 Zhan S, Ho SC. Meta-analysis of the effects of soy protein containing isoflavones on the lipid profile. Am J Clin Nutr 2005;81:397–408.
104 Dewell A, Hollenbeck PLW, Hollenbeck CB. A critical evaluation of the role of soy protein and isoflavone supplementation in the control of plasma cholesterol concentrations. Journal of Clinical Endocrinology & Metabolism 2006;91:772–80.
105 AHA Science Advisory. Soy protein and cardiovascular disease: a statement for health care professionals from the Nutrition Committee of the AHA. Circulation 2000;102:2555–9.
106 Brufau G, Canela MA, Rafecas M. Phytosterols: physiologic and metabolic aspects related to cholesterol-lowering properties. Nutr Res 2008;28:217–25.
107 Tikkanen MJ. Plant sterols and stanols. Handb Exp Pharmacol 2005;170:215–30.

108 Ikeda I, Tanabe Y, Sugano M. Effects of sitosterol and sitostanol on micellar solubility of cholesterol. J Nutr Sci Vitaminol 1989;35:361–9.
109 Subbiah MT, Kottke BA, Carlo IA. Uptake of campesterol in pigeon intestine. Biochim Biophys Acta 1971;249:643–6.
110 Ling WH, Jones PJ. Dietary phytosterols: a review of metabolism, benefits and side-effects. Life Sci 1995;57:195–206.
111 Plat J, Mensink RP. Increased intestinal ABCA1 expression contributes to the decrease in cholesterol absorption after plant stanol consumption. FASEB J 2002;16:1248–53.
112 Gylling H, Miettinen TA. Effects of inhibiting cholesterol absorption and synthesis on cholesterol and lipoprotein metabolism in hypercholesterolemic non-insulin dependent diabetic men. J Lipid Res 1996;37:1776–85.
113 Lesesne JM, Castor CW, Hoobler SW. Prolonged reduction in human blood cholesterol levels induced by plant sterols. Med Bull 1955;21:13–7.
114 Ostlund RE Jr. Phytosterols in human nutrition. Annu Rev Nutr 2002;22:533–49.
115 Clifton P. Lowering cholesterol: A review on the role of plant sterols. Australian Family Physician 2009;38:218–21.
116 Law M. Plant sterol and stanol margarines and health. BMJ 2000;320:861–864.
117 Neil HAW, Huxley RR. Efficacy and therapeutic potential of plant sterols. Athcroscler 2002;Suppl 3:11–5.
118 Lichtenstein AH. Plant sterols and blood lipid levels. Curr Opin Clin Nutr Metab Care 2002;5:147–52.
119 Simons LA. Additive effect of plant sterol-ester margarine and cerivastatin in lowering low-density lipoprotein cholesterol in primary hypercholesterolemia. Am J Cardiol 2002;90: 737–40.
120 Micallef MA, Garg ML. The Lipid-Lowering Effects of Phytosterols and (n-3) Polyunsaturated Fatty Acids Are Synergistic and Complementary in Hyperlipidemic Men and Women. J Nutr 2008;138:1086–90.
121 Khandelwal S, Demonty S, Jeemon P. Independent and interactive effects of plant sterols and fish oil n-3 long-chain polyunsaturated fatty acids on the plasma lipid profile of mildly hyperlipidaemic Indian adults. British Journal of Nutrition 2009; EPub ahead of print doi:10.1017/ S0007114509297170.
122 AbuMweis SS, Jones PJ. Cholesterol-lowering effect of plant sterols. Curr Atheroscler Rep 2008;10: 467–72.
123 Plana N, Nicolle C, Ferre R, et. al. Plant sterol-enriched fermented milk enhances the attainment of LDL-cholesterol goal in hypercholesterolemic subjects. Eur J Nutr 2008;47:32–9.
124 Moruisi KG, Oosthuisen W, Opperman AM. Phytosterols/stanols lower cholesterol concentrations in familial hypercholesterolemic subjects: a systematic review with meta-analysis. J Am Coll Nutr 2006;25:41–8.
125 O'Connor PJ, Quiter ES, Rush WA, et. al. Relative effectiveness of niacin and lovastatin for treatment of dyslipidemias in a health maintenance organisation. J Family Pract 1997;44:462–7.
126 Illingworth D, Stein EA, Mitchel YB, et. al. Comparative effects of lovastatin and niacin in primary hypercholesterolemia: a prospective trial. Arch Intern Med 1994;154:1586–95.
127 Vega G, Grundy S. Lipoprotein responses to treatment with lovastatin, gemfibrozil and nicotinic acid in normolipidemic patients with hypoalphalipoprotein. Arch Intern Med 1994;154:73–82.
128 Guyton JR, Blazing MA, Hagar J, et. al. Extended-release niacin vs gemfibrozil for the treatment of low levels of high-density lipoprotein cholesterol. Niaspan-Gemfibrozil Study Group. Arch Intern Med 2000;160:1177–84.
129 Linke A, Sonnabend M, Fasshauer M, et. al. Effects of extended-release niacin on lipid profile and adipocyte biology in patients with impaired glucose tolerance. Atherosclerosis 2009;Epub prior to print, doi:10.1016/j.atherosclerosis.2008.11.026.
130 Wolfe ML, Vartanian SF, Ross JL, et. al. Safety and effectiveness of Niaspan when added sequentially to a statin for treatment of dyslipidemia. Am J Cardiol 2001;87:476–9.
131 Wink J, Giacoppe G, King J. Effect of very-low-dose naicin on high-density lipoprotein in patients undergoing long-term statin therapy. Am Heart J 2002;143:514–8.
132 Brown BG, Zhao XQ, Chait A. Simvastatin and niacin, antioxidant vitamins, or the combination for the prevention of coronary disease. N Engl J Med 2001;345:1583–93.
133 Kamanna VS, Kashyap ML. Nicotinic acid (niacin) receptor agonists: will they be useful therapeutic agents? Am J Cardiol. 2007;100:S53–S61.
134 Digby JE, Lee JM, Choudhury RP. Nicotinic acid and the prevention of coronary artery disease. Curr Opin Lipidol. 2009;Epub ahead of print doi: 10.1097/ MOL.0b013e32832d3b9d.
135 Robinson JG. Management of complex lipid abnormalities with a fixed dose combination of simvastatin and extended release niacin. Vasc Health Risk Manag. 2009;5:31–43.
136 Karas RH, Kashyap ML, Knopp RH. Long-term safety and efficacy of a combination of niacin extended release and simvastatin in patients with dyslipidemia: the OCEANS study. Am J Cardiovasc Drugs 2008;8:69–81.
137 Plaisance EP, Mestek L, Mahurin AJ, et. al. Postprandial triglyceride responses to aerobic exercise and extended-release niacin. American Journal of Clinical Nutrition 2008;88:30–37.
138 Kamanna VS, Ganji SH, Kashyap ML. Niacin: an old drug rejuvenated. Curr Atheroscler Rep 2009;11: 45–51.
139 Kamanna VS, Vo A, Kashyap ML. Nicotinic acid: recent developments. Curr Opin Cardiol 2008;23:393–8.
140 Kamanna VS, Kashyap ML. Nicotinic acid (niacin) receptor agonists: will they be useful therapeutic agents? Am J Cardiol 2007;100:S53–S61.
141 Theuwissen E, Mensink RP. Water-soluble dietary fibres and cardiovascular disease. Physiology & Behavior 2008;94:285–92.
142 Braaten JT, Wood PJ, Scott FW, et. al. Oat beta-glucan reduces blood cholesterol concentration in hypercholesterolemic subjects. Eur J Clin Nutr 1994;48:465–74.
143 Anderson JW. Dietary fibre, complex carbohydrate and coronary artery disease. Can J Cardiol 1995;11(Suppl G):55G-62G.
144 Swain J, Rouse I, Curley C, et. al. Comparison of the effects of oat bran and low-fibre wheat on serum lipoprotein levels and blood pressure. N Engl J Med 1990;322:147–52.

145 Leadbetter J, Ball MJ, Mann JI. Effects of increasing quantities of oat bran in hypercholesterolemic people. Am J Clin Nutr 1991;54:841–5.
146 Lovegrove JA, Clohessy A, Milon H, et. al. Modest doses of betaglucan do not reduce concentrations of potentially atherogenic lipoproteins. Am J Clin Nutr 2000;72:49–55.
147 Ripsin CM, Keenan JM, Jacobs DR, et. al. Oat products and llipid-lowering. A meta-analysis. JAMA 1992;267:3317–25.
148 Glore SR, Van Treeck D, Knehans AW, et. al. Soluble fibre and serum lipids: a literature review. J Am Diet Assoc 1994;94:425–36.
149 Brown L, Rosner B, Willett WW, et. al. Cholesterol-lowering effects of dietary fibre: a meta-analysis. Am J Clin Nutr 1999;69:30–42.
150 Talati R, Baker WL, Pabilonia MS, et. al. The Effects of Barley-Derived Soluble Fibre on Serum Lipids. Ann Fam Med 2009;7:157–63.
151 Sprecher DL, Harris BV, Goldberg AC, et. al. Efficacy of psyllium in reducing serum cholesterol levels in hypercholesterolemic patients on high- or low-fat diets. Ann Intern Med 1993;199:545–54.
152 Anderson JW, Zettwoch N, Feldman T, et. al. Cholesterol-lowering effects of psyllium hydrophilic mucciloid for hypercholesterolemic men. Arch Intern Med 1988;148:292–6.
153 Olson BH, Anderson SM, Becker MP, et. al. Psyllium-enriched cereals lower blood total cholesterol & LDL-cholesterol, but not HDL-cholesterol in hypercholesterolemic adults: results of a metanalysis. J Nutr 1992;127:1973–80.
154 Anderson JW, Riddell-Mason S, Gustafson NJ, et. al. Cholesterol-lowering effects of psyllium enriched cereal as an adjunct to a prudent diet in the treatment of mild to moderate hypercholesterolemia. Am J Clin Nutr 1992;56:93–5.
155 Keys A, Grande F, Anderson JT. Fibre and pectin in the diet and serum cholesterol concentration in man. Proc Soc Exp Biol Med 1961;106:555–8.
156 Schwab U, Louheranta A, Torronen A, et. al. Impact of sugar beet pectin and polydextrose on fasting and postprandial glycemia and fasting concentrations of serum total and lipoprotein lipids in middle-aged subjects with abnormal glucose metabolism. Eur J Clin Nutr 2006;60:1073–80.
157 Mahalko JR, Sandstead HH, Johnson LK, et. al. Effect of consuming fibre from corn bran, soy hulls, or apple powder on glucose tolerance and plasma lipids in type II diabetes. Am J Clin Nutr 1984;39:25–34.
158 Fahrenbach MJ, Riccardi BA, Saunders JC, et. al. Comparative effetcs of guar gum and pectin on human serum cholesterol levels. Circulation 1965;55:767–72.
159 Martino F, Martino E, Morrone F, et. al. Effect of dietary supplementation with glucomannan on plasma total cholesterol and low density lipoprotein cholesterol in hypercholesterolemic children. Nutr Metab Cardiovasc Dis 2005;15:174–80.
160 Arvill A, Bodin L. Effect of short-term ingestion of konjac glucomannan on serum cholesterol in healthy men. Am J Clin Nutr 1995;61:585–9.
161 Zhang MO, Huang CY, Wang X, et. al. The effect of foods containing refined konjac meal on human lipid metabolism. Biomed Environ Sci 1990;3:99–105.
162 Chen HL, Huey-Herng Sheu W, Tai TS, et. al. Konjac supplement alleviated hypercholesterolemia and hyperglycemia in type 2 diabetic subjects—a randomised double-blind trial. J Am Coll Nutr 2003;22:36–42.
163 Sood N, Baker WL, Coleman CI. Effect of glucomannan on plasma lipid and glucose concentrations, body weight, and blood pressure: systematic review and meta-analysis. Am J Clin Nutr 2008;88:1167–75.
164 Weintraub MS, Zechner R, Brown A, et. al. Dietary polyunsaturated fats of the w-6 and w-3 series reduce postprandial lipoprotein levels: chronic and acute effects of fat saturation on postprandial lipoprotein metabolism. J Clin Invest 1988;82:1884–93.
165 Woodman RJ, Mori TA, Burke V, et. al. Effects of purified eicosapentaenoic and docosahexaenoic acids on glycemic control, blood pressure, and serum lipids in type 2 diabetic patients with treated hypertension. Am J Clin Nutr 2002;76:1007–15.
166 Grimsgaard S, Bonaa KH, Hansen JB, et. al. Highly purified eicosapentaenoic acid and docosahexaenoic acid in humans have similar triacylglycerol-lowering effects but divergent effects on serum fatty acids. Am J Clin Nutr 1997;66:649–59.
167 Connor WE. Dietary sterols: their relationship to atherosclerosis. J Am Diet Assoc 1968;52:202–8.
168 Eslick GD, Howe PRC, Smith C, et. al. Benefits of fish oil supplementation in hyperlipidemia: a systematic review and meta-analysis. Int J Cardiol 2009; doi:10.1016/j.ijcard.2008.03.092.
169 Studer M, Briel M, Leimenstoll B, et. al. Effects of different antilipidemic agents and diet on mortality. Arch Intern Med 2005;165:725–30.
170 GISSI-HF investigators. Effect of n-3 polyunsaturated fatty acids in patients with chronic heart failure (the GISSI-HF trial): a randomised, double-blind, placebo-controlled trial. Lancet 2008;372:1223–30.
171 Nambi V, Ballantyne CM. Combination therapy with statins and omega-3 fatty acids. Amer J Cardiol 2006;98:43i-38i.
172 Agarwal RC, Singh SP, Saran RK, et. al. Clinical trial of Guggulipid new hypolipidemic agent of plant prigin in primary Hyperlipidemia. Indian J Med Res 1986;84:626–34.
173 Nityanand S, Srivastava JS, Asthana OP. Clinical trials with Guggulipid – A new hyperlipidemic agent. J Assoc Phys India 1989;37:323–8.
174 Singh RB, Niaz MA, Ghosh S. Hypolipidemic and antioxidant effects of *Commiphora mukul* as an adjunct to dietary therapy in patients with hypercholesterolemia. Cardiovasc Drug Ther 1994;8:659–64.
175 Szapary PO, Wolfe ML, Bloedon LT, et. al. Guggulipid for the treatment of Hypercholesterolemia: A randomised controlled trial. JAMA 2003;290:765–72.
176 Nohr LA, Rasmussen LB, Straand J. Resin from the mukul myrrh tree, guggul, can it be used for treating hypercholesterolemia? A randomised, controlled study. Complement Ther Med 2009;17:16–22.
177 Kraft K. Artichoke leaf extract: recent findings reflecting effects on lipid metabolism, liver and gastrointestinal tracts. Phytomedicine 1997;4: 369–78.
178 Bundy R, Walker RF, Middleton RW, et. al. Artichoke leaf extract (Cynara scolymus) reduces plasma cholesterol in otherwise healthy hypercholesterolemic adults: A randomised, double-blind placebo-controlled trial. Phytomedicine 2008;15:668–75.
179 Nazni P, Vijayakumar TP, Alagianambi P, et. al. Hypoglycemic and hypolipidemic effect of cynara scolymus among selected type 2 diabetic individuals. Pakistan J Nutrition 2006;5:147–51.

180 Pittler MH, Ernst E. Artichoke leaf extract for treating hypercholesterolaemia. Cochrane Database of Systematic Reviews, 2002; Art. No.: CD003335. doi: 10.1002/14651858.CD003335.

181 Englisch W, Beckers C, Unkauf M, et. al. Efficacy of artichoke dry extract in patients with hyperlipoproteinemia. Arzneim.-Forsch. / Drug Res 2000;50:260–65.

182 Petrowicz O, Gebhardt R, Donner M, et. al. Effects of artichoke leaf extract (ALE) on lipoprotein metabolism in vitro and in vivo. Atherosclerosis 1997;129:147.

183 Jain A, Vargas R, Gotzkowsky S, et. al. Can garlic reduce the levels of serum lipids? A controlled clinical study. Am J Med 1993;94:632–5.

184 Alder AJ, Holub BJ. Effect of garlic and oil supplementation on serum lipid and lipoprotein concentrations in hypercholesterolemic men. Am J Cli Nutr 1997;65:445–50.

185 Steiner M, Khan AH, Holbert D, et. al. A double-blind crossover study in moderately hypercholesterolemic men that compared the effect of aged garlic extract and placebo administration on blood lipids. Am J Clin Nutr 1996;64:866–70.

186 Byrne DJ, Neil HA, Vallance DT, et. al. A pilot study of garlic consumption shows no significant effect on markers of oxidation or sub-fraction composition of low-density lipoprotein including lipoprotein (a) after allowance for non-compliance and the placebo effect. Clin Chim Acta 1999;285:21–33.

187 Berthold HK, Sudhop T, Von Bergman K. Effect of garlic oil preparation on serum lipoproteins and cholesterol metabolism: A randomised controlled trial. JAMA 1998;279:1900–2.

188 Warshafsky S, Kamer RS, Sivak SL. Effect of garlic on total serum cholesterol. A meta-analysis. Ann Intern Med 1993;119:599–605.

189 Stevinson C, Pittler MH, Ernst E. Garlic for treating hypercholesterolemia. A meta-analysis of randomised clinical trials. Ann Intern Med 2001;135:65–66.

190 Khoo YSK, Azis Z. Garlic supplementation and serum cholesterol: a meta-analysis. J Clin Pharm Ther 2009;34:133–45.

191 Castano G, Mas R, Arruzazabala ML, et. al. Effects of Policosanol and Pravastatin on lipid profile, platelet aggregation and endothelaemia in older hypercholesterolemic patients. Int. J. Clin. Pharm. Res. 1999;XIX(4):105–16.

192 Castano G, Cannetti M, Moreira M, et. al. Efficacy and tolerability of policosanol compared with lovastatin in patients with type II hypercholesterolemia and concomitant coronary risk factors. Current Therapeutic Research 2000;61: 137–46.

193 Fernandez JC, Mas R, Castano G, et. al. Comparison of the efficacy, safety and tolerability of policosanol versus fluvastatin in elderly hypercholesterolaemic women. Clinical Drug Invest. 2001;21:103–13.

194 Marcello S, Gladstein J, Tesone P, et. al. Effects of bezafibrate plus policosanol or placebo in patients with combined dyslipidaemia: a pilot study. Current Therapeutic Research. 2000;61:346–57.

195 Nikitin I, Slepchenko NV, Gratsianski NA, et. al. Results of the multicentre controlled study of the hypolipidemic drug polycosanol in Russia. Ter Arkh 2000;72:7–10.

196 Prat H, Roman O, Pino E. Comparative effects of polycosanol and two HMG-CoA reductase inhibitors on type II hypercholesterolemia. Rev Med Chil 1999;127:286–94.

197 Francini-Pesenti F, Beltramolli D, Dall'acqua S, et. al. Effect of sugar cane policosanol on lipid profile in primary hypercholesterolemia. Phytother Res 2008;22:318–22.

198 Berthold HK, Unverdorben S, Degenhardt R, et. al. Effect of policosanol on lipid levels among patients with hypercholesterolemia or combined hyperlipidemia: a randomised controlled trial. JAMA 2006;295:2262–9.

199 Cubeddu LX, Cubeddu RJ, Heimowitz T, et. al. Comparative lipid-lowering effects of policosanol and atorvastatin: a randomised, parallel, double-blind, placebo-controlled trial. Am Heart J 2006;152:982–5.

200 Keller S, Gimmler F, Jahreis G. Octacosanol administration to humans decreases neutral sterol and bile acid concentration in feces. Lipids 2008;43:109–15.

201 Chen JT, Wesley R, Shamburek RD, et. al. Meta-analysis of natural therapies for hyperlipidemia: plant sterols and stanols versus policosanol. Pharmacotherapy 2005;25:171–83.

202 Kassis AN, Jones PJ. Changes in cholesterol kinetics following sugar cane policosanol supplementation: a randomised control trial. Lipids Health Dis. 2008;7:17

203 Kassis AN, Jones PJ. Lack of cholesterol-lowering efficacy of Cuban sugar cane policosanols in hypercholesterolemic persons. Am J Clin Nutr 2006;84:1003–8

204 Kassis AN, Kubow S, Jones PJ. Sugar cane policosanols do not reduce LDL oxidation in hypercholesterolemic individuals. Lipids 2009;44:391–6.

205 Greyling A, De Witt C, Oosthuisen W, et. al. Effects of a policosanol supplement on serum lipid concentrations in hypercholesterolaemic and heterozygous familial hypercholesterolaemic subjects. Br J Nutr 2006;95:968–75

206 Heber D, Yip I, Ashley JM, et. al. Cholesterol-lowering effects of a proprietary Chinese red-yeast-rice dietary supplement. Am J Clin Nutr 1999;69:231–6.

207 Wang J, Lu A, Chi J. Multicenter clinical trial of the serum lipid-lowering effects of a monascus purpureus (red yeast) rice preparation from traditional Chinese medicine. Cur Ther Res 1997;58:964–78.

208 Kou W, Lu Z, Guo J. Effect of xuezhikang on the treatment of primary hyperlipidemia. [Article in Chinese]. Chung Hua Nei Ko Tsa Chih 1997;36:529–31.

209 Blisnakov EG. More on the Chinese red-yeast-rice supplementanditscholesterol-loweringeffect.AmJClin Nutr 2000;71:152–7.

210 Heber D, Lembertas A, Lu QY, et. al. An analysis of nine proprietary Chinese red yeast rice dietary supplements: implications of variability in chemical profile and contents. J Altern Complement Med 2001;7:133–9.

211 Keithley JK, Swanson B, Sha BE, et. al. A pilot study of the safety and efficacy of cholestin in treating HIV-related dyslipidemia. Nutrition 2002;18:201–4.

212 Bianchi A. Extracts of Monascusus purpureus beyond statins--profile of efficacy and safety of the use of extracts of Monascus purpureus. Chin J Integr Med. 2005;11:309–13.

213 Prasad GV, Wong T, Meliton G, et. al. Rhabdomyolysis due to red yeast rice (Monascus purpureus) in a renal transplant recipient. Transplantation 2002;74:1200–1.

214 Mueller PS. Symptomatic myopathy due to red yeast rice. Ann Intern Med 2006;145:474–5.
215 Roselle H, Ekatan A, Tzeng J, et. al. Symptomatic hepatitis associated with the use of herbal red yeast rice. Ann Intern Med 2008;149:516–7.
216 Wigger-Alberti W, Bauer A, Hipler UC, et. al. Anaphylaxis due to Monascus purpureus-fermented rice (red yeast rice). Allergy 1999;54:1330–1.
217 Huang CF, Li TC, Lin CC, et. al. Efficacy of Monascus purpureus Went rice on lowering lipid ratios in hypercholesterolemic patients. Eur J Cardiovasc Prev Rehabil 2007;14:438–40.
218 Lin CC, Li TC, Lai MM. Efficacy and safety of Monascus purpureus Went rice in subjects with hyperlipidemia. Eur J Endocrinol 2005;153:679–86.
219 Gheith O, Sheashaa H, Abdelsalam M, et. al. Efficacy and safety of Monascus purpureus Went rice in subjects with secondary hyperlipidemia. Clin Exp Nephrol 2008;12:189–94.
220 Liu J, Zhang J, Shi Y, et. al. Chinese red yeast rice (Monascus purpureus) for primary hyperlipidemia: a meta-analysis of randomised controlled trials. Chin Med 2006;1:4.
221 Becker DJ, Gordon RY, Halbert SC, et. al. Red yeast rice for dyslipidemia in statin-intolerant patients: a randomised trial. Annals of Internal Medicine 2009;150:830–9.

Chapter 19

Hypertension

Introduction

Hypertension (HT) is a major risk factor for cardiovascular diseases (CVDs).

Estimates from the World Health Organization show that CVD accounted for approximately 17 million deaths in 2001, this being approximately 30% of the total 57 million deaths due to chronic diseases.[1] This in fact represents approximately the total current population of the Australian continent. It is now a disease that is not restricted to the affluent Western world alone but the developing countries as well.[2] Hence, as of the mid-1990s, CVD is also the leading cause of death in developing countries. In fact, a global CVD epidemic has been predicted based on the epidemiologic transition in which control of infectious, parasitic, and nutritional diseases allows most of the population to reach the ages in which CVD manifests itself. Moreover, diet and lifestyle changes contribute to an increase in overweight and obesity and in the incidence of type 2 diabetes in Western countries, both of which are risk factors for CVD.[3] It then becomes possible to predict that disability from CVD will be a world leader by the year 2010.[1]

The medical profession must implement comprehensive preventative programs that address lifestyle and nutritional issues if it is to achieve a significant reversal of this adverse trend.[1] The major emphasis currently is on treatment of CVD however, there is increasing interest in dealing with the factors responsible for this disease.

The cornerstone to the management of essential HT is lifestyle advice, including diet, smoking avoidance, reduced salt and caffeine intake, exercising, reducing stress and correcting sleep problems.[4] Nutraceuticals have been reported to be beneficial in the prevention and risk management of CVD and may be broadly classified as those used in prevention or treatment of congestive heart failure, arrhythmias, hypertension, angina and hyperlipidemias.[5] This chapter will explore these areas and look at the scientific evidence for non-drug approaches to help prevent and treat HT.

Lifestyle interventions

Numerous lifestyle and nutritional factors can prevent, delay the onset of, reduce the severity of, assist to treat, and control HT in many patients from diverse population groups.[6] Lifestyle protective factors against HT are:

- stress reduction and management
- adequate sleep and sleep restoration
- physical activity
- smoking cessation
- healthy diet and nutrition
- maintaining healthy body weight and/or weight loss management
- salt restriction
- sun exposure and fresh air
- moderate restriction of alcohol and caffeine intake
- chocolate
- breast feeding.

Recently updated National Heart Foundation guidelines recommend that advice on reducing and ceasing smoking, nutrition, reducing alcohol use, promoting regular physical activity and achieving a healthy body weight are effective methods in lowering blood pressure (BP) and should be part of routine management of HT for all patients, regardless of drug therapy. Smoking cessation is recommended to reduce overall cardiovascular risk.[7]

Mind–body medicine

Stress reduction and management

A population-based, prospective, observational study using participant data from the Coronary Artery Risk Development in Young Adults (CARDIA) study (3308 young adults aged 18–30) showed that those who rushed, were impatient and hostile had nearly double the risk of developing HT over 15 years, compared with their peers.[8] Lifestyle stressors are important markers for the development of HT. Recently the results of a further study suggest that cumulative stressful life events have a negative effect on mental health and quality of life in young black men with high BP.[9]

A US study has reported that people who felt they had no control over an unpleasant stimulus had significantly higher BP and peripheral artery resistance than those who believed they were in control.[10]

A number of studies have demonstrated techniques used to lower stress levels can assist to lower BP, such as progressive muscle relaxation, psycho-education, biofeedback and self-hypnosis.[11–14]

A small trial of stress reduction demonstrated that 70% of the participants who had mild to moderate HT and who were taught stress reduction techniques, were able to reduce their medication after 6 weeks and, after 1 year, 55% required no medication.[15]

A meta-analysis including 29 randomised control trials (RCTs) indicated that relaxation resulted in small but statistically significant reductions in systolic and diastolic BP compared to control although most trials were of poor quality. Consequently the authors concluded 'the evidence in favour of causal association between relaxation and BP reduction is weak'.[16]

Individual psychological therapy, including anger management and stress management techniques, reduced BP by more than 5mmHg in half of the hypertensive patients with BP greater than 140/90.[17] The men and women were randomised to 10 1-hour individual sessions of therapy or a waiting list for 3 months and then therapy. However, as only half of all treated patients showed major improvement, the study recommendations were to 'consider patients for psychological treatment when they report a great deal of subjective stress and/or find psychological interventions appealing'.[17]

Given that psychosocial stress has been implicated in disproportionately higher rates of HT among African Americans, a recent RCT of stress reduction in African Americans treated for HT for over 1 year showed that a selected stress reduction approach, through a transcendental meditation program, may be useful as an adjunct in the long-term treatment of HT in African Americans.[18]

Also note that studies have been undertaken to determine the extent of the white-coat phenomenon in patients with resistant hypertension. It is estimated that about 25% of patients with HT due to white-coat HT actually have normal BP.[19, 20]

Transcendental meditation

A review on the effectiveness of the transcendental meditation program in treatment and prevention of CVD has concluded that this technique reduces BP, carotid artery intima-media thickness, myocardial ischemia, left ventricular hypertrophy, mortality, and other relevant outcomes.[21] The magnitudes of these effects compare favourably with those of conventional interventions for secondary prevention.

Sleep

Clinical research demonstrates that BP increases in hypertensive patients results from insufficient sleep.[22] Researchers suggested this may be due to increased sympathetic nervous activity at night. A recent review has concluded that a healthy amount of sleep is paramount to leading a healthy and productive lifestyle. Further, that under strict experimental conditions, short-term restriction of sleep results in a variety of adverse physiologic effects, including hypertension, activation of the sympathetic nervous system, impairment of glucose control, and increased inflammation.[23]

A recent US cross-sectional study of 1741 adults found chronic insomnia and shortened duration of sleep significantly increased the risk of HT by 2.4 times compared with those of normal sleep.[24] This risk increased by fivefold when the sleep duration was less than 5 hours.

The researchers hypothesised that poor sleep activates the sympathetic nervous system, resulting in the increased BP and concluded that insomnia is an independent risk factor on par to age, sex, alcohol use, depression and sleep-disordered breathing, although findings needed further confirmation.

Environment

An innovative study demonstrated that outdoor temperature and seasonal variations strongly correlated with BP fluctuations, particularly in elderly over 80 years of age. Systolic BP decreased with increasing temperature, with an 8.0mmHg decrease between the lowest (<7.9°C) and the highest (21.2°C) temperature quintile.[25] Consequently, the elderly should be cautious with extreme temperatures and monitor their BP and medication dosage carefully to avoid complications.

Physical activity

Epidemiologic studies demonstrate that men who lead a physically active life can reduce their risk of developing HT by approximately 35% to 70%, compared to sedentary individuals.[5] A review of the literature shows that, on average, 75% of hypertensive patients can decrease their systolic blood pressure (SBP) and diastolic blood pressure (DBP) by 11mmHg and 8mmHg respectively within 1 to 10 weeks of starting physical activity regimens (i.e. exercise training).[26] A recent epidemiological study has reported that regular physical activity was negatively associated with HT in women.[27]

Tai chi

A systematic review of 47 studies that looked at the effects of tai chi on cardiovascular and BP found overall beneficial effects for healthy people, including increased muscle strength, flexibility, less falls, and improved mood.[28] The reviewers concluded that more well-designed studies were necessary.

Qigong

A recent review suggests that there is encouraging evidence of qigong having efficacy in lowering SBP.[29] A recent study of self-practiced qigong for less than 1 year demonstrated that it was better in decreasing BP in patients with essential HT than in no-treatment controls, but is not superior to that in active controls. More methodologically strict studies are needed to prove real clinical benefits of qigong, and to explore its potential mechanism.[30]

Nutritional influences

Diets, weight loss and weight management

The scientific evidence is strong for dietary changes that promote weight reduction in overweight hypertensive individuals, irrespective of age.[31–35] This is significant because recently it was emphasised how important the prevention of obesity was in order to prevent future related problems such as HT in children and adolescents.[36]

DASH diet

Large epidemiological studies investigating dietary intake, such as that from the Dietary Approaches to Stop HT (DASH),[37] and also the ATTICA study carried out in the Greek region of Attica,[38, 39] report significant health benefits. The DASH trial was a landmark, multi-centre, randomised study (n>400) that investigated the effects of a diet rich in fruits, vegetables, and low-fat dairy on people with and without HT.[40] This study reported that adherence to the DASH-style diet is associated with a lower risk of chronic heart disease (CHD) and stroke among middle-aged women, during 24 years of follow-up. Further, the researchers found that either a significantly reduced sodium intake (below 2.4g/day) or the DASH diet substantially lowered BP. Combining the 2 interventions had an even greater effect, comparable to first-line antihypertensive medications. The DASH diet that is rich in fruit and vegetables assists with reducing BP.[41]

Similarly, a Mediterranean style diet is reported to be protective. It was reported that older people, with low education, abdominal obesity, lower adherence to the Mediterranean diet, and increased inflammation, constitute a model of pre-hypertensive individuals that are prone to develop HT.[38, 39]

Oats

A US study of 88 people being treated for HT were randomised to a daily serving of wholegrain oat-based cereal (equivalent 3gm soluble fibre) or refined grain wheat-based cereal (less than 1gm soluble fibre) for 12 weeks.[42] Participants receiving the oats had a significant positive change in BP with 73% needing to stop or reduce their medication by half during the study, compared to 42% of the participants in the wheat group. The participants who were unable to reduce their medication still had substantial improvement in BP. Furthermore, those in the oats group also had improved glucose levels, a 15% decrease in total cholesterol, and 16% decrease in LDL-cholesterol.

Weight loss

A further US study of 1000 hypertensive patients without cardiovascular disease demonstrated that with weight loss and salt reduction, up to 80% of patients could have their BP controlled without drugs a year after withdrawal of their antihypertensives.[43] Although the lifestyle changes were challenging for the patients, the goals included weight loss of at least 4.5kg and maintaining a 24-hour urinary sodium excretion of 80mmol or less.

A recent Cochrane review of 18 trials concluded that weight-reducing diets in overweight hypertensive persons with a weight loss in the range of 3–9% of body weight caused only modest BP decreases of roughly 3mmHg systolic and diastolic but it was noted that weight-reducing diets 'may decrease dosage requirements for persons taking antihypertensive medications'.[44]

A combination of dietary changes that promotes weight loss with physical activity may have significant additive effects in reducing BP in both men and women with mild HT.[45]

Salt reduction

A moderate restriction of salt intake has been associated with approximately a 5mmHg reduction in SBP and a 2–3mmHg reduction in DBP in adults diagnosed as hypertensive.

A recent Cochrane review that included 20 RCTs with 822 otherwise untreated hypertensive adult patients compared the effect on BP of a modest restricted intake of dietary salt with that of usual salt intake.[46] Modest dietary salt restriction was equal to 2.4gm/day decrease in salt intake measured by net change in 24-hour urinary sodium — by definition. Median reduction of salt intake across the trials was 4.6g/day. This regimen was maintained for 4 weeks (median, 5 weeks; range, 4 weeks–1 year). This dietary intervention produced an average decrease of 5.06 mmHg in SBP (95% confidence interval [CI], 4.31–5.81mmHg) and 2.76mmHg in DBP (95% CI, 1.97–3.55mmHg).[46]

There was also demonstrated a significant dose-response relationship between dietary salt restriction and BP decreases. Namely, a 6g/day decrease in salt intake resulted in a reduction of 7.2mmHg SBP (95% CI, 5.6–8.8mmHg) and 3.8mmHg DBP (95% CI, 2.8-4.7mmHg).[46] The study results showed that a modest decrease in dietary salt intake in adults with diagnosed HT could prevent approximately 14% of deaths due to stroke and 9% of deaths due to ischemic heart disease.[46]

A more recent meta-analysis of 7 RCTs with 491 hypertensive adult patients compared an intervention that advised dietary salt reduction of 4–6g/day with that of usual salt intake. This intervention was associated with a documented reduction in SBP and DBPs of 4.7mmHg (95% CI, 2.2–7.2mmHg) and 2.5mmHg (95% CI, 1.8– 13.3mmHg), respectively, at a follow-up of 8 weeks or more.[47]

A further recent meta-analysis of 10 RCTs with 966 normotensive and hypertensive children (median age, 13 years; range, 8–16 years) reported that a 42% decrease in salt intake was associated with a 1.17mmHg (95% CI, 0.56–1.78mmHg) reduction in SBP and a 1.29mmHg (95% CI, 0.65–1.94 mmHg) reduction in DBP.[48] This important finding suggests that significantly reducing the intake of dietary salt may also be an effective approach for lowering BP among children with HT.

Nutritional effects of Hypertension

There are numerous foods and nutraceuticals that have been shown to have angiotensin enzyme inhibitor activity and hence influence and better regulate BP.[49]

Macronutrients

Proteins

Observational and epidemiological studies demonstrate a consistent association between a high protein intake and a reduction in BP in Japanese rural farmers, Japanese–American men in Hawaii, American men in 2 cohort studies, British men and women, Chinese men and women, and American children as well as children in other countries where the degree of reduction is dependent on the protein source.[50–53] The protein source is an important factor in the BP effect, animal protein (e.g. red meat and chicken) being less effective than non-animal protein (e.g. soy, legumes, nuts and seeds).[54] However, it has been reported that lean or wild animal protein, such as fish, rabbit, kangaroo and turkey, with less saturated fat and more essential n-3 and n-6 fatty acids (FAs) may reduce BP, lipids, and CHD risk.[53, 54, 55]

The Intermap Study, a large international observational study, showed an inverse correlation of BP with total protein intake and with protein intake from non-animal sources.[54] The INTERSALT Study supported the hypothesis that higher dietary protein intake has favourable influences on BP.[51] The study evaluated 10 020 men and women in 32 countries worldwide and found that the average SBP and DBP were 3.0 and 2.5mmHg lower, respectively, for those whose dietary protein was 30% above the overall mean than for those 30% below the overall mean (81gm/day versus 44gm/day).

A study of 41 men and women with SBP between 130–160 on 1 antihypertensive medication were randomised to diets of low-protein (12.5% of energy from protein), low-fibre (15gm/day), then high-fibre diet or both high-protein (25% energy as protein) and high-fibre (30gm/day) diet. The results showed that there was a significant reduction in BP of nearly 6mmHg in the high protein/fibre diet in 2 months.[56]

Milk and soy protein

Fermented milk supplemented with whey protein concentrate significantly reduced BP in animal models (rats) and human studies.[56] Kawase et. al.[57] studied 20 healthy men given 200 mL of fermented milk supplemented with 4.4% of whey protein twice daily for 8 weeks. The SBP was reduced ($P<.05$), HDL-C increased and triglycerides fell in the treated group compared with the control group. Natural bioactive substances in milk and colostrum including minerals, vitamins, and peptides have been demonstrated to reduce BP.[58,59] Milk ingestion increases protein, vitamins A, D, and B12, riboflavin, pantothenate, Ca^{++}, phosphorous, Mg^{++}, Zn^{++}, and K^{+}.[55] These findings are consistent with the combined diet of fruits, vegetables, grains, and low-fat dairy in the DASH-I and DASH-II studies in reducing BP.[40, 60] Soy protein at intakes of 25–30g/day lowers BP and increases arterial compliance[61, 62] and reduces LDL-cholesterol and total cholesterol by 6% to 7% and LDL-cholesterol oxidation.[61,62] Soy contains many active compounds that produce these antihypertensive and hypolipidemic effects including isoflavones, amino acids, saponins, phytic acid, trypsin inhibitors, fibre, and globulins.[61, 62] Numerous foods are abundant in genistein and daidzein such as currants, raisins, hazelnuts, peanuts, coconuts, passion fruit, prunes, as well as many other fruits and nuts.[63]

Whey protein

In a study by Pins and Keenan,[64] who administered 20g of hydrolysed whey protein to 30 hypertensive participants, noted a BP reduction of 11/7mmHg compared with control participants at 1 week, that was sustained throughout the study. The antihypertensive effect was thought to be mediated by an angiotensin converting enzyme inhibitor (ACEI) mechanism. These data indicate that the whey protein must be hydrolysed to exhibit an antihypertensive effect and that the maximum BP response is dose dependent. Bovine casein-derived peptides and whey protein-derived peptides exhibit ACEI active-B-caseins, B-Ig fractions, B2-microglobulin, and serum albumin. Whey protein hydrolysates exhibit both *in vitro* and *in vivo* ACEI and antihypertensive activity in *in vivo* animal and human studies.[57, 58, 59, 64, 65]

Fish protein

Sardine muscle protein, which only contains valyl-tyrosine (VAL-TYR), significantly lowers BP in hypertensive participants.[66] Kawasaki et. al. treated 29 hypertensive participants with 3mg of VAL-TYR sardine muscle-concentrated extract for 4 weeks and lowered BP by 9.7/5.3mmHg.[66]

In addition to ACEI effects, protein intake may also alter catecholamine responses and induce natriuresis.[67] The optimal protein intake, depending on level of activity, renal function, stress, and other factors, is about 1.0–1.5g per kg per day.[68, 69]

Fats

Epidemiological studies that include observational, biochemical, cross-sectional studies and clinical trials on the effect of fats on BP have been inconsistent.[70–73] However, many of these studies have suffered from inaccurate measurements of dietary components through recall or recording and most probably have missed small associations. Some also had inadequate or incorrect BP measurements, and did not correct for numerous dietary or non dietary confounding factors.[70]

A comprehensive meta-analysis and review of these studies is reported by Morris.[70] In the National Diet Heart Study, there was no change in BP with a polyunsaturated to saturated fat ratio (P/S ratio) in the range of 0.3 to 4.5 in 1218 participants over a 52-week study period.[71] The Multiple Risk Factor Intervention Trial demonstrated that consumption of an extra 6g of trans-fatty acids (TFAs) per day increased SBP 1.4mmHg and DBP 1.0mmHg.[68] However, the addition of 2g/day of linolenic acid reduced mean BP by 1.0mmHg. Two large prospective clinical studies, the Nurses Health Study[69] and the US Male Study (USMS),[72] showed a neutral effect on BP by all the fats (total fat, saturated fat, and polyunsaturated fat) or TFAs studied.

A recent randomised control 8-week study of 80 obesity-related hypertensive patients on Ramipril found that supplementation with dietary conjugated linoleic acid (CLA) significantly enhanced the antihypertensive effect on BP.[74]

Briefly:

- n-3 FAs and n-6 FAs are EFA families
- n-9 FAs (oleic acid) can be manufactured by the body from the dietary precursor stearic acid.

See Table 19.1 for a list of common essential fatty acids.

n-3 PUFAs α-Linolenic acid (ALA), eicosapentaenoic acid (EPA), and docosahexaenoic acid (DHA) are primary members of the n-3 PUFA family.[75, 76] n-3 fatty acids are found in coldwater fish (herring, haddock, Atlantic salmon, trout, tuna, cod, and mackerel) and the contamination with mercury, which is always a concern, varies based on where the fish are caught. Fish oils, flax, flax seed, flax oil, and nuts, with flax seed and walnuts having the highest content[72, 73] n-3 PUFAs, significantly lower BP in observational,

Table 19.1 Commonly encountered essential fatty acids[71–79]

Common name	Lipid name	Chemical name
Omega-3		
cc–Linolenic acid (ALA)	18:3 (n-3)	*all cis-9,12,15 octadecatrienoic acid*
Eicosapentaenoic acid (EPA)	20:5 (n-3)	*all cis-5,8,11,14,17 eicosapentaenoic acid*
Docosahexaenoic acid (DHA)	22:6 (n-3)	*all cis-4,7,10,13,16,19 docosahexaenoic acid*
Omega-6		
Linoleic acid (LA)	18:2 (n-6)	9,12-octadecadienoic acid
Gamma linolenic acid (GLA)	18:3 (n-6)	6,9,12-octadecatrienoic acid
Dihomo gamma linolenic acid (DGLA)	20:3 (n-6)	8,11,14-eicosatrienoic acid
Arachidonic acid (AA)	20:4 (n-6)	5,8,11,14-eicosatetraenoic acid
Omega-9		
Oleic acid (OA)	18:1 (n-9)	9-octadecenoic acid

epidemiological and some small prospective clinical trials.[72, 75–83]

Two meta-analyses of controlled trials concluded that approximately 3g/day of n-3 fatty acids of fish oil (containing on average 160mg DHA, 90mg EPA per 1000mg capsule) can significantly lower BP in hypertensive, but not normotensive, individuals.[84, 85] It is possible to consume this amount of fish oil by eating fish daily, but this would depend on the amount and type of fish consumed.[75]

The meta-analysis by Appel et. al.[84] was of 17 controlled clinical trials of n-3 supplementation with an average dose > 3g/day. Significant reductions in systolic BP and diastolic BP were observed in normotensive individuals and untreated hypertensives. Side-effects included nausea and a fishy taste. The researchers concluded that a diet supplementation with a relatively high dose of n-3FAs, generally more than 3g/day, can lead to clinically relevant BP reductions in individuals with untreated HT.

A meta-analysis of 31 studies of the effects of fish oil on BP has shown that there is a dose-related response in HT as well as a relationship to the specific concomitant diseases associated with HT.[86] At fish oil doses of 4g/day, there was no change in BP in the mildly hypertensive participants. At 4–7g/day, BP fell 1.6 to 2.9mmHg; at 15g (2.04 gm EPA and 1.4 gm DHA) of fish oil from salmon per day and greater, BP decreased 5.8 to 8.1mmHg.[86] There was no change in BP in the normotensive participants. There are no known major studies that indicate that too much fish oil supplementation adversely affect the BP of some people except some trials indicating a possible tendency to bleed with dose >10gm/day.

Small trials, such as that by Knapp and FitzGerald,[83] have demonstrated a significant reduction in BP in a group of hypertensive participants given 15g/day of fish oil. There was inadequate data relating to side-effects. Bao et. al.[87] studied 69 obese hypertensive participants for 16 weeks randomised to 3 groups. The treatments included fish oils only (3.65g n-3 FAs per day), a combination with a weight loss regimen and a weight loss regimen only. Group I participants taking 3.65g/day of n-3 FAs alone reduced BP by 6/3mmHg. Group II participants who lost an average of 5.6kg of weight, but received no fish oil, had a 5.5/2.2mmHg reduction in BP. The best BP results were seen in group III participants, with combined fish oil n-3 FAs and weight loss, whose BP and HR decreased by 13.0/9.3mmHg and an average of 6 beats/min respectively.

Mori et. al.[88] studied 63 hypertensive and hyperlipidemic participants treated with n-3 FAs (3.65gg/day for 16 weeks) and found significant reductions in BP, increase in HDL2-C, decrease in HDL3-C, decrease in triglycerides (29%), but no change in LDL-C, TC, or total HDL-C. Serum glucose and insulin levels also declined. Recent studies indicate that DHA is very effective in reducing BP and HR.[88, 89]

Reports also indicate that eating coldwater fish 3 times per week (150g fish weight) is as effective as high-dose fish oil by reducing BP in hypertensive patients, and the protein in the fish may also have antihypertensive effects.[84] The BP is usually unaffected in healthy non-hypertensive patients.[84, 86] Formation of EPA and ultimately DHA from ALA is decreased in the presence of increased linoleic acid (LA) in the diet (n-6 FAs), increased dietary saturated fats and TFAs, alcohol, and ageing through inhibitory effects or reduced activity of delta-6-desaturase, delta-5-desaturase, or delta-4-desaturase.[88, 89]

A recent randomised controlled study[90] demonstrated that in dyslipaedemic patients supplementation with ALA (flaxseed oil at a dose of 8g/day) resulted in significantly lower systolic and DBP levels compared with LA (P = 0.016 and P = 0.011, respectively.

Dosage

The reported dosage of n-3 fatty acids for a significant reduction in BP is at least 4g/day.[6] There is no concern in relation to high doses of fish oil except possible bleeding tendency with dose >10gm/day.[75]

Toxicity

Fish oil capsules available in Australia have zero or near zero methyl-mercury content. Fish oil capsules in Australia contain very low levels of dioxins (polychlorinated biphenyl.[75]

For more information on fish oil supplementation refer to The Australian Heart Foundation website: http://www.heartfoundation.org.au/document/NHF/HW_FS_FishOils_PS_FINAL.pdf

n-6 FAs (sunflower, safflower oils and margarines)

The n-6 FAs family, which includes LA, GLA, DGLA, and AA (Table 19.1), have been reported to not significantly lower BP directly,[71] but that may prevent increases in BP induced by saturated fats.[91] The ideal ratio of n-3 FAs to n-6 FAs is between 1:1 and 1:2, with a polysaturated fat ratio greater than 1:5 to 2:0.[92] Hydrogenated or partially hydrogenated vegetable oils, which all contain variable amounts of TFAs, should be avoided because they will increase BP and CHD risk.[93]

n-9 FAs (olive oil)

Olive oil is rich in monounsaturated FAs (MUFAs) (~72% oleic acid) which have been associated with BP and lipid reduction in Mediterranean and other diets.[92] Ferrara and colleagues[93] studied 23 hypertensive participants in a double-blind, randomised, cross-over study for 6 months, comparing MUFAs with PUFAs. Extra virgin olive oil (MUFAs) — using 40g in males (about 4 spoonfuls) and 30g in females (about 3 spoonfuls) — was compared with sunflower oil (PUFAs) rich in LA (n-6 FAs). The SBP fell 8mmHg and the DBP fell 6mmHg in the MUFA-treated participants compared with the PUFA-treated participants. In addition, the need for antihypertensive medications was reduced by 48% in the MUFA group versus 4% in the PUFA (n-6 FAs) group.

Strazzullo and colleagues[94] found an increase in SBP and DBP in patients when olive oil was replaced with saturated FAs. Thomsen et. al.[95] compared hypertensive type II diabetics in a cross-over study comparing MUFAs (olive oil) with PUFAs. There was a significant reduction in clinic BP and 24-hour ambulatory blood pressure measurement (ABM). However, in normotensive healthy participants given an olive oil-rich diet versus a carbohydrate-rich diet, no change in BP was observed.[96]

Extra virgin olive oil is a rich source of polyphenolic compounds and has 5mg of phenols per 10g, which equates to a dose of 4 tsp of olive oil.[89, 97] Approximately 4 teaspoons of extra virgin olive oil is equal to 40g.[88] The MUFAs tend to increase HDL-cholesterol more than PUFAs,[94] and the oleate-rich LDL-cholesterol is more resistant to oxidation than to oxidised LDL-cholesterol (oxLDL-C).[98]

Recent studies on Mediterranean diet have further confirmed the additive value of olive oil in reducing HT.[99, 100] The data suggested a significant sub-additive effect of the combined consumption of wine, fruit and vegetables and the anti-lipid effect of MUFAs from olive oil.

Other foods

Caffeine and alcohol

Patients with HT or cardiovascular disease should be advised to limit their intake of caffeine as even 2 cups of caffeine or 250mg caffeine can result in prolonged deterioration in aortic elasticity and increase in SBP and DBP.[101]

However, a recent review in contrast to early studies concludes that habitual moderate coffee intake does not represent a health hazard and may even be associated with beneficial effects on cardiovascular health.[102]

However, moderate restriction of alcohol and caffeine in addition to other lifestyle modifications can prevent, delay the onset of, reduce the severity of, treat, and control HT in many patients.[51]

Chocolate

Chocolate has been shown to have beneficial effects on lowering BP[103] in a trial of 13 hypertensive elderly people. Two weeks of eating 100g of dark chocolate daily resulted in a 5.1mmHg drop in SBP and a 1.8mmHg drop in DBP. The BP returned to pre-trial levels 2 days after stopping the chocolate. The researchers reported that the *polyphenols* present in cocoa solids were responsible for the BP drop. Moreover, a small sample study of otherwise healthy individuals with above-optimal BP indicated that inclusion of small amounts of polyphenol-rich dark chocolate as part of a usual diet efficiently reduced BP and improved formation of vasodilative nitric oxide.[104]

Breastfeeding

A UK study assessed 7276 7-year old children and found mean SBP was 1.2mmHg lower and mean DBP 0.9mmHg lower in children who had been breastfed, compared with children who had not.[105] According to the researchers the significance of a 1% reduction in population SBP levels is associated with an approximate 1.5% reduction in all-cause mortality. A recent systematic review and meta-analysis concluded that the small reduction in BP associated with breastfeeding could confer important benefits on cardiovascular health at a population level.[106]

Nutritional supplements

Vitamins

Vitamin C

Numerous epidemiological, observational, and clinical studies have demonstrated that the dietary intake of vitamin C or plasma ascorbate concentration in human beings is inversely correlated with SBP, DBP, and HR.[107–112]

Controlled intervention trials have been inconclusive though as to the relationship between vitamin C administration and BP.[113–116] The systematic review by Ness et. al. on HT and vitamin C concluded that if vitamin C has any effect on BP, it is small.[116] In the 18 studies that were reviewed worldwide, 10 of 14 showed a significant BP reduction with increased plasma ascorbate levels and 3 of 5 demonstrated a decreased BP with increased dietary vitamin C.[116] Moreover, in 4 small RCTs of 20–57 participants, 1 had significant BP reduction, 1 had no significant BP reduction, and 2 were not interpretable. In 2 uncontrolled trials, there was a significant reduction in BP. The conclusion was that further studies were required. Duffy et. al. evaluated 39 hypertensive participants (DBP, 90-110mmHg) in a placebo-controlled 4-week study.[108] A 2000g loading dose of vitamin C was given initially, followed by 500g/day. The SBP was reduced 11mmHg, DBP decreased by 6mmHg and mean arterial pressure (MAP) fell 10mmHg.

Ceriello and colleagues[107] administered intravenous vitamin C to hypertensive patients with DM and reduced BP significantly. Further a randomised placebo-controlled trial demonstrated that 500mg of daily vitamin C significantly reduced SBP by 13mmHg in 45 patients with mild or moderate HT compared with placebo after 1 month of treatment.[108] Mean SBP reduced from 155 to 142mmHg. Vitamin C also reduced DBP but this was not different to the placebo group.

The variation in the published data can be explained by numerous deficits in methodological design that included: lack of a control group; no baseline BP; small study population; short trial duration; variable vitamin C doses; variable demographics and study population; unknown premorbid vitamin C status or pre-morbid general vitamin or antioxidant status; concomitant or unknown multivitamin intake; and unknown nutritional status. In addition, existing concomitant diseases — confounding factors such as stress, smoking, alcohol, weight changes, and fibre, among others — were not stated or evaluated, plasma ascorbic acid levels were not measured, the P value and CIs were not reported, variable BP measurement techniques were used (clinic or office, home, 24-hour ABM), unknown genetic polymorphisms exist, or there was publication bias.[111]

Vitamin E

There are several human clinical studies that have investigated the relationship between vitamin E intake and BP.[117–120] The results report that α-tocopherol has an antihypertensive effect, and that it is probably small and may be limited to untreated hypertensive patients or those with known vascular disease or other concomitant problems such as diabetes or hyperlipidemia.[120]

Vitamin D

Epidemiological and clinical investigations demonstrate a relationship between plasma levels of 1,25 $(OH)_2$ D3 (1,25-dihydroxychol ecalciferol), the active form of vitamin D and BP,[121–125, 130–134] including vitamin D-mediated reduction in BP in hypertensive patients.

It has been difficult to dissociate the effects of calcium from vitamin D on BP in humans.[127,128] Numerous studies have verified the finding of an inverse relationship between dietary calcium intake and BP.[127, 128, 129] In The Tromso Study there was a negative association between calcium intake from dairy products and BP.[129] Calcium and vitamin D intake was assessed in 7542 men and 8053 women and the study found a significant linear decrease in SBP and DBP with increasing dietary calcium intake in both sexes; however, vitamin D intake had no significant effect on BP. It should be noted that this group did not measure blood vitamin D levels. The relationship between vitamin D, calcium and HT showed that intakes of low-fat dairy products, calcium, and vitamin D were each inversely associated with risk of HT in middle-aged and older women. This study suggested the potential roles vitamin D and calcium may have in the primary prevention of HT.[130]

It has been documented that higher calcium levels can decrease vitamin D levels.[136]

Vitamin D may have an independent and direct role in the regulation of BP and insulin metabolism.[131,135] A study of 34 middle-aged men demonstrated that serum levels of 1,125 $(OH)_2$ D3 were inversely correlated with BP ($P<.02$), very LDL cholesterol ($P<.005$) and triglyceride removal after intravenous fat tolerance test ($P<.05$).[134] Serum levels of 25 $(OH)_2$ D3 were correlated with fasting insulin ($P<.05$), insulin sensitivity during clamp ($P<.001$), and lipoprotein lipase activity in adipose tissue ($P<.005$) and skeletal muscle ($P<.03$). Scragg and colleagues, found no difference in serum 25 $(OH)_2$ D3 levels in a group of hypertensive versus normotensive participants.[133] Further, a recent study reported that calcium plus vitamin D3 supplementation did not reduce the risk of developing diabetes over 7 years of follow-up in this randomised placebo-controlled trial.[135] Higher doses of vitamin D may be required it was suggested to affect diabetes risk, and/ or associations of calcium and vitamin D intake with improved glucose metabolism observed in non-randomised studies. Earlier reported positive outcomes may be the result of confounding or of other components of foods containing these nutrients.[135]

B Group vitamins

Animal and human studies have demonstrated that low serum vitamin B6 levels were associated with HT.[137–143] However, the effect of homocysteine-lowering vitamins on BP has not been well studied.

A recent clinical trial measured blood pressure in older people with elevated baseline homocysteine and reported that SBP and DBP as well as pulse pressure in the vitamin-supplemented group did not differ from the placebo group. However, over the duration of the trial plasma homocysteine decreased. The mean differences in BPs, adjusted for baseline values, did not exceed 1mmHg.[143] B-vitamins supplemented group lowered plasma homocysteine but had no effect on blood pressure.[144]

Minerals

Sodium (Na^+)

Epidemiological, observational, and controlled clinical trials demonstrate that an increased Na^+ intake is associated with higher BP.[145] A reduction in Na^+ intake in hypertensive patients, especially the salt-sensitive patients, will significantly lower BP by 4 to 6/2 to 3mmHg.[146–149] The BP reduction is proportional to the severity of Na^+ restriction.[150, 151] In the TOHP-I Trial,[151] a 100mmol Na^+ intake per day (2400mg) reduced the incidence of HT by 20% in a group of high-risk participants, improved HT control in elderly participants taking medication in the TONE Study,[152] reduced cardiovascular disease in obese participants,[153, 154, 155] and reduced proteinuria and progression of renal disease.[150, 156, 157] The TOHP-II Trial had a mean BP reduction of 2.9 F 1.6mmHG with moderate Na^+ restriction.[156] A Cochrane review concludes that evidence from large and small trials show that a low sodium diet helps in maintenance of lower BP following withdrawal of antihypertensives.[158] Recent reports on observational follow-up of the trials of HT prevention (TOHP) and others strongly suggest that Na^+ reduction, previously shown to lower BP, also reduce long-term risk of cardiovascular events.[159, 160] The TOHP study found that the low-salt group 10–15 years later had 25% lower heart disease and stroke.[160]

Potassium (K^+)

Numerous epidemiological, observational, and clinical trials have demonstrated a significant reduction in BP with increased dietary K^+ intake.[161, 162, 163] The magnitude of BP reduction with a K^+ supplementation of 60–120mEq/d is approximately 4.4/2.5mmHg in hypertensive patients and 1.8/1.0mmHg in normotensive patients.[164, 165] A meta-analysis of all K^+ supplementation clinical trials in the treatment of HT demonstrated a racial difference, with black participants having a more substantial reduction in BP compared with white participants.[163] A high K^+ intake is most effective in reducing BP in patients with diuretic-induced hypokalemia, in those with a high Na^+ intake,[163–166] in patients with salt-sensitive HT, severe HT, or a positive family history,[164] as well as in non-white populations such as Chinese,[165] and African Americans.[166]

It has been suggested that alteration of the K^+/Na^+ ratio to a higher level is important for both antihypertensives as well as cardiovascular and cerebrovascular effects.[168] High K^+ intake reduces the incidence of cardiovascular and CVAs independent of BP reduction.[168]

Proposed mechanisms include improvements in vascular smooth muscle function and structure, natriuresis, modulation of baroreflex sensitivity, direct vasodilation, reduced vasoconstrictive sensitivity to norepinephrine (NE) and A-II, increased serum and urinary kallikrein, increased Na^+/K^+ adenosine triphosphatase activity, and DNA synthesis and proliferation in VSMCs and SNS cells.[167, 168]

Gu and colleagues recently demonstrated for the first time that K^+ supplementation at 60mmol of KCI per day for 12 weeks significantly reduced SBP<5.0mmHg in 150 Chinese men and women aged 35 to 64 years.[165] This study confirmed that the higher the initial BP, the greater the response. In addition, K^+ may have a Ca^{++} conserving effect that would further minimise the effects of a high Na^+ intake.[170] The interactions of Na^+, Ca^{++}, K^+, and Mg^{++} are more important in BP control than isolated changes in 1 mineral.[167, 168, 169]

Care should be taken in advising K^+ supplementation as too much or too little can have serious life-threatening consequences, such as arrhythmias.

Calcium (Ca^{++})

Epidemiological studies show a link between HT and Ca^{++},[49, 170] but clinical trials that administer Ca^{++} supplements to patients have shown inconsistent effects on BP.[171–180] Higher dietary Ca^{++} is not only associated with a lower BP, but also with a decreased risk of developing HT.[165] A 23% reduction in the risk of developing HT was noted in those individuals taking a dose higher than 800mg/day compared with those taking 1 lower than 400mg/day.[165] A meta-analysis of the effect of Ca^{++} supplementation in hypertensive patients found a reduction in the SBP of 4.3/1.5mmHg.[176] Foods high in Ca^{++} were more effective than supplements in reducing BP.[176]

Karanja and colleagues[177] assessed the effects of $CaCO_3$ versus Ca^{++} contained in the diet and found significant increases in magnesium (Mg^{++}), riboflavin, and vitamin D in the dietary group that correlated with Ca^{++} intake. There is an additive or synergistic effect on BP reduction with a combination of minerals and vitamins as compared with Ca^{++} alone. Also, the heterogeneous responses to Ca^{++} supplementation have been explained, by Resnick,[178] as being dependant on the population or hypertensive subtype. Those patients with the greatest reduction in BP with Ca^{++} supplements include black patients, those with low-renin HT, ageing adults and pregnant women (pregnancy-induced HT).[179]

In a Cochrane review of 12 trials the risk of pre-eclampsia was reduced with calcium supplementation rather than placebo (11 trials, n = 14 946 women).[180] This review supports the potential role of Ca^{++} supplementation for gestational HT, especially high-risk women and in communities with low-dietary calcium intake.

Of interest, a 2-year RCT that assessed the long-term effect of calcium and vitamin D3 fortified milk on BP and serum lipid concentrations in healthy older men found no added benefit on BP and lipid concentrations compared with the control group (ingesting non-fortified milk).[181]

A dose of calcium carbonate or citrate 1000–3000mg/day is recommended.

Magnesium (Mg^{++})

Several studies have indicated there may be a role for Mg^{++} supplementation for its relaxation effects on smooth muscles of blood vessels causing vasodilation and therefore lowering BP. According to a double-blind, cross-over study,[182] 365mg of Mg^{++} per day with beta-blockers significantly reduced BP compared with beta-blockers alone.

According to Japanese researchers, Mg^{++} supplements may have a valid role in BP control.[183] The study randomised 60 hypertensive volunteers with daily small doses of magnesium oxide (20mmol) for 8 weeks. Office, home and ambulatory BP measurements all showed small but significant reductions in BP. There appears to be a positive correlation between low levels of serum and erythrocyte Mg^{++} levels and HT, only if there is a family history.[184]

In another double-blind controlled trial,[185] 91 middle-aged and elderly women with mild to moderate HT who were not on antihypertensive medication were randomly assigned to treatment with magnesium aspartate-HCl (20mmol Mg^{++}/day) or placebo for 6 months. Magnesium was well tolerated and not associated with an increased frequency of diarrhoea compared with placebo at this dose. At the end of the study, SBP had fallen by 2.7mmHg and DBP by 3.4mmHg more in the magnesium group than in the placebo group. BP response was not associated with baseline Mg^{++} status, as measured by dietary magnesium intake and urinary magnesium excretion.

Another double-blind, placebo-controlled study[186] involved 33 participants who were allocated to undergo either a 4-week treatment with oral Mg^{++} supplementation ($Mg[OH]_2$; 411–548mg/day) or a placebo. The SBP and DBP values decreased significantly in the magnesium group, but not in the placebo group. The results suggested that Mg^{++} supplementation may lower BP through the suppression of the adrenergic activity and possible natriuresis.

A recent review summarises the evidence for benefits of Mg^{++} on metabolic abnormalities, inflammatory parameters, and cardiovascular risk factors.[187] In conclusion, the review states that there is strong biological plausibility for the direct impact of Mg^{++} intake on metabolic and cardiovascular risk factors, but *in vivo* Mg^{++} deficiency might play only a modest role.

A dose of magnesium orotate 400–800mg/day is recommended.

Dosages for magnesium and potassium

A high dietary intake of Mg^{++} of at least 500–1000mg/day reduces BP in most of the reported epidemiological, observational, and clinical trials.[6]

The recommended intake of K^+ is 650 mEq/day with a K^+/Na^+ ratio of more than 5:1. Numerous epidemiological, observational, and clinical trials have demonstrated a significant reduction in BP with increased dietary K^+ intake. The magnitude of BP reduction with a K^+ supplementation of 60–120 mEq/day is 4.4/2.5mmHg in hypertensive patients and 1.8/1.0mmHg in normotensive patients.[6]

Zinc (Zn^{++})

Low serum Zn^{++} levels in observational studies correlate with HT as well as CHD, type II diabetes mellitus, hyperlipidemia (especially hypertriglyceridemia, low-density lipoprotein cholesterol [LDL-cholesterol] and elevated lipoprotein a), 2-hour postprandial increased plasma insulin levels, and insulin resistance.[188] In elderly hypertensive patients with very low plasma renin activity there is a high urinary excretion of Zn^{++} and low serum levels that are partially corrected by the administration of oral Ca^{++} in a dose greater than 800mg/day.[189] There is a close relationship between Zn^{++}, Ca^{++}, Na^+, Mg^{++}, and K^+ in various hormonal systems (renin–angiotensin–aldosterone system) that modulate BP.[190]

A dose of zinc orotate of 20–150mg/day is recommended.

Antioxidants

Galley and colleagues[191] administered antioxidants to 40 hypertensive and normotensive adult participants in a randomised, double-blind, cross-over design placebo-controlled study for 8 weeks. The antioxidants administered were zinc sulfate 200mg/day, ascorbic acid 500mg/day, α-tocopherol 600mg/day, and β carotene 30mg/day. The SBP decreased significantly in the hypertensive participants but not in the normotensive participants. Increases in plasma levels of antioxidants and increased urine nitrate excretion occurred in the hypertensive participants, suggesting an increased bioavailability of nitrous oxide.[191]

Bergomi and colleagues evaluated Zn^{++} and Ca^{++} status in 60 hypertensive compared with 60 normotensive control participants.[192] An inverse correlation of BP and serum Zn^{++} was observed, but there was a direct correlation with serum Ca^{++}.

Other nutritional supplements

Coenzyme Q_{10} (CoQ_{10})

Despite several studies[193–200] demonstrating that CoQ_{10} may be of benefit for HT, the mechanism of how it works at this stage and its potential use in HT is not clear and larger controlled trials are required to confirm its clinical efficacy.

In 1 study, 80 type 2 diabetics with dyslipidaemia were entered into a randomised double-blind, placebo-controlled interventional trial over 12 weeks.[201] The groups received 200mg CoQ_{10} and 200mg fenofibrate (FF) per day. The other 3 groups received: CoQ_{10} plus FF placebo; CoQ_{10} placebo plus FF; or all placebo capsules. The CoQ_{10} had no effect on lipid levels but a significant effect on SBP and DBP.

In a further study, 109 patients with essential HT were supplemented with an average oral dose of 225mg/day CoQ_{10} in addition to their existing antihypertensive drug regimen.[202] Patients were able to reduce their antihypertensive drug therapy gradually during the first 1–6 months. Fifty-one percent of patients completely discontinued between 1 and 3 antihypertensive drugs on average over 4.4 months after starting CoQ_{10}.

A meta-analysis of 12 clinical trials concluded that CoQ_{10} had the potential in hypertensive patients to lower SBP by up to 17mmHg and DBP by up to 10mmHg without significant side-effects.[203]

Dosage coenzyme Q_{10}

Human studies have also demonstrated significant and consistent reductions in BP in hypertensive subjects after oral administration of 100–225mg/day of coenzyme Q_{10}.[6]

Adverse reactions

No reported side-effects are known.

Lycopene

Lycopene has recently been shown to produce a significant reduction in BP, and serum lipids.[204, 205] Paran and Engelhard evaluated

30 patients with grade 1 HT and raised lipids, aged 40–65 years, taking no antihypertensive, or anti-lipid medication treated with a tomato lycopene extract, for 8 weeks.[204] The mean SBP was reduced from 144 to 135mmHg (9mmHg reduction) and DBP fell from 91 to 84mmHg (7mmHg reduction) in supplemented group. A similar study with 35 patients with grade 1 HT showed similar results with reduction of SBP but not on DBP.[205] Serum lipids were significantly improved in both studies without any change in serum homocysteine.

Herbal medicines

Garlic (*Allium sativum*)

Good clinical trials using the correct type and dose of garlic have shown consistent reductions in BP in hypertensive patients.[206–222] However, not all garlic preparations are processed similarly and are not comparable in antihypertensive potency.[215, 216] Moreover, cultivated garlic (*Allium sativum*), wild uncultivated garlic or bear garlic (*Allium urisinum*),[49, 215, 216] and aged[216] or fresh garlic will have variable effects.[207, 208] Cooking garlic, for instance, will reduce allicin compounds in the garlic and thus reduce its hypotensive properties. Raw garlic is preferred but usually causes garlic breath and odour. Hence, garlic preparations in capsules improve compliance and are usually preferred as they reduce these unwanted side-effects. According to a recent meta-analysis of garlic on HT, most studies used garlic powder dosages of 600–900mg/day, providing potentially 3.6–5.4mg of allicin, the active compound in garlic.[218] This compares to fresh garlic cloves (~2g) yielding about 5–9mg allicin. The authors concluded the 'meta-analysis suggests that garlic preparations are superior to placebo in reducing BP in individuals with HT'.[217] A further meta-analysis also confirms this conclusion.[219]

Most positive studies have used quantities of garlic beyond typical dietary levels (equivalent to 5–20 average-sized cloves/day or dried garlic powder preparation, average 900mg/day). An older meta-analysis of 8 randomised trials (n = 415) suggested some effect in mildly hypertensive patients, but not enough to recommend its routine clinical use and more rigorous trials were encouraged.[212] Of the 7 trials that compared the effect with that of placebo, 3 showed a significant reduction in SBP and 4 in DBP.

Hawthorn berries

A review reports that hawthorn may reduce systemic vascular resistance and BP, decrease the pressure-rate product in the myocardium, improve ejection fraction and congestive heart failure (CHF), improve arrhythmias, lower cholesterol, dilate coronary arteries, and improve myocardial perfusion and angina.[220] The mechanism of some of these effects is the ACE inhibitor effect of hawthorne. Doses of about 160–900mg/day of a standardised extract of hawthorn have been used to achieve these cardiovascular effects, which appear to be safe. The first RCT investigated the effects of hawthorn for HT in patients with type 2 diabetes and demonstrated a hypotensive effect.[221]

Indian snakeroot (*Rauwolfia serpentine*)

Rauwolfia serpentine is a Hindu Ayurvedic herb known since ancient times and is the natural source of the alkaloid reserpine, one of the first commercially available antihypertensive drugs. It works by depleting catecholamines in the central and peripheral nervous system. However, adverse effects, including depression, sedation and peptic ulceration were common.[220]

Rauwolfia serpentine has been studied in a 10-year intervention trial.[222] It was concluded that the overall effectiveness of lowering BP and in reducing complications and treatment failure was 60%. Further, given the low level of excess risk in mild uncomplicated HT, the use of *Rauwolfia serpentine* may be a reasonable alternative in lowering BP.

Contraindicated in HT

Liquorice herb *Glycyrrhiza glabra* and *Glycyrrhiza uralensis*

Excessive doses of liquorice preparations should be avoided in cases of HT, cardiac and renal problems, and oedema. The active component of liquorice, glycyrrhisinica acid (GA), is recognised as contributing to sodium and water retention, hypokalemia, HT and suppression of aldosterone and rennin levels.

Conclusion

Lifestyle change, including diet, exercise, stress management, weight reduction and alcohol and caffeine restriction contribute significantly to lowering BP.

There is a role for the selected use of single and component nutraceuticals, such as vitamins, antioxidants, minerals, fish oils and herbs in the treatment of HT based on scientifically controlled studies as a complement to optimal nutritional, dietary intake from food and other lifestyle modifications.

Herbs and supplements such as magnesium, calcium, CoQ_{10}, omega-3 fatty acids, and vitamins have the potential to be used in the adjuvant treatment of HT.

A recent review has concluded that there is a significant amount of evidence to support the use of various evidence based CAM modalities in the treatment of HT (Table 19.2).[223]

Table 19.2 Levels of evidence for lifestyle and complementary medicines/therapies in the management of hypertension

Modality	Level I	Level II	Level IIIa	Level IIIb	Level IIIc	Level IV	Level V
Lifestyle	x						
Sleep				x			
Environment							
Extreme temperature				x			
Physical therapies							
Exercise		x					
Tai chi	x						
Qigong	x						
Mind–body medicine							
Transcendental meditation			x				
Relaxation therapy	x						
Dietary changes							
DASH diet		x					
Mediterranean diet		x					
Proteins (high intake)				x			
Polyunsaturated fats	x(-)						
n-3 FAs	x						
Fish oils	x						
n-6 FAs					x		
Olive oil (n-9 FAs)	x						
Caffeine restriction				x			
Chocolate (cocoa)		x					
Breastfeeding	x						
Weight reduction	x						
Salt reduction	x						
Nutritional supplements							
Vitamin C		x					
Vitamin E		x					
Vitamin D		x					
B Group vitamins						x	
Sodium restriction	x						
Potassium	x						
Calcium	x						
Magnesium		x					

Continued

Table 19.2 Levels of evidence for lifestyle and complementary medicines/therapies in the management of hypertension—cont'd

Modality	Level I	Level II	Level IIIa	Level IIIb	Level IIIc	Level IV	Level V
Zinc						x	
Antioxidants		x					
Coenzyme Q_{10}	x						
Lycopene						x	
Herbal medicines							
Garlic	x						
Hawthorn		x					
Rauwolfia serpentine			x				

Level I— from a systematic review of all relevant randomised controlled trials — meta-analyses.
Level II— from at least 1 properly designed randomised controlled clinical trial.
Level IIIa— from well-designed pseudo-randomised controlled trials (alternate allocation or some other method).
Level IIIb— from comparative studies (including systematic reviews of such studies) with concurrent controls and allocation not randomised, cohort studies, case-control studies, or interrupted time series with a parallel control group.
Level IIIc— from comparative studies with historical control, 2 or more single-arm studies or interrupted time series without a parallel control group.
Level IV— opinions of respected authorities based on clinical experience, descriptive studies or reports of expert committees.
Level V— represents minimal evidence that represents testimonials.

Clinical tips handout for patients — hypertension

1 Lifestyle advice

Sleep

- Restore normal sleep patterns. Most adults require about 7 hours sleep a day. (See Chapter 22 for more advice.)
- Disrupted and less sleep can raise blood pressure.

Sunshine

- Amount of exposure varies with local climate.
- At least 15 minutes of sunshine needed daily for vitamin D an melatonin production — especially before 10 a.m. and after 3 p.m. when the sun exposure is safest during summer. Much more exposure required in winter when supplementation needs to be considered.
- Ensure gradual, adequate skin exposure to sun; avoid sunscreen and excess clothing to maximise levels of vitamin D.
- More time in the sun is required for dark skinned people and people with vitamin D deficiency.
- Direct exposure to about 10% of the body (hands, arms, face), without sunscreen and not through glass.
- Vitamin D is obtained in the diet from fatty fish, eggs, liver and fortified foods (some milks and margarines); diet alone is not a sufficient source of vitamin D.

2 Physical activity/exercise

- Exercise 30-60 minutes daily. If exercise is not regular, commence with 5 minutes daily and slowly build up to at least 30 minutes.
- Outdoor exercise in nature, with fresh air and sunshine, is ideal (e.g. brisk walking, light jogging, cycling, swimming, stretching, resistance or weight-bearing exercises). The more time you spend outdoors the better.
- Tai chi, qigong and yoga may be particularly helpful.

3 Mind-body medicine

- Stress management program — for example, 6 x 40 minute sessions for patients to understand the nature of their symptoms, the symptoms' relationship to stress, and the practice of regular relaxation exercises.
- Regular meditation practice at least 10-20 minutes daily, especially transcendental, mindfulness meditation and autogenic training.
- Anger management may be of help.
- Psychological therapy may help to deal with stressors.

Breathing

- Be aware of breathing from time to time. Notice if tendency to hold breath or over-breathe.
- Snoring and irregular breathing during sleep needs to be reported and further investigated.
- Avoid exposure to polluted air as much as possible.

Rest and stress management

Recurrent stress may cause a return of symptoms. Relaxation is important for a full and lasting recovery.

- Reduce workload and resolve conflicts. Contact family, friends, church or social groups for support.
- Listening to relaxation music and daily baths may help.
- Relaxation massage therapy is helpful.
- Listening to relaxation music helps.
- Relaxation massage therapy may help.
- Hypnotherapy, biofeedback, cognitive behavioural therapy, and psychotherapy may be of help.

Fun

- It is important to have fun in life.
- Joy can be found even in the simplest tasks, such as funny movies/videos, comedy, hobbies, dancing, playing with pets and children.

4 Environment

- Avoid environmental pollutants and chemicals — at work and in the home.
- Avoid artificial sweeteners.
- Avoid exposure to extreme temperatures, such as very cold or hot days, as this may alter your blood pressure (e.g. high temperatures can reduce your blood pressure).
- Aviod smoking and smoking environments.

5 Dietary changes

- Do not rush your meals; relax before meals; chew your food thoroughly before swallowing as this aids digestion and promotes regular, relaxed eating patterns.

- Aim to lose weight if you or your health practitioner believes you are overweight.
- Eat more fruit (>2/day) and vegetables (>5/day); a variety of colours and those that are in season.
- A vegetarian diet high in legumes is particularly helpful (e.g. soy; vegetables; garlic, nuts and fruit); for example, the Mediterranean diet.
- Increase fibre; for example, add psyllium fibre (husks) to your cereal.
- Consume fresh garlic 2g/day yields 5–9mg allicin (note: may cause garlic breath and body odour); use 5–20 average-sized cloves per day, or dried garlic powder preparation (average 900mg/day).
- Eat more nuts, seeds, beans, sprouts (e.g. alfa, mung bean, lentils). Try soy 25–30g/day.
- Consume more fish (sardines, tuna, salmon, cod, mackerel) especially deep sea fish.
- Reduce red meat intake (preferably eat lean red meat e.g. lamb, kangaroo) and white meat (e.g. free range organic chicken fillet).
- Consume cold pressed olive oil, 4 teaspoons, and flaxseed oil, 1 tablespoon (uncooked), daily. Use avocado.
- Use dark chocolate (100g/day) unless not tolerated.
- Eat a variety of wholegrains/cereals. Cooked traditional rolled oats for breakfast are particularly helpful, as is rice (brown, basmati, Mahatma, Dongara), buckwheat flour, wholegrain organic breads (rye bread, Essene, spelt, Kamut) — when toasting make hot and crisp, not brown, to avoid acrylamide — brown pasta, couscous, millet, amaranth, etc.
- Consume low-fat dairy products, such as low-fat yoghurt, unless there is a dairy intolerance. Soy milk (organic) is an alternative.
- Consume whey protein (20g/day).
- Increase potassium-rich foods (see Chapter 2).
- Drink more water, 1–2 litres a day, and teas (especially green tea, chamomile, peppermint and black tea).
- For alternative sweetener try honey (e.g. manuka, yellow box and stringy bark have the lowest GI).
- Avoid sea salt.
- Avoid hydrogenated, saturated fats and trans-fatty acids such as butter, margarines, crispy potato chips, dairy fat (e.g. yellow cheeses and cream), fat in meat and poultry, commercial biscuits, most cakes, pastries and takeaway foods, fast foods, sugar (such as soft drinks, lollies) and processed foods (e.g. white bread, white pasta).
- Reduce or avoid coffee.
- Minimise alcohol intake to no more than 1–2 glasses daily.
- Avoid chemical additives — preservatives, colourings and flavourings.

6 Physical therapies

- Acupuncture and relaxation massage may help.

7 Supplements

Fish oils

- Indication: may reduce blood pressure and help prevent heart and vascular disease.
- Dosage: 3–7g/day as tolerated and as indicated for high blood pressure (e.g. EPA 180/DHA 120mg).
- Results: 4–7 days.
- Side-effects: often well tolerated especially if taken with meals. Very mild and rare side-effects (e.g. gastrointestinal upset; reflux); allergic reactions (e.g. rash, breathing problems if allergic to seafood); blood thinning effects in very high doses > 10g/day (may need to stop fish oil supplements 2 weeks prior to surgery).
- Contraindications: sensitivity reaction to seafood; drug interactions; caution when taking high doses of fish oils >4g/day together with warfarin (your doctor will check your INR test).

Vitamins and minerals

Vitamin C

- Indication: may reduce blood pressure.
- Dosage: 500–1000mg/day, or as tolerated.
- Results: unknown.
- Side-effects: gastrointestinal irritation such as nausea, heartburn, abdominal cramps, loose stools, diarrhoea, especially in high doses.
- Contraindication: avoid if you have renal impairment or kidney stones.

Vitamin D3 (cholecalciferol 1000 international units)

- Doctors should check blood levels and suggest supplementation if levels are low.
- Increase sun exposure.

Magnesium and calcium (best provided together)

- Indication: lowers blood pressure; may also be useful in anxiety, restless sleep, cramps and insomnia.
- Dosage: children up to 65–120mg/day in divided doses. Adults 350–400mg/day including pregnant and lactating women.
- Results: 2–3 days.
- Side-effects: oral magnesium can cause gastrointestinal irritation, nausea, vomiting, and diarrhoea. The dosage varies from person to person. Although rare, toxic levels can cause low blood pressure, thirst, heart arrhythmia, drowsiness and weakness. Calcium can cause gastrointestinal upset (e.g. constipation).
- Contraindications: patients with kidney disease; patients with high blood calcium or magnesium levels (e.g. in cancer or kidney diseases).

Coenzyme Q_{10} (CoQ_{10})

- Indication: lowers blood pressure; may also be useful in heart disease, fatigue, muscle aches, breast cancer.
- Dosage: adults 100–200mg in divided doses, 2–3 times per day.
- Results: 7–14 days.
- Side-effects: generally well tolerated. May cause gastrointestinal side-effects such as nausea, vomiting, diarrhoea.
- Contraindications: avoid in pregnancy and lactating women and if allergic.

Herbal medicines

Garlic (*Allium sativum*)

- Indication: hypertension; may help with atherosclerosis and heart disease, and also helps boost immune system.
- Dosage: 600–900mg/day (3.6–5.4mg of allicin); avoid aged garlic extract or heat-treated garlic as they are less effective for blood pressure.
- Results: 4–7 days.
- Side-effects: breath and body odour; mouth, stomach and gastrointestinal burning or irritation, heartburn, flatulence, nausea, vomiting and diarrhoea. May increase risk of bleeding as garlic can affect platelet function. Some people are allergic to garlic (by ingestion or even topically) and it may cause asthma, runny nose, skin irritation and, in rare cases, severe allergic reactions.
- Contraindications: avoid if allergic to garlic; beware if taking any blood thinning medication such as warfarin; avoid at least 2 weeks prior to any surgery to minimise risk of bleeding; avoid high doses during pregnancy and lactation.

Hawthorn berries

- Indication: hypertension; may help with heart failure and heart disease.
- Dosage: adult: 500mg 3 times daily.
- Results: 14–21 days.
- Side-effects: generally well tolerated; may cause arrhythmias, palpitations, dizziness and vertigo.
- Contraindications: pregnancy and lactation; arrhythmias.

Warning: avoid licorice as this herb can raise blood pressure.

References

1 World Health Organization – Cardiovascular disease: prevention and control 2003. Online. Available: http://www.who.int/dietphysicalactivity/media/en/gsfs_cvd.pdf (accessed April 2008)

2 Flegal KM, Carroll MD, Ogden CL, et. al. Prevalence and trends in obesity among US adults, 1999-2000. JAMA 2002;288(14):1723–7.

3 Bonow RO, Eckel RH. Diet, obesity, and cardiovascular risk. N Engl J Med 2003;348(21):2057–8.

4 Kokkinos PF, Papademetriou V. Exercise and hypertension. Coronary Artery Dis. 2000;11: 99–102.

5 Sali A, Vitetta L. Nutritional supplements and cardiovascular disease. Heart Lung Circ 2004;13(4):363–6.

6 Chockalingam A. Healthy weight, healthy blood pressure. Canadian J Cardiology 2010;26(5):259–60.

7 Huang N, Duggan K, Harman J. Lifestyle management of hypertension Australian Prescriber 2008;31:150–3.

8 Yan LL, Liu K, Matthews KA, et. al. Psychosocial factors and risk of hypertension: the Coronary Artery Risk Development in Young Adults (CARDIA) study. JAMA 2003;290(16):2138–48.

9 Han HR, Kim MT, Rose L, et. al. Effects of stressful life events in young black men with high blood pressure. Ethn Dis 2006 Winter;16(1):64–70.

10 Weinstein SE, Quigley KS, Mordkoff JT. Influence of control and physical effort on cardiovascular reactivity to a video game task. Psychophysiology 2002;39:591–98.

11 Nakao M, Nomura S, Shimosawa T, et. al. Clinical Effects of Blood Pressure Biofeedback Treatment on Hypertension by Auto Shaping. Psych Med 1997;59:331–8.

12 Raskin R, Raps C, Luskin F, et. al. Pilot study of the effect of self-hypnosis on the medical management of essential hypertension. Stress Med 1999;15:243–7.

13 Shufan Z. Effects of patient education and biofeedback: interim results. J of Human Hypertension. 1995;9(1):51.

14 Yung PM, Keltner AA. A controlled comparison on the effects of muscle and cognitive relaxation procedures on blood pressure: implications for the behavioral treatment of borderline hypertensives. Behav Res Ther 1996;34:821–826.

15 Shapiro D, Hui KK, Oakley ME, et. al. Reductions in drug requirements for hypertension by means of a cognitive-behavioural intervention. Am J Hypertens1997;10:9–17.
16 Dickinson HO, Campbell F, Beyer FR, et. al. Relaxation therapies for the management of primary hypertension in adults. Cochrane Database Syst Rev 2008 Jan 23;(1):CD004935.
17 Linden W, Lenz JW, Con AH. Individualised Stress Management for Primary Hypertension: A Randomised Trial. Arch Internal Med 2001;161:1071–80.
18 Schneider RH, Alexander CN, Staggers F, et. al. A randomised controlled trial of stress reduction in African Americans treated for hypertension for over one year. Am J Hypertens 2005;18(1):88–98.
19 Brown MA, Buddle ML, Martin A. Is resistant hypertension really resistant? American Journal of Hypertension 2001;14:1263–69.
20 Björklund K, Lind L, Vessby B, et. al. Different metabolic predictors of white-coat and sustained hypertension over a 20-year follow-up period: a population-based study of elderly men. Circulation 2002;106:63–8.
21 Walton KG, Schneider RH, Nidich SI, et. al. Psychosocial stress and cardiovascular disease Part 2: effectiveness of the Transcendental Meditation program in treatment and prevention. Behav Med. 2002 Fall;28(3):106–23.
22 Lisard P, et. al. Effects of insufficient sleep on blood pressure in hypertensive patients: a 24 hour study. Am J Hypertension 1999;12:63–68.
23 Alvarez GG, Ayas NT. The impact of daily sleep duration on health: a review of the literature. Prog Cardiovasc Nurs 2004 Spring;19(2):56–9.
24 Vgontzas AN, Liao D, Bixler ED, et. al. Insomnia with objective short sleep duration is associated with high risk of hypertension. Sleep 2009;32:491–7.
25 Alpérovitch A, Lacombe J, Hanon O, et. al. Relationship Between Blood Pressure and Outdoor Temperature in a Large Sample of Elderly Individuals. The Three-City Study. Arch Intern Med 2009;169(1):75–80.
26 Hagberg JM, Park JJ, Brown MD. The role of exercise training in the treatment of hypertension: an update. Sports Med. 2000;30:193–206.
27 Carlsson AC, Wändell PE, de Faire U, et. al. Risk Factors Associated With Newly Diagnosed High Blood Pressure in Men and Women. Am J Hypertens 2008 Apr 17;[Epub ahead of print].
28 Wang C, Collet JP, Lau J. The effect of Tai Chi on health outcomes in patients with chronic conditions: a systematic review. Arch Intern Med 2004;164: 493–501.
29 Guo X, Zhou B, Nishimura T, et. al. Clinical effect of qigong practice on essential hypertension: a meta-analysis of randomised controlled trials. J Altern Complement Med 2008;14(1):27–37.
30 Lee MS, Pittler MH, Guo R, et. al. Qigong for hypertension: a systematic review of randomised clinical trials. J Hypertens 2007;25(8):1525–32.
31 Appel LJ, et. al. A clinical trial of the effects of dietary patterns on blood pressure. NEJM 1997;336:1117–1124.
32 Ascherio A, Hennekens C, Willet WC, et. al. Prospective study of nutritional factors, blood pressure, and hypertension among US women. Hypertension 1996;27:1065–1072.
33 Heyka R. Lifestyle management and prevention of hypertension. In: Rippe J. Lifestyle Medicine (1st edn). Blackwell Science, Malden, Mass, 1999:109–119.
34 Yong LC, Kuller LH, Rutan G, et. al. Longitudinal study of blood pressure: changes and determinants from adolescence to middle age. The Dormont High School follow-up study, 1957-1963 and 1989-1990. Am J Epidemiol 1993;138:973–83.
35 Lopes HL, Martin KL, Nashar K, et. al. DASH diet lowers blood pressure and lipid-induced oxidative stress in obesity. Hypertens 2003;41:422–30.
36 Gundogdu Z. Relationship between BMI and blood pressure in girls and boys. Public Health Nutr 2008; April 22:1–4.
37 Fung TT, Chiuve SE, McCullough ML, et. al. Adherence to a DASH-Style Diet and Risk of Coronary Heart Disease and Stroke in Women. Arch Intern Med 2008;168(7):713–20.
38 Pitsavos C, Chrysohoou C, Panagiotakos DB, et. al. Abdominal obesity and inflammation predicts hypertension among prehypertensive men and women: the ATTICA Study. Heart Vessels 2008;23(2):96–103.
39 Pitsavos C, Panagiotakos DB, Tzima N, et. al. Diet, exercise, and C-reactive protein levels in people with abdominal obesity: the ATTICA epidemiological study. Angiology 2007;58(2):225–33.
40 Sacks FM, Svetkey LP, Volmer WM, et. al. Effects on blood pressure of reduced dietary sodium and the Dietary Approaches to Stop Hypertension (DASH) Diet. N Engl J Med 2001;344:3–10.
41 Conlin PR, Chow D, Miller ER III, et. al. The effect of dietary patterns on blood pressure control in hypertensive patients: results from the Dietary Approaches to Stop Hypertension (DASH) trial. Am J Hypertens 2000;13:949–55.
42 Pins JJ, Geleva D, Keenan JM, et. al. Do whole-grain oat cereals reduce the need for antihypertensive medications and improve blood pressure control? Fam Pract 2002;51(4):353–9.
43 Espeland MA, Whelton PK, Kostis JB, et. al. Predictors and mediators of successful long-term withdrawal from antihypertensive medications. TONE Cooperative Research Group. Trial of Nonpharmacologic Interventions in the Elderly. Arch Fam Med 1999;8(3):228–36.
44 Mulrow CD, Chiquette E, Angel L, et. al. Dieting to reduce body weight for controlling hypertension in adults. The Cochrane Library 2004(1).
45 Blumenthal JA, Sherwood A, Gullette EC, et. al. Exercise and weight loss reduce blood pressure in men and women with mild hypertension: effects on cardiovascular, metabolic, and hemodynamic functioning. Arch Intern Med 2000;160(13):1947–58.
46 He FJ, MacGregor GA. Effect of longer-term modest salt reduction on blood pressure. Cochrane Database Syst Rev 2004; 3):CD004937.
47 Dickinson HO, Mason JM, Nicolson DJ, et. al. Lifestyle interventions to reduce raised blood pressure: a systematic review of randomised controlled trials. J Hypertens 2006;24:215–33.
48 He FJ, MacGregor GA. Importance of salt in determining blood pressure in children: meta-analysis of controlled trials. Hypertension 2006; 48:861–69.
49 Houston MC. Nutraceuticals, vitamins, antioxidants, and minerals in the prevention and treatment of hypertension. Prog Cardiovasc Dis 2005;47(6):396–449.
50 Obarzanek E, Velletri PA, Cutler JA. Dietary protein and blood pressure. JAMA 1996;274:1598–1603.
51 Stamler J, Elliott P, Kesteloot H, et. al. Inverse relation of dietary protein markers with blood pressure. Findings for 10,020 men and women in the Intersalt Study. Intersalt Cooperative Research Group. International study of salt and blood pressure. Circulation 1996;94:1629–34.

52 He J, Welton PK. Effect of dietary fiber and protein intake on blood pressure: A review of epidemiologic evidence. Clin Exp Hypertens 1999;21:785–96.

53 Zhou B. The relationship of dietary animal protein and electrolytes to blood pressure. A study on three Chinese populations. Int J Epidem 1994;23:716–22.

54 Elliott P, Dennis B, Dyer AR, et. al. Relation of dietary protein (total, vegetable, animal) to blood pressure: INTERMAP epidemiologic study. Presented at the 18th Scientific Meeting of the International Society of Hypertension, Chicago, IL, August 20-24, 2000.

55 Wolfe BM. Potential role of raising dietary protein intake for reducing risk of atherosclerosis. Can J Cardiol 1995;11:127G-131G.

56 Burke V, Hodgson JM, Beilin LJ, et. al. Dietary protein and soluble fiber reduce ambulatory blood pressure in treated hypertensives. Hypertension 2001;38:821–26.

57 Kawase M, Hashimoto H, Hosoda M, et. al. Effect of administration of fermented milk containing whey protein concentrate to rats and healthy men on serum lipids and blood pressure. J Dairy Sci 2000;83: 255–63.

58 Groziak SM, Miller GD. Natural bioactive substances in milk and colostrum: Effects on the arterial blood pressure system. Br J Nutr 2000;84:S119-S125.

59 Barr SI, McCarron DA, Heaney RP, et. al. Effects of increased consumption of fluid milk on energy and nutrient intake, body weight, and cardiovascular risk factors in healthy older adults. J Am Diet Assoc 2000;100:810–17.

60 Appel LJ, Moore TJ, Obarzanek E, et. al. A clinical trial of the effects of dietary patterns on blood pressure. N Engl J Med 1997;336:1117–24.

61 Hasler CM, Kundrat S, Wool D. Functional foods and cardiovascular disease. Curr Atheroscler Rep 2000;2:467–75.

62 Tikkanen MJ, Adlercreutz H. Dietary soy–derived isoflavone phytoestrogens: Could they have a role in coronary heart disease prevention? Biochem Pharmacol 2000;60:1–5.

63 Liggins J, Bluck LJC, Runswick S, et. al. Daidzein and genistein content of fruits and nuts. J Nutr Biochem 2000;11:326–31.

64 Pins J, Keenan J. The antihypertensive effects of a hydrolyzed whey protein supplement. Cardiovasc Drugs Ther 2002;16(Suppl):68.

65 Yamamoto N, Akino A, Takano T. Antihypertensive effect of different kinds of fermented milk in spontaneously hypertensive rats. Biosci Biotechnol Biochem 1994;58:776–78.

66 Kawasaki T, Seki E, Osajima K, et. al. Antihypertensive effect of valyl-tyrosine, a short chain peptide derived from sardine muscle hydrolysate, on mild hypertensive subjects. J Hum Hypertens 2000;14:519–23.

67 Kuchel O. Differential catecholamine responses to protein intake in healthy and hypertensive patients. Am J Physiol 1998;275:R1164-R1173.

68 Millward DJ. Optimal intakes of protein in the human diet. Proc Nutr Soc 1999;58:403–13.

69 Lemon PWR. Is increased dietary protein necessary or beneficial for individuals with a physically active lifestyle? Nutr Rev 1996;54:S169-S175.

70 Morris MC. Dietary fats and blood pressure. J Cardiov Risk 1994;1:21–30.

71 Ueshima H, Stamler J, Elliott P, et. al. Food omega-3 fatty acid intake of individuals (total, linolenic acid, long-chain) and their blood pressure: INTERMAP study. Hypertension 2007;50(2):313–9.

72 Witteman J, Willett W, Stampfer M, et. al. A prospective study of nutritional factors and hypertension among US women. Circulation 1989;80:1320–1327.

73 Ascherio A, Rimm EB, Giovannucci EL, et. al. A prospective study of nutritional factors and hypertension among US men. Circulation 1992;86:1475–1484.

74 Zhao WS, Zhai JJ, Wang YH, et. al. Conjugated Linoleic Acid Supplementation Enhances Antihypertensive Effect of Ramipril in Chinese Patients With Obesity-Related Hypertension. Am J Hypertens. 2009 Mar 19. Epub ahead of print.

75 Vitetta L, Sali A. Omega–3 Fatty Acids PUFA - A Review PART I. Journal of Complementary Medicine 2006; 5(6):52–9.

76 Vitetta L, Sali A. Omega–3 Fatty Acids PUFA - A Review PART II. Journal of Complementary Medicine 2007;6(1):48–52.

77 Bao DQ, Mori TA, Burke V, et. al. Effects of dietary fish and weight reduction on ambulatory blood pressure in overweight hypertensives. Hypertension 1998;32:710–717.

78 Mori TA, Bao DQ, Burke V, et. al. Docosahexaenoic acid but not eicosapentaenoic acid lowers ambulatory blood pressure and heart rate in humans. Hypertension 1999;34:253–60.

79 DeBusk RM. Dietary supplements and cardiovascular disease. Curr Atheroscler Rep 2000;2:508–14.

80 Alexander JW. Immunonutrition: The role of omega-3 fatty acids. Nutrition 1998;14:627–33.

81 Toff I, Bønaa KH, Ingebretsen OC, et. al. Effects of n-3 polyunsaturated fatty acids on glucose homeostasis and blood pressure in essential hypertension: A randomised, controlled trial. Ann Intern Med 1995;123:911–18.

82 Bønaa KH, Bjerve KS, Straume B, et. al. Effect of eicosapentaenoic and docosahexaenoic acids on blood pressure in hypertension: A population-based intervention trial from the Tromso study. N Engl J Med 1990;322:795–801.

83 Knapp HR, FitzGerald GA. The antihypertensive effects of fish oil: A controlled study of polyunsaturated fatty acid supplements in essential hypertension. N Engl J Med 1989;320:1037–43.

84 Appel LJ, Miller ER, Seidler AJ, et. al.: Does supplementation of diet with fish oil reduce blood pressure? A meta-analysis of controlled clinical trials. Arch Intern Med 1993;153:1429–38.

85 Morris M, Sacks F, Rosner B. Does fish oil lower blood pressure? A meta-analysis of controlled trials. Circulation 1993;88:523–33.

86 Prisco D, Paniccia R, Bandinelli B, et. al. Effect of medium term supplementation with a moderate dose of n-3 polyunsaturated fatty acid on blood pressure in mild hypertensive patients. Thromb Res 1998;91:105–112.

87 Bao DQ, Mori TA, Burke V, et. al. Effects of dietary fish and weight reduction on ambulatory blood pressure in overweight hypertensives. Hypertension 1998;32:710–17.

88 Mori TA, Bao DQ, Burke V, et. al. Docosahexaenoic acid but not eicosapentaenoic acid lowers ambulatory blood pressure and heart rate in humans. Hypertension 1999;34:253–60.

89 Mori TA, Woodman RJ. The independent effects of eicosapentaenoic acid and docosahexaenoic acid on cardiovascular risk factors in humans. Curr Opin Clin Nutr Metab Care 2006;9:95–104.

90 Paschos GK, Magkos F, Panagiotakos DB, et. al. Dietary supplementation with flaxseed oil lowers blood pressure in dyslipidaemic patients. Eur J Clin Nutr 2007;61(10):1201–6.

91 Eaton SB, Eaton III SB, Konner MJ. Paleolithic nutrition revisited: A twelve-year retrospective on its nature and implications. A review. Eur J Clin Nutr 1997;51:207–16.
92 Mozaffarian D, Willett WC. Trans fatty acids and cardiovascular risk: a unique cardiometabolic imprint? Curr Atheroscler Rep 2007;9(6):486–93.
93 Ferrara LA, Raimondi S, d'Episcopa I, et. al.: Olive oil and reduced need for antihypertensive medications. Arch Intern Med 2000;160:837–42.
94 Strazzullo P, Ferro-Luzzi A, Siani A, et. al. Changing the Mediterranean diet: Effects on blood pressure. J Hypertens 1986;4:407–12.
95 Thomsen C, Rasmussen OW, Hansen KW, et. al. Comparison of the effects on the diurnal blood pressure, glucose, and lipid levels of a diet rich in monounsaturated fatty acids with a diet rich in polyunsaturated fatty acids in type 2 diabetic subjects. Diabet Med 1995;12:600–606.
96 Mensink RP, Janssen MC, Katan MB. Effect on blood pressure of two diets differing in total fat but not in saturated and polyunsaturated fatty acids in healthy volunteers. Am J Clin Nutr 1988;47:976–80.
97 Papadopoulos G, Boskou D. Antioxidant effect of natural phenols in olive oil. J Am Oil Chem Soc 1991;68:669–71.
98 Mensink RP, Katan MB. Effect of dietary fatty acids on serum lipids and lipoproteins: A meta-analysis of 27 trials. Arterioscler Thromb 1992;12:911–19.
99 Nuñez-Cordoba JM, Alonso A, Beunza JJ, et. al. Role of vegetables and fruits in Mediterranean diets to prevent hypertension. Eur J Clin Nutr 2008 Feb 27. Epub ahead of print.
100 Papamichael CM, Karatzi KN, Papaioannou TG, et. al. Acute combined effects of olive oil and wine on pressure wave reflections: another beneficial influence of the Mediterranean diet antioxidants? J Hypertens 2008;26(2):223–9.
101 James JE. Critical review of dietary caffeine and blood pressure: a relationship that should be taken more seriously. Psychosom Med 2004;66(1):63–71.
102 Sudano I, Binggeli C, Spieker L. Cardiovascular effects of coffee: is it a risk factor? Prog Cardiovasc Nurs. 2005 Spring;20(2):65–9.
103 Taubert D, Berkels R, Roesen R, et. al. Chocolate and blood pressure in elderly individuals with isolated systolic hypertension. JAMA 2003;290:1029–30.
104 Taubert D, Roesen R, Lehmann C, et. al. Effects of low habitual cocoa intake on blood pressure and bioactive nitric oxide: a randomised controlled trial. JAMA 2007;298(1):49–60.
105 Martin RM, Ness AR, Gunnell D, et. al. Does breast-feeding in infancy lower blood pressure in childhood? The Avon Longitudinal Study of Parents and Children (ALSPAC). Circulation 2004;109:1259–66.
106 Martin RM, Gunnell D, Smith GD. Breastfeeding in infancy and blood pressure in later life: systematic review and meta-analysis. Am J Epidemiol 2005;161(1):15–26.
107 Ceriello A, Giugliano D, Quatraro A, et. al. Antioxidants show an antihypertensive effect in diabetic and hypertensive subjects. Clin Sci 1991;81:739–42.
108 Duffy SJ, Gokce N, Holbrook M, et. al. Treatment of hypertension with ascorbic acid. Lancet 1999;354:2048–49.
109 Plantiga Y, Ghiadoni L, Magagna A, et. al. Supplementation with vitamins C and E improved arterial stiffness and endothelial function in essential hypertensive patients. Am J Hypert 2007:20(4):392–7.
110 Bates CJ, Walmsley CM, Prentice A, et. al. Does vitamin C reduce blood pressure? Results of a large study of people aged 65 or older. J Hypertens 1998;16:925–32.
111 Ness AR, Khaw K-T, Bingham S, et. al. Vitamin C status and blood pressure. J Hypertens 1996;14:503–508.
112 Osilesi O, Trout DL, Ogunwole J, et. al. Blood pressure and plasma lipids during ascorbic acid supplementation in borderline hypertensive and normotensive adults. Nutr Res 1991;11:405-12.
113 Simon JA. Vitamin C and cardiovascular disease: A review. J Am Coll Nutr 1992;11:107–25.
114 Lovat LB, Lu Y, Palmer AJ, et. al. Double-blind trial of vitamin C in elderly hypertensives. J Hum Hypertens 1993;7:403–405.
115 Duffy SJ, Gokce N, Holbrook M, et. al. Treatment of hypertension with ascorbic acid. Lancet 1999;354:2048–49.
116 Ness AR, Chee D, Elliot P. Vitamin C and blood pressure—an overview. J Hum Hypertens 1997;11:343–50.
117 Palumbo G, Avanzini F, Alli C, et. al. Effects of vitamin E on clinic and ambulatory blood pressure in treated hypertensive patients. Am J Hypertens 2000;13:564–67.
118 Mottram P, Shige H, Nestel P. Vitamin E improves arterial compliance in middle-aged men and women. Atherosclerosis 1999;145:399–404.
119 Skyrme-Jones RA, O'Brien RC, Berry KL, et. al. Vitamin E supplementation improves endothelial function in type I diabetes mellitus: A randomised, placebo-controlled study. J Am Coll Card 2000;36:94–102.
120 Lino K, Abe K, Kariya S, et. al. A controlled, double blind study of DL-alpha-tocopheryl nicotinate for treatment of symptoms in hypertension and cerebral arteriosclerosis. Jpn Heart J 1977;18:277–86.
121 Dakshinamurti K, Lal KJ. Vitamins and hypertension. In: Simopoulos AP. Nutrients in the Control of Metabolic Diseases. World Rev Nutr Diet, vol 69. Basal, Karger, 1996:40–73.
122 Lind L, Wengle BO, Junghall S. Blood pressure is lowered by vitamin D (alphacalcidol) during long-term treatment of patients with intermittent hypercalcemia. Acta Med Scand 1987;222:423–27.
123 Lind L, Lithell H, Skarfos E, et. al. Reduction of blood pressure by treatment with alphacalcidol. Acta Med Scand 1988;223:211–17.
124 Lind L, Wengle BO, Wide L, et. al. Hypertension in primary hyperparathyroidism—reduction of blood pressure by long-term treatment with vitamin D (alphacalcidol). A double-blind, placebo-controlled study. Am J Hypertens 1988;1:397–402.
125 Pfeifer M, Begerow B, Minne HW, et. al. Effects of a short-term vitamin D(3) and calcium supplementation on blood pressure and parathyroid hormone levels in elderly women. J Cli Endocr Metab 2001;86:1633–37.
126 McCarron DA. Calcium metabolism and hypertension. Kidney Int 1989;35:717–36.
127 McCarron DA. Low serum concentrations of ionised calcium in patients with hypertension. N Engl J Med 1982;307:226–28.
128 Resnick LM. Dietary calcium and hypertension. J Nutr 1987;117:1806–08.
129 Jorde R, Bonaa KH. Calcium from dairy products, vitamin D intake and blood pressure: The Tromso Study. Am J Clin Nutr 2000;71:1530–35.
130 Wang L, Manson JE, Buring JE, et. al. Dietary intake of dairy products, calcium, and vitamin D and the risk of hypertension in middle-aged and older women. Hypertension 2008;51(4):1073–9.

131 Boucher BJ. Inadequate vitamin D status. Does it contribute to the disorders comprising syndrome X? Br J Nutr 1998;79:315–27.
132 Scragg R, Holdaway SR, Singh V, et. al. Serum 25-hydroxycholecalciferol concentration in newly detected hypertension. Am J Hypertens 1995;4: 429–32.
133 Scragg R, Sowers M, Bell C; Third National Health and Nutrition Examination Survey. Serum 25-hydroxyvitamin D, diabetes, and ethnicity in the Third National Health and Nutrition Examination Survey. Diabetes Care 2004;27(12):2813–8.
134 Lind L, Hanni LL, Huarfner LH, et. al. Vitamin D is related to blood pressure and other cardiovascular risk factors in middle-aged men. Am J Hypertens 1995;8:894–901.
135 de Boer IH, Tinker LF, Connelly S, et. al. Calcium plus vitamin D supplementation and the risk of incident diabetes in the Women's Health Initiative. Diabetes Care 2008;31(4):701–7.
136 Bai S, Favus MJ. Vitamin D and calcium receptors: links to hypercalciuria. Curr Opin Nephrol Hypertens 2006;15(4):381–5.
137 Fregly MJ, Cade JR. Effect of pyridoxine and tryptophan, alone and in combined, on the development of deoxycorticosterone acetate–induced hypertension in rats. Pharmacology 1995;50: 298–306.
138 Lal KJ, Krishnamurti D, Thliverv J. The effect of vitamin B6 on the systolic blood pressure of rats in various animal models of hypertension. J Hypertens 1996;14:355–63.
139 Keniston R, Enriquez JI, Sr. Relationship between blood pressure and plasma vitamin B6 levels in healthy middle-aged adults. Ann N Y Acad Sci 1990;585:499–501.
140 Dakshinamurti K, Lal KJ. Vitamins and hypertension. World Rev Nutr Diet 1992;69:40–73.
141 Bender DA. Non-nutritional uses of vitamin B-6. Br J Nutr 1999;81:7–20.
142 Dakshinamurti K, Paulose CS, Viswanathan M: Vitamin B6 and hypertension. Ann N Y Acad Sci 1990;575:241–49.
143 Sali A, Vitetta L. Nutritional supplements and cardio-vascular disease. Heart Lung Circ 2004;13(4):363–6.
144 McMahon JA, Skeaff CM, Williams SM, et. al. Lowering homocysteine with B vitamins has no effect on blood pressure in older adults. J Nutr 2007;137(5):1183–7.
145 Kotchen TA, McCarron DA. AHA Science Advisory. Dietary electrolytes and blood pressure. Circulation 1998;98:613–17.
146 Midgley JP, Matthew AG, Greenwood CM, et. al. Effect of reduced dietary sodium on blood pressure: A meta-analysis of randomised controlled trials. JAMA 1996;275:1590–97.
147 Cutler JA, Follman D, Allender PS. Randomised trials of sodium reduction: An overview. Am J Clin Nutr 1997;65:643S-651S.
148 Graudal NA, Galloe AM, Garred P. Effects of sodium restriction on blood pressure, renin, aldosterone, catecholamines, cholesterols, and triglyceride: A meta-analysis. JAMA 1998;279:1383–91.
149 Svetkey LP, Sacks FM, Obarzanek E, et. al. The DASH diet, sodium intake and blood pressure (the DASH-Sodium Study): Rationale and design. J Am Diet Assoc 1999;99:S96-S104.
150 Egan BM, Lackland DT. Biochemical and metabolic effects of very-low-salt diets. Am J Med Sci 2000;320:233–39.
151 The Trials of Hypertension Prevention Collaborative Research Group: Effects of weight loss and sodium reduction intervention on blood pressure and hypertension incidence in overweight people with high normal blood pressure: The Trials of Hypertension Prevention, Phase II. Arch Intern Med 1997;157:657–67.
152 Whelton PK, Appel LJ, Espeland MA, et. al. Efficacy of sodium reduction and weight loss in the treatment of hypertension in older persons: Main results of the randomised, controlled trial of nonpharmacologic interventions in the elderly (TONE). JAMA 1998;279:839–46.
153 He J, Ogden LG, Vupputuri S, et. al. Dietary sodium intake and subsequent risk of cardiovascular disease in overweight adults. JAMA 1999;282:2027–34.
154 Steven VJ, Obarzanek E, Cook NR, et. al. Long-term weight loss and changes in blood pressure: Results of the trials of hypertension prevention, phase II. Ann Intern Med 2001;134:1–11.
155 Kostis JB, Shindler DM, Lacy CR. Non-drug therapy for hypertension: Do effects on weight and sodium intake persist after discontinuation of intervention. Am J Med 2000;109:734–35.
156 Lasser VI, Raczynski JM, Stevens VJ, et. al. Trials of Hypertension Prevention, phase II. Structure and content of the weight loss and dietary sodium reduction interventions. Trials of Hypertension Prevention (TOHP) Collaborative Research Group. Ann Epidemiol 1995;5(2):156–64.
157 Cianciaruso B, Belliszi V, Minutolo R, et. al. Salt intake and renal outcome in patients with progressive renal disease. Miner Electrolyte Metab 1998;24:296–301.
158 Hooper L, Bartlett C, Davey SG, et. al. Advice to reduce dietary salt for prevention of cardiovascular disease. Cochrane Database Syst Rev 2004;(1):CD003656.
159 Penner SB, Campbell NR, Chockalingam A, et. al. Dietary sodium and cardiovascular outcomes: a rational approach. Can J Cardiol 2007;23(7):567–72. Review.
160 Cook NR, Cutler JA, Obarzanek E, et. al. Long-term effects of dietary sodium reduction on cardiovascular disease outcomes: observational follow-up of the trials of hypertension prevention (TOHP). BMJ 2007;334:885.
161 Whelton PK, He J. Potassium in preventing and treating high blood pressure. Semin Nephrol 1999;19:494–99.
162 Siani A, Strazzullo P, Giacco A, et. al. Increasing the dietary potassium intake reduces the need for antihypertensive medication. Ann Intern Med 1991;115:753–9.
163 Whelton PK, He J, Cutler JA, et. al. Effects of oral potassium on blood pressure: Meta-analysis of randomised controlled clinical trials. JAMA 1997;227:1624–32.
164 McCarron DA, Reusser ME. Nonpharmacologic therapy in hypertension: From single components to overall dietary management. Prog Cardiovasc Dis 1999;41:451–60.
165 Gu D, He J, Xigui W, et. al. Effect of potassium supplementation on blood pressure in Chinese: A randomised, placebo-controlled trial. J Hypertens 2001;19:1325–31.
166 Barri YM, Wingo CS. The effects of potassium depletion and supplementation on blood pressure: A clinical review. Am J Med Sci 1997;3:37–40.
167 Ma G, Mamaril JLC, Young DB, et. al. Increased potassium concentration inhibits stimulation of vascular smooth muscle proliferation by PDGF-BB and bFGF. Am J Hypertens 2000;13:1055–60.

168 Karanja N, Roullet JB, Aickin M, et. al. Mineral metabolism, blood pressure, and dietary patterns: Findings from the DASH trial. J Am Soc Nephrol 1998;9:151A.
169 Hamet P, Daignault-Gelinas M, Lambert J, et. al. Epidemiological evidence of an interaction between calcium and sodium intake impacting on blood pressure: A Montreal study. Am J Hypertens 1992;5:378–85.
170 Saito K, Sano H, Furuta Y, et. al. Effect of oral calcium on blood pressure response in salt-loaded borderline hypertensive patients. Hypertension 1989;13:219–26.
171 Cappuccio FP, Elliott P, Allender PS, et. al. Epidemiologic association between dietary calcium intake and blood pressure: A meta-analysis of published data. Am J Epidemiol 1995;142:935–45.
172 Allender PS, Cutler JA, Follmann D, et. al. Dietary calcium and blood pressure: A meta-analysis of randomised clinical trials. Ann Intern Med 1996;124:825–31.
173 McCarron DA. Calcium metabolism in hypertension. Keio J Med 1995;44:105–14.
174 Witteman JCM, Willett WC, Stampfer MJ, et. al. A prospective study of nutritional factors and hypertension among US women. Circulation 1989;80:1320–27.
175 Bucher HC, Cook RJ, Guyatt GH, et. al. Effects of dietary calcium supplementation on blood pressure. A meta-analysis of randomised controlled trials. JAMA 1996;275:1016–22.
176 Griffith L, Guyatt GH, Cook RJ, et. al. The influence of dietary and non-dietary calcium supplementation on blood pressure: An updated meta-analysis of randomised clinical trials. Am J Hypertens 1999;12:84–92.
177 Karanja N, Morris CD, Rufolo P, et. al. The impact of increasing dietary calcium intake on nutrient consumption, plasma lipids and lipoproteins in humans. Am J Hypertens 994;59:900–7.
178 Resnick LM. Calcium metabolism in hypertension and allied metabolic disorders. Diabetes Care 1991;14:505–20.
179 Hofmeyr GJ, Roodt A, Atallah AN, et. al. Calcium supplementation to prevent pre-eclampsia–a systematic review. S Afr Med J 2003;93:224–8.
180 Atallah AN, Hofmeyr GJ, Duley L. Calcium supplementation during pregnancy for preventing hypertensive disorders and related problems. Cochrane Database Syst Rev 2006;3:CD001059.
181 Daly RM, Nowson CA. Long-term effect of calcium-vitamin D3 fortified milk on blood pressure and serum lipid concentrations in healthy older men. European Journal of Clinical Nutrition advance online publication 21 January 2009; doi: 10.1038/ejcn.2008.79.
182 Wirell MP, Wester PO, Stegmayr BG. Nutritional dose of magnesium in hypertensive patients on beta blockers lowers systolic blood pressure: a double blind, cross-over study. J Intern Med 1994;236: 189–95.
183 Kawano Y, Matsuoka H, Takishita S, et. al. Effects of magnesium supplementation in hypertensive patients: assessment by office, home, and ambulatory blood pressures. Hypertension 1998;32:260–5.
184 Shibutani Y, Sakamoto K, Katsuno S, et. al. Relation of serum and erythrocyte magnesium levels to blood pressure and a family history of Hypertension. A follow-up study in Japanese children, 12-14 years old. Acta Paediatr Scand 1990;79(3):316–21.
185 Witteman JC, Grobbee DE, Derkx FH, et. al. Reduction of blood pressure with oral magnesium supplementation in women with mild to moderate hypertension. Am J Clin Nutr 1994;60(1): 129–35.
186 Itoh K, Kawasaka T, Nakamura M. The effects of high oral magnesium supplementation on blood pressure, serum lipids and related variables in apparently healthy Japanese subjects. Br J Nutr 1997;78(5):737–50.
187 Bo S, Pisu E. Role of dietary magnesium in cardiovascular disease prevention, insulin sensitivity and diabetes. Curr Opin Lipidol 2008; 19(1):50–6.
188 Singh RB, Niaz MA, Rastogi SS, et. al. Current zinc intake and risk of diabetes and coronary artery disease and factors associated with insulin resistance in rural and urban populations of North India. J Am Coll Nutr 1998;17:564–70.
189 Zozaya JL. Nutritional factors in high blood pressure. J Hum Hypertens 2000;1:S100-S104.
190 Garcia Zozaya JL, Padilla Viloria M. Alterations of calcium, magnesium, and zinc in essential hypertension: Their relation to the renin-angiotensinaldosterone system. Invest Clin 1997;38:27–40.
191 Galley HF, Thornton J, Howdle PD, et. al. Combination oral antioxidant supplementation reduces blood pressure. Clin Sci 1997;92:361–65.
192 Bergomi M, Rovesti S, Vinceti M, et. al. Zinc and copper status and blood pressure. J Trace Elem Med Biol 1997;11:166–69.
193 Langsjoen PH, Langsjoen AM. Overview of the use of CoQ10 in cardiovascular disease. Biofactors 1999;9:273–84.
194 Langsjoen H, Langsjoen P, Langsjoen P, et. al. Usefulness of coenzyme Q10 in clinical cardiology: a long-term study. Mol Aspects Med 1994; 15:S165-S175.
195 Langsjoen PH, Langsjoen PH, Folkers K. Isolated diastolicdysfunctionofthemyocardiumanditsresponseto CoQ10 treatment. Clin Investig 1993;71:S140-S144.
196 Folkers K, Drzewoski J, Richardson PC, et. al. Bioenergetics in clinical medicine. XVI. Reduction of hypertensioninpatientsbytherapywithcoenzymeQ10. ResCommunChemPatholPharmacol1981;31:129–40.
197 Yamagami T, Shibata N, Folkers K. Bioenergetics in clinical medicine. VIII. Adminstration of coenzyme Q10 to patients with essential hypertension. Res Commun Chem Pathol Pharmacol 1976;14: 721–27.
198 Langsjoen P, Langsjoen P, Willis R, et. al. Treatment of Essential Hypertension with Coenzyme Q10. Mol Aspects Med 1994;15:s265-s272.
199 McCarty MF. Coenzyme Q versus hypertension: does CoQ decrease endothelial superoxide generation? Med Hypoth. 1999;53:300–304.
200 Digiesi V, Cantini F, Oradei A, et. al. Coenzyme Q10 in essential hypertension. Mol Aspects Med 1994;15:S257-S263.
201 Hodgson JM, Watts GF, Playford DA, et. al. Coenzyme Q10 improves blood pressure and glycaemic control: a controlled trial in subjects with Type 2 diabetes. European Journal of Clinical Nutrition 2002;56:1137–42.
202 Shah SA, Sander S, Cios D, et. al. Electrocardiographic and hemodynamic effects of coenzyme Q10 in healthy individuals: a double-blind, randomised controlled trial. Ann Pharmacother 2007;41(3):420–5.

203 Rosenfeldt FL, Haas SJ, Krum H, et. al. Coenzyme Q10 in the treatment of hypertension: a meta-analysis of the clinical trials. J Hum Hypertens 2007;21(4):297–306.
204 Paran E, Engelhard YN. Effect of lycopene, an oral natural antioxidant on blood pressure. J Hypertens 2001;19:S74.
205 Paran E, Engelhard Y. Effect of tomato's lycopene on blood pressure, serum lipoproteins, plasma homocysteine and oxidative stress markers in grade I hypertensive patients. Am J Hypertens 2001;14:141A.
206 DeBusk RM. Dietary supplements and cardiovascular disease. Curr Atheroscler Rep 2000;2:508–14.
207 Auer W, Eiber A, Hertkorn E, et. al. Hypertension and hyperlipidaemia: Garlic helps in mild cases. Br J Clin Pract 1990;69:3–6.
208 McMahon FG, Vargas R. Can garlic lower blood pressure? A pilot study. Pharmacotherapy 1993;13:406–407.
209 Pedraza-Chaverri J, Tapia E, Medina-Campos ON, et. al. Garlic prevents hypertension induced by chronic inhibition of nitric oxide synthesis. Life Sci1999;62:71–77.
210 Orekhov AN, Grunwald J. Effects of garlic on atherosclerosis. Nutrition 1997;13:656–663.
211 Ernst E. Cardiovascular effects of garlic (Allium savitum): A review. Pharmatherapeutica 1987;5:83–89.
212 Silagy CA, Neil AW. A meta-analysis of the effect of garlic on blood pressure. J Hypertens 1994;12:463–68.
213 Silagy C, Neil A. Garlic as a lipid lowering agent: A meta analysis. J R Coll Physicians Lond 1994;28:39–45.
214 Kleinjnen J, Knipschild P, Ter Riet G. Garlic, onions and cardiovascular risk factors: A review of the evidence from human experiments with emphasis on commercially available preparations. Br J Clin Pharmacol 1989;28:535–44.
215 Reuter HD, Sendl A. Allium sativum and Allium ursinum: Chemistry, pharmacology and medicinal applications. Econ Med Plant Res 1994;6:55–113.
216 Mohamadi A, Jarrell ST, Shi SJ, et. al. Effects of wild versus cultivated garlic on blood pressure and other parameters in hypertensive rats. Heart Dis 2001; 2:3–9.
217 Budoff M. Aged garlic extract retards progression of coronary artery calcification. J Nutr 2006;136(3 Suppl):741S-744S.
218 Ried K, Frank OR, Stocks NP, et. al. Effect of garlic on blood pressure: a systematic review and meta-analysis. BMC Cardiovasc Disord 2008;8:13.
219 Reinhart KM, Coleman CI, Teevan C, et. al. Effects of garlic on blood pressure in patients with and without systolic hypertension: a meta-analysis. Ann Pharmacother 2008;42(12):1766–71.
220 Mashour NH, Lin GI, Frishman WH. Herbal Medicine for the Treatment of Cardiovascular Disease. Arch Intern Med 1998;158:2225–34.
221 Walker AF, Marakis G, Simpson E, et. al. Hypotensive effects of hawthorn for patients with diabetes taking prescription drugs: a randomised controlled trial. Br J Gen Pract 2006;56(527): 437–43.
222 Smith WM. Treatment of mild hypertension: results of a ten-year intervention trial. Circ Res 1977;40:198–205.
223 Nahas R. Complementary and alternative medicine approaches to blood pressure reduction: An evidence-based review. Can Fam Physician 2008;54(11): 1529–33.

Chapter 20

Infections and immunity

With contribution from Dr Lily Tomas

Introduction

The immune system is a complex of tissues, cells and molecules with specialised roles in defence against infection. There are 2 fundamentally different types of responses to invading microbes — innate (natural) immunity responses that occur to the same extent however many times the infectious agent is encountered, whereas acquired (adaptive) immune responses improve on repeated exposure to a given infection or antigen.

The mediators of the innate immune response include phagocytic cells (i.e. neutrophils, monocytes, and macrophages), cells that release inflammatory mediators (i.e. basophils, mast-cells and eosinophils), and natural killer cells. The molecular components of innate immune responses include complement, acute-phase proteins and cytokines such as the interferons.

Acquired responses involve the proliferation of antigen-specific B- and T-cells, which occurs when the surface receptors of these cells bind to antigen. Specialised cells, called antigen-presenting cells, display the antigen to lymphocytes and collaborate with them in the response to the antigen. The B-cells secrete immunoglobulins, the antigen-specific antibodies responsible for eliminating extracellular microorganisms.

T-cells help B-cells to make antibody and can also eradicate intracellular pathogens by activating macrophages and by killing virally infected cells. Innate and acquired responses usually cooperate to eliminate pathogens.

The immune system hence distinguishes entities within the body as *self* or *non-self* and acts to eliminate those that are *non-self*. Microorganisms are the principal *non-self* entities, but neoplasms, transplants, and certain foreign substances (e.g. some toxins) are also important.

A paradox shift has recently been established, between those known functions of the immune system and bacterial species. This shift has challenged the idea that all infections are adverse to health. This was the instinctive documented observations of Elie Metchnikoff from the early 20th century. There has been much interest in the beneficial effects of commensal bacteria on human health. The effect of commensal bacteria on the innate immune system of humans has changed the way we view infections with bacteria that favourably influence the health of the host by improving the indigenous microflora.

Studies of mucosal immunity and age suggest that mucosal immunity evolves with age and it is obvious that the loss of innate immunity to process, eliminate and present antigens could compromise the development of adaptive immunity.

Of significant importance is that humans represent a scaffold on which diverse microbial ecosystems are established. Immediately after birth, all mammals are initiated into a lifelong process of colonisation by foreign microorganisms that inhabit all mucosal surfaces as well as the skin. Fashioned by millennia of evolutionary inputs, some host–bacterial associations have developed into beneficial relationships, creating an environment for mutual benefit and endowing the human immune system with advantageous signalling capacities that can control pathogenic insults throughout a lifetime of interactions. This then raises the possibility that, rather than the mammalian immune system being designed to control microorganisms, it is in fact controlled by microorganisms.[1]

Lifestyle factors

Lifestyle factors can significantly influence the state of the immune system. Whilst conservative approaches such as rest and fluids, and pharmaceutical treatments such as antibiotics, anti-fungal and anti-viral medication have played a very important role in the treatment of infections, it is vital to explore factors, in particular lifestyle factors, that may be contributing to lowered or altered immunity, and enhancing susceptibility to diseases of infections, chronic fatigue or even cancers.

For example, recurring infections such as recurrent ear, urinary and sinus infections are a common presentation to medical practitioners. These can be quite distressing for families to deal with, not only in its treatment but also its impact physically, psychologically and socially, such as in time away from work and school, and dependency on others such as grandparents to care for sick children.

Table 20.1 summarises the lifestyle factors that may impact adversely on the immune system. These factors will be discussed throughout the chapter. Prevention is the best method to help maintain a healthy immune system.

Mind–body medicine

Humans as well as all other organisms have a requisite to maintain a complex dynamic equilibrium (homeostasis), which is constantly challenged by internal or external adverse stressor events. The brain's stressor-handling system that constitutes the limbic-hypothalamic-pituitary-adrenal axis is one of the most thoroughly studied circuitry systems of the central nervous system. As a result of stressor–axis activation, different behavioural and physical changes can develop which allow the organism to adapt. These are the domains of psychoneuroimmunology (PNI) and psychoneuroendocrinology (PNE).[2, 3]

Psychoneuroimmunology (PNI)

The emerging specialty fields of PNI and PNE are justification enough that stress and/or adverse stressors have a profound impact upon every system within the body.[2, 3, 4]

There is a wealth of evidence demonstrating that psychological stress can adversely affect the development and progression of almost every known disease. Both acute and chronic stressful states produce documentable changes in the innate and adaptive immune responses, which are predominantly mediated via neuroendocrine mediators from the hypothalamic-pituitary-adrenal (HPA) axis and the sympathetic-adrenal axis.[5–13]

Indeed, this is an elaborate multi-directional communication system which continually and simultaneously relays multiple messages between the immune, gastrointestinal, neurological, endocrinological, dermatological and cardiovascular systems in an ongoing attempt to restore and maintain homeostasis.[14–24]

Neurotransmitters, hormones and neuropeptides all regulate the cells of the immune system, subsequently communicating with all other systems through the secretion of a wide variety of different cytokines.[14] It is beyond the scope of this chapter to discuss such complex and intricate interactions, however, there is sufficient literature available today specifically dealing with PNI.

Table 20.1 Risk factors that impact on the immune system

Stress — chronic • Depression
Environment • Climate change — overheating that promotes vector-borne illnesses (e.g. malaria, gastroenteritis); poor housing and/or living conditions • Overcrowding • Environmental syndrome, electromagnetic radiation, Multiple Chemical Sensitivity, Sick Building Syndrome
Chemical exposure and/or pollutants • Occupational • Industrial • Pollution • Smoking
Medications • For example, immunosuppressive, chemotherapy medications
Exposure to infection(s) • For example, hygiene, poor water and/or food quality • Bacterial, fungal, viral, parasites
Lack of sleep
Lack of sunshine • Vitamin D deficiency
Exercise • Lack of exercise • Too much exercise (e.g. marathon runners)
Obesity Underweight, cachectic, anorexic
Poor nutritional intake
Nutrient deficiencies • For example, vitamin A, C, D, E, B6, B12, folate, zinc, iron, copper

Acute stress has been shown to have a stimulating effect on the immune system whereas chronic stress down-regulates the immune system.[12, 16] Chronic stress has been associated with increased susceptibility of the patient to infectious diseases and cancer.[6, 7, 9] It is also linked with worse outcomes in many immune-related disorders, including cancer, inflammatory and infectious diseases, indicating that the effects of mental states on our immune system are directly and clinically relevant to disease expression.[10, 16, 18]

Psychological interventions

There is certainly considerable variability in each individual's immune response to stress. Encouraging particular activities that increase that person's ability to cope with stress may therefore have a significantly beneficial effect on immune function with subsequent modification in the development and progression of many different diseases.[12, 14, 21, 23]

It is also important to note that stress during fetal and neonatal development can alter the programming of the neuro-endocrine-immune axis, influencing stress, immune-responsiveness and even disease resistance in later life.[16] Therefore identification and treatment of suboptimal moods in pregnant women is imperative.

Various behavioural strategies, psychological and psychopharmacotherapeutic interventions that enhance effective coping and reduce affective distress show beneficial effects in many disease, including cancer.[15, 25]

A recent Australian survey of women with breast cancer indicates that 87.5% of surveyed women had used complementary therapies in order to improve their physical health (86.3%), emotional wellbeing (83.2%) and to boost their immune system (68.8%). Support groups and meditation were commonly used therapies.[26]

Mindfulness-based stress reduction (MBSR)

There have been many recent studies, including a systematic review, which demonstrate the efficacious potential of MBSR in the management of cancer, particularly breast and prostate, and Human Immunodeficiency Virus (HIV).[27–35]

Those with breast and prostate cancer not only showed improvements in mood but also improved cytokine parameters with a reduction in levels of pro-inflammatory cytokines.[28, 29, 31] In comparison with controls, MBSR practised by those with HIV showed an increase in natural killer (NK) cells and stable CD4+ lymphocyte counts.[33, 34]

Hypnosis, relaxation and guided imagery

These therapies have been shown to be effective in improving immunity in cases of breast cancer, viral illnesses including chronic herpes simplex and the common cold, and in 1 case of the auto-immune condition dermatomyositis when combined with meditation.[36, 37, 38]

Six weeks of training was found to almost halve the recurrence of herpes simplex outbreaks as well as reduce levels of anxiety and depression. Immune functions were upregulated, notably functional NK-cell activity to HSV-1.[39]

In those with breast cancer, significant effects have been found with respect to NK-cell activity, mixed lymphocyte responsiveness and the number of peripheral blood lymphocytes when compared with controls.[40, 41, 42] Thus, there appears to be a role for hypnotic guided imagery as an adjuvant therapy to breast cancer.

Cognitive behavioural therapy (CBT)

There have been several studies demonstrating the effectiveness of CBT with regard to immune parameters in HIV positive men. Significantly greater numbers of T-cytotoxic/suppressor lymphocytes, reduced urinary cortisol output and significantly reduced HSV-2 IgG titres in HIV-positive men with concomitant herpes simplex virus have all been documented.[43, 44, 45]

Autogenic training and group psychotherapy for women with breast cancer have also resulted in improved immune parameters.[46, 47]

A Cochrane systematic review of 15 studies, inclusive of 1043 chronic fatigue syndrome (CFS) sufferers found CBT is effective in reducing the symptoms of fatigue at post-treatment compared with usual care, and may be more effective in reducing fatigue symptoms compared with other psychological therapies.[48]

Environment

Epidemiological studies have reported that the hygiene hypothesis suggests that early life exposure to a non-hygienic environment that contains endotoxin reduces the risk of developing allergic diseases. Moreover, it is increasingly recognised that microbial colonisation of the gastrointestinal tract, linked with lifestyle and/or additional geographic factors, may be important determinants of the heterogeneity in disease prevalence observed throughout the world.

Developmental immuno-toxicology (DIT) and/or Early Life Immune Insult (ELII)

Many chronic diseases of increasing incidence are now recognised to have immune dysregulation as an important underlying component of the disease process.[49] These include many childhood illnesses such as asthma, allergic disease, leukaemia, autoimmunity and certain infections.[50]

The developing immune system is extremely sensitive to environmental toxins, such as infectious agents, allergens, maternal smoking, maternally administered drugs, exposure to xenobiotics, diesel exhaust and traffic-related particles, antibiotics, environmental oestrogens, heavy metals, chemicals and other prenatal/neonatal stressors.[51–58] Dysfunctional immune responses to infections in childhood have been postulated to play a role in childhood leukaemia.[56, 57] Furthermore, many prenatal and postnatal neurological lesions are now also being recognised as being linked to prenatal immune insult and inflammatory dysregulation.[57] Evidence for an association between environmentally associated childhood immune dysfunction and autistic spectrum disorders also suggests that ELII and DIT may contribute to these conditions.[53, 54, 56, 57]

Indeed, ELII have been proposed to be pivotal in producing chronic symptoms in later life. In particular, the period from mid-gestation until 2 years seems to be one of particular concern, with this critical maturational window displaying a heightened sensitivity to chemical disruption with the outcome of persistent immune dysfunction and/or misregulation.[57] It is also important to note that the same toxin may result in different immune maturational processes according to the dose and timing of the insult.[57] The important emerging field of epigenetics (combined environmental and genetic history) is also relevant in this situation.

T Helper lymphocytes

Available data indicates that ELII results in a shift from T-helper (Th) lymphocytes 1 towards Th2 predominance, alterations in regulatory T-cell function and problematic regulation of inflammatory cell function leading to hyper-inflammatory responses and perturbation of cytokine networks. The resulting health risks may extend far beyond infectious diseases, cancer, allergy and auto-immunity to pathologies in the neurological, cardiovascular, endocrinological, respiratory and reproductive systems.[53-55, 57]

Environmental syndromes

There is also strong evidence indicating that complex syndromes such as Multiple Chemical Sensitivity, Gulf War Syndrome, Sick Building Syndrome and Chronic Fatigue Syndrome, that often have no clear underlying medical explanation, may have an environmental component to their aetiology.[59]

Electromagnetic radiation

There is currently much debate regarding the potential health risks from extremely low frequency electromagnetic fields (ELF) and radiofrequency/microwave radiation emissions from wireless communications (RF). In addition to immune system dysregulation, other risks may include childhood leukaemia, brain tumours, genotoxic effects, neurodegenerative diseases, allergic and inflammatory responses, breast cancer, miscarriage and some cardiovascular effects.[60, 61, 62]

Specific reports on immunological dysfunction are scarce, however, 1 earlier study demonstrated that people who worked in close proximity to transformers and high tension cables full-time for 1–5 years experienced a significant decrease in total lymphocytes and CD2, CD3 and CD4 lymphocytes as well as an increase in NK-cells. Leukopaenia and neutropaenia were observed in 2 people who were permanently exposed to 1.2–6.6microT.[63]

The recent Bioinitiative Report has concluded that a 'reasonable suspicion of risk exists based on clear evidence of bioeffects at environmentally relevant levels which, with prolonged exposures, may reasonably be presumed to result in health impacts'.[64]

Multiple chemical sensitivity (MCS)

Another topic of debate, MCS is characterised by various signs including neurological disorders, allergy and immune dysregulation. MCS is now becoming well recognised as a disease state affecting a number of people worldwide (see: www.nicnas.gov.au/currentissues/mcs.asp). Exposure may occur through a major event, such as a chemical spill, or from chronic exposure to chemicals at low levels. Animal studies have demonstrated immune changes and allergic reactions to different chemicals including the well-known Th2 type sensitisers TMA (trimetallic anhydride) and TDI (toluene diisocyanate) and the Th1 sensitiser DNCB (2, 4-dinitrochlorobenzene).[65, 66, 67]

Sick Building Syndrome

This is another poorly understood syndrome whereby immunological dysfunction, neuro-toxicity and allergies may arise from exposure to bioaerosols, especially moulds, in the indoor environment of water-damaged buildings.[68] Epidemiological and toxicological studies have demonstrated an increase in auto-antibodies (IgA, IgM, IgG) to neural-specific antigens with resulting neuro-physiological abnormalities, including peripheral neuropathy, in exposed individuals.[69] Mould exposure has also been shown to initiate inflammatory and allergic (IgE) processes with significant alterations in B- and T-lymphocyte counts as well as NK-cells.[51, 52, 70, 71]

Infections and vitamin D

The spectrum of human diseases caused by infective agents can be extensive. There are 7 categories of biological agents that can cause infectious diseases. Each has its own particular characteristics. The types of agents are — metazoa, protozoa, fungi, bacteria, rickettsia, viruses and prions.

Tuberculosis still kills more people than any other pathogen-associated disease, with approximately one-third of the world's population being infected. Among these, however, only 10% will actually develop the disease. Recently identified genetic polymorphisms in the vitamin D receptor and the vitamin D-binding protein are believed to generate either susceptibility or resistance to *M. Tuberculosis* infection.[70]

Vitamin D deficiency has also been found to be associated with *bacterial vaginosis* in the first trimester of pregnancy. The prevalence of vaginosis continued to reduce with treatment as the serum 25(OH)D concentration increased to 80nmol/L.

Current investigations are also focused on the role of vitamin D for the prevention of upper respiratory tract infections. In 1 study, 162 adults were randomly given 2000 IU D3 daily for 3 months. No benefits were seen in decreasing the incidence or severity of upper respiratory tract infections during winter.[71] Results of trials with higher doses of vitamin D3 are currently underway.

Maternal vitamin D supplementation is also extremely important as low prenatal vitamin D levels may also increase susceptibility to the same diseases later in life.[72]

Auto-immune diseases and vitamin D

There are a multitude of studies associating vitamin D deficiency with the development and progression of auto-immune diseases such as multiple sclerosis (MS), rheumatoid arthritis, insulin dependent diabetes mellitus (IDDM) and inflammatory bowel disease (IBD). The immune-regulatory role of vitamin D affects both the innate and the adaptive immune systems.[73]

The discoveries that activated macrophages produce active vitamin D and immune system cells express the vitamin D receptor, both initially suggested how the vitamin D endocrine system influenced immune system function.[74] Auto-immune diseases occur because of an inappropriate immune-mediated attack against self-tissue. Without vitamin D, auto-reactive T-cells develop whereas in the presence of vitamin D, the enhanced activity of immune cells is suppressed, balance in the T-cell response is restored and the process of autoimmunity is subsequently avoided.[75, 76]

Experimental animal studies have demonstrated that vitamin D deficiency accelerates the development and progression of both auto-immune diseases and cancers.[77]

Recent evidence also strongly suggests that supplementation with vitamin D may be beneficial, especially for Th1-mediated auto-immune disorders. By decreasing the Th1-immune driven response, the severity of symptoms is decreased. Some reports indicate that vitamin D may even be preventative in such disorders as MS and type 1 diabetes mellitus (T1DM).[49, 78-82]

Sleep

Good sleep is essential for physical and mental health.[83] There is strong evidence demonstrating that inadequate sleep is associated with a multitude of health problems, including cognitive impairment, mood disorders, parasitical infections, cardiovascular diseases and compromised immunity.[84–87] Unfortunately, frequently disrupted and restricted sleep is a common problem in today's society with more than 50% adults over 65 years reporting at least 1 chronic complaint.[83, 85] Many younger adults also suffer chronic sleep deprivation secondary to occupational hazards such as shift work or mental disorders such as anxiety.[88]

Both animal and human studies have revealed that sleep restriction/deprivation can result in mild temporary increases in the activity of the major neuroendocrine stress systems — the autonomic sympatho-adrenal system and the HPA axis. Chronic sleep deprivation may also affect the reactivity of these systems to future stresses and challenges, such as physical and mental illness.[85, 89] Chronic sleep deprivation tends to cause a gradual and persistent desensitisation of the 5-HT 1A receptor system, thus altering serotonergic neurotransmission.[90] As expected, these changes in neurotransmitter receptor systems and neuroendocrine reactivity are extremely similar to those seen with chronic stress/depression.[86]

Poor sleep quality has recently been confirmed to increase susceptibility to the common cold.[91] Atypical time schedules such as shift-work has also been associated with breast cancer, due to a circadian disruption and to a nocturnal suppression in melatonin production.[88]

Melatonin is our natural sleep hormone and it is known to decrease with increasing age.

Recent studies have shown that melatonin, itself, has an immune-modulating effect, stimulating the production of NK-cells and CD4+ cells and inhibiting CD8+ cells. It also stimulates the production of granulocytes and macrophages, as well as the release of various cytokines from NK-cells and T-helper lymphocytes. Thus, enhancement of the production of melatonin, or melatonin itself, has the potential therapeutic value to enhance immune function.[92]

The recognition and treatment of sleep dysfunctions can therefore be an important part of management of many health-related conditions.[88]

Physical activity

Exercise

There is a wealth of evidence supporting the beneficial effects of exercise upon the immune system. In particular, exercise has beneficial effects on many chronic diseases. It is known to have an anti-inflammatory effect, reducing body fat percentage and macrophage accumulation in adipose tissue as well as muscle-released IL-6 inhibition of TNF-alpha and the cholinergic anti-inflammatory pathway.[93, 94] In particular, exercise training improves macrophage innate immune function in both a beta(2) adrenergic receptor dependent and independent manner.[95]

NK-cells have been found to be the most responsive immune cell to acute exercise. Their sensitivity to physiological stress combined with their important role in innate immune defences indicate that these cells are 1 link between regular physical activity and general health status.[96]

Anaerobic exercise in animal studies has been shown to increase both innate and adaptive immune function, decreasing tumour growth and cancer cachexia.[97] Secretory IgA, which is the predominant immunoglobulin in mucosal secretions providing first-line of defence against pathogens and antigens presented at the mucosa, have also been shown to be increased after exercise in elderly people over 75 years.[98, 99]

It is important to note, however, that exercise needs to be performed in moderation. Multiple effects of over-training resulting in impaired immune response have been documented in the literature.[100–104] Unlike moderate exercise, intense habitual exercise can cause chronic suppression of mucosal immune parameters, especially salivary IgA and IgM.[105, 106] This can result in increased susceptibility to respiratory infections.[95, 105]

Vigorous exercise or activity may exacerbate chronic conditions such as chronic fatigue syndrome by promoting immune dysfunction, which in turn increases symptoms. It is vital that patients with chronic fatigue syndrome are provided with a well designed individualised graded exercise program to cater for individual's physical capabilities and should take into account the fluctuating nature of symptoms. Patients should be encouraged to pace their activities and respect their physical and mental limitations with the ultimate aim of improving their everyday functioning.[106]

A Cochrane systematic review of the literature identified 9 studies but only 5 randomised control studies were included in the review.[107]

In general, at 12 weeks, subjects participating in an exercise therapy program were less fatigued and experienced significantly better physical functioning compared with control groups. However, there were more drop outs in the exercise groups compared with control groups. Moods of CFS sufferers improved in the exercise group and performed better than the group receiving the antidepressant fluoxetine. Furthermore, when the exercise program was combined with patient education, patients experienced less fatigue overall. The authors concluded that patients may benefit from an exercise therapy program and could not find evidence that exercise worsens outcomes.

An interesting recent study has shown that heavy exercise in early post-partum months may be associated with elevated pro-inflammatory cytokines in breast milk. More studies are required to confirm these findings.[103]

Yoga

There have been limited studies on the efficacy of yoga practice on the immune system. Most have been focused on the breathing disciplines within yoga, namely Pranayama and Sudarshan Kriya, that are both rhythmic breathing processes traditionally used to reduce stress and improve the immune system.[108]

Studies on healthy individuals practicing the above techniques have shown a better anti-oxidant status (increased glutathione peroxidise, SOD; reduced lactic acid) at the enzyme and RNA level accompanied by improved immune status secondary to the prolonged lifespan of lymphocytes by up-regulation of anti-apoptotic genes and pro-survival genes in the subjects.[109, 110]

Cancer patients who were either undergoing or had completed their conventional therapy also showed a significant increase in NK-cells at 12 and 24 weeks after practicing the above yogic breathing techniques compared with controls.[111, 112]

Qigong

Qigong is an ancient Chinese psychosomatic exercise that integrates movement, meditation and breathing into a single exercise. All studies have been on healthy people and most demonstrate that after 1 month, there are significant changes in immune parameters.[113] Neutrophil phagocytosis and lifespan was significantly increased whilst the inflammatory neutrophils displayed accelerated apoptosis. The changes in gene expression compared with controls were characterised by enhanced immunity, down-regulation of cellular metabolism and alteration of apoptotic genes in favour of rapid inflammation resolution.[114] There is also evidence in some, but not all, studies of reduced cortisol and changes in the number of cytokine-secreting cells (increased IFN-gamma and reduced IL-10).[115, 116]

It is possible that qigong may regulate immunity, metabolic rate and apoptosis, perhaps at the transcriptional level.[114] Further studies are required to validate these findings.

Obesity

The prevalence of obesity has reached epidemic levels in many parts of the world and therefore represents a major public health problem.[117] The accumulation of visceral fat has well-established links with chronic low-grade systemic inflammation (metaflammation), cellular metabolic imbalances and impaired immunity.[118–122]

Through different biochemical cascades leading to immune cell senescence, obesity can promote a multitude of chronic diseases.[123–125] Amongst many others, these include metabolic syndrome, inflammatory diseases, bronchial asthma, Type II diabetes and insulin resistance, depression, cardiovascular disease (CVD), osteoarthritis, fatty liver disease and cancer.[2, 9, 126, 127] Leptin is increased in states of obesity and can influence mediators of innate immunity, such as IL-6. Leptin-resistance can therefore injure numerous tissues, including the liver, pancreas, platelets, vasculature and myocardium.

Major endogenous endocrine and steroid hormones can combine with lifestyle factors (low exercise, excess weight, poor diet etc) to heighten the risk of many diseases, including cancer. Indeed, obesity has been associated with increased mortality from all cancers combined and there is an accumulating body of research regarding all mechanisms by which obesity can contribute to the carcinogenesis process.

White adipose tissue actively participates in many physiological and pathological processes, including immunity and inflammation, playing a major role in the development of leptin, adrenaline and insulin resistance. There are, indeed, complex links between the metabolic and immune systems, with multiple neuroendocrine peptides, cytokines and chemokines interacting in order to integrate energy balance with immune function. Such interactions are heightened in obesity and lessened with caloric restriction (CR).[126]

Ghrelin and leptin are 2 important hormones and cytokines that both regulate energy balance and influence immune function.[13] Ghrelin regulates immune function by reducing pro-inflammatory cytokines and promoting thymopoiesis during ageing and is found to be reduced in states of obesity. Thus, this provides 1 mechanism by which obesity can be associated with a state of immunodeficiency and chronic inflammation which can contribute to an increased risk of premature death.

In stark contrast, CR, which increases ghrelin and reduces leptin, can reduce oxidative stress and is a potentially immune-enhancing state which has prolonged a healthy lifespan in all species studied to date.[10, 16, 127, 128]

Nutrition

Dietary modulation

Pro-inflammatory foods

There is strong evidence regarding the pro-inflammatory effects of *fast–foods* that contain high amounts of saturated fatty and trans-fatty acids, refined carbohydrates with a high glycaemic index.[122, 123, 129–142]

The presence of these substances, in particular trans-fatty acids, fructose, glucose (sugars) in the diet negatively impacts on immunity and induces inflammation, creating a pro-inflammatory state, which contributes to many diseases.[143–158]

Protective foods

Likewise, there is a wealth of evidence concerning the anti-inflammatory and immune-enhancing properties of foods such as fish, fruits, vegetables, nuts, seeds, cocoa / dark chocolate, low GI foods, white button, maitake, oyster and shiitake mushrooms, high fibre intake, dairy calcium, green tea, and lean game meats.[158–177]

Spices, herbs, garlic and ginger

Spices, garlic, ginger and herbs have traditionally been highly regarded in cooking for many centuries by many cultures who believe they play an important role in health enhancement and protecting the immune system.[178–183]

For instance, curcumin and capsaicin are known to protect the immune system and re-regulate the systemic inflammatory responses.[179, 184, 187]

Grape polyphenols

Polyphenols have diverse biological effects.[188] Polyphenolic compounds found in red wine are a complex mixture of flavonoids (predominantly anthocyanins and flavan-3-ols) and non-flavonoids such as resveratrol and gallic acid. Flavan-3-ols are the most abundant, with oligomeric and polymeric procyanidins often representing 25–50% of the total phenolic constituents.[189] Inflammation is the process by which the immune system deals with infections or injury due to pathogenic bacteria, viruses and other pathogens. Recently it has been reported that the daily moderate consumption of alcohol and of red wine for 2 weeks at doses which inversely correlate with CVD risk had no adverse effects on human immune cell functions.[190] Polyphenol-rich beverages such as red grape juice and de-alcoholised red wine did not suppress immune responses in healthy men.

Cocoa and/or dark chocolate

Cacao liquor polyphenols have been reported to affect human immune system cells *in vitro*. The results demonstrated that at least *in vitro*, treatment of normal peripheral blood lymphocytes inhibited mitogen-induced proliferation of T-cells and polyclonal Ig production by B-cells in a dose-dependent manner. Also the treatment inhibited both IL-2 mRNA expression of and IL-2 secretion by T-cells. These results suggest that cacao derived polyphenolic compounds have immuno-regulatory effects.[191] The effects of polyphenolic compounds from chocolate may be due to the modulation of cellular metabolic functions (re-regulation of inflammatory responses) that are synergistic with immunological functions.[192] A number of phenolic compounds can be found in a variety of food sources (see Table 20.2).

Dairy calcium

A recent study provides significant *in vivo* evidence that dietary calcium and dairy may regulate metabolic processes associated with inflammatory responses in a mouse model of diet-induced obesity and redox metabolism aberration as well as in obese adult humans. Dietary calcium-induced suppression of circulating 1alpha, 25-dihydroxycholecalciferol may be responsible for calcium-induced suppression of inflammatory responses, although further effects of dairy foods on oxidative stress appear to be mediated by additional mechanisms.[193]

Table 20.2 Flavonoid types, representative flavonoids in food and beverages sources

Class	Representative flavonoids	Food and beverage sources
Flavonols	• Quercetin • Kaempferol • Myricetin	• Tea • Apples • Onions
• Catechins • Procyanidins	• Tea • Red wine • Red grapes • Grape seeds • Cocoa	Flavones
• Apigenin • Luteolin	• Herbs • Vegetables	Flavanones
• Hesperidin • Naringenin	• Citrus fruits (i.e. oranges and lemons)	Anthocyanins
• Cyanidin	• Berries	Isoflavones
• Genistein • Daidzein	• Soy protein-containing foods	

Lactoferrin from milk

Lactoferrin is an iron-binding glycoprotein of the transferrin family with a molecular mass of about 80 kilodalton (kDa). It is a component of milk, saliva, tears, airway mucus and secondary granules of neutrophils.[194, 195] It is also a major component of mammals' innate immune system. Lactoferrin has a range of protective effects from direct antimicrobial activities — in relation to bacteria, viruses, fungi, and parasites — and anti-inflammatory and anti-cancer activities.[196] In addition, lactoferrin has demonstrated activities that are immuno-modulatory/anti-inflammatory (down-regulating cytokines)[197] and that regulate cell proliferation[198] and intestinal iron absorption.[199]

Similar to human lactoferrin, bovine lactoferrin has been shown to induce proliferation and differentiation of human enterocytes and to modulate their cytokine production.[200] The beneficial effects of orally administered bovine lactoferrin on infections and iron status have also been recently demonstrated in clinical trials in human adults and infants.[201–206] The protective effect of lactoferrin towards microbial and viral infections has been widely demonstrated in a large number of *in vitro* studies, although the number of clinical trials so far completed is not extensive. Nevertheless, lactoferrin can be considered not only a primary defence factor against mucosal infections but also a polyvalent regulator, which interacts with several microbial, viral and host components involved in infectious processes. The capability of lactoferrin to exert antiviral activity through its binding to host-cells and/or viral particles strengthens the hypothesis that this glycoprotein constitutes a significant barrier in the mucosal wall of the GI tract, which has been demonstrated to be effective against both microbial and viral insults.

Essential fatty acids; omega-3 fish oils

Inflammation is part of the body's immediate response to infection or injury. It is typified by redness, swelling, heat and pain. These occur as a result of increased blood flow, increased permeability across blood capillaries, which allows large molecules (e.g. complement, antibodies, pro-inflammatory cytokines) to leave the bloodstream and cross the endothelial wall, and increased movement of leukocytes from the bloodstream into the surrounding tissue. Inflammation functions to begin the immunological process of elimination of pathogenic and toxin insults and to repair damaged tissue. The key link between fatty acids and inflammation is that the eicosanoid family of inflammatory mediators is generated from 20 carbon polyunsaturated fatty acids (PUFAs) liberated from cell membrane phospholipids. The membrane phospholipids of inflammatory cells taken from humans consuming typical Western diets usually contain approximately 20% of fatty acids as the n-6 PUFA arachidonic acid.[207, 208] The proportions of other 20 carbon PUFAs such as the n-6 PUFA linolenic acid and the n-3 PUFA eicosapentaenoic acid are typically about 2% and approximately 1% of fatty acids, respectively. Therefore arachidonic acid is usually the dominant substrate for eicosanoid synthesis promoting and sustaining the inflammatory response. Addition of n-3 PUFAs to the diet adds potentially useful anti-inflammatory agents that can regulate the inflammatory response by directly replacing arachidonic acid as an eicosanoid substrate, by inhibiting arachidonic acid metabolism, and by giving rise to anti-inflammatory resolvins, and indirectly, by altering the expression of inflammatory genes through effects on transcription factor activation.[209, 210]

Mediterranean diet, portfolio diet, healthy diet

Different dietary regimes have been reported to be useful in influencing immune function.[180, 211–217]

Recently it was demonstrated that adherence to a Mediterranean type diet with addition of virgin olive oil resulted in down-regulation of cellular and circulating inflammatory biomarkers.[218] Additional dietary strategies that focus on healthy food consumptions, such as the portfolio diet, reduced low-density lipoprotein cholesterol by approximately 30% and produced clinically significant reductions in CHD risk.[219] Consequently it would be expected that pro-inflammatory mediators would be reduced and re-regulated to normal levels.

Nuts

The consumption of nuts (i.e. almonds, brazil nuts, cashews, chestnuts, hazelnuts, macadamias, pecans, pine nuts, pistachios, walnuts) in the diet can significantly down regulate inflammatory responses of the immune system.[220–222] Nuts are an excellent source of phytochemicals (phyotsterols, phenolic acids, flavonoids, stilbenes, and carotenoids). The total phenolic constituents probably contribute to the overall metabolic regulation of immune function anti-inflammatory responses.[220]

Soy protein

The intestines are an important organ responsible for nutrient absorption, metabolism and recognition of food signals.[223] Soy proteins have been reported to modulate immune function pro-inflammatory activity.[224, 225] Recently it was demonstrated that soy milk and supplemental isoflavones modulated B-cell populations and appeared to be protective against DNA damage in post-menopausal women.[226]

Teas

Green tea

EPG (Epigallocatechin-3-gallate), present in green tea, is well-known for its ability to reduce the risk of a variety of immunodeficiency disorders.[227] Green tea possesses anti-oxidant, anti-inflammatory, anti-carcinogenic and immune enhancing properties. They have also been found to be photo-protective in nature, having the potential to be used for the prevention of photo-ageing, melanoma and non-melanoma skin cancers.[228] In a recent randomised, double-blind, placebo-controlled trial, healthy adults were given green tea capsules or placebo twice daily for 3 months. Those taking the active formulation had enhanced gammadelta T-cell function with 32% fewer subjects experiencing symptoms of cold and flu. Those who did become unwell experienced a significantly shorter duration of symptoms.[229–232]

Black tea

Habitual consumption of tea has been associated with improved immune system function.[233–235]

A recent review has concluded that the current scientific evidence supports the concept that dietary intervention with tea or L-theanine leads to T-cell priming. Such priming is beneficial because it is associated with an enhancement of the magnitude and the breadth of early responses to microbial and neoplastic disease. Small clinical trials in normal volunteers have demonstrated that increased intake of tea or a supplement containing the bioactive tea components L-theanine and epigalenocatechins affect T-cell activity and the latter was associated with a decrease in cold and flu symptoms.[236]

Food intolerance

It is important to realise that any food, however, may be pro-inflammatory for an individual who is intolerant to that food. Adverse reactions to foods can have a significant impact on the immune system and general wellbeing of an individual's life. Immune-mediated adverse reactions may be roughly divided into IgE-mediated and non IgE-mediated. Non IgE-mediated food reactions are not well understood and their negative effects on wellbeing and immune efficiency may be highly underestimated. In the first few years of life, humans gradually develop an intricate balance between tolerance and immune reactivity in the gut mucosa along with a tremendous expansion of the gut-associated lymphoid tissue (GALT), which is profoundly affected by changes in commensal flora.[237]

The simplest test to determine which foods contribute to gastrointestinal or other symptoms is to perform a food elimination diet (FED), with initial avoidance then separate re-introduction of individual foods (see: www.integrative-medicine.com.au for details). Some of the most common dietary intolerances are due to wheat, dairy and soy. In such cases, immune reactivity may be associated with apparent dietary protein intolerance (gliadin, cow's milk protein, soy) and gastrointestinal inflammation that may be partly associated with an aberrant innate immune response against endotoxin, a product of specific gut bacteria.[238]

Alcohol

Alcohol in light-moderate amounts (1 glass for women, 2 glasses for men, every second day) has been shown to be particularly beneficial for the immune system when compared with both non-drinkers and heavy drinkers.[239] Resveratrol, a polyphenol from red wine, is able to stimulate both innate and adaptive immune responses; in particular, the release of cytokines such as IL-12, IL-10 and IFN-gamma and immunoglobulins that may be important for host protection in different immune-related disorders.[240, 241] Its effects may be also related to cytokine production by both CD4+ and CD8+ T-cells.[242]

Nutritional supplementation

Nutrition is a critical determinant of immunity and malnutrition is the most common cause of immunodeficiency worldwide.[243] Nutrients either enhance or depress immune function depending on the nutrient and level of its intake.[244] Indeed, both insufficient and excess nutrient intakes can have negative consequences on immune status and susceptibility to a variety of pathogens.[245] Deficiency of nutrients may suppress immunity by affecting innate, T-cell mediated and adaptive antibody responses, leading to dysregulation of the host response. This can subsequently lead to increased susceptibility to infections which can then lead to further nutrient deficiency and so on.[246]

Available data indicates that vitamins A, B6, B12, C, D, E, folic acid and the trace elements Fe, Zn, Cu and Se all work synergistically to support the protective activities of the immune cells. With the exception of iron and vitamin C, they are all also intricately involved in antibody production.[245, 246] Antioxidant vitamins and trace elements (vitamins C, E, Se, Cu, Zn) counteract damage to tissues secondary to reactive oxygen species whilst simultaneously modulating immune cell function by affecting the production of cytokines and prostaglandins. Adequate intakes of vitamin B6, B12, C, E, folic acid and trace elements Se, Zn, Cu and Fe all support a Th1 cytokine-mediated immune response with sufficient production of pro-inflammatory cytokines. This maintains an effective immune response,[246] avoiding a shift to an anti-inflammatory Th2 immune state and an increased risk of extracellular infections. Supplementation with these nutrients reverses the Th2 cell-mediated immune response to Th1, thereby enhancing innate immunity.[247–249]

Presented below is a summary of evidence for the most recently studied nutrients, supplements and herbs with regard to immune system enhancement.

Probiotics

The gastrointestinal mucosa is the major contact area between the host and the external world of microflora. Over 400 square metres in size, it is colonised by an immense number of bacteria that are in constant communication with our immune cells.[250] In fact, it is the GALT itself that houses the largest number of immune cells in the body.[251]

Although the intestinal immune system is fully developed after birth, the actual protective function of the gut requires the microbial stimulation of bacterial colonisation. Breast milk naturally contains prebiotic oligosaccharides, designed to feed and proliferate specific resident bacteria with important protective functions (probiotics), primarily *Lactobacillus* and *Bifidobacterium*, in the infant's gut.[251] However, the nature and species of microflora is also determined by many other factors, including external environment microflora, use of antibiotics and immuno-modulatory agents and early introduction of cow's milk.[252]

Until recently, the gut bacteria were regarded as residents without any specific functions.[251] However, it now appears that altered mucosal microflora in early childhood alters signalling reactions which determine T-helper cell differentiation and/or the induction of tolerance.[253–254] Thus, the nature of mucosal microflora acquired in early infancy determines the outcome of mucosal inflammation and the subsequent development of mucosal disease, autoimmunity and allergic diseases later in life.[254]

Probiotics are recognised for their roles in nutrient absorption, mucosal barrier function, angiogenesis, morphogenesis and postnatal maturation of intestinal cell lineages, intestinal motility and, most importantly, the maturation of the GALT.[256]

An important adjustment of the immune system to bacterial colonisation of the gut is the production of secretory immunoglobulin A (sIgA) by B-cells in the GALT.[248, 255, 256] Probiotics stimulate both the production and secretion of polymeric IgA, the antibody that coats and protects mucosal surfaces against harmful bacterial invasion.[253] Secretory IgA also promotes an anti-inflammatory environment by neutralising immune stimulatory antigens.[250] Thus, sIgA plays a significant role in the regulation of bacterial communities and maintenance of immune homeostasis.[255]

In addition, appropriate colonisation with probiotics helps to produce a balanced T-helper cell response and prevent an imbalance which can contribute in part to clinical disease. For example, Th2 imbalance may contribute to atopic disease and Th1 imbalance may contribute to Crohn's disease and *Helicobacter pylori*-induced gastritis.[253] Th1>Th2 cytokine expression in the respiratory tract associated with increased allergic disease has been correlated with reduced exposure to microbial agents associated with Th1 responses. In contrast, reduced exposure to helminths in the gut associated with reduced Th2 expression appears to correlate well with dominant Th1 cytokine expression and IBD.[249, 254, 255]

Pre and probiotics are certainly attractive options for maintaining the steady nutritional state of the host with defective gut barrier functions. Prebiotics (inulin from chicory root, fructooligosaccharides, arabinogalactans) resist enzymatic digestion in the upper GI tract and therefore reach the colon virtually intact where they undergo bacterial fermentation. The consumption of prebiotics favours the growth of probiotics and impedes growth of pathogenic organisms, thereby modulating immune parameters in the GALT, secondary lymphoid tissues and peripheral circulation.[257] The change in gut microflora may decrease intestinal permeability, consequently influencing both intestinal and systemic body functions.[258]

Adverse reactions to foods can have a significant impact on an individual's life. In the first few years of life, humans gradually develop an intricate balance between tolerance and immune reactivity in the gut mucosa along with a tremendous expansion of the GALT, which is profoundly affected by changes in commensal flora.[237]

Probiotics modify the structure of potentially harmful food antigens and thereby alter their immunogenicity.[258] Both IgE and non IgE-mediated food allergy are frequently seen in the early years of life, with cow's milk and soy proteins being the most common causative dietary proteins for non IgE-mediated food allergy.[237] Certain probiotics have recently been found to release low-molecular-weight peptides into milk products using bacterial-derived proteases that degrade milk casein, and thereby generate peptides, triggering immune responses. Thus the intestinal microbial communities contribute to the processing of food antigens in the gut.[259]

Abnormalities in Th1 function may not only play a role in some patients with non IgE-mediated food allergy in whom decreased Th1 function is seen, but also in patients with coeliac disease in whom an increased Th1 is seen. Lymphonodular hyperplasia may also be a hallmark histologic lesion in patients with non IgE-mediated food allergy.[260] In such patients, a localised IgE-mediated response rather than a systemic food-specific IgE response may be responsible for these gastrointestinal symptoms.[261]

The pathogenesis of IBD involves an interaction between genetically determined host susceptibility, dysregulated immune response and the enteric microbiota.[262, 263] Inappropriate secretion of quorum sensing molecules by certain gut bacteria may alter the GALT and thereby deregulate the immune tolerance normally present.[264, 265] Thus manipulation of the luminal contents with antibiotics, prebiotics or probiotics represents a potentially effective therapeutic option.[266] Both inulin and oligofructose stimulate the colonic production of short chain fatty acids and favour the growth of lactobacilli and/or bifidobacteria, which are associated with reduced mucosal inflammation, particularly in relapsing pouchitis.[267] Clinical trials using specific probiotics to treat IBDs have demonstrated that the multi-agent mixture *VSL3#* is particularly beneficial for ulcerative colitis and pouchitis whereas *Escherichia coli Nissle 1917* is effective in the prevention of recurrence of ulcerative colitis.[268, 269] Thus far, probiotics seem to be less effective in patients with Crohn's disease.[270] *Lactobacillus rhamnosus GG* is another strain that has been effectively used for the prevention and treatment of rotavirus and antibiotic-associated diarrhoea, the prevention of cow's milk-induced food allergy and pouchitis.[271–275]

Some gluten peptides are able to induce an innate immune response in intestinal mucosa and gluten intake is linked to the production of pro-inflammatory cytokines IL-15, IL-18 and IL-21. The failure to control this inflammatory response may also be one of the factors underlying gluten intolerance in individuals with coeliac disease.[274]

Zinc

Zinc is an essential trace element that is critical for cellular function and structural integrity.[276] Normal zinc homeostasis is required for a functional immune system (both innate and adaptive), metabolic homeostasis (energy utilisation and hormone turnover), anti-oxidant activity, glucose homeostasis and wound healing.[276, 277] Zinc is known to regulate the immune system systemically as well as having direct T-cellular effects resulting in the regulation of gene expression, bioenergetics, metabolic pathways, signal transduction and cell invasion, proliferation and apoptosis.[278]

Furthermore, zinc is an essential cofactor for the structure and function of a wide range of cellular proteins including enzymes, structural proteins, transcription and replication factors. It is now known that nearly 2000 of these transcription factors require zinc for their structural integrity.[279–282] Zinc also affects entire functional networks of genes that are related to pro-inflammatory cytokines and cellular survival.[282, 283] Thus an individual's zinc status has a significant impact on their immune system, with zinc deficiency having the ability to profoundly modulate immune function and zinc supplementation, the ability to prevent and treat many acute and chronic diseases.[284–288]

Even a mild deficiency of zinc in humans results in immune dysfunction by decreasing serum thymulin activity, which is required for the maturation of T-helper cells. In particular, Th1 cytokines are decreased whilst Th2 cytokines remain relatively unaffected.[287, 288] This shift of Th1 to Th2 function results in cell-mediated immune dysfunction. Decreased Th1 results in decreased IL-2 production, which leads to decreased activities of NK-cells and T-cytolytic cells, in turn enhancing susceptibility to malignancies and infections with viruses and bacteria.[289] Ageing is associated with the same Th1/Th2 imbalance and moderate zinc supplementation has been shown to alter these proportions.[290–292]

Recent research has shown that zinc can either activate or inhibit several signalling pathways that interact with the signal transduction of pathogen-sensing receptors, the so-called toll-like receptors (TLR), which, upon activation, lead to secretion of pro-inflammatory cytokines. Thus zinc can play a major regulatory role in the immune system.[293]

Zinc also directly influences GALT, contributing to host defence by maintaining the integrity of the gut mucosal barrier and thereby controlling inflammatory cell infiltration.[294]

Oxidative stress is known to be an important contributing factor in many chronic diseases and zinc deficiency is constantly observed in states of chronic inflammation.[295] Zinc supplementation has been shown to decrease the gene expression and production of both pro-inflammatory cytokines and oxidative stress markers.[296] Metallothionein increase in ageing and chronic inflammation allows a continuous sequestration of intracellular zinc with subsequent low zinc ion availability against stressor agents and inflammation. This phenomenon influences NF-kappaB and the inhibitory protein A20, leading to an impaired inflammatory/immune response.[295] Zinc deficiency also induces vascular pro-inflammatory parameters associated with NF-kappaB and PPAR signalling, markedly modulating mechanisms of the pathology of inflammatory diseases such as atherosclerosis.[297] As such, zinc may prove to be a useful chemo-preventative agent for many chronic diseases, including neurodegenerative disorders, rheumatoid arthritis, macular degeneration, IBD and cancer.[298]

Many studies have demonstrated the beneficial effects of zinc supplementation in the management of the common cold, cold-sores, influenza, acute and chronic diarrhoea and acute respiratory infections. Average daily doses were 15–30mg elemental zinc for adults, 7.5–20mg for children and 10mg for infants < 6 months.[297–301] Zinc gluconate lozenges, in particular, have been shown to significantly decrease common cold duration and number of antibiotics required whereas prophylactic use significantly decreased cold frequency.[302–306] The formulation of the lozenge also appears to be important because the addition of citric or tartaric acid may reduce the efficacy due to chelation of the zinc ions.[307, 308] Current evidence also shows that zinc (and selenium) improve humoral immunity in elderly subjects after an influenza vaccination.

Serum levels of zinc are significantly lower in HIV+ individuals and an imbalance between Th1 and Th2 responses in these patients has been implicated in the immune dysregulation. Researchers have proposed that resistance to infection and/or progression to AIDS is dependent on a Th1>Th2 dominance.[309, 310]

Several recent animal studies have also demonstrated a link between zinc deficiency and several auto-immune diseases, including systemic lupus erythematosus (SLE) and type 1 diabetes. Egr-2 is a zinc-finger transcription factor which controls the self-tolerance of T-cells preventing the development of auto-immunity.[311] Another zinc-finger transcription factor, Gfi1, is also emerging as a novel master regulator restricting B-cell mediated autoimmunity.[312] The zinc transporter ZnT8 is targeted by 60–80% new-onset type 1 diabetics compared with <2% controls and <3% Type 2 diabetics. It is also targeted in up to 30% patients with other auto-immune diseases associated with T1DM.[313–316]

Vitamin A

Vitamin A has received particular attention in recent years. It is now recognised that it modulates a wide range of immune functions, such as lymphocyte activation and proliferation, T-helper cell differentiation, tissue-specific lymphocyte homing, the production of specific antibody isotypes and regulation of the immune response.[317]

Retinoic acid is produced naturally from intestinal dendritic cells.[318] The presence of high levels of retinoic acid in the intestine and GALT can promote B-cell class switching to IgA, hence boosting the production of IgA in the intestinal mucosa.[318] When B- and T-cells are activated in the GALT, gut-homing receptors are induced on these cells via the actions of retinoic acid. These gut-homing B- and T-cells play essential roles in protecting the digestive tract from pathogens i.e. the development of *'oral tolerance'*. Furthermore, retinoic acid is also[318] required for the maturation of phagocytes in the bone marrow.[318, 319]

Superfluous activation of natural immune system cascades is now thought to be one of the underlying mechanisms in psoriasis. vitamin A derivatives are currently being investigated in the treatment of *psoriasis*.[320]

Vitamin A deficiency is also a risk factor for low antibody production. In countries where vitamin A deficiency is endemic, many children are receiving retinol as an adjunct in their vaccinations, especially polio, DPT and measles. This is because vitamin A appears to *promote the vaccine antibody response*. In particular, the oral polio seroconversion rate is increased by vitamin A in those children who are deficient in this nutrient.[321]

Current evidence does not support vitamin A supplementation to pregnant HIV+ women to reduce transmission to their child, however, there is an indication that supplementation improves birth weight.[322] Periodic vitamin A supplementation of *HIV-infected infants and children* is recommended as it has been shown to be beneficial in reducing all-cause mortality and morbidity.[323, 324]

Current recommendations for vitamin A intake are based simply on the maintenance of *normal vision*. However, it has been realised that higher levels may in fact be necessary in order to optimise innate immune function.[325] Vitamin A supplementation above dietary requirements has been shown to enhance inflammatory responses with decreased Th1 and increased mucosal responses in animals.[326]

Selenium

Selenium is a potent nutritional antioxidant that influences immune responses through its incorporation into selenoproteins. Given that these selenoproteins play crucial roles in regulating reactive oxygen species in nearly every tissue in the body, it is hardly surprising that selenium significantly influences inflammatory and immune responses.[327–329]

Evidence is accumulating that selenium levels lower than previously thought can cause adverse health effects, such that the RDA levels have recently been increased to 150ug/day. Furthermore, it has also been demonstrated that higher levels of selenium may give additional protection from many diseases by significantly enhancing immune responses.[330] Perhaps these higher levels are required for the full expression of protective selenoproteins.[331, 332]

Selenium is a key nutrient in the protection from certain viral infections, including the *Coxsackie virus and Influenza virus*. Selenium plus zinc has been found to improve humoral immunity in elderly subjects after the influenza vaccination. Many individuals with HIV are deficient in selenium, and it is in the selenium deficient host, that *HIV infection* progresses more rapidly to AIDS.[333, 334]

A recent clinical study investigated a high selenium yeast supplement (200mcg/day) in a double-blind, randomised, placebo-controlled trial. Intention-to-treat analyses assessed the effect on HIV-1 viral load and CD4 count after 9 months of treatment. This study concluded that a daily selenium supplement suppressed the progression of HIV-1 viral burden and provided indirect improvement of CD4 T lymphocyte count. Hence the results support the use of selenium as a simple, inexpensive, and safe adjunct therapy in HIV spectrum disease.[335]

Just as an inadequate status of selenium is linked to an increased risk of cancer, there is also growing evidence that an elevated selenium intake may be associated with a reduced risk of cancer. [336–339] Interventions with selenium (at least 200mcg/day) have shown benefit in reducing both the incidence of cancer and the mortality in all cancers combined. This has been shown to be particularly relevant in liver, prostate, colorectal, lung, oesophageal and stomach cancers, the effect of which is most pronounced in those that are most deficient in selenium. There is also some new evidence that selenium may also affect the risk of cancer progression and metastasis.[337] It should be noted that the dose and form of selenium are critical factors in cancer prevention.[338]

The protective roles of selenium are still not entirely clear. Selenium is essential for the proper functioning of neutrophils, macrophages, NK-cells and T lymphocytes.[318] Other proposed mechanisms include the protective role of selenoproteins/ selenoenzymes, the induction of apoptosis, immune system effects, detoxification of antagonistic metals, inactivation of nuclear transcription factor, regulation of lipoxygenases, reduction of oxidative stress, induction of Phase II enzymes, androgen receptor down-regulation, inhibition of DNA adduct formation and cell cycle arrest.[335, 337, 338]

Vitamin C

The human body is not able to synthesize vitamin C, hence we are entirely dependent upon dietary sources and/or nutritional supplementation to maintain adequate levels of this important water-soluble anti-oxidant.[340, 341] It has long been known that vitamin C concentrations in the plasma and leukocytes rapidly decline during infections and stress, subsequently resulting in a reduced resistance to pathogens.[342, 343] For this reason, vitamin C has traditionally been used as a *cure for the common cold.*

Supplementation of vitamin C has, indeed, been found to improve components of the immune system such as antimicrobial and NK-cell activities, lymphocyte proliferation, chemotaxis and delayed-type hypersensitivity. It also contributes to the maintenance of the redox activity of cells, thereby protecting them from reactive oxygen species generated during the inflammatory response.[342]

There has been a large number of RCTs that indicate vitamin C supplementation (up to 1g/day) with zinc (up to 30mg/day) can ameliorate the symptoms and shorten the duration of respiratory infections when used prophylactically. However, there has been no reduced incidence of the common cold.[340, 342] It is important to note that optimal dosing is critical to intervention studies using vitamin C.[340]

When combined with zinc, vitamin C has also been found to reduce the incidence and improve the outcome of pneumonia, malaria and diarrhoeal infections, especially in children in developing countries.[340]

A recent Cochrane review has concluded that supplementation of vitamin C is only effective in preventing the common cold in cases of excess physical activity or in cold environments.[343] Intense exercise is known to increase lipid peroxidation and cause muscle damage. Supplementation with anti-oxidant vitamins, including vitamin C, reduces these without blocking the cellular adaptation to exercise.[344, 345]

Smoking-induced oxidative stress impairs the function of peripheral mononuclear cells. Results are mixed as to the efficacy of vitamin C in reducing the oxidative stress and ameliorating the impaired migratory activity of these mononuclear cells.[346–348]

Whilst the efficacy of vitamin C supplementation is still controversial, it is argued by some authors that to achieve an optimal daily allowance of vitamin C, we require 1g daily supplementation accompanied by a diet high in fruits and vegetables.[342]

Vitamin D

Vitamin D has been rediscovered in recent years and there is a now a plethora of studies regarding the serious health consequences due to deficiency of vitamin D. Very few foods naturally contain vitamin D, so sun exposure is the primary source of vitamin D.[349]

Indeed, vitamin D deficiency is now a recognised global pandemic, in both developing and developed countries.[350–352] As such, there are a growing number of diseases which are associated with vitamin D deficiency.[353] Originally, vitamin D deficiency was only regarded to be important for bone health, however, it is now understood that this 'vitamin' is actually a complex hormone that is intricately involved in the integrity of the innate immune system.[354]

The deficiency of vitamin D is strongly associated with an increased risk of common cancers, auto-immune diseases (e.g. MS), rheumatoid arthritis (RA), IDDM, IBD, SLE, infectious diseases (e.g. TB), mental health disorders, cardiovascular disease (hypertension), skin disorders (psoriasis) and bone disorders (osteoporosis, osteomalacia, rickets).[355–361] In the third National Health and Nutrition Survey linked mortality files, the lowest quartile of 25(OH)D level (<17.8ng/mL) was found to be independently associated with all-cause mortality in the general population.[362]

Most tissues, including the breast, colon and prostate, not only have a vitamin D receptor, but also have the ability to make 1,25-dihydroxyvitamin D(3). This active form of vitamin D influences the modulation of the immune system, acting in an autocrine fashion to regulate cell growth and decrease the risk of cells becoming malignant. It is believed that the local production of 1,25-dihydroxyvitamin D(3) may be responsible for the anti-carcinogenic benefits of vitamin D. It enhances innate immunity by inducing the cathelicidin antimicrobial peptide (hCAP).[355, 363–369] Furthermore, 1,25-dihydroxyvitamin D is now known to either directly or indirectly regulate more than 200 different genes in the human body that are responsible for a wide range of biological processes.[367, 368]

Cancer

Vitamin D deficiency has now been linked to 17 different types of cancer.[368, 370] It has been estimated that there is a 30–50% reduction in the risk of developing breast, colorectal and prostate cancer by increasing one's vitamin D intake to at least 1000IU/day. Women who are vitamin D deficient are estimated to have a 253% increased risk for developing colorectal cancer. Furthermore, women who consume 1500mg/day calcium and 1100IU/day vitamin D3 for 4 years, reduce their risk of developing cancer by more than 60%.[361]

In a recent study, patients with head and neck squamous cell carcinoma were treated with vitamin D3 for 3 weeks before surgery. This resulted in reduced levels of immune inhibitory CD34+ cells with increased maturation of dendritic cells, demonstrating intra-tumoural immune competence.[369]

Inflammatory bowel disease (IBD)

Crohn's disease is associated with a higher Th1 cytokine expression, whereas ulcerative colitis appears to express a modified type 2 response. Studies have demonstrated that calcitriol, the hormonally active form of vitamin D, exerts immuno-regulatory effects such as modulation of the Th1/Th2 cytokine balance on these conditions.[371]

Both vitamin D deficiency and vitamin D receptor deficiency result in acceleration of IBD. Dietary calcium is an important additional factor that determines the effect of vitamin D status on immune function. Animal studies show that treatment with vitamin D3 to animals with high calcium levels improves symptoms of IBD more than the same treatment administered to animals on low-calcium diets.[372]

Herbal Medicines

Astragalus membranaceus

Astragalus membranaceus (astragalus) is a common traditional Chinese medicinal plant that has been widely used to enhance the body's natural defence mechanisms for centuries.[373, 374] It is a chemically complex herb which contains over 60 components, including polysaccharides, B-sitosterol, glycosides, saponins, plants acids, choline, betaine, isoflavones, amino acids and various micro-elements.[375]

There have been numerous studies in recent years demonstrating the immuno-modulating and immuno-restorative effects, both *in vitro* and *in vivo*, of the roots of astragalus.[373–378] It appears that the immuno-potentiating effect of astragalus is primarily due to the polysaccharide fraction (APS), as it increases both cellular and humoral immune responses.[377] Studies have shown that astragalus can stimulate immune cells within 24 hours of ingestion and continue for at least 7 days.[378]

Astragalus can reverse the Th2 dominant status of many common illnesses.[379] For instance, Th1 cell subset dysfunction may exist in children with recurrent tonsillitis at the remission stage, suggesting that this may play an important role in its pathogenesis. *In vitro* studies demonstrate that astragalus can improve Th1 status, thereby displaying an important significance in the treatment of recurrent tonsillitis.[376] Although astragalus has been used traditionally for respiratory tract infections, there is a paucity of good quality studies demonstrating its effectiveness for this particular condition.

In contrast to this, however, there are many studies showing that astragalus has the potential to reverse the Th2 predominant status in patients with asthma. It appears to do this by increasing the expression of T-bet mRNA and Th1 cytokines such as IFNgamma.[381, 382, 383]

Th2 cytokines are also predominant in cancer patients and have been found to be associated with tumour progression. *In vitro* studies have shown that astragalus is able to enhance gene expression levels of Th1 cytokines (IFNgamma and IL-2) and reverse the predominance of Th2 cytokines and their up-stream transcript factors in lung cancer patients, making it a possible CAM therapy for the future.[379]

Levels of Th1 cytokines (IFNgamma, IL-2) are significantly lower and Th2 cytokines (IL-4, IL-10) are significantly higher in patients with herpes simplex keratitis (HSK). Astragalus is able to modulate this imbalance state of Th1/Th2 in such patients, improving their immune system dysfunction, again suggesting that it may be an effective treatment for treating HSK.[384]

There have also been multiple animal studies on the effects of astragalus as an effective preventative and treatment for T1DM. This is a chronic auto-immune disease that is also related to the disequilibrium state of Th1 and Th2 subgroups of T-helper lymphocytes and their cytokines. Here it has been shown that astragalus can correct the imbalance between the Th1/Th2 cytokines with a lower incidence rate of developing T1DM in those animals treated with astragalus.[385] Astragalus has also been shown to down-regulate the Th1/Th2 cytokine ratio in mice that already have T1DM.[386] Astragalus ameliorates both the clinical and histological parameters of these mice in a long-lasting fashion, demonstrating that it can both attenuate insulitis and preserve beta cells from apoptosis. This is most likely through its immuno-regulatory actions on the Th1/Th2 ratio, which is strongly associated with PPAR gamma gene expression in spleens.[387, 388]

Astragalus has also been shown to be capable of restoring the impaired T-cell functions in cancer patients. It exhibits anti-tumour effects both *in vitro* and *in vivo*, which appear to be achieved through activating the host's anti-tumour immune mechanisms.[389] Thus patients may use astragalus to help inhibit tumour growth or to boost resistance to infections.[390] In 1 recent trial children with acute leukaemia were given conventional chemotherapy alone or with 90g astragalus daily for 1 month. It was found that large doses of astragalus increased the dendritic cell induction of peripheral mononuclear cells and enhanced the antigen-presenting ability of dendritic cells in children with acute leukaemia.[391]

A recent Cochrane review has concluded that astragalus can stimulate immuno-competent T-cells and significantly reduce side-effects such as nausea and vomiting in patients treated with chemotherapy.[392] There was no evidence of harm arising from the use of astragalus.[393] Another meta-analysis has also demonstrated that astragalus may increase the effectiveness of platinum-based chemotherapy drugs used for treating non-small-cell lung cancer. Furthermore, high dose astragalus injection used together with cyclophosphamide (CTX) is more effective than CTX alone in decreasing infection rate and urine protein and improving immune function for patients with lupus nephritis.[393]

Studies have revealed that astragalus also has diuretic, anti-oxidant and anti-inflammatory activities.[394]It has tissue generating effects and improves the inflammatory reaction in wound healing.[395] It may also suppress the development of atopic dermatitis by reducing IFN-gamma production and inhibit the enzyme 5-lipoxygenase which is important in the treatment of psoriasis.[396, 397] Furthermore, astragalus polysaccharides and astragalosides have strong promoting effects on the phagocytosis of mycobacterium tuberculosis by macrophages and the secretion of IL-1beta, IL-6 and TNF alpha by activated macrophages.[398]

Cranberry

The proanthocyanidins in cranberry juice (*vaccinium macrocarpon*) are thought to reduce susceptibility to urinary tract infections (UTIs) by preventing bacteria from attaching to uroepithelial cells.[399] Recent *in vitro* studies of the non-dialysed material of cranberry indicate the possibility that cranberry acts as an anti-adhesive agent upon bacteria through decreasing the secretion of extracellular fructosyltransferase (FTF), an extracellular enzyme associated with the pathogenesis of oral bacteria.[400] In the same study cranberry was also noted to decrease the genetic expression of FTF in a dose dependent manner. The resulting effect may explain the demonstrated disruption of bacterial ligand-uroepithelial cell binding that has been observed to occur in the presence of cranberry juice.[401]

Indeed investigations of the ability of the uropathic bacteria, *Esherichia coli* and *Enterococcus fecalis*, to adhere to biomaterials in the presence proanthocyanidins extracted from cranberry[402] demonstrates that is does reduce the binding capacity of this bacteria. Similar *in vitro* examinations identified that diluted cranberry juice inhibited the growth of *Staphylococcus aureus*, *Escherichia coli* (up to a 20:1 dilution), *Salmonella spp*, and *Pseudomonus aureus*, however having a less inhibitory influence on *Pseudomona aeruginosa*.[403] This decrease in bacterial adherence has been noted to occur in a dose dependent relationship in which *Escherichia coli* loses its adherence the higher the dosage of cranberry given to a subject (36mg vs 108mg of cranberry capsule).[404]

The clinical efficacy of the use of cranberry juice for UTIs has been reviewed by the Cochrane Database (2008) with a supportive conclusion that use of cranberry over a 12-month period may decrease the incidence of recurrent infections amongst women.[401] Earlier reviews have clarified that the use of cranberry juice in other groups susceptible to urinary tract infections (children, elderly men and women and patients that require catheterisation) remained presently unsubstantiated.[406, 407] However, continuing studies indicate the potential for cranberry to be effective in these groups, notable amongst older women as evidenced by a 2009 RCT in which the use of trimethoprim (100mg) was only found to have very limited advantage when compared to 500mg of cranberry extract in instances in which the women had experienced 2 or more antibiotic treated UTIs in the previous 12 months.[406] Notably, there was almost double the rate of withdrawal from the trimethoprim group (16%) compared to the cranberry group (9%) suggesting cranberry may be better tolerated.[406] While multiple daily cranberry juice cocktails may be effective in reducing UTIs in pregnancy, as demonstrated in a 2008 randomised pilot study of only low statistical weighting, concern might be raised by the 38.8% of active participants who withdrew from the trial, many due to gastrointestinal upset.[408]

It should be noted that many commercial cranberry juices contain high levels of sugar, a concern that can be avoided by using cranberry extract capsules.

Echinacea purpurea

Clinical evaluation of the herb *Echinacea* and its influences upon the immune system are problematic due to the disparate use of different preparations across studies. Unfortunately only 1 extract, using the aerial components of *Echinacea purpurea*, has been evaluated in more than a single study preventing the pooling of data on specific extracts, [409] which may in itself explain the varied results achieved from *Echinacea* use. There is, however, preliminary evidence that the use of the aerial component of *Echinacea purpurea* may be beneficial in the early treatment of the common cold in adults, as concluded by a Cochrane review in 2006.[410]

Interestingly, *in vitro* studies of different extracts and forms of *Echinacea* consumed orally suggest that root components have an increased effect on phagocytosis when compared with aerial.[411]

In regards to safety, whilst concern has been raised regarding the long term use of *Echinacea* in depressing the immune system, a 2001 study of immune parameters demonstrated that 6 months oral use of *Echinacea* did not alter these measures. Furthermore, a critical evaluation of drug interaction with *Echinacea* (*angustifolia, pallida* and *purpurea* extracts) concluded that the use of *Echinacea* did not presently appear of risk to the consumer.[412] There have been allergic reactions to Echinacea reported in susceptable individuals, although this is rare.

Other herbs

A number of other herbs have also been claimed to be immune enhancers, such as:

- olive leaf extract
- green tea extract
- H48 combined Chinese herbs
- *Coriolus versicolor* raw water extract, purified polysaccharide-K
- Maitake extract
- *Echinacea* lipophilic, neutral and acidic extracts
- turmeric
- yeast β-glucan.

However, more research is required to clarify the evidence that these herbs are able to augment immunological responses against defined antigens.[413]

Medicinal foods

Manuka honey

The use of specific honey forms as derived from the tree origins, *Leptospermum scoparium* (New Zealand manuka) and *Leptospermum polygalifolium* (Australian jelly bush) are suggested to have therapeutic effects on wound and ulcer healing when applied with dressings.[414, 415] These forms of honey would appear to have antibacterial qualities as demonstrated by *in vitro* studies in which it has been demonstrated that manuka honey can inhibit several oral bacterial pathogens including *Escherichia coli*, *Salmonella typhimurium*, *Shigella sonnei*, *Listeria monocytogenes*, *Staphylococcus aureus* (including wound-associated methicillin resistance strains),[416] *Bacillus cereus*, and *Streptococcus mutans*.[415, 417, 418]

Due to this antibacterial quality, clinical evidence as reported by a 2008 Cochrane review indicates honey may reduce wound healing times as compared to conventional dressings in partial thickness burns, [419] however, it does not appear to provide additional benefit to compression bandages for leg ulcers when measured over a 12-week period.[420] Recent studies continue to report the benefits of medicinal honeys. An RCT of wounds healing by secondary intention identified that, when compared to conventional dressings, honey was effective in reducing healing times (100 v 140 days).[421]

Manuka honey (Woundcare 18+) appears to have benefit in reducing MRSA infections in patients with sloughy venous leg ulcers when compared to hydrogel (IntraSite Gel) over a 4-week period but may be less effective in wounds with *Pseudomonas aeruginosa*, although the results of this RCT are derived from a small population (n = 10 for honey; n = 6 for hydrogel).[422] Manuka honey was also reported to decrease mean slough area, wound size and infection rates when compared to hydrogel.[423] An examination of wound pH indicates Manuka honey dressings have the potential to lower pH in association with improved wound healing for chronic wounds.[424]

It must be noted that honey used in medical practice should be of 'medical grade' — that is, it has been sterilised by gamma irradiation and has standardised antibacterial activity.[425]

Physical therapies

Massage

There are mixed results as to the benefits of massage for immune enhancement. Two earlier studies have noted increases in dopamine, serotonin, NK-cells and lymphocytes in women with breast cancer after thrice weekly massage for 5 weeks. Depression, anxiety and anger were also significantly reduced.[426, 427] However, a more recent randomised control trial (RCT) showed that effleurage massage had no significant effect on immune and neuroendocrine parameters.[428]

Acupuncture

Acupuncture has been used for centuries to prevent and treat various conditions and to simply maintain good health.[429] In addition to its known effects on the nervous system, emerging evidence suggests that it may also effectively modulate the innate immune system which plays important roles in inflammation, pain, metabolism, cell proliferation and apoptosis.[430, 431] There is now experimental evidence that the electrical stimulation of the vagus nerve inhibits macrophage activation and the production of pro-inflammatory cytokines including TNF, IL-1 beta, IL-6 and IL-18, indicating a possible underlying neuro-immune basis to acupuncture.[432]

A small study involving healthy volunteers has shown a statistically significant increase in the number of CD2+, CD4+, CD8+, CD11b+, CD16+, CD19+, CD56+ cells in addition to IL-4, IL-1beta and IFN-gamma levels after acupuncture stimulation of meridian points. Another small study on HIV+ individuals demonstrated an increase in the total lymphocyte count after moxibustion at specific points in the treatment group compared with controls. Such observations suggest that acupuncture may regulate the immune system by promoting both humoral and cellular immunity as well as NK-cell activity.[433, 434]

Acupuncture may therefore be used as an adjunct to conventional medical treatment for a number of chronic inflammatory and auto-immune diseases. More studies are again required.

Conclusion

The immune system is a network of interacting cellular and soluble components. It is subject to multiple modulatory factors that include lifestyle factors, dietary and nutritional factors, sun exposure for vitamin D, pollutants, chemical exposure, life stressors and physical activity. In addition, there are a number of nutraceuticals and herbal medicines that have been reported to influence immune function.

Foods in particular contain various substances that can control the physiological functions of the body, and modulating immune responses is one of the most important functions of foods. Immune functions are indispensable for defending the body against attack by pathogens or cancer cells, and thus play a pivotal role in the maintenance of health. However, immune functions are disturbed by malnutrition, ageing, physical and mental stress or undesirable lifestyles. Therefore, the consumption of foods with immune-modulating activities is a beneficial and efficient way to prevent immune functions from declining and reduce the risk of infection or cancer.

The consumption of foods does not always change immune parameters. Therefore, it is useful to define those immune parameters affected by foods. Vitamins (such as vitamin C), minerals (such as selenium), amino acids, proteins, carbohydrates or lipids, for example, enhance parameters of acquired immunity. In contrast, supplementing with functional foods such as probiotics, that include lactic acid bacteria, mainly augment parameters of innate immunity.

These findings support the notion that food-derived materials act on different immune cells or distinct molecules of the cells and improve at least 1 parameter of either innate or acquired immunity. These results mean that one can evaluate the immune-modulating abilities of foods by analysing parameters of either innate or acquired immunity.

The neural and endocrine changes that accompany changes in behavioural states and the network of brain-immune system connections that have been elaborated provide numerous pathways through which behavioural processes could influence immune responses. The domain of the central premise underlying these processes that relates to psychoneuroimmunology is that the nervous, endocrine, and immune system are components of an integrated system of defences. Therefore, the integrative approach to managing infections and improving immune function outcomes also requires lifestyle stressor management.

Table 20.3 summarises the level of evidence for some CAM therapies for the management of immune deficiencies and infections.

Note: Parts of this chapter were extracted with permission from the article 'Immunity' by Dr Lily Tomas in *The Journal of Complementary Medicine* 2009;8(3):12–8.

Table 20.3 Levels of evidence for lifestyle and complementary medicines/therapies in the management of immune deficiencies and infections

Modality	Level I	Level II	Level IIIa	Level IIIb	Level IIIc	Level IV	Level V
Lifestyle modification		x					
Mind-body medicine							
Meditation and/or relaxation			x				
Hypnosis and/or guided imagery				x			
Cognitive behaviour therapy	x						
Sleep restoration			x				
Nutrition							
Diets — weight management			x				
Mediterranean diet			x				
Alcohol			x				
Tea			x				
Physical activity							
Exercise therapy	x						
Yoga				x			
Qigong				x			
Nutritional supplements							
Probiotics		x					
Zinc		x					
Vitamin A				x			
Vitamin C				x			
Vitamin D				x			
Selenium				x			
Manuka honey				x			
Herbal medicines				x			
Cranberry	x						
Echinacea purpurea	x						
Astragalus membranaceus	x						
Physical therapies							
Massage					x		
Acupuncture				x			

Level I — from a systematic review of all relevant randomised controlled trials — meta-analyses.
Level II — from at least 1 properly designed randomised controlled clinical trial.
Level IIIa — from well-designed pseudo-randomised controlled trials (alternate allocation or some other method).
Level IIIb — from comparative studies (including systematic reviews of such studies) with concurrent controls and allocation not randomised, cohort studies, case-control studies, or interrupted time series with a parallel control group.
Level IIIc — from comparative studies with historical control, 2 or more single-arm studies or interrupted time series without a parallel control group.
Level IV — opinions of respected authorities based on clinical experience, descriptive studies or reports of expert committees.
Level V — represents minimal evidence that represents testimonials.

Clinical tips handout for patients — infections and immunity

1 Lifestyle advice

Smoking

- Quit smoking through whatever means are available. Support is often essential as smoking cessation over the long term is a challenge.

Sunshine

- At least 15 minutes of sunshine needed daily for vitamin D and melatonin production — especially before 10 a.m. and after 3 p.m. when the sun exposure is safest in summer.
- Ensure adequate skin exposure (back of hands or face) during this period. Apply sun protection after adequate exposure has been achieved.
- More time in the sun is required for dark skinned people and in winter.
- Vitamin D is obtained in the diet from fatty fish, eggs, liver and fortified foods (some milks and margarines), however it is unlikely that adequate vitamin D concentrations can be obtained from diet alone.

Sleep

- Good sleep is essential to improving the immune system.
- Attempt to establish healthy sleep patterns. Wake with the sun and go to sleep between 9–10 p.m. (For more information see Chapter 22.)

2 Physical activity/exercise

- Aerobic exercise 30–60 minutes daily, within the limits of functional ability. If exercise is not regular, commence with 5 minutes at a time and slowly build up increment length towards 30 minutes. Exercising several short manageable sessions per day that total 30 minutes while increasing increment time is also beneficial. Outdoor exercise is also encouraged, with nature, fresh air and safe sunshine whenever possible.
- Strengthening programs may be beneficial, performed 2–3 sessions per week involving all major muscle groups.
- Yoga and tai chi may also be considered for balance and flexibility.
- Qigong may improve immune system function.
- Start slowly and respect fatigue in all forms of exercise.
- Do not over exercise. Excessive exercise has a negative influence on the immune system, increasing the risk of chronic cold and other infective processes.

3 Mind-body medicine

- Cognitive behavioural therapy maybe useful.
- Mindfulness-based stress reduction programs and meditation have been demonstrated to improve outcomes (e.g. mood) in immune-related diseases such as breast and prostate cancer and HIV.
- Hypnosis, relaxation and guided imagery have been demonstrated to improve outcomes in breast cancer, viral illnesses (e.g. chronic herpes simplex) and incidences of the common cold.

Breathing

- Be aware of breathing from time to time. Notice if tendency to hold breath or over-breathe.
- Always aim to relax breath and the muscles around chest wall.

Rest and stress management

Recurrent stress may cause a return of symptoms. Relaxation is important for a full and lasting recovery.

- Reduce workload and resolve conflicts.
- Contact family, friends, church, social or other groups for support.
- Listening to relaxation music and daily baths help.
- Massage therapy helps.
- Regular exercise reduces stress.
- Stress management program might be useful. For example, 6 x 40 minute sessions for patients to understand the nature of their symptoms, the symptoms' relationship to stress, and the practice of regular relaxation exercises.

Fun

- It is important to have fun in life. Joy can be found even in the simplest tasks, such as being with friends with a sense of humour, funny movies/videos, comedy, hobbies, dancing, playing with pets and children.
- Try to maintain an 'easy-going approach to life'; avoid feeling time-pressured or rushed.

4 Environment

- Reduce your exposure to chemicals wherever possible, including household cleaning agents, paints and solvents, petrochemical fumes, passive smoking, drinking water bottles exposed to the sun, over-medication with pharmaceutical drugs (review with your doctor) etc.

- Reduce your exposure to electromagnetic radiation wherever possible. Carry your mobile phone away from the body rather than in your pocket. Turn off home appliances at the power point when not in use.
- Investigate whether there are any sources of mould in your environment and remove wherever possible.

5 Dietary changes

- Due to the relationship between obesity and the immune system, it is important to aim to reach an ideal weight through an effective long-term weight loss and maintenance program.
- Consider undertaking a food elimination regime to establish if you have any food intolerances/allergies (grain, milk, beef, eggs, salicylates, etc.) that affect your digestive and, hence, your immune system. This should be done under medical supervision (see www.integrative-medicine.com.au for details).
- Presentations (particularly in children) with *recurrent tonsillitis*, *otitis media*, *asthma*, *eczema* or adults with *chronic sinusitis* should always be trialled with a cow's milk and chocolate-free diet for 1 month to determine whether food intolerances are contributing to or causing the above symptoms. Note: avoid everything with dairy (e.g. bread/biscuits) that contains cow's milk to give a true result. Reintroduce each component separately to determine which component(s) is/are the culprit.
- Eat regular balanced healthy meals; ideally 3 main meals and 2 snacks per day, each containing protein.
- Increase fish intake (sardines, tuna, salmon, cod, mackerel) especially deep sea fish. Consume at least 3 fish meals per week.
- Two *small* serves of red meat per week should be consumed to ensure adequate iron levels.
- Consume high quantities of coloured (in particular red) fruit and vegetables.
- Use extra virgin cold pressed olive oil and avocado in dressings.
- Increase intake of nuts (especially brazil nuts), seeds, bean sprouts (e.g. alfalfa, mung beans, lentils).
- Eat shiitake and oyster mushrooms.
- Enjoy dark chocolate.
- If not intolerant/allergic to dairy products, consume full-fat varieties to increase vitamin D intake from fat soluble sources.
- Consume 1–2 glasses of red wine every other day, however, assess whether it affects your symptoms.
- Drink green tea.
- Drink 1–2 litres of water per day.
- For sweeteners try honey (e.g. manuka, yellow box and stringy bark have lowest GI).
- Avoid hydrogenated fats, salt, fast foods and sugar, such as in soft drinks, lollies, biscuits, cakes and other processed foods (e.g. white breads, white pasta, pastries).
- Moderate coffee consumption; 1–2 cups per day. Assess whether it affects your symptoms.
- Avoid chemical additives — preservatives, colourings and flavourings.

6 Physical therapies

- Regular massages may provide short- and long-term benefits in immune system improvements, although the scientific evidence is lacking.
- Acupuncture may be used as an additional therapy in instances of inflammatory or immune system disease.

7 Supplementation

Broad-based multi-vitamin with high anti-oxidant value

Due to the synergistic manner in which vitamins and minerals support the immune system, it is recommended that a broad-based, high-strength multivitamin is used to support the immune system.

Vitamin A

- Indications: Reducing infection severity (measles and infectious diarrhoea), very low birth weight infants, chemo-prevention, night blindness, retinitis pigmentosa, xerophthalmia, glaucoma and cataract prevention, acne, psoriasis, icythyoses, skin cancers, improving dental health, Crohn's disease, asthma, sinusitis and rhinitis.
- Dosage: Australian recommended dietary intake:
  - 1–3 years: 300ug/day
  - 4–8 years: 400ug/day
  - 9–13 years: 600ug/day

  - 14 years and over (females): 700ug/day
  - 14 years and over (males): 900ug/day
  - upper level of intake: 3000ug/day
  - pregnancy <18 years: 700ug/day
  - pregnancy > 18 years: 800ug/day
  - lactation: 1100ug/day.
- Dosage: treatment doses:
  - 10 000–50 000IU/day in short term
  - 200 000IU on 2 consecutive days can reduce secondary infection in children with measles who are vitamin A deficient
  - 15–000IU/day for retinitis pigmentosa.
- Results: depends on form of vitamin A and condition being treated.
- Side-effects: none at appropriate doses.
- Contraindications: caution with concurrent use of isotretinoin, minocycline, OCP or with liver and/or renal disease. Toxicity may occur at doses >10 000IU vitamin A/day or >2000IU/day when pregnant. Early signs: Dry rough skin, cracked lips, course or sparse hair, alopecia of eyebrows, diplopia, dryness of mucous membranes, peeling of skin, bone and joint pain, fatigue, nausea and vomiting.

Vitamin C

- Indications: upper respiratory tract infections, sinusitis, atopy, asthma (exercise-induced), to enhance the efficacy of some medications (cisplatin, cyclophosphamide, doxorubicin, etoposide, fluorouracil, L-dopa, tamoxifen, vincristine), to improve connective tissue integrity, wound healing, sunburn prevention, anti-histamine, cancer prevention and treatment, prevention of cardiovascular disease, diabetes complications.
- Dosage: for acute infections, short-term use (3–6g/day) or until bowel tolerance then reduce dose. For cancer, 10–30g IV 2–3 times weekly.
- Side-effects: reversible diarrhoea at high doses when given orally.
- Contraindications: use with caution in haemochromatosis, thalassemia major, sideroblastic anaemia, erythrocyte G6P deficiency.

Vitamin D3 (cholecalciferol)

- Indications: auto-immune diseases (IBD), cancer, infectious diseases.
- Dosage: in the absence of sun exposure, at least 800–1000IUD3/day may be needed for adequate vitamin D levels in children and adults, respectively. Treatment doses vary considerably depending on condition: generally, 2000–6000IU/day vitamin D3. Up to 50 000IU D2 twice weekly for 5 weeks has been shown to be safe. Check blood levels with your doctor for correct dosage of vitamin D.
- Results: 3-month trial.
- Side-effects: mild and rare when used appropriately.
- Contraindications: hypersensitivity to vitamin D, SLE, hypercalcaemia, Caution in sarcoidosis and hyperparathyroidism. Possible interaction with calcium channel blockers and digitalis.

Zinc

- Indication: to improve immunity, reduce severity and frequency of infections and reduce oxidative stress.
- Dosage: 35–45mg elemental zinc nocte.
- Results: 3-month trial. Cease earlier if nausea occurs.
- Side-effects: nausea, vomiting, reduced copper after long-term use.
- Contraindications: high zinc levels, sideroblastic anaemia, severe kidney disease. Caution with amiloride.

Selenium

- Indication: to improve immunity, chemo-prevention.
- Dosage: up to 150ug/day.
- Results: 3-month trial.
- Side-effects: nausea, vomiting, irritability, fatigue, nail changes at doses > 1mg.
- Contraindications: sensitivity to selenium.

Herbs

Immune support

Astragalus herbs (*A. membranaceus*)

- Indications: general immune system support, from viral upper respiratory tract infections to synergistic effects with various forms of chemotherapy.
- Dosage:
  - 2–30g/day dried root
  - (1:2) 4.5–8.5 mL/day liquid extract or solid dose equivalent
  - Decoction: 8–12g divided in 2 doses daily on empty stomach.
- Results: may notice effects within 2 weeks.
- Side-effects: none known.
- Contraindications: caution with immunosuppressive agents. May have additive effects with inotropic drugs.

Echinacea (*E. Purpurea*)

- Indications: shorten duration of the cold; skin infections.
- Dosage:
  - 1–3g/day *E. Angustifolia* or *E. Purpurea*
  - 2.5–6g/day *E. Purpurea* dried aerial part
  - 6–9mL/day *E. Purpurea* expressed juice of fresh plant
  - 2–4 mL/day *E. Pallida* ethanolic extract of root.
- Results: early results for acute infections.
- Side-effects: rash can occur if allergic; rare cases of anaphylaxis reported.
- Contraindications: if allergic to *Compositae* family of plants (chamomile, ragweed). Caution with immunosuppressive medications and long-term use (>8 weeks). Avoid if on immunosuppressive medication.

Probiotics

- Indications: to enhance gut-associated lymphoid tissue (GALT), thereby providing balance between Th1 and Th2 cytokines in order to prevent and treat auto-immune and infectious diseases.
- Dosage: depending upon condition, different probiotics may be required. Generalised treatment dose before breakfast:
  - *Lactobacillus rhamnosus*: 12 billion CFU
  - *Lactobacillus acidophilus*: 4 billion CFU
  - *Lactobacillus casei*: 2 billion CFU
  - *Bifidobacterium bifidum*: 1 billion CFU
  - *Bifidobacterium longum*: 1 billion CFU.
- Results: from a few days to a few weeks depending on condition.
- Side-effects: gastrointestinal disturbance if taking the wrong probiotic.
- Contraindications: true cow's milk allergy if contained in the product.

Throat infection and wound healing

Manuka honey

- Indications: coughs; partial thickness burns, ulcerations, wound healing; throat infections. Use under medical supervision.
- Dosage: topical application as directed; 1tsp of honey for sore throats.
- Results: within a week; may have immediate soothing effect on throat.
- Side-effects: none.
- Contraindications: allergy to honey.

Urinary tract infection and/or Helicobactor pylori

Cranberry (*V. Macrocarpon*)

- Indications: prevention of urinary tract infections (UTIs); helps prevent *Helicobacter pylori* to gastrointestinal cells.
- Dosage: 10 000–17 000mg/day to prevent UTIs. If becoming symptomatic, may increase dose to 20 000mg bd in the short-term. A urine M/C/S is recommended due to possible masking of symptoms with concurrent UTI.
- Results: 3-month trial for prevention. At higher doses, results may be noticed in less than 1 week if symptomatic.
- Side-effects: gastrointestinal discomfort and diarrhoea at very large doses.
- Contraindications: caution with warfarin and if a history of oxalate kidney stones. Diabetics should avoid commercial cranberry juice which is high in sugar.

References

1 Round JL, Mazmanian SK. The gut microbiota shapes intestinal immune responses during health and disease. Nat Rev Immunol 2009;9(5):313–23.

2 Irwen MR. Human Psychoneuro-immunology: 20 years of discovery. Brain Behav Immun 2008;22(2):129–39.

3 Ziemssen T, Kern S. Psychoneuro-immunology-cross-talk between the immune and nervous systems. J Neurol 2007;254(Suppl 2):II8–II11.

4 Tausk F, Elenkov I, Moynihan J. Psychoneuro-immunology. Dermatol Ther 2008;21(1):22–31.

5 Kemeny ME, Schedlowski M. Understanding the interaction between psychological stress and immune-related diseases: a stepwise progression. Brain Behav Immun 2007;21(8):1009–18.

6 Reiche EM, Nunes SO, Morimoto HK. Stress, depression, the immune system and cancer. Lancet Oncol 2004;5(10):617–25.

7 Reiche EM, Morimoto HK, Nunes SM. Stress and depression-induced immune dysfunction: implications of the development and progression of cancer. Int Rev Psych 2005;17(6):515–27.

8 Alves GJ, Palermo-Neto J. Neuroimmunomodulation: the cross-talk between nervous and immune systems. s.l.: Rev Bras Psiquiatr 2007;29(4):363–9.

9 Leonard B. Stress, depression and the activation of the immune system. World J Biol Psychiatry 2000;1(1):17–25.

10 Mawdsley JE, Rampton DS. Psychological stress in IBD: new insights into pathogenic and therapeutic implications. Gut 2005;54(10):1481–91.

11 Gareau MG, Silva MA, Perdue MH. Pathophysiological mechanisms of stress-induced intestinal damage. Curr Mol Med 2008;8(4):274–81

12 Olff M. Stress, depression and immunity: the role of defense and coping styles. Psychiatry Res 1999;85(1):7–15.

13 Miller AH. Neuroendocrine and immune system interactions in stress and depression. Psychiatr Clin North Am 1998;21(2):443–63.

14 Tausk F, Elenkov I, Moynihan J. Psychoneuro–immunology. Dermatol Ther 2008;21(1):22–31.
15 Karrow NA. Activation of the HPAA and ANS during inflammation and altered programming of the neuroendocrine-immune axis during foetal and neonatal devt: lessons learned from the model inflammagen, lipopolysaccharide. Brain Behav Immun 2006;20(2):144–58.
16 Raison CL, Miller AH. The neuroimmunolgy of stress and depression. Semin Clin Neuropsychiatry 2001;6(4):277–94.
17 Stasi C, Orlandelli E. Role of the brain-gut axis in the pathophysiology of Crohns disease. Dig Dis 2008;26(2):156–66.
18 Maunder RG, Levelstein S. The role of stress in the devt and clinical course of IBD: epidemiological evidence. Curr Mol Med 2008;8(4):247–52.
19 Maunder RG. Evidence that stress contributes to IBD: evaluation, sntheis and future directions. IBD 2005;11(6):600–8.
20 Boye B, Jahnson J, Mokleby K, et. al. The INSPIRE study: are different personality traits related to disease-specific QOL in distressed patients with UC and Crohns disease? IBD 2008;14:680–6.
21 Grippo AJ, Johnson AK. Stress, depression and CV dysregulation: a review of neurobiological mechanisms and the integration of research from preclinical disease models. Stress 2009;12(1):1–21.
22 Grippo AJ. Mechanisms underlying altered mood and CV dysfunction: trhe value of neurobiological and behavioural research with animal models. Neurosci Biobehav Rev 2009;33(2):171–80.
23 Gold SM, Irwin MR. Depression and immunity: inflammation and depressive symptoms in MS. Neurol Clin 2006;24(3):507–19.
24 Mawdsley JE, Rampton DS. The role of psychological stress in IBD. s.l.: Neuroimmunomodulation 2006;13(5–6):327–36.
25 McGregor BA, Antoni MH. Psych intervention and health noutcomes among women treated for breast cancer: a review of stress pathways and biological mediatore. Brain Behav Immun 2009;23(2):159–66.
26 Kremser T, Evans A, Moore A, et. al. Use of CAM by Australian women with breast cancer. Breast 2008;17(4):387–94.
27 Smith JE, Richardson J, Hoffman C, et. al. MBSR as supportive therapy in cancer care: a systematic review. J Adv Nurs 2005;52(3):315–27.
28 Witek-Janusek L, Albuquerque K, Chroniak KR, et. al. Effect of MBSR on immune function, QOL and coping in women newly-diagnosed with early stage breast cancer. Brain Beh Immun 2008;22:969–81.
29 Carlson LE, Speca M, Faris P, et. al. 1 year pre-post intervention follow-up of psychological, immune, endocrine and BP outcomes of MBSR in breast and prostate cancer outpatients. Brain Behav Immun 2007;21(8):1038–49.
30 Carlson LE, Speca M, Patel KD, et. al. MBSR in relation to QOL, mood, symptoms of stress and levels of cortisol, DHEA and melatonin in breast and prostate cancer outpots. Psychoneuroendocrinology 2004;29(4):448–74.
31 Carlson LE, Speca M, Patel KD, et. al. MBSR in relation to QOL, mood, symptoms of stress and immune parameters in breast and prostate cancer outpatients. Psychosom Med 2003;65(4):571–81.
32 Ott MJ, Norris RL, Bauer-Wu SM. Mindfulness meditation for oncology pts: a discussion and critical review. Integr Cancer Ther 2006'5(2):98–108.
33 Creswell JD, Myers HF, Cole SW, et. al. Mindfulness meditation training effects on CD4+ lymphocytes in HIV+ adults: a small RCT. Brain behav Immun 2009;23(2):184–8.
34 Robinson FP, Mathews HL, Witek-Janusek L. Psycho-endocrine-immune response to MBSR in individulals infected with HIV: a quasiexperimental study. J Altern Comp Med 2003;9(5):683–9.
35 Taylor DN. Effects of a behavioural stress management program on anxiety, mood, self-esteem and T count in HIV positive men. s.l.: Psychol Rep 1995;76(2):451–7.
36 Collins MP, Dunn LF. The effects of meditation and visual imagery on an immune system disorder: dermatomyositis. J Alt Comp Med 2005;11(2): 275–84.
37 Gruzelier J, Smith F, Nagy A. Cellular and humoral immunity, mood and exam stress: the influences of self-hypnosis and personality predictors. Int J Psychphysiol 2001;42(1):55–71.
38 Whitehouse WG, Dinges DF, Orne EC, et. al. Psychosocial and immune effects of self-hypnosis training for stress management throughout the first semester of medical school. Psychsom Med 1996;58(3):249–63.
39 Gruzelier JH. A review of the impact of hypnosis, relaxation, guided imagery and individual differences on aspects of immunity and health. Stress 2002;5(2):147–63.
40 Gruber BL, Hersh SP, Hall NR, et. al. Immunological responses of breast cancer patients to behavioual interventions. Biofeedback Self Regul 1993;18(1):1–22.
41 Lengacher CA, Bennett MP, Gonzalez L, et. al. Immune reponses to guided imagery during breast cancer treatment. Biol Res Nurs 2008;9(3):205–14.
42 Bakke AC, Purtzer MZ, Newton P. The effect of hypnotic guided imagery on psychological wellbeing and immune function in patients with prior breast cancer. J Psychosom Res 2002;53(6):1131–7.
43 Cruess S, Antoni M, Cruess D, et. al. Reductions in HSV-2 antibody titres after CBT and relationships with neuroendocrine function, relaxation skills and social support in HIV positive men. Psychosom Med 2000;62(6):828–37.
44 Antoni MH, Cruess S, Cruess DG, et. al. CBT reduces distress and 24 hr urinary cortisol output among symptomatic HIV positive gay men. Ann Behav Med 2000;22(1):29–37.
45 Antoni MH, Cruess Dg, Cruess S, et. al. CBT effects on anxiety, 24 hour urinary norepinephrine output and T-cytotoxic/suppressor cells over time among symptomatic HIV positive gay men. J Consult Clin Psychol 2000;68(1):35–45.
46 Hidderley M, Holt M. A pilot RCT assessing the effects of autogenic training in early stage cancer pts in relation to psychological status and immune system responses. Eur J Oncol Nurs 2004;8:61–5.
47 van der Pompe G, Antoni MH, Duivenvoorden HJ, et. al. An exploratory study into the effects of group psychotherapy on cardiovascular and immunoreactivity to acute stress in breast cancer patients. Psychther Psychosom 2001;70(6):307–18.
48 Price JR, Mitchell E, Tidy E, et. al. Cognitive behaviour therapy for chronic fatigue syndrome in adults. Cochrane Database of Systematic Reviews 2008, Issue 3. Art. No.: CD001027. DOI: 10.1002/14651858.CD001027.pub2.
49 Dietert RR. DIT: focus on health risks. Chem Res Toxicol 2009;22(1):17–23.

50 Dietert RR. DIT in drug safety testing: matching DIT testing to adverse outcomes and childhood disease risk. Curr Drug Saf 2008;3(3):216–26.
51 Kilburn HK. Summary of the 5th Int Conf on Bioaerosols, Fungi, Bacteria, Mycotoxins and Human Health. Arch Environ Health 2003;58(8):538–42.
52 Edmondson DA, Nordness ME, Zacharisen MC, et. al. Allergy and toxic mould syndrome. Ann Allergy Asthma Immun ol 2005;94(2):234–9.
53 Dietert RR, Zelikoff JT. Early-life environment, DIT and the risk of paediatric allergic disease including asthma. Birth Defects Res B Dev Reprod Toxicol 2008;83(6):547–60.
54 Dietert RR, Dietert JM. Possible role for ELII inc DIT in CFS or ME. Toxicology 2008;247:61–72.
55 Dietert RR, Dierert JM. ELII and DIT-associated diseases: potential of herbal and fungal derived medicinals. Curr Med Chem 2007;14(10): 075–85.
56 Dietert RR. DIT, postnatal immune dysfunction and childhood leukaemia. Blood Cells Mol Dis 2009;42(2):108–12.
57 Dietert RR, Dietart JM. Potential for ELII inc DIT in autism and ASD: focus on critical windows of immune vulnerability. J Toxicol Environ Health B Crit Rev 2008;11(8):660–80.
58 Kipen HM, Fiedler N. Envt'al factors in medically unexplained symptoms and related syndromes: the evidence and the challenge. Environ Health Perapect 2002;110(Suppl 4):597–9.
59 Krewski D, Glickman BW, Habash RW, et. al. Recent advances in research on RF fields and health: 2001–2203. J Toxicol Environ Health B Crit Rev 2007;10(4):287–318.
60 Valberg PA, van Deventer TE, Repacholi MH. Worgroup report: base stations and wireless networks RF exposures and health consequences. Environ Health Perspect 2007;115(3):416–24.
61 Knave B. EMF and health outcomes. Ann Acad Med Singapore 2001;30(5):489–93.
62 Bonhomme-Fivre L, Marion S, Bezie Y, et. al. Study of human neurovegetative and haematological effects of envt'al low frez (50Hz) EMF produced by transformers. Arch Env Health 1998;53:87–92.
63 Hardell L, Sage C. Biological effects from EMF exposure and public exposure standards. Biomed Pharmacother 2008;62(2):104–9.
64 Fukuyama T, Ueda H, Hayashi K, et. al. Detection of low-level envt'al chemical allergy by a long-term sensitisation method. Toxicol Lett 2008;180(1):1–8.
65 Dietert RR, Hedge A. Chemical sensitivity and the immune system: a paradigm to approach potential immune involvement. Neurotoxicology 1998;19(2):253–7.
66 Bernstein DI. MCS: state of the art symposium. the role of chemical allergens. Regul Toxicol Pharmacol 1996;24(1 Pt 2):S28–31.
67 Laumbach RJ, Kipen HM. Bioaerosols and SBS:particles, inflammation and allergy. Curr Opin Allergy Clin Immunol 2005;5(2):135–9.
68 Campbell AW, Thrasher JD, Madison RA, et. al. Neural auto-antibodies and neurophysiological abnormalities in patients exposed to mould in water-damaged buildings. Arch Environ Health 2003;58(8):464–74.
69 Gray MR, Thrasher JD, Crago R, et. al. Mixed mould mycotoxicosis: immunological changes in humans following exposure in water-damaged buildings. Arch Environ Health 2003;58(7):410–20.
70 Lander F, Meyer HW, Norn S. Serum IgE specific to indoor moulds, measured by basophil histamine release, is associated with building-related symptoms in damp buildings. Infl amm Res 2001;50(4):227–31.
71 Li-Ng M, Aloia JF, Pollack S, et. al. A RCT of D3 supplements for the prevention of symptomatic URTIs. Epidemiol Infect 2009 Mar 19:1–9.
72 Lucas RM, Ponsonby AL, Pasco JA, et. al. Future health implications of prenatal and early-life vitamin D status. Nutr Rev 2008;66(12):710–20.
73 Szodoray P, Nakken B, Gaal J, et. al. The complex role of Vit D in auto-immune disease. Scand J Immunol 2008;68(3):261–9.
74 Hayes CE, Nashold FE, Spach KM, et al. The immunological functions of the vitamin D endocrine system. Cell Mol Biol 2003; 29(2): 277–300.
75 Cantorna MT. vitamin D and its role in immunology: MS and IBD. Prog Biophys Mol Biol 2006;92(1):60–4.
76 Lips P. Vit D Physiology. Prog Biophys Mol Biol 2006;92(1):4–8.
77 Kurylowicz A, Bednarczuk T, Nauman J. The influence of Vit D deficiency on cancers and auto-immune disease development. Endokrynol Pol 2007;58(2):140–52.
78 Cantorna MT. Vitamin D and its role in immunology: multiple sclerosis, and inflammatory bowel disease. Prog Biophys Mol Biol 2006;92(1):60–4.
79 Arnson Y, Amital H, Shoenfeld Y. vitamin D and Autoimmunity: new aetiological and therapeutic considerations. Ann Rheum Dis 2007;66(9):1137–42.
80 Cantorna MT, Mahon BD. Mounting evidence for Vit D as an environmental factor affecting auto-immune disease prevalence. Exp Biol Med 2004;229(11):1136–42.
81 Du T, Zhou ZG, You S, et. al. Regulation by Vit D3 on altered TLRs expression and response to ligands of monocyte from AI diabetes. Clin Chim Acta 2009;402(1–2):133–8.
82 Smolders J, Damoiseaux J, Menheere P, et. al. Fok-1 Vit D receptor gene polymorphism and Vit D metabolism in MS. J Neuroimmunol 2009; 207(1–2):117–21.
83 Cantorna MT. Vit D and Autoimmunity: is Vit D status an environmental factor affecting auto-immune disease prevalence? Proc Soc Exp Biol Med 2000;223(3):230–3.
84 Imeri L, Opp MR. How (and why) the immune system makes us sleep. Nat Rev Neurosci 2009;10(3):199–210.
85 Smyth CA. Evaluating sleep quality in older adults: the Pittsburgh Sleep Quality Index can be used to detect sleep disturbances or deficits. Am J Nurs 2008;108(5):42–50.
86 Meerlo P, Sgoifo A, Suchecki D. Restricted and disrupted sleep: effects on ANS function, neuroendocrine stress systems and stress responsitivity. Sleep Med Rev 2008;12(3):197–210.
87 Novati A, Roman V, Cetin T, et. al. Chronically restricted sleep leads to depression-like changes in NT receptor sensitivity and neuroendocrine stress reactivity in rats. Sleep 2008;31(11):1579–85.
88 Preston BT, Capellini I, McNamara P, et. al. Parasite resistance and the adaptive significance of sleep. BMC Evol Biol 2009;9:7.
89 Spaggiari MC. Sleep medicine in occupational health. G Ital Med Lav Ergon 2008;30(3):276–9.
90 Bentivoglio M, Kristensson K. Neural-immune interactions in disorders of sleep-wakefulness organisation. Trends Neurosci 2007;30(12):645–52.

91 Roman V, Walastra I, Luiten PG, et. al. Too little sleep gradually desensitises the serotonin 1A receptor system. Sleep 2005;28(12):1505–10.
92 Cohen S, Doyle WJ, Alper CM, et. al. Sleep habits and susceptibility to the common cold. Arch Intern Med 2009;169(1):62–7.
93 Cardinali DP, Esquifino AI, Srinivasan V, et. al. Melatonin and the IS in ageing. Neuroimmunomodulation 2008;15(4–6):272–8.
94 Woods JA, Vieira VJ, Keylock KT. Exercise, inflammation and innate immunity. Immunol Allergy Clin North Am 2009;29(2):381–93.
95 Schedlowski M, Schmidt RE. Stress and the immune system. s.l.: Naturwissenschaften 1996;83(5):214–20.
96 Kisaki T, Takemasa T, Sakurai T, et. al. Adaptation of macrophages to exercise training improves innate immunity. Biochem Biophys Res Commun 2008;372(1):152–6.
97 Timmons BW, Cieslak T. Human NK-cell subsets and acute exercise: a brief review. Exerc Immunol Rev 2008;14:8–23.
98 de Lima C, Alves LE, Iagher F, et. al. Anaerobic exercise reduces tumour growth, cancer cachexia and increases macrophage and lymphocyte response in Walker 256 tumour-bearing rats. s.l.: Eur J Appl Physiol 2008;104(6):957–64.
99 Sakamoto Y, Ueki S, Kasai T, et. al. Effect of exercise, ageing and functional capacity on acute sIgA response in elderly people over 75 years of age. Geriatr Gerontol Int 2009;9(1):81–8.
100 Bishop NC, Gleeson M. Acute and chronic effects of exercise on markers of mucosal immunity. Front Biosci 2009;14:4444–56.
101 Matsuzawa-Nagata N, Takamura T, Ando H, et. al. Increased oxidative stress precedes the onset of high-fat diet-induced insulin resistance and obesity. Metabolism 2008;57(8):1071–77.
102 Gleeson M, Pyne DB. Special feature for the Olympics: effects of exercise on the immune system: exercise effects on mucosal immunity. Immunol Cell Biol 2000;78(5):536–44.
103 Nijs J, Paul L, Wallman K. Chronic fatigue syndrome: an approach combining self-management with graded exercise to avoid exacerbations. J Rehabil Med 2008;40(4):241–7
104 West NP, Pyne DB, Kyd JM, et. al. The effect of exercise on innate mucosal immunity. Br J Sports Med 2008 May 22.
105 Nieman DC, Henson DA, McMahon M, et. al. Beta-glucan, immune function and URTI in athletes. Med Sci Sports Exerc 2008;40(8):1463–71.
106 Close P, Thielen V, Bury T. Mucosal immunity in elite athletes. Rev Med Liege 2003;58:548–53.
107 Groer MW, Shelton MM. Exercise is associated with elevated proinflammatory cytokines in human milk. J Obstet Gynaec Neonatal Nurs 2009;38(1):35–41.
108 Edmonds M, McGuire H, Price J. Exercise therapy for chronic fatigue syndrome. Cochrane Database of Systematic Reviews 2004, Issue 3. Art. No.: CD003200. DOI: 10.1002/14651858.CD003200.pub2
109 Kjellgren A, Bood SA, Axelsson K, et. al. Wellness through a comprehensive yogic breathing program-a controlled pilot trial. BMC Comp Altern Med 2007;7;43.
110 Sharma H, Datta P, Singh A, et. al. Gene expression profiling in practitioners of SK. J Psychosom Res 2008;64(2):213–8
111 Sharma H, Sen S, Singh A. SK practitioners exhibit better antioxidant status and lower blood lactate levels. Biol Psychol 2003;63(3):281–91.
112 Kochupillai V, Kumar P, Singh D, et. al. Effect of rhythmic breathing (SK and P) on immune functions and tobacco addiction. Ann N Y Acad Sci 2005;1056:242–52.
113 Rao RM, Tellas S, Nagendra HR, et. al. Effects of yoga on NK-cell counts in early breast cancer pts undergoing conventional treatment. Med Sci Monit 2008;14(2):LE3–4.
114 Manzaneque JM, Vera FM, Maldonado EF, et. al. Assessment of immunological parameters following a Q training program. Med Sci Monit 2004;10(6):CR264–70.
115 Li QZ, Li P, Garcia GE, et. al. Genomic profiling of neutrophil transcripts in Asian Qigong practitioners: a pilot study in gene regulation by MB interaction. J Altern Complement Med 2005;11(1):29–39.
116 Jones BM. Changes in cytokine production in healthy subjects practicing Guolin Qigong: a pilot study. BMC Comp Altern Med 2001;1:8.
117 Manzanaque JM, Vera FM, Rodriguez FM et al. Serum cytokines, mood and sleep after a Qigong program: Is Qigong an effective psychobiological tool? J Health Psychol 2009;14(1):60–7.
118 Devaraj S, Wang-Polagruto J, Polagruto J, et. al. High-fat, energy-dense, fast-food-style breakfast results in an increase in oxidative stress in metabolic syndrome. Metabolism. 2008 Jun;57(6):867–70.
119 Okamatsu Y, Matsuda K, Hiramoto I, et. al. Ghrelin and leptin modulate immunity and liver function in overweight children. Pediatr 2009;51(1):9–13.
120 Aeberli I, Beljean N, Lehmann R, L'allemand D, Spinas GA, Zimmermann MB. The increase of fatty acid-binding protein aP2 in overweight and obese children: interactions with dietary fat and impact on measures of subclinical inflammation. Int J Obes (Lond). 2008 Aug 5. [Epub ahead of print]
121 Moreira A, Arsati F, Cury PR, et. al. The impact of a 17 day training period for an international championship on mucosal immune parameters in top-level basketball players and staff members. Eur J Oral Sci 2008;116(5):431–7.
122 Fung, TT, Rimm EB, Spiegelman D, Rifai N, Tofler GH, Willett WC, Hu FB. Association between dietary patterns and plasma biomarkers of obesity and cardiovascular disease risk. Am J Clin Nutr 2001;73:61–7.
123 Matsuzawa-Nagata N, Takamura T, Ando H, et. al. Increased oxidative stress precedes the onset of high-fat diet-induced insulin resistance and obesity. Metabolism 2008;57(8):1071–1077.
124 Basdevant A, Ciangura C. [Obesity, a disease] Bull Acad Natl Med 2010;194(1):13-20; discussion 20–4.
125 Bulló M, Casas-Agustench P, Amigó-Correig P, Aranceta J, Salas-Salvadó J. Inflammation, obesity and comorbidities: the role of diet. Public Health Nutr 2007t;10(10A):1164–72
126 Epel ES. Psychological and metabolic stress: a recipe for accelerated cellular ageing? Hormones (Athens) 2009;8(1):7–22.
127 Miranda-Garduno LM, Reza-Albarran A. Obesity, inflammation and diabetes. Gac Med Mex 2008;144(1):39–46.
128 Hofer T, Fontana L, Anton SD, et. al. Long-term effects of caloric restriction or exercise on DNA and RNA oxidation levels in WBCs and urine in humans. Rejuvenation Res 2008;11(4):793–9.
129 Fontana L, Villareal DT, Weiss EP, et. al. Caloric restriction or exercise: effects on coronary heart disease RFs. A RCT. Am J Physiol Endocrinol Metab 2007;293(1):E197–202.

130 Crujeiras AB, Parra D, Milagro FI, et. al. Differential expression of ox stress and indflammation related genes in peripheral MNCs on response to a low-calorie diet: a nutrigenomics study. OMICS 2008;12(4):251–61.

131 Aljada A, Mohanty P, Ghanim H, Abdo T, Tripathy D, Chaudhuri A, Dandona P. Increase in intranuclear nuclear factor B and decrease in inhibitor B in mononuclear cells after a mixed meal: evidence for a proinflammatory effect. AJCN 2004; 79: 682–90.

132 Devaraj S, Wang-Polagruto J, Polagruto J, et. al. High-fat, energy-dense, fast-food-style breakfast results in an increase in oxidative stress in metabolic syndrome. Metabolism. 2008 Jun;57(6):867–70.

133 Esmaillzadeh A, Kimiagar M, Mehrabi Y, Azadbakht L, Hu FB, Willett WC. Dietary Patterns and Markers of Systemic Inflammation among Iranian Women. J Nutr 2007; 137:992–998.

134 Kechagias S, Ernersson A, Dahlqvist-Lundberg P, et. al. Fast food based hyper-alimentation can induce rapid and profound elevation of serum alanine aminotransferase in healthy subjects. Gut 2008 0: 200713179

135 Lopez-Garcia, E, SchulzeMB, Fung TT, Meigs JB, Rifai N, Manson JE, Hu FB. Major dietary patterns are related to plasma concentrations of markers of inflammation and endothelial dysfunction. Am J Clin Nutr 2004;80:1029 –35.

136 Delgado-Lista J, Lopez-Miranda J, Cortes B, Perez-Martinez P, Lozano A, Gomez-Luna R, Gomez P, Gomez MJ, Criado J, Fuentes F, Perez-Jiminez F. Chronic dietary fat intake modifies the postprandial response of hemostatic markers to a single fatty test meal. AJCN 2008; 87:317–22.

137 Erridge C, Attina T, Spickett CM, Webb DJ. A high-fat meal induces low-grade endotoxemia: evidence of a novel mechanism of postprandial inflammation. AJCN 2007; 86(5):1286–92.

138 Håversen L, Danielsson KN, Fogelstrand L, Wiklund O. Induction of proinflammatory cytokines by long-chain saturated fatty acids in human macrophages. Atherosclerosis. 2008 May 28. [Epub ahead of print]

139 Jakulj F, Zernicke K, Bacon S, et. al. A high fat meal increases cardiovascular reactivity to psychological stress in healthy young adults. J Nutr 2007;137: 935–9.

140 Mohanty P, G.H., Hamouda W. Both lipid and protein intakes stimulated increased generation of reactive oxygen species by polymorphonuclear leukocytes and mononuclear cells. Am J Clin Nutr, 2002. 75(767–72).

141 O'Keefe J, Bell D. The post-prandial hyperglycemia/ hyperlipemia hypothesis: a hidden cardiovascular risk factor? Am J Cardiol 2007;100: 899 –904.

142 Petersson H, Lind L, Hulthe J, Elmgren A, Cederholm T, Risérus U. Relationships between serum fatty acid composition and multiple markers of inflammation and endothelial function in an elderly population. Atherosclerosis. 2008 Jul 1. [Epub ahead of print].

143 Tschop M, Thomas G. Fat fuels insulin resistance through toll-like receptors. Nature 2006;12(12):1359–61.

144 Velloso LA, Araújo EP, de Souza CT. Diet-Induced Inflammation of the Hypothalamus in Obesity. Neuroimmunomodulation. 2008 Sep 9;15(3):189–193.

145 Han NS, Leka LS, Lichtenstein AH, Ausman LM, Schaefer EJ, Meydani SN. Effect of hydrogenated and saturated, relative to polyunsaturated, fat on immune and inflammatory responses of adults with moderate hyper-cholesterolemia. J Lipid Res 2002; 43: 445–52.

146 Mozaffarian D, Katan MB, Ascherio A, et. al. Trans Fatty Acids and Cardiovascular Disease. NEJM, Volume 354:1601–1613

147 Parks EJ, Skokan LE, Timlin MT, Dingfelder CS. Dietary sugars stimulate fatty acid synthesis in adults. J Nutr 2008; 138(6):1039–1046.

148 Galgani J, Aguirre C, Diaz E. Acute effect of meal glycaemic index and glycaemic load on blood glucose and insulin response in humans. Nutr J 2006; 5: 22–8

149 Kallio P, Kolhmainen M, Laaksonen DE, Pulkkinenen L, Atalay M, Mykkanen H, Uusitupa m, Poutanen K, Niskanen L. Inflammation markers are modulated by responses to diets differing in postprandial responses in individuals with the metabolic syndrome. AJCN 2008;87:1497–503.

150 Qi L, Hu FB. Dietary glycaemic load, whole grains and systemic inflammation in diabetes: the epidemiological evidence. Curr Opin Lipidol 2007;18(3):3–8.

151 Rayssiguier Y, Gueux E, Nowacki W, Rock E, Mazur A. High fructose consumption combined with low dietary magnesium intake may increase the incidence of the metabolic syndrome by inducing inflammation. Magnes Res 2006; 19(4): 237–43.

152 Rebolledo OR, Marra CA, Raschia A, et. al. Abdominal Adipose Tissue: Early Metabolic Dysfunction Associated to Insulin Resistance and Oxidative Stress Induced by an Unbalanced Diet. Horm Metab Res. 2008 Jul 11. [Epub ahead of print]

153 Vinayagamoorthi R, Bobby Z, Sridharmg. Antioxidants preserve redox balance and inhibit c-Jun-N-terminal kinase pathway while improving insulin signaling in fat-fed rats: evidence for the role of oxidative stress on IRS-1 serine phosphorylation and insulin resistance. J Endocrin 2008;197:287–96

154 Dickinson S, Hancock DP, Petocz P, Ceriello A, Brand-Miller J. High-glycemic index carbohydrate increases nuclear factor-kappaB activation in mononuclear cells of young, lean healthy subjects. AJCN 2008;87(5):1188–93.

155 Kallio P, Kolhmainen M, Laaksonen DE, et. al. Inflammation markers are modulated by responses to diets differing in postprandial responses in individuals with the metabolic syndrome. AJCN 2008;87:1497–503.

156 Nareika A, Im YB, Game BA, et. al. High glucose enhances lipopolysaccharide-stimulated CD14 expression in U937 mononuclear cells by increasing nuclear factor kappaB and AP-1 activities. J Endocrinol 2008;196:45–55.

157 Beulens JW, de Bruijne LM, Stolk RP, et. al. High dietary glycaemic load and glycaemic index increase risk of cardiovascular disease among middle-aged women. J Am Coll Cardiol 2007;50:14–21.

158 Galgani J, Aguirre C, Diaz E. Acute effect of meal glycaemic index and glycaemic load on blood glucose and insulin response in humans. Nutr J 2006; 5: 22–8.

159 Ye X, Franco OH, Yu Z, et. al. Associations of inflammatory factors with glycaemic status among middle-aged and older Chinese people. Clin Endocrinol (Oxf). Sep 2. [Epub ahead of print]

160 Yu S, Weaver V, Martin K, et. al. The Effects of whole mushrooms during inflammation. BMC Immunol 2009;10:12.

161 Florentino RF. Symposium on diet, nutrition and immunity. Asia Pac J Clin Nutr 2009;18(1):137–42.

162 Chun OK, Chung S-J, Claycombe KJ, Song WO. Serum C-reactive protein concentrations are inversely associated with dietary flavonoid intake in U.S. adults. J Nutr 2008;138:753–760.

163 Ock, K.C., Chung, S.-J., Claycombe, K.J., Song, W.O. Serum C-reactive protein concentrations are inversely associated with dietary flavonoid intake in U.S. adults. J Nutr 2008;138:753–760

164 Murakami A, Ohigashi H. Targeting NOX, INOS and COX-2 in inflammatory cells: chemoprevention using food phytochemicals. Int J Cancer 2007;121(11):2357–63.

165 Middleton E Jr, Kandaswami C, Theoharides TC. The effects of plant flavonoids on mammalian cells: implications for inflammation, heart disease, and cancer. Pharmacol Rev 2000;52(4):673–751.

166 Calder PC. Polyunsaturated fatty acids, inflammatory processes and inflammatory bowel diseases. Mol Nutr Food Res. 2008 May 26. [Epub ahead of print

167 Yokoyama M, Origasa H, Matsuzaki M, et. al. Effects of eicosapentaenoic acid on major coronary events in hypercholesterolaemic patients (JELIS): a randomised open-label, blinded endpoint analysis. Lancet 2007; 369: 1090–8.

168 Bo S, Ciccone G, Guidi S, Gambino R, Gentile L, Cassader M, Cavallo-Perin P, Pagano G. Diet or exercise: what is more effective in preventing or reducing metabolic alterations? Eur J Endocrinol. 2008 Sep 4. [Epub ahead of print]

169 Esposito K., Nappo F, Giugliano F et. al. Meal modulation of circulating interleukin 18 and Adiponectin concentrations in healthy subjects and in patients with type 2 diabetes mellitus. Am J Clin Nutr 2003;78:1135–40.

170 King DE, Egan BM, Woolson RF, Mainous AG 3rd, Al-Solaiman Y, Yesri A. Effect of a high fibre diet vs a fiber supplemented diet on C-reactive protein level. Arch Intern Med 2007;167:502–6.

171 Ma Y, Griffith J, Chasan-Taber L, et. al. Association between dietary fiber and serum C-reactive protein. Am J Clin Nutr 2006; 83: 760–6.

172 Ma Y, Hébert JR, Li W, Bertone-Johnson ER, Olendzki B, Pagoto SL, Tinker L, Rosal MC, Ockene IS, Ockene JK, Griffith JA, Liu S. Association between dietary fiber and markers of systemic inflammation in the Women's Health Initiative Observational Study. Nutrition 2008 Jun 16.

173 Oi L, Meigs JB, Liu S, Manson JE, Mantzoros C, Hu FB. Dietary fibers and glycaemic load, obesity, and plasma Adiponectin levels in women with type 2 diabetes. Diabetes Care 2006;29:1501–05.

174 Lichtenstein AH, Appel LJ, Brands M, et. al. Summary of American Heart Association Diet and Lifestyle Recommendations revision 2006. Arterioscler Thromb Vasc Biol. 2006;26(10): 2186–91.

175 Puglisi MJ, Vaishnav U, Shrestha S, Torres-Gonzalez, M,Wood,RJ, Volek, JS, Fernandez,ML Raisins and additional walking have distinct effects on plasma lipids and inflammatory cytokines. Lipids in Health and Disease. 7:14 doi:10.1186/1476-511X-7-14

176 Zern TL, Fernandez ML. Cardioprotective effects of dietary polyphenols. J Nutr 2005;135:2291–4.

177 Zern TL, Wood RJ, Greene C, et. al. Grape polyphenols exert a cardioproteictive effect in pre and post-menopausal women by lowering plasma lipids and reducing oxidative stress. J Nutr 2005;135:1911–1917.

178 Hodgson JM, Ward NC, Burke V, Beilin L, Puddy IB. Increased lean red meat intake does not elevate markers of oxidative stress and inflammation in humans. J Nutr 2007; 137(2): 363–7.

179 Hickling S, Hung J, Knuiman M, Divitini M, Beilby J. Are the associations between diet and C-reactive protein independent of obesity? Prev Med 2008; doi:10.1016/j.ypmed.2008.02.007.

180 Franco OH, Bonneux L, de Laet C, Peeters A, Steyerberg EW, Mackenbach JP. The Polymeal: a more natural, safer, and probably tastier (than the Polypill) strategy to reduce cardiovascular disease by more than 25%. BMJ 2004;329;1447–1450.

181 Krishnaswamy K. Traditional Indian spices and their health significance. Asia Pac J Clin Nutr. 2008;17(Suppl 1):265–8.

182 Tapsell LC, Hemphill I, Cobiac L, et. al. Health benefits of herbs and spices: the past, the present, the future. Med J Aust. 2006 Aug 21;185(Suppl 4):S4–S24

183 Shukla Y, Singh M. Cancer preventive properties of ginger: a brief review. Food Chem Toxicol 2007;45:683–690.

184 Surh YJ. Anti-tumor promoting potential of selected spice ingredients with anti-oxidative and anti-inflammatory activities: a short review. Food Chem Toxicol 2002;40:1091–1097.

185 Gonzales AM, Orlando RA. Curcumin and resveratrol inhibit Nuclear Factor-kappaB-mediated cytokine expression in adipocytes. Nutr Metab (Lond). 2008;5(1):17

186 Anand P, Sundaram C, Jhurani S, et. al. Curcumin and cancer: an 'old-age' disease with an 'age-old' solution. Cancer Lett 2008; 267(1):133–64.

187 Kang J-H, Kim C-S, Han I-S, Kawada T, Yu R. Capsaicin, a spicy component of hot peppers, modulates adipokine gene expression and protein release from obese-mouse adipose tissues and isolated adipocytes, and suppresses the inflammatory responses of adipose tissue macrophages FEBS Letters 2007; 581: 4389–96.

188 Yoon JH, Baek SJ. Molecular targets of dietary polyphenols with anti-inflammatory properties. Yonsei Med J. 2005;46(5):585–96

189 Waterhouse AL. Wine phenolics. Ann N Y Acad Sci 2002;957:21–36.

190 Watzl B, Bub A, Pretzer G, et. al. Daily moderate amounts of red wine or alcohol have no effect on the immune system of healthy men. Eur J Clin Nutr 2004;58(1):40–5.

191 Sanbongi C, Suzuki N, Sakane T. Polyphenols in chocolate, which have antioxidant activity, modulate immune functions in humans in vitro. Cell Immunol 1997;177(2):129–36.

192 Faridi Z, Njike VY, Dutta S, Ali A, Katz DL. Acute dark chocolate and cocoa ingestion and endothelial function: a randomised controlled crossover trial. AJCN 2008;88:58–63

193 Zemel MB, Sun X. Dietary Calcium and Dairy Products Modulate Oxidative and Inflammatory Stress. J Nutr 2008;138:1047–1052.

194 Lönnerdal B, Iyer S. Lactoferrin: molecular structure and biological function. Annu Rev Nutr 1995;15:93–110.

195 Yamauchi K, Wakabayashi H, Shin K, Takase M. Bovine lactoferrin: benefits and mechanism of action against infections. Biochem Cell Biol 2006;84(3):291–6.

196 Shin K, Yamauchi K, Teraguchi S, et. al. Antibacterial activity of bovine lactoferrin and its peptides against enterohaemorrhagic Escherichia coli O157:H7. Lett Appl Microbiol 1998;26(6):407–11.

197 Shin K, Wakabayashi H, Yamauchi K, et. al. Effects of orally administered bovine lactoferrin and lactoperoxidase on influenza virus infection in mice. J Med Microbiol 2005;54(Pt 8):717–23.

198 Buccigrossi V, de Marco G, Bruzzese E, et. al. Lactoferrin induces concentration-dependent functional modulation of intestinal proliferation and differentiation. Pediatr Res 2007;61(4):410–4.
199 Suzuki YA, Shin K, Lönnerdal B. Molecular cloning and functional expression of a human intestinal lactoferrin receptor. Biochemistry 2001;40(51):15771–9.
200 Berlutti F, Schippa S, Morea C, et. al. Lactoferrin downregulates pro-inflammatory cytokines upexpressed in intestinal epithelial cells infected with invasive or noninvasive Escherichia coli strains. Biochem Cell Biol 2006;84(3):351–7.
201 Di Mario F, Aragona G, Dal Bò N, et. al. Use of bovine lactoferrin for Helicobacter pylori eradication. Dig Liver Dis 2003;35(10):706–10.
202 Paesano R, Torcia F, Berlutti F, et. al. Oral administration of lactoferrin increases hemoglobin and total serum iron in pregnant women. Bioch Cell Biol 2006;84(3):377–80.
203 Trümpler U, Straub PW, Rosenmund A. Antibacterial prophylaxis with lactoferrin in neutropenic patients. Eur J Clin Microbiol Infect Dis 1989;8(4):310–3.
204 Tanaka K, Ikeda M, Nozaki A, etal. Lactoferrin inhibits hepatitis C virus viremia in patients with chronic hepatitis C: a pilot study. Jpn J Cancer Res 1999;90(4):367–71.
205 Yamauchi K, Hiruma M, Yamazaki N,et. al. Oral administration of bovine lactoferrin for treatment of tinea pedis. A placebo-controlled, double-blind study. Mycoses 2000;43(5):197–202.
206 King JC Jr, Cummings GE, Guo N, Trivedi L, et. al. A double-blind, placebo-controlled, pilot study of bovine lactoferrin supplementation in bottle-fed infants. J Pediatr Gastroenterol Nutr 2007;44:245–51.
207 Yaqoob P, Pala HS, Cortina-Borja M, et. al. Encapsulated fish oil enriched in a-tocopherol alters plasma phospholipid and mononuclear cell fatty acid compositions but not mononuclear cell functions, Eur. J. Clin Invest 2000;30:260–274.
208 Healy DA, Wallace FA, Miles EA, et. al. The effect of low to moderate amounts of dietary fish oil
209 Simopoulos AP. Essential fatty acids in health and chronic disease. AJCN 1999; 70: 560S-569S.
210 Calder PC. Polyunsaturated fatty acids and inflammation. Prostaglandins Leukot Essent Fatty Acids 2006;75(3):197–202.
211 Badia E, Sacanella E, Fernadez-Sola J, Nicolas JM, Antunez E, Rotilio D, de Gaetano G, Urbano-Marquez A, Estruch R. Decreased tumor-necrosis factor-induced adhesion of human monocytes to endothelial cells after moderate alcohol consumption. AJCN 2004;80: 225–230.
212 Blum S, Aviram M, Ben-Amotz A, Levy Y. Effect of a Mediterranean meal on post-prandial carotenoids, paraoxonase activity and C-reactive protein levels. Ann Nutr Metab 2006; 50: 20–4.
213 Esmaillzadeh A, Kimiagar M, Mehrabi Y, et. al. Dietary patterns and markers of systemic inflammation among Iranian women. J Nutr. 2007 Apr;137(4):992–8.
214 Giugliano D, Esposito K. Mediterranean diet and metabolic diseases. Curr Opin Lip 2008;19: 63–8.
215 Jenkins DJ, Josse AR, Wong JM, Nguyen TH, Kendall CW. The portfolio diet for cardiovascular risk reduction. Curr Atheroscler Rep 2007;9(6):501–7.
216 Lopez-Garcia, E, SchulzeMB, Fung TT, Meigs JB, Rifai N, Manson JE, Hu FB. Major dietary patterns are related to plasma concentrations of markers of inflammation and endothelial dysfunction. Am J Clin Nutr 2004;80:1029 –35.
217 Nanri, A., Yoshida, D., Yamaji, T., Misoue, T., Takayanagi, R., Kono, Dietary patterns and C-reactive protein in Japanese men and women. Am J Clin Nut 2008; 87 (5), pp. 1488–1496.
218 Mena MP, Sacanella E, Vazquez-Agell M, et. al. Inhibition of circulating immune cell activation: a molecular anti-inflammatory effect of the Mediterranean diet. AJCN 2009;89(1):248–56.
219 Kendall CW, Jenkins DJ. A dietary portfolio: maximal reduction of low-density lipoprotein cholesterol with diet. Curr Atheroscler Rep 2004;6(6):492–8.
220 Jenkins D, Kendall C, Josse A, et al. Almonds decrease post-prandial glycemia, insulinemia, and oxidative damage in healthy individuals. J Nutr 2006; 136:2987-92.
221 Josse A, Kendall C, Augustin L, Ellis P, Jenkins D. Almonds and post-prandial glycemia—a dose-response study. Metabolism 2007;56:400–4.
222 Salas-Salvadó J, Casas-Agustench P, Murphy MM, et. al. The effect of nuts on inflammation. 1: Asia Pac J Clin Nutr 2008;17(Suppl 1):333–6.
223 Shimizu M, Son DO. Food-derived peptides and intestinal functions. Curr Pharm Des 2007;13(9):885–95.
224 Cupisti A, Lorenzo G, D'Alessandro C, et. al. Soy protein diet improves endothelial dysfunction in renal transplant patients. Nephrol Dial Transplant 2007;22:229–234.
225 Chako BK, Chandler RT, Mundhekar A, et. al. Revealing anti-inflammatory mechanisms of soy isoflavones by flow: modulation of leukocyte-endothelial interaction. Am J Physiol Heart Circ Physiol 2005;289:H908-H915.
226 Ryan-Borchers TA, Park JS, Chew BP, et. al. Soy isoflavones modulate immune function in healthy post-menopausal women. AJCN 2006;83(5): 1118–25.
227 Monobe M, Ema K, Kato F, et. al. Immunostimulating activity of a crude polysaccharide derived from green tea extract. J Agric Food Chem 2008;56(4):1423–7.
228 Katiyer SK. Skin photoprotection by green tea: antioxidant and immunomodulatory effects. Curr Drug Targets Immune Endocr Metabol Disord 2003;3(3):234–42.
229 Rowe CA, Nantz MP, Bukowski JF, et. al. Specific formulation of CS prevents cold and flu symptoms and enhances gamma,delta T-cell function: a RCT. J Am Coll Nutr 2007;26(5):445–52.
230 Babu PV, Liu D. Green tea catechins and cardiovascular health: an update. Curr Med Chem. 2008;15(18):1840–50.
231 Cao H, Kelly MA, Kari F, Dawson HD, Urban JF Jr, Coves S, Roussel AM, Anderson RA. Green tea increases anti-inflammatory tristetraprolin and decreases pro-inflammatory tumor necrosis factor mRNA levels in rats. J Inflamm (Lond). 2007 Jan 5;4:1.
232 Chen L, Zang HY. Cancer protective mechanisms of the green tea polyphenol (-) –epigallocatchin-3-gallate. Molecules 2007; 12:946–957.
233 Byrans JA, Judd PA, Ellis PR. The effect of consuming instant black tea on postprandial plasma glucose and insulin concentrations in healthy humans. J Am Coll Nutr 2007;26: 471–7.
234 De Bacquer D, Clays E, Delanghe J, De Backer G. Epidemiological evidence for an association between habitual tea consumption and markers of chronic inflammation. Atherosclerosis 2006; 189(2): 428–35

235 Suganuma M, Sueoka E, Sueoka N, Okabe S, Fujiki H. Mechanisms of cancer prevention by tea poyphenols based on inhibition of TNF-alpha expression. Biofactors 200;13(1–4):67–72.
236 Bukowski JF, Percival SS. L-theanine intervention enhances human gammadeltaT lymphocyte function. Nutr Rev 2008;66(2):96–102.
237 Jyonouchi H. Non-IgE mediated food allergy. Inflamm Allergy Drug targets 2008;7(3):173–80.
238 Jyonoucchi H, Sun S, Itokazu N. Innate immunity associated with inflammatory responses with cytokine production against common dietary proteins in patients with ASD. Neuropsychobiologgy 2002;46(2):76–84.
239 Diaz LE, Montero A, Gonzalez-Gross M, et. al. Influence of alcohol consumption on immumological status: a review. Eur J Clin Nutr 2002;56(Suppl 3):S50–3.
240 Magrone T, Candore G, Caruso C, et. al. Polyphenols from red wine modulate immune responsiveness: biological and clinical significance. Curr Pharm Des 2008;14(26):2733–48.
241 Putics A, Vegh EM, Csermely P, et. al. Resveratrol induces the heat-shock response and protects human cells from severe heat stress. Antiox Redox Signal 2008;10(1):65–75.
242 Falchetti R, Fuggetta MP, Lanzilli G, et. al. Effects of resveratrol on human immune cell function. Life Sci 2001;70(1):81–96.
243 Chandra RK. Nutrition and the immune system: an introduction. AJCN 1997;66(2):260S-63S.
244 Harbige LS. Nutrition and immunity with emphasis on infection and AI disease. Nutr Health 1996;10(4):285–312.
245 Ferencik M, Ebringer L. Modulatory effects of Se and Zn on the immune system. Folia Microbiol (Praha) 2003;48(3):417–26.
246 Maggini S, Wintergerst ES, Beveridge S, et. al. Selected vitamins and trace elements support immune function by strengthening epithelial barriers and cellular and humoral immune responses. Br J Nutr 2007;98(Suppl 1):S28–S35.
247 Wintergerst ES, Maggini S, Hornig DH. Contribution of selected vitamins and trace elements to immune function. Ann Nutr Metab 2007;51(4):301–23.
248 Tsuji M, Suzuki K, Kinoshita K, et. al. Dynamic interactions between bacteria and immune cells leading to IgA synthesis. Semin Immunol 2008;20(1):59–66.
249 Van Eden W, Van der Zee R, Van Kooten P, et. al. Balancing the Immune System: Th1 and Th2. Ann Rheum Dis 2002;61(Suppl 2):25–8.
250 Mason KL, Huffnagle GB, Noverr MC, et. al. Overview of Gut immunology. Adv Exp Med Biol 2008;635:1–14.
251 Forschelli ML, Walker WA. The role of GALT and mucosal defence. Br J Nutr 2005;93:S41–8.
252 Ogra PL, Welliver RC Sr. Effects of early environment on mucosal immunologic homeostasis, subsequent bimmune responses and disease outcome. Nestle Nutr Workshop Ser Pediatr Program 2008;61:145–81.
253 Pai R, Kang G. Microbes in the Gut: A digestable account of host-symbiont interactions. Indian J Med Res 2008;128(5):587–94.
254 Walker WA. Mechanisms of action of probiotics. Clin Infect Dis 2008;46(Suppl 2): S87–S91.
255 Suzuli K, Fagarasan S. How host-bacterial interactions lead to IgA synthesis in the gut. Trends Immunol 2008 [Epub ahead of print].
256 Mora JR, von Andrian UH. Role of retinoic acid in the imprinting of gut-homing IgA-secreting cells. Semin Immunol 2009;21(1):28–35.
257 Bodera P. Influence of probiotics on the human immune system (GALT). Recent Pat Inflamm Allergy Drug Discov 2008;2(2):149–53.
258 Bodera P, Chcialowski A. Immunomodulatory effect of probiotic bacteria. Recent Pat Inflamm Allergy Drug Discov 2009;3(1):58–64.
259 Singh V, Singh K, Amdekar S, et. al. Innate and specific gut-associated immunity and microbial interference. FEMS Immunol Med Microbiol 2009;55(1):6–12.
260 Bellanti JA, Zeligs BJ, Malka-Rais J, et. al. Abnormalities of Th1 function in non IgE food allergy, coeliac disease and ileal lymphonodular hyperplasia: a new relationship? Ann Allergy Asthma Immunol 2003;90(6 Suppl 3):84–9.
261 Lin XP, Magnusson J, Ahlstedt S, et. al. Local allergic reaction in food-hypersensitive adults despite a lack of systemic food-specific IgE. J allergy Clin Immun 2002;109(5):879–87.
262 Seksik P, Dray X, Sokol H, et. al. Is there any place for alimentrary probiotics, prebiotics or synbiotics for patients with IBD? Mol Nutr Food Res 2008;52(8):906–12.
263 Famularo G, Mosca L, Minisola G, et. al. Probiotic lactobacilli: a new perspective for the treatment of IBD. Curr Pharm Des 2003;9(24):1973–80.
264 Chandran P, Satthaporn S, Robins A, et. al. IBD: dysfunction of GALT and gut bacteria flora (II). Surgeon 2003;1(3):125–36.
265 Mora JR. Homimg imprinting and immunomodulation in the gut: role of dendritic cells and retinoids. Inflamm Bowel Dis 2008;14(2): 275–89.
266 Mach T. Clinical usefulness of probiotics in IBD. J Physiol Pharmacol 2006;57(Suppl 9):23–33.
267 Guarner F. Inulin and oligofructose: impact on intestinal diseases and disorders. Br J Nutr 2005;93(Suppl 1):S61–5.
268 Heilpern D, Szilagyi A. Manipulation of intestinal microbial flora for therapeutic benefit in IBD: Review of clinical trials of probiotics, prebiotics and synbiotics. Rev Recent Clin Trials 2008;3(3): 167–84.
269 Bohm SK, Kruis W. Probiotics: do they help to control intestinal inflammation? Ann NY Acad Sci 2006;1072:339–50.
270 Vitetta L, Sali A. Probiotics, prebiotics and gastrointestinal health. Medicine Today 2008;9(9):65-70.
271 Goldin BR, Gorbach SL. Clinical indications for probiotics: an overview. Clin Infect Dis 2008;46(Suppl 2):S96–S100.
272 Santosa S, Farnworth E, Jones PJ. Probiotics and their potential health claims. Nutr Rev 2006;64(6):265–74.
273 Gosselink MP, Schouten WR, van Lieshout LM, et. al. Delay of the first onset of pouchitis by oral intake of the probiotic strain Lactobacillus rhamnosus GG. Dis Colon Rectum 2004;47(6): 876–84.
274 Garrote JA, Gomez-Gonzalez E, Bernardo D, et. al. Coeliac disease pathogenesis: the proinflammatory cytokine network. J Pediatr Gastrointerol Nutr 2008;47(Suppl 1):S27–S32.
275 du Toit G, Meyer R, Shah N, et al. Identifying and managing cow's milk protein allergy. Arch Dis Child Educ Pract Ed 2010;95(5):134–44.

276 Mazzatti DJ, Uciechowski P, Hebel S, et. al. Effects of long-term zinc supplementation and deprivation on gene expression in human THP-1 mononuclear cells. J Trace Elem Med Biol 2008;22(4):325–36.
277 Prasad AS. Impact of the discovery of human zinc deficiency on health. J Am Coll Nutr 2009;28(3):257–65.
278 Heyland DK, Jones N, Cvijanovich NZ, et. al. Zinc supplementation in critically ill patients: a key pharmaconutrient? JPEN J Parenter Enteral Nutr 2008;32(5):509–519.
279 Mocchegiani E, Malavolta M, Muti E, et. al. Zinc, metallothioneins and longevity: inter-relationships with niacin and selenium. Curr Pharm Des 2008;14(26):2719–32.
280 Franklin RB, Costello LC. The important role of the apoptotic effects of zinc in the development of cancers. J Cell Biochem 2009 Jan 21 [Epub ahead of print].
281 Prassad AS, Zinc in Human Health: Effect of Zinc on Immune Cells. Mol Med 2008;14(5–6):353–7.
282 Prasad AS. Zinc: Mechanisms of Host Defence. AJN 2007;137:1345–49.
283 Overbeck S, Uciechowski P, Ackland ML, et. al. Intracellular zinc homeostasis in leukocyte subsets is regulated by different expression of zinc exporters ZnT-1 to ZnT-9. J Leukoc Biol 2008;83:368–80.
284 Haase H, Mazzatti DJ, White A, et. al. Differential gene expression after zinc supplementation and deprivation in human leukocyte subsets. Mol Med 2007;13(7–8):362–70.
285 Haase H, Overbeck S, Rink L. Zinc supplementation for the treatment or prevention of disease: current status and future perspectives. Exp Gerontol 2008;43(5):394–408.
286 Wang L, Wildt KF, Castro E, et. al. The zinc-finger transcription factor Zbtb7b represses CD*-lineage gene expression in peripheral CD4+ T-cells. Immunity 2008;29(6):876–87.
287 Hermann-Kleiter N, Gruber T, Lutz-Nicoladoni C, et. al. The nuclear orphan receptor NR2F6 suppresses lymphocyte acrivation and T-helper 17-dependent autoimmunity. s.l.: Immunity 2008;29(2):205–16.
288 Haase H, Ober-Blobaum JL, Engelhardt G, et. al. Zinc signals are essential for lipopolysaccharide-induced signal transduction in monocytes. J Immunol 2008;181(9):6491–502.
289 Prasad AS. Clinical, immunological, anti-inflammatory and anti-oxidant roles of zinc. Exp gerontol 2008;43(5):370–7.
290 Uciechowski P, Kahmann L, Plumakers B, et. al. Th1 and Th2 cell polarisation increases with ageing and is modulated by zinc supplementation. Exp Gerontol 2008;43(5):493–8.
291 Varin A, Larbi A, Dedoussis GV, et. al. In vitro and in vivo effects of zinc on cytokine signalling in human T-cells. Exp Gerontol 2008;43(5):472–82.
292 Mariani E, Neri S, Cattini L, et. al. Effect of zinc supplementation on plasma IL-6 and MCP-1 production and NK-cell function in healthy elderly: interactive influence of +647 MT1a and _174 IL-6 polymorphic alleles. Exp gerontol 2008;43(5):462–71.
293 Haase H, Rink L. Signal transduction in monocytes: the role of zinc ions. Biometals 2007;20(3–4): 579–85.
294 Finamore A, Massimi M, Conti Devirgillis L, et. al. Zinc deficiency induces membrane barrier damage and increases neutrophil transmigration in Caco-2 cells. J Nutr 2008;138(9):1664–70.
295 Vasto S, Mocchegiani E, Malavolta M, et. al. Zinc and the inflammatory/immune response in ageing. Ann N Y Acad Sci 2007;1100:111–22.
296 Scrimgeour AG, Lukaski HC. Zinc and diarrhoeal disease: current status and future perspectives. Curr Opin Clin Nutr Metab care 2008;11(6):711–7.
297 Shen H, Oesterling E, Stromberg A, et. al. Zinc deficiency induces vascular pro-inflammatory parameters associated with NF-kappa B and PPAR signalling. J Am Coll Nutr 2008'27(5):577–87.
298 Plum LM, Rink L, Haase H. The essential toxin: impact of zinc on human health. Int J Environ Res Pub Health 2010;7(4):1342–65.
299 Wintergerst ES, Maggini S, Hornig DH. Immune-enhancing role of Viamin C and zinc and effect on clinical conditions. Ann Nutr Metab 2006;50(2): 85–94.
300 Lukacik M, thomas RL, Aranda JV. A meta-analysis of the effects of oral zinc in the treatment of acute and persistent diarrhoea. Pediatrics 2008;121(2):326–36.
301 Walker CL, Black RE. Zinc for the treatment of diarrhoea: effect on diarrhoea morbidity, mortality and incidence of future episodes. Int J Epidemiol 2010;39 Suppl 1:i63–9.
302 Cuevas LE, Koyanagi A. Zinc and Infection: A review. Ann Trop Paediatr 2005;25(3):149–60
303 McElroy BH, Miller SP. Effectiveness of zinc gluconate glycine lozenges (Cold-Eeze) against the common cold in school-aged subjects: a retrospective chart review. Am J Ther 2002;9(6):472–5.
304 Silk R, LeFante C. Safety of zinc gluconate glycine (Cold-Eeze) in a geriatric population: a randomised placebo-controlled double-blind trial. Am J Ther 2005;12(6):612–7.
305 McElroy BH, Miller SP. An open-label single-centre, phase IV clinical study of the effectiveness of zinc gluconate glycine lozenges (Cold-Eeze) in reducing the duration and symptoms of the common cold in school-aged subjects. Am J Ther 2003;10(5):424–9.
306 Marshall S. Zinc gluconate and the common cold. review of RCTs. Can Fam Physician 1998;44: 1037–42.
307 Garland ML, Hagmeyer KO. The role of zinc lozenges in treatment of the common cold. Ann Pharmacother 1998;32(1):63–9.
308 Eby GA.Zinc ion availability - the determinant of efficacy in zinc lozenge treatment of common colds. J Antimicrobial Chemether 1997;40(4):483–93.
309 Khalili H, Soudbakhsh A, Hajiabdolbaghi M, et. al. Nutritional status and serum zinc and selenium levels in Iranian HIV infected individuals. BMC Infect Dis 2008;8:165.
310 Becker Y. The changes in Th1 and Th2 cytokine balance during HIV-1 infection are indicative of an allergic response to viral proteins that may be reversed by Th2 cytokine inhibitors and immune response modifiers-a review and hypothesis. Virus Genes 2004;28(1):5–18.
311 Zhu B, Symonds AL, Martin JE, et. al. Early growth response gene (Egr-2) controls the self-tolerance of T-cells and prevents the development of lupus-like auto-immune disease. J Exp Med 2008;2005:2295–307.
312 Rathinam C, Lassmann H, Mengel M, et. al. Transcription factor Gfi1 restricts B-cell mediated autimmunity. J Immunol 2008;181(9):6222–9.
313 Wenzlau JM, Juhl K, Yu L, et. al. The cation efflux transporter ZnT8(Slc30A8) is a major auto-antigen in human Type 1 DM. Proc Natl Acad Sci USA 2007;104(43):17040–5.

314 Knip M, Siljander H. Auto-immune mechanisms in Type 1 DM. Autoimmun Rev 2008;7(7):550–7.
315 Egefjord L, Petersen AB, Rungby J. Zinc, alpha cells and glucagon secretion. Curr Diabetes Rev 2010;6(1):52–7.
316 Gyulkhandanyan AV, Lu H, Lee SC, et al. Investigation of transport mechanisms and regulation of intracellular Zn2+ in pancreatic alpha-cells. J Biol Chem 2008;283(15):10184–97.
317 Moro JR, Iwata M, von Andriano UH. Vitamin effects on the immune system: vitamin A and D take centre stage. Nat Rev Immunol 2008;8(9):685–98.
318 Pino-lagos K, Benson MJ, Noelle RJ. Retinoic acid in the immune system. Ann N Y Acad Sci 2008;1143:170–87.
319 Kim CH. Roles of retinoic acid in induction of immunity and immune tolerance. Endocr Metab Immune Disord Drug Targets 2008;8(4):289–94.
320 Bos JD, Spuls PI. Topical treatments in psoriasis: today and tomorrow. Clin dermatol 2008;26(5): 432–7.
321 Strober W. vitamin A rewrites the ABCs of oral tolerance. Mucosal Immunol 2008;1(2):92–5.
322 Ross AC. Vit A supp and retinoic acid treatment in the regulation of antibody responses in vivo. Vitamin Horm 2007;75:197–222.
323 Wiysonge CS, Shey MS, Sterne JA, et. al. Vit A supp for reducing the risk of mother-to-child transmission of HIV infection. Cochrane Database Syst Rev 2005;(4):CD003648.
324 Mehta S, Fawzi W. Effects of vitamins, inc Vit A, on HIV/AIDS patients. vitamin Horm 2007;75:355–83.
325 Ahmad SM, Haskell MJ, Raqib R, et. al. Markers of innate immune fn are associated with vitamin A stores in men. J Nutr 2009;139(2):377–85.
326 Albers R, Bol M, Bleumink R, et. al. Effects of suppl with vitamins A, C, E, Se and Zn on immune function in a murine sterilised model. Nutrition 2003;19(11–12):940–6.
327 Hoffman PR, Berry MJ. The influence of selenium on immune responses. Mol Nutr Food Res 2008;52(11):1273–80.
328 Hoffman PR. Mechanisms by which selenium influences immune responses. Arch Immunol Ther Exp 2007;55(5):289–97.
329 Beck MA, Levander OA, Handy J. Selenium deficiency and viral infection. J Nutr 2003;133(5 Suppl 1):1463S-7S.
330 Rayman MP. The argument for increasing selenium intake. Proc Nutr Soc 2002;61(2):203–15.
331 Rayman MP. Selenium in cancer prevention: a review of the evidence and mechanism of action. Proc Nutr Soc 2005;64(4):527–42.
332 Combs GF Jr, Gray WP. Chemopreventative agents: Se. Pharmacol Ther 1998;79(3):179–92.
333 Rayman MP. The importance of selenium to human health. Lancet 2000;356(9225):233–41.
334 Luty-Frackiewicz A. The role of selenium in cancer and viral infection prevention. Int J Occup Med Environ Health 2005;18(4):305–11.
335 Hurwitz BE, Klaus JR, Llabre MM, et L. Suppression of human immunodeficiency virus type 1 viral load with selenium supplementation: a randomised controlled trial. Arch Intern Med 2007;167:148–54.
336 Naithani R. Organoselenium compounds in cancer chemoprevention. Mini Rev Med Chem 2008;8(7):657–68.
337 Combs GF Jr, Clark LC, Turnball BW. An analysis of cancer prevention by selenium. Biofactors 2001;14(1–4):153–9.
338 Sinha R, El-Bayoumy K. Apoptosis is a critical cellular event in cancer chemoprevention by selenium compounds. Curr Cancer Drug Targets 2004;4(1):13–28.
339 Rikiishi H. Apoptotic cellular events for selenium compounds involved in cancer prevention. J Bioenerg Biomembr 2007;39(1):91–8.
340 Deruelle F, Baron B. vitamin C: Is supplementation necessary for optimal health? J Altern Comp Med 2008;14(10):1291–8.
341 Padayatty SJ, Katz A, Wang Y, et. al. Vit C as an anti-oxidant: evaluation of its role in disease prevention. J Am Coll Nutr 2003;22(1):18–35.
342 Strohle A, Hahn A. vitamin C and immune function. Med Monatsschr Pharm 2009;32(2):49–54.
343 Douglas RM, Hemilia H, Chalker E, et. al. Vit C for preventing and treating the common cold. Cochrane Database Syst Rev 2007;(3):CD000980.
344 Sureda A, Tauler P, Aguilo A, et. al. Influence of an anti-oxidant vitamin enriched drink on pre and post lymphocyte antiox system. Ann Nutr Metab 2008;52(3):233–40.
345 Nakhostin-Roohi B, Babaei P, Rahmani-Nia F, et. al. Effect of Vit C suppl on lipid peroxidation, muscle damage and inflammation after 30 min exercise at 75%VO2max. J Sports Med Phys Fitness 2008;48(2):217–24.
346 Takeshita Y, Katsuki Y, Katsuda Y, et. al. Vit C reversed malfunction of peripheral blood-derived MNCs in smokers through antiox properties. Circ J 2008;72(4):654–9.
347 Van Hoydonck PG, Schouten EG, Manuel-Keenoy B, et. al. Does Vit C supp influence the levels of circulating oxidised LDL, slCAM-1,sVCAM-1 and vWF-antigen in healthy male smokers? Eur J Clin Nutr 2004;58(12):1587–93.
348 Moyad MA, Combs MA, Vrablic AS, et. al. Vit C metabolites, independent of smoking status, sig enhance leukocyte, but not plasma ascorbate concentrations. Adv Ther 2008;25(10):995–1009.
349 Holick MF, Chen TC. Vit D Deficiency: a world-wide problem with health consequences. AJCN 2008;87(4):1080S-6S.
350 Holick MF. Sunlight and Vit D for bone health and prevention of AI diseases, cancers and CVD. AJCN 2004;80(Suppl 6):1678S-88S.
351 Holick MF. Vit D: Importance in the prevention of cancers, Type 1 DM, heart disease and osteoporosis. AJCN 2004;79(3):362–71.
352 Kurylowicz A, Bednarczuk T, Nauman J. The influence of Vit D deficiency on cancers and AI disease devt. Endokrynol Pol 2007;58(2):140–52.
353 Wagner CL, Taylor SN, Hollis BW. Does Vit D make the world go round? Breastfeed Med 2008;3(4): 239–50.
354 Bruce D, Ooi JH, Yu S, Cantorna MT. Vitamin D and host resistance to infection? Putting the cart in front of the horse. Exp Biol Med 2010;235(8): 921–7.
355 Holick MF. Vitamin D: extraskeletal health. Endocrinol Metab Clin North Am 2010;39(2): 381–400.
356 Holick MF. Vitamin D: a D-Lightful health perspective. Nutr Rev 2008;66(10 Suppl 2): S182–94.
357 Holick MF. vitamin D: important for prevention of OP, CVD, IDDM,AI diseases and some cancers. South Med J 2005;98(10):1024–7.
358 DeLuca HF. Evolution of our understanding of vitamin D. Nutr Rev 2008;66(10 Suppl 2):S73–87.

359 Reichrath J. The challenge resulting from + and - effects of sunlight: how much solar UV exposure is appropriate to balance between risks of vitamin D deficiency and skin cancer? Prog Biophys Mol Biol 2006;92(1):9–16.
360 Peyrin-Biroulet L, Oussalah A, Bigard MA. Crohn's Disease: the hot hypothesis . Med Hypotheses 2009;73(1):94–6.
361 Kamen DL, Cooper GS, Bouali H, et. al. Vitamin D deficiency in systemic lupus erythematosus. Autoimmunity Reviews 2006;5:114–117.
362 Melamid ML, Michos ED, Post W, et. al. 25(OH) D levels and the risk of mortality in the general population. Arch Intern Med 2008;168(15):1629–37.
363 Holick MF. Vit D and sunlight: strategies for Ca prevention and other health benefits. Clin J Am Soc Nephrol 2008;3(5):1548–54.
364 Holick MF. vitamin D: its role in cancer prevention and treatment. Prog Biophys Mol Biol 2006;92(1):49–59.
365 Mullin GE, Dobs A. vitamin D and its role in Ca and immunity: a prescription for sunlight. Nutr Clin Pract 2007;22(3):305–22.
366 Adams JS, Ren S, Liu PT, et. al. vitamin D directed rheostatic regulation of monocyte antibacterial responses. J Immunol 2009;182(7):4289–95.
367 Enioutina EY, Bareyan D, Daynes RA. TLR-induced local metabolism of D3 plays an important role in the diversification of adaptive immune responses. J Immunol 2009;182(7):4296–305.
368 van Etten E, Stoffels K, Gysemans C, et. al. Regulation of Vit D homeostasis: implications for the immune system. s.l.: Nutr Rev 2008;66(10 Suppl 2):S125–34.
369 Holick MF. The vitamin D deficiency pandemic and consequences for nonskeletal health. Mol Aspects Med 2008;29(6):361–8.
370 Autler P, Gandini S. Vitamin D supplementation and total mortality: a meta-analysis of randomized controlled trials. Arch Int Med 2007;167:1730-7.
371 Ardiszone S, Cassinotti A, Trabattoni D, et. al. Immunomodulatory effects of vitamin D3 on Th1/Th2 cytokines in IBD: an in vitro study. Int J Immunopathol Pharmacol 2009;2291):63–71.
372 Cantorna MT, Zhu Y, Froicu M, et. al. Vit D status, 1, 25(OH)D3 and the Immune system. AJCN 2004;80(6 Suppl):1717S-20S.
373 Cho WC, Leung KN. In vitro and in vivo immunomodulating and imunorestorative effects of A. membranaceus. J Ethnopharmacol 2007;113(1):132–41.
374 Braun L. Astragalus membranaceous. JCM 2008; 7(3):44–7).
375 Liu QY, Yao YM, Zhang SW, Sheng ZY. Astragalus polysaccharides regulate T cell-mediated immunity via CD11c(high)CD45RB(low) DCs in vitro. J Ethnopharmacol 2010 Jul 8.
376 Tan BK. Immunomodulatory and antimicrobial effects of some TCM herbs: a review. Curr Med Chem 2004;11(11):1423–30.
377 Shao BM, Xu W, Dai H, et. al. A study on the immune reseptors for polysaccharides from the roots of A. mem, a TCM herb.
378 Brush J, Mendenhall E, Guggenheim A, et. al. The effect of Echinacea, Astragalus and Glycyrrhisa on CD69 expression and immune cell activation in humans. Phytother res 2006;20(8):687–95.
379 Wei H, Sun R, Xiao W, et. al. TCM Astragalus reverses predominance of Th2 cytokines and their up-stream transcript factors in lung cancer patients. Oncol Rep 2003;10(5):1507–12.
380 Yang Y, Wang LD, Chen ZB. Effects of A. membranaceus on TH cell subset function in children with recurrent tonsillitis. Zhongguo Dang Dai Er Ke Za Zhi 2006;8(5):376–8.
381 Wang G, Liu CT, Wang ZL, et. al. Effects of A. membranaceus inproducing T-helper cell type 1 polarisation and IFNgamma production by upregulating T-bet expression in patients with asthma. Chin J Integr Med 2006;12(4):262–7.
382 Shan HH, Wang K, Li W, et. al. A. membranaceus prevents airway hyperreactivity in mice related to Th2 inhibition. J Ethnopharmacol 2008;116(2): 363–9.
383 Du Q, Chen Z, Zhou LF, et. al. Inhibitory effects of astragaloside IV on ovalbumin-induced chronic experiemental asthma. Can J Physiol Pharmacol 2008;86(7):449–57.
384 Mao SP, Cheng KL, Zhou YF. Modulatory effects of A. membranaceus on Th1/Th2 cytokine in patients with herpes simplex keratitis. Zhongguo Zhong Xi Yi Jie He Za Zhi 2004;24(2):121–3.
385 Chen W, Li YM, Yu MH. Astragalus polysaccharides: an effective treatment for diabetes prevention in NOD mice. Exp Clin Endocrinol Diabetes 2008;116(8):468–74.
386 Li RJ, Qiu SD, Chen HX, et. al. Effect of A polysaccharide on pancreatic cell mass in type I diabetic mice. Zhongguo Zhong Yao Za Zhi 2007;32(20):2169–73.
387 Li RJ, Qiu SD, Chen HX, et. al. The Immunotherapeutic effects of A polysaccharide in Type I diabetic mice. Biol Pharm Bull 2007;30(3):470–6.
388 Li RJ, Qiu SD, Chen HX, et. al. Immunomodulatory effects of A polysaccharide in diabetic mice. Zhong Xi Yi Jie He Xue Bao 2008;6(2):166–70.
389 Cho WC, Leung KN. In vitro and in vivo anti-tumour effects of AM. Cancer Lett 2007;252: 43–54.
390 Block KI, Mead MN. Immune system effects of echinacea, ginseng and astragalus: a review. Integr Cancer Ther 2003;2(3):247–67.
391 Dong J, Gu HL, Ma CT, et. al. Effects of large dose of AM on the dendritic cell induction of peripheral mononuclear cell and antigen -presenting ability of dendritic cells in children with acute leukaemia. Zhongguo Zhong Xi Yi Jie He Za Zhi 2005;25(10):872–5.
392 Taixang W, Munro AJ, Guanjian L. Chinese medical herbs for chemotherapy side-effects in colorectal cancer patients. Cochrane database Syust Rev 2005;(1):CD004540.
393 McCulloch M, See C, Shu XJ, et. al. Astragalus-based Chinese herbs and platinum-based chemotherapy for advanced non-small-cell lung cancer: meta-analysis of randomised trials. J Clin Oncol 2006;24(3): 419–30.
394 Su L, Mao JC, Gu JH. Effect of IV drip infusion of CTX with high-dose Astraglus injection in treating lupus nephritis. Zhong Xi Yi Jie He Xue Bao 2007;5(3):272–5.
395 Hao Y, Qiu QY, Wu J. Effect of Astragalus polysaccharides in promting neutophil-vascular endothial cell adhesion and expression of related adhesive molecules. Zhongguo Zhong Xi Yi Jie He Za Zhi 2004;24(5):427–30.
396 Lee SJ, Oh SG, Seo SW, et. al. Oral administration of A. membranaceus inhibits the development of DNFB-induced dematitis in NC/Nga mice. Biol Pharm Bull 2007;30(8):1468–71.

397 Prieto JM, Recio MC, Giner RM, et. al. Influence of traditional Chinese anti-inflammatory medicinal plants on leukocyte and platelet functions. J Pharm Pharmacol 2003;55(9):1275–82.

398 Xu HD, You CG, Zhang RL, et. al. Effects of A polysaccharides and astragalosides on the phagocytosis of M. tuberculosis by macrophages. J Int Med Res 2007;35(1):84–90.

399 Nergard CS, Solhaug V. Cranberries for prevention of recurrent urinary tract infections Tidsskr Nor Laegoforen 2009;129(4): 303–4.

400 Feldman M, Weiss E, Shemesh, et. al. Crnberry constituents affect fructosyltransferase expression in Streptococcus mutans Altern Ther Health Med 2009;15(2): 32–8.

401 Liu Y, Gallardo-Moreno AM, Pinzon-Arango PA, et. al. Cranberry changes the physicochemical surface properties of E. coli and adhesion with uroepithelial cells Colloids Surf B Biointerfaces 2008; 65(1): 35–42.

402 Eydelnant IA, Tufenkji N. Cranberry derived proanthocyanidins reduce bacterial adhesion to selected biomaterials Langmuir 2008;24(18): 10273–81.

403 Magarinos HL, Sahr C, Selaive SD, et. al. Prikl Biokhim Mikrobiol 2008; 44(3):333–6.

404 Lavigne JP, Bourg G, Combescure C, et. al. In vitro and in vivo evidence of dose-dependent decrease of uropathogenic Escherichia coli virulence after consumption of commercial Vaccinium macrocarpon (cranberyy) capsules Clin Microbiol Infect 2008;14(4): 350–5.

405 Jepson RG, Craig JC. Cranberries for preventing urinary tract infections. Cochrane Database Systematic Reviews 2008 Jan 23(1): CD001321.

406 Jepson RG, Craig JC A systematic review of the evidence for cranberries and blueberries in UTI prevention Mol Nutr Food Res 2007;51(6): 738–45.

407 McMurdo ME, Argo I, Phillips et al J Antimicrob Chemother 2009;63(2): 389–95.

408 Wing DA, Rumney PJ, Preslicka CW et al Daily cranberry juice for the prevention of asymptomatic bacteriura in pregnancy: a randomised, controlled pilot study J Urol 2008;180 (4): 1367–72.

409 Linde k, Barrett B, Wolkart K. Echinacea for preventing and treating the common cold Cochrane Database Systematic Reviews 2006 Jan 25; (1): CD000530.

410 Barrett B. Medicinal properties of Echinacea: a critical review. Phytomedicine 2003;10: 66–86.

411 Vonau B, Chard S, Mandalia S, Wilkinson D, Barton SE. Does the extract of the plant Echinacea purpurea influence the clinical course of recurrent gnital herpes? Int STD AIDS 2001;12:154–8.

412 Freeman C, Spelman L. A critical evaluation of drug interactions with Echinacea spp. Mol Nutr Food Res 2008; 52(7): 789–98.

413 Ragupathi G, Yeung KS, Leung PC,et. al. Evaluation of widely consumed botanicals as immunological adjuvants. Vaccine 2008;26:4860–5.

414 Braun L, Honey. J Complem Med 2003 V2 N1;54–56.

415 Lusby PE, Coombes A, Wilkinson JM J. Wound Ostomy Continence Nurse 2002; 29(6): 296–300.

416 Blair S. Honey and drug resistant pathogens. Paper presented at the Joint Scientific Meeting of the Australian Society for Microbiology, Cairns, 8–13 July 2000.

417 Taormine Pj, Niermira BA, Beuchat LR, et. al. Inhibitory activity of honey against foodborne pathogens as influenced by the presence of hydrogen peroxide and level of antioxidant power Int J Food Microbiology 2001; 69(3): 217–25.

418 Steinberg D, Kaine G, Gedalia I. Antibacterial effect of propolis and honey on oral bacteria. Am J Dent 1996; 9(6): 236–9.

419 Jull AB, Rodgers A, Walker N. Honey as a topical treatment for wounds. Cochrane Database of Systematic Reviews 2008; Oct 8; (4):CD 05083.

420 Jull AB, Rodgers A, Paraq V et al. Randomized trial of honey-impregnated dressing for venous ulcers Br J Surg 2008;95(2):175–82.

421 Robson V, Dodd S, Thomas D. Standardised antibacterial honey (Medihoney) with standard therapy in wound care: a randomised clinical trial. J Adv Nurs 2009; 65(3): 565–75.

422 Gethin G, Cowman S. Bacteriological changes in sloughy venous leg ulcers treated with manuka honey or hydrogel: an RCT. Journal of wound care 2008;17(6): 241–4.

423 Gethin G, Cowman S. Manuka honey versus hydrogel- a prospective, open label, multicentre, randomised controlled trial to compare desloughing efficacy and healing outcomes in venous ulcers J Clin Nurs 2009;18(3): 466–74.

424 Gethin G, Cowman S, Coroy R. The impact of Manuka honey dressings on the surface pH of chronic wounds Int Wound J 2008; 5(2): 185–94.

425 Evans J, Flavin S. Honey: a guide for healthcare professionals Br J Nurs 2008 Aug 14-Sep 10; 17(15): S24, S26, S28–30.

426 Hernandez-Reif M, Field T, Ironson G, et. al. NK-cells and lymphocytes increase in women with breast cancer following massage therapy. Int J Neurosci 2005;115(4):495–510.

427 Hernandez-Reif M, Ironson G, Field T, et. al. Breast cancer patients have improved immune and neuroendocrine functions following massage therapy. J Psychosom Res 2004;57(1):45–52.

428 Billhult A, Lindholm C, Gunnarsson R, et. al. The effect of massage on cellular immunity, endocrine and psycholigical factors in women with BC- a RCT. Auton Neurosci 2008;140(1–2):88–95.

429 Cabioglu MT, Cetin BE. Acupuncture and immune modulation. Am J Chin Med 2008;36(1):25–36.

430 Peng G. Acupuncture and innate immunity. Zhen Ci Yan Jiu 2008;33(1):49–52.

431 Du J. The messengers from PNS to CNS: involvement of neurotrophins and cytokines in the mechanisms of A. Zhen Ci Yan Jiu 2008;33(1):37–40.

432 Kavoussi B, Ross BE. The neuroimmune basis of anti-inflammatory acupuncture. Integr Cancer Ther 2007;6(3):251–7.

433 Yamaguchi N, Takahashi T, Sakuma M, et. al. A regulates leukocyte subpopulations in human peripheral blood. Evid Based Comp Altern Med 2007;4(4):447–53.

434 Wang JR, Chen XR, Zhang Q, et. al. Effect of moxibustion on immunological fn in the patient of AIDS in spleen-kidney yang deficiency. Zhongguo Zhen Jiu 2007;27(12):892–4.

Chapter 21

Infertility

Introduction

Infertility, defined as the inability to conceive after 1 year of trying, differs from sterility, as many couples are able to conceive after a 1-year period. Sterility is the total inability to produce offspring; that is, the inability to conceive (female sterility) or to induce conception (male sterility),[1] summarised in Table 21.1. Sterility is estimated to occur in 1% of cases. In about 80% of couples, the cause of infertility can be found.[2] Infertility affects 10–15% of couples, 35% of which is attributed to female infertility and 30% to male infertility.[3] This figure is now as high as 1 in 6 couples suffering infertility in New South Wales (Australia).[4] It is essential infertile couples are investigated thoroughly to exclude reversible organic causes such as infections requiring antibiotics, or polyps requiring surgery.

Causes of infertility

Males

Causes of infertility in men include:

- idiopathic/unknown
- lifestyle — diet, exercise, smoking
- sperm defects — concentration, morphology
- low sperm count
- low percentage of progressively motile sperm
- low percentage of good sperm morphology
- high degree of sperm with abnormal morphology: teratozoospermia index
- high percentage of chromosome fragmentation: sperm chromosome structural assay (SCSA) abnormality
- infection — pelvic/testicular (e.g. mumps, genital infection)
- illness (e.g. haemochromatosis)
- environmental, chemical, toxin exposure
- weight — obese or underweight
- nutritional disorders
- structural (e.g. varicocoele malformation)
- hormonal imbalance (e.g. testosterone or thyroid deficiency)
- raised scrotal temperature (e.g. excessive driving, use of hot tubs)
- drugs (e.g. recreational drugs, antidepressants)
- age.

Females

Causes of infertility in women include:

- idiopathic/unknown
- lifestyle — diet, exercise, smoking
- ovulation disorders (e.g. irregular ovulation, polycystic ovary syndrome [PCOS], amenorrhoea)
- hormonal disorders (e.g. endometriosis, thyroid disease)
- disorders of the fallopian tubes and/or uterus (e.g. fibroids and cervical pathology, such as polyps)
- immune problems; anti-sperm antibodies, auto-immune thyroid disease
- age
- infection — pelvic (e.g. PID, STDs such as chlamydia trachomata, ureaplasma urealyticum)
- illness (e.g. coeliac disease, malignancy, thyroid disease)
- environmental, chemical, toxin exposure
- medication (e.g. hormonal, anti-epileptics [may cause folate and B12 deficiency], chemotherapy)
- weight — obese or underweight
- nutritional disorders
- lactational amenorrhoea.

The following factors contribute to female infertility

- non-specific immune factors such as vaginal pH, as well as specific immunity such as antibodies to sperm and auto antibodies to proteins in the phospholipid bilayer such as cardiolipin and beta 2 glycoprotein plus natural killer cells
- steroid hormone levels influenced by:
  - thyroid function
  - insulin secretion
  - body fat percentage
  - exposure to xeno-estrogens and stress

Table 21.1 Causes of infertility

Origin of sterility	Cause
No eggs	Due to: • menopause • radiation damage • auto-immune disease
No sperm	Due to: • arrested development • infectious causes • immature sperm
Fallopian tube obstruction	Due to: • infections, particularly *Chlamydia* • surgery • endometriosis
No uterus	Medically recommended hysterectomy

(Source: adapted from Jansen R, 1998 *Getting Pregnant*. Allen and Unwin, Sydney)

- incompatible endometrial environment due to:
  - hormonal imbalance
  - abnormal uterine structure
  - fibroids
  - presence of infections.

Genetic variations

A significant number of infertility cases in both men and women relate to exposure to toxins in the environment, and nutritional disorders and deficiencies. In men, these factors can influence major causes of infertility such as sperm count, decreased sperm motility, sperm agglutination, impotence and ejaculatory disorders. In the last 50 years, the prevalence of male infertility disorders has doubled, and sperm counts have declined by about one-third. In the 1940s typical sperm count was estimated to be 60 in 1 million. Today the average sperm count is around 20 in 1 million. In women, over-exposure to toxins and nutritional deficiencies can lead to incorrect weight balance and body mass ratio for conception, underproduction of ova and altered hormone levels and processes.

General CM use

Complementary medicine use amongst infertile couples is common. In an Australian study of 100 women at a fertility clinic, 66% were using complementary medicines alongside prescribed medication, namely multivitamins, mineral and herbal supplements.[5]

Lifestyle risk factors

Lifestyle risk factors for infertility include:

- age
- poor lifestyle factors
- psychological factors
- emotional stress
- excessive exposure to toxins
- smoking
- lack of physical exercise
- underweight or overweight
- poor dietary habits
- nutrient deficiencies.

Age as a risk factor

The risk of infertility in women and men increases with age and this is becoming a bigger problem as more women choose to delay childbearing. Infertility increased from 8% amongst women aged 19–26 and up to 18% in those aged 35–39 according to a European survey.[6] Male age was significant after 30 years of age with estimated incidence of infertility of 18–28% between the ages of 35–40 years. The authors concluded that whilst older couples may have increased infertility, they may conceive if they keep trying for an additional year.

In a more recent study in the UK, data from a total of 7172 women at a fertility clinic, found there was an association between female age and the cause of female infertility and more women over 35 had unexplained infertility.[7]

Hormonal imbalance as a risk factor

Hormonal abnormalities, such as those caused by significant, prolonged stress, or through weight or dietary imbalances can play a role in infertility, particularly in women.

Thyroid disorders

Thyroid autoimmunity (TAI) has also been associated with infertility in women. TAI in women of a reproductive age frequently leads to hypothyroidism, associated with reproductive complications such as irregular menstrual cycles.[8, 9]

Ovarian and uterine disorders

Other disorders include endometriosis plus ovarian causes of infertility including polycystic ovary syndrome (PCOS), which is commonly linked with autoimmune thyroid disorders.[9]

Nutrient deficiencies as risk factors

Deficiencies in essential vitamins and minerals can contribute to infertility by affecting sperm count and motility in men, and hormonal processes in women.

Males

Antioxidants

It has been reported that in approximately 25% of couples, infertility can be attributed to decreased semen quality. In a recent convenience sample of healthy non-smoking men from a non-clinical setting, it was concluded that higher antioxidant intake was associated with higher sperm numbers and motility.[10]

Also, antioxidant deficits in males can lead to a decline in sperm motility. Spermatozoa cell membranes contain high concentrations of fatty acids, which are highly susceptible to oxidative damage. Adequate levels of antioxidants are required in order to maintain healthy cell membranes.[11]

Selenium

Selenium is an important nutrient for male fertility. Two of the proteins found to be structurally important in sperm require adequate levels of selenium.[12] Deficiency is associated with decreased sperm motility and increased abnormal sperm.[13]

Vitamin B12

Vitamin B12 deficiency can cause male infertility as it affects both sperm count and motility.[14]

Zinc

High concentrations of zinc are present in ejaculatory fluid. Frequent ejaculation, can contribute to zinc deficiency. This is associated with oligospermia, decreased serum testosterone levels and decreased sperm count and motility.[11,13]

Females

Folate

An early study has suggested that blood folate level recovery in women following a normal pregnancy delivery and 1 year of breastfeeding may require supplementation with a multivitamin in order to re-establish blood folate levels before further conceiving.[15] Folic acid deficiency can play a role in ovulatory infertility.[16] Women trying to conceive within this 2-year period of folate replenishment may continue to experience difficulty with conception. Deficiency may also be caused by digestive disorders such as celiac disease.

Vitamin B12

Pernicious anaemia leading to vitamin B12 deficiency can lead to female infertility.[16]

Vitamin B2

Insufficient levels of vitamin B2 can lead to altered levels of oestrogen and progesterone, often causing irregular menstruation. Treatment of menstrual problems, such as irregular periods, PMT and general menstrual difficulties, often results in a correction of infertility issues also.[17]

Iron

Conception can be difficult in women with low iron stores.[18]

Zinc

The effect of zinc deficiency on female fertility has not been extensively studied, however animal trials have linked low zinc levels with impaired ovulation and an increased amount of deteriorated ovocytes.[19] Zinc supplementation can be beneficial for women experiencing fertility problems however an excessive presence of zinc also appears to be detrimental.[20]

General signs

Hormonal signals and Billings Ovulation Method (BOM)

For sub-fertile couples, the BOM can be useful to help identify the time of maximum fertility in the women's cycle. BOM allows a woman to familiarise herself with the cyclical changes that are happening in her body, such as cervical mucous and temperature changes (basal body temperature) and timing of menstrual cycle. A useful multilingual website to assist couples to learn the BOM is available free to the public at:

- http://www.woomb.org/bom/index.html.

By mastering the BOM, a couple can time sexual activity during peak ovulation period to maximise the risk of conceiving.

A trial conducted by the World Health Organization in 5 different countries demonstrated up to 97% of women had an excellent or good interpretation of the BOM. However, couples should be encouraged not to use this method alone to assist conception. Similarly, the BOM can be used to help prevent conception as a natural method of contraception and if used correctly, can achieve a failure rate as low as 0.5–1.0% with accurate teaching and vigilant implementation.[21, 22] However, higher reported failure rates, up to 3%, have been documented worldwide and occurred due to factors such as inadequate teaching, poor compliance and poor understanding of the BOM.[23, 24, 25]

Urinary ovulation predictors can be useful in identifying urinary LH surges at the time of ovulation, but requires the woman to estimate the timing of the ovulation and a LH surge is not necessarily followed up with an ovulation, as commonly occurs in PCOS and in luteinised unruptured follicle where some LH is released by the follicle but not enough to cause an ovulation. This method can be expensive for couples wanting to identify time of ovulation.

Scent of a woman

Interestingly studies indicate that the scent of a woman may provide a clue as to when she is ovulating and alert men to her current state of fertility. A study demonstrated that men could detect differences in body odour in women correlating to different stages of their menstrual cycle.[26] Women menstruating were rated as the most intense and least attractive odour; whilst during the most fertile period they were rated by men as least intense smelling and the most attractive.

Lifestyle and diet

Lifestyle factors play an important part in successful fertility outcomes.[27]

A recent study has reported that couples who succeed in becoming fertile, especially those diagnosed with unexplained infertility, do so by adhering to lifestyle changes.[28] Only those couples who sought information to help them conceive found the experience empowering.

Females

A cohort of 17 544 women monitored over an 8-year period found that women who adhered to a healthy lifestyle and *fertility diet* pattern were associated with a lower risk of ovulatory infertility disorder.[29] This risk was reduced to 69% for women in the highest quintile group compared to those in the lowest quintile for adherence to the *fertility diet* pattern in healthy women. Furthermore, women's age (older than 35 years of age), parity and body weight (Body Mass Index ≥ 25) were inversely associated with infertility.

The following lifestyle factors were protective towards infertility for women:

- *high fertility diet* — lower intake of trans fat, greater intake of monounsaturated fat, lower intake of animal protein, greater vegetable protein intake, higher intake of high-fibre, low-glycaemic carbohydrates, preference for high-fat dairy products, higher non-haeme iron intake (found in fruits, vegetables, grains, eggs, milk, meat)
- higher frequency of multivitamin or iron supplement use
- vigorous physical activity 30 minutes or more daily
- weight control; Body Mass Index between 20–25.

Of interest, fertile women were more likely to consume tea, coffee, drink alcohol, be physically active and less likely to smoke, have long menstrual cycles and be recent past users of the oral contraceptive pill. High-fat dairy food reduced the risk of anovulatory infertility by more than 50% in contrast to low-fat dairy food that reduced risk of successful conception by 11%.

Mind–body medicine

Psychological factors

Psychological factors such as stress alone do not cause infertility, however they can play a role in factors such as impotence and menstrual problems. In the brain, the 2 major organs involved in the production of stress hormones and reproductive hormones LH and FSH are the pituitary gland and the hypothalamus. The brain is connected through fibres in the spinal cord to the reproductive organs. The ordinary sequence for the release of reproductive hormones can be severely disrupted during times of significant stress, leading to irregularities with menstruation and ovulation. In some cases, ovulation may come to a compete halt. In men, fertility problems contributed to by emotional stress include erectile dysfunction and hormonal imbalances.

Treating infertility in both men and women often involves psychological intervention. As trouble conceiving can itself be an extremely stressful situation, a stress–infertility cycle may be created. This can be aided with activities which have been shown to reduce stress, anxiety and depression. These include regular exercise, meditation, relaxation breathing, guided visualisation and, most commonly, counselling.

The therapeutic dilemma is how to use psychotherapy.[30] Recently it was reported that medical and psychosexual therapies are not 2 distinct therapeutic entities to be used in different clinical settings. They are, however, 2 important tools to be simultaneously considered (as well as often simultaneously employed) to fully rescue the sexual satisfaction of the couple that is trying to conceive.

In vitro fertilisation (IVF) can be quite a stressful experience for many couples. Women who undergo IVF are more likely to have parenting difficulties and be admitted into a special unit for postnatal mood disturbance or infant sleeping disorder compared with women conceiving naturally.[31] Couples undergoing IVF require additional support.

Support groups

A randomised controlled trial (RCT) was conducted to assess the benefits of a web-based education and support program for women with infertility and assessed for psychological outcomes such as infertility distress, infertility self-efficacy, decisional conflict, marital cohesion and coping style.[32] At 4-weeks follow-up women exposed to the online program were observed to significantly improve in the area of social concerns related to infertility distress, and felt better informed about a challenging medical decision and experienced less global stress, sexual concerns, distress related to child-free living, increased infertility self-efficacy and decision-making clarity. Those women who spent more time online (>60 minutes) gained more psychological benefits.[32]

Stress reduction and/or meditation

Relaxation therapy

In a study measuring the effects of stress reduction on fertility, 54 women were enrolled in a behavioural treatment program and taught a relaxation response technique over 10 weeks. The women were instructed to utilise this practice twice daily for 20 minutes at home. At the end of the trial the women were reported as experiencing significantly less stress, depression and fatigue. Within months of completion of the study, 34% of the women became pregnant — a figure much higher than what is expected in women undergoing typical infertility treatment.[33]

Transcendental meditation (TDM)

An early study of TDM and infertility reported that TDM was useful in infertility.[34]

Sexual activity

Infrequent or lack of sexual activity and difficulties with sex, such as erectile dysfunction in males, can interfere with fertility. Lifestyle factors such as overwork, exhaustion and night-shift can all impact on the frequency of sex and the chances of conception. Erectile dysfunction is a common problem in men over 60 years of age. Researchers in Finland found in over 1000 middle-aged men, that those who had infrequent intercourse (less than once weekly) were more likely to experience sexual dysfunction compared with men who had sex weekly.[35] Stress and fatigue is a large contributor to lack of sexual activity.

Sleep

Shiftwork is associated with menstrual irregularities, reproductive disturbances, risk of adverse pregnancy outcome and sleep disturbances in women. A study of 68 nurses, aged less than 40 years, evaluated sleep, menstrual function, and pregnancy outcome and found 53% of the women noted menstrual changes when working shiftwork; menstrual irregularities which may impact on fertility.[36]

Sunshine

A number of animal studies have demonstrated vitamin D deficiency can cause infertility.[37] Vitamin D is an important factor in the biosynthesis of both female and male gonads. No reliable human data are available yet to recommend vitamin D for infertility. Nevertheless, in view of the multiple health benefits of vitamin D from safe sun exposure, if blood levels are reduced then vitamin D supplementation should be advised in order to improve overall wellbeing.

Environment

Smoking

Smoking is well documented as contributing to problems with fertility in both men and women.[38] Smoking reduces fertility in women by having a direct detrimental effect on the uterus, on the oocytes and embryos by increasing the zona pellucida thickness.[39] Of interest, in a study of women who received donated eggs through an IVF program, those that smoked or had a history of smoking did not affect pregnancy outcome.[40] Nevertheless, it is still advisable to instruct women to avoid smoking due to harmful effects on the fetus.

Infertile men who smoke have higher levels of seminal oxidative stress and sperm DNA damage[41] and lower levels of antioxidant levels in the seminal fluid.[42] Smoking was associated with a 48% increase in seminal leukocyte concentrations and a 107% increase in seminal oxidative stress compared with infertile non-smokers, suggesting men who smoke should quit.

Smoking increases the risk of impotence and erectile dysfunction in men who smoke or have a past history of smoking compared with those who have never smoked.[43]

External heat

Men should avoid high scrotal temperatures such as the use of hot tubs, long hours of sitting, and tight clothing as heat can inversely impact on sperm quality and count.[44] Men who drove for more than 2 hours a day recorded significant scrotal temperature rises by 1.7–2.2°C than that recorded while walking. This rise in scrotal temperature indicates a potential cause for male infertility in some professions; for example, taxi drivers and office workers.

Chemicals and toxins

Exposure to environmental toxins such as radiation, heavy metals and chemicals can cause oxidative stress and sperm DNA damage.[45–48] Oxidative damage to DNA may also impact on female fertility.[49]

Increased industrialisation and use of agricultural chemicals in the 20th century has contributed to exposure of thousands of chemicals which has contributed to impaired fertility in both men and women.[50]

Males

Semen quality, concentration and counts have declined significantly in a number of countries implicating exogenous oestrogens, heavy metals and pesticides as causes.[51, 52]

Exposure of xenobiotics and oestrogen-mimicking chemicals in the environment and food such as beef ingested by mothers has been implicated as a possible cause of poor testicular development in male fetuses *in-utero* leading to poor reproductive ability and low sperm concentration later in life.

A US study of males found that sperm concentration was inversely related to the number of maternal beef meals per week.[53] Son's of mothers who consumed more than 7 beef meals per week had lower sperm concentration by up to 24% than in men whose mothers ate less beef. No other meat intake, such as lamb, was associated with low sperm. Also sperm concentration was lowest in men who ate more beef.[53]

A multi-faceted therapeutic approach to improve male fertility involves identifying harmful environmental and occupational risk factors, while correcting underlying nutritional imbalances to encourage optimal sperm production and function.

Heavy metals

Exposure to heavy metals, such as lead and mercury, can interfere with fertility processes in men. For example, mercury can decrease the ability of the sperm to penetrate the ova for fertilisation, and causes breakages in sperm DNA strands. In women, lead can contribute to infertility, as well as other reproductive disorders such as premature membrane rupture, pregnancy-related disorders and premature delivery.[54, 55]

Cadmium exposure has also been associated with altered concentrations of serum estradiol, FSH and testosterone, the latter can lead to a decrease in testicular size.[19]

A study assessing heavy metals in premenopausal women found an association between cadmium and endometriosis.[56] The study concluded that further investigations in properly designed studies were needed.

Exposure to these toxins can occur with regular contact with heavy metal. Other chemicals which can affect fertility can be found in adhesives, cleaning compounds and cigarette smoke. Treatment for infertility, especially in males, should limit contact with these substances plus the use of antioxidants, in the hope of reversing the damage caused by over-exposure.

Seasonal and regional variations in sperm quality

Researchers noted regional variation in sperm quality across European nations and higher levels of sperm concentration noted over the winter period compared to summer (summer about 70% of winter).[57] For instance, Finnish men have higher sperm counts than in Danish men. Environmental exposures and lifestyle factors may be contributors to these regional differences.

Physical activity

Exercise

Exercise plays an important role in fertility. Obese women with PCOS who suffered anovulatory infertility demonstrated a significant improvement in menstrual cycles and fertility equally in a structured exercise training (SET) program and to dietary interventions.[58] Both the frequency of menses and the ovulation rate were significantly higher in the SET group than in the dietary group but the increased cumulative pregnancy rate was not significant.

However, a study of women undergoing IVF found that regular exercise before IVF may negatively affect outcome, especially in women who exercised 4 or more hours per week.[59]

Yoga

Many postures are designed to help with hormone balance and impact positively on fertility and assist with relaxation for both men and women.[60]

Nutritional influences

As stated earlier under lifestyle, the *high fertility diet* has been shown to promote fertility.[29] It includes a lower intake of trans fat, greater intake of monounsaturated fat, lower intake of animal protein, greater vegetable protein intake, higher intake of high-fibre, low glycaemic carbohydrates, preference for high-fat dairy products, and higher non-haeme iron intake (found in fruits, vegetables, grains, eggs milk, meat).

Alcohol

Excessive alcohol consumption can cause hyperprolactinemia which is associated with female infertility.[61] In males, a high intake of alcohol has been shown to have a negative effect on Leydig cells, and therefore possibly on testosterone production.[62] This is specifically caused by the ethanol in alcohol, and the degree of damage depends on the length of exposure and quantity ingested.[63]

Of interest, some alcohol consumption (1–20 standard drinks per week) is associated with reduced incidence of erectile dysfunction by 25–30% compared with non-drinkers.[64]

Caffeine

Caffeine promotes dopamine production, and this in turn inhibits the production of prolactin, a deficiency or excess of which increases the risk of infertility in women. Consuming as little as 1 caffeinated drink per day is associated with a temporary reduction in conception.[65, 66]

Underweight or overweight

Excessive or insufficient body weight in women is associated with infertility. For conception, the ideal body fat percentage in women is between 20% and 25%. A body fat percentage below 17% can result in anovulation and, following correction of body fat ratio, it may take as long as 2 years before regular ovulation resumes.[67]

A study of about 4000 pregnant women recruited from antenatal clinics or hospitals at least at 20 weeks of gestation, found after adjustment for socio-demographic, biologic and lifestyle-related factors, for women smokers there was a strong association between obesity (BMI of > or = 30 kg/m^2) and women whose BMI was <20 kg/m^2 and delayed conception. Of interest, the same analysis conducted for women non-smokers showed no association. The authors concluded that women who are underweight or obese require a longer time to conceive if they also smoke.[67] A recent study demonstrated obesity is a clear risk factor reducing chances of spontaneous conception in sub-fertile, ovulatory women.[68]

In men, obesity (BMI >30kg/m^2) is associated with hypogonadism, and therefore with infertility.[69] Studies have shown a correlation between increased BMI and decreased testosterone levels, sperm motility and sperm concentrations.[70–74]

Trans-fatty acids (TFA)

TFA such as those found in commercially baked and fried products (e.g. French fries, fish burgers, chicken nuggets, corn chips, pies, Danish rolls and doughnuts) is linked to increased risk of infertility. A prospective cohort study of over 18 000 women demonstrated that for every 2% increase in energy intake from TFAs, there was a significant increase in risk of ovulatory infertility by up to 73% compared with no TFA intake. The study reported[75] that this association was similar to that seen with fat intake and insulin in Polycystic Ovary Syndrome.

Males

Soy consumption

Soy contains isoflavones which are known to have mild estrogenic activity. Men who consume high dietary soy theoretically may suffer reduced sperm concentration consequently impacting on their fertility. Over a 3-month period, men who consumed isoflavone-rich foods (the equivalent of 1 cup of soy milk or 1 serving of soy product every second day), had on average less sperm concentration of 41 million/millilitre than men who didn't eat soy.[76] This inverse association was more evident in overweight and obese men. Soy products did not impact other parameters of sperm quality such as motility, morphology, total sperm count or ejaculate volume.

Nutritional supplements

Antioxidants

Antioxidants may be of benefit in infertility although there is mixed debate about their potential role. [77, 78] The general weight of evidence is supportive of the use of antioxidants for infertility.

Males

Antioxidants

Male sperm membranes are rich in polyunsaturated fatty acids and are sensitive to oxygen-induced damage mediated by lipid peroxidation and free radicals. Seminal plasma contains a rich source of antioxidants and mechanisms which are likely to quench the free radicals and protect against any likely damage to spermatozoa. Antioxidants such as vitamin C, vitamin E, glutathione, and coenzyme Q_{10} have some proven beneficial effects in treating male infertility.[79] Men who took just 1 multivitamin daily during IVF program recorded a statistically significant improvement in viable pregnancy rate (38.5% of transferred embryos resulting in a viable fetus at 13 weeks gestation) compared to the control group (16% viable pregnancy) of taking a placebo.[80]

Supplementation with antioxidant vitamins C and E, selenium and coenzyme Q_{10} can prevent and reverse oxidative damage to sperm and therefore increase sperm motility and quality.[81] Sperm improved with antioxidant supplements (1g vitamin C and 1g vitamin E daily) even in short periods of time given over a 2-month period.[82] The percentage of DNA-fragmented spermatozoa was markedly reduced in the antioxidant treatment group after treatment compared with pre-treatment levels.

High diet and supplement in vitamin C is associated with higher sperm number; vitamin E intake improved motility and sperm count; beta-carotene improved sperm concentration and motility.[83]

Vitamin C

An open trial of infertile male patients with oligospermia received 1000mg of vitamin C twice daily for a maximum of 2 months. Results showed that the mean sperm count increased from 14 x 10^6 sperms/ml to an average of 33 x10^6 sperms/mL, the mean sperm motility increased significantly from 31% to 60%, and mean sperms with normal morphology increased significantly from 43% to 67%. This study demonstrated that vitamin C supplementation in infertile men improves semen quality.[84]

Vitamin B12

Infertility disorders arising from B12 deficiency can be treated with B12 supplementation. Oral vitamin B12 can also be used provided that the patient does not have pernicious anaemia, where sublingual or injections of B12 are required. It may be wise to supplement with B12 where decreased sperm count and motility are present, even if no symptoms of deficiency are obvious.[85]

Folate

Folate did not demonstrate any benefits on sperm quality.[86] However high total folate intake in diet and as supplements may lower the risk of genetically abnormal sperm known as aneuploidy but not for other micronutrients (zinc, vitamin C, vitamin E and beta-carotene).[87]

Glutathione

Glutathione is also instrumental in the defence against oxidative stress in the spermatogenic epithelium. It has been shown to be particularly important in the treatment of oligozoospermia due to its antioxidant effect during spermiogenesis.[88] Glutathione has to be supplemented intramuscularly as it is destroyed in the stomach.[89] Further, glutathione levels cannot be increased to a clinically beneficial extent by orally ingesting a single dose of glutathione.[90] That is glutathione is manufactured intracellularly from its precursor amino acids, glycine, glutamate and cystine.

Hence food sources or supplements that increase glutathione must either provide the precursors of glutathione, or enhance its production. Consuming foods rich in sulfur-containing amino acids can help increase glutathione levels.

Asparagus is a leading source of glutathione. Foods such as broccoli, avocado and spinach are also known to boost glutathione levels. Raw eggs, garlic and fresh unprocessed meats contain high levels of sulfur-containing amino acids and can also significantly assist to maintain optimal glutathione levels.

Minerals

Selenium

Supplementation with selenium has been shown in some trials to increase sperm count and motility. A small study of infertile men supplemented daily by vitamin E (400mg) and selenium (225μg) or vitamin B (4.5gm/day) over 3 months demonstrated the vitamin E and selenium treatment group produced a significant improvement of sperm motility and sperm quality in comparison to the vitamin B group.[91] However, an excessive presence of selenium can have the opposite effect.[92]

Zinc

Supplementation with zinc can increase fertility, particularly in oligospermic men.[93] Combined 66mg zinc and 5mg folate supplements improved sperm concentration by 18% in men who were sub-fertile compared with those on placebo.[94]

Another study demonstrated zinc supplementation did not benefit sperm quality.[84]

Amino acids

Arginine

Arginine deficiency can contribute to low sperm count and motility, but can be reversed with supplementation.[95]

Carnitine

A recent systematic review has concluded that supplementation with carnitine increased both sperm count and motility.[96] The administration of L-carnitine and/or L-acetyl carnitine may be effective in improving pregnancy rate and sperm kinetic features in patients affected by male infertility. However, it was also reported that the exact efficacy of carnitines on male infertility needs to be confirmed by further investigations.[96]

Patients with abacterial prostato-vesiculoepididymitis (PVE) and elevated seminal and leukocyte concentrations and on non-steroidal anti-inflammatory drugs for 2 months were followed by treatment with carnitine for 2 months. Men demonstrated significant reduction in reactive oxygen species associated with increased sperm motility and viability.[97]

Coenzyme Q_{10} (CoQ_{10})

CoQ_{10} may play a role in male infertility by increasing sperm motility. An open, uncontrolled pilot study of infertile men with abnormal sperm motility resulted in a significant increase in sperm motility compared with baseline.[98] Similarly an RCT has found that CoQ_{10} treatment improves sperm motility in men with idiopathic asthenozoospermia.[99, 100]

Lycopene

A small preliminary trial of lycopene (2000mg twice a day) for 3 months may play a role in the management of idiopathic male infertility, by improving sperm concentration.[101] However, larger RCTs are essential before definitive therapeutic guidelines can be made for the use of lycopene.

Female

Antioxidants

The evidence is a lot less for the use of antioxidants in the treatment of infertility and care should be undertaken especially with excessive or imbalanced use of antioxidants in women of child-bearing years aiming to fall pregnant.

Use of antioxidants together with a good diet improves fertility in women.[5] A Cochrane review of the studies also found that women given any type of vitamin(s) compared with controls were significantly less likely to develop pre-eclampsia and more likely to have a multiple pregnancy.[102]

Folate

Folate deficiency can be corrected with folic acid supplementation and is recommended as routine for at least 3 months for any woman planning a pregnancy.[103]

Vitamin B2 and B6

Supplementation with vitamin B2 to achieve optimal hormone levels, and vitamin B6 to alleviate PMT can lead to improved fertility.

Minerals

Iron

Relative iron deficiency is common in women in reproductive years. Taking iron supplements up to 40mgs or more can reduce risk of anovulatory infertility by up to 60% and improve chances of conception compared with women who did not take iron supplements.[104] Potential side-effects of iron supplements need to be weighed against any decision to supplement women with iron.

Herbal medicine

Herbal remedies can be used to assist with infertility however, many herbs have also been trialled to deal specifically with secondary causes of infertility, such as irregular cycles, PCOS and erectile dysfunction. Generally it is difficult to research herbs for infertility, particulary in women, due to there unknown effect on the fetus.

Males

The herbs discussed below have been used in the treatment of male infertility but there is incomplete evidence regarding their use.[5, 105]

Tribulus terrestris

Preparations based on the saponin fraction of *Tribulus terrestris* are used for treatment of infertility and libido disorders in men and women.[106] Tribulus terrestris may increase testosterone levels, sperm count and sperm morbility.[105, 106]

Pygeum africanum,[107, 108, 109] *Plantago ovata*[111] and *Serenoa repens*[111] may also be useful in infertility remedies.

Serenoa repens may be useful for testicular atrophy.[106]

Korean red ginseng (KRG) (*Panax ginseng)*

A double-blind cross-over study of 45 patients randomised to KRG or placebo over a 2-month period demonstrated improved penile rigidity and erectile function, and better penetration maintenance and erection during sex in the treatment group compared with the placebo group.[112]

Panax ginseng may be useful for increased sperm production.[108, 109]

Panax ginseng and *Siberian ginseng* may be useful for sexual dysfunction.[113, 114]

Pycnogenol

A small French study with 19 sub-fertile men given 200mg of pycnogenol daily (orally) for 90 days resulted in significant improvement in capacitated sperm morphology and mannose receptor binding.[115] The study concluded that the increase in morphologically and functionally normal sperm could allow couples diagnosed with teratozoospermia to forgo IVF and either experience improved natural fertility or undergo less invasive and less expensive fertility promoting procedures (such as intrauterine insemination).[106]

Japanese herbal medicine — *sairei-to*

The Japanese herbs called *sairei-to* (9g/day) significantly increased sperm concentration and motility, and the pulsatility index of the testicular artery in men with oligospermia in a trial period over 3 months.[116]

Maca *(Lepidium meyenii)*

The root of the Peruvian plant Maca has traditionally been used as an aphrodisiac and its fertility-enhancing properties.[117] Also, Maca appears to improve sexual performance in men with mild erectile dysfunction.[118]

Other herbs

Other herbs that may assist male infertility but warrant further research include: astragalus, schisandra, *Ginkgo biloba*, turmeric and ginger.

Females

Vitex agnus castus

A randomised double-blind control trial of a registered product called Mastodynon® containing *Vitex agnus castus* preparation demonstrated improved hormone balance, recurrence of menstruation in women with amenorrhoea and pregnancy outcome in women with fertility problems compared with a placebo group.[119] In women with amenorrhoea or luteal insufficiency, pregnancy occurred in the Mastodynon group more than twice as often as in the placebo group with minimal adverse effects.

Maca *(Lepidium meyenii)*

A randomised double-blind, placebo controlled cross-over trial demonstrated that 3.5g/day of Maca reduced anxiety, depression and sexual dysfunction in post-menopausal women independent of estrogenic and androgenic activity when compared with placebo over a 12-week period.[121] Another study found Maca to alleviate SSRI-induced sexual dysfunction in women suffering aggression.[122]

The following herbs have been used for the treatment of female infertility but there is incomplete evidence regarding their use and uncertain effect on the fetus:

- chamaelirium as an ovarian stimulant
- false unicorn root for PCOS and anovulatory cycles
- berberis — although considered a liver tonic, is used to treat oestrogen excess
- herbs that impact on glycaemic index may be of assistance (see Chapter 14)
- schisandra
- ginger
- chaste tree
- cinnamon
- corydalis.

It is advisable that women avoid herbs during conception and pregnancy.

Physical therapies

Acupuncture for females

Acupuncture, as an adjunctive treatment for infertility in women, has produced promising results. In trials involving IVF, women receiving adjunctive acupuncture had higher rates of pregnancy than those receiving conventional treatment.[122, 123]

A recent Cochrane review of 13 RCTs involving acupuncture and assisted conception found there is evidence that acupuncture does increase the live birth rate with IVF treatment when acupuncture is performed within 1 day of embryo transfer (ET) but not when it is performed 2–3 days after ET.[124] There were no adverse effects from acupuncture.

Some studies demonstrated that acupuncture in the luteal phase doubled IVF pregnancy rates[125] and acupuncture did not have any adverse outcomes.[126]

Conclusion

The integrated medicine approach should incorporate both nutritional and lifestyle management to attain a state of optimal health conducive for conception, concurrent with pharmaceutical treatment of acute conditions such as infection and hormonal dysfunction.

Complementary therapies such as mind–body medicine and acupuncture can be implemented in alleviating psychological distress, help balance hormones and in conjunction with general treatment to enhance effectiveness and help promote fertility.

Table 21.2 summarises the level of evidence for some CAM therapies for infertility.

Table 21.2 Levels of evidence for lifestyle and complementary medicines/therapies in the management of infertility

Modality	Level I	Level II	Level IIIa	Level IIIb	Level IIIc	Level IV	Level V
Lifestyle modification			x				
Mind–body medicine							
Counselling				x			
TD meditation and/or relaxation				x			
Support groups				x			
Diets							
Weight management				x			
Fertility diet		x					
Alcohol over-consumption avoidance				x			
Caffeine avoidance					x		
Trans fatty acid avoidance					x		
Environment							
Chemical and toxin avoidance				x			
Physical activity							
Exercise		x					
Yoga					x		
Nutritional supplements							
Males							
Antioxidant multivitamins			x				
Zinc				x			
Vitamin C				x			
Vitamin E				x			
Folate				x			
Selenium				x			
Coenzyme Q_{10}				x			
Glutathione			x				
L–Carnitine	x						
Arginine				x			
Lycopene				x			
Vitamin B12				x			
Females							
Antioxidant multivitamin				x			
Iron				x			
Folate				x			

Continued

Table 21.2 Levels of evidence for lifestyle and complementary medicines/therapies in the management of infertility—cont'd

Modality	Level I	Level II	Level IIIa	Level IIIb	Level IIIc	Level IV	Level V
Herbal medicines							
Males							
Japanese herbal medicine					x		
Tribulus terrestris						x	
Panax ginseng				x			
Pycnogenol					x		
Maca (*Lepidium meyenii*)				x			
Females							
Vitex agnus castus		x					
Maca (*Lepidium meyenii*)		x					
Physical therapies							
Acupuncture	x						

Level I — from a systematic review of all relevant randomised controlled trials — meta-analyses.
Level II — from at least 1 properly designed randomised controlled clinical trial.
Level IIIa — from well-designed pseudo-randomised controlled trials (alternate allocation or some other method).
Level IIIb — from comparative studies (including systematic reviews of such studies) with concurrent controls and allocation not randomised, cohort studies, case-control studies, or interrupted time series with a parallel control group.
Level IIIc — from comparative studies with historical control, 2 or more single-arm studies or interrupted time series without a parallel control group.
Level IV — opinions of respected authorities based on clinical experience, descriptive studies or reports of expert committees.
Level V — represents minimal evidence that represents testimonials.

Clinical tips handout for patients — infertility

1 Lifestyle advice

Sleep

- Females should avoid shift work. Adequate sleep is essential to help reduce stress.

Sunshine

- Amount of exposure varies with local climate.
- At least 15 minutes of sunshine needed daily for vitamin D and melatonin production — especially before 10 a.m. and after 3 p.m. when the sun exposure is safest during summer. Much more exposure is required in winter, when supplementation needs to be considered.
- Ensure gradual adequate skin exposure to sun; avoid sunscreen and excess clothing to maximise levels of vitamin D.
- More time in the sun is required for dark skinned people.
- Direct exposure to about 10% of body (hands, arms, face), without sunscreen and not through glass.
- Vitamin D is obtained in the diet from fatty fish, eggs, liver and fortified foods (some milks and margarines); however, it is unlikely that adequate vitamin D concentrations can be obtained from diet alone.

2 Physical activity/exercise

- Exercise at least 30 minutes per day with a maximum of less than 4 hours per week.
- Outdoor exercise with nature, fresh air and sunshine is ideal (e.g. walks in parks).
- Yoga may be of help.

3 Mind–body medicine

- Stress management program; for example, initially 6 x 40 minute sessions for patients: to understand the nature of their symptoms, the symptoms' relationship to stress and the practice of regular relaxation exercises.
- Regular meditation practice, at least 10–20 minutes daily, can be most helpful.
- Support groups can be beneficial for women with infertility and pregnancy issues (e.g. contact family, friends, church, social or other groups for support).

Breathing

- Be aware of breathing at all times. Notice if tendency to hold breath or over-breathe. Always aim to relax breath and the muscles around the chest wall.

Rest and stress management

Recurrent stress may cause a return of symptoms. Relaxation is important for a full and lasting recovery.

- Reduce workload and resolve conflicts. Contact family, friends, church or social groups for support.
- Listening to relaxation music helps.
- Relaxation massage therapy is helpful.
- Sex should be enjoyable and relaxing for couples; make plenty of time for sex.
- Cognitive behavioural therapy and psychotherapy are extremely helpful.
- Focus on wellness, not just the condition.

Fun

- It is important to have fun in life.
- Joy can be found even in the simplest tasks, such as funny movies/videos, comedy, hobbies, dancing, playing with pets and children.

Billings ovulation method

Women should familiarise themselves with the cyclical changes happening in their bodies to time sexual activity during the peak ovulation period for conception. Refer to www.womb.org/bom/index.html

4 Environment

- The office or home environment is enhanced with a view overlooking garden or park.
- Don't smoke and avoid smoking environments.
- Avoid environmental pollutants, especially mercury, lead and cadmium, and chemicals — both at work and in the home.
- Men should avoid excess heat around scrotal area; for example, from spas, hot baths, continuous long drives (e.g. taxi and truck driving).

5 Dietary changes

- Eat a high fertility diet: organic fruit, vegetables, eggs, yoghurt/milk, high fibre, low glycaemic index foods, meat (fish is best), fats from olive oil, avocados and nuts.
- A high fertility diet in females includes a lower intake of trans-fats (e.g. French fries, fish burgers, chicken nuggets, corn chips, pies, Danish rolls and donuts).

- Eat more nuts (e.g. walnuts, peanuts), seeds, beans (e.g. soy in women) and sprouts (e.g. alfalfa, mung bean sprouts).
- Eat more vegetable protein compared to animal protein, but avoid excess soy intake, especially in men.
- Eat more unprocessed carbohydrate with lower GI (e.g. wholegrain bread, wholemeal pasta and wholegrain rice).
- Eat more legumes (e.g. beans, lentils).
- Increase fish intake, daily if possible, especially deep sea fish; canned fish is okay (mackerel, salmon, sardines, cod, tuna).
- Avoid large predatory fish e.g. shark, marlin, broadbill and swordfish (containing highest levels of mercury).
- Reduce red meat intake (preferably use red lean meat e.g. lamb, kangaroo). White meat is okay (e.g. free range organic chicken).
- Do not rush your meals; chewing your food thoroughly as this aids digestion.
- If overweight or underweight, aim to normalise weight.
- For sweetener try honey (e.g. yellow box and stringy bark have the lowest GI).
- Drink more water (1–2 litres a day) and teas (especially organic green tea and black tea) plus vegetable juices.
- Chamomile tea may help aid relaxation. Drink 1 cup of 30–60 minutes before meals.
- Women should avoid coffee.
- Avoid excess soy intake, especially in men.
- Avoid hydrogenated fats, salt, fast foods, added sugar (such as in soft drinks), lollies, biscuits, cakes and processed foods (e.g. white bread, white pasta, pastries).
- Reduce alcohol intake.
- Avoid chemical additives — artificial sweeteners, preservatives, colourings and flavourings.

6 Physical therapies

- Acupuncture can be useful for aiding conception in women.
- Kegel penile exercises can help improve erectile dysfunction in men. These exercises can improve muscle tone within the penis. Apply a wet towel over an erect penis and swing it up and down (similar to weight-bearing exercises). Frequent sexual intercourse also helps.

7 Supplements

Males and females — daily consumption of a multivitamin/mineral supplement, containing vitamin C, vitamin E, selenium, coenzyme Q_{10} and beta-carotene may be useful.

Folate

- Indication: improves quantity and quality of sperm. Improves risk of conception in women and reduces risk of neural tube defects.
- Dosage: 500mcg daily in women 3 months prior to planned conception; 5–15mg daily in men.
- Result: 3 months.
- Side-effects: very mild and rare.
- Contraindications: avoid in anaemias until assessed by a doctor.

Females

Multivitamin

- Indication: improves risk of conception in women; nutritional deficiency states (e.g. vegetarians, teenagers, substance misusers of drugs, tobacco and alcohol).
- Dosage: 1 multivitamin (containing a mixture of multivitamin B, antioxidants, minerals and fish oils) daily.
- Result: 3 months.
- Side-effects: very mild and rare; gastrointestinal irritation can be avoided if taken after meals.
- Contraindications: avoid any multivitamin with herbal ingredients and when vitamin A content greater than 2000IU daily.

Warning: Vitamin A requirements increase during pregnancy but excessive intake of vitamin A above 3000IU daily may cause birth deformities.

Iron

- Indication: improves risk of conception in women, particularly in deficiency states, including borderline levels.
- Dosage: 25–40mg daily.
- Result: 3 months.
- Side-effects: very mild and rare; constipation; digestive disorders.
- Contraindications: avoid in anaemias, hemosiderosis or haemochromatosis until assessed by a doctor.

Males

Vitamin C

- Indication: improve sperm quantity and quality.
- Dosage: 200mg daily.
- Results: 3 months.
- Side-effects: with high doses can cause nausea, heartburn, abdominal cramps and diarrhoea.

- Contraindications: can increase iron absorption. Use with caution if glucose-6-phosphate dehydrogenase deficiency.

Vitamin E (natural)

- Indication: can improve sperm quantity and quality.
- Dosage: 200mg daily.
- Side-effects: doses below 1500IU daily are very unlikely to result in haemorrhage, diarrhoea, flatulence, nausea, heart palpitations.
- Contraindications: use with caution if bleeding disorder or if taking with blood thinning medication. If using very high dose, reduce dose before surgery.

Vitamin B12

- Indication: can improve sperm quantity and quality, especially in those with vitamin B12 deficiency.
- Dosage: between 600–1000mcg daily.
- Result: 3 months.
- Side-effects: does not cause side-effects even in large doses.
- Contraindications: concurrent use with vitamin C may decrease vitamin B12 absorption therefore best if taken at least 2 hours apart. Several drugs can reduce serum vitamin B12 levels. Excess alcohol intake can also decrease vitamin B12 absorption. Likely to be safe during pregnancy although there is insufficient data.

Zinc

- Indication: improves sperm quantity and quality.
- Dosage: 60mg zinc sulfate once or twice daily combined with 2mg copper daily.
- Results: 3 months.
- Side-effects: nausea, vomiting, metallic taste in mouth. Avoid long-term use and high dosage as this may cause copper deficiency, impair the immune system and cause anaemia.
- Contraindications: sideroblastic anaemia, above normal blood levels of zinc, severe kidney disease.

Selenium

- Indication: can improve sperm quantity and quality.
- Dosage: 100mcg daily given together with vitamin C and vitamin B complex.
- Result: 3 months.
- Side-effects: no risk at this dose.
- Contraindications: pregnant women.

Glutathione

- Indication: can improve sperm quality.
- Dosage: 600mg daily intramuscularly on alternate days.
- Result: 2 months.
- Side-effects: safe to use at this dose.
- Contraindications: none known at this dose.

Acetyl-L-carnitine

- Indication: can improve sperm quantity and quality.
- Dosage: 1g 3 times daily.
- Result: 6 months.
- Side-effects: rare, but can cause nausea, vomiting, abdominal pain, heartburn and diarrhoea.
- Contraindications: pregnant women — insufficient evidence. Can decrease effectiveness of thyroid hormone replacement.

L-arginine

- Indication: can improve quantity and quality of sperm when arginine deficiency is present.
- Dosage: 4g daily.
- Result: 3–6 months.
- Side-effects: rare, but can cause abdominal pain and bloating, diarrhoea and gout. Can exacerbate airway inflammation in asthmatics.
- Contraindications: none reported. Theoretically could enhance anti-hypertensive drugs, nitrates and sildenfal. Discontinue 2 weeks before surgery because it might interfere with blood pressure control.

Coenzyme Q_{10}

- Indication: can improve quality of sperm.
- Dosage: 200mg daily.
- Result: 6 months.
- Side-effects: rare.
- Contraindications: none reported.

Herbs for males and females

Maca (*Lepidium meyenii*)

- Indication: improves sexual performance.
- Dosage: 3.5gm/day.
- Result: 4–6 weeks.
- Contraindications: none known.

Males

Korean red ginseng (*Panax ginseng*)

- Indication: may improve sperm count and may also be helpful for erectile dysfunction.
- Dosage: 200mg daily.
- Result: 2–4 hours for erectile dysfunction, but approximately 3 months for sperm count improvement.

- Side-effects: very rarely occurs. Possible insomnia. Even more rarely and with higher doses — breast discomfort, vaginal bleeding, amenorrhea, tachycardia and palpitations.
- Contraindications: avoid stimulants such as excess caffeine and nicotine. There are a number of theoretical interactions with drugs.

Pycnogenol

Indication: can improve sperm count.

Dosage: 200mg daily.

Result: 90 days.

Side-effects: rarely occur, but include dizziness and gastrointestinal problems plus headache and mouth ulcers.

Contraindicated: theoretical evidence only that it could interfere with immunosuppressive drugs.

Sairei-to

Indication: improve sperm quantity and quality.

Dosage: 9g daily.

Result: 3 months.

Side-effects: information unavailable.

Contraindicated: information unavailable.

Females

Vitex agnus castus

- Indication: improves PMS, hormone balance, fertility.
- Dosage: 20mg VAC extract.
- Side-effects: rare; skin rashes; nausea; gastrointestinal disturbances and headaches.
- Interactions: use cautiously with oral contraceptive pill. Consult your doctor.
- Contraindications: individuals with oestrogen sensitive tumours.

References

1 http://cancerweb.ncl.ac.uk/cgi-bin/omd/?query = sterility (accessed January 2009).

2 Mosher WD and Pratt WF. Fecundity and infertility in the United States: incidence and trends. Fertil Steril 1991;56:192–93.

3 Healy DL et. al. Female infertility: causes and treatment. Lancet 1994;343:1539–44.

4 Laws P, Abeywardana S, Walker J, Sullivan EA.2007 Australian Mothers and Babies 2005 Perinatal Statistics Unit. No 20. Cat. No. PER 40 Sydney: Australian Institute of Health and Welfare National Perinatal Statistics Unit. http://www.npsu.unsw.edu.au/ (accessed January 2009).

5 Stankiewicz M, Smith C, Alvino H, Norman R. The use of complementary medicine and therapies by patients attending a reproductive medicine unit in South Australia: a prospective survey. Aust NZ J Obstet Gynaecol 2007;47(2):145–9.

6 Dunson DB, Baird DD, Colombo B. Increased infertility with age in men and women. Obstetrics and Gynecology 2004;103(1):51–6.

7 Maheshwari A, Hamilton M, Bhattacharya S.Effect of female age on the diagnostic categories of infertility. Hum Reprod 2008;23(3):538–42.

8 Hollowell JG et. al. Serum TSH, T, and thyroid antibodies in the Unite States population (1988–1994): National Health and Nutrition Examination Survey (NHANES III). J Clin Endocr Metab 2002:87;489–99.

9 Janssen OE et. al. High prevalence of autoimmune thyroiditis in patients with polycystic ovary syndrome. Eur J Endocrinol 2004:150;363–69.

10 Eskenazi B, Kidd SA, Marks AR, et. al. Antioxidant intake is associated with semen quality in healthy men. Hum Reprod 2005;20(4):1006–12.

11 Ebisch IM, Thomas CM, Peters WH, et. al. The importance of folate, zinc and antioxidants in the pathogenesis and prevention of subfertility. Hum Reprod Update 2007;13(2):163–74.

12 Shrauzer GN. Benefits of natural selenium. Anabolism 1988:7(4):5.

13 Bedwal R. et. al. Zinc, copper and selenium in reproduction. Experientia 1994;50:626–40.

14 Boxmeer JC, Smit M, Weber RF, et. al. Seminal plasma cobalamin significantly correlates with sperm concentration in men undergoing IVF or ICSI procedures. J Androl 2007;28(4):521–7.

15 Bruinse HW, van der Berg H, Haspels AA. Maternal serum folacin levels during and after normal pregnancy. Eur J Obstet Gynecol Reprod Biol 1985;20(3):153–8.

16 Chavarro JE, Rich-Edwards JW, Rosner BA, Willett WC. Use of multivitamins, intake of B vitamins and risk of ovulatory infertility. Fertil Steril 2008;89(3):668–76.

17 Barron ML. Light exposure, melatonin secretion, and menstrual cycle parameters: an integrative review. Biol Res Nurs 2007;9(1):49–69.

18 Allen LH. Multiple micronutrients in pregnancy and lactation: an overview. AJCN 2005;81(5):1206S-1212S.

19 Favier A. The role of zinc in reproduction: Hormonal mechanisms. Biol Trace Elem Res 1992;32:363–82.

20 Favier A. Current aspects about the role of zinc in nutrition. Rev Prat 1993;43(2):146–51.

21 Weissmann MC et. al. A trial of the Ovulation Method of family planning in Tonga. Lancet 1972;2:813–16.

22 Qian SZ, et. al. Evaluation of the effectiveness of a natural fertility regulation program in China. The Woman of Today and Her Identity: Femininity, Fecundity and Procreation congress, Centre for Study and Research in the Natural Regulation of Fertility. Universita Cattolica del Sacro Cuore. Rome, 8 September 2000.

23 World Health Organisation. A prospective multicentre trial of the Ovulation Method of natural family planning. I: The teaching phase. Fertility and Sterility 1981;36:152–58.

24 World Health Organisation. A prospective multicentre trial of the Ovulation Method of natural family planning. I: The effectiveness phase. Fertility and Sterility 1981;36:591–98.

25 Ball, M. A Prospective field trial of the ovulation method of avoiding conception. European Journal of Obstetrics and Gynecology Reprod Biol 1976, 6/2;63–66.

26 Jan Havlícek, Radka Dvoráková, Ludek Bartoš, & Jaroslav Flegr. Non-Advertised does not Mean Concealed: Body Odour Changes across the Human Menstrual Cycle. Ethology 2006;112:81–90.
27 House SH. Nurturing the brain nutritionally and emotionally from before conception to late adolescence. Nutr Health 2007;19(1–2):143–61.
28 Porter M, Bhattacharya S. Helping themselves to get pregnant: a qualitative longitudinal study on the information-seeking behaviour of infertile couples. Hum Reprod 2008;23(3):567–72.
29 Chavarro, JE, Rich-Edwards JW, Rosner, BA, Walter CW. Diet and Lifestyle in the Prevention of Ovulatory Disorder Fertility. Obstetrics and Gynecology 2007;110;1050–8.
30 Giommi R, Corona G, Maggi M. The therapeutic dilemma: how to use psychotherapy. Int J Androl 2005;28(Suppl 2):81–5.
31 Fisher, K. Hammarberg, H. Baker. Assisted conception is a risk factor for postnatal mood disturbance and early parenting difficulties. Fertility and Sterility, 2005;84:426–430.
32 Cousineau TM et. al. Online psychoeducational support for infertile women: a randomised controlled trial. Hum Reprod 2008;23(3):554–66.
33 Domar AD, Seibel MM, Benson H. The mind/body program for infertility: a new behavioral treatment approach for women with infertility. Fertil Steril 1990;53(2):246–9.
34 Lovell-Smith HD. Transcendental meditation and infertility. N Z Med J 1985;98(789):922.
35 Koskimäki J, Shiri R, Tammela T, et. al. Regular intercourse protects against erectile dysfunction: Tampere Ageing Male Urologic Study. American Journal of Medicine 2008;21:592–96.
36 Labyak S, Lava S, Turek F, et. al. Effects of shift-work on sleep and menstrual function in nurses. Health Care for Women International 2002;23:703–14.
37 Kinuta, K, Tanaka H, Moriwake T, et. al. Vitamin D Is an Important Factor in Estrogen Biosynthesis of Both Female and Male Gonads. Endocrinology 2000;141:1317–1324.
38 Tiboni GM, Bucciarelli T, Giampietro F, et. al. Influence of cigarette smoking on vitamin E, vitamin A, beta-carotene and lycopene concentrations in human pre-ovulatory follicular fluid. Int J Immunopathol Pharmacol 2004;17(3):389–93.
39 Shiloh H, Lahav Baratz S, Koifman M, et. al. The impact of cigarette smoking on zona pellucida thickness of oocytes and embryos prior to transfer into the uterine cavity. Human Reproduction, Vol. 19, No. 1, 157–159, January 2004
40 K.P. Wright, J.R. Trimarchi, J. Allsworth and D. Keefe The effect of female tobacco smoking on IVF outcomes. Human Reproduction 2006 21(11): 2930–34. Online. Available: http://humrep.oxfordjournals.org/cgi/content/full/21/11/2930 (accessed 19 June 2009).
41 Saleh RA, Agarwal A, Sharma RK, et. al. Effect of cigarette smoking on levels of seminal oxidative stress in infertile men: a prospective study. Fertil Steril 2002;78(3):491–9.
42 Tiboni GM, Bucciarelli T, Giampietro F, et. al. Influence of cigarette smoking on vitamin E, vitamin A, beta-carotene and lycopene concentrations in human pre-ovulatory follicular fluid. Int J Immunopathol Pharmacol 2004;17(3):389–93.
43 Gades NM et. al. Association between smoking and erectile dysfunction: a population-based study. Am J Epidemiol 2005;161:346–51.
44 Louis Bujan, Myriam Daudin, Jean-Paul Charlet, Patrick Thonneau and Roger Mieusset. Increase in scrotal temperature in car drivers. Human Reproduction 2000;15:1355–1357.
45 Appasamy M. et. al. Relationship between male reproductive hormones, sperm DNA damage and markers of oxidative stress in infertility. Reprod Biomed Online. 2007 Feb;14(2):159–65.
46 Appasamy M, Muttukrishna S, Piszey AR, et. al. Relationship between male reproductive hormones, sperm DNA damage and markers of oxidative stress in infertility. Online. Available: http://www.ncbi.nlm.nih.gov/pubmed/17298717?dopt = Abstract (accessed 19 June 2009).
47 Sanocka D, Kurpisz M. Reactive oxygen species and sperm cells. Reprod Biol Endocrinol 2004;2:12.
48 Aitken RJ, Krausz C. Oxidative stress, DNA damage and the Y chromosome. Reproduction 2001;122(4):497–506.
49 Agarwal A, Gupta S, Sharma R. Oxidative stress and its implications in female infertility - a clinician's perspective. Reprod Biomed Online 2005;11(5): 641–50.
50 Bhatt RV. Environmental influence on reproductive health. Int J Gynaecol Obstet 2000;70(1):69–75
51 De Kretser DM. Declining Sperm counts. Environmental Chemicals may be to blame. BM J 1996;312:457–8.
52 Irvine S, Cawood E, Richardson D, Mac Donald E, Aitken J. Evidence of deteriorating semen quality in the United Kingdom: birth cohort study in 577 men in Scotland over 11 years. BMJ 1996;312:467–71.
53 S.H.Swan1, F.Liu1, J.W.Overstreet, C.Brazil and N.E.Skakkebaek. Semen quality of fertile US males in relation to their mothers' beef consumption during pregnancy. Human Reproduction Vol.22, No.6 pp. 1497–1502, 2007 doi:10.1093/humrep/dem068.
54 Winder C. Lead, reproduction and development. Neurotoxicology, 1993;14(2–3):303–17.
55 Triche EW, Hossain N. Environmental factors implicated in the causation of adverse pregnancy outcome. Semin Perinatol 2007;31(4):240–2.
56 Jackson LW, Zullo MD, Goldberg JM. Hum Reprod. 2008 The association between heavy metals, endometriosis and uterine myomas among premenopausal women: National Health and Nutrition Examination Survey 1999–2002;23(3):679–87.
57 Jørgensen N, Andersen AG, Eustache F, et. al. Regional differences in semen quality in Europe. Human Reproduction 2001;16:1012–19.
58 Palomba S et. al. Structured exercise training program versus hypocaloric hyperproteic diet in obese polycystic ovary syndrome patients with anovulatory infertility: a 24-week pilot study Hum Reprod 2008;23(3):642–50.
59 Morris SN, et. al. Effects of Lifetime Exercise on the Outcome of In Vitro Fertilisation. Obstet Gynecol 2006;108(4):938–45.
60 Khalsa HK. Yoga: an adjunct to infertility treatment. Fertil Steril 2003;80(Suppl 4):46–51.
61 Mendelson JH. Alcohol effects on reproductive function in women. Psychiatry Letter. 1986;4(7): 35–8.
62 Van Thiel DH et. al. Ethanol, a Leydig cell toxin: evidence obtained in vivo and in vitro. Pharmacol Biochem behave, 1983;18(Suppl 1):317–23.
63 Anderson RA Jr et. al. Spontaneous recovery from ethanol induced male infertility. Alcohol, 1985;2(3):479–84.

64 Chew K-K, Bremner A, Stuckey B, Earle C, and Jamrozik K. Alcohol consumption and male erectile dysfunction: An unfounded reputation for risk? Journal of Sexual Medicine. 8 Jan 2009.
65 Casas M et. al. Dopaminergic mechanism for caffeine induced decrease in fertility? Letter. Lancet, 1989; i:731.
66 Homan GF, Davies M, Norman R. The impact of lifestyle factors on reproductive performance in the general population and those undergoing infertility treatment: a review. Hum Reprod Update 2007;13(3):209–23.
67 Bolúmar F, Olsen J, Rebagliato M, et. al. Body mass index and delayed conception: a European Multicenter Study on Infertility and Subfecundity. Am J Epidemiol 2000;151(11):1072–9.
68 Van der Steeg JW, Steures P, Eijkemans MJ, et. al. Obesity affects spontaneous pregnancy chances in subfertile, ovulatory women. Hum Reprod. 2008 Feb;23(2):324–8.
69 Hedley et. al. Prevalance of overweight and obesity among US children, adolescents and adults 1999–2002. JAMA 2004:291;2847–2850
70 Hammoud AO et. al. Obesity and male reproductive potential. J Androl 2006:27;619–26.
71 Jensen TK et. al. Body mass index in relation to semen quality and reproductive hormones among 1,558 Danish men. Fertil Steril 2004;82:863–70.
72 Aggerholm AS et. al. Is overweight a risk factor for reduced semen quality and altered serum sex hormone profile? Fertil Steril 2007: doi:10.1016/j.fertnstert.2007.10.011.
73 Nguyen RH et. al. Men's body mass index and infertility. Hum Reprod 2007:22;2488–2493.
74 Hammoud AO et. al. Male obesity and alteration in sperm parameters. Fertil Steril [doi: 10.1016/j.fertnstert.2007.10.011].
75 Chavarro JE, Rich-Edwards JW, Rosner BA, et. al. Dietary fatty acid intakes and the risk of ovulatory infertility. AJCN 2007;85:231–7.
76 Chavarro JE, Toth TL, Sadio SM, et. al. Soy food and isoflavone intake in relation to semen quality parameters among men from an infertility clinic. Hum Reprod.2008;23(11):2584–90.
77 Juan J.Tarı´n1, Juan Brines and Antonio Cano Is antioxidant therapy a promising strategy to improve human reproduction? Antioxidants may protect against infertility. Human Reprod 1998;13:1415–24.
78 Martin-Du Pan RC. et. al. Is antioxidant therapy a promising strategy to improve human reproduction? Are antioxidants useful in the treatment of male infertility? Hum Reprod 1998;13(11):2984–5.
79 Sheweita SA, Tilmisany AM, Al-Sawaf H. Mechanisms of male infertility: role of antioxidants. Curr Drug Metab 2005;6(5):495–501.
80 Tremellen K, Miari G, Froiland D, Thompson J. A randomised control trial examining the effect of an antioxidant (Menevit) on pregnancy outcome during IVF-ICSI treatment. Aust N Z J Obstet Gynaecol. 2007 Jun;47(3):216–21.
81 Ermanno Greco, Stefania Romano, Marcello Iacobelli, Susanna Ferrero, Elena Baroni, Maria Giulia Minasi, Filippo Ubaldi, Laura Rienzi and Jan Tesarik. ICSI in cases of sperm DNA damage: beneficial effect of oral antioxidant treatment. Human Reproduction 2005 20(9):2590–2594.
82 Ermanno Greco, Marcello Iacobelli, Laura Rienzi, et. al. Reduction of the Incidence of Sperm DNA Fragmentation by Oral Antioxidant Treatment. Journal of Andrology 2005;26:
83 B.Eskenazi1, S.A.Kidd, A.R.Marks, et. al. Antioxidant intake is associated with semen quality in healthy men. Human Reproduction 2005;20:1006–12.
84 Mohammed Akmal, J.Q. Qadri, Noori S. Al-Waili, Shahiya Thangal, Afrozul Haq, Khelod Y. Saloom. Improvement in human semen quality after oral supplementation of vitamin C. Journal of Medicinal Food 2006;9(3):440–2.
85 Chen Q, Ng V, Mei J, Chia SE. Comparison of seminal vitamin B12, folate, reactive oxygen species and various sperm parameters between fertile and infertile males. Wei Sheng Yan Jiu 2001;30(2):80–2.
86 Eskenazi B, Kidd SA, Marks AR, et. al. Antioxidant intake is associated with semen quality in healthy men. Hum Reprod 2005;20(4):1006–12.
87 Young SS, Eskenazi B, Marchetti FM, et. al. The association of folate, zinc and antioxidant intake with sperm aneuploidy in healthy non-smoking men. Human Reproduction Vol.23, No.5 pp. 1014–1022, 2008 doi:10.1093/humrep/den036. Advance Access publication on March 19, 2008.
88 Lenzi, A, Culasso F, Gandini L, et. al. Placebo-controlled, double-blind, cross-over trial of glutathione therapy in male infertility. Hum Reprod 1993;8:1657–62.
89 Anderson ME. Glutathione: an overview of biosynthesis and modulation. Chem Biol Interact 1998;111–112:1–14.
90 Witschi A, Reddy S, Stofer B, Lauterburg BH. The systemic availability of oral glutathione. Eur J Clin Pharmacol 1992;43(6):667–9.
91 Keskes-Ammar L, Feki-Chakroun N, Rebai T, et. al. Sperm oxidative stress and the effect of an oral vitamin E and selenium supplement on semen quality in infertile men. Arch Androl 2003;49(2):83–94.
92 Hansen JC et. al. Selenium and fertility in animals and man – a review. Acta Vet Scand 1996;37(1): 19–30.
93 Tikkiwal M et. al. Effect of zinc administration on seminal zinc and fertility of oligospermic males. Indian J Physiol Pharmacol 1987;31(1):30–4.
94 International Journal of Andrology, November 2005.
95 Lewis SE et. al. Nitric oxide synthase and nitrite production in human spermatozoa: evidence that the endogenous nitric oxide is beneficial to sperm motility. Mol Hum Reprod 1996;2(11):873–8.
96 Zhou X, Liu F, Zhai S. Effect of L-carnitine and/or L-acetyl-carnitine in nutrition treatment for male infertility: a systematic review. Asia Pac J Clin Nutr 2007;16(Suppl 1):383–90.
97 Vicari E, La Vignera S, Calogero AE. Antioxidant treatment with carnitines is effective in infertile patients with prostatovesiculoepididymitis and elevated seminal leukocyte concentrations after treatment with nonsteroidal anti-inflammatory compounds. Fertil Steril 2002;78(6):1203–8.
98 Balercia G, et. al. Coenzyme q10 supplementation in infertile men with idiopathic asthenozoospermia: an open, uncontrolled pilot study. Fertility and Sterility 2004;81:93–8.
99 Coenzyme Q_{10} treatment improves sperm motility. Nature Clinical Practice Urology 2008;5:412 doi:10.1038/ncpuro1163
100 Balercia G, et. al. Coenzyme q10 supplementation in infertile men with idiopathic asthenozoospermia: an open, uncontrolled pilot study. Fertility and Sterility 2008;02:119.
101 Gupta NP, Kumar R. Lycopene therapy in idiopathic male infertility--a preliminary report. Int Urol Nephrol 2002;34(3):369–72.

102 Rumbold A, Middleton P, Crowther CA. Vitamin supplementation for preventing miscarriage. Cochrane Database of Systematic Reviews 2005, Issue 2. Art. No.: CD004073. doi: 10.1002/14651858.CD004073.pub2.
103 Forges T, Monnier-Barbarino P, Alberto JM, et. al. Impact of folate and homocysteine metabolism on human reproductive health. Hum Reprod Update 2007;13(3):225–38.
104 Chavarro JE, Rich-Edwards JW, Rossner BA, Willett WC. Iron intake and risk of ovulatory infertility. Obstetrics Gynecology 2006;108:1145–52.
105 Tempest HG, Homa ST, Routledge EJ, et. al. Plants used in Chinese medicine for the treatment of male infertility possess antioxidant and anti-oestrogenic activity. Syst Biol Reprod Med 2008;54(4–5):185–95.
106 Rowland DL, Tai W. A review of plant-derived and herbal approaches to the treatment of sexual dysfunctions. J Sex Marital Ther 2003;29(3): 185–205.
107 Lucchetta G, Weill A, Becker N, et al: Reactivation from the prostatic gland in cases of reduced fertility. Urol Int 1984;39:222–4.
108 Menchini-Fabris GF, Giorgi P, Andreini F, et al: New perspectives of treatment of prostato-vesicular pathologies with *Pygeum africanum*. Arch Int Urol 1988;60:313–22.
109 Clavert A, Cranz C, Riffaud JP, et al: Effects of an extract of the bark of *Pygeum africanum* on prostatic secretions in the rat and man. Ann Urol 1986;20:341–3.
110 Dhar MK, Kaul S, Sareen S, Gill BS. *Plantago ovata*: genetic diversity, cultivation, utilisation and chemistry. Plant Genetic Resources 2005;3:252–63.
111 Bennett BC, Hicklin JR. Uses of saw palmetto (Serenoa repens, Arecaceae) in Florida. Economic botany 1998;52:381–393.
112 Hong B, Ji YH, Hong JH, et. al. A double-blind crossover study evaluating the efficacy of Korean red ginseng in patients with erectile dysfunction: A preliminary report. The Journal of Urology 2002;168:2070–3.
113 Mkrtchyan A, Panosyan V, Panossian A, et. al. A phase I clinical study of Andrographis paniculata fixed combination Kan Jang versus ginseng and valerian on the semen quality of healthy male subjects. Phytomedicine 2005;12(6–7):403–9.
114 Salvati G, Genovesi G, Marcellini L, et. al. Effects of Panax Ginseng C.A. Meyer saponins on male fertility. Panminerva Med 1996;38(4):249–54.
115 Roseff SJ. Improvement in sperm quality and function with French maritime pine tree bark extract. J Reprod Med 2002;47(10):821–4.
116 Suzuki M, Kurabayashi T, Yamamoto Y, et. al. Effects of antioxidant treatment in oligozoospermic and asthenozoospermic men. J Reprod Med 2003;48(9):707–12.
117 Gonzales GF et. al. Effect of Lepidium meyenii (maca), a root with aphrodisiac and fertility-enhancing properties on serum reproductive hormone levels in adult healthy men. Journal of Endocrinology 2003;176:163–8.
118 Zenico T, Cicero AFC, Valmorr L, Mercuriali M, Berocovish E. Subjective effect of maca on wellbeing and sexual performance in patients with mild erectile dysfunction. Andrologia 2008;41:95–9.
119 Gerhard II, Patek A, Monga B, et. al. Mastodynon(R) bei weiblicher Sterilität. Forsch Komplementarmed. 1998;5(6):272–8.
120 Brooks NA, Wilcox G, Walkerk K, et. al. Beneficial effects of Lepidium meyenii (maca) on psychological symptoms and measures of sexual dysfunction in menopausal women are not related to oestrogen of androgen content. Menopause: Journal of American Menopause Society 2008;15(6):115–162.
121 Pording C, Fisher L, Papakostas G, et. al. A double-blind randomised, pilot dose finding study of maca root (L. meyenii) for the management of SSRI-induced sexual dysfunction. CNS Neuroscience & Therapeutics 2008;14:182–91.
122 Stener-Victorin E, et. al. A prospective randomised study of electro-acupuncture versus alfentanil as anaesthesia during oocyte aspiration in in-vitro fertilisation. Hum Reprod 1999:14;2480–4.
123 Paulus WE, et al. Influence of acupuncture on the pregnancy rate in patients who undergo assisted reproduction therapy. Fertil Steril 2002:77;721–4.
124 Cheong YC, Hung Yu Ng E, Ledger WL. Acupuncture and assisted conception. Cochrane Database of Systematic Reviews 2008, Issue 4. Art. No.: CD006920. doi: 10.1002/14651858. CD006920.pub2. Online. Available: http://www.cochrane.org/reviews/en/ab006920.html (accessed 19 June 2009).
125 Dieterle S, Ying G, Hatzmann W, et. al. Effect of acupuncture on the outcome of in vitro fertilisation and intracytoplasmic sperm injection: a randomised, prospective, controlled clinical study.Fertil Steril 2006;85(5):1347–51.
126 C. Smith, M. Coyle, R. Norman. Influence of acupuncture stimulation on pregnancy rates for women undergoing embryo transfer. Fertility and Sterility 2006;85:1352–8.

Chapter 22

Insomnia and sleep disorders

Epidemiology of insomnia

Insomnia is the most common sleep disorder across all stages of adulthood, and is often associated with significant medical, psychological and social disturbances.[1, 2] It is a prevalent health complaint associated with daytime impairments, reduced quality of life, and increased health care costs. The epidemiological data indicate occasional episodes of insomnia symptoms are reported by one-half of all adults in the US,[3, 4] while multiple studies have documented the prevalence of chronic insomnia in 10–15% of the US adult population, and that an additional 25–35% has transient or occasional insomnia identified in various countries.[4–7] Reported rates of insomnia in other countries include 21% in Japan,[8] 19% in France,[9] and 18% in Canada.[10] Among those people who experience insomnia at least a few nights per week, the most frequent symptoms reported are 1) waking up feeling unrefreshed (34%) and 2) awakening often during the night (32%).[3, 4] Less often, adults with insomnia report difficulty falling asleep or awakening early (23–24%).[4] Furthermore, up to 25% of children seen in general practice[11] and 60% of adults older than 60 years of age experience sleep problems.[12, 13]

In a telephone survey about sleep and insomnia, in randomly selected French-speaking adults in Quebec, of the total sample 25% were dissatisfied with their sleep, 30% reported insomnia symptoms, and 10% met criteria for an insomnia syndrome.[3] Of the respondents, 13% had consulted a health care provider specifically for insomnia in their lifetime, with general practitioners being the most frequently consulted. Daytime fatigue (48%), psychological distress (40%) and physical discomfort (22%) were the main determinants prompting individuals with insomnia to seek treatment. Fifteen percent had used at least 1 herbal/dietary products to facilitate sleep and 11% had used prescribed sleep medications in the year preceding the survey. Other self-help strategies used to facilitate sleep included reading, listening to music and relaxation.[3]

Symptoms of insomnia

Insomnia is a common symptom caused by a variety of health problems or lifestyle situations. Poor sleep can have major adverse effects on daily functioning due to fatigue, poor concentration and memory problems.

As insomnia is a frequent symptom in the general population, classifications have gradually given more emphasis to its daytime repercussions and to their consequences on social and cognitive functioning.[14] The criteria for the diagnosis of insomnia include at least 1 of the following complaints:

- difficulty with initiating and/or maintaining sleep
- sleep that is poor in quality
- trouble sleeping despite adequate opportunity and circumstances for sleep
- waking up too early.

(For reviews see Ramakrishnan and Scheid;[15] American Academy of Sleep Medicine.[16])

Moreover, at least 1 of the following types of daytime-impaired activities that is related to sleep difficulty should be documented:

- attention, concentration, or memory impairment
- concerns or worries about sleep
- daytime sleepiness
- errors or accidents at work or while driving
- fatigue or malaise
- gastrointestinal symptoms
- lack of motivation
- mood disturbance or irritability
- social or vocational dysfunction or poor school performance in children
- tension headaches.

Risk factors

General

There are various root causes of insomnia, such as drugs and stimulants that are known to cause insomnia, hormonal problems (e.g. menopause and pregnancy), adjustment sleep disorder (e.g. grief and major stress), environmental changes (e.g. moving house, excessive noise) and limit-setting sleep disorder (e.g. children who need clear boundaries for sleep).[4] These need to be addressed and treated in their own right.

Psychological factors

One study exploring sleep patterns in 472 children aged 4–12 years found a higher incidence of depression, anxiety, somatic complaints, attention problems, enuresis, frequent falls, ADHD, pica and fatigue in children suffering insomnia compared with those who do not suffer insomnia.[17]

School transition

Data from a longitudinal study of 4460 children aged 4–5 years and 6–7 years found sleep problems during school transition are common and are significantly associated with poor health-related quality of life, behaviour, language and learning scores compared with children reported not to have sleep problems.[18]

Pain

Clearly pain is a common cause of insomnia and is best treated by controlling the pain. Opiates are valuable in pain-associated insomnia.[15]

Smoking

In a randomly selected sample of 769 individuals (379 men and 390 women, aged 20–98), participants completed 2 weeks of sleep diaries.[19] They provided a global report on their sleep, indicated the number of cigarettes smoked per day, and supplied information on health, depressive symptoms, anxiety, caffeine and alcohol use. After controlling for demographic, health, psychological and behavioural variables, light smoking (< 15 cigarettes per day), but not heavier smoking, was associated with self-reported chronic insomnia and reduced sleep (diary recorded as total sleep time and time in bed). Smokers did not differ significantly from non-smokers on diary measures of sleep–onset latency, number of awakenings during the night, wake-time after sleep onset, or sleep efficiency.[19]

The ARIC study[20] is a well-characterised population-based study that specifically correlated sleep complaints in adults to differing covariates. Difficulty falling asleep and difficulty staying asleep was demonstrated to have different causes and outcomes and smoking was a significant correlate. Table 22.1 summarises some of the risk factors for insomnia.

Pharmacological treatments

The most common treatment for sleep disorders (particularly insomnia) is pharmacological. The efficacy of non-drug interventions has been suggested to be slower than pharmacological methods, but with no risk of drug-related tolerance or dependency. A recent meta-analysis of 24 studies[21] of more than 2400 patients found that whilst improvements in sleep with sedative use are statistically significant *the magnitude of this effect is small.* The analysis demonstrated risk of adverse events as statistically significant particularly in older people at risk of falls and cognitive impairment. In people using any sedatives, the risk of adverse events compared with placebo, was 4.78 times more common for cognitive events, 2.61 times more common for adverse psychomotor events and daytime fatigue was 3.82 times greater than placebo.[21] Based on these concerns, the authors concluded that, in people over 60, *the benefits of these drugs may not justify the increased risk, particularly if the patient has additional risk factors for cognitive or psychomotor adverse events.*

A survey of 100 insomnia cases in hospital found 51% were younger than age 65 and 40% of patients had started experiencing insomnia whilst in hospital.[22] Short-acting benzodiazepine medication was used in 88% of the cases and only 11% of patients received information about non-drug alternatives for insomnia. Eighty-two patients felt that the alternatives were *healthier*, and the majority (n = 67) responded that if an alternative were offered in the hospital, they would be willing to accept it. Female patients were more willing to consider alternatives ($P<0.01$). First time users of benzodiazepines were more receptive to alternatives compared with chronic users ($P<0.002$). Preferred alternatives for insomnia included massage therapy, sleep hygiene, music and relaxation techniques ($P<0.001$). The authors concluded that educational programs are needed for appropriate evidence-based management protocols for insomnia.

Behavioural interventions such as developing healthy sleep patterns, avoiding over-stimulation before sleep, such as watching too much TV[14, 20, 23] good sleep hygiene tips, reducing stress levels, and avoiding over-work would appear to be useful first-line advice.

Table 22.1 Risk factors for insomnia

Risk factors
Life stages Elderly Teenagers Menopause
Travel and work Jet lag Night shift work
Drugs and stimulants Pseudoephedrine, caffeine, cola drinks, smoking, alcohol
Sleep disturbance Post-natal period: newborns frequently waking up at night; snoring partners
Grief and stress Personal loss School transition
Poor sleep habits and patterns
Environmental Excessive noise, smells, lights
Mind–body Depression, anxiety, preoccupied thoughts, stress
Medical illness Chronic pain, fatigue, sleep apnoea, enuresis, ADHD, autism, restless leg syndrome, headache, viral illness, cardiac or respiratory disease

This chapter explores the scientific evidence for useful non-pharmacological and integrative approaches to the management of insomnia.

Insomnia and health risks

Cardiovascular

Long-term sleep deprivation may also increase risk of coronary heart disease (CHD) due to sympathetic overdrive and increases in blood pressure according to data from 71 617 women.[24] The association between sleep and CHD persisted after adjusting for age, smoking, obesity, hypertension, diabetes and other cardiovascular risk factors. According to this study, women who were getting 5 or fewer hours of sleep per night had a 39% increased risk of CHD at 10 week follow-up compared to those on 8 hours sleep. Sleep of 6–9 hours was linked to an 18% increase link of CHD.

General poor quality of health

Children who do not sleep well are more likely to suffer ill health compared with children who do sleep well.[18]

Insomnia can also contribute to depression and anxiety (see Chapters 4 and 12), fatigue, poor memory, and headaches.[16]

The integrative approach to the management of insomnia

Lifestyle and behavioural changes

Developing good sleep habits can help. These include:

- avoiding sleeping in and daytime naps
- developing a relaxing bedtime routine, such as having a warm bath before bed, and avoid arguments and worrying during this time
- going to bed early and when sleepy
- developing a regular routine, going to bed and rising at the same time every day
- avoiding excessive sleep
- avoiding watching TV and bright lights before bed
- using the bedroom for sex and sleep only
- ensuring a comfortable temperature and creating a quiet, dark environment suitable for sleep
- exercising regularly but not before bed
- avoiding heavy late meals and overeating in the evenings
- reducing stimulants such as cola, caffeine and smoking before sleep
- if hungry, resort to small snacks before bed.

In a trial of 36 community-dwelling patients with Alzheimer's disease and their family caregivers, all received written materials describing age- and dementia-related changes in sleep and standard principles of good sleep hygiene.[25] The patients and caregivers were then randomised to either an active group (n = 17) receiving specific recommendations about setting up and implementing a sleep hygiene program for the dementia patient or a control group, receiving training in behaviour management skills. Also, the patients in the active group were instructed to walk daily and increase daytime light exposure with the use of a light box. Control participants (n = 19) received general dementia education and caregiver support. Sleep outcomes were derived at baseline, post-test (2 months), and 6-month follow-up. Patients in the active group showed significantly greater (P<.05) post-test reductions in number of night-time awakenings, total time awake at night, and depression, and increases in weekly exercise days than control subjects. At 6-month follow-up, treatment benefit was maintained, with further improvement in reduced night awakenings. The control subjects were noted to spend more time in bed at 6 months than the active group. The authors' concluded:

> this study provides the first evidence that patients with Alzheimer's Disease who are experiencing sleep problems can benefit from behavioural techniques (specifically, sleep hygiene education, daily walking, and increased light exposure).[25]

Mind–body medicine

Behaviour modification

It has been recently reported that non-drug therapies, such as using sleep diaries and dispelling dysfunctional beliefs about sleep patterns, may be as effective as hypnotics.[26] It is important to educate patients about normal sleep patterns for age. For example, the elderly can function on sleep of up to 6 hours per night. Actually counting the number of hours patients sleep can be reassuring. For instance, waking up in the early hours such as 5 a.m. might be considered abnormal for a person, but when counting the total hours of sleep, this might actually be adequate. Also, establishing a proper bedtime routine and avoiding daytime naps might help (see clinical tips at the end of this chapter).

Cognitive behaviour therapy (CBT)

A recent Cochrane review identified 6 trials to examine the effectiveness of CBT for sleep problems.[27] The final total of participants included in the meta-analysis was 224. The data suggests only a mild effect of CBT for sleep problems in older adults, best demonstrated for sleep maintenance insomnia. The authors' concluded that, whilst more research is required, 'when the possible side-effects of standard treatment (hypnotics) are considered, there is an argument to be made for clinical use of cognitive behavioural treatments'.[27]

Despite these findings, a recent randomised, double-blinded placebo-controlled trial that was not included in the Cochrane review but published in *JAMA*,[28] found CBT was superior to a hypnotic. The study compared CBT with the pharmaceutical zopiclone for the treatment of chronic primary insomnia in older adults (mean age 61 years). The participants (n = 46) were randomised over 6 weeks to either CBT (sleep hygiene, sleep restriction, stimulus control, cognitive therapy, and relaxation; n = 18), sleep medication (7.5mg zopiclone each night; n = 16), or placebo medication (n = 12). The 2 active treatments were followed up at 6 months. CBT resulted in improved short- and long-term outcomes compared with zopiclone and, overall for most outcomes, zopiclone did not differ from placebo. Participants receiving CBT improved their sleep efficiency from 81.4% at pre-treatment to 90.1% at 6-month follow-up compared with a decrease from 82.3% to 81.9% in the zopiclone group. Participants in the CBT group spent much more time in slow-wave sleep (stages 3 and 4) compared with those in other groups, and spent less time awake during the night. Total sleep time was similar in all 3 groups; at 6 months, patients receiving CBT had better sleep efficiency using polysomnography than those taking zopiclone. Based on these results CBT is superior to zopiclone treatment both in short- and long-term management of insomnia in older adults.

Another study compared, for 8 weeks, CBT alone with the pharmaceutical agent zolpidem alone, a CBT/zolpidem combination, and a placebo in 63 adults, aged 25–64.[29] Therapists taught CBT participants how to identify and curb thoughts that elevate arousal and interfere with sleep. They were advised to reserve the bedroom for sleep and sex, to go to bed only when drowsy, arise at the same time each day, and use other behavioural tactics known to benefit sleep. At 1-year follow-up, the CBT group demonstrated marked improvement with sleep, superior to the zolpidem group, and combination treatment offered no advantage over CBT alone.

Hypnosis

Several studies suggest hypnosis may be useful in managing insomnia, however most of these trials are dated and of poor quality.[30] A small study randomised 45 participants and compared hypnotic relaxation technique to stimulus control and placebo as a means of reducing sleep onset latency (SOL).[31]

The hypnotic group involved 4 weekly sessions of 30-minutes duration and compared stimulus control and placebo from baseline assessment. The subjects in this group were able to sleep more quickly. A similar case study also found hypnotherapy to assist with insomnia.[32] Factors that seemed to contribute to long-term response in this small group of patients included a report of sleeping at least half of the time while in bed, increased hypnotic susceptibility and no history of major depression.

A recent study reported on a retrospective chart review performed for 84 children and adolescents with insomnia, excluding those with central or obstructive sleep apnoea.[33]

All children (mean age 12 years) were offered and accepted instruction in self-hypnosis for treatment of insomnia, and for any other symptoms that was suitable for hypnosis. Seventy-five patients returned for follow-up after the first hypnosis session. If the first session was not useful, patients were offered the opportunity to use hypnosis to gain insight into the cause of their insomnia. The younger children were more likely to report that the insomnia was related to fears. Two or fewer hypnosis sessions were provided to 68% of the patients. Of the 70 patients reporting a delay in sleep onset of more than 30 minutes, 90% reported a reduction in sleep onset time following hypnosis. Of the 21 patients reporting night-time awakenings more than once a week, 52% reported resolution of the awakenings and 38% reported improvement. Of the 41% of children with somatic complaints such chest pain, dyspnoea, functional abdominal pain, habit cough, headaches, and vocal cord dysfunction, 87% reported improvement or resolution of the somatic complaints following hypnosis. The authors concluded the use of 'hypnosis appears to facilitate efficient therapy for insomnia in school-age children'.[33]

Meditation and relaxation

Relaxation techniques may be useful when stress and worry cause sleep disruption. An assessment of the literature by an expert panel found a number of well-defined behavioural and relaxation interventions now exist and are effective in the treatment of chronic pain and insomnia.[34] The panel found strong evidence for the use of relaxation techniques in reducing chronic pain conditions and behavioural techniques (relaxation and biofeedback) for sleep improvement. However, they concluded 'it is questionable whether the magnitude of the improvement in sleep onset and total sleep time are clinically significant'.[34]

A recent pilot study of 14 patients aimed to test mindfulness-based meditation for persistent insomnia.[35] Despite methodological limitations, meditation had significant benefit on improving quality of sleep.

Music therapy

Several studies have explored the effect of music on sleep patterns. One study of 28 abused women residing in domestic violence shelters was assessed for anxiety and sleep quality.[36] They were randomised to music therapy procedure (music listening paired with progressive muscle relaxation) or to a control. Results from pre- and post-testing indicated that music therapy constituted an effective method for reducing anxiety levels and had a significant effect on sleep quality for the music therapy group, but not for the control group. In another study, 60 Taiwanese elderly men and women aged 60–83, with difficulty sleeping, were randomised to a music group or a control group.[37] The music group involved participants listening to their choice of six 45-minute sedative music tapes at bedtime for 3 weeks. Sleep quality was measured before the study and at 3-weekly post-tests. Groups were comparable on demographic variables, anxiety, depressive symptoms, physical activity, bedtime routine, herbal tea use, napping, pain, and pre-test overall sleep quality. Music resulted in significantly better sleep quality, better perceived sleep quality, longer sleep duration, greater sleep efficiency, shorter sleep latency, less sleep disturbance and less daytime dysfunction in the music group compared with the control and pre-testing groups. Sleep improved weekly, indicating a cumulative dose effect.

Physical activity

Exercise

A number of studies with healthy participants have documented the benefits on sleep patterns of exercise during the day. Whilst several reasons are provided, regular physical exercise may promote relaxation and raise core body temperature in ways that are beneficial to initiating and maintaining sleep. A study that surveyed a randomly selected population of adults (mean 54–59 years of age, n = 319 men and 403 women), found that when participating in an exercise program and walking at a normal pace for more than 6 blocks per day, both women and men had significantly reduced risk of developing sleep disorders.[38] The findings suggest that a program of regular exercise may be a useful therapeutic modality in the treatment of sleep disorders. A small randomised controlled trial (RCT) conducted over 16 weeks reported that participants with sedentary lifestyles and moderate sleep problems experienced significant improvement in sleep from baseline with an exercise program comprised of four 30–40 minutes of endurance training per week when compared with wait-listed controls.[39]

Exercise for the elderly

Exercise for the elderly may be more difficult, but may also enhance sleep and contribute to an increased quality of life. An early study demonstrated that in older adults with moderate sleep complaints self-rated sleep quality was improved by initiating a regular moderate-intensity exercise program.[39]

A recent Cochrane review identified 1 trial of 43 participants over 60 years of age with insomnia, to examine the effectiveness of exercise.[40] The findings at post-treatment found that total sleep duration, sleep onset latency and scores on a scale of global sleep quality showed significant improvement, but improvements in sleep efficiency were not significant. The Cochrane reviewers conclude:

> ... when the possible side-effects of standard treatment (hypnotics) are considered, there is an argument to be made for clinical use of alternative treatments in the elderly. Research involving exercise programs designed with the elderly in mind are needed.[40]

It is also advisable to wind down and have quiet time before bed and avoid strenuous exercise in the evening.

Yoga

A small 8-week trial of 20 people suffering chronic insomnia found a simple daily yoga treatment was useful in statistically improving sleep-onset, sleep efficiency, total sleep time and sleep quality compared with pre-treatment values.[41] Participants practiced the treatment on their own following a single training session with subsequent brief interview and telephone follow-ups. In a recent study with 120 residents from a home for the aged, 69 were stratified based on age (5-year intervals) and randomly allocated to 3 groups, namely the yoga group (physical postures, relaxation techniques, voluntarily regulated breathing and lectures on yoga philosophy), a group for Ayurveda herbal preparation, and a wait-list control (no intervention). The groups were evaluated for self-assessment of sleep over a 1-week period at baseline, and after 3 and 6 months of the respective interventions.[42] It was concluded that yoga practice improved different aspects of sleep in a geriatric population as compared to herbal and control groups.

Sunshine and bright light therapy (BLT)

Exercise combined with sunshine may provide additional benefit for sleep disorders. It is generally advisable to increase daytime exposure to the sun and avoid bright lights at night. Darkness and daylight help to control the natural circadian rhythm and the production and release of the pineal hormone melatonin (N-acetyl-5-methoxytryptamine). Rest–activity and sleep–wake cycles are controlled by the endogenous circadian rhythm generated by the suprachiasmatic nuclei (SCN) of the hypothalamus. According to a Cochrane review,[43] degenerative changes in the SCN may be a biological basis for circadian disturbances in people with dementia, and might be reversed by stimulation of the SCN by light.

A randomised, prospective trial compared the efficacy of 20-minutes versus 45-minutes bright light exposure (10 000 lux for 60 days) for relieving insomnia in the elderly.[44] Compared with baseline, improvement was significantly higher in the 45-minutes versus 20-minutes exposure group at 3 months. At 6 months, variables returned toward baseline in the 20-minutes but not in the 45-minutes group. Another study found 2 evenings of BLT (2500 lux bright light) compared with control (dim red light) improved early morning awakening in insomniacs and day-time functioning up to 1 month after treatment.[45]

Findings are not so positive for the effectiveness of BLT in managing sleep, behaviour, or mood disturbances associated with dementia, according to a recent Cochrane review that found most studies were of poor quality and revealed inadequate evidence.[46] The Cochrane review concluded when:

> the possible side-effects of standard treatment (hypnotics) are considered, there is a reasonable argument to be made for clinical use of non-pharmacological treatments. In view of the promising results of bright light therapy in other populations with problems of sleep timing, further research into their effectiveness with older adults would seem justifiable.[46]

Nutritional influences

Diet

Recently it has been demonstrated that changes in lifestyle behaviours after attending an educational program significantly reduced sleep and stress disorders in as little as 4 weeks, primarily explained by decreasing Body Mass Index (BMI) and/or increasing exercise.[47] These are lifestyle modifications that take into significant deliberation nutritional practices.

It is generally advisable to avoid a heavy late meal and over-eating in the evening.

It has been suggested that night eating syndrome may be related to sleep disorders.[48] Reducing caffeine intake during the day, particularly close to bedtime, found in colas, some teas (e.g. black and green) and coffee is beneficial and limiting the intake of alcohol.[49] Eliminating and or reducing cigarette smoking is also of benefit, as nicotine is a stimulant to the brain.[19]

Tryptophan and melatonin – food sources

Tryptophan has a long research history for sleep disorders, spanning some 3 decades. There are foods and plants rich in tryptophan and melatonin that are considered as being helpful in inducing sleep. Studies have identified indolamines such as serotonin, tryptamine, and melatonin in some edible and medicinal plants that can assist with sleep.[50] For example, the pulp of under-ripe and ripe yellow banana contains 5-hydroxytryptamine at concentrations of 31.4 and 18.5ng/g respectively.[51] Corn, rice, barley grains, and ginger showed the highest concentrations of melatonin, at 187.8, 149.8, 87.3, 142.3ng/100g, respectively. Pomegranate and strawberry also showed a low level of indolamines (8–12μg/g serotonin, 4–9μg/g tryptamine, and 13–29ng/100g melatonin).

The amino acid tryptophan is necessary for the pineal gland to make both serotonin and melatonin. In animal models, consumption of L-tryptophan can cause a rise in blood melatonin levels by fourfold. Pyridoxine (vitamin B6) is also necessary for the production of serotonin from tryptophan (see Figure 22.1). Protein food sources of tryptophan can be comparable to pharmaceutical grade tryptophan for the treatment of insomnia.

Melatonin is naturally produced by the pineal gland in the brain from tryptophan and requires various minerals and vitamins as co-factors for each pathway. Deficiency of any of these co-factors may lead to reduced production of melatonin.

Tryptophan

A double-blind placebo-controlled study of 57 insomniacs were randomly assigned to 1 of 3 conditions:[52] protein source tryptophan (de-oiled gourd seed; an extremely rich source of tryptophan, 22mg tryptophan/1g protein) in combination with carbohydrate; pharmaceutical grade tryptophan in combination with carbohydrate; or carbohydrate alone. Only 49 patients completed the 3-week protocol. Both protein source tryptophan with carbohydrate and pharmaceutical grade tryptophan, but not carbohydrate alone, resulted in significant improvement on subjective and objective measures of insomnia. Protein source tryptophan with carbohydrate alone proved effective in significantly reducing time awake during the night.[52]

Foods high in amino acid tryptophan include:

- dairy products: cottage cheese, cheese, milk
- soy products: soy milk, tofu, soybean nuts
- seafood
- meats
- poultry
- whole grains
- beans
- rice
- hummus
- lentils
- hazelnuts, peanuts
- eggs
- sesame seeds, sunflower seeds.

Proteins

Peptic HCl ↓ Zinc, B1, B6

L-Tryptophan

Tryptophan hydroxylase ↓ Folate, Fe, Ca, B3

5-Hydroxytryptophan

Dopa Decarboxylase ↓ B6, Zn,mg, Vit C

5-Hydroxytryptamine (serotonin)

Proteins ⟶ Methionine ⟶ SAMe ↓ B5

Melatonin

Figure 22.1 Production of melatonin from tryptophan

Melatonin supplement

Melatonin is a pineal hormone that plays a central part in regulating bodily rhythms and has been used as a drug to re-adjust to the changes in time with travel. It shows promise for the treatment of insomnia but it does present with some concerns. Adopting a lifestyle that maximises the body's production of melatonin through safe sun exposure and dietary sources of tryptophan is the safest approach.

A recent Cochrane review identified 9 placebo-controlled trials to assess the efficacy of melatonin supplement for jet lag.[53]

Eight trials found if melatonin was taken close to the target bedtime at the destination (10 p.m. to midnight), this resulted in decreased jetlag from flights crossing 5 or more time zones.[53] Whilst daily doses of between 0.5 and 5mg are similarly effective, people fall asleep faster and sleep better with dosages greater than 5mg than 0.5mg. Slow-release melatonin (2mg) was relatively ineffective, suggesting that a short-lived higher peak concentration of melatonin works better. Benefit is greater the more time zones are crossed and less for westward flights. Adverse events are low but case reports suggest epileptics and patients with depression taking warfarin should avoid its use. The authors' concluded 'melatonin is remarkably effective in preventing or reducing jet lag, and occasional short-term use appears to be safe'.[53]

Melatonin has been trialled in the elderly and children who suffer insomnia. Results indicate melatonin is generally well tolerated and beneficial for insomnia.

A double-blind, placebo-controlled trial involving 62 children with idiopathic chronic sleep-onset insomnia were randomised to either 5mg melatonin or placebo at 7 p.m.[54] The study consisted of a 1-week baseline period, followed by a 4-week treatment. Total sleep improved significantly with melatonin treatment compared to placebo. Melatonin treatment also significantly advanced sleep onset by 57 minutes, sleep offset by 9 minutes, and melatonin onset by 82 minutes, and decreased sleep latency by 17 minutes. Lights-off time and total sleep time did not change. The authors' concluded melatonin 'improves health status and advances the sleep-wake rhythm in children with idiopathic chronic sleep-onset insomnia'.[54]

A prospective, double-blind, placebo-controlled, cross-over trial of 22 elderly people (over 65) with a history of sleep disorder complaints were randomised to 2 months of melatonin (5mg/day) or placebo.[55] Melatonin significantly improved sleep quality, behavioural disorders and mood levels (depression and anxiety) compared with placebo. Melatonin administration also facilitated discontinuation of therapy with conventional hypnotic drug. Another trial of a night-time milk containing ultra-low dosage (10–40 nanogram/litre) melatonin drink may benefit institutionalised elderly by increasing their daytime activity.[56]

A very small trial of 7 children with Autism Spectrum Disorder (ASD) were randomised to melatonin or placebo. For those who completed the trial, sleep improved significantly with melatonin supplementation resulting in reduced waking per night, earlier onset of sleep and increased duration of sleep.[57]

Recent research found 3mg of melatonin at bedtime was effective for the treatment of sleep problems in children with ASD and fragile X syndrome.[58]

Melatonin also plays a role in facilitating withdrawal of addictive medication such as benzodiazepines, which can cause significant adverse events such as drowsiness and falls in the elderly, whilst improving sleep quality.[59, 60]

A double-blind placebo-controlled study of 45 elderly patients taking low-dose anxiolytic benzodiazepines, randomised to melatonin 3mg or placebo for 6 weeks, found no benefit of melatonin compared with placebo.[61]

A systematic review of the literature found an overall trend towards efficacy of melatonin on sleep quality in the elderly, including those with Alzheimer's dementia.[62]

More long-term studies are required for the treatment of insomnia. Its use for jet lag is more established.

Nutritional supplements

Magnesium

Periodic limb movements during sleep (PLMS), with or without symptoms of restless leg syndrome (RLS), may cause sleep disturbances. A small, open, clinical and polysomnographic study researched 10 patients (mean age 57 years; 6 men, 4 women) suffering from insomnia related to PLMS (n = 4) or mild-to-moderate RLS (n = 6).[63] Following oral magnesium treatment (dose of 12.4mmol in the evening) over a period of 4 to 6 weeks, PLMS associated with arousal significantly decreased, PLMS without arousal were also moderately reduced and sleep efficiency improved. In 7 of the patients, estimating their sleep and/or symptoms of RLS as improved after therapy, the effects of magnesium on PLMS and PLMS-A were even more pronounced. The study indicates that magnesium treatment may be a useful therapy in patients with mild or moderate RLS or PLMS-related insomnia.[63]

Herbal medicine

An excellent review article assesses the efficacy and safety of stimulants and sedatives in sleep disorders.[64] The authors postulated that herbal sedatives may have evidence of efficacy based on observation studies that certain plant flavonoid compounds bind to benzodiazepine receptors. Caution is required with their use combined with other sedatives as they may have an overall additive effect. Withdrawal symptoms such as delirium have also been reported with chronic valerian use.[65] Whilst these herbs have a mild sedative effect, the effect can be strong in sensitive people.

Overall, valerian, hops and kava have received the most research attention, and have shown efficacy in some studies.

Kava also displays anti-anxiolytic effects.[66] The ethanolic form and use in high doses has been associated with hepatotoxicity.[67, 68] Consequently this preparation is banned in Australia with limitations in dosage.[69] (See Chapter 4 for more detail.)

Valerian (*Valerian officinalis*)

A recent systematic review and meta-analysis of an extensive literature search identified 16 eligible studies examining a total of 1093 patients.[70] The available evidence suggests that valerian may improve sleep quality without producing serious side-effects, although most studies have significant methodologic problems, with considerable variations in the valerian doses and preparations used, and with the length of treatment. Another systematic review of RCTs also suggests that valerian might improve sleep quality without producing significant side-effects,[71] although 1 systematic review whilst supporting that valerian as being a safe herb associated with rare adverse events, did not support the clinical efficacy of valerian as a sleep aid for insomnia.[72]

One randomised, double-blind trial found valerian was shown to have positive benefit on sleep although trial quality was generally low.[73] Two studies found valerian to be equally effective to oxazepam and triazolam in randomised, double-blind, clinical comparative studies.[74, 75] When compared with triazolam in the small, randomised control trial of 9 healthy individuals, valerian had less adverse effects on cognitive function.[75] In another study the effect of an aqueous extract of valerian root was assessed on subjectively rated sleep measures studied on 128 people.[76] Each person received 9 samples to test (3 containing placebo, 3 containing 400mg valerian extract and 3 containing a proprietary over-the-counter valerian preparation) presented in random order, and were taken on non-consecutive nights.

> Valerian produced a significant decrease in subjectively evaluated sleep latency scores and a significant improvement in sleep quality especially among people who considered themselves poor or irregular sleepers, smokers, and people who thought they normally had long sleep latencies.[76]

Another double-blind study of valerian compared with placebo also showed benefit for insomnia, however more robust quality studies are required.[77]

Valerian and kava (*Kava Kava*) combined

A combined formula consisting of valerian and kava herbs were compared in a pilot study of 24 patients suffering from stress-induced insomnia.[78] Patients were treated for 6 weeks with kava 120mg daily, followed by 2 weeks off treatment and then (5 having dropped out) 19 received valerian 600mg daily for another 6 weeks. Overall stress severity and insomnia were significantly relieved by both compounds ($P < 0.01$) equally. Side-effect profile was similar for both; 58% with each herb respectively and the commonest effect was vivid dreams with valerian (16%), followed by dizziness with kava (12%).[78]

Valerian and hops (*Humulus lupulus*) extract

The herb hops is well known as a bitter agent in the brewing industry and has a long traditional history in medicine to treat sleep disturbances.[79]

A pilot study of 30 patients with insomnia resulted in better quality sleep with the fixed valerian–hop extract combination (Ze 91019 extract) after 2 weeks of treatment, with no adverse events noted.[80] The exact mechanism for its pharmacological activity is not clear, but it is postulated from *in vitro* studies that partial agonistic activity on adenosine receptors (A1Ars) for the fixed extract and valerian extract may be contributing to its sleep-inducing effect.[81]

A randomised placebo-controlled trial (n = 184) of a valerian–hops combination versus diphenhydramine showed a modest hypnotic effect relative to placebo for adults suffering mild insomnia.[82]

Also, sleep improvements with a valerian–hops combination were associated with improved quality of life, did not produce rebound insomnia upon discontinuation of use, and both treatments appeared safe.[82]

Another randomised, placebo-controlled, double-blind sleep-EEG study in a parallel design using electrohypnograms of 42 subjects found time spent in sleep was significantly higher for subjects who took a single dose of valerian–hops fluid extract compared with placebo.[83]

Other herbs

German chamomile, lavender, lemon balm, *Panax ginseng*[84, 85] and passionflower[86] also have mild sedative effects, but more human studies are warranted for these herbs.

Physical therapies

Massage therapy

A study aimed to examine the effects of massage therapy versus relaxation therapy on sleep, substance P, and pain in fibromyalgia patients.[87] Twenty-four adult fibromyalgia patients were randomised to a massage therapy or relaxation therapy group. They received 30-minute massage treatments twice weekly for 5 weeks. Of interest, both groups displayed a decrease in anxiety and depressed mood immediately after the first and last therapy sessions, however, only the massage therapy group reported an increase in the number of sleep hours and a decrease in their sleep movements. In addition, substance P levels decreased, and the patients' physicians assigned lower disease and pain ratings and rated fewer tender points in the massage therapy group.

A recent Cochrane review[88] identified studies in which babies under the age of 6 months were randomised to an infant massage or a no-treatment control group. Twenty-three studies were included in the review. Fourteen studies were excluded, 13 of which were regarded at high risk of bias. The results of 9 studies suggest that infant massage has no effect on growth, but provided some evidence suggestive of improved mother–infant interaction, sleep and relaxation, reduced crying and a beneficial impact on a number of hormones controlling stress. The authors' concluded:

> some evidence of benefits on mother-infant interaction, sleeping and crying, and on hormones influencing stress levels. In the absence of evidence of harm, these findings may be sufficient to support the use of infant massage in the community, particularly in contexts where infant stimulation is poor.

Further research is needed.[88]

Acupuncture

A recent Cochrane review conducted to investigate the effectiveness of acupuncture in treating insomnia that included 7 eligible studies for review, involving 590 participants, found most studies were of low methodological quality and were diverse in the types of participant, acupuncture treatments and sleep-outcome measures used.[89] This severely limited the ability to pool the findings and draw conclusions. Therefore the review concluded that currently there is a lack of high quality clinical evidence supporting the treatment of people with insomnia using acupuncture.

A recent study of 40 patients suffering insomnia aimed to evaluate the efficacy of an acupressure device, 'H7-insomnia control', positioned on Heart-7 (HT-7) points of both wrists during the night, and assessed general health, anxiety levels, sleep quality and the urinary melatonin metabolite 6-hydroxymelatonin sulfate determination.[90]

Compared with the placebo group, the H7-treated patients demonstrated improved quality of sleep, reduced anxiety levels in insomniacs to a higher extent. Furthermore, the 24 hours urinary melatonin metabolite rhythm obtained at the end of treatment was found to be of normal levels in a higher percentage of H7-treated patients compared with placebo group.[90]

A similar trial assessing HT-7 point acupressure in cancer patients with insomnia was also beneficial in improving quality of sleep.[91]

Considering the relative safety of acupuncture and acupressure, more rigorous studies are warranted to assess the efficacy of these therapies for treating people with insomnia.

Aromatherapy

A number of essential oils from fragrant plants, such as lavender, have been reported to help promote relaxation and sleep in a pilot study.[92] A recent Cochrane review identified 3 small trials for aromatherapy, but only 1 trial had useable data. This trial showed a statistically significant treatment effect in favour of aromatherapy intervention on measures of agitation and neuropsychiatric symptoms in patients with dementia and thus may play a role in inducing sleep.[93]

Obstructive sleep apnoea/hypopnoea (OSAH)

Sleep apnoea can be a serious sleep disorder. People who exhibit sleep apnoea stop breathing for 10 to 30 seconds at a time while they are sleeping.[94] These short stops in breathing can happen up to 400 times every night, disrupting sleep patterns, hence we have briefly included it in our compilation of disordered sleep patterns.

A Cochrane review[95] aimed to determine whether weight loss, sleep hygiene and exercise were effective in the treatment of obstructive sleep apnoeas. No completed RCTs were identified for this analysis and the authors' concluded a need for RCTs of these commonly used treatments in obstructive sleep apnoeas.[95]

Jaw splint — sleep apnoea

A recent Cochrane review included 16 studies (745 participants) that assessed oral appliances (OA) with a control and in several trials compared with continuous positive airway pressure (CPAP).[96]

Overall, the authors' concluded there is:

> increasing evidence suggesting that OA improves subjective sleepiness and sleep disordered breathing compared with a control. CPAP appears to be more effective in improving sleep disordered breathing than OA. The difference in symptomatic response between these 2 treatments is not significant, although it is not possible to exclude an effect in favour of either therapy.[96]

Until there is more definitive evidence available, the reviewers recommend:

> with regard to symptoms and long-term complications, it would appear to be appropriate to recommend OA therapy to patients with mild symptomatic OSAH, and those patients who are unwilling or unable to tolerate CPAP therapy.[96]

Long-term data on more severe symptoms of sleep disorder, quality of life and cardiovascular health are required.

Summary

There is a strong scientific rationale for the use of an integrative approach to assist with the management of insomnia. The integrative approach may include a combination of modalities that also promote and sustain a healthy lifestyle, particularly correcting diet, reducing caffeine, restoring sleep, sun exposure, reducing stress levels and exercise which are essential in the management of insomnia. Table 22.2 summarises the evidence for complementary medicine/therapies.[97]

Table 22.2 Levels of evidence for lifestyle and complementary medicines/therapies in the management of insomnia

Modality	Level I	Level II	Level IIIa	Level IIIb	Level IIIc	Level IV	Level V
Lifestyle behaviour modification		x					
Sleep hygiene program		x					
Jaw splint for sleep apnoea	x						
Sunshine				x			
Avoid excessive television						x	
Listen to music						x	
Mind–body medicine							
Music therapy		x					
Hypnosis						x	
Reading						x	
Cognitive behaviour therapy	x						
Relaxation therapy	x						
Bright light therapy	x						
Environment							
Avoid excessive noise						x	
Avoid smoking				x			
Physical activity							
Exercise	x	x					
Nutritional supplements							
Food and supplement sources of tryptophan		x					
Food and supplement sources of melatonin		x					

Continued

Table 22.2 Levels of evidence for lifestyle and complementary medicines/therapies in the management of insomnia—cont'd

Modality	Level I	Level II	Level IIIa	Level IIIb	Level IIIc	Level IV	Level V
Magnesium supplement						x	
Melatonin supplement	x						
Herbal medicines							
Valerian	x						
Valerian–hop extract herbs		x					
Valerian–kava herbs		x					
Panax ginseng						x	
Passionflower						x	
Physical therapies							
Massage therapy	x						
Acupuncture/ acupressure		x					
Yoga		x	x			x	
Aromatherapy		x					

Level I — from a systematic review of all relevant randomised controlled trials — meta-analyses.
Level II — from at least 1 properly designed randomised controlled clinical trial.
Level IIIa — from well-designed pseudo-randomised controlled trials (alternate allocation or some other method).
Level IIIb — from comparative studies (including systematic reviews of such studies) with concurrent controls and allocation not randomised, cohort studies, case-control studies, or interrupted time series with a parallel control group.
Level IIIc — from comparative studies with historical control, 2 or more single-arm studies or interrupted time series without a parallel control group.
Level IV — opinions of respected authorities based on clinical experience, descriptive studies or reports of expert committees.
Level V — represents minimal evidence that represents testimonials.

Clinical tips handout for patients — insomnia

1 Lifestyle advice

General advice about sleep

- Restore normal sleep patterns. Develop a regular routine; that is, early to bed (about 9–10 p.m.). Try to wake up at the same time every day.
- Developing good sleep habits can help. These include:
  - avoiding sleeping in and daytime naps
  - developing a relaxing bedtime routine such as having a warm bath before bed and avoiding arguments and worrying during this time
  - going to bed early and when sleepy
  - avoiding excessive sleep
  - avoiding watching TV and bright lights before bed (e.g. computer use)
  - using the bedroom for sex and sleep only
  - ensuring a comfortable temperature and creating a quiet, dark environment suitable for sleep
  - exercising regularly, but not before bed
  - avoiding heavy, late meals and overeating in the evenings
  - reducing stimulants such as cola, caffeine and smoking before sleep
  - if hungry, resorting to small snacks before bed.
  - using clean sheets and bedding
  - avoiding worrying in bed; keep a sheet of paper and pen nearby and jot down your worries so you can attend to them in the morning; avoid ruminating and going over problems in your head.

Sunshine

- At least 15 minutes of sunshine is needed daily for vitamin D and melatonin production — especially before 11 a.m. and after 4 p.m. in summer when the sun exposure is safest.
- In winter, you may need more sunshine >1 hour per day.
- Dark-skinned people require longer sun exposure for adequate vitamin D production.
- Melatonin is a hormone made in the part of the brain called the pineal gland; it is produced from the amino acid tryptophan. Sunshine stimulates its production and darkness stimulates its release from the pineal gland. So before retiring turn off all lights in the household.

2 Physical activity/exercise

- Exercise at least 30–60 minutes daily. If exercise is not regular, commence with 5 minutes daily and slowly build up to at least 30 minutes. Outdoor exercise in nature, with fresh air and sunshine, is ideal (e.g. brisk walking, light jogging, cycling, swimming, stretching, weight-bearing exercises).
- Yoga may be of help, as may qigong and tai chi.

3 Mind–body medicine

- Stress management program; for example, initially 6 x 40 minute sessions for patients so they can understand the nature of their symptoms, the relationship to stress and the practice of regular relaxation exercises.
- Regular meditation practice: at least 10–20 minutes daily.
- Hypnosis, including self-hypnosis.
- Cognitive behaviour therapy or counselling to attend to any stress or psychological difficulties.
- If you suffer chronic pain that wakes you at night ensure you seek pain relief; for example, medication, acupuncture etc.

Breathing

- Be aware of breathing at all times. Notice if tendency to hold breath or over-breathe. Always aim to relax breath and the muscles around the chest wall.

Rest and stress management

Recurrent stress may cause a return of symptoms. Relaxation is important for a full and lasting recovery.

- Reduce workload and resolve conflicts. Contact family, friends, church or social groups for support.
- Listening to relaxation music during the day helps reduce anxiety and stress, and can aid sleep.
- Relaxation massage therapy is helpful.
- A relaxing bath and reading a happy book before bed may help.
- Sex may help with bringing on sleep induction.
- Hypnotherapy, biofeedback, cognitive behavioural therapy, and psychotherapy may be of help.

Fun

- It is important to have fun in life.
- Joy can be found even in the simplest tasks, such as funny movies/videos, comedy, hobbies, dancing, playing with pets and children.

4 Environment

- Ensure your bedroom is quiet, safe and free of smells and chemicals.
- Use heavy curtains if too much light enters the room.
- Aromatherapy with a few drops of lavender sprinkled on your pillow may help.
- Avoid environmental pollutants and chemicals — at work and in the home.
- Avoid smoking as nicotine acts as a stimulant.
- Avoid artificial sweeteners.

5 Dietary changes

- Do not rush your meals; relax before meals; chew your food thoroughly.
- Eat more fruit and vegetables — variety of colours and those in season.
- Eat more nuts; for example, walnuts, peanuts; seeds, beans (e.g. soy), sprouts (e.g. alfalfa, mung bean, lentils).
- Increase fish intake — canned is okay (mackerel, salmon, sardines, cod, tuna, salmon), and especially deep sea fish — daily if possible.
- Reduce red meat intake — preferably eat lean red meat (e.g. lamb, kangaroo) and white meat (e.g. free range organic chicken).
- Use cold pressed olive oil and avocado oil.
- Eat low GI wholegrains/cereals (variety): rice (brown, basmati, Mahatmi, Doongara), traditional rolled oats, buckwheat flour, wholegrain organic breads (rye bread, Essene, spelt, Kamut), brown pasta, millet, amaranth etc.
- Avoid artificial sweeteners. For sweetener try honey (e.g. manuka, yellow box and stringy bark have lowest GI).
- Tryptophan-rich foods that help production of melatonin. Examples are: dairy products such as cottage cheese, cheese, milk; soy products such as soy milk, tofu, soybeans, nuts; seafood; meats; poultry; whole grains; beans; rice; hummus; lentils; hazelnuts, peanuts; eggs; sesame seeds, sunflower seeds.
- Drink more water (1–2 litres a day) and teas particularly calming herbal teas such as chamomile and valerian, especially 1 hour before bed. Note some people are sensitive or allergic to chamomile or valerian. Avoid if you react to these.
- Avoid hydrogenated fats, salt, fast foods, sugar (e.g. in soft drinks, lollies, biscuits, cakes) and processed foods (e.g. white bread, white pasta, pastries).
- Avoid coffee, stimulants and drugs.
- Minimise alcohol intake to no more than 1–2 glasses daily.
- Avoid chemical additives — preservatives, colourings and flavourings.

6 Physical therapies

- Acupuncture may help — improves general wellbeing and can help with relaxation
- Regular relaxation aromatherapy massage may help.

7 Supplements

Melatonin

- Melatonin is derived from tryptophan and requires various minerals and vitamins for its production. Deficiency of any of these may lead to reduced production of melatonin.
- Indication: helps insomnia by improving circadian rhythm sleep disorders; reduces the time to fall asleep; jet lag.
- Dosage: adult: 0.3–6mg at 6 p.m. or closer to bedtime; for short-term use. Requires a prescription from your doctor. Children — smaller doses required, up to 3mg.
- Results: within 1–3 hours.
- Side-effects: usually well tolerated. Avoid long-term use. May cause drowsiness, dizziness, depressive symptoms, reduced alertness, irritability, headaches; all these symptoms can be transient.
- Contraindications: children, pregnant, lactating mothers; epilepsy sufferers; with alcohol, sedating medication such as benzodiazepines and use with narcotics; depression.

Vitamin D3 (cholecalciferol 1000 international units)

Doctors should check blood levels and suggest supplementation if levels are low.

Magnesium and calcium (best taken together)

- Indication: insomnia; may lower blood pressure; may be useful in anxiety, restless sleep and cramps.
- Dosage: children up to 65–120mg daily in divided doses. Adults 350–400mg daily including pregnant and lactating women.
- Results 2–3 days.
- Side-effects: oral magnesium can cause gastrointestinal irritation, nausea, vomiting, and diarrhoea. The dosage varies from person to person. Although rare, toxic levels can cause low blood pressure, thirst, heart arrhythmia, drowsiness and weakness.
- Contraindications: patients with kidney disease; if you have high blood calcium or magnesium levels (e.g. in cancer or kidney diseases).

Multivitamins, especially B-group

- Indication: Vitamin supplement containing low doses of B1, B3, B5, B6, folate and the minerals zinc, iron, calcium and magnesium may be of help in the production of melatonin.
- Side-effects: avoid single vitamin B supplementation and high doses of vitamin B6 >50mg daily for prolonged periods of time. Vitamin B6 toxicity may cause neurological problems such as tingling sensation and balance problems that are often reversible but can be permanent.

Herbs

Valerian

- Indication: insomnia; helps reduce time taken to fall asleep and improves sleep quality; may help with anxiety.
- Dosage: adults 400–900mg 1–2 hours before bed.
- Results: same evening.
- Side-effects: may cause paradoxical hyperactivity reaction, agitation, restlessness, hyperactivity, insomnia. May cause drowsiness, dizziness, reduced concentration and alertness the following morning.
- Contraindications: young children, pregnancy and lactating mothers. Avoid concomitant use with alcohol, analgesia or hypnotic medication.

Valerian and kava combined

- Indication: insomnia; helps reduce time taken to fall asleep and improves sleep quality; may help with anxiety.
- Dosage: kava 120mg daily; valerian 600mg daily.
- Side-effects: may cause paradoxical hyperactivity reaction, agitation, restlessness, hyperactivity, insomnia. May cause drowsiness, dizziness, reduced concentration and alertness following morning.
- Contraindications: young children, pregnancy and lactating mothers. Avoid concomitant use with alcohol, analgesia or hypnotic medication.

Hops

- Indication: insomnia; helps reduce time taken to fall asleep and improves sleep quality.
- Dosage: adults: hops (fruit dry) 100–1500mg 1–2 hours before bed.
- Results same evening.
- Side-effects: may cause allergic reactions, drowsiness, dizziness, reduced concentration and alertness following morning. May exacerbate depression.
- Contraindications: young children, pregnancy and lactating mothers. Avoid concomitant use with alcohol, analgesia or hypnotic medication. Depression. Avoid at least 2 weeks before surgery.

Other herbs

German chamomile, lavender, lemon balm, *Panax ginseng* and passionflower also have mild sedative effects, but more studies are warranted for these herbs.

References

1 NIH State-of-the-Science Conference Statement on Manifestations and Management of Chronic Insomnia in Adults. NIH Consens Sci Statements 2005 Jun 13-15;22(2)1–30.

2 Becker PM. Insomnia: prevalence, impact, pathogenesis, differential diagnosis, and evaluation. Psychiatr Clin North Am 2006;29(4):855–70.

3 Morin CM, Le Blanc M, Daley M, et. al. Epidemiology of insomnia: prevalence, self-help treatments, consultations, and determinants of help-seeking behaviours. Sleep Med. 2006;7(2): 123–30.

4 Zammit GK. The prevalence, morbidities, and treatments of insomnia. CNS Neurol Disord Drug Targets. 2007;6(1):3–16. Review.

5 Drake CL, Roehrs T, Roth T. Insomnia causes, consequences, and therapeutics: an overview. Depress Anxiety 2003;18(4):163–76. Review.

6 Ancoli-Israel S, Roth T. Characteristics of insomnia in the United States: results of the 1991 National Sleep Foundation Survey. I. Sleep. 1999;22(Suppl 2): S347-53.

7 Ford DE, Kamerow DB. Epidemiologic study of sleep disturbances and psychiatric disorders. An opportunity for prevention? JAMA1989;262:1479–84.

8 Kim K, Uchiyama M, Okawa M, et. al. An epidemiological study of insomnia among the Japanese general population. Sleep 2000;23:41–7.
9 Leger D, Guilleminault C, Dreyfus JP, et. al. Prevalence of insomnia in a survey of 12,778 adults in France. Sleep Res 2000;9:34–42.
10 Ohayon MM, Caulet M, Guilleminault C. How a general population perceives its sleep and how this relates to the complaint of insomnia. Sleep 1997;20(9):715–23.
11 Blunden S, Lushington K, Lorenzen B, et. al. Are sleep problems under-recognised in general practice? Arch Dis Child 2004;89(8):708–12.
12 Neckelmann D, Mykletun A, Dahl AA. Chronic insomnia as a risk factor for developing anxiety and depression. Sleep 2007;30(7):873–80.
13 Almeida OP, Pfaff JJ. Sleep complaints among older general practice patients: association with depression British Journal of General Practice 2005;55:864–66.
14 Thompson MD, Christakis DA. The Association Between Television Viewing and Irregular Sleep Schedules Among Children Less Than 3 Years of Age. Pediatrics 2005;116:851–56.
15 Ramakrishnan K, Scheid DC. Treatment options for insomnia. Am Fam Physician. 2007;76(4):517–26. Review.
16 American Academy of Sleep Medicine. International Classification of Sleep Disorders: Diagnostic and Coding Manual. 2nd ed. Westchester, Ill.: American Academy of Sleep Medicine, 2005.
17 Leger D, Poursain B. An international survey of insomnia: under-recognition and under-treatment of a polysymptomatic condition. Curr Med Res Opin 2005;21(11):1785–92.
18 Quach J, Hiscock H, Canterford L, et. al. Outcomes of Child Sleep Problems Over the School-Transition Period: Australian Population Longitudinal Study. PEDIATRICS 2009 May;123(5):1287-1292. doi:10.1542/peds.2008-1860.
19 Riedel BW, Durrence HH, Lichstein KL, et. al. The relation between smoking and sleep: the influence of smoking level, health, and psychological variables. Behav Sleep Med. 2004;2(1):63–78.
20 Phillips B, Mannino D. Correlates of sleep complaints in adults: the ARIC study. J Clin Sleep Med 2005;1(3):277–83.
21 Glass J, Lanctôt KL, Herrmann N, et. al. Sedative hypnotics in older people with insomnia: meta-analysis of risks and benefits. British Medical Journal 2005;331:1169.
22 Azad N, Byszewski A, Sarazin FF, et. al. Hospitalised patients' preference in the treatment of insomnia: pharmacological versus non-pharmacological. Can J Clin Pharmacol. 2003 Summer;10(2):89–92.
23 Johnson JG, Cohen P, Kasen S, et. al. Association between television viewing and sleep problems during adolescence and early adulthood. Arch Pediatr Adolesc Med 2004;158(6):562–68.
24 Ayas NT, White DP, Manson JE, et. al. A prospective study of sleep duration and coronary heart disease in women. Archives of Internal Medicine 2003;163:205–9.
25 McCurry SM, Gibbons LE, Logsdon RG, et. al. Nighttime insomnia treatment and education for Alzheimer's disease: a randomised, controlled trial. J Am Geriatr Soc 2005;53(5):793–802.
26 Becker PM. Sleep diaries and dispelling dysfunctional beliefs may be as effective as hypnotics. Current Psychiatry 2008;7:13–20.
27 Montgomery P, Dennis J. Cognitive behavioural interventions for sleep problems in adults aged 60+. The Cochrane Database of Syst Rev 2003;(1):CD003161.
28 Sivertsen B, Omvik S, Pallesen S, et. al. Cognitive behavioural therapy vs zopiclone for treatment of chronic primary insomnia in older adults: a randomised controlled trial. JAMA. 2006;295(24):2851–8.
29 Lamberg L. CBT outperforms hypnotics in sleep-disorder patients. Psychiatr News 2005;40:30.
30 Anderson JA, Dalton ER, Basker MA. Insomnia and hypnotherapy. J Roy Soc Med 1979;72:734–739.
31 Stanton HE. Hypnotic relaxation and the reduction of sleep onset insomnia. Int J Psychosom 1989; 36(1-4):64–8.
32 Becker PM. Chronic insomnia: outcome of hypnotherapeutic intervention in six cases. Am J Clin Hypn. 1993;36(2):98–105.
33 Anbar RD, Slothower MP. Hypnosis for treatment of insomnia in school-age children: a retrospective chart review. BMC Pediatrics 2006;6:23.
34 NIH Technology Assessment Panel on Integration of Behavioural and Relaxation Approaches into the Treatment of Chronic Pain and Insomnia. Integration of behavioural and relaxation approaches into the treatment of chronic pain and insomnia. JAMA 1996;276(4):313–8.
35 Heidenreich T, Tuin I, Pflug B, et. al. Mindfulness-based cognitive therapy for persistent insomnia: a pilot study. Psychother Psychosom 2006;75(3):188–9.
36 Hernandez-Ruiz E. Effect of music therapy on the anxiety levels and sleep patterns of abused women in shelters. J Music Ther 2005;42(2):140–58.
37 Lai HL, Good M. Music improves sleep quality in older adults. J Adv Nurs 2005;49(3):234–44.
38 Sherrill DL, Kotchou K, Quan SF. Association of Physical Activity and Human Sleep Disorders. Archive of Internal Medicine 1998;158:1894–8.
39 King AC, Oman RF, Brassington GS, et. al. Moderate-intensity exercise and self-rated quality of sleep in older adults. A randomised controlled trial. JAMA 1997;277:32–7.
40 Montgomery P, Dennis J. Physical exercise for sleep problems in adults aged 60+. Cochrane Database Syst Rev 2002;(4):CD003404.
41 Khalsa SB. Treatment of chronic insomnia with yoga: a preliminary study with sleep-wake diaries. Appl Psychophysiol Biofeedback. 2004;29(4):269–78.
42 Manjunath NK, Telles S. Influence of Yoga and Ayurveda on self-rated sleep in a geriatric population. Indian J Med Res 2005;121(5):683–90.
43 Forbes D, Morgan DG, Bangma J, et. al. Light Therapy for Managing Sleep, Behaviour, and Mood Disturbances in Dementia. The Cochrane Database of Syst Rev 2004;(2):CD003946.
44 Kirisoglu C, Guilleminault C. Twenty minutes versus forty-five minutes morning bright light treatment on sleep onset insomnia in elderly subjects. J Psychosom Res. 2004;56(5):537–42.
45 Lack L, Wright H, Kemp K, et. al. The treatment of early-morning awakening insomnia with 2 evenings of bright light. Sleep 2005;28(5):616-23.
46 Montgomery P, Dennis J. Bright light therapy for sleep problems in adults aged 60+ The Cochrane Database of Syst Rev 2002;(2):CD003403.
47 Merrill RM, Aldana SG, Greenlaw RL, et. al. The effects of an intensive lifestyle modification program on sleep and stress disorders. J Nutr Health Ageing 2007;11:242–8.

48 Winkelman JW. Sleep-related eating disorder and night eating syndrome: sleep disorders, eating disorders, or both? Sleep 2006;29(7):876–7.
49 Philip P, Taillard J, Moore N, et. al. The effects of coffee and napping on nighttime highway driving: a randomised trial. Ann Intern Med 2006;144(11):785–91.
50 Reiter RJ, Reiter RJ, Tan DX, et. al. Melatonin in plants. Nutr Rev. 2001;59(9):286–90.
51 Badria FA. Melatonin, Serotonin, and Tryptamine in Some Egyptian Food and Medicinal Plants. Journal of Medicinal Food 2002;5:153–57.
52 Hudson C, Hudson SP, Hecht T, et. al. Protein source tryptophan versus pharmaceutical grade tryptophan as an efficacious treatment for chronic insomnia. Nutr Neurosci 2005;8(2):121–7.
53 Herxheimer A, Petrie KJ. Melatonin for the prevention and treatment of jet lag. The Cochrane Database of Syst Rev 2002;(2):CD001520.
54 Smits MG, van Stel HF, van der Heijden K, et. al. Melatonin improves health status and sleep in children with idiopathic chronic sleep-onset insomnia: a randomised placebo-controlled trial. J Am Acad Child Adolesc Psychiatry 2003;42(11):1286–93.
55 Garzón C, Guerrero JM, Aramburu O, et. al. Effect of melatonin administration on sleep, behavioural disorders and hypnotic drug discontinuation in the elderly: a randomised, double-blind, placebo-controlled study. Ageing Clin Exp Res 2009 Feb;21(1):38–42.
56 Valtonen M, Niskanen L, Kangas AP, et. al. Effect of melatonin-rich night-time milk on sleep and activity in elderly institutionalised subjects. Nord J Psychiatry. 2005;59(3):217–21.
57 Garstang J, Wallis M. Randomised controlled trial of melatonin for children with autistic spectrum disorders and sleep problems. Child Care Health Dev. 2006 Sep;32(5):585–9.
58 Wirojanan J, Jacquemont S, Diaz R, et. al. The Efficacy of Melatonin for Sleep Problems in Children with Autism, Fragile X Syndrome, or Autism and Fragile X Syndrome. J Clin Sleep Med 2009;5:145–150.
59 Garfinkel D, Zisapel N, Wainstein J, et. al. Facilitation of benzodiazepine discontinuation by melatonin: a new clinical approach. Arch Intern Med. 1999 Nov 8;159(20):2456–60.
60 Peles E, Hetzroni T, Bar-Hamburger R, et. al. Melatonin for perceived sleep disturbances associated with benzodiazepine withdrawal among patients in methadone maintenance treatment: a double-blind randomised clinical trial. Addiction. 2007 Dec;102(12):1947-53. Epub 2007 Oct 4.
61 Cardinali DP, Gvozdenovich E, Kaplan MR, et. al. A double-blind-placebo-controlled study on melatonin efficacy to reduce anxiolytic benzodiazepine use in the elderly Neuro Endocrinol Lett. 2002 Feb;23(1):55–60.
62 Olde Rikkert MG, Rigaud AS. Melatonin in elderly patients with insomnia. A systematic review. Z Gerontol Geriatr. 2001 Dec;34(6):491–7.
63 Hornyak M, Voderholzer U, Hohagen F, et. al. Magnesium therapy for periodic leg movements-related insomnia and restless legs syndrome: an open pilot study. Sleep 1998;21(5):501–5.
64 Gyllenhaal C, Merritt SL, Peterson SD, et. al. Efficacy and safety of herbal stimulants and sedatives in sleep disorders. Sleep Medicine Reviews 2000;4(3):229–51.
65. Garges HP, Varia I, Doraiswarmy PM. Cardiac Complications and Delirium Associated with Valerian Root Withdrawal. JAMA 1998;280:1566–67.
66 Pittler MH, Ernst E. Kava extract versus placebo for treating anxiety. The Cochrane Database of Syst Rev 2002;(2):CD003383.
67 Russmann S, Lanterburg BH, Helbling A. Kava Hepatotoxicity. Annals of Internal Medicine, 2001;135:68–69.
68 Escher M, Desmeulus J, Giostra E, et. al. hepatitis Associated with Kava, a Herbal Remedy for Anxiety. BMJ 2000;322(7279):139.
69 Therapeutic Goods Administration (TGA) Web page last updated on 21 August 2006. Available: http://www.tga.gov.au/cm/kavafs0504.htm (accessed August 2007).
70 Bent S, Padula A, Moore D, et. al. Valerian for sleep: a systematic review and meta-analysis. Am J Med. 2006;119(12):1005–12.
71 Stevenson C, Ernst E. Valerian for insomnia: a systematic review of randomised clinical trials. Sleep Med 2000;1:91–99.
72 Taibi DM, Landis CA, Petry H, et. al. A systematic review of valerian as a sleep aid: safe but not effective. Sleep Med Rev 2007 Jun;11(3):209–30.
73 Dorn M. Efficacy and tolerability of Baldrian versus oxazepam in non-organic and non-psychiatric insomniacs: a randomised, double-blind, clinical, comparative study. Forsch Komplementarmed Klass Naturheilkd 2000;7:79–84.
74 Ziegler G, Ploch M, Miettinen-Baumann A, et. al. Efficacy and tolerability of valerian extract LI 156 compared with oxazepam in the treatment of non-organic insomnia- a randomised, double-blind, comparative clinical study. Eur J Med Res 2002;7(11):480–86.
75 Hallam KT, Olver JS, McGrath C, et. al. Comparative cognitive and psychomotor effects of single doses of Valerian officinalis and triazolam in healthy volunteers. Hum Psychopharmacol 2003;18:619–25.
76 Leathwood PD, Chauffard F, Heck E, et. al. Aqueous extract of valerian root (Valeriana officinalis L.) improves sleep quality in man. Pharmacol Biochem Behav 1982;17(1):65–71.
77 Lindahl O, Lindwall L. Double blind study of a valerian preparation. Pharmacol Biochem Behav 1989;32(4):1065–6.
78 Wheatley D. Kava and valerian in the treatment of stress-induced insomnia. Phytother Res 2001;15(6):549–51.
79 Zanoli P, Zavatti M. Pharmacognostic and pharmacological profile of Humulus lupulus L. J Ethnopharmacol.2008Mar28;116(3):383–96.Epub2008 Jan 20.
80 Fussel A, Wolf A, Brattstrom A. Effect of a fixed valerian-Hop extract combination (Ze 91019) on sleep polygraphy in patients with non-organic insomnia: a pilot study. Eur J Med Res 2000;5:385–90.
81 Müller CE, Schumacher B, Brattström A, et. al. Life Sciences 2002;71:1939–49.
82 Morin CM, Koetter U, Bastien C, et. al. Valerian-hops combination and diphenhydramine for treating insomnia: a randomised placebo-controlled clinical trial. Sleep. 2005 Nov 1;28(11):1465–71.
83 Dimpfel W, Suter A. Sleep improving effects of a single dose administration of a valerian/hops fluid extract - a double blind, randomised, placebo-controlled sleep-EEG study in a parallel design using electrohypnograms. Eur J Med Res. 2008 May 26;13(5):200–4.

84 Takagi K, Saito H, Tsuchiya M. Pharmacological studies of Panax Ginseng root: pharmacological properties of a crude saponin fraction. Japanese Journal of Pharmacology 1972;22(3):339–46.

85 Lee SP, Honda K, Rhee YH, et. al. Chronic intake of panax ginseng extract stabilises sleep and wakefulness in food-deprived rats. Neurosci Lett 1990;111(1-2):217–21.

86 Speroni E, Minghetti A. A NeuroPharmacological Activity of extracts from Passiflora Incarnata. Planta Medica 1988;54:488–491.

87 Field T, Diego M, Cullen C, et. al. Fibromyalgia Pain and Substance P Decrease and Sleep Improves After Massage Therapy. J Clin Rheumatol 2002;8(2):72–76.

88 Underdown A, Barlow J, Chung V, et. al. Massage intervention for promoting mental and physical health in infants aged under six months. The Cochrane Database of Syst Rev 2006;(4):CD005038.

89 Cheuk DKL, Yeung WF, Chung KF, et. al. Acupuncture for insomnia. Cochrane Database of Systematic Reviews 2007, Issue 3. Art. No.: CD005472. doi: 10.1002/14651858.CD005472.pub2.

90 Nordio M, Romanelli F. Efficacy of wrists overnight compression (HT 7 point) on insomniacs: possible role of melatonin? Minerva Med 2008 Dec;99(6):539–47.

91 Cerrone R, Giani L, Galbiati B, et. al. Efficacy of HT 7 point acupressure stimulation in the treatment of insomnia in cancer patients and in patients suffering from disorders other than cancer. Minerva Med. 2008 Dec;99(6):535–7.

92 Lewith GT, Godfrey AD, Prescott P. A single-blinded, randomised pilot study evaluating the aroma of Lavandula augustifolia as a treatment for mild insomnia. J Altern Complement Med 2005;11(4):631–7.

93 Thorgrimsen L, Spector A, Wiles A, et. al. Aroma therapy for dementia. Cochrane Database Syst Rev 2003;(3):CD003150.

94 American Family Physician. http://familydoctor.org /online/famdocen/home/articles/212.html Accessed October 2007.

95 Shneerson J, Wright J. Lifestyle modification for obstructive sleep apnoea. The Cochrane Database of Syst Rev 2001;(1):CD002875.

96 Lim J, Lasserson TJ, Fleetham J, et. al. Oral appliances for obstructive sleep apnoea. The Cochrane Database of Syst Rev 2006;(1):CD004435.

97 National Health and Medical Research Council. A guide to the development, implementation and evaluation of clinical practice guidelines. Commonwealth of Australia, Canberra, 1999.

Chapter 23

Irritable bowel syndrome

Introduction

The prevalence of irritable bowel syndrome (IBS) has been reported to be 9–22% in the US and 4–35% worldwide.[1–5] In the US this burden accounts for 12% of primary care provider visits and 28% of visits to a gastroenterologist.[6–8] IBS is a disorder of the brain–gut interactions with both physical and psychosocial components. Key factors appear to be mind–body, nutrition, bacterial flora and immunity.

The common symptoms of IBS include abdominal discomfort, abdominal pain, bloating and irregular bowel habits (Table 23.1).[9] Several non-gastrointestinal somatic symptoms, including lethargy, backache, headache, urinary symptoms, irritability of the uterus and dyspareunia suggest a generalised disorder. Usually there is no weight loss or weight gain and pain does not disturb sleep. It is vitally important that the patient has been well screened to exclude other pathological causes for their symptoms, such as coeliac disease, Crohn's disease, ulcerative colitis, diverticulitis and parasite infection such as *Blastocystis Hominis* and *Giardia*, as a clear diagnosis that offers treatment options can offer reassurance to patients. Management should include a positive diagnosis with an explanation of symptoms and their possible causes, and listening to patient's concerns, thereby addressing any underlying fears and beliefs which may help reduce patient anxiety.

IBS is a significant problem in general practice, as treatment options are limited and can frequently develop into a chronic condition. Many patients turn to alternative health care to seek symptomatic relief.[10] Given the frequency and disabling nature of IBS symptomatology, resorting to complementary and alternative medicine (CAM) remedies and therapies has long been a frequent encounter among IBS patients.[11] A recent study reports that IBS is poorly understood by patients.[12] There is evidence that some IBS patients in primary care experience dissatisfaction and negative attitudes in GP interactions.[12] GPs may be the first avenue for IBS patients to voice their frustrations, and hence appropriate education programs for optimal management of patients with IBS may be needed in primary care.[12] The health care practitioner is ideally suited to provide comprehensive lifestyle advice including diet, exercise and stress management to assist patients with IBS.

Healthy lifestyles

A healthy lifestyle approach of diet, exercise and stress management is of benefit in adult patients with IBS.[13–15] According to a prospective longitudinal study of 52 adult outpatients with IBS, patients attended a structured class that taught health-promoting lifestyle by completing a Health-Promoting Lifestyle Profile (HPLP). According to symptom scores on questionnaires, improved response rates to the HPLP at 1 and 6 months were 75% and 83%, respectively. Results revealed significant improvements in pain and overall IBS symptoms such as bloating and discomfort.[14]

Moreover, in a study that investigated the effects of multidisciplinary education on outcomes in patients with IBS, it was demonstrated that a one-time, multidisciplinary education class for patients with IBS was significantly associated with improvement in symptoms and health-promoting lifestyle behaviors.[15]

Mind–body medicine

Meditation and/or relaxation

Patients with IBS do well when they are taught to understand the nature of their symptoms, the symptom's relationship to stress and the practice of regular relaxation exercises. A controlled trial with 35 patients diagnosed with IBS who were randomised to a stress management program involving six 40-minute sessions with a physiotherapist, or to conventional care, demonstrated that two-thirds of the intervention group improved symptomatically, including less episodes of abdominal pain and cramps.[16] The benefits persisted over 12 months.

A small controlled treatment study of 16 adults revealed that meditation was superior to control ($P = 0.04$) in relieving symptoms of

Table 23.1 The criteria for diagnosing irritable bowel syndrome

Manning criteria[(a)]
• Abdominal pain relieved by defecation • Looser stools with onset of pain • More frequent stools with onset of pain • Abdominal distension • Passage of mucus in stools • Sensation of incomplete evacuation
Rome I criteria[(b)]

At least 3 months of recurrent symptoms of:
• abdominal pain or discomfort relieved with defecation, or associated with a change in stool frequency, or associated with a change in stool consistency and
• two or more of the following on at least 25% of occasions or days of:*
  • altered stool
    • frequency
    • form
    • passage
  • passage of mucus
  • bloating and or distension.

Rome II criteria[(c)]

• Twelve weeks or more in the last 12 months of abdominal discomfort or pain that has 2 of the following 3 features
  1 relieved by defecation
  2 associated with a change in frequency of stool
  3 associated with a change in consistency of stool.

* The second group of criteria included in Rome I are now considered supportive rather than mandatory in the diagnosis.
(a) Manning AP, Thompson WG, Heaton KW, et. al. Towards a positive diagnosis of the irritable bowel. BMJ 1978;2:653–4.
(b) Drossman DA, Thompson WG, Talley NJ, et. al. Identification of sub-groups of functional gastrointestinal disorders. Gastroenterol Int 1990;3:159–72.
(c) Thompson WG, Longstreth GF, Drossman DA, et. al. Functional bowel disorders and functional abdominal pain. Gut 1999;45:II43–7.
(Source: adapted and modified from the British Society of Gastroenterology guidelines for the management of the irritable bowel syndrome)[9]

IBS.[17] A symptom diary at 3-month follow-up, showed significant improvements in flatulence ($P<0.01$), belching ($P = 0.02$), bloating ($P = 0.05$), and diarrhoea ($P = 0.03$). Further follow-up at 1 year by the same group demonstrated additional improvement in reducing symptoms of pain and bloating with regular meditation practice.[18] At the 1-year follow-up they examined changes from the original 3-month follow-up point and noted significant additional reductions in pain ($P = 0.03$) and bloating ($P = 0.04$), which tended to be the most distressing symptoms reported of IBS. Hence, it appears that:

- the continued use of meditation was particularly effective in reducing the symptoms of pain and bloating
- that relaxation response meditation was a beneficial treatment for IBS in both the short- and long-terms of follow-up.[18]

Cognitive behaviour therapy (CBT)

There exists research demonstrating the efficacy of CBT in the treatment of IBS. An early published study on a multi-component delivery design that included relaxation, thermal biofeedback, and CBT treatments for IBS compared to an ostensible attention-placebo control (pseudo-meditation and EEG alpha suppression biofeedback) and to a symptom-monitoring control, showed that participants in both treatment conditions showed significant reductions in gastrointestinal (GI) symptoms, as measured by daily symptom diaries, and significant reductions in trait anxiety and depression compared with control group.[19] The gastrointestinal tract (GIT) symptom reductions held up over a 6-month follow-up. However, this same group in a more recent randomised study of 210 patients with Rome II diagnosed

IBS, of at least moderate severity, were randomised to 1 of 3 groups that consisted of:

- group-based CBT (n = 120)
- psycho-educational support groups (n = 46) as an active control, or
- intensive symptom and daily stress monitoring (n = 44).

The results demonstrated that the CBT and psycho-educational support groups continued not to differ on any measure. It was hence concluded that group CBT is not superior to an attention placebo-control condition.[20]

Hypnosis

There are numerous clinical reports and a body of research on the effectiveness of hypnotherapy in the treatment of IBS. Early randomised clinical trials have demonstrated that hypnotherapy provided a small but significant improvement in abdominal pain, abdominal distension and general wellbeing with lasting benefits in the treatment of IBS.[21, 22] Both individual and group hypnotherapy have been reported to be equally effective in alleviating symptoms in patients with IBS. Thirty-three patients were treated with either four 40-minute sessions of hypnotherapy over 7 weeks alone or in a group of 8 patients.[23] Twenty improved and 11 participants were virtually asymptomatic. This improvement was maintained at 3 months without further formal treatment.

In a recent study, a large scale audit was conducted on the first 250 unselected patients at a UK centre undergoing hypnosis for IBS.[24] Patients underwent 12 sessions of hypnotherapy over a 3-month period and were required to practice at home. Questionnaires before and after treatment demonstrated greater than 70% improvement in all symptom measures, improved quality of life, anxiety and depression (all $P < 0.001$), fewer consultations and less medication. These benefits persisted for greater than 5 years. It was less useful in males with diarrhoea-predominant IBS, suggesting differences in pathophysiology.[24]

A recent Cochrane review has concluded that more high-quality research is required.[25] The review found that 4 studies including a total of 147 patients met the inclusion criteria. Only 1 study compared hypnotherapy to an alternative therapy (psychotherapy and placebo pill), 2 studies compared hypnotherapy with waiting-list controls and the final study compared hypnotherapy to usual medical management. Data were not pooled for meta-analysis due to differences in outcome measures and study design. The therapeutic effect of hypnotherapy was found to be superior to that of a waiting list control or usual medical management, for abdominal pain and composite primary IBS symptoms, in the short term in patients who fail standard medical therapy. Harmful side-effects were not reported in any of the trials.

Physical activity/exercise

A recent study has reported that associations between GIT symptoms and exercise as well as dietary behaviours may have implications for the treatment of GIT symptoms that includes IBS.[26] Lack of exercise is considered as a contributor to the development of IBS although it is not clear what level and duration of exercise would be helpful.[13]

Yoga

In a controlled study of 22 males (mean age 35 years) with diarrhoea-predominant IBS, the participants were randomised to yoga treatment 2 times a day or symptomatic treatment with loperamide 2–6mg/day for 2 months.[27] Both the pharmaceutical and yogic interventions showed a significant decrease of bowel symptoms and anxiety state. However, there was an increase in electro-physiologically recorded gastric activity and enhanced sympathetic reactivity, as measured by heart rate parameters, in the loperamide intervention group suggesting concerns with safety. In a more recent study with 25 adolescents aged 11 to 18 years with IBS who were randomly assigned to either a yoga or wait list control group, it was demonstrated that yoga held promise as an intervention for adolescents with IBS.[28] In a recent review it was concluded that non-drug options such as yoga may be proposed to some patients.[29]

Nutritional influences

Diet

It has been reported that the prevalence of IBS has increased over the last 50 years in countries where a Western-style diet has been prominent or introduced and that 20–65% of patients with IBS attribute their symptoms to something in their food consumption that activates an abnormal response.[30]

The role of high fibre in the diet — from fruit, vegetables, nuts and seeds — adequate fluid intake, and establishing normal relaxed eating patterns is well established for the maintenance of good gastrointestinal function. This approach is best in those with mainly constipation and less likely to be useful in those with diarrhoea. The role of food sensitivity is not as well established.

A review of the evidence from 12 studies concluded that whilst more research is required, the history of adverse reactions to food in patients with IBS is common.[31] The reviewers concluded that there was a high placebo response of 30%, a small fraction of patients with IBS showed immunoglobulin E (IgE)-mediated food allergy and that there was evidence of an increase in the inflammatory cells present in the gut of some IBS patients. A recent study of 150 outpatients with IBS found elimination diets provided considerable relief in individuals who demonstrated raised immunoglobulin G (IgG) food antibodies by an ELISA test.[32] The commonest foods identified were wheat, milk, cashew nuts, whole eggs and yeast. The elimination diet led to 26% greater improvement in fully compliant patients compared with a sham diet after 12 weeks.[32]

In general, blood tests are of limited value. Food intolerances can be IgG-mediated particularly to wheat, milk, cashew nuts, whole eggs and yeast. Food allergies are less common and are IgE-mediated. These are particularly seen in patients suffering diarrhoea-predominant IBS; commonest foods include milk, wheat, eggs and amines.

An Australian systematic review of the literature included 7 studies which demonstrated positive response rates to an elimination diet ranging from 15–71% improvement in IBS symptoms.[33] Of the double-blind placebo-controlled challenges, food contributed from 6% to 58% of cases. Patients with diarrhoea-predominant IBS showed a higher likelihood of adverse food reactions. The foods most commonly identified as exacerbating symptoms of IBS from the studies included milk, wheat, eggs and amines. Carefully designed controlled clinical trials are reported to be warranted. It is suspected that there is increased immunological activity, perhaps due to stress and poor digestive flora.

Bulk-producing agents

Bulking agents include various types of fibre including psyllium, methylcellulose, corn fibre, calcium polycarbophil, and ispaghula husk.[1] Fibre provides bulk to the stool and is prescribed to increase stool frequency and improve stool passage in those who have constipation as a key symptom of IBS.

Whilst some research demonstrates benefit with bulk-producing agents such as psyllium and ispaghula husk (*Plantago ovata*) in IBS, a recent meta-analysis of 51 double-blind clinical trials found the evidence weak for the use of bulking agents in the treatment of constipation-predominant IBS.[34] A recent Cochrane review further concluded that bulking agents may improve constipation and can be used empirically, but should be evaluated at an early stage for individual benefit.[35]

Herbal medicines

Traditionally a number of herbs such as meadowsweet, golden seal, *Aloe vera*, German chamomile, slippery elm, marigold, ginger root, passiflora and wild yam have been used for digestive problems such as IBS, but little or no scientific evidence exists to support their efficacy and safety.[36] In 1 small study, *Aloe vera* appeared to be useful in the short-term treatment of constipation, but not IBS.[37] Long-term use of *Aloe vera* should be avoided and has been linked with melanosis coli.

There are only a few herbs that have been clinically trialled for IBS.

Peppermint oil

Peppermint oil is known to have anti-spasmodic properties.[38] A 1998 meta-analysis reviewed the use of peppermint oil for IBS but only 5 double-blind, randomised controlled trials (RCTs) were suitable for assessment.[39] Collectively the studies indicated that peppermint oil could be efficacious for symptom relief in IBS, however, in view of the methodological flaws associated with most studies, no definitive conclusions on efficacy were possible.

In a more recent review[40] of 4 of the 5 trials published and reported earlier by Pittler and Ernst there was sufficiently comparable methodologies to attempt a meta-analysis.[41] The result of this analysis modestly favoured peppermint oil over placebo (odds ratio [OR], 2.70; 95% confidence interval [CI], 1.56–4.76). This was consistent with the earlier analysis.[37] However, this latter analysis showed significant heterogeneity, which limited interpretability ($\chi^2 = 20.81$; $P<.001$).

Recent studies have used enteric-coated peppermint oil capsules. Not included in the meta-analysis, was a randomised, double-blind controlled trial of 42 children (mean age of 12 years) with IBS that were supplemented with enteric-coated peppermint oil capsules or placebo.[42] After 2 weeks, 76% of the children receiving peppermint oil had reduced symptoms of IBS and resolution of abdominal pain compared with 19% improvement in the placebo group. In a randomised study performed on a Taiwanese population consisting of 66 men and 44 women (aged 18–70 years) with symptoms of IBS, it was reported that peppermint oil was superior to placebo in improving symptoms after 1 month of therapy.[42]

Peppermint oil appears to be relatively safe,[43] however, side-effects such as heartburn and peri-anal burning/itch have been documented in the literature.

Iberogast (STW 5-II)

Iberogast is a complex herbal preparation.[44] Composed of a mixture of aqueous-ethanolic plant extracts from *Iberis amara*, chamomile leaves, caraway seeds, peppermint leaves, greater celandine, liquorice root, lemon balm leaves, angelica root and St Mary's thistle. Iberogast has a long history of use in Europe for over 40 years and is newly available in Australia. In a multi-centre study of 208 patients with IBS, the patients were randomised to treatment with Iberogast (STW 5), modified Iberogast (STW 5-II) or placebo.[45] STW 5-IIa is a mixture of 6 herbs of Iberogast excluding greater celandine, angelica and milk thistle, but with added bitter candytuft extract or placebo. STW5 was better in reducing the total abdominal symptoms by 54% compared with 27% in the placebo group at 4 weeks. There were no statistical differences between the STW 5-IIa group and the placebo group. Iberogast (STW 5) and STW 5-II were significantly better than placebo in reducing the total abdominal pain score (Iberogast, P = 0.0009; STW 5-II, P = 0.0005 versus placebo) and the IBS symptom score (Iberogast, P = 0.001; STW 5-II, P = 0.0003 versus placebo) at 4 weeks.[45] Further studies are warranted to assess the long term effects of treatment and the mechanism of action.

Chinese herbal medicines (CHMs)

An Australian study demonstrated strong scientific support for the traditional use of Chinese herbs in the treatment of IBS.[46] Patients diagnosed with IBS (n = 116) were randomised to receive a standard Chinese herbal formula, an individualised herbal formula or placebo. Significant improvement in IBS symptoms were reported in patients receiving either the Chinese herbal supplement or the individual preparation, compared with those receiving placebo. The average improvement of symptoms was 64%, 76% and 33% respectively. This improvement continued for 14 weeks after therapy was ceased. The group receiving individualised therapy did not relapse after treatment was discontinued, suggesting a change in the person being treated.[46]

A recent systematic review reports that herbal medicines have therapeutic benefit in IBS.[47] A total of 22 studies with 25 CHMs met the inclusion criteria. Four of these studies were of good quality, while the remaining 18 studies involving 17 CHM formulas were of poor quality. Eight of these reports using 9 CHMs showed global improvement of IBS symptoms, 4 studies with 3 CHMs were efficacious in diarrhoea-predominant IBS, and 2 studies with 2 CHMs showed improvement in constipation-predominant IBS. Out of a total of 1279 patients, 15 adverse events in 47 patients were reported with CHMs. No serious adverse events or abnormal laboratory tests were observed. Thus the incidence of the adverse events was low (2.97%; 95% CI: 2.04%–3.90%).[47]

However, a recent study that investigated the therapeutic efficacy of an ancient herbal Chinese formula in patients with diarrhoea-predominant IBS did not lead to global symptom improvement.[48] There was no significant difference in the proportion of patients with global symptom improvement between the herbal preparation and placebo groups at week 8 (35% versus 44.1%, P = 0.38) and at week 16 (31.7% versus 33.9%, P = 0.62). Moreover, there was no difference in individual symptom scores and the quality-of-life assessment between the 2 groups at all time points.[48]

Supplements

Probiotics and prebiotics

To date, there are more than half a dozen randomised, double-blind, cross-over trials that demonstrate the usefulness of probiotics in the management of IBS.[49]

A recent trial of 50 patients, mean age 40 years with IBS, were randomly assigned to receive either combined probiotics *lactobacillus plantarum* and *bifidobacterium breve* or placebo powder for 4 weeks.[50] Abdominal pain score after treatment decreased in probiotics group of 38% versus 18% of placebo group after 14 days and of 52% versus 11% after 28 days respectively. The severity of symptoms significantly decreased in probiotic group versus placebo group after 14 days 49.6% versus 9.9% (P<0.001) and these data were confirmed after 28 days (44.4% versus 8.5%, P<0.001).[50]

A further randomised, double-blind, placebo-controlled trial of 19 patients with Rome II criteria-defined IBS failed to show benefit after treatment with *lactobacillus GG*.[51] There was a trend toward improvement for a reduction in the number of unformed bowel motions in treated patients with diarrhoea.

Prebiotic agents such as oligofructose and inulin are reported to increase *bifidobacteria* in faeces and increase stool weight, which makes them attractive in the management of constipation.[52] A randomised, controlled, double-blind cross-over study of oligofructose in 21 patients with IBS, however, failed to detect any effects on symptoms, whole-gut transit time, faecal weight, or pH.[53]

Three recent reviews report that there is substantial biological plausibility as well as research evidence for the use of probiotics in the treatment of IBS.[54, 55, 56] However, recommendations for the use of probiotics for IBS are still limited as results of controlled clinical trials are contradictory because they have been performed using different species, dosages, treatment durations and end-points for effective result evaluation. Nevertheless, the role of the enteric flora is an area of great potential in IBS and requires additional trials to further confirm efficacy.

Physical therapies

Acupuncture

Several small studies suggest that acupuncture may be of value for IBS.[57, 58] A pilot study of 7 people with IBS found that acupuncture improved general wellbeing and symptoms of bloating.[59] Recent Cochrane and systematic reviews for IBS show it is still inconclusive whether acupuncture is more effective than sham acupuncture or other interventions for treating IBS.[59, 60]

Conclusion

The treatment difficulties encountered with IBS often lead clinicians and patients to seek alternative therapies for the management of IBS-associated symptoms. A number of therapies offer limited scientific support from the existing evidence. The exceptions are the use of diet modification, peppermint oil, Iberogast (STW-5) Chinese herbs, probiotics and psychotherapy which present the best evidence. While Chinese medicine offers only 1 study of high quality, psychological and relaxation therapies offer many studies of lesser quality.[40] However these studies have methodological deficits. Many of the studies are further disadvantaged by the absence of a defined control group.

Moreover, while dietary factors play an important role in symptom generation for many patients with IBS, food allergy is extremely uncommon, while food intolerance is quite common. Elimination of offending foods is a reasonable therapeutic adjunct if a clear trigger is seen, however, elimination diets are difficult and may have adverse nutritional consequences if not conducted properly under expert supervision.

From the current evidence what appears scientifically plausible and feasible is that the treatment of IBS symptoms requires an integrative (multi-modal) approach for symptom management that may, in the first instance, require an individualised approach. This is clearly evident in the high-quality Chinese herb study that hints at a subset of responsive patients with similar needs.[46] However, details of what this individualised therapy was were not given.[46] A holistic approach to treating IBS should at least include lifestyle changes such as exercise, stress management and dietary adjustments. Table 23.2 summarises the evidence for complementary medicine/therapies.

Table 23.2 Levels of evidence for lifestyle and complementary medicines/therapies in the management of irritable bowel syndrome

Modality	Level I	Level II	Level IIIa	Level IIIb	Level IIIc	Level IV	Level V
Lifestyle modification							
Diet,exercise and stress management					x		
Mind–body medicine							
CBT			x				
Meditation and relaxation				x			
Hypnosis		x					
Physical activity					x		
Yoga				x			
Nutritional influences							
Diet elimination (allergy)	x						
Bulk-producing agents	x*						
Herbal medicines							
Peppermint	x						
Iberogast (STW-5)		x					
Traditional Chinese Medicines	x						
Supplements							
Probiotics		x					
Prebiotics		x					
Physical therapy							
Acupuncture	x(+/-)	x					

*Efficacy reported for constipation only.

Level I — from a systematic review of all relevant randomised controlled trials — meta-analyses.
Level II — from at least 1 properly designed randomised controlled clinical trial.
Level IIIa — from well-designed pseudo-randomised controlled trials (alternate allocation or some other method).
Level IIIb — from comparative studies (including systematic reviews of such studies) with concurrent controls and allocation not randomised, cohort studies, case-control studies, or interrupted time series with a parallel control group.
Level IIIc — from comparative studies with historical control, 2 or more single-arm studies or interrupted time series without a parallel control group.
Level IV — opinions of respected authorities based on clinical experience, descriptive studies or reports of expert committees.
Level V — represents minimal evidence that represents testimonials.

Clinical tips handout for patients — irritable bowel syndrome

1 Lifestyle advice

Allow adequate and suitable time for regular defecation.

Sleep

- Restore normal sleep patterns. Early to bed (about 9–10 p.m.) and awakening upon sunrise. (See Chapter 22 for more advice.)

Sunshine

- At least 15 minutes of sunshine needed daily for vitamin D and melatonin production — especially before 10 a.m. and after 3 p.m. when the sun exposure is safest in summer.
- Ensure adequate skin exposure to sun; avoid sunscreen and excess clothing to maximise levels of vitamin D.
- More time in the sun is required for dark skinned people.

2 Physical activity/exercise

- Yoga may be of help. Other examples: qigong, tai chi.
- Exercise 30–60 minutes daily. If exercise is not regular, commence with 5 minutes daily and slowly build up to at least 30 minutes. Outdoor exercise with nature, fresh air and sunshine is ideal (e.g. brisk walking, light jogging, cycling, swimming, stretching, weight-bearing exercises). The more time you spend outdoors the better.

3 Mind–body medicine

- Hypnotherapy, biofeedback, cognitive behavioural therapy, and psychotherapy may be of help.
- Stress management program — for example, six 40 minute sessions for patients to understand the nature of their symptoms, the symptoms' relationship to stress, and the practice of regular relaxation exercises.
- Regular meditation practice, at least 10–20 minutes daily.

Breathing

- Be aware of breathing at all times. Notice if tendency to hold breath or over-breathe. Always aim to relax breath and the muscles around the chest wall.

Rest and stress management

Recurrent stress may cause a return of symptoms. Relaxation is important for a full and lasting recovery.

- Reduce workload and resolve conflicts. Contact family, friends, church or social groups for support.
- Listening to relaxation music helps.
- Relaxation massage therapy is helpful.
- Cognitive behavioural therapy and psychotherapy are extremely helpful in dealing with stress.
- Hypnotherapy, biofeedback may be of help.

Focus on wellness, not just the disease.

Fun

- It is important to have fun in life.
- Joy can be found even in the simplest tasks, such as funny movies/videos, comedy, hobbies, dancing, playing with pets and children.

4 Environment

- Avoid smoking, environmental pollutants and chemicals — at work and in the home.

5 Dietary changes

Do not rush your meals. Relax before meals; chew your food thoroughly before swallowing as this aids digestion. Maintain regular relaxed eating patterns.

- Eat regular balanced healthy meals, ideally 3 small meals, and 2 snacks, each containing protein in order to avoid fluctuating blood sugar levels and provide amino acids for nerve transmitters such as tryptophan.
- For some individuals, raw food or steaming food is better; increasing dietary fibre if you predominately suffer constipation.
- Bran may be of benefit for some patients; if you are intolerant of wheat you can use alternative bran such as oat bran.
- Eat more fruit (>2/day) and vegetables (>5/day) — a variety of colours and those in season.
- Eat more nuts, seeds, beans, sprouts (e.g. alfalfa, mung, bean, lentil).
- Increase fish intake (sardines, tuna, salmon, cod, mackerel) especially deep sea fish >3 servings per week.
- Reduce red meat intake — preferably eat lean red meat (e.g. lamb, kangaroo) and white meat (e.g. free range organic chicken).

- Use cold pressed olive oil and avocado.
- Eat dark chocolate.
- Eat wholegrains/cereals (variety): rice (brown, basmati, Mahatmi, Doongara), traditional rolled oats, buckwheat flour, wholegrain organic breads (rye bread, Essene, spelt, Kamut), brown pasta, couscous, millet, amaranth etc. Avoid wheat if intolerant.
- Reduce dairy intake; consume low fat dairy products such as yoghurt and cheeses, unless there is a dairy intolerance.
- Drink more water (1–2 litres a day) and teas (especially green tea, black tea).
- Ginger, chamomile and peppermint aid digestion. Drink 1 cup of either tea 30–60 minutes before meals.
- Avoid hydrogenated fats, salt, fast foods, sugar (such as in soft drinks), lollies, biscuits, cakes and processed foods (e.g. white bread, white pasta, pastries).
- Minimise coffee no more than 1cup per day as it can cause restlessness and agitation in high doses.
- Minimise alcohol intake to no more than 1–2 glasses daily as it is a brain depressant and can disturb sleep.
- Avoid chemical additives — preservatives, colourings and flavourings.
- For sweetener try honey (e.g. manuka, yellow box and stringy bark have lowest GI).

Food intolerance

- Intolerance of poorly absorbed carbohydrate, especially lactose and fructose, is well recognised and can be checked by your doctor by doing a breath test.
- Exclusion diets, performed under supervision of a dietitian or experienced health practitioner, may be helpful to a limited number of patients.
- Exclusion diets are particularly helpful for food allergies when diarrhoea is a predominant feature of IBS, especially for milk, wheat, eggs and amines.
- Common food intolerances include wheat, milk, cashew nuts, whole eggs and yeast.
- Your doctor will advise you accordingly.

6 Physical therapies

- Acupuncture may be of help — it improves general wellbeing and reduces abdominal bloating.

7 Supplements

Bulk-producing agents

Psyllium and ispaghula husk (*Plantago ovata*)
Indication: reduces symptoms of constipation-dominant IBS and resolution of abdominal pain; flatulence; softens stools; used for constipation.

- Dosage for IBS: adult: psyllium seed husk, 10–30g in 2–3 divided doses with >250mls water.
- Results: 1–4 days.
- Side-effects: often well tolerated. Very mild and rare side-effects; transient abdominal discomfort (e.g. pain, bloating); bowel obstruction may occur with inadequate fluid intake; allergic reactions.
- Contraindications: faecal impaction or bowel obstruction, previous occupation exposure to psyllium (sensitivity reaction); diarrhoea; drug interaction; lower blood glucose levels; avoid taking same time as other pharmaceutical medication — check with your doctor.

Other bulk-producing agents include methyl cellulose, corn fibre, calcium polycarbophil.

Probiotics: *lactobacillus plantarum* and *bifidobacterium breve*

- Indication: reduces symptoms of IBS such as abdominal pain and bloating.

***Lactobacillus GG* (acidophilus)**

- Indication: reduces number of unformed stools; IBS, treating and preventing diarrhoea (e.g. rotaviral diarrhoea in children, relapsing Clostridium difficile colitis and traveller's diarrhoea); antibiotic-associated diarrhoea; inflammatory bowel syndrome (Crohn's disease, ulcerative colitis), bacterial overgrowth in short-bowel syndrome and *Helicobacter pylori* infection; vaginal and Candida-related (yeast) infections.
- Dosage: *lactobacillus* combined with *bifidobacterium breve* preparations are quantified by the number of living organisms per capsule. Typical doses range from 1 to 10 billion viable organisms taken daily in 3–4 divided doses (e.g. 1–2 capsules or 1tsp mixed in warm water before meals).
- Results: 1–14 days.

- Side-effects: often well tolerated. Very mild and rare side-effects; transient abdominal discomfort (e.g. bloating, flatulence).
- Contraindications: severely ill and/or immuno-compromised patients.

Prebiotics — oligofructose and inulin to increase *bifidobacteria*

- Indications: prebiotics promote the growth and activity of specific strains of bacteria (e.g. *bifidobacetrium*) in the gut. Oligofructose is used for constipation, traveller's diarrhoea, increasing faecal mass. Inulin is used for constipation-predominant IBS.
- Dosage: 20g x 2, daily mixed with water before meals.
- Results: 15–20 days.
- Side-effects: often well tolerated. Very mild and rare side-effects; transient abdominal discomfort (e.g. bloating, flatulence).
- Contraindications: severely ill and/or immuno-compromised patients. Allergies to any of the food sources from which inulin and oligofructose are derived.

Inulin is derived from wheat, onions, bananas, leaks, artichokes, asparagus, and hot water extraction from chicory root.

Oligofructose are plant sugars from a wide variety of fruits, vegetables, and cereals.

Consisting of amylase, lipase, protease, tilactase, and cellulose.

- Indications: IBS; may help aid digestion (belching, reflux, flatulence, abdominal pain and bloating).
- Dosage: 1 capsule with each meal.
- Side-effects: very safe.
- Contraindications: nil known

Digestive enzymes

Consisting of amylase, lipase, protease, tilactase, and cellulose.

- Indications: IBS; may help aid digestion (belching, reflux, flatulence, abdominal pain and bloating).
- Dosage: 1 capsule with each meal.
- Side-effects: very safe.
- Contraindications: nil known.

Herbs

Traditional use with little or no evidence

Meadow sweet, golden seal, *Aloe vera* (short-term use only as long-term may cause damage to lining of your gut), German chamomile, slippery elm, marigold, ginger root, passiflora, wild yam.

Peppermint oil (enteric coated capsules)

Indication: reduces symptoms of IBS and resolution of abdominal pain; flatulence; dyspepsia.

- Dosage for IBS: adult: 0.2–0.4 mL 3 times daily in enteric-coated capsules. Children > 8 years of age: 0.1–0.2 mL 3 times daily in enteric-coated capsules. Dyspepsia, peppermint oil 90mg/day combined with caraway oil.
- Results: 1–4 days.
- Side-effects: very mild and rare; heartburn, stomach upset, peri-anal burning/itch; sensitivity to herb; burning mouth.
- Contraindications: diarrhoea, drug interaction; avoid use with pharmaceutical medication such as anti-ulcer medication — check with your doctor.

Iberogast or STW-5

(Mixture of low-dose herbs in alcoholic extract: *Iberis amara*, chamomile leaves, caraway seeds, peppermint leaves, greater celandine, liquorice root, lemon balm leaves, angelica root, St Mary's thistle.)

- Indication: IBS for reduction of abdominal symptoms.
- Dosage: 10–20 drops before meals.
- Results: 1–4 days.
- Side-effects: very mild and rare. Includes sensitivity to any of the herbs.
- Contraindications: avoid if any sensitivity to alcohol — check with your doctor.

Traditional Chinese herbal medicine (most helpful)

- Indication: benefit appeared to be better sustained in the individualised group. No relapse of IBS symptoms occurred after individual herbal therapy. Must be provided by an experienced Chinese herbalist in accordance with the published study. Note: some imported Chinese herbs are tainted with heavy metals.
- Dosage: 9g/day of raw powdered herbs.
- Results: uncertain.
- Side-effects: very mild and rare; nausea, vomiting, diarrhoea, sensitivity reactions to any of the herbs; no liver damage occurred in study although this may rarely occur with any herb.
- Contraindications: avoid if any liver or kidney problems.

References

1 Podovei M, Kuo B. Irritable bowel syndrome: a practical review. South Med J 2006;99(11):1235–42.
2 Cash BD, Chey WD. Advances in the management of irritable bowel syndrome. Curr Gastroenterol Rep 2003;5(6):468–75.
3 Saito YA, Locke GR, Talley NJ, et. al. A comparison of the Rome and Manning criteria for case identification in epidemiological investigations of irritable bowel syndrome. Am J Gastroenterol 2000;95(10):2816-24.
4 Drossman DA, Li Z, Andruzzi E, et. al. U.S. householder survey of functional gastrointestinal disorders. Prevalence, sociodemography, and health impact. Dig Dis Sci 1993;38(9):1569–80.
5 Drossman DA, Whitehead WE, Camilleri M. Irritable bowel syndrome: a technical review for practice guideline development. Gastroenterology 1997;112:2120–2137.
6 Mitchell CM, Drossman DA. Survey of the AGA membership relating to patients with functional gastrointestinal disorders. Gastroenterol 1987; 92(5 Pt 1):1282–4.
7 Schuster MM. Defining and diagnosing irritable bowel syndrome. Am J Manag Care. 2001;7(8 Suppl):S246–51.
8 Switz DM. What the gastroenterologist does all day: a survey of a state society's practice. Gastroenterology 1976;70:1048–50.
9 Jones J, Boorman J, Cann P, British Society of Gastroenterology guidelines for the management of the irritable bowel syndrome. Gut 2000;47(Suppl 2):ii1–ii19.
10 Hussain Z, Quigley EM. Systematic review: Complementary and alternative medicine in the irritable bowel syndrome. Aliment Pharmacol Ther 2006;23(4):465–71.
11 Langmead L, Chitnis M, Rampton DS. Use of complementary therapies by patients with IBD may indicate psychosocial distress. Inflamm Bowel Dis 2002;8(3):174–9.
12 Dhaliwal SK, Hunt RH. Doctor-patient interaction for irritable bowel syndrome in primary care: a systematic perspective. Eur J Gastroenterol Hepatol 2004;16(11):1161–6.
13 Wald A, Rakel D. Behavioral and complementary approaches for the treatment of irritable bowel syndrome. Nutr Clin Pract 2008;23(3):284–92.
14 Colwell LJ, Prather CM, Phillips SF, et. al. Effects of an irritable bowel syndrome educational class on health-promoting behaviors and symptoms. Am J Gastroenterol 1998;93(6):901–5.
15 Saito YA, Prather CM, Van Dyke CT, et. al. Effects of multidisciplinary education on outcomes in patients with irritable bowel syndrome. Clin Gastroenterol Hepatol 2004;2(7):576–84.
16 Shaw, et. al. Stress management for irritable bowel syndrome: a controlled trial. Digestion 1991;50(1):36–42.
17 Keefer L, Blanchard EB.The effects of relaxation response meditation on the symptoms of irritable bowel syndrome: results of a controlled treatment study. Behav Res Ther 2001;39(7):801–11.
18 Keefer L, Blanchard EB. A one year follow-up of relaxation response meditation as a treatment for irritable bowel syndrome. Behav Res Ther 2002;40(5):541–6.
19 Blanchard EB, Schwarz SP, Suls JM, et. al. Two controlled evaluations of multicomponent psychological treatment of irritable bowel syndrome. Behav Res Ther 1992;30(2):175–89.
20 Blanchard EB, Lackner JM, Sanders K, et. al. A controlled evaluation of group cognitive therapy in the treatment of irritable bowel syndrome. Behav Res Ther 2007;45(4):633–48.
21 Whorwell PJ, Prior A, Colgan SM. Hypnotherapy in severe irritable bowel syndrome: further experience. Gut 1987;28(4):423–5.
22 Whorwell PJ, Prior A, Faragher EB. Controlled trial of hypnotherapy in the treatment of severe refractory irritable-bowel syndrome. Lancet 1984;2(8414):1232–4.
23 Harvey RF, Hinton RA, Gunary RM, et. al. Individual and group hypnotherapy in treatment of refractory irritable bowel syndrome. Lancet 1989;1(8635):424–5.
24 Gonsalkorale WM, Houghton LA, Whorwell PJ. Long term benefits of hypnotherapy for irritable bowel syndrome. Gut 2003;52:1623–29.
25 Webb AN, Kukuruzovic RH, Catto-Smith AG, et. al. Hypnotherapy for treatment of irritable bowel syndrome. Cochrane Database Syst Rev 2007;(4):CD005110.
26 Levy RL, Linde JA, Feld KA, et. al. The association of gastrointestinal symptoms with weight, diet, and exercise in weight-loss program participants. Clin Gastroenterol Hepatol 2005;3(10):992–6.
27 Taneja I, Deepak KK, Poojary G, et. al. Yogic versus conventional treatment in diarrhea-predominant irritable bowel syndrome: a randomised control study. Appl Psychophysiol Biofeedback 2004;29(1):19–33.
28 Kuttner L, Chambers CT, Hardial J, et. al. A randomised trial of yoga for adolescents with irritable bowel syndrome. Pain Res Manag 2006 Winter;11(4):217–23.
29 Ducrotté P.(Irritable bowel syndrome: current treatment options) Presse Med 2007;36(11 Pt 2):1619–26.
30 Wächtershäuser A, Stein JM. Nutritional factors and nutritional therapy for irritable bowel syndrome—what is worthwhile? Z Gastroent 2008;46(3):279–91.
31 Ortolani C, Bruijnzeel-Koomen C, Bengtsson U, et. al. Controversial aspects of adverse reactions to food. Allergy 1999;54:27–45.
32 Atkinson W, et. al. Food elimination based on IgG antibodies in irritable bowel syndrome: a randomised controlled trial. Gut 2004;53:1391–1393.
33 Niece AM, Frankum B, Talley N. Are adverse food reactions linked to irritable bowel syndrome? Am J Gastroenterol 1998;93(11):2184–90.
34 Lesbros-Pantoflickova D, Michetti P, Fried M, et. al. Meta-analysis: The treatment of irritable bowel syndrome. Aliment Pharmacol Ther 2004;20(11–12):1253–69.
35 Quartero AO, Meineche-Schmidt V, Muris J, et. al. Bulking agents, antispasmodic and antidepressant medication for the treatment of irritable bowel syndrome. Cochrane Database Syst Rev 2005;(2):CD003460.
36 Langmead L, Rampton DS. Herbal treatment in gastrointestinal and liver disease—benefits and dangers. Aliment Pharmacol Ther 2001;15:1239–52.
37 Davis K, Philpott S, Kumar D, et. al. Randomised double-blind placebo-controlled trial of aloe vera for irritable bowel syndrome. Int J Clin Pract 2006;60(9):1080–6.
38 Hills JM, Aaronson PI. The mechanism of action of peppermint oil on gastrointestinal smooth muscle: an analysis using patch clamp electrophysiology and isolated tissue pharmacology in rabbit and guinea pig. Gastroenterology 1991;101:55–65.

39 Pittler MH, Ernst E. Peppermint oil for irritable bowel syndrome: a critical review and metaanalysis. Am J Gastroenterol 1998;93:1131–5.
40 Spanier JA, Howden CW, Jones MP. A systematic review of alternative therapies in the irritable bowel syndrome. Arch Intern Med 2003;163(3):265–74.
41 Kline RM, Kline JJ, Di Palma J, et. al. Enteric-coated, pH-dependent Peppermint oil capsules in the treatment of Irritable Bowel Syndrome in children. Journal of Pediatrics 2001;138:125–8.
42 Liu JH, Chen GH, Yeh HZ, et. al. Enteric-coated peppermint-oil capsules in the treatment of irritable bowel syndrome: a prospective, randomised trial. J Gastroenterol 1997;32:765–8.
43 McKay DL, Blumberg JB. A review of the bioactivity and potential health benefits of peppermint tea (Mentha piperita L.). Phytother Res 2006;20(8):619–33.
44 Saller R, Pfister-Hotz G, Iten F, et. al. Iberogast: a modern phytotherapeutic combined herbal drug for the treatment of functional disorders of the gastrointestinal tract (dyspepsia, irritable bowel syndrome)-from phytomedicine to "evidence based phytotherapy." Forsch Komplementarmed Klass Naturheilkd 2002;9(Suppl 1):1–20.
45 Madisch A, Holtmann G, Plein K, et. al. Treatment of irritable bowel syndrome with herbal preparations: results of a double-blind, randomised, placebo-controlled, multicentre trial. Aliment Pharmacol Ther 2004;19:271–9.
46 Bensoussan A, Talley NJ, Hing M, et. al. Treatment of Irritable Bowel Syndrome with Chinese Herbal Medicine. JAMA 1998;280:1585–9.
47 Shi J, Tong Y, Shen JG, et. al. Effectiveness and safety of herbal medicines in the treatment of irritable bowel syndrome: a systematic review. World J Gastroenterol 2008;14(3):454–62.
48 Leung WK, Wu JC, Liang SM, et. al. Treatment of diarrhea-predominant irritable bowel syndrome with traditional Chinese herbal medicine: a randomised placebo-controlled trial. Am J Gastroenterol 2006;101(7):1574–80.
49 Vitetta L, Sali A. Probiotics, Prebiotics and Gastrointestinal Health. Medicine Today 2008;9(8):65–70.
50 Saggioro A. Probiotics in the treatment of irritable bowel syndrome. J. Clin Gastroenterol. 2004;38 (6 Suppl):S104–6.
51 O'Sullivan MA, O'Morain CA. Bacterial supplementation in the irritable bowel syndrome: a randomised double-blind placebo-controlled cross-over study. Dig Liver Dis 2000;32:294–301.
52 Gibson GR, Beatty ER, Wang X, et. al. Selective stimulation of bifidobacteria in the human colon by oligofructose and inulin. Gastroenterology 1995;108:975–82.
53 Hunter JO, Tuffnell Q, Lee AJ. Controlled trial of oligofructose in the management of irritable bowel syndrome. J Nutr 1999;129:1451S–1453S.
54 Guslandi M. Probiotic agents in the treatment of irritable bowel syndrome. J Int Med Res 2007;35(5):583–9.
55 Borowiec AM, Fedorak RN. The role of probiotics in management of irritable bowel syndrome. Curr Gastroenterol Rep 2007;9(5):393–400.
56 Quigley EM. Probiotics in irritable bowel syndrome: an immunomodulatory strategy? J Am Coll Nutr 2007;26(6):684S–690S.
57 Li Y, Tougas G, Chiverton SG, et. al. The effect of acupuncture on gastrointestinal function and disorders. Am J Gastroenterol. 1992;87: 1372–81.
58 Chan J, Carr I, Mayberry JF. The role of acupuncture in the treatment of irritable bowel syndrome: a pilot study. Hepatogastroenterology. 1997;44(17): 1328–30.
59 Schneider A, Streitberger K, Joos S. Acupuncture treatment in gastrointestinal diseases: a systematic review. World J Gastroenterol 2007;13(25): 3417–24.
60 Lim B, Manheimer E, Lao L, et. al. Acupuncture for treatment of irritable bowel syndrome. Cochrane Database Syst Rev 2006;(4):CD005111.

Chapter 24

Large bowel cancer

Introduction

Bowel cancer screening

Colorectal cancer (CRC) is one of the most common forms of cancers in the Western world. Lifetime risk to age 75 in the general population is 1:17 for men and 1:26 for women in Australia and is the second leading cause of death.[1]

Research shows that the risk of developing bowel cancer rises significantly from the age of 50 and accounts for 85% of sporadic cancers.[2]

Most cancers of the bowel arise from polyps (adenomas) and removal of polyps markedly reduces the subsequent risk of disease.[3]

Various countries are in the process of introducing national screening programs, and in Australia a population of greater risk are invited to take part in the program.[1]

The eligible population in Australia is those turning 50, 55 and 65 years of age between January 2008 and 31 December 2010. In the US, screening will commence at a similar age (50).[4] People eligible to participate in the program will receive an invitation through the mail to complete a faecal occult blood test (FOBT) and no cost is involved. There is controversy as to which is the best screening method and also which is the best FOBT.[2,5,6] In the US, FOBT will also be used.

There is also increasing evidence to support the use of virtual colonoscopy as an initial screening test.[7]

If the FOBT is positive, the participant will be advised to discuss the result with their doctor who will generally refer them for a colonoscopy.[4] Doing an FOBT every 2 years can reduce the risk of dying from bowel cancer by up to one-third.[2]

High-risk patients such as those with familial adenomatous polyposis and hereditary non-polyposis CRC need to be screened more frequently. As with all other screening tests, there needs to be an emphasis on combining screening with prevention, in particular with CRC where there is considerable research data on prevention.[8]

Lifestyle and prevention

The importance of prevention has been highlighted by Baker and Wardle, even suggesting that lifestyle changes could prevent more colorectal than screening.[8] Key lifestyle and dietary factors for primary prevention are:

- behavioural factors
- exercise
- diet
- weight
- alcohol
- smoking.

Behavioural factors

Personality factors, especially emotional suppression and loss (and a feeling of hopelessness), have been linked to the occurrence and progression of cancer. Hence, as with almost all chronic illness, behavioural factors have been reported to be important in CRC.[9, 10]

Recently a population-based prospective cohort study from Denmark investigated associations between personality traits and cancer survival.[11] This study showed that neuroticism was negatively associated with cancer survival. A further recent study reported that certain personality factors may not be a risk factor for CRC in the Japanese population. However the report concluded that an ambivalent connection and egocentricity may be protective.[12]

The relationship between personality traits and cancer remains contentious. However, it should also be noted that behavioural factors play a key factor in influencing other risk factors such as disregard for prudent eating and physical activity regimens which may increase the risk for the development of large bowel cancer.

Physical activity/exercise

Regular and vigorous physical exercise has been scientifically established as being a strong preventative factor against cancer with the potential to reduce incidence by 40%.[13] With respect to bowel cancer, physical activity can decrease its incidence by 50%, independent of diet and body weight.[14]

Mind-body medicine

The diagnosis of cancer presents a major and stressful life event that necessitates an adaptive adjustment to sustain quality of life. A fundamental goal is to enhance quality of life while striving to prolong life. Quality of life has been reported to predict survival in patients with advanced large bowel cancer.[15]

Surveys of patients with cancer repeatedly identify information provision as a major unmet need. Research has shown that the provision of adequate information is related to an increase in psychological wellbeing.[16] Effective communication skills ensure that this information is clearly explained and understood.

There is incontrovertible evidence from 3 meta-analysis of the benefits of psychological interventions in patients with cancer. Such interventions improve emotional adjustment (including anxiety and depression, sense of control, self-esteem), functional status (including daily living activitics, social and disease-related symptoms (e.g. like nausea. vomiting, pain) and overall quality of life.[17, 18, 19]

There are wide benefits from relaxation-based therapies in reducing anxiety, treatment-related phobias, conditioned nausea and vomiting and insomnias.[13]

Both cognitive behavioural therapy (CBT) and supportive expressive therapy are effective in countering existential fears of dying, aloneness, meaninglessness, and unrealistic fears about the processes of treatment.[13–16]

Nutritional influences

Diet

Excess energy intake/fat and carbohydrates

Execss energy intake has been shown to be consistently associated with bowel cancer.[20]

Fat intake is closely associated with energy intake, it has been difficult to differentiate between the two, to add to this confusion a meta-analysis found little evidence of any energy-independent effect of either total or saturated fat.[21]

Several prospective, observational studies have shown that diet is a major factor in the aetiology of large bowel cancer, with high fish consumption highlighted as decreasing CRC risk. A problem with most of the older studies has been that fats, such as those from fish fats which have been shown to be protective in more recent studies, were not differentiated from other fats.[22, 23]

A recent randomised clinical trial (RCT) objectively investigated the effects of a 6-month intervention with oil-rich or lean fish versus dietary advice only, on apoptosis and mitosis within the colonic crypt. The participants had either colorectal polyps, inactive ulcerative colitis, or no macroscopic signs of disease.[24] The results of the trial showed that the total number of mitotic cells per crypt decreased non-significantly in the salmon group and in the cod group compared with the dietary-advice-only group. The study concluded that an increase in the consumption of either oil-rich or lean fish to 2 portions weekly over 6-months did not markedly change apoptotic and mitotic rates in the colonic mucosa. Moreover it should be noted that fish fats consumption may be a lifetime strategy, not just a short-term solution. A recent review unequivocally concludes that intake of fish fats has a favourable effect on lowering cancer risk.[25]

High consumption of trans-fatty acids is linked to colorectal adenomas.[26]

There is confusion as to whether carbohydrate intake can influence CRC, but it would be very unlikely that refined carbohydrates were not a risk factor.[27, 28]

Meat

A meta-analysis of studies on meat and CRC risk showed that it is a risk factor. Much of the risk was associated with processed meat.[29]

Dietary fibre

An inverse correlation between plant food and intake in cancer risk in 8 of 10 case-controller cohort studies has been published.[30]

A systematic review of case-control studies found that 12 out of 13 showed a decreased risk of CRC with increased fibre intake.[31]

A huge and morc rccent study of 519 978 participants also showed that fibre intake reduced risk.[32]

Vegetables and fruit

Vegetables and fruit are more consistently protective against CRC than cereals in case-control cohort studies.[25] It is unknown whether vegetable or fruit offer most protection. In general, cruciferous vegetables appear to offer special protection.[33]

It is likely that the non-fibre vegetable components such as phytonutrients, and vitamins and minerals offer special protection.

Resistance starch

Resistance starch includes those carbohydrates that escape digestion in the small intestine.[34]

Resistance starch produces the highest level of faecal butyrate which is protective against large bowel polyp/cancer formation.[35]

Weight/body mass index (BMI)

Obesity and high BMI has been shown to have a direct association with bowel cancer risk independent of physical activity.[36]

Smoking

A huge study of 1 million adults showed strong evidence linking cigarette smoking and CRC adenomatous polyps.[37]

Alcohol

In general, total alcohol intake is more consistently associated with CRC risks than specific types of alcohol.[38]

This positive association of alcohol intake and development of CRC is not as strong for wine intake, especially in women, and wine drinking is not related to rectal cancer.[33]

Nutritional supplements

Micronutrients

Folic acid

The Nurses Health Study of nearly 90 000 nurses showed an inverse relationship between incidence of colon cancer and dietary folate intake.[39] A strong association of alcohol intake with CRC cancers and adenomas have been shown to be associated with low folate and methionine.[40]

Dietary folate can modify the risk of alcohol consumption on breast cancer, and hence it is possible that folate supplementation could also protect for CRC.[41]

There is controversial evidence indicating that folate supplementation, later in life, may increase the risk of CRC and possibly other cancers.[42]

Vitamin B6

An inverse association between intake of dietary vitamin B6 and CRC were shown in a longitudinal study especially in women consuming moderate to excess alcohol.[43]

Another study has confirmed the importance of vitamin B6.[44]

Vitamin D/calcium

An inverse association has been shown with vitamin D and CRC.[45]

It is likely that vitamin D is essential for calcium to reduce recurrence of CRC polyps.[46]

The most important source of vitamin D production is from skin exposure to sunshine. Vitamin D can be obtained from food sources such as fatty fish, eggs, liver, and fortified foods, but it is unlikely that adequate vitamin D concentrations can be obtained from diet alone.

Magnesium/calcium

In the placebo-controlled calcium/polyp prevention study, calcium supplementation only reduced the risk of colorectal adenoma recurrence in subjects with low calcium/magnesium ratios.[47] In this study 1000mg calcium was given for a period of 4 years.

Probiotics/prebiotics

Probiotics and prebiotics are likely to be protective, in particular as they greatly influence the internal bowel environment.[48]

A number of studies demonstrate that probiotics alter bowel microflora and decrease premalignant and malignant lesions in laboratory experiments in animal studies.[49, 50]

Radiation enteritis is a severe problem in patients receiving irradiation of the abdomen or pelvis in the course of cancer treatment. Experimental studies in animal models and clinical trials of patients with inflammatory bowel disease (IBD) have consistently shown that the use of probiotic organisms may effectively down-modulate the severity of intestinal inflammation by altering the composition and metabolic and functional properties of indigenous flora of the gut.[51] Recently a multi-centre randomised study demonstrated that nutritional intervention with the probiotic drink containing L. casei DN-114 001 does not reduce the incidence of radiation-induced diarrhoea as defined by a Common Toxicity Criteria Grade 2 or greater. However, it had a significant effect on stool consistency as measured by the Bristol scale.[52] However an earlier study with 490 patients who underwent adjuvant postoperative radiation therapy after surgery for sigmoid, rectal, or cervical cancer and who were assigned to either the high-potency probiotic preparation VSL#3 (one sachet 3 times a day [tid]) or placebo starting from the first day of radiation therapy showed that with a multi-strain preparation it protected cancer patients against the risk of radiation-induced diarrhoea.[53]

Phytonutrients

There are several naturally occurring compounds on foods of plant origin (vegetables, fruit, cereals and tea) that have strong protective effects against CRC in addition to their protection from their fibre content.[54, 55] Of particular interest are the cruciferous vegetables, onion family, leafy vegetables, tomatoes, as well as fruits and cereals containing carotenoids, vitamin C and E.[46] Phytonutrients include carotenoids, vitamin C, vitamin E, folate, indoles, allylic sulphides and lycopene.

Selenium

A multi-centre, double-blind, randomised placebo-controlled cancer-prevention trial was designed to investigate if selenium supplementation could decrease skin cancer incidence.[56] This trial found a highly significant reduction of CRC when using a daily dose of selenium of 200mcg.

Another study has shown that selenium levels related inversely to the large adenomas, but this has been confirmed in a nested case-controlled study.[57, 58]

Vitamins E and C

Several dietary antioxidants such as tea polyphenols, curcumin, genistein, resveratrol, lycopene, pomegranate and lupeol can re-stabilise and modulate cellular metabolic function. A case-control study from Melbourne (Australia) found that dietary micronutrients involved in DNA methylation (folate, methionine and vitamins B6 and B12) and some of those with antioxidant properties (selenium and vitamins E and C) may have a role to play in lowering colorectal cancer risk.[59]

Stone and Papas highlight the difference between alpha-tocopherol and gamma-tocopherol, and that the latter may be more protective.[60]

Gamma-tocopherol is a major form of vitamin E in Western diets and has found to be an anti-inflammatory agent plus directly inhibits cyclooygenase-2 (COX-2) activity and this may be another way in which it could be protective.[61] These authors highlight the important difference between the synthetic dl-alpha-tocopherol acetate and the natural form.

An earlier meta-analysis of 5 prospective nested, case-control studies indicated that high serum levels of alpha-tocopherol were associated with a modest decrease in subsequent incidence of CRC.[62] A more recent study, the large Nurses Health Study, found that 300IU/day of supplemented vitamin E mainly protects CRC in men but not in women.[63] A population-based control study of patients with rectal cancer from the US showed that vitamin E and lycopene may reduce the risk of rectal cancer.[64]

More recently, in 4 major trials involving beta-carotene, vitamin C and synthetic alpha-tocopherol vitamin E, or vitamin C and E or beta-carotene, and vitamin C and E, the latter study involved those with familial adenomatous polyposis. All studies showed no benefit.[65–68]

All of these latter studies supplemented with the synthetic form of alpha-tocopherol, and also did not use gamma-tocopherol.

Fibre supplements

Soluble fibre (which includes oats as well as a maize extract-hi maize) is fermented into fatty acids including butyrate, which is the major energy source of colonocytes. Other fatty acids include propionate, which is taken up by the liver, and acetate, which enters the peripheral circulation.

Butyrate can activate a colonic receptor with cancer-killing potential. It also has an anti-inflammatory effect.[69]

Herbs

Liquorice

A recent study found that liquorice prevented CRC in mice.[70] COX-2 derived PGE2 promotes CRC regression, and both non-selective COX inhibitors (non-steroidal anti-inflammatory drugs [NSAIDs]) and selective COX-2 inhibitors (Celecoxib) reduces the size and numbers of colonic adenomas. However, increased gastrointestinal side-effects of NSAIDs and increased cardiovascular risk of selective COX-2 inhibitors limit their use in chemo-prevention of CRC.

A derivative of liquorice root reduces tumour COX-2 activity, tumour growth, and metastases in mice without the adverse effects associated with NSAIDs and selective COX-2 inhibitors.

The findings of Zhang et. al. suggest that the enzyme inhibition may be a potentially therapeutic option in CRC.[71]

Conclusion

Lifestyle changes are important for large bowel cancer prevention and management. Lifestyle changes go further than disease-specific concerns and can potentially improve overall health and wellbeing plus significantly reduce the burden of the disease. It is clearly documented in the scientific literature that people whose diets are low in fibre, fruit and vegetables, with high energy and GI intake, and who do not exercise regularly appear to be at an increased risk of developing large bowel cancer.

Clinicians cannot only provide assistance with early detection but may also provide significant input into the prevention of large bowel cancer by helping people with lifestyle factors that have an overall effect of reducing the risks as well as allay unreasonable and perceived fears associated with treatments. Table 24.1 summarises the current evidence for CAM treatments.

Table 24.1 Levels of evidence for lifestyle and complementary medicines/therapies in the management of large bowel cancer

Modality	Level I	Level II	Level IIIa	Level IIIb	Level IIIc	Level IV	Level V
Lifestyle modification							
Behavioural factors				x			
Exercise (↓ risk)				x			
Alcohol (↑ intake, ↑risk)				x			
Smoking (↑risk)				x			
Weight management/ BMI				x			
Mind–body medicine							
Mindfulness-based stress reduction	x						
Relaxation	x						
Psycho-educational interventions	x						
Cognitive behavioural therapy		x					
Education			x				
Nutritional influences							
High energy intake				x			
Dietary saturated and trans fats (↑ risk)				x			
Processed meat consumption (↑ risk)				x			
Mediterranean diet (↓ risk)				x			
Vegetarian diet (↓ risk)				x			
Alcohol reduction especially from beer (↓ risk)				x			
High glycaemic load (↑risk)				x			
Dietary fibre (↓ risk)				x			
Vegetables and fruit (↓ risk)				x			
Physical activity (protective)			x				
Nutritional Supplements							
Folate				x			
Vitamin B6				x			
Vitamin E (alpha-tocopherol)	x(–)						
Vitamin E (gamma-tocopherol)		x					
Vitamin D/calcium			x				
Magnesium					x		
Selenium		x					

Continued

Table 24.1 Levels of evidence for lifestyle and complementary medicines/therapies in the management of large bowel cancer—cont'd

Modality	Level I	Level II	Level IIIa	Level IIIb	Level IIIc	Level IV	Level V
Functional foods							
Probiotics		x					
Prebiotics/fibre supplements					x		
Herbal medicines							
Liquorice						x	

Level I — from a systematic review of all relevant randomised controlled trials, meta-analyses.
Level II — from at least 1 properly designed randomised controlled clinical trial.
Level IIIa — from well-designed pseudo-randomised controlled trials (alternate allocation or some other method).
Level IIIb — from comparative studies (including systematic reviews of such studies) with concurrent controls and allocation not randomised, cohort studies, case-control studies, or interrupted time series with a parallel control group.
Level IIIc — from comparetive studies, with historities control, 2 or more single-arm studies or interrupted time series without a parallel control group.
Level IV — opinions of respected authorities based on clinical experience, descriptive studies or experts of expert committees.
Level V — represents minimal evidence that represents testimonials.

Clinical tips handout for patients — large bowel cancer

1 Lifestyle advice

Sleep

- Ensure 7–8 hours sleep and regular sleep pattern. Avoid shift work at night as this can be a risk for cancer. (See Chapter 22 for more advice.)

Sunshine

- Eye protection should be worn in the form of sunglasses at all times when exposed to the sun for prolonged periods of time.
- Amount of exposure varies with local climate.
- At least 15 minutes of sunshine needed daily for vitamin D and melatonin production — especially before 10 a.m. and after 3 p.m. when the sun exposure is safest during summer. Much more exposure is required in winter, when supplementation needs to be considered.
- Ensure gradual adequate skin exposure to sun; avoid sunscreen and excess clothing to maximise levels of vitamin D.
- More time in the sun is required for dark skinned people.
- Direct exposure to about 10% of body (hands, arms, face), without sunscreen and not through glass.
- Vitamin D is obtained in the diet from fatty fish, eggs, liver and fortified foods (some milks and margarines); however, it is unlikely that adequate vitamin D concentrations can be obtained from diet alone.

2 Physical activity/exercise

- Exercise is important for cancer prevention and during treatment. (If in treatment discuss appropriate exercise regimens with your doctor.)
- Exercise for 30–60 minutes daily. If exercise is not regular, commence with 5 minutes daily and slowly build up to at least 30 minutes. Outdoor exercise, in nature, fresh air (avoid polluted air) and sunshine is ideal.
- Brisk walking, light jogging, cycling, swimming, stretching, and weight-bearing exercises are all good forms of physical activity/exercise.
- Tai chi, qigong and yoga may be particularly helpful.

3 Mind–body medicine (most helpful)

- Stress management program — for example, six 40 minute sessions for patients to understand the nature of their symptoms, the symptoms' relationship to stress, and the practice of regular relaxation exercises.
- Regular meditation practice at least 10–20 minutes daily, especially transcendental, mindfulness meditation and autogenic training.
- Anger management may be of help.
- Psychological therapy may help to deal with stressors.

Breathing

- Be aware of breathing from time to time. Notice if tendency to hold breath or over-breathe.
- Snoring and irregular breathing during sleep needs to be reported and further investigated.
- Avoid exposure to polluted air as much as possible.

Rest and stress management

Relaxation is important for a full and lasting recovery.

- Reduce workload and resolve conflicts. Contact family, friends, church or social groups for support. Full-time work can increase breast cancer risk whereas part-time work does not.
- Listening to relaxation music helps.
- Relaxation massage therapy helps.
- Hypnotherapy, biofeedback, cognitive behavioural therapy, and psychotherapy may be of help.

Fun

- It is important to have fun in life.
- Joy can be found even in the simplest of tasks.
- Treat yourself by watching funny movies/videos, comedy, hobbies, dancing, playing with pets and children.
- Creative tasks, such as knitting, can help with distressing thoughts.

Focus on wellness, not just the disease.

4 Environment

- Don't smoke and avoid smoking environments.
- Avoid environmental pollutants and chemicals — at work and in the home.
- Avoid artificial sweeteners.

5 Dietary changes

- Do not rush your meals; relax before meals; chew your food thoroughly before swallowing as this aids digestion and promotes regular, relaxed eating patterns.
- Aim to lose weight if you or your health practitioner believes you are overweight.
- Eat more fruit (>2/day) and vegetables (>5day); a variety of colours and those that are in season.
- A vegetarian diet high in legumes is particularly helpful (e.g. soy; vegetables; garlic, nuts and fruit); for example, the Mediterranean diet.
- Increase fibre; for example, cooked oats for breakfast, and add psyllium fibre (husks) to your cereal.
- Fresh garlic and other members of the onion family offer protection.
- Cruciferous or Brassica group of vegetables are protective; they include broccoli, cabbage, brussel sprouts, cauliflower and bok choy.
- Eat more nuts, seeds, beans, sprouts (e.g. alfalfa, mung bean, lentils). Try soy 25–30g/day.
- Consume more fish (sardines, tuna, salmon, cod, mackerel) especially deep sea fish.
- Reduce red meat intake (preferably eat lean red meat e.g. lamb, kangaroo) and white meat (e.g. free range organic chicken fillet).
- Consume cold pressed olive oil, 4 teaspoons, and flaxseed oil, 1 tablespoon (uncooked), daily. Use avocado.
- Use dark chocolate (25–50g/day) unless not tolerated.
- Eat a variety of wholegrains/cereals (best if not toasted). Cooked traditional rolled oats for breakfast are particularly helpful, as is rice (brown, basmati, Mahatma, Dongara), buckwheat flour, wholegrain organic breads (rye bread, Essene, spelt, Kamut) — when toasting make hot and crisp, not brown, to avoid acrylamide — brown pasta, couscous, millet, amaranth, etc.
- Consume low-fat dairy products, such as low-fat yoghurt, unless there is a dairy intolerance. Soy milk (organic) is an alternative.
- Drink more water, 1–2 litres a day, and teas (especially green tea, chamomile, peppermint and black tea).
- For alternative sweetener try honey (e.g. manuka, yellow box and stringy bark have the lowest GI).
- Avoid sea salt.
- Avoid hydrogenated, saturated fats and trans-fatty acids such as butter, margarines, crispy potato chips, dairy fat (e.g. yellow cheeses and cream), fat in meat and poultry, commercial biscuits, most cakes, pastries and takeaway foods, fast foods, sugar (such as soft drinks, lollies) and processed foods (e.g. white bread, white pasta).
- Avoid coffee.
- Minimise alcohol intake to no more than 1–2 glasses daily; red wine may be best.
- Avoid chemical additives — preservatives, colourings and flavourings.

6 Physical therapies

- Acupuncture may help with pain and naused (including chemotherapy-induced nausea).

7 Supplements

Fish oils

- Indication: may reduce LBC risk, may reduce inflammation and blood stickiness. Can reduce chemotherapy toxicity and normalise immunity.
- Dosage: 4–10g of 1000mg capsules daily as tolerated (e.g. EPA 180/DHA 120mg/1000mg capsule).
- Results: 4–7 days.
- Side-effects: often well tolerated especially if taken with meals. Very mild and rare side-effects (e.g. gastrointestinal upset); allergic reactions (e.g. rash, breathing problems if allergic to seafood); blood thinning effects in very high doses > 10g daily (may need to stop fish oil supplements 2 weeks prior to surgery).
- Contraindications: sensitivity reaction to seafood; drug interactions; caution when taking high doses of fish oils >4g per day together with warfarin (your Doctor will check your INR test).

Vitamins and minerals

Folate

- Indication: can reduce large bowel cancer (LBC) risk and also adenomas.
- Dosage: 0.5–1mg daily.
- Result: probably years.
- Side effects: no toxicity, best to use in combination with vitamin B6 and vitamin B12.
- Contraindications: high doses commenced later in life may increase risk of LBC later in life.

Vitamin B6

Indication:can reduce LBC risk.

- Dosage: best if dosage is no more than 50mg daily.
- Result: probably years.
- Side-effects: none if recommended dose not exceeded.
- Avoid doses exceeding 50mg/day as high doses and prolonged use can cause B6 toxicity such as neuropathy (e.g. nerve shooting pains, numbness).
- Contraindications: generally safe.

Vitamin C

- Indication: can reduce LBC risk; may reduce thrombosis and improve immunity when combined with natural vitamin E and selenium.
- Dosage: 500–1000mg daily.
- Results: combined with natural vitamin E and selenium, can reduce blood stickiness in 1 week.
- Side-effects: with high doses can cause nausea, heartburn, abdominal cramps and diarrhoea.
- Contraindications: can increase iron absorption. Use with caution if glucose-6-phosphate dehydrogenase deficiency.

Natural vitamin E

- Indication: may reduce thrombosis plus improve immunity when combined with vitamin C and selenium.
- Dosage: 200–400IU/day.
- Results: can reduce blood stickiness in 1 week.
- Side-effects: rare, but can cause nausea, vomiting, abdominal pain, heartburn and diarrhoea. Doses below 1500IU/day are very unlikely to result in haemorrhage; rarely causes diarrhoea, flatulence, nausea, heart palpitations.
- Contraindications: use with caution if bleeding disorder or if taking with blood-thinning medication. If using very high dose, reduce dose before surgery.
- Contraindications: pregnancy (insufficient evidence). Can reduce effectiveness of thyroid hormone replacement.

Vitamin D3 (cholecalciferol)

- Indication: low levels are a risk factor for LBC.
- Dosage: safe sunshine exposure of skin is the safest source of vitamin D. Vitamin D3, cholecalciferol 1000IU. Doctors should check blood levels and suggest supplementation if levels are low.
    - Adults: 400–1000IU/day for maintenance; 3000–5000IU/day for 1 month then 1000IU/day if vitamin D level below normal. Ensure repeat blood measurement.
    - Children at risk: 200–400IU/day under medical supervision.
    - Pregnant and lactating women at risk: under medical supervision.
- Results: unknown.
- Side-effects: very high doses can cause vitamin D toxicity; raised calcium levels in the blood. Can increase aluminium and magnesium absorption; prolonged heparin therapy can increase reabsorption and reduce formation of bone and hence more vitamin D and calcium required.
- Contraindications: thiazide diuretics decrease urinary calcium and hence hypercalcaemia possible with vitamin D supplementation.

Magnesium and calcium (best provided together)

- Indication: calcium and magnesium may decrease LBC risk.
- Dosage: magnesium: children, up to 65–120mg daily in divided doses. Adults, 400–800mg daily including pregnant and lactating women.
- Calcium citrate: 800mg/day or calcium carbonate 1000mg/day in adults. Children 30–40mg daily.
- Results: unknown.
- Side-effects: oral magnesium can cause gastrointestinal irritation, nausea, vomiting, and diarrhoea. The dosage varies from person to person. Although rare, toxic levels can cause low blood pressure, thirst, heart arrhythmia, drowsiness and weakness. Calcium can cause gastrointestinal irritation and constipation.
- Contraindications: patients with kidney disease.

Selenium (sodium selenite, organic selenium found in yeast)

- Indication: may help prevent LBC. May reduce thrombosis plus improve immunity when combined with vitamin C and vitamin E.
- Dosage: 50–100mcg/day daily; do not exceed >600mcg/day (health professional supervision required to avoid toxicity).
- Results: uncertain.
- Side-effects: very mild and rare; nausea, vomiting, rash, sensitivity reactions, toxicity in high doses; nail changes, irritability, fatigue.

Contraindications: pregnancy, lactation, children <12 years of age.

Probiotics

- Indications: may help prevent LBC, can improve immunity. May assist in preventing radiation therapy induced diarrhoea.
- Dosage: variable dose before breakfast (multi-strain formula is best). One capsule or 1tsp pf powder twice daily (mixed in water) before meals.
- Results: few days to a few weeks.
- Side-effects: gastrointestinal disturbance can occur.
- Contraindications: true cow's milk allergy if contained in product.

Prebiotics/fibre

- Indications: may help prevent LBC; prebiotics promote the growth and activity of specific strains of bacteria in the gut and are best given with a probiotic. Inulin and oligofructose usually used.
- Dosage: variable dose.
- Results: few days to a few weeks.
- Side-effects: often well tolerated. Very mild and rare side-effects; transient abdominal discomfort (e.g. bloating; flatulence).
- Contraindications: severely ill and/or immuno-compromised patients. Allergies to any of the food sources from which inulin and oligofructoses are derived.

Inulin is derived from wheat, onions, bananas, leaks, artichokes, asparagus, hot water extraction from chicory root.

Oligofructoses are plant sugars from a wide variety of fruits, vegetables, and cereals.

References

1 Dept Health and Ageing. Bowel cancer screening. Cancerscreening. Online. Available: www.cancerscreening.gov.au/internet/screening/publishing.nsf/content/bowel-a (accessed July 2009)

2 Bolin T, Cowen AE, Korman MG. Colorectal cancer prevention. MJA 2002;176:145–6.

3 Winawer SJ, Zauber AG, Ho MN, et. al. Prevention of colorectal cancer by colonoscopic polypectomy. The National Polyp Study Workgroup. N Eng J Med 1993;329:1977–81.

4 Dept Health and Ageing. Colorectal cancer. Cancer topics. Online. Available: www.cancer.gov/cancertopics/pdq/prevention/colorectal (accessed July 2009).

5 Ahlquist DA, Sargent DJ, Loprinzi CL. Stool DNA and occult blood testing for screen detection of colorectal neoplasia. Ann Int Med 2008;149:4412–450.

6 Young GP, Cole SR. Which faecal occult blood test is best to screen for colorectal cancer? Nat Clin Pract Gastroenterol Hepatol 2009;6:140–41.

7 Summers R, Yao J, Pickhardt P, et. al. Computer tomographic virtual colonoscopy computer-aided polyp detection in a screening population. Gastroenterology 2005;129:1832–44.

8 Baker AH, Wardle J. Increasing fruit and vegetable intake among adults attending colorectal cancer screening: the efficacy of a brief tailored intervention. Cancer Epidemiol Biomarkers Prev 2002;11:203–06.

9 Kune S, Kune GA, Watson LF, et. al. Recent life change and large bowel cancer. Data from the Melbourne Colorectal Cancer Study. J Clin Epidemiol 1991;44:57–68.

10 Kune GA, Kune S, Watson LF, et. al. Personality as a risk factor in large bowel cancer: data from the Melbourne Colorectal Cancer Study. Psychol Med 1991;21:29–41.

11 Nakaya N, Hansen PE, Schapiro IR, et. al. Personality traits and cancer survival: a Danish cohort study. Br J Cancer 2006;95(2):146–52.

12 Nagano J, Kono S, Toyomura K, et. al. Personality and colorectal cancer: the Fukuoka colorectal cancer study. Jpn J Clin Oncol 2008;38(8):553–61.

13 Newton RU, Galvao DA. Exercise in prevention and management of cancer. Curr Treat Options Oncol 2008;9(2–3):135–46.

14 Colditz GA, Cannuscicc CC, Frazier AL. Physical activity and reduced risk of colon cancer: implications for prevention. Cancer Causes Control 1997;8:649–67.

15 Maisey NR, Norman A, Watson M, et. al. Baseline quality of life predicts survival in patients with advanced colorectal cancer. Eur J Cancer 2002;38(10):1351–7.

16 Smith JR, Mugford M, Holland R, et. al. A systematic review to examine the impact of psycho-educational interventions on health outcomes and costs in adults and children with difficult asthma. Health Technol Assess. 2005;9(23):iii-iv.

17 Devine EC, Westlake SK. The effects of psychoeducational care provided to adults with cancer: meta-analysis of 116 studies. Oncol Nurs Forum 1995;22(9):1369–81.

18 Sheard T, Evans J, Cash D, et. al. A CAT-derived one to three session intervention for repeated deliberate self-harm: a description of the model and initial experience of trainee psychiatrists in using it. Br J Med Psychol 2000;73:179–96.

19 Spiegel D, Bloom JR, Kraemer HC, et. al. Effect of psychosocial treatment on survival of patients with metastatic breast cancer. Lancet 1989;2(8668):888–91.

20 Willett WC, Stampfer MJ, Colditz GA, et. al. Relation of meat, fat, and fibre intake to the risk of colon cancer in a prospective study among women. N Engl J Med 1990;323:1664–72.

21 Howe GR, Aronson KJ, Benito E, et. al. The relationship between dietary fat intake and risk of colorectal cancer: evidence from the combined analysis of 13 case-control studies. Cancer Causes Control 1997;8:15–28.

22 Hall MN, Chavarro JE, Lee IM, et. al. A 22–year prospective study of fish, n-3 fatty acid intake, and colorectal cancer risk in men. Cancer Epidemiol Biomarkers Prev 2008;17:1136–43.

23 Norat T, Bingham S, Ferrari P, et. al. Meat, fish, and colorectal cancer risk: the European Prospective Investigation into cancer and nutrition. J Natl Cancer Inst 2005;97:906–16.

24 Pot GK, Majsak-Newman G, Geelen A, et. al. Fish consumption and markers of colorectal cancer risk: a multicenter randomised controlled trial. AJCN 2009;90(2):354–61.

25 Pauwels EK, Kairemo K. Fatty acid facts, part II: role in the prevention of carcinogenesis, or, more fish on the dish? Drug News Persp 2008;21(9):504–10.

26 Vinikoor LC, Schroeder JC, Millikan RC, et. al. Consumption of trans-fatty acid and its association with colorectal adenomas. Am J Epidemiol 2008;168:289–97.
27 Higginbotham S, Zhang ZF, Lee IM, et. al. Dietary glycemic load and risk of colorectal cancer in the Women's Health Study. J Natl Cancer Inst 2004;96:229–33.
28 Fuchs CS, Giovannucci EL, Colditz GA, et. al. Dietary fibre and the risk of colorectal cancer and adenoma in women. N Engl J Med 1999;340:169–76.
29 Sandhu MS, White IR, McPherson K. Systematic review of the prospective cohort studies on meat consumption and colorectal cancer risk: a meta-analytical approach. Cancer Epidemiol Biomarkers Prev 2001;10:439–46.
30 Potter JD. Nutrition and colorectal cancer. Cancer Causes Control 1996;7:127–46.
31 Howe GR, Benito E, Castelleto R, et. al. Dietary intake of fibre and decreased risk of cancers of the colon and rectum: evidence from the combined analysis of 13 case-control studies. J Natl Cancer Inst 1992;84:1887–96.
32 Bingham SA, Day NE, Luben R, et. al. Dietary fibre in food and protection against colorectal cancer in the European Prospective Investigation into Cancer and Nutrition (EPIC): an observational study. Lancet 2003;361:1496–501.
33 IARC (International Agency for Cancer on Research). Cruciferous vegetables, Isothiocyanates and Indoles. IARC Handbooks of Cancer Prevention 2004:9 (Leon IARC).
34 Cassidy A, Bingham SA, Cummings JH. Starch intake and colorectal cancer risk: an international comparison. Br J Cancer 1994;69:937–42.
35 Muir JG, Yeow EGW, Keough J, et. al. Combining wheat bran with starch resistance has more beneficial effects on fecal indixes than does wheatbran alone. AJCN 2004;79:1020–28.
36 Giovannucci E, Ascherio A, Rimm EB, et. al. Physical activity, obesity, and risk for colon cancer and adenoma in men. Ann Intern Med 1995;122:327–34.
37 Chao A, Thun MJ, Jacobs EJ, et. al. Cigarette smoking and colorectal cancer mortality in the cancer prevention study II. J Natl Cancer Inst 2000;92:1888–96.
38 American Institute for Cancer Research, World Cancer Research Fund. Food, nutrition and the prevention of cancer. A global prospective, London: American Institute for Cancer Research and World Cancer Research Fund 1997.
39 Giovannucci E, Stamfer MJ, Colditz GA, et. al. Multivitamin use, folate, and colon cancer in women in the Nurses' Health Study. Ann Intern Med 1998;129:517–24.
40 Giovannucci E. Epidemiologic studies of folate and colorectal neoplasia: a review. J Nut 2002;132:2350S-2355S.
41 Baglietto L, English DR, Gertig DM, et. al. Does dietary folate intake modify effect of alcohol consumption on breast cancer risk? Prospective cohort study. BMJ 2005;331:807–14.
42 Hubner RA, Houlston RS. Folate and colorectal cancer prevention. Br J Cancer 2009;100:233–9.
43 Larsson SC, Giovannucci E, Wolk A. Vitamin B6 intake, alcohol consumption, and colorectal cancer: a longitudinal population-based cohort of women. Gastroenterology 2005;128:1830–7.
44 Wei EK, Giovannucci E, Salhub J, et. al. Plasma vitamin B6 and the risk of colorectal cancer and adenoma in women. J Natl Cancer Inst 2005;97:684–92.
45 Peters U, Hayes RB, Chatterjee M, et. al. Circulating vitamin D and metabolites, polymorphism in vitamin D receptor, and colorectal adenoma risk. Cancer Epidemiol Biomarkers Prev 2004;13:546–52.
46 Harris DM, Go VL. Vitamin D and colon carcinogenesis. J Nutr 2004;134 (12 Suppl): 3463S–3471S.
47 Dai Q, Shrubsole MJ, Sess RM, at al. The relation of magnesium and calcium intakes and a genetic polymorphism in the magnesium transporter to colorectal neoplasia risk. AJCN 2007;86:743–51.
48 Otte JM, Mahjurian-Namari R, Brand S, et. al. Probiotics regulate the expression of COX-2 in intestinal epithelial cells. Nutr Cancer 2009;61: 103–13.
49 Wollowski I, Rechkemmer G, Pool-Zobel BL. Protective role of probiotics and prebiotics in colon cancer. Am J Clin Nutr 2001;73:451S-455S.
50 Mai V, Draganov PV. Recent advances and remaininggapsinourknowledgeofassociationsbetween gutmicrobiotaandhumanhealth.WorldJGastroenterol. 2009;15:81–5.
51 Blanarova C, Galovicova A, Petrasova D. Use of probiotics for prevention of radiation-induced diarrhea. Bratisl Lek Listy 2009;110(2):98–104.
52 Giralt J, Regadera JP, Verges R, et. al. Effects of probiotic Lactobacillus casei DN-114 001 in prevention of radiation-induced diarrhea: results from multicenter, randomised, placebo-controlled nutritional trial. Int J Radiat Oncol Biol Phys 2008;71(4):1213–9.
53 Delia P, Sansotta G, Donato V, et. al. Use of probiotics for prevention of radiation-induced diarrhea. World J Gastroenterol 2007;13(6):912–5.
54 Kune GA. Causes and control of colorectal cancer: model of cancer protection. Boston Kluwer Academic Publishers, 1996.
55 Il'yasova D, Hodgson ME, Martin C, et. al. Tea consumption, apoptosis, and colorectal adenomas. Eur J Cancer Prev 2003;12:439–43.
56 Clark LC, Combs GFJr, Turnbull BW, et. al. Effects of selenium supplementation for cancer prevention in patients with carcinoma of the skin. A randomised controlled trial. Nutritional Prevention of Cancer Study Group. JAMA 1996;276:1957–63.
57 Fernández-Bañares F, Cabré E, Esteve M, et. al. Serum selenium and risk of large size colorectal adenomas in a geographical area with a low selenium status. Am J Gastroenterol. 2002;97:2103–8.
58 Wallace K, Byers T, Morris JS, et. al. Prediagnostic serum selenium concentration and the risk of recurrent colorectal adenoma: a nested case-control study. Cancer Epidemiol Biomarkers Prev 2003;12:464–7.
59 Kune G, Watson L. Colorectal cancer protective effects and the dietary micronutrients folate, methionine, vitamins B6, B12, C, E, selenium, and lycopene. Nutr Cancer 2006;56:11–21.
60 Stone WL, Papas AM. Tocopherols and the etiology of colon cancer. J Natl Cancer Inst 1997;89:1006–14.
61 Jiang Q, Elson-Schwab I, Courtemanche C, et. al. gamma-tocopherol and its major metabolite, in contrast to alpha-tocopherol, inhibit cyclooxygenase activity in macrophages and epithelial cells. Proc Natl Acad Sci U S A 2000;97:11494–9.

62 Longnecker MP, Martin-Moreno JM, Knekt P, et. al. Serum alpha-tocopherol concentration in relation to subsequent colorectal cancer: pooled data from five cohorts. J Natl Cancer Inst 1992;84:430–5.
63 Wu K, Willett WC, Chan JM, et. al. A prospective study on supplemental vitamin E intake and risk of colon cancer in women and men. Cancer Epidemiol Biomarkers Prev. 2002;11:1298–304.
64 Murtaugh MA, Ma K, Benson J, et. al. Antioxidants, carotenoids, and risk of rectal cancer. Am J Epidemiol 2004;159:32–41.
65 Greenberg ER, Baron JA, Tosteson TD, et. al. A clinical trial of antioxidant vitamins to prevent colorectal adenoma. Polyp Prevention Study Group. N Engl J Med 1994;33:141–7.
66 McKeown-Eyssen G, Holloway C, Jazmaji V, et. al. A randomised trial of vitamins C and E in the prevention of recurrence of colorectal polyps. Cancer Res 1988;48:4701–5.
67 MacLennan R, Macrae F, Bain C, et. al. Randomised trial of intake of fat, fibre, and beta carotene to prevent colorectal adenomas. Australian Polyp Prevention Project. J Natl Cancer Inst 1995;87:1760–6.
68 DeCosse JJ, Miller HH, Lesser ML. Effect of wheat fibre and vitamins C and E on rectal polyps in patients with familial adenomatous polyposis. J Natl Cancer Inst. 1989;81:1290–7.
69 Thangaraju M, Cresci GA, Liu K, et. al. GPR109A is a G-protein-coupled receptor for the bacterial fermentation product butyrate and functions as a tumor suppressor in colon. Cancer Res 2009;69:2826–32.
70 Zhang MZ, Xu J, Yao B, et. al. Inhibition of 11beta-hydroxysteroid dehydrogenase type II selectively blocks the tumor COX-2 pathway and suppresses colon carcinogenesis in mice and humans. J Clin Invest 2009;119:876–85.
71 Stewart PM, Prescott SM. Can licorice lick colon cancer? J Clin Invest 2009;119:760–63.

Chapter 25

Menopause

Introduction

The definition of menopause is when there is no menstruation over a 12-month period. That is, when menstrual periods permanantly stop. Women undergo significant reproductive transitional and physiological changes which are accompanied by the additional effects of ageing and social adjustment. This phase known as the climacteric or perimenopause describes the time leading up to a woman's final menstruation, along with the endocrinological, biological, and clinical features of the approaching menopause. The length of this transition is usually about 4 years, but is shorter in smokers than non-smokers.[1] Ten percent of women may not experience this phase and menses may stop abruptly. The median age for menopause is 51 years, over an age range of 39–59 years.[1, 2]

This transitional phase is associated with a number of vasomotor, urinary symptoms and psychological tribulations (Table 25.1). There is a variation in symptoms experienced.

The severity of symptoms that women may experience range from mild to severe. Approximately 40–65% of women experience hot flushes or night sweats, 30–60% disturbed sleep, and 25–35% vaginal dryness which leads women to consult health professionals.[3] The duration of these symptoms may vary from 2–20 years.[4]

The most effective treatments for hot flushes include oestrogens and progestagens.[2] Current evidence supports short-term use of hormone replacement therapy (HRT) as the standard therapy for hot flushes.[5, 6] Since the Women's Health Initiative and Millenium study findings with long-term use of HRT in menopausal women, demonstrated increased risk of breast cancer[7] more women are turning to non-pharmacological and various complementary medicines (CMs) for the relief of menopausal symptoms. Many women are reluctant to accept hormonal treatments, except when symptoms are severe, as they see this stage of their lives as a *natural event*, and not a disease. Menopause is an opportunity for lifestyle changes and it is worthwhile exploring prevention strategies, as women who commence HRT for hot flushes are likely to re-experience them after stopping HRT, even after 5 years.[8]

This chapter explores the scientific evidence base and safety concerns for lifestyle, non-pharmacological approaches to the management of menopausal symptoms.

Lifestyle changes

Reduced physical activity, low socioeconomic status and cigarette smoking (past and current) are contributors documented to increase the relative risk of hot flushes in menopausal women.[9] A recent review has reported that lifestyle and diet adjustment interventions have the potential to significantly improve menopausal symptoms.[10, 11] Hence, lifestyle behaviours are important determinants of menopausal symptoms. The available literature suggests that smoking and greater body weight are risk factors for vasomotor symptoms; women with vasomotor symptoms who smoke may benefit from smoking cessation, and women who are heavier than ideal body weight may benefit from weight reduction.[12]

Body mass/overweight

Very obese women have significantly higher odds of experiencing hot flushes compared with normal weight women. Whilst the mechanism is not clear, oestrogen levels may partly explain this relationship.[13]

Cigarette smoking

A case-control study of 611 middle-aged women (45–54 years) demonstrated that past and current smokers have higher odds of experiencing hot flushes compared with never smokers.[14] Past and current smoking and duration of smoking influenced frequency and the severity of hot flushes. The longer the women smoked, the more severe the symptoms. Smoking did not influence blood levels of estradiol and estrone and the risk persisted even when women were treated with hormones. Cigarette smoking is therefore a strong predictor of experiencing hot flushes, including the severity of hot flushes.

Cultural differences

There are many cultures where the prevalence of menopausal symptoms is reported as low. Prevalence rates for vasomotor symptoms in

Table 25.1 Physical, vasomotor and urogenital symptoms, and psychological problems encountered by women approaching and during menopause

Physical/vasomotor symptoms	Urogenital symptoms	Psychological problems
Hot flushes	Vaginal dryness • dyspareunia • vaginitis	Loss of confidence
Night sweats	Urinary problems • frequency • urgency • dysuria	Depressed mood
Palpitations	Lack of libido	Irritability/anxiety
Headaches		Forgetfulness
Amenorrhoea		Difficulty in concentrating
Dry skin		Panic attacks
Hair loss		Insomnia
Joint pains		Fatigue
Breast tenderness		
Skin irritation 'creepy-crawly feelings'		

surveys of women (on average 2-week recall of symptoms) conducted between 2000–2005 include:[15]

- Mayan–Mexico/peasant Greek women — negligible
- Taiwan (Han Chinese) — 15.1%
- China/Singapore/Malay/India — 17.6%
- Hong Kong China — 23%
- Japan — 22–46.6%
- US Caucasian — 36.6–37.8%
- US African-American — 46.5%
- Australian — 26.2–44.7%
- Lebanese — 49%
- Slovenian — 55%
- Morrocan — 61%

Of interest, the lowest reported symptoms are found in peasant Greek women and Mayan women from Mexico.[15, 16]

Under-reporting of symptoms by women in surveys may also contribute to low prevalences. It is not clear why the incidence of menopausal symptoms vary in different geographical areas. A recent review has reported that the prevalence variation of these symptoms may be influenced by a range of factors, including climate, diet, lifestyle, women's roles, and attitudes regarding the end of reproductive life and ageing.[17] Women's attitude and expectations that can influence the experience of the perimenopause are determined by a number of factors including cultural attitudes and expectations, medicalisation (menopause viewed as an illness), their reproductive history, general health, mother's experience, marital status, relationships with and attitude by their husbands/partners, extended family, social support, career and religious belief. In general, a healthy lifestyle, namely diet (e.g. foods high in phytoestrogens and isoflavones), exercise and avoiding smoking, and strong support from friends and family can positively impact on menopausal symptoms.[15]

Health practitioners and other caregivers should recognise that variations exist and ask patients specific questions about symptoms and their impact on usual functioning.[17–20]

Core body temperature

Possible mechanisms for hot flushes include the effects of oestrogen on norepinephrine/noradrenaline and serotonin receptors in the hypothalamus[21] and genetics may also play a role.[22] Research evidence suggests that small temperature elevations preceding hot flushes may constitute a triggering mechanism.[20, 23] In addition, higher body core temperature prior to and during sleep is significantly associated with poorer quality of sleep and higher luteinizing hormone (LH) levels.[24]

This may explain why many women describe more hot flushes in bed and in hot weather conditions such as summer. Therefore lowering core body temperature may help to prevent hot flushes. Cooler environments, lowering air temperature within the household, swimming, avoiding spicy and hot foods or drinks may be useful adjuncts to managing small temperature elevations.

Mind–body medicine

Psychological support

In a study of 78 menopausal women suffering hot flushes and breast cancer, the women were randomised to education and psychosocial support groups or a control group.[25] A significant improvement in symptoms was found with the active treatment.[25] A recent pilot trial demonstrated a possible effectiveness of cognitive behavioural interventions for the treatment of climacteric syndrome.[26] A further pilot investigating cognitive behavioural group therapy (CBGT) supported the notion that CBGT interventions aimed at reducing vasomotor symptoms may be of value for menopausal hot flushes when administered in a small-group format.[27] A recent systematic review has concluded that psycho-educational interventions seem to alleviate hot flushes in menopausal women and breast cancer survivors.[28]

Relaxation therapies

Nervous tension may cause instability of the thermoregulatory centre leading to sudden, transient, and erratic peripheral vasodilation in the skin blood vessels causing the sensation of flushing.[29] Interestingly, even excitement, such as laughter, can stimulate the nervous system and bring on more hot flushes. Relaxation can alleviate menopausal symptoms.[28]

Three randomised control trials (RCTs) identified by the North American Menopausal Society,[30] demonstrated paced respiration (slow, controlled, diaphragmatic breathing) reduced hot flushes by 50%, particularly if performed at the onset of a hot flush when compared with controls. A pilot study of mindfulness-based stress reduction for hot flushes has shown a positive result in improving both quality of life and reducing severity of hot flushes in 15 women experiencing severe hot flushes over the course of treatment.[31]

Physical activity/exercise

Aerobic exercise and customised exercise programs

Physical activity may ameliorate hot flushes and insomnia by influencing opioid levels.[32] It is known that opioid levels are lowered in menopause and that exercise can increase opioid levels such as endorphins and activity.[33] Although data supporting physical activity are still preliminary recent studies suggest that women who exercise regularly are less likely to experience severe hot flushes.[34] A customised exercise program is valuable for improving the health related quality of life of menopausal women compared to those who do not perform any form of physical activity.[35]

A Cochrane review of RCTs identified 1 small trial that compared exercise with HRT and found both interventions were effective in reducing vasomotor symptoms, although HRT was more effective than exercise.[36]

A recent systematic review of the literature of RCTs found aerobic exercise improves psychological health and quality of life in vasomotor symptomatic women.[37] The review also identified several RCTs of middle-aged menopausal women and found aerobic exercise can invoke significant improvements in this age group of menopause-related symptoms such as mood, health-related quality of life and insomnia compared with middle-aged women who did not exercise.[37]

Yoga

Yoga can play an important role in the management of menopausal symptoms. A number of trials support the recommendation of specific yoga exercises as an evidence-based prescription for menopausal symptoms.[38, 39, 40]

A recent randomised control study of 180 perimenopausal women comparing yoga comprised of breathing practises, sun salutation and meditation was found to be significantly beneficial for reducing hot flushes and night sweats and improving cognitive functions such as memory, mental balance, attention, concentration and recall when compared with control group; a set of simple physical exercises, under supervision.[41]

A trial of 120 women (aged 40–55 years) with menopausal symptoms randomised women into 2 study arms: yoga and an exercise (control) group.[42] In the yoga therapy group, women were instructed to practise various yoga postures such as sun salutation that consists of 12 postures, pranayama (breathing practices) and avartan dhyan (cyclic meditation). Women in the control group were instructed a set of simple physical exercises (supervision by trained teachers). Women in both groups practised either yoga or physical exercises 1 hour daily, 5 days per week over the 8-week study period.

The perimenopausal women in the yoga therapy group demonstrated significantly reduced perceived stress, climacteric symptoms, and neuroticism traits compared with controls.[42]

A systematic review that explored the role of meditation and yoga for treating diseases concluded the strongest evidence for efficacy was found for epilepsy, symptoms of the premenstrual syndrome and menopausal symptoms.[43]

However, a recent systematic review of 7 studies reported mixed results and the evidence at present is insufficient to suggest that yoga is effective in menopause.[44]

Some studies did not demonstrate any benefit of yoga on menopausal symptoms, sleep or self-esteem in menopausal women.[44, 45, 46]

More rigorous studies are required to assess the role of specific yoga and breathing practises for the management of menopausal symptoms.

Nutritional influences

It is essential that women consume a healthy well-balanced diet and are aware of the importance of exercise (weight-bearing) and sunshine for vitamin D synthesis well before menopause to prevent health problems accelerated after the menopause, such as cardiovascular disease and osteoporosis. Women presenting with menopausal symptoms provide an opportunity to discuss and educate them about the importance preventative advice, the importance of lifestyle changes, and a healthy diet (see clinical tips at the end of this chapter).

Calcium and vitamin D for menopausal women

There is a role for the recommendation of calcium and vitamin D (cholecalciferol) supplementation by menopausal women with demonstrated vitamin D deficiency for the prevention of osteoporosis. Routine use, however, is questionable. (See Chapter 30 for osteoporosis.)

A Cochrane review of 45 trials, found vitamin D alone is not effective in preventing hip fracture, vertebral fracture or any new fracture.[47] Vitamin D with calcium reduced hip fractures especially in people in institutional care, but not significantly in the community-dwelling subgroup.[47]

The World Health Initiative for the calcium/vitamin D RCT of 36 282 post-menopausal women (aged 51–82 years) from 40 US clinical centres assigned to 1000mg of elemental calcium carbonate and 400IU of vitamin D(3) daily or placebo with average follow-up of 7 years, found that supplementation did not have a statistically significant effect on mortality rates but may reduce mortality rates in post-menopausal women.[48]

Furthermore, findings from the Women's Health Initiative study also found adherence to calcium and vitamin D supplements over 4 years did not produce any favourable effects compared to placebo on physical functioning or physical performance in the older women.[49]

Despite these findings, there is strong overwhelming evidence that vitamin D deficiency is associated with an increased risk of osteomalacia, fractures, falls and osteoporosis. Hence, when serum vitamin D levels are below normal range, women should be supplemented with combined calcium and cholecalciferol vitamin D3 supplements, and be encouraged to increase appropriate sun exposure.

Phytoestrogens and isoflavones in diet

Phytoestrogens are oestrogenic compounds found in plants and consist of isoflavones, lignans and coumestans (Table 25.2).[50] Isoflavones have a similar structure to oestrogen and have the capacity to exert both mild oestrogenic effects in menopausal women and anti-oestrogenic effects in pre-menopausal women.[50] Comparative surveys of Japanese women and parallel groups of women from Canada and North America determined significant differences in the incidence of hot flushes and nocturnal sweating during premenopausal, perimenopausal and post-menopausal phases.[51]

However, a diet high in phytoestrogens alone is probably less successful in addressing menopausal symptoms without a change in lifestyle and more physical activity as well as the awareness of a low-calorie diet and stress management. This notion was evident in a cross-cultural comparison of health-related quality of life in Australian and Japanese midlife women.[52] It was reported that if the women had a lowered body mass index, undertook physical activity, consumed dietary phytoestrogens, and consumed some alcohol (any regular use of alcohol) their physical functioning seemed to be better.[52]

Asians and Japanese ingest on average 25–45mgs isoflavones per day over long periods

Table 25.2 Foods rich in phytoestrogen content

Phytoestrogen food sources	Phytoestrogen content (µg/100g)
Flax seed	379380
Soy beans	103920
Tofu	27150.1
Soy yoghurt	10275
Sesame seed	8008.1
Flax bread	7540
Black bean sauce	5330.3
Multigrain bread	4798.7
Soy milk	2957.2
Hummus	993
Soy bean sprouts	789.6
Garlic	603.6
Mung bean sprouts	495.1
Dried apricots	444.5
Alfalfa sprouts	441.4
Pistachio nuts	382.5
Dried dates	329.5
Sunflower seed	216
Chestnuts	210.2
Dried prunes	183.5
Olive oil	180.7
Walnuts	139.5
Almonds	131.1
Green beans	105.8
Broccoli	94.1
Cabbage	80
Peaches	64.5
Strawberry	51.6
Peanuts	34.5
Onion	32
Blueberry	17.5
Corn	9
Coffee with cow's milk	6.3
Watermelon	2.9
Milk, cow	1.2

(Source: adapted and modified from Thompson LU, Boucher BA, Lui Z, et. al. Phytoestrogen content of foods consumed in Canada, including isoflavones, lignans and coumestan. Nutrition and Cancer 2006; 54:184–201.)

of time. Just 40mg of isoflavones alone is sufficient to reduce menopausal symptoms which are up to 50 000 times higher than levels of endogenous estradiol.[15]

High phytoestrogen consumption in Asian women is thought to contribute to the low incidence of menopausal symptoms such as hot flushes, and exert protective effects on the cardiovascular system, reduce reproductive-related cancer risk, cardiovascular risk, reduce total cholesterol lipid levels and the risk of osteoporosis.

Furthermore, a high-phytoestrogen diet especially if initiated before puberty is associated with reduced risk of breast, colon and prostate cancer.[53, 54]

Middle-aged Japanese women are generally healthier than North American women, have lower rates of heart disease, breast cancer and osteoporosis, and have one of the longest life expectancy in the world (mean 85.33 yrs).[51]

The incidence of breast cancer is one-third compared with North American women, for osteoporosis less than half of Caucasian women in North America, even though Asian women have lower bone density, and 28% suffer a chronic health problem such as diabetes, allergies, asthma, arthritis and hypertension compared with 45% of Canadian (Manitoban) women and 53% of US (Massachusetts) women.[15]

The authors attribute these results to exercise, including weight-bearing exercise, no smoking, minimal consumption of alcohol and coffee, and a low-fat diet high in soybeans, vegetables and herbal teas (phytoestrogen-rich).[15]

Comparative studies of Japanese-oriental women, US and Finnish women proved that the Japanese women had a 60 to 110 times higher amount of isoflavones excreted in the urine while the concentration of oestrone and oestradiol was nearly identical and the amount of oestradiol was slightly less.[55] The average age in both groups (Japan and Finland) was 50.4

years. Both groups came from rural regions, therefore the socio–psychological differences were less than assumed. The measured higher concentrations of isoflavones in Japanese women were attributed to high consumption of soy products such as tofu, miso, aburage, atuage, koridofu as well as cooked soy beans. It was concluded that this dietary factor was responsible for less climacteric complaints and protective effect against cancer. (See Table 25.3.)

More research on the use of foods rich in phytoestrogens for menopausal symptoms with lifestyle modifications is required. Other food groups such as high fish, vegetable, fruit, nut intake and calcium rich foods also play a role and contribute to health benefits, reducing the risk of cardiovascular disease and osteoporosis (see chapters on cardiovascular disease and osteoporosis).

Nutritional supplements

Phytoestrogens

Phytoestrogens (plant oestrogens) are found in legumes, namely soy and red clover, and are rich in isoflavones which demonstrate significant oestrogenic activity, playing a role in the management of menopausal symptoms when blood oestrogen levels are low.

Safety concerns with the use of phytoestrogen supplements have been raised,[56] but the general consensus is that they are safe except where there is still uncertainty in some situations such as in women with breast cancer.[57] Phytoestrogens can also competitively bind to oestrogen receptors, displacing more potent oestrogens, and potentially decrease the overall oestrogenic effect in the premenopausal woman.[58]

Recent evidence demonstrates that a high dietary soy intake in women with a history of oestrogen and progesterone positive receptor breast cancer, had a significantly lower risk of breast cancer recurrence while taking tamoxifen.[59]

Soy (*Glycine max L.*) isoflavone extracts

Soy supplementation may play a role in the management of menopause and cholesterol, although diet plays a bigger role here.

A randomised double-blind, placebo-controlled trial has demonstrated that supplementation of soy isoflavones up to 100mgs/day for 4 months in post-menopausal women reduced cholesterol and menopausal symptoms by 21%.[60]

In another RCT, 25g of soy protein alone was able to reduce total cholesterol and LDL-cholesterol (-29.0 and -24.0mg/dL, $p<0.001$ and $p<0.006$) after 16 weeks compared with placebo and resistance exercise.[61]

Other studies have demonstrated its effectiveness only when the diet involved increasing phytoestrogen intake. Murkies et. al.[62] demonstrated that after 3 months, the soy flour supplementation evidenced a 40% reduction in hot flushes compared with controls fed wheat flour resulting in only 25% reduction. Advising patients to add 2 tablespoons of soy grits to their diet, such as cereal, may be comparable.

A double-blind, randomised, placebo-controlled study of 80 post-menopausal

Table 25.3 Excretion of isoflavones, phystoestrogens, and endogenous oestrogens in Japanese, American and Finnish women (with Western-type nutrition)

Urinary excretion	Japanese women [ng/24 hr]	US women [ng/24 hr]	Finnish women [ng/24 hr]
Genistein	3440	–	30.1
Daidzein	2600	216	40.5
Equol	2600	62.8	44.2
Estrone (post-menopausal)	4.48	–	4.48
Estradiol (post-menopausal)	0.76	–	0.94
Estriol (post-menopausal)	4.48	–	4.44

(Source: adapted and modified from Baird DD, Umbach DM, Landsdell L, et. al. Dietary intervention study to assess estrogenicitiy of dietary soy among post-menopausal women. Clin Endocrinol Metab 1995; 80: 1685–90)

women (mean age = 55.1 years), who reported 5 or more hot flush episodes per day, were randomised to receive either 250mg of standardised soy extract (Glycine max AT) a total of 100mg/day of isoflavone or placebo.[63]

After 10 months, there was a significant reduction in severity and frequency of hot flushes among isoflavone users when compared to those on placebo. Endometrial thickness, mammography, vaginal cytology, lipids and hormonal profile did not change in both groups.

A 12-week randomised placebo-controlled trial of 84 post-menopausal women randomised to 20g of soy protein containing 160mg of total isoflavones or taste-matched placebo (20g whole milk protein) demonstrated a significant improvement in all 4 quality-of-life subscales (vasomotor, psychosexual, physical, and sexual) among the women taking isoflavones compared with no changes observed in the placebo group.[64]

However, total testosterone and HDL levels were significantly lower in the isoflavone group compared to placebo group.

Another study has also demonstrated efficacy and safety of a soy isoflavone extract in post-menopausal women.[65] The soy isoflavone extract exerted favourable effects on vasomotor symptoms and compliance was good, providing a safe and effective alternative therapy for post-menopausal women.

However, RCTs have yielded mixed results for the effectiveness of soy isoflavones for menopausal symptoms due to various factors such as small sample sizes, short-term treatment and variation in dosage used. In addition, there is sub-population and individual variation in the metabolisation of daidzein which converts to the more bioactive estrogenic product equol by the gut bacteria. Western women are only 30% equol producers compared with 50–60% of Japanese women.[15]

A recent Cochrane review[66] concluded that there was no evidence of effectiveness in the alleviation of menopausal symptoms with the use of phytoestrogen treatments.

Most trials were small, of short duration and poor quality. Some trials found a slight reduction in hot flushes and night sweats, but overall no benefit compared with no treatment. There was no evidence of harm with short-term use.

Yet another systematic review and meta-analysis of multiple RCTs using a non-random effects model, demonstrated that isoflavone therapy had a significant 30% reduction in frequency hot flushes, especially in women with frequent hot flushes.[67]

Interestingly it has also been reported that the quality of soy phytoestrogens is almost certainly likely to influence efficacy.[68]

Herbal medicine

Herbal medicines may play a role in short-term management of the symptoms of menopause.

A review of the literature found the majority of studies indicate that extract of black cohosh (*Cimicifuga racemosa*) improves menopause-related symptoms, although the quality of studies is poor.[69] Studies for isoflavone red clover (*Trifolium pratense* L.) leaf extracts to relieve menopausal symptoms are contradictory. When compared with placebo, the largest study showed no benefit for reducing menopausal symptoms for 2 different red clover isoflavone products.[69] Clinical trials for the use of dong quai (*Angelica sinensis* L.), ginseng (*Panax ginseng*), or evening primrose seed oil (*Oenothera biennis* L.) demonstrate these are ineffective for improving menopausal symptoms.[69]

Another review suggests that isoflavones found in soy foods and red clover appear to have a 'small but positive health effect on plasma lipid concentrations, bone mass density, and cognitive abilities'.[70]

Red clover (*Trifolium pratense*)

Red clover is a member of the legume family and contains high levels of isoflavones, namely genistein, and significantly less daidzein compared with soy. Daidzein converts to the more bioactive equol, which exerts stronger estrogenic effects, and may explain why red clover is less effective than soy extracts in clinical trials.[71, 72]

The majority of placebo–controlled, randomised, double-blind studies have resulted in no effect of 40–160mg isoflavones (red clover isoflavones).[73, 74]

Three blinded randomised trials with red clover supplements containing either 57mgs/day isoflavones or 40mgs/day isoflavones found no benefit for hot flushes in peri- and post-menopausal women.[75] A further trial of 30 women aged 49–65 years, after 4 weeks, reported reduced hot flushes with 80mgs/day of red clover propriety extract compared with placebo.[76] Another similar trial demonstrated red clover to reduce symptoms of menopause with up to 73% of women experiencing a significant improvement, 50% reduction of hot flushes and 47% reduction in night sweats within 6 weeks of treatment.[76] However, a systematic review identified 5 trials measuring the effects of *T. pratense* isoflavones on vasomotor symptoms in menopausal women.[77] The meta-analysis only indicates a small reduction in hot flush frequency in women receiving active treatment (40–80mg/day) compared with those receiving placebo. A recent, large US clinical trial concluded that the red clover extract had no clinically important effect on hot flashes or other symptoms of menopause.[78]

A more recent systematic review and meta-analysis confirms efficacy of red clover extract.[79] It was concluded that there was evidence (albeit small) from *T. pratense* isoflavones for treating hot flushes in menopausal women. Minimal side-effects and no serious safety concerns were associated with short-term use of red clover, although technically one would avoid its use in estrogenic related health problems such as breast and endometrial cancers due to its high oestrogenic content, although this is not well established. A double-blinded placebo-controlled trial of 30 perimenopausal women demonstrated no proliferative effects on the endometrium by biopsy after 12 weeks of use with red clover-derived isoflavone extract, suggesting it may possibly have an anti-oestrogenic effect on the uterus.[80] A recent review of the literature confirms this finding.[81] Red clover demonstrates some efficacy in maintenance of bone health and improvement of arterial compliance.[82]

Black cohosh (*Cimicifuga racemosa*)

Black cohosh has been traditionally used in North American Indian medicine to treat gynaecological disorders including menopause. The German Commission E lists black cohosh for the treatment of menopausal symptoms, as well as PMS and dysmenorrhoea, and is only recommended for use up to 6 months because of the lack of long-term safety data.[83]

There have been numerous trials investigating the effectiveness of black cohosh to abrogate menopausal symptoms.[84, 85] A recent review has reported that black cohosh and foods that contain phytoestrogens show promise for the treatment of menopausal symptoms.[84]

Several small studies of a propriety extract of isopropanolic extract of black cohosh have revealed a trend to reducing vasomotor symptoms, however only 1 large trial with 304 post–menopausal women (mean age 54 years) has demonstrated a statistically significant reduction in hot flushes.[86] This study compared isopropanolic extract of black cohosh at 40mg twice daily versus placebo for 12 weeks. The treatment group showed significant improvement with hot flushes, urinary symptoms, vaginal dryness and mood. Liver function tests did not alter in both groups. A recent review came to similar conclusions.[83] The authors concluded that the isopropanolic extract of black cohosh root stock is effective in relieving climacteric symptoms, especially in early climacteric women.

None of the studies in the review investigated adverse events with black cohosh but other studies have reported that it is generally well tolerated and the commonest adverse reaction reported is gastrointestinal symptoms (nausea, dyspepsia and abdominal upset).[87, 88]

A multi-centre, randomised, placebo-controlled, double-blind, parallel group study conducted on 122 menopausal women treated over 12 weeks found *Cimicifuga racemosa* dried ethanolic extract significantly reduced hot flushes in women with severe symptoms by 47% compared with 21% in the placebo group.[89]

Another trial found isopropanolic *Cimicifuga racemosa* (iCR) therapy just as effective as tibolone for alleviation of moderate to severe climacteric symptoms.[90]

In an RCT 64 post-menopausal women (45–55 years old) with severe hot flushes, at least 5 daily, were randomised in a 3-month trial to 40mg isopropanolic aqueous iCR extract daily or 25mcg low dose transdermal estradiol (TTSE2) plus dihydrogesterone 10mg/day for the last 12 days of the 3-month estradiol treatment.[91]

At the end of 3 months, both groups significantly reduced hot flushes with no difference between them. Also symptoms of anxiety and depression reduced but no change in urogenital symptoms in either group. The overall trend for improvement was in the TTSE2 group. Other findings included reduction in total cholesterol in the TTSE2 group, significant reduction in low-density lipoprotein cholesterol (LDL-cholesterol) in both groups and black cohosh group significantly increased high-density lipoprotein cholesterol (HDL-cholesterol). There was no change in liver function tests, serum triglyceride levels or endometrial thickness in either group. A rise in prolactin and oestradiol was noted in the TTSE2 group but not the black cohosh group. No significant adverse effects were observed in either group.[91]

When compared with fluoxetine, black cohosh was more effective for treating hot flushes and night sweats in post-menopausal women.[92]

In the prospective randomised trial, when compared with fluoxetine treatment, supplementation with black cohosh was more effective for treating hot flushes and night sweats in post-menopausal women.

At the end of the 6-month trial, black cohosh reduced the hot flush score by 85%, compared with a 62% in the fluoxetine.[92]

There are also a number of trials that demonstrated black cohosh was not effective for the alleviation of menopausal and vasomotor symptoms.[93, 94]

One trial demonstrated black cohosh (1 capsule, *Cimicifuga racemosa* 20mg BID) was less efficacious than placebo in alleviating symptoms of menopause in women with breast cancer.[95]

Black cohosh and breast cancer

The relationship of phytoestrogen herbs and breast cancer is not well established. There have been conflicting reports about black cohosh having estrogenic properties.[96]

It appears that black cohosh does not exert oestrogenic properties. The main active ingredients of black cohosh are triterpenes. The activity and mechanism of action of these compounds are largely unknown. One study aimed to compare the effects of 2 black cohosh preparations, analysed for triterpene content and compared this to their efficacy for menopausal symptoms.[97]

One black cohosh product contained trace amounts and the other 2.5% triterpenes. The black cohosh product with 2.5% triterpenes resulted in relief of menopausal symptoms, compared with no benefit with the black cohosh with trace triterpenes. Also, it had no effect on estrogenic markers in serum and systemic or breast-specific estrogenic effects. Triterpene content varies in commercially available black cohosh preparations and may explain variations in efficacy in trials.

A population-based retrospective case-control study in 3 US counties (Philadelphia area), looked at 949 menopausal women with breast cancer cases and 1524 controls. It concluded the use of black cohosh had a 'significant breast cancer protective effect (adjusted odds ratio [OR] 0.39, 95% confidence interval [CI]: 0.22–0.70)'.[98]

An epidemiologic observational retrospective cohort study over an average of 3.6 years of 18 861 breast cancer women, including oestrogenic dependent cancers, 1102 of these women were on iCR therapy. The study endpoint was disease-free survival following a diagnosis of breast cancer. After controlling for confounders such as tamoxifen and age, the study found 'a protractive effect of iCR on the rate of recurrence (hazard ratio [HR] 0.83, 95% CI 0.69–0.99)'.[99]

Following initial diagnosis, 14% of the control group had developed a recurrence after 2 years and the iCR group reached this proportion after 6.5 years. The authors concluded iCR is 'not associated with increased risk of recurrence of breast cancer but associated with prolonged disease-free survival'.[99] This implies that black cohosh may have a protective effect toward recurrence of breast cancer.

Adverse reactions to black cohosh

Hepato-toxicity has been reported worldwide in a number of patients who presented with serious liver problems such as hepatitis associated with the use of several herbal products containing black cohosh.[100, 101] There have also been rare reports of liver failure requiring liver transplantation, raising concern with the daily therapeutic use of the herb.[102, 103] Hepatic reactions are likely to be idiosyncratic and occur rarely compared with the overall rate of use of black cohosh internationally.

A systematic review of clinical trials suggested black cohosh to be overall relatively safe. The review included 3 post-marketing surveillance studies, 4 case series, 8 single case reports and clinical studies.[104]

Systematic reviews for black cohosh

An early review of the literature of 4 RCTs as well as many more less rigorous studies found 3 of the 4 RCTs, conducted on menopausal women taking black cohosh in Germany, were useful for the control of not only hot flushes but also mood.[104] These trials demonstrated a significant effect on menopausal symptoms over placebo with no oestrogenic effect on vaginal epithelium.

Another review of the literature of black cohosh effects on vasomotor symptoms identified 32 papers.[106]

The review found black cohosh significantly reduced frequency or severity of hot flushes, although the results of randomised, placebo-controlled, double-blind clinical trials were contradictory. Adverse symptoms have been rare (5.4%), mild and reversible, mostly gastrointestinal upsets, rashes, headaches, dizziness and mastalgia.

Another systematic review found the evidence from 6 studies with a total of 1112 perimenopausal and post-menopausal women did not consistently demonstrate an effect of black cohosh on menopausal symptoms and suggested further rigorous trials were warranted.[107]

Further research is warranted to help identify the useful extract, dosage and exactly who is at risk of adverse reactions with black cohosh therapy.

St John's wort (SJW) (*Hypericum perforatum*)

A double, blind RCT over 16 weeks of 301 women with climacteric and psychological symptoms who were randomised to ethanolic St John's wort extract and isopropanolic black cohosh extract, or a matched placebo. The study assessed both climacteric symptoms (Menopause Rating Scale mean score) and psychological complaints (Hamilton Depression Rating Scale sum score).[108] The study reported reduced symptoms of 50% in the treatment group versus 19.6% in the placebo arm. Also reduced symptoms of depression in the treatment group of 41.8% compared with the placebo group of 12.7%. The study concluded that the treatment group was significantly ($P<0.001$) superior to placebo in both measures of menopause and depression, there were no differences regarding adverse events, laboratory values, or tolerability. The fixed combination of black cohosh and St John's wort was superior to placebo in alleviating climacteric complaints, including the related psychological component.

A prospective, controlled open-label observational study of 6141 women at 1287 outpatient gynaecologists in Germany followed up over 6 months and optionally at 12 months found the combination therapy of black cohosh and St John's wort more superior for the alleviation of both psychological and menopausal symptoms compared with the use of St John's wort alone. St John's wort also alleviated psyche symptoms, but not to the same degree as the combined formula. Adverse events were rare and non-serious: rate of 0.16%.[109]

Another trial of combined black cohosh and St John's wort also demonstrated efficacy for climacteric symptoms.[110]

In a further and recent clinical trial with St John's wort combined with Vitex agnus-castus (chaste tree berry) in the management of menopausal symptoms, it was reported that the herbal combination was no more effective than placebo.[111]

Hop extract (*Humulus lupulus* L.)

A recent double-blind randomised study investigated the efficacy of a hop extract (*Humulus lupulus* L.) to alleviate menopausal discomforts. The study concluded that the daily consumption of a hop extract, standardised on 8-prenylnaringenin (8-PN, the phytoestrogen in hops, *Humulus lupulus* L.) which is a potent phytoestrogen, exerted favourable effects on vasomotor symptoms and other menopausal discomforts.[112]

Mixed herbal formula

A double-blind placebo-controlled trial of 50 post-menopausal women were randomised to a herbal mixture containing black cohosh, dong quai, milk thistle, red clover, American ginseng and chaste tree berry or placebo. After 3 months of treatment, the herbal group demonstrated reduced hot flushes (>73%), reduction in night sweats (69%), reduction in intensity of hot flushes and improved sleep quality. The hot flushes ceased completely in 47% of women compared with only 19% in placebo group. There were no changes observed on vaginal ultrasound, hormone levels (estradiol, FSH), liver enzymes or thyroid in either group.[113]

Other herbal supplements

A Mayo Clinic trial found that flaxseed reduced hot flushes.[114] Other herbs implicated in having benefit for menopausal symptoms, with little or no research, include dong quai, evening primrose oil, *Panax ginseng*, gingko, wild yam, fennel, red sage, liquorice root and sarsaparilla root.[115–118]

Gingko biloba

Gingko biloba extract contains 24% of phytoestrogens (kaempferol, quercetin and isorhamnetin) which demonstrate weak estrogenic activities through the oestrogen response pathway by an interaction with oestrogen receptors.[119]

Ginseng (*Panax ginseng*)

An extract of ginseng, ginsenoside-Rb1, a weak phytoestrogen, is also known to exhibit oestrogenic activity by binding and activating oestrogen receptors.[120, 121, 122]

Wild yam (*Dioscorea villosa*)

Wild yam is a species of plant with edible roots (called yams) and is grown in abundance in humid (tropical) conditions. Some varieties of yams are consumed as foods. Wild yam was traditionally used by the Maya and Aztec civilization for colic, rheumatism and relief of inflammation and pain (e.g. cramps and arthritis). Wild yam is rich in steroidal saponin (sapogenin). Since the 1940s, the Japanese successfully isolated diosgenin from dioscin in wild yam, used to synthesise progesterone, making it attractive for its use in menopause, although there is no research to support the use of wild yam.[118]

For a list of herbs used in the treatment of hot flushes, but with limited supporting evidence,[123] see Table 25.4.

Table 25.4 Herbs used in the treatment of hot flushes with limited supporting evidence

Herb	Study population	Dosage	Study follow-up	Results	Adverse events
Dong quai[115]	71 menopausal women	4.5g/day	6 months	No significant difference compared with placebo	Similar between groups
Evening primrose oil[116]	56 menopausal women	500mg/day	6 months	No significant difference compared with placebo	Similar between groups
Ginseng[117]	384 menopausal women	200mg/day	4 months	No significant difference compared with placebo	Similar between groups
Wild yam[118]	50 menopausal women	1 teaspoon topically twice a day	6 months	No significant difference compared with placebo	None reported

Vitamins

Vitamin E

Vitamin E is reported to be regularly used by post-menopausal women.[82] However, the data from clinical trials is controversial. In 1 small placebo control trial 125 women with a history of breast cancer were given 800IU/day vitamin E supplementation for 9 weeks. The study demonstrated that on cross-over there was a slight improvement in menopausal symptoms (reduction in hot flash frequency) compared with placebo with a similar incidence of adverse events reported in both groups.[124] A recent trial, however, has demonstrated that vitamin E at 400IU/day was effective for the treatment of hot flashes.[125]

Other non-hormonal treatments

A useful literature review identified non-hormonal treatments for menopause. Non-hormonal pharmaceuticals for menopausal symptoms include such compounds as selective serotonin reuptake inhibitors (SSRIs) (e.g. paroxetine and sertraline, venlafaxine, gabapentin) mirtazapine and trazodone.[126] (See Table 25.5.)

The review also concluded that soy isoflavones reduced hot flushes by 9–40% in some trials, but most trials showing no benefit over placebo, and black cohosh and red clover also have had inconsistent results, with some trials also showing no benefit compared with placebo.

The evidence for these compounds in abrogating menopausal symptoms is limited and further randomised trials are warranted.

Physical therapies

Acupuncture

The World Health Organization supports the use of acupuncture for the management of menopause. Recently a number of clinical trials have reported on the use of acupuncture in women with and without breast cancer for the relief of menopausal symptoms.[127–131] In one study there were no significant effects for changes in hot flush interference, sleep, mood, health-related quality of life, or psychological wellbeing.[127] The results suggested that either there was a strong placebo effect or that both traditional and sham acupuncture significantly reduce hot flash frequency.[127] The second study was a long-term follow-up of acupuncture and hormone therapy on hot flushes in women with breast cancer.[128] This study demonstrated a significant reduction in hot flushes and concluded that electro-acupuncture may be a possible treatment of vasomotor symptoms for women with breast cancer for this group of women.[128] Three further studies on the use of acupuncture for menopausal symptoms in women with breast cancer have reported efficacy.[129, 130, 131]

However, the overall studies are methodologically poor and a number of systematic reviews have demonstrated mixed

Table 25.5 Non–prescribed and prescribed non-hormonal compounds for the treatment of hot flushes

Non-prescribed compounds	Prescribed compounds (non-hormonal)
Herbal medicines/plants/foods supplements • Black cohosh • Dong quai • Evening primrose oil • Ginseng • Red clover isoflavones • Soy isoflavones • St John's wort • Wild yam Hormones • Melatonin Vitamins • Vitamin E	Pharmaceuticals • Belladonna/ergotamine tartrate [phenobarbital combination] • Clonidine (Catapres®) • Fluoxetine (Prozac®) • Gabapentin (Neurontin®) • Mirtazapine (Remeron®) • Paroxetine (Paxil®) • Trazodone (Desyrel®) • Venlafaxine (Efexor®)

(Source: adapted and modified from Carroll DG. Non-hormonal therapies for hot flashes in menopause. *Am Fam Physician* 2006;73(3):457–64)

findings and failed to demonstrate acupuncture to be beneficial over sham acupuncture for climacteric symptoms.[132, 133, 134]

Conclusion

Women are seeking alternative options for the alleviation of symptoms associated with menopause. They view this time as a natural event and are concerned by side-effects associated with HRT. Although there have been a number of observational and epidemiologic studies conducted for the relief of menopausal symptoms, there is a continued need for further research on the efficacy as well as the long-term safety of herbal medicines and dietary supplements. An emergent body of scientific literature suggests that incorporation of some form of complementary therapy that promotes lifestyle changes, including suitable dietary changes, exercise and relaxation strategies, with the use of supplements/herbal medicines may result in significant improvement in clinical outcomes.[135] Table 25.6 summarises the level of scientific evidence for lifestyle and non-drug approaches to managing menopause.

Table 25.6 Levels of evidence for lifestyle and complementary medicines/therapies in the management of menopause

Modality	Level I	Level II	Level IIIa	Level IIIb	Level IIIc	Level IV	Level V
Lifestyle modifications							
[diet, exercise, smoking cessation, stress management]			x				
Mind–body medicine							
Psychological support (e.g. CBT)			x				
Relaxation therapies			x				
Physical activity/ exercise			x				
Exercise program	x						
Yoga	x (-)	x					
Nutrition							
Phytoestrogens				x			
Dietary soy		x					
Soy Isoflavone extract		x					
Herbal medicines							
Black cohosh	x(+/-)	x					
St John's wort		x					
Red clover extract	x (+/-)	x	x				
Hops extract				x			
Chinese herbs					x		
Dietary and/ or herbal combinations							
Soy isoflavones/ black cohosh				x			
St John's Wort/ black cohosh		x					
Mixed herbal formula		x					
Other supplements							
Flaxseed				x			
Vitamin E					x		
Physical therapies							
Acupuncture	x(-)	x					

Level I — from a systematic review of all relevant randomised controlled trials — meta-analyses.
Level II — from at least 1 properly designed randomised controlled clinical trial.
Level IIIa — from well-designed pseudo-randomised controlled trials (alternate allocation or some other method).
Level IIIb — from comparative studies (including systematic reviews of such studies) with concurrent controls and allocation not randomised, cohort studies, case-control studies, or interrupted time series with a parallel control group.
Level IIIc — from comparative studies with historical control, 2 or more single-arm studies or interrupted time series without a parallel control group.
Level IV — opinions of respected authorities based on clinical experience, descriptive studies or reports of expert committees.
Level V — represents minimal evidence that represents testimonials.

Clinical tips handout for patients — menopause

1 Lifestyle advice

Sleep

- Restore normal sleep patterns. Early to bed (about 9–10 p.m.) and awakening upon sunrise.
(See Chapter 22 for more advice.)

Sunshine

- At least 15 minutes of sunshine needed daily for vitamin D and melatonin production — especially before 10 a.m. and after 3 p.m. when the sun exposure is safest in summer.
- Ensure adequate skin exposure to sun; avoid sunscreen and excess clothing to maximise levels of vitamin D.
- More time in the sun is required for dark skinned people and in winter.

2 Physical activity/exercise

- Yoga may be of help, as may qigong and tai chi.
- Exercise at least 30–60 minutes daily. If exercise is not regular, commence with 5 minutes daily and slowly build up to at least 30 minutes. Outdoor exercise in nature, with fresh air and sunshine, is ideal (e.g. brisk walking, light jogging, cycling, swimming, stretching).
- Weight-bearing exercises are essential to prevent osteoporosis. Consider carrying shopping in a backpack or wearing strapped weights (<1kg) around ankles and wrists for extra weight-bearing whilst walking. The gym can also offer individual advice on weight-bearing exercises for older women.

3 Mind–body medicine (most helpful)

- Stress management program; for example, initially 6 x 40 minute sessions for patients: to understand the nature of their symptoms, the symptoms' relationship to stress and the practice of regular relaxation exercises.
- Regular meditation practice: at least 10–20 minutes daily.
- Psychological support, psycho-education and cognitive behaviour therapy.
- Cognitive behavioural therapy and psychotherapy are extremely helpful.
- Hypnotherapy, biofeedback may be of help.

Breathing

- Be aware of breathing at all times. Notice if tendency to hold breath or over-breathe. Always aim to relax breath and the muscles around the chest wall.

Rest and stress management

- Reduce workload and resolve conflicts. Contact family, friends, church or social groups for support.
- Listening to relaxation music helps.
- Relaxation massage therapy is helpful.
- Focus on wellness, not just the disease.

Fun

- It is important to have fun in life.
- Joy can be found even in the simplest tasks, such as funny movies/videos, comedy, hobbies, dancing, playing with pets and children.

4 Environment

- Avoid smoking, environmental pollutants and chemicals — at work and in the home.
- Lowering core body temperature may help to prevent hot flushes. Cooler environments, swimming, lowering air temperature within the household, avoiding overheating whilst sleeping, and avoiding spicy and hot foods or drinks.
- Avoid artificial sweeteners.

5 Dietary changes

- Add 1–2 tablespoons of soy grit to your morning cereal.
- Consume more phytoestrogenic foods — oestrogenic compounds found in plants such as flax seed, soy beans, tofu, soy yoghurt, soy milk, soy bean sprouts, sesame seed, multigrain bread, hummus, garlic, mung bean sprouts, alfalfa sprouts, dried apricots, pistachio nuts, dried dates, sunflower seeds, chestnuts, dried prunes, fennel, yams.
- Drink more water (1–2 litres a day) and teas (especially green tea, black tea).
- Eat more fruit (>2/day) and vegetables (>5/day) — a variety of colours and those in season.
- Eat wholegrains/cereals (variety): rice (brown, basmati, Mahatmi, Doongara), traditional rolled oats, buckwheat flour,

wholegrain organic breads (rye bread, Essene, spelt, Kamut), brown pasta, couscous, millet, amaranth etc.
- For sweetener try honey (e.g. manuka, yellow box and stringy bark have lowest GI).
- Increase fish intake (sardines, tuna, salmon, cod, mackerel) especially deep sea fish >3 servings per week.
- Reduce dairy intake; consume low fat dairy products such as yoghurt and cheeses, unless there is a dairy intolerance.
- Reduce red meat intake — preferably eat lean red meat (e.g. lamb, kangaroo) and white meat (e.g. free range organic chicken).
- Use cold pressed olive oil and avocado.
- Use dark chocolate.
- Minimise alcohol intake to no more than 1 glass daily.
- Avoid chemical additives — preservatives, colourings and flavourings.
- Avoid excessive coffee.
- Avoid hydrogenated fats, salt, fast foods, sugar (such as in soft drinks), lollies, biscuits, cakes and processed foods (e.g. white bread, white pasta, pastries).
- Avoid phytoestrogenic foods if you have a history of breast cancer (especially with hormone sensitive oestrogen receptors) until more research is available to clarify this.

6 Physical therapies

- Acupuncture may help relieve menopause symptoms.

7 Supplements

Phytoestrogens

Soy

- Indication: may reduce frequency and severity of hot flushes in some menopausal women; other menopausal symptoms, preventing osteoporosis, preventing cardiovascular disease, cyclic breast pain, premenstrual syndrome (PMS).
- Dosage: 20–60g soy protein (34–76mg of isoflavones) daily.
- Results: 1–14 days.
- Side-effects: often well tolerated. Very mild and rare side-effects; transient abdominal discomfort; theoretically may stimulate estrogenic receptors, causing breast discomfort, heavy menstrual bleeding and endometrial hyperplasia.
- Contraindications: more evidence is required to determine effect of soy on patients with existing hormone sensitive cancers such as breast and uterine. One study showed it was protective toward breast cancer recurrence.

Herbs

Black cohosh

- Indication: reduces symptoms of menopause.
- Dosage: 20–40 milligrams per day (1–2–4mg triterpene glycosides).
- Side-effects: in rare instances, black cohosh may cause liver damage in some patients. Several case reports internationally have linked black cohosh to liver failure or autoimmune hepatitis. Common side-effects include: gastrointestinal upset, headache, dizziness, weight gain, breast discomfort and vaginal spotting or bleeding. Long-term safety data are not available. Check liver function tests before commencing black cohosh and repeat 2–12 weeks, although liver damage can occur at any stage. Warn patient to stop product and seek medical advice if she develops symptoms of liver disease, such as yellowing of skin or whites of eyes, dark urine, nausea, abdominal pain, tiredness, loss of appetite, diarrhoea.
- Contraindications: liver disease. Avoid in children, pregnancy and lactation.

Red clover

- Indication: may have a small reduction in frequency and severity of hot flushes in some menopausal women. The evidence is weak.
- Dosage: 40–80mg/day.
- Results: 1–14 days.
- Side-effects: often well tolerated. Very mild and rare side-effects; headache, nausea, phytoestrogen activity may stimulate estrogenic receptors causing breast discomfort, heavy menstrual bleeding, vaginal spotting and endometrial hyperplasia (although unlikely). Long-term safety data on individual isoflavones or isoflavone concentrates are not available.
- Contraindications: more evidence is required to determine effect of red clover on patients with existing hormone-sensitive cancers such as breast and uterine cancer. Due to its coumarin content, red clover may increase the risk of bleeding. Avoid use 2 weeks prior to surgery and if you suffer bleeding disorders.

Traditional herbal medicine

Dong quai, Chinese herbal medicine, evening primrose oil, *Panax ginseng*, wild yam, fennel, red sage, liquorice root and sarsaparilla root have all been used traditionally for the symptomatic relief of menopause symptoms. There is very little or no research to support the use of these herbs.

St John's wort

- Indication: mild-moderate depression; combined with black cohosh can be very effective for menopausal symptoms, especially for mood disturbance.
- Dosage: 300mg 2–3 x daily.
- Results: 1–3 weeks.
- Side-effects: very mild and rare. Includes: photo-sensitivity skin rash, digestion disturbance, dizziness, fatigue, dry mouth.
- Contraindications: pregnancy, lactation, fertility, drug interaction avoid use with most pharmaceutical medication such as the oral contraceptive pill, other antidepressants, epileptic medication. Check with your doctor.

References

1. Sowers MR, Zheng H, McConnell D, et. al. Follicle stimulating hormone and its rate of change in defining menopause transition stages. J Clin Endocrinol Metab 2008 Jul 22.
2. Nelson HD. Menopause. Lancet 2008;371(9614):760–70.
3. Shrader SP, Ragucci KR. Life after the women's health initiative: evaluation of post-menopausal symptoms and use of alternative therapies after discontinuation of hormone therapy. Pharmacotherapy 2006;26(10):1403–9.
4. Ettinger B. NIH State of the Science conference on management of menopause– related symptoms. Symptom relief versus unwanted effects: role of estrogen–progestin dosage and regime.US Department of Health and Human Services, Bathesda, MD, 2005.
5. Stephenson J. FDA orders estrogen safety warnings: agency offers guidance for HRT use. JAMA 2003;289:537–38.
6. [No authors listed] Estrogen and progestogen use in post-menopausal women: July 2008 position statement of The North American Menopause Society. Menopause. 2008 Jun 20.
7. Van Horn L, Manson JE. The Women's Health Initiative: implications for clinicians. Cleve Clin J Med 2008;75(5):385–90.
8. Ockene JK, Barad DH, Cochrane BB, et. al. Symptom experience after discontinuing use of estrogen plus progestin. JAMA 2005;294(2):183–93.
9. Position statement of the North American Menopause Society. Treatment of menopause associated vasomotor symptoms. Menopause 2004;11:11–33.
10. Blake J. Menopause: evidence-based practice. Best Pract Res Clin Obstet Gynaecol 2006;20(6):799–839.
11. McKee J, Warber SL. Integrative therapies for menopause. South Med J 2005;98(3):319–26.
12. Greendale GA, Gold EB. Lifestyle factors: are they related to vasomotor symptoms and do they modify the effectiveness or side effects of hormone therapy? Am J Med 2005;118(Suppl 12B):148–54.
13. Gallicchio L, Visvanathan K, Miller SR, et. al. Body mass, estrogen levels, and hot flashes in midlife women. Am J Obstet Gynecol 2005 Oct;193(4):1353–60.
14. Gallicchio L, Miller SR, Visvanathan K, et. al. Cigarette smoking, estrogen levels, and hot flashes in midlife women. Maturitas 2006 Jan 20;53(2):133–43.
15. Melby MK, Lock M, Kaufert P. Culture and symptom reporting at menopause. Human Reproduction Update 2005;11(5):495–512.
16. Martin MC, Block JE, Sanchez SD, et. al. Menopause without symptoms: the endocrinology of menopause among rural Mayan Indians. Am J Obstet Gynecol 1993;168(6 Pt 1):1839–43.
17. Freeman EW, Sherif K. Prevalence of hot flushes and night sweats around the world: a systematic review. Climacteric 2007;10(3):197–214.
18. Crawford SL. The roles of biologic and nonbiologic factors in cultural differences in vasomotor symptoms measured by surveys. Menopause 2007;14(4):725–33.
19. Schnatz PF, Serra J, O'Sullivan DM, et. al. Menopausal symptoms in Hispanic women and the role of socioeconomic factors. Obstet Gynecol Surv 2006;61(3):187–93.
20. Freedman RR. Physiology of hot flashes. Am J Hum Biol 2001;13(4):453–64.
21. Freedman RR. Core body temperature variation in symptomatic and asymptomatic post-menopausal women: brief report. Menopause 2002 Nov-Dec;9(6):399–401.
22. Crandall CJ, Crawford SL, Gold EB. Vasomotor symptom prevalence is associated with polymorphisms in sex steroid-metabolizing enzymes and receptors. Am J Med 2006;119:S52–S60.
23. Deecher DC, Dorries K. Understanding the pathophysiology of vasomotor symptoms (hot flushes and night sweats) that occur in perimenopause, menopause, and post-menopause life stages. Arch Womens Ment Health 2007;10(6):247–572.
24. Murphy PJ, Campbell SS. Sex hormones, sleep, and core body temperature in older post-menopausal women. Sleep 2007 Dec 1;30(12):1788–94.
25. Ganz PA, Greendale GA, Petersen L, et. al. Managing menopausal symptoms in breast cancer survivors: results of a randomised controlled trial. JNCI 2000;92(13):1054–64.
26. Alder J, Eymann Besken K, Armbruster U, et. al. Cognitive-behavioural group intervention for climacteric syndrome. Psychoth Psychosom 2006;75(5):298–303.
27. Keefer L, Blanchard EB. A behavioural group treatment program for menopausal hot flashes: results of a pilot study. Appl Psychophysiol Biofeedback 2005;30(1):21–30.
28. Tremblay A, Sheeran L, Aranda SK. Psychoeducational interventions to alleviate hot flashes: a systematic review. Menopause 2008;15(1):193–202.
29. Stearns V, Ullmer L, López JF, et. al. Hot flushes. Lancet 2002;360(9348):1851–61.

30 North American Menopause Society. Treatment of menopause-associated vasomotor symptoms: position statement of The North American Menopause Society. Menopause 2004;11(1):11–33.

31 Carmody J, Crawford S, Churchill L. A pilot study of mindfulness-based stress reduction for hot flashes. Menopause 2006;13(5):760–9.

32 Nelson DB, Sammel MD, Freeman EW, et. al. Effect of physical activity on menopausal symptoms among urban women. Med Sci Sports Exerc 2008;40(1):50–8.

33 Gannon L, Stevens J. Portraits of menopause in the mass media. Women Health 1998;27(3):1–15.

34 Stadberg E, Mattsson LA, Milsom I. Factors associated with climacteric symptoms and the use of hormone replacement therapy. Acta Obstet Gynecol Scand 2000;79(4):286–92.

35 Villaverde-Gutiérrez C, Araújo E, Cruz F, et. al. Quality of life of rural menopausal women in response to a customized exercise programme. J Adv Nurs 2006;54(1):11–9.

36 Daley A, Stokes-Lampard H, Mutrie N, MacArthur C. Exercise for vasomotor menopausal symptoms. Cochrane Database of Systematic Reviews 2007;(4).

37 Daley AJ, Stokes-Lampard HJ, Macarthur C. Exercise to reduce vasomotor and other menopausal symptoms: a review. Maturitas. 2009 Jul 20;63(3):176–80.

38 Cohen BE. Yoga: an evidence-based prescription for menopausal symptoms? Menopause. 2008 Sep-Oct;15(5):827–9.

39 Cohen BE, Kanaya AM, Macer JL, et. al. Feasibility and acceptability of restorative yoga for treatment of hot flushes: a pilot trial. Maturitas 2007 Feb 20;56(2):198–204.

40 Booth-LaForce C, Thurston RC, Taylor MR. A pilot study of a Hatha yoga treatment for menopausal symptoms. Maturitas 2007 Jul 20;57(3):286–95. Epub 2007 Mar 2.

41 Chattha R, Nagarathna R, Padmalatha V, et. al. Effect of yoga on cognitive functions in climacteric syndrome: a randomised control study. BJOG 2008;115(8):991–1000.

42 Chattha R, Raghuram N, Venkatram P, et. al. Treating the climacteric symptoms in Indian women with an integrated approach to yoga therapy: a randomised control study. Menopause 2008 Sep-Oct;15(5):862–70.

43 Arias AJ, Steinberg K, Banga A, et. al. Systematic review of the efficacy of meditation techniques as treatments for medical illness. J Altern Complement Med 2006 Oct;12(8):817–32.

44 Lee MS, Kim JI, Ha JY, et. al. Yoga for menopausal symptoms: a systematic review. Menopause. 2009 May-Jun;16(3):602–8.

45 Elavsky S, McAuley E. Lack of perceived sleep improvement after 4-month structured exercise programs. Menopause. 2007 May-Jun;14(3 Pt 1): 535–40.

46 Elavsky S, McAuley E. Exercise and self-esteem in menopausal women: a RCT involving walking and yoga. Am J Health Promot. 2007 Nov-Dec;22(2):83–92.

47 Avenell A, Gillespie WJ, Gillespie LD, et. al. Vitamin D and vitamin D analogues for preventing fractures associated with involutional and post-menopausal osteoporosis. Cochrane Database of Systematic Reviews 2008, Issue 1. Art. No.: CD000227. DOI: 10.1002/14651858.CD000227.pub3.

48 LaCroix AZ, Kotchen J, Anderson G, et. al. Calcium plus vitamin D supplementation and mortality in post-menopausal women: the Women's Health Initiative calcium-vitamin D randomised controlled trial. J Gerontol A Biol Sci Med Sci 2009 May;64(5):559–67. Epub 2009 Feb 16.

49 Brunner RL, Cochrane B, Jackson RD, et. al. Calcium, vitamin D supplementation, and physical function in the Women's Health Initiative. J Am Diet Assoc. 2008 Sep;108(9):1472–9.

50 Thompson LU, Boucher BA, Lui Z, et. al. Phytoestrogen content of foods consumed in Canada, including isoflavones, lignans and coumestan. Nutrition and Cancer 2006; 54:184–201.

51 Lock M. Menopause in cultural context. Exp Gerontol 1994 May-Aug;29(3-4):307–17.

52 Anderson DJ, Yoshizawa T. Cross-cultural comparisons of health-related quality of life in Australian and Japanese midlife women: the Australian and Japanese Midlife Women's Health Study. Menopause 2007;14(4):697–707.

53 Adlercreutz H. Phyto-oestrogens and cancer. The Lancet Oncology 2002;3:364–373.

54 Ingram D, Saunders K, Kolybaba M et. al. Case-control study of Phyto-oestrogens and Breast Cancer and Plant Oestrogen. Lancet 1997;350:990–94.

55 Baird DD, Umbach DM, Landsdell L, et. al. Dietary intervention study to assess estrogenicitiy of dietary soy among post-menopausal women. J Clin Endocrinol Metab 1995;80:1685–90.

56 Song WO, Chun OK, Hwang I, et. al. Soy isoflavones as safe functional ingredients. J Med Food 2007;10(4):571–80.

57 Kurzer MS. Phytoestrogen supplement use by women. J Nutr 2003;133(6):1983S–1986S.

58 Tham DM, Gardner CD, Haskell WL. Clinical review 97: Potential health benefits of dietary phytoestrogens: a review of the clinical, epidemiological, and mechanistic evidence. J Clin Endocrinol Metab 1998;83(7):2223–35.

59 Guha N, Kwan ML, Queensberry CP, et. al. Soy isoflavones and risk of cancer recurrence in a cohort of breast cancer survivors: the Life After Cancer Epidemology study. Treat 2009; 118(2):395–405.

60 Han KK, Soares JM Jr, Haidar MA, et. al. Benefits of soy isoflavone therapeutic regimen on menopausal symptoms. Obstet Gynecol 2002;99(3):389–94.

61 Maesta N, Nahas EA, Nahas-Neto J, et. al. Effects of soy protein and resistance exercise on body composition and blood lipids in post-menopausal women. Maturitas 2007 Apr 20;56(4):350–8.

62 Murkies AL, Lombard C, Strauss BJ, et. al. Dietary flour supplementation decreases post-menopausal hot flushes: effect of soy and wheat. Maturitas 1995;21:189–95.

63 Nahas EA, Nahas-Neto J, Orsatti FL, et. al. Efficacy and safety of a soy isoflavone extract in post-menopausal women: a randomised, double-blind, and placebo-controlled study. Maturitas 2007 Nov 20;58(3):249–58.

64 Basaria S, Wisniewski A, Dupree K, et. al. Effect of high-dose isoflavones on cognition, quality of life, androgens, and lipoprotein in post-menopausal women. J Endocrinol Invest. 2009 Feb;32(2):150–5.

65 Knight DC, Howes JB, Eden JA, et. al. Effects on menopausal symptoms and acceptability of isoflavone-containing soy powder dietary supplementation. Climacteric 2001;4(1):13–8.

66 Lethaby A, Marjoribanks J, Kronenberg F, et. al. Phytoestrogens for vasomotor menopausal symptoms. Cochrane Database of Systematic Reviews 2007,Oct 17;(4):CD001395.

67 Howes LG, Howes JB, Knight DC. Isoflavone therapy for menopausal flushes: a systematic review and meta-analysis. Maturitas 2006 Oct 20;55(3):203–11.

68 American College of Obstetricians and Gynecologists Committee on Practice Bulletins. Clinical Management Guidelines for Obstetrician/ Gynecologists: Use of Botanicals for the management of Menopausal symptoms. Obstet Gynecol 2001;97 (Suppl):1-11.

69 Low Dog T. Menopause: a review of botanical dietary supplements. Am J Med 2005 Dec 19;118(Suppl 12B):98–108.

70 Geller SE, Studee L. Soy and red clover for mid-life and aging. Climacteric 2006 Aug;9(4):245–63.

71 Setchell KD, Brown NM, Desai PB, et. al. ioavailability, disposition, and dose-response effects of soy isoflavones when consumed by healthy women at physiologically typical dietary intakes. J Nutr 2003;133, 1027–1035.

72 Setchell KD, Brown NM, Lydeking-Olsen E. The clinical importance of the metabolite equol-a clue to the effectiveness of soy and its isoflavones. J Nutr 2002;132, 3577–3584.

73 Nedrow A, Miller J, Walker M, et. al. Complementary and alternative therapies for the management of menopause-related symptoms: a systematic evidence review. Arch Intern Med 2006;166(14):1453–65.

74 Knight DC, Howes JB, Eden JA. The effect of promensil™, an isoflavone extract, on menopausal symptoms. Climacteric 1999;2:79–84.

75 Peter HM, van de Weijer PHM, Ronald Barentsen. Isoflavones from red clover (Promensil) significantly reduce menopausal hot flush symptoms compared with placebo. Maturitas 2002;42:187–193.

76 Jeri AR, Romana CD. The effect of isoflavone phytoestrogens in relieving hot flushes in Peruvian post-menopausal women. The Fem Patient 2002;27:35–37.

77 Thompson Coon JS, Pittler MH, Ernst E. The role of red clover (Trifolium pratense) isoflavones in women's reproductive health: a systematic review and meta-analysis of randomised clinical trials. Foc Altern Compl Ther 2003;8:544.

78 Tice JA. Ettinger B. Ensrud K. et. al. Phytoestrogen supplements for the treatment of hot flashes: the Isoflavone Clover Extract (ICE) Study: a randomised controlled trial. JAMA 2003;290(2):207–14.

79 Booth NL, Piersen CE, Banuvar S, et. al. Clinical studies of red clover (Trifolium pratense) dietary supplements in menopause: a literature review. Menopause 2006;13(2):251–64.

80 Hale GE, et. al. A double-blind randomised study on the effects of red clover isoflavones on the endometrium. Menopause 2001;8(5)338–346.

81 Coon JT, Pittler MH, Ernst E. Trifolium pratense isoflavones in the treatment of menopausal hot flushes: a systematic review and meta-analysis. Phytomedicine 2007;14(2-3):153–9.

82 Umland EM. Treatment strategies for reducing the burden of menopause-associated vasomotor symptoms. J Manag Care Pharm 2008;14(3 Suppl):14–9.

83 Geller SE, Studee L. Botanical and dietary supplements for mood and anxiety in menopausal women. Menopause 2007;14(3 Pt 1):541–9.

84 Kronenberg F, Fugh-Berman A. Complementary and alternative medicine for menopausal symptoms: a review of randomised, controlled trials. Ann Intern Med 2002;137(10):805–13.

85 Geller SE, Studee L. Botanical and dietary supplements for menopausal symptoms: what works, what does not. J Womens Health 2005;14(7): 634–49.

86 Osmers R, Friede M, Liske E, et. al. Efficacy and safety of isopropanolic black cohosh extract for climacteric symptoms. Obstet. Gynecol. 2005;105:1074–1083.

87 Kligler B. Black cohosh. Am Fam Physician 2003;68(1):114–6.

88 Huntley A. The safety of black cohosh (Actaea racemosa, Cimicifuga racemosa). Expert Opin Drug Saf 2004;3(6):615–23.

89 Frei-Kleiner S, Schaffner W, Rahlfs VW, et. al. Cimicifuga racemosa dried ethanolic extract in menopausal disorders: a double-blind placebo-controlled clinical trial. Maturitas 2005 Aug 16;51(4):397–404.

90 Bai W, Henneicke-von Zepelin HH, Wang S, et. al. Efficacy and tolerability of a medicinal product containing an isopropanolic black cohosh extract in Chinese women with menopausal symptoms: a randomised, double-blind, parallel-controlled study versus tibolone. Maturitas 2007 Sep 20;58(1):31–41.

91 Nappi RE, Malavasi B, Brundu B, et. al. Efficacy of Cimicifuga racemosa on climacteric complaints: a randomised study versus low-dose transdermal estradiol. Gynecol Endocrinol 2005 Jan;20(1):30–5.

92 Oktem M, Eroglu D, Karahan HB, et. al. Black cohosh and fluoxetine in the treatment of post-menopausal symptoms: a prospective, randomised trial. Adv Ther 2007 Mar-Apr;24(2):448–61.

93 Geller SE, Shulman LP, van Breemen RB, et. al. Safety and efficacy of black cohosh and red clover for the management of vasomotor symptoms: a randomised controlled trial; Menopause: The Journal of The North American Menopause Society 2009;16(6):pp. 000/000. doi: 10.1097/ gme.0b013e3181ace49b.

94 Newton KM, Reed SD, LaCroix AZ, et. al. Treatment of vasomotor symptoms of menopause with black cohosh, multibotanicals, soy, hormone therapy, or placebo: a randomised trial. Ann Intern Med 2006 Dec 19;145(12):869–79.

95 Pockaj BA, Gallagher JG, Loprinzi CL, et. al. Phase III double-blind, randomised, placebo-controlled crossover trial of black cohosh in the management of hot flashes: NCCTG Trial N01CC1. J Clin Oncol 2006 Jun 20;24(18):2836–41.

96 Liske E. Physiological investigation of a unique extract of black cohosh: a 6-month clinical study demonstrates no systemic estrogenic effect. Journal of women's health and gender-based medicine, 2002;2:163–74.

97 Ruhlen RL, Haubner J, Tracy JK, et. al. Black cohosh does not exert an estrogenic effect on the breast. Nutr Cancer 2007;59(2):269–77.

98 Rebbeck TR, Troxel AB, Norman S, et. al. A retrospective case-control study of the use of hormone-related supplements and association with breast cancer. Int J Cancer 2007 Apr 1;120(7): 1523–8.

99 Zepelin HH, Meden H, Kostev K, et. al. Isopropanolic black cohosh extract and recurrence-free survival after breast cancer. Int J Clin Pharmacol Ther 2007 Mar;45(3):143–54.
100 Chow EC, Teo M, Ring JA, et. al. Liver failure associated with the use of black cohosh for menopausal symptoms. MJA 2008;188(7):420–2.
101 Whiting PW, Clouston A, Kerlin P. Black cohosh and other herbal remedies associated with acute hepatitis. Med J Aust 2002;177:440–443.
102 Lontos S, Jones RM, Angus PW, et. al. Acute liver failure associated with the use of herbal preparations containing black cohosh. Med J Aust 2003;179(7):390–1.
103 Walji R, Boon H, Guns E, et. al. Black cohosh (Cimicifuga racemosa [L.] Nutt.): safety and efficacy for cancer patients. Support Care Cancer 2007;15(8):913–21.
104 Borrelli F, Ernst E. Black cohosh (Cimicifuga racemosa): a systematic review of adverse events. Am J Obstet Gynecol 2008 Nov;199(5):455–66.
105 Lieberman S. A review of the effectiveness of Cimicifuga Racemosa (Black Cohosh) for the Symptoms of Menopause. J Women's Health 1998;7:525–29.
106 Kanadys WM, Leszczyńska-Gorzelak B, Oleszczuk J. Efficacy and safety of Black cohosh (Actaea/ Cimicifuga racemosa) in the treatment of vasomotor symptoms--review of clinical trials. Ginekol Pol 2008 Apr;79(4):287–96.
107 Borrelli F, Ernst E. Black cohosh (Cimicifuga racemosa) for menopausal symptoms: a systematic review of its efficacy. Pharmacol Res 2008 Jul;58(1):8–14.
108 Uebelhack R, Blohmer JU, Graubaum HJ, et. al. Black cohosh and St. John's wort for climacteric complaints: a randomised trial. Obstet Gynecol 2006;107(2 Pt 1):247–55.
109 Briese V, Stammwitz U, Friede M, et. al. Black cohosh with or without St. John's wort for symptom-specific climacteric treatment--results of a large-scale, controlled, observational study. Maturitas 2007 Aug 20;57(4):405–14.
110 Chung DJ, Kim HY, Park KH, et. al. Black cohosh and St. John's wort (GYNO-Plus) for climacteric symptoms. Yonsei Med J 2007 Apr 30;48(2):289–94.
111 van Die MD, Burger HG, Bone KM, et. al. Hypericum perforatum with Vitex agnus-castus in menopausal symptoms: a randomised, controlled trial. Menopause 2008 Sep 10.
112 Heyerick A, Vervarcke S, Depypere H, et. al. A first prospective, randomised, double-blind, placebo-controlled study on the use of a standardised hop extract to alleviate menopausal discomforts. Maturitas 2006;54(2):164–75.
113 Rotem C, Kaplan B. Phyto-Female Complex for the relief of hot flushes, night sweats and quality of sleep: randomised, controlled, double-blind pilot study. Gynecol Endocrinol. 2007 Feb;23(2):117–22.
114 Pruthi S, Thompson SL, Novotny PJ, et. al. Pilot evaluation of flaxseed for the management of hot flashes. J Soc Integr Oncol 2007 Summer;5(3):106–12.
115 Hirata JD, Swiersz LM, Zell B, et. al. Does dong quai have estrogenic effects in post-menopausal women? A double-blind, placebo- controlled trial. Fertil Steril 1997;68:981–6.
116 Chenoy R, Hussain S, Tayob Y, et. al. Effect of oral gamolenic acid from evening primrose oil on menopausal flushing. BMJ 1994;308:501–3.
117 Wiklund IK, Mattsson LA, Lindgren R, et. al. Effects of standardised ginseng extract on quality of life and physiological parameters in symptomatic post-menopausal women: a double-blind, placebo-controlled trial. Swedish Alternative Medicine Group. Int J Clin Pharmacol Res 1999;19:89–99.
118 Komesaroff PA, Black CV, Cable V, et. al. Effects of wild yam extract on menopausal symptoms, lipids and sex hormones in healthy menopausal women. Climacteric 2001;4:144–50.
119 Oh SM, Chung KH. Estrogenic activities of Ginkgo biloba extracts. Life Sci 2004 Jan 30;74(11):1325–35.
120 Papapetropoulos A. A ginseng-derived oestrogen receptor beta (ERbeta) agonist, Rb1 ginsenoside, attenuates capillary morphogenesis. Br J Pharmacol 2007 Sep;152(2):172–4.
121 Cho J, Park W, Lee S, et. al. Ginsenoside-Rb1 from Panax ginseng C.A. Meyer activates estrogen receptor-alpha and -beta, independent of ligand binding. J Clin Endocrinol Metab 2004 Jul;89(7):3510–5.
122 Lee YJ, Jin YR, Lim WC, et. al. Ginsenoside-Rb1 acts as a weak phytoestrogen in MCF-7 human breast cancer cells. Arch Pharm Res. 2003 Jan;26(1):58–63.
123 Herbs2000.com. Available: http://www.herbs2000.com /herbs/herbs_wild_yam.htm (accessed 9 March 2010).
124 Barton DL, Loprinzi CL, Quella SK, et. al.Prospective evaluation of vitamin E for hot flashes in breast cancer survivors. J Clin Oncol 1998;16(2):495–500.
125 Ziaei S, Kazemnejad A, Zareai M. The effect of vitamin E on hot flashes in menopausal women. Gynecol Obstet Invest 2007;64(4):204–7.
126 Carroll DG. Nonhormonal therapies for hot flashes in menopause. Am Fam Physician 2006;73(3):457–64.
127 Avis NE, Legault C, Coeytaux RR, et. al. A randomised, controlled pilot study of acupuncture treatment for menopausal hot flashes. Menopause 2008 Jun 2.
128 Frisk J, Carlhäll S, Källström AC, et. al. Long-term follow-up of acupuncture and hormone therapy on hot flushes in women with breast cancer: a prospective, randomised, controlled multicenter trial. Climacteric 2008;11(2):166–74.
129 Filshie J, Bolton T, Browne D, et. al. Acupuncture and self acupuncture for long-term treatment of vasomotor symptoms in cancer patients-audit and treatment algorithm. Acupunct Med 2005;23(4):171–80.
130 Deng G, Vickers A, Yeung S, et. al. Randomised, controlled trial of acupuncture for the treatment of hot flashes in breast cancer patients. J Clin Oncol 2007;25(35):5584–90.
131 Hervik J, Mjåland O. Acupuncture for the treatment of hot flashes in breast cancer patients, a randomised, controlled trial. Breast Cancer Res Treat. 2008 Oct 7.
132 Lee MS, Shin BC, Ernst E. Acupuncture for treating menopausal hot flushes: a systematic review. Climacteric 2009 Feb;12(1):16–25.
133 Cho SH, Whang WW. Menopause. Acupuncture for vasomotor menopausal symptoms: a systematic review 2009 May 6.
134 Lee MS, Kim KH, Choi SM, et. al. Acupuncture for treating hot flashes in breast cancer patients: a systematic review. Breast Cancer Res Treat 2009 Jun;115(3):497–503. Epub 2008 Nov 4.
135 McBane SE. Easing vasomotor symptoms: Besides HRT, what works? JAAPA 2008;21(4):26–31.

Chapter 26

Multiple sclerosis

With contribution from Dr Lily Tomas

Introduction

Multiple sclerosis (MS) is the most common progressive, neurological disorder in most Western countries today.[1] It is an auto-immune, inflammatory, demyelinating condition of the central nervous system (CNS) that has no known cure.[2] Despite the incredible progress that has been made with modern medicine, the treatment of MS with pharmaceuticals is certainly not ideal. Presumably for this reason, many people with MS worldwide are actively involved in self-care, using complementary and alternative medicine (CAM) therapies to help with symptom management.[3, 4]

A recent review of the literature demonstrates that the primary reasons for choosing CAM include the desire to use an holistic health care approach, conventional treatment not being effective, anecdotal reports of CAM efficacy and doctor referral. It is interesting to note that many people also choose CAM because they were unsatisfied with their initial consultation with their physician lasting less than 15 minutes.[5, 6] The major symptoms being treated with CAM include pain, fatigue and stress, with the major therapies being dietary modification, nutritional and herbal supplementation, exercise, cold baths and mind–body therapies.[4, 7, 8]

Use of CAM therapies has been associated with religiosity, functional independence, female sex, white-collar jobs and higher education. Compared with conventional treatments, CAM therapies also rarely have unwanted side-effects (9% vs 59%).[5]

MS is a complex disease, perhaps encompassing more than a single aetiopathological entity and very likely subject to multi-factorial aetiology[9] with ample evidence revealing an intricate interplay from genetics and differing environmental factors. Current research strongly indicates that previous infection with Epstein-Barr virus, vitamin D deficiency and smoking are major risk factors for developing this most debilitating and unpredictable disorder.[10–14] Furthermore, it has been shown that good nutrition, sunlight exposure, exercise, stress and social factors can all influence the rate of progression and the level of disability.[1]

MS has always been considered to be more common in women and in areas further from the equator. However, recent reports indicate that the female:male ratio has increased and the latitude gradient decreased in the last 5 decades.[15]

Incidence/prevalence

MS prevalence worldwide is estimated at over 1 million cases. In the US this number is approximately 250 000–350 000.[16] It is the most frequent non-traumatic disabling neurologic disease among young adults, with 12 000 new diagnoses per year in the US alone.[17]

Lifestyle — general

It is well documented that lifestyle approaches may significantly influence the development and progression of MS, and hence offer potentially effective avenues for therapy.[1]

Patients with MS have frequent adverse health behaviours, such as lack of outdoor exercise, smoking and drinking alcohol, which increase the risk of other chronic diseases. Further research is required to determine the extent of such behaviours on the progression of MS.[18]

Mind–body medicine

As we are all aware, stress can exacerbate many pathophysiogical disease processes, including those of neurodenerative origin.[19]

Corticotropin-releasing hormone (CRH) plays a central role in the regulation of the hypothalamic–pituitary–adrenal (HPA) axis; that is, the common final pathway in the stress response.[20] Patients with MS have also been demonstrated to have HPA axis hyperactivity, therefore stress-relieving activities are considered to be particularly beneficial in this population.[21]

The discipline of psychoneuroimmunology has demonstrated that the immune system most certainly interacts with the CNS.[22]

A recent RCT has shown that telephone counselling for those with MS significantly improves physical activity, spiritual growth, stress management, fatigue and general mental health status compared with controls. There was also greater improvement in walking speed in those who chose to exercise more.[23]

As previously stated, fatigue is a frequent and disabling symptom in those with MS. Underlying psychological processes may certainly be part of this aetiology.[24] It has been shown that a challenging mental task can alter the pattern and increase the cerebral activation on an unrelated motor task in fatigued MS patients.[25, 26]

Cognitive behaviour therapy (CBT) rehabilitation in MS is in its relative infancy.[27] A recent Cochrane review has indicated that there is adversity of psychological interventions that can potentially help those with MS. CBT approaches, in particular, are beneficial in the treatment of depression, and in helping people adjust to, and cope with, having MS.[28] A recent Australian longitudinal assessment study of anxiety, depression and fatigue in MS has confirmed this finding.[29]

Sleep

Fatigue is one of the most common symptoms of MS. The mechanisms underlying such fatigue are still poorly understood and are obviously multifactorial. Eliminating sleep disorders (as well as adverse drug effects, infections, iron/vitamin B12 deficiency) is an important part of an MS work-up.[30, 31, 32] The prevalence of sleep problems in MS is significantly higher than in the general population and mostly affects women with MS more than men.[33]

Restless legs syndrome (RLS) is also significantly associated with MS, especially in patients with severe pyramidal and sensory disability. RLS is known to have a significant impact on sleep quality in patients with MS, and as such, a thorough history regarding this should always be taken.[34] Patients with RLS present with greater disability and greater levels of fatigue.[35] Anecdotal evidence strongly suggests that magnesium can assist with RLS. Restoring sleep patterns may help reduce symptoms of MS.

Sunshine

Sunlight exposure has emerged as being the most likely candidate for the explanations in geographical variations in MS prevalence; that is, increased risk of MS in populations residing at higher or lower latitudes.[36] This observation implies a protective effect of sunlight, which is reduced at higher or lower latitudes, contributing to insufficient levels of vitamin D that are frequently found in those with MS.[37]

Monthly variations in MS relapses (with more relapses occurring in colder months) have been recently documented in Australia. Relapse rates were therefore inversely associated with UV radiation and serum 25(OH)D levels and positively associated with upper respiratory tract infections.[38]

Australian research has also demonstrated that those individuals with fair skin/red hair have an increased risk of MS that is more evident in women. As a child, they tended to behaviourally avoid sun exposure. In contrast, increased sun exposure from ages 6–10 is associated with reduced MS risk in those individuals without red hair. It should be noted, however, that the interplay between melanocortin 1 receptor variants, red hair/fair skin phenotype, past sun exposure and MS is complex.[39]

Earlier studies have also shown that increased outdoor activities during summer in early life even north of the Arctic circle are associated with a reduced risk of developing MS; most pronounced age range being 16–20 years.[40, 41]

Adverse reports of high ambient temperatures in people with MS correlate significantly with the report of strong sunlight, apparently making MS worse. This appears to be worse with increasing age. In Australia, high temperatures are more likely to be reported as adverse in warmer, lower latitude regions. This apparent adverse factor therefore appears to be related to solar heat, not solar light.[8]

Environmental influences

Geographical patterns in Australia currently imply that modifiable environmental factors hold the key to preventing approximately 80% of MS cases. Genetic epidemiology demonstrates that family history has an important role. However, if these factors are held constant, the environment sets the disease threshold.[42]

Recent studies have shown that men develop MS at lower levels of environmental exposure than women. Women, however, appear to be more responsive to the recent changes in environmental exposure that have seen a change in the sex ratio prevalence of MS in recent decades.[43]

Epstein-Barr virus (EBV)

Data from studies of twins and migrants with MS certainly imply environmental factors in the development of MS.[44] There is a wealth of evidence linking EBV with MS, with the viral infection having potential roles in both initiating the auto-immune process and exacerbating disease progression.[12, 43, 45–48] Furthermore, there is evidence to suggest that there is infection with EBV in brain lesions of MS patients.[49] There is nearly a 100% sero-prevalence to EBV antibodies in MS years before clinical onset of the disease.[44, 49] It appears that individuals with EBV Nuclear antigen 1 (EBNA-1) have a 2.8 times increased risk of developing MS, independently from DR15 allele.[49] Carriers of this allele who also have elevated anti-EBNA-1 titres may have a significantly increased risk of MS.[50] Amongst those who develop MS, antibody titres were 2–3 times higher in those individual who were 25 years of age or higher, suggesting an age-dependent relationship between EBV and MS.[51] The risk is also increased after an initial symptomatic EBV infection.[44]

There is also recent evidence to suggest that Chlamydia pneumonia, which belongs to the rickettsial family of micro-organisms, is also linked to MS.[52]

Smoking

As stated previously, there is a multitude of studies demonstrating an association between smoking and MS.[53, 54] Those who begin smoking at an early age are significantly more likely to develop progressive MS at an early age compared with later debut smokers or non-smokers.[55]

Furthermore, modestly elevated cotinine levels suggestive of passive smoking are also associated with an increased risk for MS.[56, 57]

A recent Australian prospective cohort study has demonstrated that cumulative pack years smoking is associated with progressive disease course and increased progression in clinical disability.

Smoking during the cohort period was not associated with relapse.[58]

Thus far, smoking during pregnancy has not been shown to be a risk for early-onset MS amongst offspring.[59]

Heavy metal exposure

There is an observable difference in MS prevalence in particular regions with perceived clusters of MS throughout several countries. Such clusters have occurred around lead smelters, oil refineries and air pollutants. No direct associations have as yet been made.[60–63]

In contrast to immunoglobulins (IgGs) of healthy individuals, antibodies of MS patients effectively hydrolyse human myelin basic protein (MBP). Furthermore, IgG from sera of MS patients have been shown to possess metal-dependent human MBP-hydrolysing activity.[64]

Iron overload and the upregulation of iron-binding proteins in the brain have also been implicated in the pathogenesis of MS.[65] Indeed, MRIs reveal significant and pathological iron deposition in brain MS lesions.[66, 67] Urinary concentrations of iron are significantly increased in secondary progressive MS and insignificantly increased in relapsing–remitting MS (RRMS). This increased urinary iron excretion supports a role for iron dysmetabolism in MS.[68] Iron imbalance is associated with pro-inflammatory cytokines and oxidative stress, suggesting that the improvement of neuronal iron metabolism may be a future target for MS therapy.[65]

Similarly, urinary concentrations of aluminium (Al) are also significantly increased in both secondary progressive and relapsing–remitting forms of MS. These levels of urinary Al are high enough to be compared with levels observed in individuals with Al intoxication who are undergoing specific metal chelation therapy. In accordance with this, urinary excretion of silicon is lower in MS and significantly lower in secondary progressive MS. It has since been concluded that Al may be another environmental factor associated with the aetiology of MS. If this is the case, then an increased intake of its natural antagonist, silicon, may be another therapeutic option.[68]

Individuals with dental amalgam have been shown to have 2–12 times more mercury in their body tissues than those without. Mercury deposits in brain and bone tissues have a half-life lasting from several years to decades and may accumulate over time of exposure.[69] A recent systematic review and meta-analysis was performed in order to investigate the possible association between methyl mercury in dental amalgam and MS. The pooled odds ratios for the risk of MS amongst those with amalgams was consistent with a slight non–statistically significant increase between amalgam use and risk of MS. Further studies regarding amalgam restoration size and duration of exposure are needed to definitively rule out any link between amalgam and MS.[70]

Studies have also shown that Tetrathiomolybdate (TM), a potent anti-copper drug, significantly inhibits neurological damage associated with animal models of MS. TM also strongly suppresses increases in inflammatory and immune-related cytokines, reducing oxidative stress significantly.[71]

Physical activities

Exercise

The cumulative evidence supports the idea that exercise training is associated with an improvement in mobility amongst individuals with MS.[72, 73, 74] Current studies indicate that physical activity in MS patients counteracts depression and fatigue and may improve quality of life.[75, 76, 77] Aerobic treadmill activity is feasible, safe and may improve anomalies of posture and gait in early MS patients.[78] Physical activity can certainly adapt and manipulate neuronal connections and synaptic activity with natural killer (NK) cells having been shown to be the most responsive immune cell to acute exercise.[79, 80]

Physicians should be encouraged to promote individualised strategies which enhance 'perceived control over fatigue' and 'listening to your body' in order to maximise the benefits of exercise intervention for individuals with MS-related fatigue.[81] As such, it is difficult to prescribe a generalised regular exercise prescription for all those suffering with MS.[82]

Heat reactions are common in MS, such that exposure to heat may consequently result in the appearance of neurological signs. Exercise is one means that is known to increase basal body temperature. It is as yet not understood if or why thermal heat induces central fatigue in patients with MS, however, this is subjectively reported as a common phenomenon.[83]

One recent study involving MS patients who performed acute cycling has demonstrated that moderate intensity exercise was associated with reductions in anxiety and general mood disturbances. Such changes are noted to be greater in those with higher baseline anxiety.[84]

Exercise therapy was also noted to be beneficial for patients with MS not experiencing a relapse in a 2005 Cochrane review.[85]

RCTs investigating the effects of functional electrical stimulation suggest that this may also provide an orthotic benefit to those suffering with MS.[86, 87]

Further studies are still required as to the effects of whole body vibration therapy on muscle performance in people with MS.[88]

Yoga

Recent yoga studies have provided evidence that it may have some benefit for MS sufferers.[7, 89]

Nutritional influences

Diet

Diets and dietary supplements are widely used by people with MS in order to improve disease outcomes. Clinical data has suggested that certain dietary regimes may be beneficial in MS. However, a recent Cochrane review states that more research is needed to assess the efficacy of dietary interventions in MS.[90]

Caloric restriction

It is thought that caloric restriction with adequate nutrition under diligent medical supervision should be explored as a potential treatment for MS as it induces anti-inflammatory, antioxidant and neuroprotective effects that may be beneficial.[91, 92]

Fish intake

The risk of developing MS has been associated with an increased dietary intake of saturated fatty acids.[93] A recent study has indicated that a diet rich in salmon (3–4 times weekly) may provide a protective role in demyelination.[40] This is believed to be secondary to the omega-3 polyunsaturated fatty acids (PUFA) content as no protective effect was observed with a cod-liver oil-based diet.[94, 95] It is important to note, however, that cod-liver oil supplementation may provide some protection.[40] Norway appears to be a discrete exception to the prevalence of MS in higher latitudes. UV exposure is low in this country, however, vitamin D sufficiency is maintained through a traditional diet providing vitamin D as well as marine omega-3 PUFAs.[96] Indeed, recent results suggest that a low fat diet supplemented with omega-3 PUFAs may become the standard recommended therapy for those with MS.[97]

Artificial sweeteners

There is currently controversy regarding the potential toxicity of low-calorie artificial sweeteners such as aspartame, acesulfame-K (ASK) and saccharin and their possible relationship to MS. Animal studies have shown that the genotoxic potential of ASK and saccharin is greater than aspartame (ASP). However, none could act as a potential mutagen alone. These findings are important as they represent a potential health risk associated with exposure to these agents.[98, 99]

Gluten

MS and coeliac disease are both considered to be T-cell mediated auto-immune diseases. It has been postulated that the interaction of MS and coeliac disease inflammatory processes may result in an amplification of Th1 response.[100] There is some evidence that individuals with MS have highly significant increases of IgA and IgG antibodies against gliadin and gluten and significant increases against casein (cow's milk) compared with controls. It should be noted that anti-endomycium and anti-transglutaminase antibodies were negative.[101, 102] Recent studies, however, have conflicting data, showing that gluten sensitivity is not associated with MS.[103, 104]

Nutritional supplementation

Vitamin D

Supplementation with vitamin D is considered to be necessary in northern and southern latitudes to maintain adequate levels of 25(OH)D3 for optimal health and disease prevention.[105] This is certainly understandable, however, it is imperative to note that vitamin D insufficiency is also very common across a wide latitude range in Australia.

In 2007, the prevalence of vitamin D insufficiency in women in winter/spring was 40.5% in south-east Queensland, 37.4% in Geelong and 67.3% in Tasmania. In some months, a high insufficiency or even a deficiency in 25(OH)D3 was noted which correlated with recommendations in sun exposure protection on the basis of the simulated UV index, highlighting the importance of behavioural factors such as sunscreen use. Therefore:

> current Australian sun exposure guidelines do not seem to fully prevent vitamin D insufficiency, and consideration should be given to their modification or to pursuing other means to achieve vitamin D adequacy.[106]

There has been a multitude of recent studies linking low levels of vitamin D with an increased risk of MS. Initial research centred around the striking prevalence of MS in populations residing at higher latitudes. The protective effect of sunlight is reduced at these latitudes, subsequently leading to insufficiencies in vitamin D. Vitamin D is a hormone now known to be involved in far more than the protection of bones. It can regulate processes of cell proliferation, differentiation and apoptosis important in cancer prevention and can profoundly affect both the innate and adaptive immune systems providing protection against certain immune-mediated disorders.[107, 108, 109]

Recent genetic studies have also revealed important vitamin D receptor gene polymorphisms, highlighting once again the complex interaction between genetics and environment.[96, 110, 111] There is strong evidence that vitamin D is an important modifiable environmental/nutritional factor in the pathogenesis of MS with a potential role in its prevention and/or treatment.[37, 107, 112]

Epidemiological evidence supports the view that vitamin D metabolites have significant immune and disease-modulating effects in MS. Vitamin D mediates a shift to a more anti-inflammatory immune response and enhances regulatory T-cell functionality.[113] As such, vitamin D plays an important role in T-cell homeostasis during the course of MS and correcting low levels may be useful during treatment of this disease.[114]

A recent hypothesis suggests that lack of sunlight exposure and viral infections such as herpes and EBV may synergistically induce a defect in IL-10-producing regulatory lymphocytes that may undermine self-tolerance mechanisms and hence enable a pathogenic autoimmune response to neural proteins.[115]

Low serum vitamin D3 levels correlate strongly with MS risk and have been well documented in many studies.[115,116] Lower levels are seen in RRMS compared with progressive MS patients and controls, particularly during relapses.[114] Lower circulating levels of 25(OH) D have since been found to be particularly associated with higher MS-related disability in women.[117]

Supplementation with the active form of vitamin D to animal models of MS both suppresses disease development and leads to improvement of immune-mediated symptoms.[108] Complete disease prevention only occurred with extremely high doses of vitamin D3, such that calcium levels were also significantly elevated. A combination of calcitonin and a smaller dose of vitamin D3, however, synergistically suppressed MS development in animals without causing hypercalcaemia. This finding may become extremely important in the treatment of patients with MS.[118]

A recent meta-analysis has demonstrated that vitamin D supplementation significantly reduces all-cause mortality, highlighting the medical, ethical and legal implications of promptly diagnosing and treating vitamin D deficiency. Treatment in otherwise healthy patients with vitamin D supplementation should be sufficient to maintain year-round 25(OH)D3 levels at least between 40–70ng/mL. Those vitamin D deficient patients with chronic diseases such as MS often need to be investigated and treated more aggressively so that levels are at least between 55–70ng/mL.[116, 119] It is important to note, however, that with increasing knowledge of the importance of vitamin D to health, these reference ranges are likely to be increased in the future.

Long-term supplementation with vitamin D and cod-liver oil has been associated with a decreased incidence of developing MS. Osteoporosis is more common in patients with MS, such that prophylaxis with vitamin D and calcium is widely accepted by most.[120, 121, 40] Parathyroid hormone (PTH) levels have been noted to be higher during a relapse of MS and lower during remission and in winter. MS patients also have a relative hypocalcaemia in winter, thus the endocrine circuitry regulating serum calcium is altered in MS.[122]

Antioxidants

Reactive oxygen species (ROS) play a major role in various events in the pathogenesis of MS. When ROS are formed in MS and animal models of MS, products such as peroxynitrite and superoxide are generated which are highly toxic to cells.[123] ROS initially mediate the transendothelial migration of monocytes and induce dysfunction in the blood–brain barrier. They may also contribute to the formation and persistence of MS lesions by acting on distinct pathological processes. Extensive oxidative damage to proteins, lipids and nucleotides is well documented in active demyelinating lesions. Oxidative stress can be counteracted by endogenous antioxidant enzymes that confer protection against such damage.[124] Antioxidant therapy may therefore represent an attractive treatment option for those with MS with their potential to diminish symptoms by targeting specific patho-mechanisms and support recovery.[93, 125, 126]

Animal studies have demonstrated beneficial effects of antioxidants such as vitamin C and E in MS, although there is limited research as yet of the effects in humans.[125, 127] Clinical trials of more potent antioxidants, including lipoic acid (LA), are currently being trialled with promising results in humans.[123] LA works by reducing and recycling cellular antioxidants, such as glutathione and chelating zinc, copper and other transition metal ions as well as heavy metals. It also acts as a scavenger of ROS and nitrogen species.[128]

Polyunsaturated fatty acids (PUFAs)

Deregulated lipid metabolism is of particular importance in CNS disorders as the brain has the highest lipid concentration after adipose tissue.[2] Omega-3 PUFAs are known to play a significant role in nervous system activity, cognitive development, memory-related learning, neuroplasticity of nerve membranes, synaptogenesis and synaptic transformation.[129] Deficiencies in omega-3 and omega-6 PUFAs and excess levels of monounsaturated and saturated fatty acids have been observed in patients with MS whilst omega-3 and 6 supplementation, in animal models, has been shown to decrease clinical signs of disease.[93, 130]

As such, considerable interest has been shown in the potential anti-inflammatory effects of PUFAs in MS and other auto-immune and neurodegenerative disorders. There is good evidence that both omega-3 and omega-6 supplementation can reduce immune-cell activation by various pathways.[131] In particular, PUFA supplementation has been shown to dose-dependently inhibit the lipopolysaccharide-induced production of the myelinotoxic factor, MMP-9, from microglial cells. Such results suggest that supplementation with omega-3 may become recommended for the wellbeing of all MS patients under therapy.[97, 120, 132]

A recent small study of RRMS patients receiving 9.6g/day fish oil has confirmed that immune cell secretion of MMP-9 was decreased by 58% after 3 months supplementation when compared with baseline levels. This effect was coupled with a significant increase in omega-3 fatty acid levels in red blood cell (RBC) membranes. Omega-3 PUFAs may therefore act as immune modulators with potentially beneficial results in individuals with MS.[133]

Epidemiological, biochemical, animal model and clinical trial data strongly suggest that omega-6 PUFAs also play a significant role in the pathogenesis and treatment of MS. In another double-blind, placebo-controlled RCT, patients with MS were given either high-dose GLA (omega-6), low-dose GLA or placebo. High dose GLA was shown to have a marked clinical effect in RRMS, significantly decreasing the relapse rate and disease progression. Such improvements in disability suggest a beneficial effect on neuronal lipids and neural function in MS.[134]

It should be noted, however, that clinical trials in MS patients provide mixed results. There is a need for larger good quality trials, preferably with MRI investigations.[131]

B vitamins and iron

Myelin is continually regenerated in the human body. For this process to occur, adequate iron and a functional folate/vitamin B12 methylation pathway is required.[135] Homocysteine levels are often increased in those with MS and are associated with cognitive impairment, depression and abnormal electrophysiological parameters in this disease.[136–139]

In Caucasian females with RRMS, serum iron and ferritin concentrations have been found to be significantly lower than in matched controls. A small 6-month study of RRMS patients taking nutritional supplements specifically designed to promote demyelination, has shown a significant neurological improvement when compared to a control group taking multivitamins. Both groups had significantly reduced homocysteine levels at 6 months, suggesting that methylation is necessary but not sufficient for myelin regeneration.[135]

Herbal medicines

Cannabis

Endocannabinoids (eCBs) play a role in the modulation of neuro-inflammation, and experimental findings suggest that they may be directly involved in the pathogenesis of MS. Significantly reduced levels of eCBs have been found in the CSF of MS patients compared to controls. These findings support the development of drugs targeting eCBs to reduce symptoms and slow disease progression in MS.[140, 141]

A recent internet-based survey for Australian residents with MS has shown that cannabis was beneficial in reducing symptoms of MS.[8] Indeed, world-wide, many patients use cannabis to alleviate spasticity and pain. Small scale studies do indicate positive effects, however, larger RCTs are thus far negative for improvements in spasticity. It should be noted that most patients report a subjective benefit even if their objective parameters are unchanged.[120] Recently cannabis has been analysed in more controlled studies which have provided evidence that it may have some benefit.[4, 7]

It should be noted, however, that inhaled cannabis is associated with impaired mentation in MS patients, particularly in respect to cognition.[142]

Physical therapies

Acupuncture

There is preliminary evidence to suggest that acupuncture is safe and effective for improving quality of life for people with secondary progressive MS.[4, 143] However, more rigorous trials are warranted.[144]

Other supplements

Hormones

Mean DHEA levels have been found to be lower in MS patients than controls, with no significant difference between the different subgroups.[145] Those MS patients with fatigue displayed even lower levels of DHEA therefore hormone replacement is a possible option for treating fatigue-related MS.[146]

Testosterone treatment has been shown to ameliorate symptoms in animal models of MS. A small pilot study involved administering 100mg testosterone gel daily to a group of men with RRMS for 1 year. An improvement in cognitive performance and a slowing of brain atrophy was demonstrated, however, there was no significant effect on MS brain lesions. Thus, it was concluded that testosterone treatment is safe, well tolerated and has potential neuroprotective effects in men with RRMS.[147]

Bee venom therapy (BVT)

There is currently only limited supportive evidence for the use of BVT in MS. The active component has not yet been identified and there is a significant risk of anaphylaxis which has deterred its widespread use.[121]

Conclusion

MS features autoimmune inflammatory attack against the myelin insulation of neurons. Hence individuals with MS experience a variety of symptoms that may include disrupted motor, sensory and cognitive functioning. Specifically these symptoms may include speech and swallowing problems, tremors, spasticity, visual and cognitive problems, fatigue, pain or bowel and bladder problems.

Most people with MS have a normal or near-normal life expectancy, however, quality of life is often affected by the disease and its function-related changes that occur. The socio-demographic issues associated with the use of CAM modalities by patients with chronic diseases has been extensively reported over the last 2 decades.

Recently additional patterns have emerged as to why chronically ill people include CAM therapies and this is to complement conventional medicine.[148] Individuals do not tend to give up their conventional health care providers in lieu of CAM treatment. The trend is to use CAM as an adjunct to the treatment being received from a conventional clinician. Another pattern that emerged was the use of CAM to treat or manage MS symptoms. Although a small percentage of patients do seek CAM for disease-modifying purposes, research reports that significantly more patients use CAM to treat or manage the daily symptoms.[149]

The most frequently used CAM therapies include massage, acupuncture, chiropractic, vitamins/herbal medicines and nutrition, and hence this trend lends itself significantly to an integrative management approach. Lack of sunshine exposure and vitamin B deficiency are significant risk factors for MS. Table 26.1 summarises the current evidence for CAM treatments.

Table 26.1 Levels of evidence for lifestyle and complementary medicines/therapies in the management of multiple sclerosis

Modality	Level I	Level II	Level IIIa	Level IIIb	Level IIIc	Level IV	Level V
Lifestyle factors: non-modifiable							
Genetics				x			
Lifestyle factors: modifiable							
Sleep					x		
Mind–body medicine							
Cognitive behavioural therapy	x						
Sunshine/vitamin D link					x		
Environmental							
Epstein Barr virus				x			
Chlamydia pneumoniae				x			
Smoking				x			
Environmental metals							
• Aluminium					x		
• Methyl mercury					x		
• Lead					x		
Physical activity			x				
Yoga				x			
Nutrition							
Diets	x						
Calorie restriction	x						
Nutritional supplements							
vitamin D				x			
Antioxidants					x		
Omega-3 fatty acids			x				
Omega-6 fatty acids			x				
B group vitamins					x		
Other supplements							
Hormones							
• DHEA					x		
• Testosterone					x		
Herbal medicines							
Cannabis			x				
Physical therapies		x					
Acupuncture					x		
Bee venom						x	

Level I – from a systematic review of all relevant randomised controlled trials–meta-analyses.
Level II – from at least 1 properly designed randomised controlled clinical trial.
Level IIIa – from well-designed pseudo-randomised controlled trials (alternate allocation or some other method).
Level IIIb – from comparative studies (including systematic reviews of such studies) with concurrent controls and allocation not randomised, cohort studies, case-control studies, or interrupted time series with a parallel control group.
Level IIIc – from comparative studies with historical control, 2 or more single-arm studies or interrupted time series without a parallel control group.
Level IV – opinions of respected authorities based on clinical experience, descriptive studies or reports of expert committees.
Level V – represents minimal evidence that represents testimonials.

Clinical tips handout for patients — multiple sclerosis

1 Lifestyle advice

Sleep

- Eliminating underlying sleep disorders contributing to fatigue is an important part of an MS assessment.
- Restless legs syndrome is significantly associated with MS and can be effectively and easily treated with magnesium in most cases.
- Magnesium (up to 350mg elemental twice daily) can be used to assist sleep and reduce restless legs at night (3 month trial).
- L-Tryptophan (200mg bd) may be trialled for 1 month in the morning and 1 hour before bedtime.
- Melatonin (3–6mg) at bedtime may be trialled for 1 month (not with L-tryptophan).
- Herbal supplements including passionflower and valerian may be helpful in some cases.
- Herbal teas such as chamomile can be helpful in some cases.

Sunshine

- Reduced sunlight exposure is strongly associated with MS throughout the world.
- Increase outdoor activities whenever possible.
- At least 15 minutes sunshine is needed daily for vitamin D production. More sun exposure may be required in areas with higher and lower latitudes.
- Sunscreen can block the conversion to vitamin D so this should be avoided during this specified time period.
- Dark skinned people need more sun exposure.

2 Physical activity/exercise

- Regular moderate-intensity exercise can improve mobility and reduce depression, anxiety and fatigue in patients with MS.
- Aerobic treadmill activity may improve early anomalies of posture and gait.
- Yoga practice may also improve symptoms of MS.
- An individualised exercise prescription is necessary with patients needing to be aware of their own body symptoms/signs.

3 Mind-body medicine

- Stress can exacerbate symptoms of MS, therefore any healthy activities which reduce stress should be encouraged.
- Counselling can be particularly helpful in this population, having been shown to significantly improve physical activity, spiritual growth, stress management, fatigue and general mental status.
- Cognitive behaviour therapy approaches are beneficial in the treatment of depression and in helping people to adjust to, and cope with, having MS.

4 Environment

- Previous exposure to Epstein-Barr virus, particularly if it was symptomatic, is strongly associated with MS. Risk-taking behaviours with individuals infected with EBV should therefore be discouraged, whether someone has MS or not.
- Smoking is also strongly associated with MS, particularly when started at an early age. Passive smoking is also a risk factor. It is important to advise all patients to seek help to stop smoking.
- Excessive iron, aluminium, mercury and copper have all been implicated in the pathogenesis of MS. All patients with MS should therefore be tested for the presence of heavy metals, whether by plasma (copper, zinc), serum (iron studies, ceruloplasmin), hair mineral analysis or comprehensive urinary elements profiling. Where metals are detected, referral to a chelation specialist is recommended as treatment may be complex and vary according to which metals are detected.
- Generalised chelation techniques may include supplementation with chlorella, silicon (for aluminium), zinc and metallothionine promoting nutrients.

5 Dietary modification

- Supervised caloric restriction may be explored as a potential treatment for MS as it induces anti-inflammatory, antioxidant and neuroprotective effects.
- Reduce dietary intake of saturated fatty acids.
- A diet rich in salmon (3–4 times weekly) and other sources of omega-3 polyunsaturated fatty acids may provide a protective role in demyelination.
- Avoid artificial sweeteners such as aspartame, acesulfame-K and saccharin wherever possible.

- Increase dietary intake of antioxidant containing foods such as blueberries.
- There is currently conflicting data regarding the prevalence of IgA and IgG antibodies against gliadin, gluten and casein (cow's milk). Suspect patients should ideally be tested for coeliac disease and a 1-month trial without wheat and dairy may be undertaken to see if there are any improvements in mobility, depression or fatigue.

6 Physical therapies

- Acupuncture is safe and well tolerated and a trial of acupuncture may be warranted for people with secondary progressive MS.

7 Supplementation

Vitamin D3 (cholecalciferol)

- Indication: most important nutrient for MS; to improve immunity and reduce disease development and/or risk of relapses, to improve bone health.
- Dosage: requires medical supervision; 5000–10 000IU vitamin D3 daily may be needed to keep serum 25(OH)D3 levels at approximately 100ng/mL. Serum levels of 25(OH)D3, corrected calcium and parathyroid hormone need to be checked regularly and the dosage of vitamin D3 changed as required.
- Results: long-term supplementation with vitamin D3 may be required to treat and reduce incidence of developing MS.
- Side-effects: mild and rare when used appropriately.
- Contraindications: hypersensitivity to vitamin D, SLE, hypercalcaemia. Caution in sarcoidosis and hyperparathyroidism. Possible interaction with calcium channel blockers and digitalis.

Cod-liver oil

- Indication: to improve immunity and reduce disease development and or risk of relapses.
- Dosage: 5ml bd.
- Results: long-term supplementation with cod-liver oil may be required to reduce the incidence of developing MS.
- Side-effects: use high-quality pharmaceutical grade cod-liver oil to avoid possible rancidity, fishy burps, nausea and/or diarrhoea.
- Contraindications: use with caution if taking anti-coagulant medication.

Calcium/magnesium

- Indication: calcium: to improve bone health (osteoporosis is more common in people with MS); magnesium: to improve restless legs syndrome.
- Dosage: calcium citrate is the most absorbable form of calcium. 1500mg/day in combination with accessory nutrients, including magnesium.
  - Calcium/magnesium 350mg each, 1–2 tablets, 1–2 times/day.
- Results: long-term supplementation with calcium and magnesium with vitamin D are required for bone health.
- Side-effects: GI disturbances — flatulence, constipation, irritation, diarrhoea.
- Contraindications: hypercalcaemia. Caution with hyperparathyroidism and chronic renal disease.

Antioxidants

- Indication: to reduce oxidative stress, thereby modifying disease progression and reducing symptoms.
- Dosage:
  - vitamin C: 3–6g/day calcium ascorbate; reduce dose if diarrhoea occurs
  - vitamin E: 200–500IU/day (mixed tocopherols)
  - lipoic acid: 100–600mg/day.
- Results: ongoing supplementation may be required.
- Side-effects: a balanced mix of antioxidants are recommended. Side-effects are mild and rare.
- Contraindications: caution with warfarin and vitamin E at higher doses than 500IU.

Polyunsaturated fatty acids

- Indication: to improve immunity and decrease symptoms of MS. Reduces relapses of MS.
- Dosage: 6–10g EPA/DHA daily.
- Results: 3–6 month trial.
- Side-effects: fishy burps, diarrhoea, gastrointestinal discomfort.
- Contraindications: fish allergy. Caution with anticoagulants at very high doses.

References

1 Jelinek GA, Hassed CS. Managing MS in primary care: are we forgetting something? Qual Prim care 2009;17(1):55–61.

2 Adibhatia RM, Hatcher JF. Altered lipid metabolism in brain injury and disorders. Subcell Biocem 2008;49:241–68.

3 Fryze W, Mirowski-Guzel D, Wiszniewska M, et. al. Alternative methods of treatment used by MS patients in Poland. Neurol Neurochir Pol 2009;40(5):386–90.
4 Olsen SA. A review of CAM by people with MS. Occup Ther Int 2009;16(1):57–70.
5 Schwartz S, Knorr C, Geiger H, et. al. CAM for MS. Mult Scler 2008;14(8):1113–9.
6 Nayak S, Matheis RJ, Schoenberger NE, et. al. Use of unconventional therapies by individuals with MS. Clin Rehabil 2003;17(2):181–91.
7 Yadav V, Bourdette D. CAM Medicine: is there a role in MS? Curr Neurol Neurosci Rep 2006;6(3):259–67.
8 Simmons RD, Ponsonby AL, van der Mei IA, et. al. What effects you MS? Responses to an anonymous Internet-based epidemiological survey. Mult Scler 2004;10(2):202–11.
9 Willer CJ, Ebers GC. Susceptibility to multiple sclerosis: interplay between genes and environment. Curr Opin Neurol 2000;13:241–7.
10 Ascherio A, Munger K. Epidemiology of MS: from risk factors to prevention. Semin Neurol 2008;28(1):17–28.
11 Fujihara K. Update on the aetiology and pathogenesis of MS and neuromyelitis optica. Nippon Rinsho 2008;66(6):1087–91.
12 Holmey T, Hestvik AL. MS: Immunopathogenesis and controversies in defining the cause. Curr Opin Infect Dis 2008;21(3):271–8.
13 Pugliatti M, Harbo HF, Holmey T, et. al. Environmental risk factors in MS. Acta Neurol Scand Suppl 2008;188:34–40.
14 Giovannoni G, Ebers G. MS: the environment and causation. Curr Opin Neurol 2007;20(3):261–8.
15 Alonso A, Hernan MA. Temporal trends in the incidence of MS: a systematic review. Neurology 2008;71(2):129–35.
16 Anderson DW, Ellenberg JH, Leventhal CM, et. al. Revised estimate of the prevalence of multiple sclerosis in the United States. Am Neurol 1992;31:333–6.
17 Hirtz D, Thurman DJ, Gwinn-Hardy K, et. al. How common are the 'common' neurologic disorders? Neurology 2007;68:326–37.
18 Marrie R, Horwitz R, Cutter G, et. al. High frequency of adverse health behaviours in MS. Mult Scler 2009;15(1):105–13.
19 Esch T, Stafano GB, Fricchione GL, et. al. The role of stress in neurodegenerative diseases and mental disorders. Neuro Endocrinol Lett 2002;23(3):199–208.
20 Swaab DF, Bao AM, Lucassen PJ. The stress system in the human brain in depression and neurodegenration. Ageing Res Rev 2005;4(2):141–94.
21 Ysrraelit MC, Gaitan MI, Lopez AS, et. al. Impaired HPA-axis activity in patients with MS. Neurology 2008;71(24):1948–54.
22 Torem MS. MB Hypnotic imagery in the treatment of AI disorders. Am J clin Hypnosis 2007;50(2):157–70.
23 Bombardier CH, Cunniffe M, Wadwani R, et. al. The efficacy of telephone counseling for health promotion in people with MS; a RCT. Arch Phys Med Rehabil 2008;89(10):1849–56.
24 Bol Y, Duits AA, Hupperts RM, et. al. The psychology of fatigue in patients with MS: a review. J Psychosom Res 2009;66(1):3–11.
25 Tartaglia MC, Narayanan S, Arnold DL. Mental fatigue alters the pattern and increases the volume of cerebral activation required for a motor task in MS patients with fatigue. Eur J Neurol 2008;15(4):413–9.
26 White A, Lee J, Light A, et. al. Brain activation in MS: a BOLD fMRI study of the effects of fatiguing hand exercise. Mult Scler 2009 Mar 19.
27 O'Brien AR, Chiaravalotti N, Goverover Y, et. al. Evidenced-based cognitive rehabilitation for persons with MS: a review of the literature. Arch Phys Med Rehabil 2008;89(4):761–9.
28 Thomas PW, Thomas S, Hillier C, et. al. Psychological interventions for MS. Cochrane Database Syst rev 2006;(1):CD004431.
29 Brown RF, Valpiani EM, Tennant CC, et. al. Longitudinal assessment study of anxiety, depression and fatigue with MS. Psycholog Psychother 2009;82(Pt 1):41–56.
30 Dworzanska E, Mitosek-Szewczyk K, Stelmasiak Z. Fatigue in MS. Neurol Neurochir Pol 2009;43(1):71–6.
31 Attarian H. Importance os sleep in the QOL of MS patients:a long under-recognised issue. Sleep Med 2009;10(1):7–8.
32 Merlino G, Frattici L, Lenchig C, et. al. Prevalence of poor sleep amomg patients with MS: an independent predictor of mental and physical status. Sleep Med 2009;10(1):26–34.
33 Bamer AM, Johnson KL, Amtmann D, et. al. Prevalence of sleep problems in individuals with MS. Mult Scler 2008;14(8):1127–30.
34 Manconi M, Ferini-Strambi L, Filipi M, et. al. Multicentre case-control study on RLS in MS: the REMS study. Sleep 2008;31(7):944–52.
35 Moreira NC, Damasceno RS, Medieras CA, et. al. RLS, sleep quality and fatigue in MS. Braz J Med Biol Res 2008;41(10):932–7.
36 Ascherio A, Munger KL. Environmental risk factors for MS. Part II: Non-infectious factors. Ann Neurol 2007;6196):504–13.
37 Niino M, Fukazawa T, Kikuchi S, et. al. Therapeutic potential of Vit D for MS. Curr Med Chem 2008;15(5):499–505.
38 Tremiett H, vander Mei IA, Pittas F, et. al. Monthly ambient sunlight, infections and relapse rates in MS. Neuroepidemiology 2008;31(4):271–9.
39 Dwyer T, van der Mei I, Ponsonby AL, et. al. MC1R genotype, past environmental sun exposure and risk of MS. Neurology 2008;71(8):583–9.
40 Kampman MT, Wilsgaard T, Mellgren SI. Outdoor activities and diet in childhood and adolescence relate to MS risk above the Arctic circle. J Neurol 2007;254(4):471–7.
41 Ascherio A, Munger KL. Environmental risk factors for MS. part i:the role of infection. Ann Neurol 2007;61(4):288–99.
42 Ebers GC. Environmental factors and MS. Lancet Neurol 2008;7(3):268–77.
43 Goodin DS. The causal cascade to MS: a model for MS pathogenesis. PLoS ONE 2009;4(2):e4565. Epub 2009 Feb 26.
44 Ruprecht K. MS and EBV: new developments and perspectives. Nervenartz 2008;79(4):399–407.
45 Jilek S, Schluep M, Meylan P, et. al. Strong EBV-specific CD8+ T cell response in patients with early MS. Brain 2008;131(Pt 7):1712–21.
46 Posnett DN. Herpes viruses and auti-immunity. Curr Opin Investig drugs 2008;9(5):505–14.
47 Niller HH, Wolf H, Minarovits J. Regulation and dysregulation of EBV latency: implications for the development of Auto-immune Disease. Autoimmunity 2008;41(4):298–328.
48 Marrie RA. When one and one make three: HLA and EBV infection in MS. Neurology 2008;70(13 part 2):1067–8.

49 Haahr S, Hollsberg P. MS is linked to EBV infection. Rev Med Virol 2006;16(5):297–310.
50 De Jager PL, Simon KC, Munger KL. Integrating Risk factors:HLA-DRB1*1501 and EBV in MS. Neurology 2008;70 (13 Pt 2):1113–8.
51 Levin LI, Munger KL, Rubertone MV, et. al. Temporal relationship between elevation of EBV antibody titres and initial onset of neurological symptoms in MS. JAMA 2005;293(20):2496–500.
52 Frykholm B. On the question of infectious aetiologies for MS, schizophrenia and CFS and their treatment with antibiotics. Med Hypotheses 2009;72(6):736–9.
53 Marrie RA, Cutter G, Tyry T, et. al. Smoking status over 2 years in patients with MS. Neuroepidemiology 2009;32(1):72–9.
54 Di Pauli F, Reindl M, Ehling R, et. al. Smoking is a risk factor for early conversion to clinically definite MS. Mult Scler 2008;14(8):1026–30.
55 Sundstrom P, Nystrom L. Smoking worsens the prognosis in MS. Mult Scler 2008;14(8):1031–5.
56 Sundstrom P, Nystrom L, Hallmans G. Smoke exposure increases the risk for MS. Eur J Neurol 2008;15(6):579–83.
57 Tardieu M, Mikaeloff Y. MS in children: Environmental risk factors. Bull acad Natl Med 2008;192(3):507–9.
58 Pittas F, Ponsonby AL, van der Mei IA, et. al. Smoking is associated with progressive disease course and increased progression in clinical disability in a prospective cohort of people with MS. J Neurol 2009 Apr 9. Epub ahead of print.
59 Montgomery SM, Bahmanyar S, Hillert J, et. al. Maternal smoking during pregnancy and MS amongst offspring. Eur J Neurol 2008;15(12):1395–9.
60 Williamson DM. Studies of MS in communities concerned about environmental exposures. J Womens Health 2006;15(7):810–4.
61 Henry JP, Willialson DM, Schiffer DM, et. al. Investigation of a cluster of MS in 2 elementary school cohorts. J Environ Health 2007;69(10):34–8.
62 Neuberger JS, Lynch SG, Sutton ML, et. al. Prevalence of MS in a residential area bordering an oil refinery. Neurology 2004;63(10):1796–802.
63 Turabelidze G, Schootman M, Zhu BP, et. al. MS Prevalence and possible lead exposure. J Neurol Sci 2008;269(1-2):158–62.
64 Polosukhini DI, Kanyshkova TG, Doronin BM, et. al. Metal-dependent hydrolysis of MBP by IgGs from the sera of patients with MS. Immunol lett 2006;103(1):75–81.
65 Abo-Krysha N, Rashed L. The role of iron dysregulation in the pathogenesis of MS: an Egyptian study. Mult Scler 2008;14(5):602–8.
66 Haacke EM, Makki M, Ge Y. Characterising iron deposition in MS lesions using susceptibility weighted imaging. J Magn Reson Imaging 2009;29(3):537–44.
67 Hammond KE, Metcalf M, Carvajal L, et. al. Quantitative in vivo MRI of MS at 7 Tesla with sensitivity to iron. Ann Neurol 2008;64(6):707–13.
68 Exley C, Mamutse G, Korchazhkina O, et. al. Elevated urinary excretion of Al and Fe in MS. Mult Scler 2006;12(5):533–40.
69 MutterJJ, Naumann J, Guethlin C. Comments on the article 'the toxicology of mercury and its chemical compounds' by Clarkson and Magos (2006). Crit Rev Toxicol 2007;37(6):537–49.
70 Aminzadeh KK, Etminan M. Dental amalgum and MS: a SR and meta-analysis. J Public Health Dent 2007;67(1):64–6.
71 Hou G, Abrams GD, Dick R, et. al. Efficacy of TM in a mouse model of MS. Trans Res 2008;152(5):239–44.
72 Snook EM, Motl RW. Effect of exercise training on walking mobility in MS;23(2):108-16. Neurorehabil Neural Repair 2009;23(2):108–16.
73 Dettmers C, Sulzmann M, Ruchav-Plossl A, et. al. Endurance exercise improves walking distance in MS patients with fatigue. Acta Neurol Scand 2009 Jan 19. Epub ahead of print.
74 Motl RW, Snook EM, Wynn DR, et. al. Physical activity correlates with neurological impairment and disability in MS. J Nerv Ment Dis 2008;196(6): 492–5.
75 Waschbisch A, Tallner A, Pfeifer K, et. al. MS and exercise: Effects of physical activity on the immune system. Nervenartz 2009 Jan 23. Epub ahead of print.
76 Fragaso YD, Santana DL, Pinto RC. The positive effects of a physical activity program for MS patients with fatigue. NeuroRehabilitation 2008;23(2):153–7.
77 Motl RW, McAuley E, Snook EM, et. al. Physical activity and QOL in MS: Intermediary roles of disability, fatigue, mood, pain, self-efficacy and social support. Psychol Health Med 2009;14(1): 111–24.
78 Benedetti MG, Gasparroni V, Stecchi S, et. al. Treadmill exercise in early MS: a case series study. Eur J Phys Rehab Med 2009 Jan 21. Epub ahead of print.
79 Achiron A, Kalron A. Physical activity: positive impact on brain plasticity. Harefuah 2008;147(3);252–5.
80 Timmons BW, Cieslak T. Human NK cell subsets and acute exercise: a brief review. Exerc Immunol Rev 2008;14:8–23.
81 Smith C, Hale L, Dison K, et. al. How does exercise influence fatigue in people with MS? Disabil rehabil 2008:1–8.
82 Sano M, Dawes DJ, Arafah A, et. al. What does a structured review of the effectiveness of exercise interventions for persons with MS tell us about the challenges of designing trials? Mult Scler 2009;15(4):412–21.
83 Marino FE. Heat reactions in MS: an overlooked paradigm in the study of comparative fatigue. Int J Hyperthermia 2009;25(1):34–40.
84 Petruzzello SJ, Snook EM, Gliotoni RC, et. al. Anxiety and mood changes associated with acute cycling in persons with MS. Anxiety Stress Coping 2009;22(3):297–307.
85 Rietbrg MB, Brooks D, Uitdehaag BM, et. al. Exercise therapy for MS. Cochrane Database syst Rev 2005;(1):CD003980.
86 Paul L, rafferty D, Young S, et. al. The effect of FES on the physiological cost of gait in people with MS. Mult Scler 2008;14(7):954–61.
87 Barrett C, Mann G, Taylor P, et. al. A RCT to investigate the effects of FES and therapeutic exercise on walking performance for people with MS. Mult Scler 2009;15(4):493–504.
88 Jackson KJ, Merriman HL, Vanderburgh PM, et. al. Acute effects of whole-body vibration on lower extremity muscle performance in persons with MS. J Neurol Phys Ther 2008;32(4):171–6.
89 Esmonde L, Long AF. Comp therapy use by persons with MS: benefits and research priorities. Complement Ther Clin Pract 2008;14(3):176–84.
90 Farinotti M, Simi S, Di Pietrantonj C, et. al. Dietary interventions for MS. Cochrane Database Syst Rev 2007;(1):CD004192.

91 Piccio L, Stark JL, Cross AH. Chronic caloric restriction attenuates experimental AI encephalomyelitis. J Leukoc Biol 2008;84(4):940–8.
92 Fernandes G. Progress in nutritional immunology. Immunol Res 2008;40(3):244–61.
93 van meeteren ME, Teunissen CE, Dijkstra CD, et. al. Antiox and PUFAs in MS. Eur J Clin Nutr 2005;59(12):1347–61.
94 Torkildsen O, Brunberg LA, Thorson F, et. al. Effects of dietary interevntion on MRI activity, de and remyelination in the cuprizone model for demyelination. Exp Neurol 2009;215(1):160–6.
95 Torkildsen O, Brunborg LA, Milde AM, et. al. A salmon-based diet protects mice from behavioural changes in the cuprizone model for demyelination. Clin Nutr 2009;28(1):83–7.
96 Kampman MT, Brustad M. Vit D: a candidate for the environmental effect in MS; observations from Norway. Neuroepidemiology 2008;30 (3):140–6.
97 Liuzzi GM, Latronico T, Rossano R, et. al. Inhibitory effect of PUFAs on MMP-9 from microglial cells: implications for complementary MS treatment. Neurochem Res 2007;32(12):2184–93.
98 Whitehouse CR, Boullata J, McCauley LA. The potential toxicity of artificial sweeteners. AAOHN J;56(6):251–9.
99 Bandyopadhyay A, Ghoshal S, Mukherjee A. Genotoxicity testing of low-calorie sweeteners: aspartame, ASK and saccharin. Drug Chem Toxicol 2008;31(4):447–57.
100 Frisullo G, Nociti V, Iorio R, et. al. Increased expression of T-bet in circulating B cells from a patient with MS and CD. Hum Immunol 2008;69(12):837–9.
101 Reichelt KL, Jensen D. IgA antibodies against gliadin and gluten in MS. Acta Neurol Scand 2004;110(4):239–41.
102 Pengiran Tengah CD, Lock RJ, Unsworth DJ, et. al. MS and occult gluten sensitivity. Neurology 2004;62(12):2326–7.
103 Borhani Haghighi A, Ansari N, Mokhtari M, et. al. MS and gluten sensitivity. Clin Neurol Neurosurg 2007;109(8):651–3.
104 Nicoletti A, Patti F, Lo Fermo S, et. al. Frequency of coeliac disease is not increased among MS patients. Mult Scler 2008;14(5):698–700.
105 Huotari A, Herzig KH. vitamin D and living in the Northern latitudes - an endemic risk area for Vit D deficiency. Int J Circumpolar Health 2008;67 (2-3):164–78.
106 van der Mei IA, Ponsonby AL, Engelson O, et. al. The high prevalence of Vit D insufficiency across australian populations is only partly explained by season and latitude. Environ Health Perspect 2007;115(8):1132–9.
107 Raghuwanshi A, Joshi SS, Christakos S. Vit D and MS. J Cell Biocem 2008;105(2):338–43.
108 Szodoray P, Nakken B, Gaal J, et. al. The complex role of Vit D in AI diseases. Scand J Immunol 2008;68(3):261–9.
109 Holick MF. Vit D and sunlight: strategies for cancer prevention and other health benefits. Clin J Am Soc Nephrol 2008;3(5):1548–54.
110 Ramagopalan SV, Maugeri NJ, Handunnetthi L, et. al. Expression of the MS associated MHC class II Allele HLA-DRB1*1501 is regulated by Vit D. PLoS Genet 2009;5(2):e1000369. Epub 2009 Feb 6.
111 Smolders J, Damoiseaux J, Menheere P, et. al. Fok-1 Vit D receptor gene polymorphism (rs10735810) and Vit D metabolism in MS. J Neuroimmunol 2009;207(1-2):117–21.
112 Cantorna MT. Vit D and MS: an update. Nutr Rev 2008;66(10 Suppl 2):S135–8.
113 Smolders J, Damoiseaux J, Menheere P, et. al. Vit D as an immune modulator in MS: a review. Neuroimmunol 2008;194(1-2):7–17.
114 Correale J, Ysrraelit MC, Gaitan MI. Immunomodulatory effects of vitamin D in MS. Brain 2009 Mar 24. Epub ahead of print.
115 Hayes CE, Donald Acheson E. A unifying MS aetiology linking virus infection, sunlight and vitamin D through viral IL-10. Med Hypotheses 2008;71(1):85–90.
116 van der Mei IA, Ponsonby AL, Dwyer T, et. al. Vit D levels in people with MS and community controls in Tasmania, Australia. J Neurol 2007;254(5): 581–90.
117 Kragt J, van Amerongen B, Killestein J, et. al. Higher levels of 25(OH)D are assoc with a lower incidence of MS only in women. Mult Scler 2009;15(1):9–15.
118 Becklund BR, Hansen DW Jr, Deluca HF. Enhancement of 1,25(OH)D3-mediated suppression of EAE by calcitonin. Proc Natl Acad Sci USA 2009;106(13):5276–81.
119 Cannell JJ, Hollis BW. Use of vitamin D in clinical practice. Altern Med Rev 2008;13(1):6–20.
120 Schwartz S, Leweling H, Meinck HM. Alternative and Complementary therapies in MS. Fortschr Neurol Psychiatr 2005;73(8):451–62.
121 Namaka M, Crook A, Doupe A, et. al. Examining the evidence: complementary adjunctive therapies for MS. Neurol Res 2008;30(7):710–9.
122 Soilu-Hanninen M, Laaksonen M, Laitinen I, et. al. A longitudinal study of serum 25(OH)D and intact PTH levels indicate the importance of Vit D and calcium homeostasis regulation in MS. J Neurol Neurosug Psychiatry 2008;79(2):152–7.
123 Carlson NG, Rose JW. Antioxidants in MS: do they have a role in therapy? CNS Drugs 2006;20(6)433–41.
124 van Horssen J, Schreibelt G, Drexhage J, et. al. Severe ox damage in MS lesions coincides with enhanced antiox enzyme expression. Free radic Biol Med 2008;45(12):1729–37.
125 Mirshafiey A, Mohsenzadegan M. Antioxidant therapy in MS. Immunopharmacol Immunotoxicol 2009;31(1):13–29.
126 Schreibeit G, van Horssen J, van Rossum S, et. al. Therapeutic potential and biological role of endogenous antioxidant enzymes in MS pathology. Brain Res Rev 2007;56(2):322–30.
127 Gilgun-Sherki Y, Melamed E, Offen D. The role of ox stress in the pathogenesis of MS: the need for effective antioxidant therapy. J Neurol 2004;251(3):261–8.
128 Salinthone S, Yadav V, Bourdette DN, et. al. Lipoic acid: a novel therapeutic approach for MS and other chronic inflammatory diseases of the CNS. Endocr Metab Immun Disorder Drug Targets 2008;8(2):132–42.
129 Mazza M, Pomponi M, Janiri L, et. al. Omega 3 FAs and antioxidants in neurological and psychiatric diseases: an overview. Prog Neuropsychopharmacol Biol Psychiatry 2007;31(1):12–26.

130 Aupperle RP, Denney DR, Lynch SG, et. al. Omega-3 FAs and MS: relationship to depression. J Behav Med 2008;31(2):127–35.
131 Mehta LR, Dworkin RH, Schwid SR. PUFAs and their potential therapeutic role in MS. Nat Clin Pract Neurol 2009;5(2):82–92.
132 Salvati S, Attorri L, Di Benedetto R, et. al. PUFAs and neurological diseases. Mini Rev Med Chem 2006;6(11):1201–11.
133 Shinto L, Marracci G, Baldauf-Wagner S, et. al. Omega-3 FA supp decreases MMP-9 production in RRMS. Prostaglandins Leukotr Essent Fatty Acids 2009;80(2-3):131–6.
134 Harbige LS, Sharief MK. PUFAs in the pathogenesis and treatment of MS. Br J Nutr 2007;98 Suppl 1:S46–S53.
135 van Rensburg SJ, Kotze MJ, Hon D, et. al. Fe and the folate/vitamin B12 methylation pathway in MS. Metab Brain Dis 2006;21(2-3):121–37.
136 Russo C, Morabito F, Luise F, et. al. Hyperhomocysteinaemia is assoc with cognitive impairment in MS. J Neurol 2008;255(1):64–9.
137 Obeid R, McCaddon A, Herrmann W. The role of hyperhomocysteinemia and B vitamin deficiency in neuro and psychiatric diseases. Clin Chem Lab Med 2007;45(12):1590–606.
138 Kocer B, Engur S, Ak F, et. al. Serum B12, folate and HC levels and their association with clinical and electrophysiological parameters in MS. J Clin Neurosci 2009;16(3):399–403.
139 Triantafyllou N, Evangelopoulos ME, Kimiskidis VK, et. al. Increased plasma HC in patients with MS and depression. Ann Gen Psychiatry 2008;7:17.
140 Di Filippo M, Pini LA, Pelliccioli GP, et. al. Abnormalities in the CSF levels of eCBs in MS. J neurol Neurosurg Psychiatry 2008;79(11):1224–9.
141 Ashton J. Pro-drugs for indirect cannabinoids as therapeutic agents. Curr drug deliv 2008;5(4):243–7.
142 Ghaffar O, Feinstein A. MS and cannibis: a cognitive and psychiatric study. Neurology 2008;71(3):164–9.
143 Donnellan CP, Shanley J. Comparison of the effect of 2 types of acupuncture on QOL in SPMS: a preliminary single-blind RCT. Clin rehab 2008;22(3):195–205.
144 Lee H, Park HJ, Park J, et. al. Acupuncture application for neurological disorders. Neurol Res 2007;29 Suppl 1:S49–S54.
145 Ramsaransing GS, Heersema DJ, De Keyser J. Serum uric acid, DHEA and Apolipoprotein E genetype in benign vs progressive MS. Eur J Neurol 2005;12(7):514–8.
146 Tellez N, Comabella M, Julia E, et. al. Fatigue in progressive MS is associated with low levels of DHEA. Mult Scler 2006;12(4):487–94.
147 Sicotte NL, Giesser BS, Tandon V, et. al. Testosterone treatment in MS: a pilot study. Arch Neurol 2007;64(5):683–8.
148 Statistics, National Center for Health. National Health Interview Survey 2008. Online. Available: http://www.cdc.gov/nchs/about/major/nhis/quest_data_related_1997_forward.htm (accessd May 2009).
149 Pucci E, Cartechini E, Taus C, et. al. Why physicians need to look more closely at the use of complementary and alternative medicine by multiple sclerosis patients. European Journal of Neurology 2004;11:263–7.

Chapter 27

Musculoskeletal disorders

With contribution from Greg de Jong

Introduction

A survey of US adults in December 2007 found that 42% of respondents reported that they were in pain on the day of the survey, 1 in 4 experiencing acute pain, with 72% indicating they had experienced pain in the last 12 months. Of particular interest, 70% of people who reported acute pain, 45% recurrent pain and 20% of chronic pain sufferers indicated that they did not seek medical advice for their condition. The common reason given for the reluctance to seek advice included the perception that people take too many pills, a reluctance to take general medication for pain in a specific location, or that oral prescriptive medications upset their stomachs.[1]

In light of such statistics and concerns it would appear pertinent to investigate all available options in regard to the management of musculoskeletal care. Interestingly, in a further US study, knowledge of complementary health care providers and interventions specific to the most prevalent musculoskeletal conditions was found to be surprisingly low, with the exception of chiropractic treatment. However, most respondents indicated that they would be interested in accessing complementary health care for musculoskeletal injury and pain if costs were subsidised and that their doctors considered such interventions as reasonable.[2]

In Australia, national surveys indicate substantial usage of acupuncture, chiropractic and osteopathic treatments, particularly for back complaints. Approximately 1 in 4 Australians surveyed visited 1 of these providers — 16.1% chiropractors, 9.2% acupuncturists and 4.6% osteopaths — amounting to approximately 32.3 million visits per year, with over 90% considering their treatments to be somewhat helpful or very helpful.[3]

A British survey of patients with chronic musculoskeletal pain demonstrated similarly high levels of usage for all forms of complementary therapies. In the survey, 84% of participants reported having used a complementary treatment in the last year with 65% as present users. Three people used over-the-counter complementary medicines for every 2 who sought treatment from a provider with the most used products being glucosamine and fish oils. Of respondents, 69% used conventional medicines concurrently with their complementary treatment of choice.[4]

This willingness to use complementary therapies in the US, the UK and Australia coupled with reluctance in the use of pharmacological therapies for day-to-day pain management suggests it is necessary for all doctors to expand their knowledge in the use of complementary medicine in addressing musculoskeletal pain and disability. However, this increased awareness to the public's desire for complementary medicines also comes with the responsibility of addressing the efficacy of each option, keeping in mind that public interest may not always reflect best practice in medical care.

The first part of this chapter deals with acute musculoskeletal pain and the second part deals with chronic musculoskeletal pain.

Acute musculoskeletal pain and/or injury management

Acute pain is defined as pain of less than 3 months.[5, 6] It may arise as a result of injury, repetitive movement or be insidious in nature. It has been highlighted by the Australian Acute Musculoskeletal Pain Guidelines Group[7] that most incidences of acute musculoskeletal pain are of short duration (less than 3 months) and will not lead to chronic pain and disability, although mild symptoms may persist.

Furthermore, in the majority of cases the determination of cause and specific diagnosis is not required, whilst simple interventions, including information, assurance and the maintenance of appropriate levels of activity, when coupled with pharmacological and non-pharmacological approaches will be satisfactory without the need for extensive investigation. What is critical is to identify as early as possible the minority of patients who are either presenting with a serious medical condition ('red flags') or are at risk of developing chronic musculoskeletal pain due to psychosocial factors ('yellow flags').[8] (See Tables 27.1 to 27.3.)

Table 27.1 Identifying features ('red flags') of serious conditions associated with acute low back pain

Feature or risk factor	Factor/condition
Symptoms and signs of infection (e.g. fever) Risk factors for infection (e.g. underlying disease process, immunosuppression, penetrating wound)	Infection
History of trauma Minor trauma (if > 50 years, history of osteoporosis and taking corticosteroids)	Fracture
Past history of malignancy Age > 50 years Failure to improve with treatment Unexplained weight loss Pain at multiple sites Pain at rest	Tumour
Absence of aggravating features	Aortic aneurysm

(Source: Australian Acute Musculoskeletal Pain Guidelines Group 2003 *Evidence-Based Management of Acute Musculoskeletal Pain*. National Health and Medical Research Council)

Table 27.2 Identifying features of serious conditions associated with acute thoracic spinal pain

Feature or risk factor	Condition
Minor trauma (if > 50 years, history of osteoporosis and taking corticosteroids) Major trauma	Fracture
Fever Night sweats Risk factors for infection (e.g. underlying disease process, immunosuppression, penetrating wound)	Infection
Past history of malignancy Age > 50 Failure to improve with treatment Unexplained weight loss Pain at multiple sites Pain at rest Night pain	Tumour
Chest pain or heaviness Movement, change in posture has no effect on pain Abdominal pain Shortness of breath, cough	Other serious conditions

(Source: Australian Acute Musculoskeletal Pain Guidelines Group 2003 *Evidence-Based Management of Acute Musculoskeletal Pain*. National Health and Medical Research Council)

Table 27.3 Identifying features of serious conditions associated with acute neck pain

Feature or risk factor	Condition
Symptoms and signs of infection (e.g. fever, night sweats) Risk factors for infection (e.g. underlying disease process, immunosuppression, penetrating wound, exposure to infectious diseases)	Infection
History of trauma Use of corticosteroids	Fracture
Past history of malignancy Age > 50 years Failure to improve with treatment Unexplained weight loss Dysphagia, headache, vomiting	Tumour
Neurological symptoms in the limbs	Neurological condition
Cerebrovascular symptoms or signs, anticoagulant use	Cerebral or spinal haemorrhage
Cardiovascular risk factors, transient ischaemic attack	Vertebral or carotid aneurysm

(Source: Australian Acute Musculoskeletal Pain Guidelines Group 2003 *Evidence-Based Management of Acute Musculoskeletal Pain*. National Health and Medical Research Council)

Lifestyle, mind–body issues and acute musculoskeletal injury

While lifestyle and mind–body medicine interventions may not be necessary during the initial stage of acute injury management, it is the assessment of these factors that form the core tool for identifying those patients who are most likely to progress onto chronic musculoskeletal conditions ('yellow flags') and hence require greater monitoring and follow up.[8]

For instance, in regard to low back pain, psychosocial and occupational factors are considered to have greater clinical value in predicting chronicity than clinical presentation.[9, 10] A systematic review of psychosocial factors in 2008 identified that the most pertinent risks of failure to return to work after a low back injury were a low expectation of recovery and fear-avoidance behaviours.[11] Depression, job satisfaction and stress levels did not appear to have an impact on the likelihood of return to work after injury.

A variety of evaluation tools, such as the Acute Low Back Screening Tool,[8] Roland Morris Disability Questionnaire, Fear Avoidance Beliefs Questionnaire, Oswestry Low Back Pain and Disability Questionnaire and so forth, have subsequently been developed to assess various aspects of psychosocial behaviours, particularly in regard to low back pain. Where such factors are identified as pertinent during an acute episode of injury early referral to behavioural strategies outlined under chronic musculoskeletal management should be considered.

Remaining active versus bed rest and collars

Current evidence suggests remaining active after an acute musculoskeletal injury is preferable in most instances to bed rest or immobilisation. A Cochrane review in 2005[12] indicated that advice to remain active was preferable to bed rest for acute low back pain, although there was no indication of difference where sciatic symptoms were present. Fordyce[13] compared the use of analgesia, exercise, time contingent and behaviour contingent activity in addressing acute low back pain and found that the latter group who had been advised to 'let pain be your guide' were less likely to progress to chronic pain. In the instance of neck pain, remaining active was reported to be of more benefit than rest in a collar after whiplash injuries of the neck.[14] Thus it would appear that remaining as active as possible while respecting pain levels is the best encouragement for patients experiencing acute musculoskeletal pain. Exceptions, however, do apply in the instance where musculoskeletal injury is significant enough to require protection from further damage (e.g. strains of ankle and knee ligaments).[15]

Behavioural therapy

A recent review reported on the rationale and evidence supporting 3 frequently used psychosocial interventions for chronic pain; namely, cognitive behavioural therapy (CBT), operant behavioural therapy and self-hypnosis training.[16] The study concluded that CBT and operant behavioural therapy treatments have a focus on factors that exacerbate or maintain suffering in chronic pain, and should be considered as part of a multidisciplinary treatment paradigm. Whereas self-hypnosis training may be of benefit, it appears to be no more (or less) effective than other relaxation strategies that include hypnotic elements.

Education

A summary of findings on patient education from controlled trials on acute low back pain by the Australian Acute Musculoskeletal Guidelines Group[7] indicated that practitioner-delivered information was more effective than brochures and booklets. Furthermore, information provided in the mail was less effective than in person. In regard to neck pain in general, a Cochrane review indicated no strong evidence for the effectiveness of educational interventions.[17]

Exercise

A Cochrane review[18] indicated that for acute low back pain exercise was no more effective than no treatment or other conservative treatments. In the subacute phase limited evidence suggests that a graded exercise program may improve absentee rates. A literature review in 2008[19] supported this view, indicating that the most appropriate advice at an early stage was the continuation of normal activities as effectively as possible rather than an exercise program. Exercise at the subacute stage (>4 weeks) onwards was indicated to decrease pain and disability, although no specific exercise program was indicated as superior.

A Cochrane review of exercises for acute neck pain indicated limited evidence supporting active range of motion exercises or home-based exercise programs, including both mechanical and whiplash associated disorders.[20] Exercise has been found beneficial in terms of short-term recovery and long-term function in relation to rotator cuff disease of the shoulder.[21]

Nutritional supplements

Where a condition arises insidiously the division into acute/subacute/chronic is less pertinent in regard to nutritional supplementation, as length of chronicity may depend upon successful identification by the assessing practitioner. For this reason and to avoid repetition all Nutritional/Herbal interventions for musculoskeletal pain will be considered in this section, although information is also pertinent to chronic pain.

Vitamin D

Increasing evidence indicates the importance of vitamin D deficiency in muscle pain and weakness. In a study of vitamin D deficiency in a community health clinic, 93% of patients with non-specific musculoskeletal pain were found to have vitamin D deficiency, and 100% of those were under 30 years of age.[22] The authors highlighted the fact that vitamin D deficiency should be considered in all patients with non-specific muscular pain, including those not usually expected to be deficient — the young and non-house-bound.

A review of papers on vitamin D deficiency in 2006 concluded that vitamin D deficiency should be considered as a differential diagnosis in the evaluation of musculoskeletal complaints and treated accordingly.[23] Furthermore, musculoskeletal weakness (e.g. of the thigh muscles) was an additional consequence of vitamin D deficiency. A pilot study of vitamin D deficiency in chronic pain patients found that in those patients with vitamin D deficiency (26%; serum 25-hydroxyvitamin D [25(OH) D<20ng/l) using opioid drugs, the mean morphine equivalent dose and duration of use was significantly higher than non-vitamin D deficient patients.[24]

It is a misassumption that a sunny environment is necessarily protective against vitamin D deficiency. Case studies in Saudi Arabia and Egypt demonstrate significant relationships between vitamin D deficiency and chronic low back pain.[25, 26] In Saudi Arabia 83% of patients with chronic low back pain were found to be vitamin D deficient with the majority successfully treated with vitamin D supplementation over a 3-month period.[25] In the Egyptian study 81% of low back pain patients and 60% of controls were found to be vitamin D deficient indicating that despite the sunny climate many Egyptians were vitamin D deficient. Both limited duration of sun exposure and limited area of skin exposure were associated with deficiency findings.[26] A small study of urban Australian Aboriginals comparing low back pain subjects with controls also demonstrated a 100% vitamin D deficiency amongst the 8 patients with low back pain.[27]

Treatment with vitamin D has been found to be effective for many low back pain patients in several case studies. It must be noted, however, that most studies used either intramuscular injections of between 10 and 30 000IU[28,29] or high dose supplementation at levels of 50 000IU.[30, 31] The one exception was a Saudi Arabian study in which levels of 5000IU/day (<50kg) or 10 000IU/day (>50kg) were used. In all instances clinical improvements were observed in the majority of patients within 3 months.[25]

A caveat to vitamin D supplementation addresses the question as to whether vitamin D has any effect on diffuse musculoskeletal pain that may be associated with low vitamin D levels. Warner and Arnspiger[32] recently reported that low vitamin D levels were not associated with diffuse musculoskeletal pain, and treatment with vitamin D did not reduce pain in patients with diffuse pain and who have low vitamin D levels.

Magnesium and/or alkaline minerals

Anecdotally magnesium is often reported to assist in the alleviation of muscular pain and spasms. Physiologically magnesium plays a significant role in the musculoskeletal system being responsible in part for control of neuronal activity, neuromuscular transmission and muscular contraction/relaxation phases.[33]

However, whilst studies indicate successful use of magnesium sulfate for tetanic muscle spasms[34] and magnesium glycerophosphate in the reduction of muscle spasticity in multiple sclerosis,[35] there is minimal current evidence to support or reject magnesium use in the otherwise well patients with musculoskeletal pain/injury.

One open prospective study of 82 patients with chronic low back pain provided an alkaline mineral supplement demonstrated a clinically significant 49% drop on the Arhus Low Back Pain Rating Scale over a 4-week period. Interestingly, of the multi-minerals used in the formula, including potassium, calcium, iron and copper, only magnesium demonstrated changes in serum (11% increase) and plasma readings (3% decrease) after supplementation.[36] The authors also noted an increased blood buffering capacity from the alkaline formula and concluded with the view that a disturbed acid-base balance might be responsible for chronic low back pain.[36]

Omega-3 essential fatty acids

The resolution of acute inflammation is a dynamic process that requires an appropriate host response, tissue protection and resolution of inflammation. Increasing evidence recognises the role of omega-3 derived mediators (e.g. resolvin, protectin) in regulating the resolution of the acute inflammatory process.[37, 38] To date no trials have been undertaken in regard to the use of omega-3 supplements during acute inflammation.

However, given the effectiveness of non-steroidal anti-inflammatory drugs (NSAIDs) for both acute and chronic low back pain, and the assumed role of omega-3 essential fatty acids in the inflammatory process, a controlled study was undertaken amongst non-surgical neck and low back pain patients attending a neurosurgical practice.[39] Patients were requested to take 1200mg/day of omega-3 supplements (EPA/DHA) and followed up after 1 month. Although response rate to recall by mail was only 50%, 78% remained compliant to recommended dosage, with 22% doubling the dosage themselves. Sixty percent of patients reported that their overall pain had improved, 60% that joint pain had improved and 59% discontinued their NSAID. Eighty percent reported that they were satisfied with their improvement.[39] This early evidence indicates that further studies are required in this area, given the lack of complications associated with omega-3 supplementation as compared to NSAIDs.

B Vitamins

A single randomised double-blind placebo-controlled study of 60 patients with non-surgical low back pain found that an active group receiving intramuscular B12 injections showed a statistically significant decrease in pain as measured on an Visual Analogue Scale (VAS) and a disability questionnaire. The active group also had a significant decrease in paracetamol use in compare to the placebo group.[40]

Clinical trials of low back pain have also been undertaken to establish whether B group vitamins (B1 thiamine nitrate 25mg, B6 pyridoxine hydrochloride, B12 cyanocobalamin 0.25mg; 3 x 2 capsules per day for 3 weeks) added to diclofenac can shorten the need for this medication. A clinically significant difference in diclofenac use in favour of the B vitamin group was noted for patients with severe pain at the beginning of the trial.[41] However, no further trials have been undertaken to evaluate the analgesic role of the B group vitamins in this regard.

Herbal medicines

A 2007 Cochrane review of herbal medicines for the low back identified 3 herbs; *Harpagophytum procumbens* (devil's claw), *Salix alba* (white willow bark) and *Capsicum frutescens* (cayenne) as potentially beneficial in reducing low back pain, however, it was noted that the quality of studies were generally poor.[42] While other herbs are often recommended for acute and chronic musculoskeletal conditions, evidence is usually of low quality, by inference from non-human studies or lacking at present.

Devil's claw (*Harpagophytum procumbens*)

Reductions in low back pain and muscle stiffness have been reported in a series of double-blind studies using a Devil's Claw extract Ll 174.[43, 44] A double-blind study comparing devil's claw (50 or 100mg harpagogoside)/day to rofecoxib (12.5mg) found equivalent benefit over a 6 week period,[45, 46] with follow up after 1 year[47] highlighting that devil's claw was well tolerated and that treatment gains were sustained.

A recent review investigated 28 trials of which 20 reported adverse events.[48] In none of the double-blind RCTs was the incidence of adverse events during treatment with *Harpagophytum procumbens* higher than during placebo treatment. Also, minor adverse events occurred in approximately 3% of the patients, these being mainly gastrointestinal in nature. A few reports of acute toxicity were found but there were no reports of chronic toxicity. Since the dosage used in most of the studies was at the lower limit and since long-term treatment with *Harpagophytum* products was advised, more safety data are required.

White willow bark (*Salix alba*)

In a randomised placebo-controlled study of patients, 39% of active patients treated with white willow bark, standardised to 240mg salicins daily, were found to be pain free. In the control group only 6% achieved the same result over a 4-week trial period.[49] In an open trial comparing 240mg salicins daily, 120mg salicins daily and a control group of conventional treatment, results favoured the 240mg salicins daily group (40% pain free over 4 weeks compared to 19% for the 120mg salicin group and 18% for control).[50]

White willow bark, 240mg salicins daily, has been found to be equivalent to rofecoxib in use for acute episodes of chronic low back pain. The need for rescue dosages of NSAIDs or tramadol was found to be 10% in the white willow bark group and 13% with rofecoxib use.[51]

Cayenne (*Capsicum frutescens*)

As noted, a 2007 Cochrane review found 3 low quality trials supporting the use of topical preparations of *Capsicum frutescens* for low back pain. Cayenne trials were carried out in the form of plaster applications and outcomes were judged to be modest in effect.[42]

Bromelain

A single open study of the use of bromelian for acute knee pain in the absence of osteoarthritis or rheumatoid arthritis demonstrated that 400mg dosages provided significantly more benefit in pain, function and a decrease in knee joint stiffness as compared to a 200mg dosage.[52]

Topical analgesia

Arnica

Topical arnica is often advocated to reduce bruising and swelling in acute injury. Whilst no clinical trials have been performed for acute musculoskeletal injury, post-surgical trials involving wound healing after carpal tunnel syndrome (homeopathic arnica and topically applied arnica ointment) indicate reduced pain levels 2 weeks post surgery when compared to placebo subjects.[53] Further studies with this gel are required to substantiate its wide spread use for acute injury, swelling and bruising.

Topical salicylates

Salicylate is considered to work as a counter irritant in its role as a topically applied pain reducing agent. A review of the use of topical salicylates for acute injuries such as low back pain, ligamentous strains and mild athletic injuries revealed that 67% of active subjects received greater than 50% pain reduction from topical application as compared to only 18% of controls. No comparison studies have been undertaken to compare the use of such topical applications to other conventional therapies.[54]

Other herbal medicines

Whilst several other herbs are often advocated for their individual anti-inflammatory actions, such as *Boswellia serrata* (boswellia), *Curcuma longa* (turmeric), *Rosmarinus officianalis* (rosemary) and *Zingiber officianale* (ginger), no specific clinical evidence to support or refute their effects upon non-arthritic acute musculoskeletal pain and injury are presently available.

Physical therapies

Manipulation

Reviews are mixed as to the benefits of manipulation in managing acute musculoskeletal back pain. A Cochrane review in 2009 established that manipulation was only more effective when compared to sham treatments or treatments that were considered ineffective or harmful. No clinically significant advantage was noted when compared to general practice care, analgesics, physical therapy, exercise or back school.[55] Other reviews, however, have indicated that spinal manipulation may be beneficial in the first 4 weeks post injury.[56, 57] A review of the evidence by the American Pain Society/American College of Physicians in 2007 suggested that there was fair evidence for small to moderate benefits from spinal manipulation.[58]

Two systematic reviews in 2005 of manipulation for acute neck conditions indicated scant evidence for the use of cervical manipulation.[59, 60]

Massage

A Cochrane review of massage for subacute (4 weeks–3months) low back pain indicated that massage may be of benefit.[61]

A Cochrane review of massage of mechanical neck disorders made no recommendations due to methodological considerations.[62]

Cold and/or heat therapies

Despite almost universal acceptance of ice as a first-line treatment to reduce swelling after acute injury, there is a surprising paucity of studies to support or refute its use, with only marginal evidence that ice plus exercise was of benefit after ankle sprains.[63, 64] Moderate evidence from a small number of trials indicates that heat wraps may be of benefit during acute episodes of low back pain.[65]

Acupuncture

A Cochrane review (2009) of the use of acupuncture or dry needling for acute low back pain indicated insufficient evidence to make any recommendations.[66] A Cochrane review in 2006 found no trials on acupuncture for acute neck pain.[67] A Cochrane review of acupuncture for shoulder pain indicated the possibility of short-term benefit in pain and function, but that evidence was otherwise lacking in its efficacy.[68] Acupuncture may also provide short-term relief from lateral elbow pain (tennis elbow), however, no benefit lasting greater than 24 hours has been demonstrated.[69]

Moreover, a systematic review investigated the effectiveness of acupuncture for non-specific low back pain[70] in 23 trials (n = 6359). There was moderate evidence that acupuncture was more effective than no treatment, and strong evidence of no significant difference between acupuncture and sham acupuncture, for short-term pain relief. However, there was strong evidence that acupuncture could be a useful supplement to other forms of conventional therapy for non-specific lower back pain.

Conclusion — acute musculoskeletal pain and/or injury

The vast majority of acute musculoskeletal episodes are temporary, therefore the most important aspects of acute care may be educational support, reassurance to remain active and the early identification of those patients who are likely to progress to chronicity, potentially due to non-organic psychosocial factors. Furthermore, evidence for non-pharmacological treatments for acute musculoskeletal pain and injury are insufficient in most cases. Even the more universally accepted regimes of care, such as ice, lack evidence to effectiveness. While promise is shown in some treatment areas such as vitamin D and herbal interventions for acute low back pain, the evidence for other interventions such as manipulation and acupuncture are yet to be established. Furthermore, as the vast majority of acute musculoskeletal episodes are temporary, the most important aspect of acute care may be educational support, reassurance to remain active and the early identification of those patients who are likely to progress to chronicity, potentially due to non-organic psychosocial factors, rather than patient specific treatments.

Table 27.4 summarises the level of evidence for some CAM therapies for musculoskeletal pain and/or injury conditions.

Chronic musculoskeletal pain (e.g. low back pain)

The Australian Bureau of Statistics estimated that in 2004–2005 15% of the Australian population experienced low back pain at a cost of $567 million per year.[71] In fact it has been estimated that up to 70% of the community of wealthy nations will experience low back pain in their lifetime, with 2–7% of patients developing chronic low back pain (pain>12 weeks) as a result of an acute episode.[72] In approximately 85% of cases a specific diagnosis for low back pain cannot be determined despite diagnostic efforts.[72] Even in instances where an initial acute episode is resolved, low back pain often follows a recurrent pattern with re-exacerbations likely.[73]

The biopsychosocial model of pain has been adopted to explain the complexities of the pain experience (Figure 27.1).[74] Within this approach chronic pain is viewed as a composite response that results from the summation of biological, psychological and social factors individual to the

Table 27.4 Levels of evidence for lifestyle and complementary medicines/therapies in the management of musculoskeletal pain and/or injury conditions

Modality	Level I	Level II	Level IIIa	Level IIIb	Level IIIc	Level IV	Level V
Lifestyle modification and/ or mind–body medicine			x				
Remaining active versus bed rest and/or collars	x						
Patient education by clinicians			x				
Physical activity	x						
Nutritional supplements							
Vitamin D			x				
Vitamin B group					x		
Magnesium				x			
Omega-3 fatty acids				x			
Herbal medicines							
Devil's claw	x		x				
While willow	x		x				
Topical cayenne	x						
Bromelain					x		
Topical Arnica					x		
Topical salicylates	x						
Physical therapies							
Spinal manipulation	x(+/–)						
Massage	x						
Cold and/or heat therapy					x		
Acupuncture	x(+/–)						

Level I — from a systematic review of all relevant randomised controlled trials — meta-analyses.
Level II — from at least 1 properly designed randomised controlled clinical trial.
Level IIIa — from well-designed pseudo-randomised controlled trials (alternate allocation or some other method).
Level IIIb — from comparative studies (including systematic reviews of such studies) with concurrent controls and allocation not randomised, cohort studies, case-control studies, or interrupted time series with a parallel control group.
Level IIIc — from comparative studies with historical control, 2 or more single-arm studies or interrupted time series without a parallel control group.
Level IV — opinions of respected authorities based on clinical experience, descriptive studies or reports of expert committees.
Level V — represents minimal evidence that represents testimonials.

patient's pain 'experience' rather than directly correlating with tissue damage or disease. Although tissue damage may lead to nociception and a painful experience, the level of pain may be modified by many factors such as emotional response, belief structures, personal experience, cultural background, community and work environment and so forth. Alternatively in some instances tissue healing may be complete, yet pain may persist as part of a greater personal experience unique to the individual.

Hence in the context of integrative and complementary medicine the treatment of chronic low back pain may potentially involve the complete spectrum of mind–body therapies. Chronic low back pain should not be viewed solely as a musculoskeletal condition but as an experience of not only the body, but emotions, thought processes, family, social and spiritual network and, in instances of occupational injury, the work community of the patient. However, on the other hand we should not

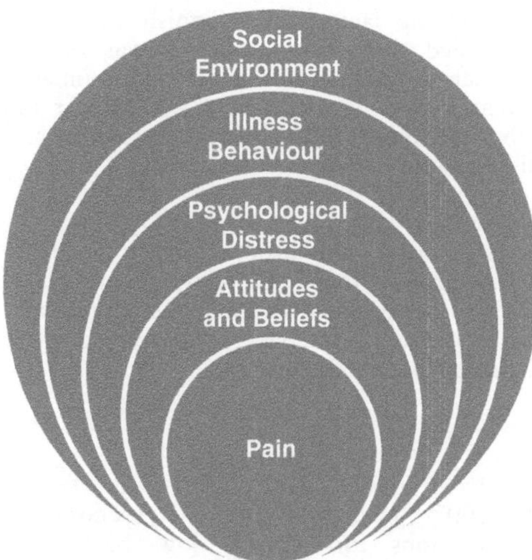

Figure 27.1 Biopsychosocial model of pain

pass over the possibility of prolonged tissue damage or organic imbalance once the patient has entered the classification of chronic pain by assuming that the pain is 'only' psychosomatic in origin, for to do so would also risk overlooking the holism that is the individual living within the pain experience.

Lifestyle factors

Genetic

Recent studies indicate genetic influence in the development of some aspects of chronic low back pain. In twin studies related to low back pain, disc height narrowing was the factor found to correlate most with low back pain history, and further found to be genetically correlated. Other genetic correlations were found with the duration of the longest episode of back pain, hospitalisation from back pain and disability from back pain in the year previous to the study.[75] Twin studies of adult women demonstrated a heritability of low back pain in adult females in the range of 52–68%, and neck pain in the range of 35–85%.[76] A Danish twin study of men and women over the age of 70 indicated a genetic association with low back pain of 25% in men. However, only a modest and non-significant concordance was noted in women such that the conclusion was that genetics did not play a role in low back pain in women over 70.[77]

Education/socioeconomic factors

Consistent findings indicate that low socioeconomic status are predictive of the risk of low back pain. The results of the 1958 British Birth Cohort Study published in 2004 indicated a 2.9 relative risk loading for widespread areas of pain with a 1.5 to 2.0 risk loading for regional pain conditions including low back pain. Childhood socioeconomic status was to a lesser extent significant in regards to most aspects of pain.[78]

Low education levels have also been consistently associated with low back pain. For instance, prospective cohort studies in Norway of 38 426 employed men and women aged 29–59 established that the most significant mediating factor for men between education and low back pain was working conditions (authority to plan own work, physically demanding work, concentration and attention and job satisfaction), while in women occupational class, working conditions and lifestyle factors (smoking, BMI, exercise, alcohol) contributed to increased risk of low back pain. However, such mediating factors only reduced the link between education and low back pain by 39%, suggesting an otherwise strong and unexplained independent effect of education on low back pain incidence.[79]

Physical activity

While physical activity is considered important in preventing and managing low back pain, recent evidence suggests that both the sedentary and over active may be at risk. A Netherlands study of 3364 adults, 25 years and older, drawn from the Dutch population-based Musculoskeletal Consequences Cohort study (1998) identified a modest increase in risk of low back pain in people with sedentary lifestyles (1.31), but also in those involved in physically strenuous activities (1.21), with the relationship being particularly true in women (sedentary = 1.44, physically strenuous = 1.36). Sporting activity was associated with less low back pain (0.78).[80]

Overweight and obesity

A 2009 systematic review and meta-analysis of the comorbidities of the overweight and obese as defined by BMI identified that both groups had a statistically significant association with chronic low back pain.[81] Amongst the elderly (>70), obese subjects (BMI 30–34.9) have twice the likelihood, and severely obese people (BMI >35) 4 times the likelihood, of chronic pain including low back pain than normals.[82] A study of the effects of bariatric weight reduction on obese patients presenting with low back pain indicated that substantial weight reduction after bariatric surgery was associated with moderate decreases in pre-existing pain and disability scores.[83]

Smoking

Analysis of a population-based sample of 29 424 twins aged 12–41 identified a definite link between smoking and incidence of low back pain. Significantly, however, data analysis demonstrated no biological gradient between levels of smoking and measures of low back pain nor did the prevalence of low back pain diminish after the cessation of smoking, suggesting the relationship between smoking and low back pain is not causal in nature.[84, 85] A similar relationship between smoking and low back pain has also been demonstrated in adolescents.[86] A study of the success rates of smokers in rehabilitation programs for low back pain showed smokers were less likely to complete such programs (dropping from a 86.3% to 75% with smokers), however, outcomes did not differ if the programs were completed.[87]

Sleep

A 2008 French study of 101 chronic low back pain patients demonstrated that low back pain patients had much poorer sleep quality and higher numbers of sleep disorders when compared to 97 age and sex matched controls. No conclusion was made on whether or not low back pain or poor sleep was the causal factor.[88]

A 2007 study of 70 chronic back pain patients and 70 gender- and age-matched pain-free controls comparing the sleep patterns of chronic low back pain patients, found that 53% of subjects were rated as insomniacs on the Insomnia Severity Index compared to only 3% of normals. Of 6 variables measured (pain intensity, sensory pain ratings, affective pain ratings, general anxiety, general depression and health anxiety) affective pain levels was found to be the most significant predictor of insomnia, remaining so after the effects of anxiety and depression were controlled for.[89]

While the preceding study suggests that aspects of low back pain may lead to sleep problems, the reverse may also be the case. A Swedish study of the causal relationship between sleep disturbances using the Malmo Shoulder Neck Cohort followed up 4140 vocationally active healthy 45–64 year olds. Of these people, 11.8% of men and 14.8% of women subsequently developed neck, shoulder or low back pain over the following year and an analysis revealed that preceding sleep problems increased the risk of pain by 1.72% in men and 1.91% in women. As a result it was estimated that 1 in 15–20 cases of newly arising chronic pain could be attributed to sleep difficulties, even after accounting for confounding factors.[90] A Finnish study also concluded that sleep problems was one of the factors predictive of developing pain in a 1-year follow up amongst a 40–49 year old subgroup, other factors being mental stress and dissatisfaction with life.[91]

Alcohol

A systematic literature review in 1999 demonstrated that no study identified a positive link between alcohol consumption and the incidence of low back pain, nor a positive dose-dependent response.[92]

Mind–body medicine

Cognitive behavioural therapies (CBTs)

A 2007 meta-analysis of psychological interventions for chronic low back pain demonstrated that such interventions lead to improvements in pain intensity, pain-related interference, health-related quality of life scores and depression. The 2 most effective therapies were found to be cognitive behavioural therapies (CBT) and self-regulatory treatments. Additionally, multidisciplinary programs that included psychological components were more effective when compared to active control groups.[93] A 2006 Cochrane review differed in its conclusions. Although commenting that CBT and progressive relaxation therapy was more effective than waiting list controls, no significant difference could be found when compared to exercise, nor did behavioural treatments provide any additional benefit to other interventions (e.g. physiotherapy, back education).[94]

Recently, electromyographic biofeedback — a therapeutic modality used along with other interventions in the treatment of pain — has been suggested to be effective as an adjunct therapy for pain management.[95] The review concluded that electromyographic biofeedback was comparable to CBT and relaxation techniques. When added to an exercise program in patients with patellofemoral pain or acute sciatic pain, the reviewers noted no further pain reduction was achieved. However, electromyographic biofeedback may promote active participation and thus in turn may motivate patients to adopt an active role in establishing and reaching goals in rehabilitation. Further research is required to investigate its efficacy on musculoskeletal pain.

Back schools

A Cochrane review of back schools (2004) identified that this form of intervention is often used for chronic low back pain, however, content may vary considerably. This said, there is moderate evidence of improvements in pain and function from back schools provided in the primary and secondary health settings or amongst the general public. Back schools also appear to offer benefits superior to exercise, manipulation, myofascial therapies or advice when performed in an occupation environment. Measures of gain include pain, functional statue and return to work.[96]

A systematic review in 2007 of back schools with a specific focus on fear-avoidance training concluded that the evidence on back schools was conflicting due to variant inclusion criteria and evidence rules. Brief education in a clinical setting was concluded to have strong evidence of effectiveness, whilst limited or conflicting evidence existed for back books and internet discussions. Interestingly, a review of 3 high quality RCTs found that fear avoidance training as a component of a rehabilitation program was an equally valid intervention as compared to spinal fusion.[97]

Individual patient education

A Cochrane review of individual education concluded that it was a less effective intervention than more intensive programs of education and rehabilitation for chronic low back pain and no more effective than many single forms of therapy (e.g. CBT, acupuncture, physiotherapy, chiropractic, massage and so forth). No one form of education (written, video, in person) was found to be more effective than another.[98]

Other mind–body medicine

A structured review of 8 complementary mind-body therapies in older patient groups (>50) with chronic pain suggested that although more evidence was required regarding their efficacy, treatment was feasible to the elderly population. The 8 mind–body therapies included in the review were biofeedback, meditation, progressive muscle relaxation, guided imagery, hypnosis, tai chi, qigong and yoga.[99]

Meditation

Low-level evidence suggests the possibility that meditation is beneficial for chronic low back pain. A qualitative study of mind–body medicine amongst 27 elderly patients (> 65) with moderate chronic low back pain or worse found that they reported numerous benefits, including less pain, greater attention, improved sleep, increased wellbeing and quality of life. The authors recommended further research to establish why mindfulness meditation works and additional benefits to other medical conditions.[100]

Progressive muscle relaxation/hypnotherapy

A Cochrane review of behavioural therapies indicated moderate evidence from 2 trials in favour of significant positive short-term benefits from progressive muscle relaxation.[24] A 1984 study of progressive relaxation found that applied relaxation can significantly improve pain ratings, whilst the addition of an operant conditioning program did not improve outcomes.[101]

A comparison of relaxation to hypnotherapy demonstrated equivalent benefits in a small trial of 17 patients (relaxation n = 8), with improvements in pain scores and depression noted for both active groups. A placebo group showed no improvements. Hypnotherapy patients (n = 9) also demonstrated less difficulties with getting to sleep, whilst their doctors noted less problems with their use of medication.[102]

Physical activity/exercise

A Cochrane review of exercise therapy in the treatment of non-specific low back pain indicated that for chronic low back pain exercise was slightly effective in reducing pain and increasing function.[103] There was no comment on which form of exercise was preferable.

Work conditioning (work hardening/ functional restoration)

Work conditioning programs are intensive exercise regimes (strengthening, aerobic capacity, stretching) intended to mimic work conditions. Such programs have also been defined as consisting of a full day program of activities lasting from 3 to 6 weeks.[104] Programs are often multi-modal and include various interventions other than exercise, in particular, cognitive behavioural components. The aim of work conditioning programs is usually specific to return-to-work goals.[105]

A Cochrane review (2003) found significant evidence that these programs do enhance return to work and work days off in the year following treatment as compared to usual care and advice when a cognitive behavioural approach is undertaken. Evidence is lacking in programs in which a cognitive behavioural approach is not included.[105]

It is questionable whether results are as impressive when less rigorous programs are undertaken. For instance, a UK study of active exercise (2 hour sessions), education and CBT, 8 sessions over 6 weeks, concluded only a small and non-significant reduction in pain and disability when patients were reassessed after a year. Interestingly, those patients who allocated a preference to such a program prior to the study demonstrated clinically significant improvements in pain and dysfunction, suggesting patient preference was important in outcomes of such a program.[106] A study in the Netherlands similarly demonstrated no difference between standard physiotherapy and an intensive group training exercise program at 6, 13 and 52 weeks (at 26 weeks a difference was noted).[107]

Specific exercise regimes

Core stability exercises

The use of what is known as 'core stability' or inter-segmental spinal stabilisation exercises have been advocated for the treatment of low back pain. However, there is no clear evidence that core stability exercises are any more effective than standard physiotherapy treatment (general exercise and manual therapy) or physiotherapy-led pain management classes[108, 109] even if they may be more beneficial than daily walks when combined with a graded exercise program.[110]

Pilates

Pilates is a form of rehabilitative exercise with a relationship to core stability principles. Clinical studies suggest that Pilates exercises performed on specific equipment report significant decreases in pain scores compared to a control group defined as usual care (physician attendance and other health professionals as required).[111] However, when Pilates exercises were compared to a standard back school only, equivalent gains in pain and disability were registered in both groups.[112]

Swiss ball

A single pilot study suggests that a 12-week program of Swiss ball exercises may potentially have benefit in reducing low back pain and disability after a 3 month follow-up period.[113]

High intensity lumbar exercises

Although it has been hypothesised that high intensity lumbar extension exercises should improve low back pain, the evidence is not clear. A physiotherapy led study comparing high intensity isolated extension exercises to a non-progressive low intensity regime demonstrated that at 8 weeks back symptoms had improved by 39%, however, no other differences were noted at either 8 weeks or at 26 week follow up.[114] This outcome has been replicated in a further study where little difference was observed between standard physiotherapy and the lumbar extension group.[115] Thus there does not appear to be sufficient evidence to advocate isolated lumbar extension exercises over other interventions.

Aquatic exercises

A systematic review of aquatic exercises performed in 2009 indicates that while aquatic exercises do assist in managing low back pain, the effects are no more advantageous than other interventions.[116]

Alexander technique

A single 2008 randomised controlled trial (RCT) of the Alexander technique concluded that it was beneficial for reducing chronic low back pain after a 1-year period. It was established that 6 sessions of one-to-one therapy followed by exercise was as effective as 24 sessions.[117]

Yoga

Preliminary evidence suggests yoga may be of benefit in chronic low back pain. Yoga has been found to be of more benefit than a self-care book in reducing disability and pain after 26 weeks but equivalent to conventional exercise.[118] Iyengar yoga has been observed to be beneficial compared to an educational group at 3 months follow up after a 16-week program. Significant reductions were observed in pain intensity, functional disability and medication usage.[119] A small pilot study demonstrated Hatha yoga was of benefit compared to a control group over a 6-week period (2 sessions, 2 hour/week) in reducing disability.[120] A study of veterans also supports the potential for yoga in aiding back care, however, as with all the above studies, design and numbers make conclusions tentative.[121]

Breath therapy

A single RCT of breath therapy (n = 36) demonstrated improvements in low back pain after 12 sessions of breath therapy and a benefit compared to physiotherapy at completion of the sessions, however, at 6 months patients in the physiotherapy group showed greater gains.[122]

Physical therapies

Manipulation

Manipulation is a therapy predominantly associated with chiropractic treatment, although performed also by physiotherapists and osteopaths.[123] A Cochrane review (2004) indicated that although spinal manipulation was more effective than sham and other therapies already shown to be ineffective, manipulation showed no comparative advantage when compared to normal general practitioner care, medication, physical therapy, exercises or back schools.[124]

However, a review by the American Pain Society/American College of Physicians found that there was good evidence of moderate efficacy for spinal manipulation.[125] A further review suggested that spinal manipulation was as efficacious as a prescription of NSAIDs (moderate evidence), effective in the short-term compared to general practitioner care and placebo and over the long-term to physical therapy.[126] Chiropractic manipulation was considered efficacious in reducing chronic low back pain in a literature synthesis in 2008, however, it was suggested that additional exercise in conjunction with spinal manipulation would enhance treatment gains.[127]

Little evidence exists as to the preferred provider of manipulations services (chiropractor, physiotherapist, osteopath). Interestingly, the UK BEAM trial that sought to investigate spinal manipulation concluded that there was more similarities between practices than differences, although a precondition of the trial was that no attempt would be made to define efficacy between programs.[128] The finding of this trial was that spinal manipulation for back pain (general) was the most cost-effective tool,[129] although the benefits to pain and disability outcomes to the individual were only small to moderate at 3 months and small at 12 months (as compared to exercise; small effect at 3 months, no effect after 12 months).[130]

The aforementioned trials and reviews suggest differences of opinion exist amongst reviewers when evaluating the benefit of spinal manipulation. It has been argued that the variances in conclusions may be related to not only methodological weaknesses but interpretational bias. A review of reviews on manipulation in 2005 came to the conclusion that there was statistically significant correlations amongst reviews between direction of conclusion (positive towards manipulation), methodological quality (low) and authorship by osteopaths and chiropractors as compared to negative results being associated with quality reviews from other professions.[131] Thus it appears that care needs to be taken in interpreting the available evidence for the effectiveness of manipulation for chronic low back pain.

Massage

A Cochrane review (2008) found that massage appeared to be effective in reducing pain and increasing function when compared to a sham treatment. It further found that massage provided similar benefits to exercise and superior benefits to joint mobilisation, relaxation therapy, physical therapy, acupuncture and self-care education. Benefits could last up to a year after the end of massage sessions. Acupuncture massage appeared to provide better results to Swedish massage, while Swedish massage demonstrates similar results to Thai massage.[132]

Interestingly, neuro-reflexotherapy has been found to be efficacious in low back pain according to a 2006 Cochrane review, however, only as performed in specialist clinics in Spain. No inference can be made at present as to whether this form of treatment is successful away from this environment.[133]

Acupuncture

A 2009 Cochrane review of acupuncture and dry needling for low back pain demonstrated that acupuncture was more effective than no or sham treatments yet no more beneficial than other therapies. However, acupuncture has been found to be of small benefit in providing short-term pain relief in combination with other therapies. Dry needling also appears to be of benefit when added to other conventional treatments. Studies, however, were of low methodological value, and further investigations are required.[134]

Prolotherapy

A 2009 Cochrane review of prolotherapy concluded that there was insufficient evidence to indicate whether prolotherapy had a role in the management of chronic low back pain.[135]

Conclusion — chronic musculoskeletal pain and/or injury

Multi-modal programs that include patient education, and an exercise and stress reduction program appear to provide the most benefit for chronic low back pain, particularly when they involve a psychological component. Encouragement for positive behavioural and lifestyle changes is essential to the rehabilitation of patients with chronic musculoskeletal pain. There appears to be insufficient evidence to conclude that any one intervention provides significant benefits over any other, and many questions remain to be answered through further quality research, which potentially may require additional work on subgroups of low back pain conditions and presentations, before clearer guidelines are established. Furthermore, individual preference for an intervention and, indeed, relative cost will have a significant part to play in each personal scenario, and decisions need be made on a case-by-case basis.

Clinicians should be aware that in the absence of evidence of harm, a range of options are potentially useful to the individual patient given that one of the strengths of integrative medicine is its application to individual patients. Table 27.5 summarises the levels of evidence for some CAM therapies for chronic musculoskeletal pain/injury conditions.

Table 27.5 Levels of evidence for lifestyle and complementary medicines/therapies in the management of chronic musculoskeletal pain/injury conditions

Modality	Level I	Level II	Level IIIa	Level IIIb	Level IIIc	Level IV	Level V
Lifestyle unmodifiable							
Genetics				x			
Lifestyle modifiable							
Patient education and/or low				x			
sociodemography							
Sedentary				x			
Overweight and/or obese	x						
Sleep				x			
Smoking				x			
Mental stress				x			
Alcohol	x(+/–)						
Mind–body medicine							
Cognitive behavioural therapy	x						
Back schools	x						
Individual patient education	x						
Meditation					x		
Progressive muscle relaxation and/or	x						
hypnotherapy		x					
Biofeedback		x					
Guided imagery		x					
Hypnosis		x					
Physical activity	x						
Work conditioning	x						
Specific exercise programs					x		
Core stability exercises		x					
Pilates		x					
Swiss Ball					x		
High intensity lumbar exercises					x		
Aquatic exercises	x						
Alexander technique			x				
Yoga			x				
Breath exercise			x				

Continued

Table 27.5 Levels of evidence for lifestyle and complementary medicines/therapies in the management of chronic musculoskeletal pain/injury conditions—cont'd

Modality	Level I	Level II	Level IIIa	Level IIIb	Level IIIc	Level IV	Level V
Physical therapies							
Spinal manipulation	x						
Massage	x						
Acupuncture	x						
Prolotherapy	x						

Level I — from a systematic review of all relevant randomised controlled trials — meta-analyses.
Level II — from at least 1 properly designed randomised controlled clinical trial.
Level IIIa — from well-designed pseudo-randomised controlled trials (alternate allocation or some other method).
Level IIIb — from comparative studies (including systematic reviews of such studies) with concurrent controls and allocation not randomised, cohort studies, case-control studies, or interrupted time series with a parallel control group.
Level IIIc — from comparative studies with historical control, 2 or more single-arm studies or interrupted time series without a parallel control group.
Level IV — opinions of respected authorities based on clinical experience, descriptive studies or reports of expert committees.
Level V — represents minimal evidence that represents testimonials.

Clinical tips handout for patients — acute injury

1 Reassurance

- If you have been assessed by your doctor and cleared of serious injury you should be reassured that in most instances (85% or more) your injury will not be long-term.
- Therefore as you recover *let pain be your guide* as to the amount of activity you engage in.
- While relative rest according to your pain guidelines is advised, absolute rest is not.
- Unless you have been advised to by your doctor or therapist do not use a back brace, neck collar or other device as it may limit your progress.
- *You should not fear movements that your body allows.* Fear and subsequent avoidance of activity can be a significant factor in whether or not acute injury develops into chronic pain, irrespective of how serious your injury is.

Ice/compression/elevation

- For peripheral injuries (foot, ankle, knee, upper limb) where swelling is of concern, ice, compression (moderately restrictive bandaging) and elevation should be used.
- Ice may be applied for 20 minutes every 2 hours.

2 Physical activity/exercise

- Return to your normal exercise program as you feel comfortable.
- *Range of motion exercise* may be of benefit at an early stage of treatment.
- Specific condition exercise programs may be of benefit after the initial stages of injury (inflammation, bruising etc.) have resolved (2–4 weeks), but as long as you are increasing your activity with respect to pain. Exercises do not need to be rapidly progressed.

3 Physical therapies

- Manipulation, massage, acupuncture and other physical therapies may be of assistance, however, you should assess for yourself whether you experience worthwhile gains from therapy.
- Your therapist should be motivating you towards independence throughout therapy. You should not become convinced that these treatments are necessary over the long term. Responsibility for healing is your own.

4 Supplementation

While most episodes of acute pain or injury should be self-limiting, the following supplements may be of benefit.

Omega-3 (fish oils)

- Indications: may provide an anti-inflammatory effect and reduce the pain of acute conditions.
- Dosage: between 1 and 4g per day maximum (depending on dietary intake of fish) during exacerbations or beginning treatment.
- Side-effects: care should be taken at higher dosage if you have a clotting disorder or are using a blood thinning drug (e.g. Coumadin).

Vitamin D3 (Cholecalciferol)

- Indications: may be indicated where your pain develops without any prior injury or cause. Recommendation should be based on clinical tests performed by doctor.
- Dosage: may begin with supplementation up to 50 000IU per week (7500IU/day) until levels normalise, after which 1000IU maintenance dosage.
- Side-effects: some people may be sensitive to vitamin D supplementation. Potentially vitamin D may reduce the effectiveness of calcium channel blockers and therefore need to be used under medical supervision (patients with cardiac conditions).
- Contraindication: patients with systemic lupus erythmatosis, hypercalcemia, sarcoidosis, hyperparathyroidism and patients taking digitalis should take care with high doses, and therefore require medical supervision.

Magnesium

- Indications: acute muscular spasm, myofascial trigger points, muscle twitches, heart palpitations.
- Dosage: 300–600mg/day.
- Side-effects: some people have gastrointestinal side-effects from high dosages.
- Contraindications: not to be used in patients with severe kidney disease or heart blocks.

Herbs

Devil's claw *(Harpagophytum procumbens)*

- Indications: may provide an anti-inflammatory effect and reduce the pain of acute conditions.

- Dosage: devil's claw (50 or 100mg harpagogoside)/day over 6–12 weeks to note effects.
- Side-effects: may interact with warfarin. Care should be taken in case of diarrhoea, gallstones, stomach ulcers or pregnancy.

Willow bark *(Salix alba)*

- Indications: may provide an anti-inflammatory effect and reduce the pain of acute conditions.
- Dosage: 240mg/day in divided doses.
- Side-effects: minimal.
- Contraindications: should not be taken by aspirin or salicylate-sensitive individuals.

Curcumin (Tumeric)

- Indications: may have an anti-inflammatory affect allowing a reduction in the use of NSAIDs.
- Dosage: 1200mg/day recommended.
- Side-effects: may increase the risk of bleeding in high doses. Contradicted in cases of bile duct obstruction. May negatively affect chemotherapy in breast cancers so should not be used. Suspend use 1 week prior to major surgery.

Topical gels

- Topically applied gels containing methyl salicylate may provide short-term relief.

Clinical tips handout for patients — chronic musculoskeletal pain and/or injury

1 Lifestyle advice

Sunshine

- At least 15 minutes of sunshine needed daily for vitamin D and melatonin production — especially before 10 a.m. and after 3 p.m. when the sun exposure is safest in summer.
- Ensure adequate skin exposure (back of hands or face) during this period. Apply sun protection after adequate exposure has been achieved.
- More time in the sun is required for dark skinned people in winter.

Sleep

- Attempt to establish healthy sleep patterns. Wake with the sun and go to sleep between 9–10 p.m. (For more information see Chapter 22.)

Weight loss

- If you are overweight participate in a formalised weight loss program as any loss of weight will reduce the load on your spine.

2 Physical activity/exercise

- Exercise 30–60 minutes daily. If exercise is not regular, commence with 5 minutes daily and slowly build up to at least 30 minutes. Outdoor exercise with nature, fresh air and sunshine is ideal (e.g. brisk walking, light jogging, cycling, swimming, stretching, weight-bearing exercises). The more time you spend outdoors the better.
- There is no present evidence that any specific form of exercise (Pilates, Swiss ball, gym etc.) is superior to any other.
- They are all helpful. The key, therefore, is to find a form of exercise that you enjoy.
- Yoga and tai chi may be helpful approaches as long as exercise is assessed for risk. Some positions (e.g. inverted postures) may not be appropriate, and indeed dangerous, so monitoring by a qualified instructor is essential.

3 Mind–body therapies

- Cognitive behavioural therapies, hypnosis, biofeedback and other psychological interventions may be of benefit for some people. You should assess the benefits on an individual basis.
- Back exercise classes may be of assistance in increasing your knowledge as to how to best take care of your condition.
- Stress management programs may be helpful, including journaling/verbal disclosure of emotions. The use of a counsellor does not appear to provide additional benefit.
- Regular meditation practice, at least 10–20 minutes daily.
- Meditation and/or relaxation of at least 10–20 minutes per day can be helpful.

Breathing

- Be aware of breathing at all times. Notice if tendency to hold breath or over-breathe. Always aim to relax breath and the muscles around the chest wall and overall body.

Fun

- It is important to have fun in life.
- Joy can be found even in the simplest tasks, such as funny movies/videos, comedy, hobbies, dancing, playing with pets and children.

4 Environment

- Quit smoking through whatever means are available. Support is often essential as smoking cessation over the long-term is a challenge.
- Actively engage in your community in order to increase your support networks.

5 Dietary changes

- Eat regular balanced healthy meals; ideally 3 main meals and 2 snacks per day, each containing protein.
- Increase fish intake (sardines, tuna, salmon, cod, mackerel) especially deep sea fish > 3 meals per week.
- Two small serves of red meat per week should be consumed to ensure adequate iron levels.
- Consume high quantities of fruit and vegetables (in particular red fruit and vegetables).
- Use extra virgin cold pressed olive oil and avocado in dressings.
- Consume more nuts, seeds, bean sprouts (e.g. alfalfa, mung beans, lentils).
- Enjoy dark chocolate.
- Reduce dairy intake but consume full-fat varieties to increase vitamin D intake from fat-soluble sources.
- Eat a variety of wholegrains/cereals (best if not toasted). Cooked traditional rolled oats for breakfast are particularly helpful, as is rice (brown, basmati, Mahatma, Dongara), buckwheat flour, wholegrain organic breads (rye bread, Essene, spelt, kamut) — when toasting make hot and crisp, not brown, to avoid acrylamide — brown pasta, couscous, millet, amaranth, etc.
- Drink 1–2 litres of water per day.
- Short-term fasting may be of benefit during symptom exacerbation.
- Avoid hydrogenated fats, salt, fast foods, sugar such as soft drinks, lollies, biscuits, cakes and other processed foods e.g. white breads, white pasta, pastries.
- Moderate coffee and alcohol consumption; 1–2 serves per day. Assess whether either affect your symptoms.
- Avoid chemical additives — preservatives, colourings, flavourings.
- For sweeteners try honey (e.g. manuka, yellow box and stringy bark).

6 Physical therapies

- Manipulation, massage, acupuncture and other physical therapies may be of assistance, however, you should assess for yourself whether you experience worthwhile gains from therapy.
- Your therapist should be motivating you towards independence throughout therapy. You should not become convinced that these treatments are necessary over the long-term. Responsibility for healing is your own.

7 Supplementation

While most episodes of acute pain or injury should be self-limiting, the following supplements may be of benefit.

Omega-3 (fish oils)

- Indications: may provide an anti-inflammatory effect and reduce the pain of acute exacerbations of chronic pain.
- Dosage: 1–4g/day maximum (depending on dietary intake of fish) during exacerbations or beginning treatment.
- Side-effects: care should be taken at higher dosage if you have a clotting disorder or are using a blood thinning drug (e.g. Coumadin).
- Contraindications: sensitivity to seafood; drug interactions; caution when taking high doses of fish oils >4g per day together with warfarin (your doctor will check your INR test).

Vitamin D3 (cholecalciferol)

- Indications: may be indicated where your pain develops without any prior injury or cause. Recommendation should be based on clinical tests performed by doctor.
- Dosage: may begin with supplementation up to 50 000IU per week (7500IU/day) until levels normalise, after which 1000IU maintenance dosage.
- Side-effects: some people may be sensitive to vitamin D supplementation.

Potentially vitamin D may reduce the effectiveness of calcium channel blockers and therefore need to be used under medical supervision (patients with cardiac conditions).

Patients with systemic lupus erythmatosis, hypercalcemia, sarcoidosis, hyperparathyroidism and patients taking digitalis should take care with high doses, and therefore require medical supervision.

Magnesium + malic acid

- Indications: acute muscular spasm, myofascial trigger points, muscle twitches, heart palpitations.
- Dosage: 300–600mg magnesium with 1200–2400mg malic acid/day.
- Side-effects: some people have gastrointestinal side-effects from high dosages.

- Contraindications: not to be used in patients with severe kidney disease or heart blocks.

Herbs

Devil's claw *(Harpagophytum procumbens)*

- Indications: may provide an anti-inflammatory effect and reduce the pain of acute exacerbations of chronic pain.
- Dosage: 50 or 100mg harpagogoside/day over 6–12 weeks to note effects.
- Side-effects: may interact with warfarin. Care should be taken in case of diarrhoea, gallstones, stomach ulcers or pregnancy.

Willow bark *(Salix alba)*

- Indications: may provide an anti-inflammatory effect and reduce the pain of acute exacerbations of chronic pain; has aspirin-like properties.
- Dosage: 240mg daily in divided doses.
- Side-effects: should not be taken by salicylate-sensitive individuals.
- Contraindications: digestive upset, allergies to aspirin.

Curcumin (Tumeric)

- Indications: may have an anti-inflammatory affect allowing a reduction in the use of NSAIDs.
- Dosage: 1200mg/day recommended.
- Side-effects: may increase the risk of bleeding in high doses.
- Contraindications: in cases of bile duct obstruction. May negatively affect chemotherapy in breast cancers so should not be used. Suspend use 1 week prior to major surgery.

Topical gels

- Topically applied gels containing capsaicin or methyl salicylate may provide short-term relief.

References

1 New Survey Finds Majority of Americans in Pain. Online. Available: www.reuters.com.article/press Release/idUS157460+23-Jan-2008+PRN20080123 (accessed 9 June 2009).
2 Sherman KJ, Cherkin DC, Connelly MT, et. al. Complementary and alternative medical therapies for chronic low back pain: What treatments are patients willing to try? BMC Complement Alt Med, 2004 Jul 19;4:9.
3 Xue CC, Zhang AL, Lin V. Acupuncture, chiropractic and osteopathy use in Australia: a national population survey. BMC Public Health 2008 Apr 1;8:105.
4 BMV Family Practice. The use of complementary and alternative medicine, and conventional treatment, among primary care consulters with chronic musculoskeletal pain. BMV Family Practice 4 May 2007, 8:26. doi:10.
5 Bonica JJ. The Management of Pain. Lea and Febiger 1953. doi:0.1186/1471-2296-8-26.
6 Merskey H. Pain terms: a list with definitions and notes on usage recommended by the IASP Subcommittee on Taxonomy. Pain 1979;6:249–52.
7 Australian Acute Musculoskeletal Pain Guidelines Group. Evidence Based Management of Acute Musculoskeletal Pain. National Health and Medical Research Council 2003.
8 New Zealand Guidelines Group. New Zealand Acute Low Back Pain Guide 2004.
9 Truchon M, Fillion L. Biopsychosocial determinants of chronic disability and low back pain: a review. Journal of Occupational Rehabilitation 2000;10:117–42.
10 Wessels T, van Tulder M, Sigl T, et. al. What predicts outcome in non-operative treatments of chronic low back pain? A systematic review. Eur Spin J. 2006 Nov;15(11):1633-44.
11 Iles RA, Davidson M, Taylor NF. Psychosocial predictors of failure to return to work in chronic no-specific low back pain: a systematic review. Occup Environ Med 2008 Aug 65(8):507–17. Epub 2008 Apr 16.
12 Hagen KB, Jamtevedt G, Hilde G, et. al. The updated Cochrane review of bed rest for low back pain. Spine 2005 Mar 1;30(5):542–6.
13 Fordyce WE, Brockway JA, Bergman JA, et. al. Acute back pain: a control group comparison of behavioural vs traditional management methods. Journal of Behavioral Medicine 1986;9:127–40.
14 Borchgrevink GE, Kaasa A, McDonagh D, et. al. Acute treatment of whiplash neck sprain injuries. A randomised trial of treatment during the first 14 days after a car accident. Spine 1998;23:25–31.
15 Kerkhoffs GM, Struijs PA, Assendelft WJ, et. al. Different functional treatment strategies for acute lateral ankle ligaments. Cochrane Database of Systematic Reviews 2002, Issue 3, Art. No CD002938. doi: 10.1002/14651858.CD002938.
16 Molton IR, Graham C, Stoelb BL, et. al. Current psychological approaches to the management of chronic pain. Curr Opin Anaesthesiol 2007;20(5):485–9.
17 Haines T, Gross A, Goldsmith CH, et. al. Patient education for neck pain with or without radiculopathy. Cochrane Database of Systematic Reviews 2008 Issue 4. Art. No CD005106. doi: 1002/14651868. CD005106.pub2.
18 Hayden JA, van Tulder MW, Malmivarra A, et. al. Exercise Therapy for treatment of non-specific low back pain. Cochrane Database Systematic Review, 2005 Jul 20;3:CD000335.
19 Henchoz Y, Kai Lik So. A Exercise and non-specific low back pain: a literature review. Joint Bone Spine 2008 Oct;75(5):533–9. Epub 2008 Sep 17.
20 Kay TM, Gross A, Goldsmith CH, et. al. Exercise for mechanical neck disorders. Cochrane Database of Systematic Reviews 2005, Issue 3. Art. No. CD004250. doi: 10.1002/14651858.CD004250.pub3.
21 Green S, Buchbinder R, Hetrick SE. Physiotherapy interventions for shoulder pain. Cochrane Database of Systematic Reviews 2003, Issue 2. Art. No; CDOO4258. doi. 10.1002/14651858.CD004258.
22 Plotnikoff GA, Qigley JM. Prevalence of severe hypovitaminosis D in patients with persistent, non-specific musculoskeletal pain. Mayo Clinic Proc 2003;78:1463–70.
23 Heath KN, Elovic EP. Vitamin D deficiency: implications in the rehabilitation setting. Am J Phys Med Rehabil 2006;85:916–23.

24 Turner MK, Hooten WM, Schmidt JE, et. al. Prevalence and clinical correlates of Vitamin D inadequacy among patients with chronic pain. Pain Med 2008 Nov;9(8):979–84.

25 Al Faraj S, Al Mutairi K. Vitamin D deficiency and chronic low back pain in Saudi Arabia. Spine 2003 Jan 15;28(2):177–9.

26 Lofti A, Abdel-Nasser AM, Hamdy A, et. al. Hypovitaminosis D in female patients with chronic low back pain. Clin Rheumatol 2007 Nov; 26(11):1895–901.

27 Benson J, Wilson A, Stocks N, et. al. Muscle pain as an indicator of vitamin D in an urban Australian Aboriginal population. MJA 2006 July 17;185(2):76–77.

28 De Torrente de la Jara, Precund A, Favrat B. Musculoskeletal pain in female asylum seekers and hypovitaminosis D3. BMJ 2004:329:156–7.

29 Glerup H, Mikkelsen L, Poulser L, et. al. Hypovitaminosis myopathy without biochemical signs of osteomalacic bone involvement. Calcif Tissue Int 2000;66:419–24.

30 Gloth FM, Lindsay Jm, Zelesnick LB, et. al. Can vitamin D deficiency produce an unusual pain syndrome. Arch Intern Med 1991;151:1662–4.

31 Prabhala A, Garg R, Dandona P. Severe myopathy associated with vitamin D deficiency in western New York. Arch Intern Med 2000;160:1199–203.

32 Warner AE, Arnspiger SA. Diffuse musculoskeletal pain is not associated with low vitamin D levels or improved by treatment with vitamin D. J Clin Rheumatol 2008;14(1):12–6.

33 Altura BM, Altura BT. Roel of Magnesium in pathophysiological processes and the clinical utility of magnesium ion selective electrodes Scand. J Clin Lab Invest Suppl 1996;226:211–34.

34 Attgalle D, Rodrigo N. Magnesium as first line therapy in the management of tetanus: a prospective study of 40 patients. Anaesthesia 2002 Aug;57(8):811–7.

35 Rossier P, van Erven S, Wade DT. Effect of magnesium oral therapy on spasticity in a patient with multiple sclerosis. Eur J Neurol 2000 Nov;7(6):741–4.

36 Vormann J, Worlitschek M, Goedecke T, et. al. Supplementation with alkaline minerals reduces symptoms in patients with chronic low back pain. J Trace Elem Med Biol 2001;15(2-3):179–83.

37 Schwab JN, Chiang N, Arita M, Serhan CN. Resolvin E1 and protectin D1 activate inflammation resolution programmes. Nature 2007 Jun 14;447(7146):869–74.

38 Serhan CN. Novel eicosanoid and ocosanoid mediators: resolvins, docosatrienes, and neuroprotectins. Curr Opin Clin Nutr Metab Care 2005 Mar 8(2):115–21.

39 Maroon JC, Bost JW. Omega-3 fatty acids (fish oils) as an anti-inflammatory: an alternative to nonsteroidal anti-inflammatory drugs for discogenic pain. Surg Neur 2006 April;65(4):326–31.

40 Mauro GL, Martorana U, Cataldo P, et. al. Vitamin B12 in low back pain: a randomised, double-blind, placebo-controlled study. Eur Med Pharmacol Sci 2000 May-Jun;4(3):53–8.

41 Bruggemann G, Koehler CO, Koch EM. Results of a double-blind study of diclofenac + vitamin B1,B6,B12 versus diclofenac in patients with acute pain of the lumbar vertebrae. A multicenter study Klin Wochenschr 1990 Jan 19;68(2):116–20.

42 Gagnier JJ, van Tulder MW, Berman B, et. al. Herbal Medicine for low back pain: a Cochrane review. Spine 2007 Jan 1;32(1):82–92.

43 Laudahn D, Walper A. Efficacy and tolerance of Harpogophytum extract Ll 174 in patients with chronic non-radicular back pain. Phyto Res 2001: 15(7):621–4.

44 Gobel HA, et. al. Effects of Harpogophytum procumbens Ll 174 (devil's claw) on sensory, motor and vascular muscle reagibility in the treatment of unspecific back pain. Schmertz 2001;15(1):10–18.

45 Chrubasik S, et. al. Effectiveness of Harpogophytum extract WS1531 in the treatment of exacerbation of low back pain: a randomised placebo-controlled, double-blind study. Eur J Anaesthesiol 1999;16(2):118–29.

46 Chrubasik S, et. al. A randomised double-blind pilot study comparing Doloteffin(R) and Vioxx(R) in the treatment of low back pain. Rheumatology 2003b;42(1):141–8.

47 Chrubasik S, et. al. A 1 year follow up after a pilot study with Doloteffin(R) for low back. Pain Phytomedicine 2205; 12(1-2):1–9.

48 Vlachojannis J, Roufogalis BD, Chrubasik S. Systematic review on the safety of Harpagophytum preparations for osteoarthritic and low back pain. Phytother Res 2008;22(2):149–52.

49 Chrubasik S, et. al. Treatment of low back pain exacerbations with willow bark extract: a randomised double-blind study. Am J Med 2000; 109(1):9–14.

50 Chrubasik S, et. al. Potential economic impact of using a proprietary willow bark extract in outpatient treatment of low back pain: an open non randomised study. Phytomedicine 2001; 8(4):241–51.

51 Chrubasik S, et. al. Treatment of low back pain with a herbal synthetic ant-rheumatic: a randomised control study: willow bark extract for low back pain. Rheumatology (Oxford) 2001; 40(12):1388–93.

52 Walker AF, Bundy R, Hicks SM, et. al. Bromelain reduces mild acute knee pain and improves well being in a dose dependent fashion in an open study of otherwise healthy adults. Phytomedicine 2002 Dec;9(8):681–6.

53 Jeffrey SL, Belcher HJ. Use of arnica to relieve pain after carpal tunnel release surgery. Alter Ther Health Med 2002 Mar-April;8(2):66–8.

54 Mason L, Moore RA, Edwards JE, et. al. Systematic review of efficacy of topical rubefacients containing salicylates for the treatment of acute and chronic pain. BMJ 2004;328:995–8.

55 Assendelft WJ, Morton SC, Yu EI, et. al. Spinal manipulation therapy for low back pain Cochrane Database of Systematic Reviews 2004 Issue 1 Art No. CD000447. doi: 10. 1002/14651858. CD000447.pub 2.

56 Smith D, McMurray N, Disler P. Early Intervention for acute back injury: can we finally develop an evidence based approach? Clin Rehabil 2002 Feb;16(1):1–11.

57 Swenson R, Haldeman A. Spinal manipulative therapy for low back pain. J Am Acad Orthop Surg 2003 Jul-Aug;11(4):228–37.

58 Chou R, Huffman LH. American Pain Society, American College of Physicians Nonpharmacological therapies of acute and chronic low back pain: a review of the evidence for an American Pain Soceity/American College of Physicians clinical practice guideline Ann Intern Med 2007 Oct 2;147(7):492–504.

59 Vernon HJ, Humphreys BK, Hagino CA. A systematic review of conservative treatments for acute pain not due to whiplash. J Manipulative Physiol Ther 2005 Jul-Aug;28(6):443–8.

60 Haneline MT. Chiropractic manipulation and acute neck pain: a review of the evidence. J Manipulative Physiol Ther 2005 Sep;28(7):520–5.
61 Furlan AD, Imamura M, Dryden T. Massage for low back pain Cochrane Database for Systematic Reviews 2008, Issue 4. Art.No.: CD001929. doi 10.1002/14651858.CD001929.pub2.
62 Haraldsson B, Gross A, Myers, et. al. Massage for mechanical neck disorders. Cochrane Database of Systematic Reviews 2006, Issue 3. Art. No.:CD004871. doi:10.1002/14651858.CD004871. pub3.
63 Bleakley C, NcDonough S, MacCauley D. The use of ice in the treatment of acute soft tissue injury: a systematic review of randomised controlled trials. Am J Sports Med 2004 Jan-Feb;32(1):251–61.
64 Collins NC. Is ice right? Does cryotherapy improve outcome for acute soft tissue injury? Emerg Med J 2008 Feb;25(2):65–8.
65 French SD, Cameron M, Walker BF, et. al. Superficial heat or cold for low back pain Cochrane Database Systematic Review 2006 Jan 25; (1): CD004750.
66 Furian AD, van Tulder MW, Cherkin D, et. al. Acupuncture and dry-needling for low back pain Cochrane Database of Systematic Reviews 2005, Issue 1. Art. No:CDOO1351. doi: 10.1002/14651858.CD001351.pub2.
67 Trinh KV, Graham N, Gross AR, et. al. Acupuncture of neck disorders Cochrane Data Base of Systematic Reviews 2006 Issue 3 Art. No.:CD004870. doi: 10.1002/14651858.CD004870.pub.3.
68 Green S, Buchbinder R, Hetrick SE. Acupuncture for shoulder pain Cochrane Database of Systematic Reviews 2005, Issue 2. Art. No.: CD005319. doi: 10.1002/14651858.CD005319.
69 Green S, Buchbinder R, Barnsley L, et. al. Acupuncture for lateral elbow pain pain Cochrane Database of Systematic Reviews 2002, Issue 1. Art. No.: CD003527. doi: 10.1002/14651858. CD003527.
70 Yuan J, Purepong N, Kerr DP, et. al. Effectiveness of acupuncture for low back pain: a systematic review. Spine 2008;33(23):E887-E900.
71 Musculoskeletal conditions in Australia: a snapshot 2004-2005 2004-2005. Australian Bureau of Statistics 2006.
72 Deyo RA, Rainville J, Kent DL. What can the history and physical examination tell us about low back pain? JAMA 1992;268:760–5.
73 Waddell G. The clinical course of low back pain. In: The back pain revolution. Edinburgh, Churchill Livingstone, 1998:103–17.
74 Engel G. The need for a new medical model: a challenge for biomedicine. Science 1977,196: 129–136.
75 Battie MC, Vidernan T, Levalahti E, et. al. Heritability of back pain and the role of disc degeneration. Pain 2007 Oct;131(3):272-80.
76 MacGregor AJ, Andrew T, Sambrook PN, et. al. Structural, psychological, and genetic influences on low back and neck pain: a study of adult female twins. Arthrititis Rheum 2004 Apr 15;51(2): 160–167.
77 Hartvigsen J, Christensen K, Frederiksen H, et. al. Genetic and environmental contributions to back pain inold age: a study of 2108 danish twins aged 70 and older. Spine 2004 Apr 15;29(8):897–901. Discussion 092.
78 McFarlane GJ, Norris G, Atherton, et. al. The influence of socioeconomic status on reporting of regional and widespread musculoskeletal pain: results from the 1958 British Birth Cohort Study. Ann Rheum Dis 2008 Oct 24.
79 Hagen KB, Tambs K, Bjerkedal T. What mediates the inverse association between education and occupational disability from back pain? – a prospective cohort study from the Nord-Trondelag health study in Norway. Soc Sci Med 2006 Sep;63(5):1267–75.
80 Heneweer H, Varness L, Pricavet HS. Physical activity and low back pain: a U shaped relationship. Pain 2009 May;143(1-2);21–5.
81 Guh DP, Zhang W, Barnsback N, et. al. The incidence of co-morbidities related to obesity and overweight: a systematic review and meta analysis. BMC Public Health 2009 Mar 25;9:88.
82 McCarthy LH, Bigal ME, Katz M, et. al. Chronic pain and obesity in elderly people: results from the Einstein study. J Am Geriatric Soceity 2009 Jan;57(1):115–9.
83 Khouier P, Black MH, Crookes PF, et. al. Prospective assessment of axial pain symptoms before and after bariatric weight reduction surgery. Spine J 2009 Apr 6.
84 Leboeuf-Yde C, Kyvik KO, Bruun NH. Low back pain and lifestyle: Part 1. Information from population based sample of 29,424 twins. Spine 1998 Oct 15;23(20):2207–13.
85 Leboeuf–Yde C. Smoking and low back pain. A systematic literature review of 41 journal articles reporting epidemiological studies. Spine 1999 Jul 15;24(14):1463–70.
86 Mikkonen P, Leinos-Arjas P, Remes J, et. al. Is smoking a risk factor for low back pain in adolescents? A prospective cohort study. Spine 2008 Mar 11:33(5):527–32.
87 McGeary D, Mayer T, Gatchel R, et. al. Smoking status and psychosocioeconomic outcomes of functional restoration in patients with chronic spinal stability. Spine 2004;4(2):170–5.
88 Marty M, Rozenberg S, Duplan B, et. al. Quality of sleep in patients with chronic low back pain: a case control study. Eur Spine J 2008 June;17(6):839–44.
89 Tang NK, Wright KJ, Salkovskis PM. Prevalence and correlates of clnical insomnia co-occurring with chronic back pain. PJ Sleep Res 2007;16(1)85–95.
90 Carnivet S, Ostergren Po, Chroi B. Sleeping Problem as a risk factor for subsequent musculoskeletal pain and the role of job strain: results from a one year follow up of the Malmo Neck Study. Cohort Int j Beh Med 2008;15(4):254–62.
91 Miranda H, Viikari-Juntura E, Punnett L, et. al. Occupational loading, health behaviour and sleep disturbances as a predictor of low back pain. Scand J Work Environ Health 2008 Dec;34(6):411–9.
92 Leboeuf-Yde. Alcohol and low back pain: a systematic review J Manipulative. Therapy 2000 June;23(5):343–6.
93 Hoffman BM, Papas RK, Chatkoff DK, et. al. Meta-analysis of psychological interventions for chronic low back pain. Health Psychol 2007 Jan;26(1):1–9.
94 Ostelo R, van Tulder M, Vlaeyen J. Behavioural Treatment for chronic pain. The Cochrane Database of Systematic Reviews 2006 Issue 3
95 Angoules AG, Balakatounis KC, Panagiotopoulou KA, et. al. Effectiveness of electromyographic biofeedback in the treatment of musculoskeletal pain. Orthopedics 2008;31(10). pii: orthosupersite.com/ view.asp?rID=32085.

96 Heymans M, van Tulder M, Esmail R, et. al. Back schools for non-specific low back pain. Cochrane Database for Systematic Reviews 2004 Issue 4 Art. No. CDoooo261 doi: 10.1002/14651858. CD000261.pub 2.
97 Brox I, Reikeras O, Nygaard O, et. al. Lumbar instrumented fusion compared with cognitive intervention and exercise in patients with chronic back pain after previous surgery for disc herniation: a prospective randomised controlled study. Pain 2006 May;122(1-2):145–55.
98 Engers AJ, Jellerma P, Wensing M, et. al. Individual Patient Education for low back pain Cochrane Database of Systematic Reviews 2008 Issue 1 Art. No.: CD004057. doi: 1002/14651858.CD004047. pub.3.
99 Morone NE, Greco CM. Mind-body interventions for chronic pain in older adults: a structured review. Pain Med 2007 May-Jun;8(4):359–75.
100 Morone NE, Lynch CS, Greco SM, et. al. 'I felt like a new person.' The effect of mindfulness on older patients with chronic pain: qualitative narrative analysis of diary entries. J Pain 2008 Sep;9(9): 841–8.
101 Linton SJ, Gotestam KG. A controlled study of the effects of applied relaxation and applied relaxation plus operant procedures in the regulation of chronic pain. BR J Clin Psychol 1984 Nov;23(Pt 4):291–9.
102 McCauley JD, Thelan MH, Frank RG. Hypnosis compared to relaxation in the outpatients management of chronic low back pain. Arch Phys Med Rehabil 1983 Nov; 64(11):548–52.
103 Hayden JA, van Tulder MW, Malmivaara A, et. al. Exercise therapy for treatment of non-specific low back pain. Cochrane Database of Systematic Reviews 2005 Issue 3 CD000335.
104 Poiraudeau S, Rannou F, Revel M. Functional Restoration for low back pain: a systematic review. Ann Readapt Med Phys 2007 Jul;50(6):425–9, 419–24.
105 Schonstein E, Kenny DT, Keating JL, et. al. Work conditioning, work hardening and functional restoration for workers with back and neck pain. Cochrane Database of Systematic Reviews 2003, Issue 3. Art. No.: CD001822. doi 10.1002/14651858.CD001822.
106 Johnson Re, Jones Gt, Wiles NJ. Active exercise, education and cognitive behavioural therapy for persistent disabling low back pain: a randomised controlled trial. Spine 2007 Jul 1;32(15):1578–85.
107 Van der Roer N, van Tulder M, Barendse J, et. al. Intensive group training protocol versus guideline physiotherapy for patients with chronic low back pain: a randomised controlled trial. Eur Spine J 2008 Sep;17(9):1193–200.
108 Cairns MC, Foster NE, Wright C. Randomised controlled trial of specific spinal stabilisation exercises and conventional physiotherapy for recurrent low back pain. Spine 2006 Sep 1;31(19):E670-81.
109 Critchley D, Ratcliffe J, Noonan, et. al. Effectiveness and cost effectiveness of three types of physiotherapy used to reduce chronic low back pain disability: a pragmatic randomized trial with economic evaluation. Spine 2007 June 15,32(14):1474–81.
110 Rasmussen-Barr E, Ang B, Arvidsson I, et. al. Graded exercise for recurrent low back pain: a randomised, controlled trial with 6, 12, and 36 months follow ups. Spine 2009 Feb 1;34(3):221–8.
111 Rydeard R, Leger A, Smith D. Pilates-based therapeutic exercise: effect on subjects with non-specific chronic low back pain and functional disability: a randomised controlled trial. J Orthop Sports Phys Ther 2006 Jul;36(7):472–84.
112 Donzelli S, Di Domenico E, Cova Am, et. al. Two differential techniques in the rehabilitation of low back pain: a randomised controlled trial. Eura Medicophys 2006 Sep;42(3):205–10.
113 Marshall PW, Murphy BA. Evaluation of functional and neuromuscular changes after exercise rehabilitation for low back pain using a Swiss Ball: a pilot study. J Manipulative Physiol Ther 2006 Sep;29(7):550–60.
114 Harts CC, Helmhout Ph, de Rie RA. A high intensity lumbar extensor strengthening program is little better than a low intensity program or a waiting list control group for chronic low back pain: a randomised control clinical trial. Aust J Physiother 2008;54(1):23–31.
115 Helmhout PH, Harts CC, Viechtbauer W, et. al. Isolated lumbar extensor strengthening versus regular physical therapy in an army working population with nonacute low back pain: a randomised controlled trial. Arch Phys Med Rehabil Sep; 89(9):1675–85.
116 Waller B, Lambeck J, Daly D. Therapeutic aquatic exercise in the treatment of low back pain: a systematic review. Clin Rehabil 2009 Jan;23(1): 3–14.
117 Little P, Lewith G, Webley F, et. al. Randomised controlled trial of Alexander technique lessons, exercise, and massage (ATEAM) for chronic and recurrent back pain. BMJ 2008;337:884.
118 Sherman KJ, Cherkin DC, Erro J, et. al. Comparing yoga, exercise, and a self care book for chronic low back pain: a randomised controlled trial. Ann Intern Med 2005 Dec 20;143(12):849–56.
119 William KA, Petronis J, Smith D, et. al. Effect of Iyengar yoga therapy for chronic low back pain. Pain 2005 May;115(1-2):107–17.
120 Galantino ML, Bzdewka TM, Eisser-Russo JL, et. al. The impact of modified Hatha Yoga on chronic low back pain. Altern Ther health Med 2004 Mar-April;10(2):56–9.
121 Grossel EJ, Weingart KR, Aschbacher K, et. al. Yoga for veterans with chronic low back pain. J Altern Complement Med 2008 Nov;14(9):1123–9.
122 Mehling We, Hamel KA, Acree M, et. al. Randomized, controlled trial of breath therapy for patients with chronic low back pain. Altern Ther Health Med 2005 Jul-Aug;11(4):44–52.
123 Swenson R, Haldeman S. Spinal Manipulation therapy for low back pain. A Am Acad Orthop Surg 2003 Jul-Aug;11(4):228–37.
124 Assendelft WJ, Morton SC, Yu EI, et. al. Spinal manipulation therapy for low back pain. Cochrane Database of Systematic Reviews 2004 Issue 1 Art No. CD000447 doi: 10. 1002/14651858. CD000447.pub 2.
125 Assendelft WJ, Morton SC, Yu EI, et. al. Spinal manipulation therapy for low back pain Cochrane Database of Systematic Reviews 2004 Issue 1 Art No. CD000447 doi: 10. 1002/14651858. CD000447.pub 2.
126 Bronfort G, Haas M, Evans, et. al. Efficacy of spinal manipulation and mobilization for low back pain and neck pain: a systematic review and best evidence synthesis. Spine 2004 May-June;4(3):335–56.

127 Lawrence DJ, Meeker W, Branson R, et. al. Chiropractic management of low back pain and low back pain related leg complaints: a literature review. J Manipulative Physiol Ther 2008 Nov-Dec;31(9):659–74.

128 Harvey E, Burton AK, Moffet JK, et. al. Spinal manipulation for low back pain: a treatment package agreed to by the UK chiropractic, osteopathy and physiotherapy professional associations. Man Ther 2003 Feb;8(1):46–51.

129 UK BEAM Trial Team United Kingdom back pain exercise and manipulation (UK BEAM) randomised trial: cost effectiveness of physical treatments for back pain in primary care. BMJ 2004 Dec 11;329(7479):1381.

130 UK BEAM Trial Team United Kingdom back pain exercise and manipulation (UK BEAM) randomised trial: cost effectiveness of physical treatments for back pain in primary care. BMJ 2004 Dec 11;329(7479):1377.

131 Canter PH, Ernst E. Sources of bias in reviews of spinal manipulation for back pain. Wien Klin Wochenschr 2005 May;117(9-10):333–41.

132 Furlan Ad, Imamura M, Dryden T. Massage for low back pain. Cochrane Database for Systematic Reviews 2008, Issue 4. Art.No.: CD001929. doi 10.1002/14651858.CD001929.pub2.

133 Urrutia G, Burton AK, Morral A. Neuroreflexotherapy for non-specific low back pain. Cochrane Data base of Systematic Reviews 2006(3).

134 Furian Ad, van Tulder MW, Cherkin D, et. al. Acupuncture and dry-needling for low back pain. Cochrane Database of Systematic Reviews 2005, Issue 1. Art. No:CDOO1351. doi: 10.1002/14651858.CD001351.pub2.

135 Dagenais S, Yelland MJ, Del Mar C. Prolotherapy injections for chronic low back pain. Cochrane Database of Systematic. Reviews 2007 Issue 2 Art. No.: CDoo4059 doi: 10.1002/14651858. CD004059.pub3.

Chapter 28

Oral health disorders

Introduction

Holistic dentistry is defined as the practice of dental medicine, the core principle of which is: oral health and the body's health are intimately connected.[1] Holistic dentistry focuses on the whole person and supports their physical, social, psychological, emotional and spiritual wellbeing. It is health promoting and emphasises lifestyle advice such as behaviour modification, dietary changes, stress management, exercise, appropriate sunshine exposure, environmental advice, and integrates appropriate complementary therapies where necessary to improve dental and oral health. Good communication and providing clear education guidelines to dental patients to promote good dental care, especially healthy behaviour patterns (e.g. regular teeth brushing and flossing) to encourage adherence to oral hygiene, is an important aspect of dental treatment.

Lifestyle factors, other than dietary factors, can play an important role in the prevention and management of oral health and dentists and health practitioners are in a unique position to reinforce lifestyle advice to complement dental care. Many dentists worldwide are already reinforcing the importance of maintaining good oral health through a healthy diet, regular brushing, teeth flossing and mouth washes. A small growing number of dentists in Australia and worldwide are practising holistic dentistry, however very few integrate complementary therapies that include acupuncture and homeopathy.[1–4]

Communication with dental practitioners

Communication plays an important role in the practitioner-patient relationship and contributes to positive health outcomes. Dentists who communicate with patients about their dental fears can help to significantly alleviate dental anxiety. A trial of anxious patients (n = 119) who completed Spielberger's State Anxiety Inventory (STAI-S) pre- and post-treatment, were randomly allocated to intervention (dentist informed of anxiety score) and control (dentist not informed) groups. Communication was able to reduce the patients' level of anxiety and significantly reduce anxiety scores during dental procedure.[5] The study concluded that providing the dentist with information regarding the high level of a patient's dental anxiety prior to treatment and involving the patient with this, helped reduce the patient's overall anxiety with dental treatment.

Relationship between oral and general health

It is well recognised that ageing and a number of drugs and medical diseases such as cancers, blood disorders, lung disease, infections, gut and/or malabsorption diseases can impact on oral and dental health. So attending to general health issues and treatment of diseases, particularly chronic diseases, may assist in improving oral health.

What is less well recognised is that dental health may actually impact and affect physical health and medical diseases that can then go on to affect the rest of the body. A new growing body of evidence now suggests that oral health can potentially impact on general health.[6] For example, periodontal disease appears to be associated with increased risk of cardiovascular disease (CVD).

Periodontal disease (PD) and risk of diseases

Periodontal disease, also known as periodontitis, is a chronic bacterial infection of the gums and teeth.

PD and CVD

Recent research suggests that PD may have a systemic effect and increase the risk of CVD, including coronary heart disease, myocardial infarction, peripheral vascular disease and stroke.[6–11] The exact mechanism to explain this correlation is not clear, but may be linked to bacterial infections associated with PD and atherosclerotic plaque formation.[12]

PD and diabetes mellitus

There is also an association of PD with poorly controlled diabetes in patients with

Type 2 diabetes mellitus (T2DM). Improved periodontal health may benefit diabetes and metabolic control in type 2 diabetes mellitus.[13, 14, 15] For example, in a study, non-surgical periodontal treatment involving a full-mouth scaling and root planing led to a statistically significant improvement in plaque index, gingival index, probing pocket depth, clinical attachment levels and bleeding on probing, and improved HbA1c levels and glycaemic control in type 2 diabetic patients compared with the control group that received no periodontal treatment. Similarly, a recent randomised control trial (RCT) also demonstrated improved glycaemic control with periodontal treatment in type 2 diabetic patients.[16] However, the difference in improved glycaemic control for type 1 diabetics was not as significant compared with control group following PD treatment.[17] The benefits appear to be confined to type 2 diabetics.

PD and effect on other diseases

An epidemiological study suggests PD may increase the risk of chronic obstructive pulmonary disease,[18] and may also increase the risk of adverse pregnancy outcomes and osteoporosis, although further research is warranted.[19]

Prevention

Tooth brushing

According to a Cochrane review of 42 trials involving 3855 participants, compared to manual toothbrushes, powered toothbrushes with a rotation oscillation action provides better protection against gum inflammation (gingivitis) and plaque removal.[20]

Chewing gum

Mastic or chewing gum can play an important role in prevention of caries. The benefits of chewing gum are based on its ability to stimulate salivary flow which helps promote food clearance from the mouth and reduce bacterial growth in saliva, such as *Streptococcus mutans*, and consequent plaque formation on teeth.[21, 22] A study found the total number of bacterial colonies was significantly reduced during the 4 hours of chewing mastic gum compared to the placebo gum and significantly reduced plaque index and gingival index compared to the placebo group.[23]

Chewing gums containing sugar substitute products such as xylitol are very effective for preventing dental caries by stimulating the salivary flow, although an antimicrobial effect cannot be excluded. Xylitol appears to be superior to the other sugar alcohols such as sorbitol, mannitol, maltitol, lactitol and the products Lycasin and Palatinit for caries control. Xylitol is a polyol sugar alcohol and is naturally sourced from plums, strawberries, raspberries and rowan berries. A number of trials suggest xylitol is more effective than those sweetened with sorbitol for reduction of caries[24, 25, 26] however, another review of all clinical trials concluded that chewing sugar-free gum 3 or more times daily for prolonged periods of time may reduce caries incidence irrespective of the type of sugar alcohol used.[27] Xylitol is not fermented by bacteria and causes a fall in plaque pH by having an inhibitory effect on *mutans streptococci*.

One study found a significant statistical reduction in the number of bacteria *mutans streptococci* found in saliva and plaque with a chewing program using xylitol-only chewing gums compared with xylitol-sorbitol chewing gum or control in 8-year old children over a 39-month period.[28] Another study suggested a different mechanism for xylitol chewing gum benefit in preventing caries in children.[29] This study demonstrated 5 grams of xylitol-containing chewing gums in children over a 14-day period reduced the glucose-initiated lactic acid formation in supragingival plaque by up to 22% compared with baseline and the control group. The authors concluded reducing lactic acid formation may play a more important role in reducing plaque formation, as the numbers of salivary mutans streptococci were unaffected in this study.[29]

Chewing gum combined with vitamin C

An RCT of chewing gum containing vitamin C (60mg) and gum containing vitamin C and carbamide (30mg + 30mg) were compared to placebo.[30] A significant reduction in the total calculus score was observed after the use of vitamin C (33%) and vitamin C + carbamide (12%) gums compared with no gum use, especially in the heavy calculus formers. Vitamin C also reduced the number of bleeding sites (37%) and a reduced amount of visible plaque was observed after use of vitamin C and non-vitamin C gum. Carbamide added to vitamin C in chewing gum did not offer more benefit.[30]

Halitosis

Mouth rinses for halitosis

A Cochrane review of 5 RCTs found mouth rinses containing antibacterial agents such as chlorhexidine and cetylpyridinium chloride may play an important role in reducing the levels of halitosis-producing bacteria on the tongue, and mouth rinses containing chlorine dioxide or zinc can be effective in neutralisation of odoriferous sulfur compounds.[31] However, there is sufficient evidence to suggest that alcohol-based mouth rinses should be avoided due to their association with oral and pharyngeal cancer, and should not be recommended.[32–36]

Warm salt water rinses are a safer option.

Tongue scraping for treating halitosis

A Cochrane review of 2 trials involving 40 participants found tongue scrapers or cleaners are slightly more effective than toothbrushes as a means of controlling halitosis in adults.[37]

Sunlight

Sunshine is the main source of vitamin D produced by the body in response to direct skin exposure to ultraviolet B (UVB). Consequently, nil or minimal exposure to sun can contribute to vitamin D deficiency as seen in many community groups with dress codes (e.g. wearing veils), those living in geographically prone areas, especially over winter (southern or northern latitudes), those working indoors (e.g. office work), institutionalisation, prolonged hospitalisation and the bed-bound (e.g. stroke, elderly), and particularly in dark-skinned people who need longer sun exposure.[38, 39] Vitamin D plays an important role in dental health (see the section on vitamin D below).

Environment

Mercury exposure

Dental amalgam is the most commonly used material in restorative dentistry. Dental amalgam is an alloy of silver, tin, copper and mercury.[40] Mercury vapour absorption through the lungs (by dental practitioners or patients) or accidental oral ingestion of mercury from cracked teeth containing amalgams (by patients) are the main sources of mercury exposure in dentistry. The safety of mercury exposure from amalgam fillings has been explored in Australia.[41] The findings of the National Health and Medical Research Council (NHMRC) working party concluded there was a lack of evidence to confirm dangers associated with mercury toxicity from amalgams and no studies exploring health outcomes amongst dental patients with and without amalgams and neurotoxicity. Based on current evidence, the NHMRC working party also concluded there is no role for removal protocols and concomitant therapeutic regimens, such as chelation therapy, for patients attributing symptoms to mercury from dental amalgam restorations. The NHMRC working party claim that the release of mercury is at a slow rate from dental amalgams, generally of a few micrograms per person per day among adults dependent upon variables such as number and shape of fillings, eating habits, and bruxism. For the current mean numbers of amalgam fillings in Australian children and adults (0.5 and 8, respectively), daily mercury absorption per person is about 0.3μg and 3.5μg, respectively, which is tenfold and twofold (respectively) higher than dietary sources of mercury retained in the body.[19]

However, there have since been more studies exploring effects of amalgam in children. A study of 507 children (aged 8–10 years) with at least 1 carious lesion on a permanent tooth and no previous exposure to amalgam were randomised to receive routine dental care during the 7-year trial period, 1 group receiving amalgam restorations (n = 253) and the other group receiving resin composite restorations (n = 254). Baseline mean creatinine-adjusted urinary mercury levels were 1.0–1.5mg/g higher in the amalgam group than in the composite group ($P<0.001$) at the 7-year follow-up. This study found no significant differences in measures of memory, attention, visuomotor function or nerve-conduction velocities for the groups over the 7 years of follow-up.[42]

A recent RCT of 534 children (aged 6–10 years) involving 5 community health settings compared neuropsychological and renal function of children whose dental caries were restored using amalgam or mercury-free materials.[43] Children with no prior amalgam restorations and ≥2 posterior teeth with caries were randomised to receive dental restoration during a 5-year follow-up period using either amalgam or resin composite (non-amalgam) materials. The researchers found higher mean urinary mercury levels in children with amalgams at 5- and 7-year follow-up respectively but no significant differences in IQ, memory, attention/concentration and motor and visuomotor performance in either group.

Amalgam use in children and renal concerns

A study of 403 children in Shanghai found minimal differences in mean urinary mercury concentration for children with and without amalgam fillings, and no differences for either renal function biomarker, or on neurobehavioural, neuropsychological, or intelligence tests.[44]

However, in the New England Children's Amalgam Trial there was a significantly increased prevalence of microalbuminuria among children in the amalgam group in years 3–5 (adjusted odds ratio [OR] 1.8; 95% confidence interval [CI], 1.1–2.9) compared with the composite group (p = 0.04) with no differences in levels of renal tubular markers — alpha1-microglobulin (A1M), gamma-glutamyl transpeptidase (gamma-GT) and for N-acetyl-beta-D-glucosaminidase (NAG).[45] A sub-study of the New England Children's Amalgam Trial collected 82 pairs of urine samples from children aged 10–16 years and found the creatinine-corrected excretions of albumin, gamma-GT, and NAG were significantly higher in daytime samples than in overnight samples, with a non-significant trend for A1M.[46] Another study also found significantly higher levels of mercury in blood and urine and higher urinary excretion of NAG, gamma-GT and albumin in persons with dental amalgams than those without.[47] Albuminuria and urinary excretion of NAG significantly correlated with the number of fillings. The authors concluded from:

> ... the nephrotoxicity point of view, dental amalgam is an unsuitable filling material, as it may give rise to Hg toxicity' and based on the mercury levels in blood and urine 'renal damage is possible.[47]

There is considerable international controversy over the safety of mercury amalgam (fillings). In 2008, Norway, Denmark and Sweden totally banned the use of mercury products, including fillings, in their countries.[48, 49, 50]

Mercury in food

It is well recognised that mercury enters the food chain from naturally occurring mercury (as sulfides) or from air pollutants (e.g. industrial or vehicle exhaust pollution) deposited in sea, rivers and lakes and is transformed into methyl mercury by bacteria in the water. The methyl mercury is ingested by small fish and algae and consequently accumulates and builds up in larger and older predatory fish that are at the top of the food chain. Foods Standards Australia New Zealand (FSANZ) advises pregnant women, women planning pregnancy and young children should limit their intake of shark (flake), broadbill, marlin and swordfish to no more than 1 serve per fortnight with no other fish to be consumed during that fortnight due to risks of mercury toxicity.[51] Those at risk of mercury toxicity are children, the unborn infant of pregnant women and newborns who are breastfeeding (exposure via the breast milk) from mothers who frequently (more than once a week) eat large predator species of fish. The developing nervous system of a fetus and children are particularly susceptible to the ill effects of high methyl mercury levels that can cause a multitude of symptoms such as nausea, vomiting, lack of appetite, weight loss, kidney failure, skin irritations, respiratory distress, swollen gums, mouth sores, neurological symptoms such as paraesthesia, numbness, seizures, tremors and incoordination, and mental retardation.[52]

Conclusion on mercury

Concerns associated with direct mercury toxicity via accidental inhalation and ingestion are real. Amalgams may be best avoided in pregnant women and young children, especially those with kidney disease or renal impairment, although there are very few studies exploring long-term health concerns. Dentists and dental health practitioners may also be at risk, although there are strict guidelines for discarding solid waste from lost or extracted teeth with amalgam fillings and amalgam-contaminated waste, which are carefully contained and in most instances incinerated. Proper collection of mercury-contaminated solid waste using high-frequency suction (while wearing a mask) prevents the release of mercury vapour during combustion. The use of rubber dams stops contaminated saliva secretions and amalgam debris from entering the oral cavity of the patient, minimising mercury exposure.[53]

Cadmium (Cd) exposure

Periodontal disease

Environmental cadmium (Cd) exposure is known to adversely affect bone remodelling and is associated with higher odds of periodontal disease. Analysis of data from the 3rd National Health and Nutrition Examination Survey (NHANES III) of 11 412 participants included in the study found 15.4% of participants had periodontal disease with a mean urine Cd concentration significantly higher among participants with periodontal disease [0.50; 95% CI, 0.45–0.56] compared with participants without periodontal disease [0.30; 95% CI, 0.28–0.31].[54] After adjusting for tobacco exposure, there was a further significant threefold increase in creatinine-corrected urinary Cd concentrations from the 25th (0.18 mug/g) to the 75th (0.63 mug/g) percentile associated with a significant 54% greater risk of prevalent periodontal disease (OR = 1.54; 95% CI, 1.26–1.87).

Smoking

Cigarette smoking, cigar and pipe use in smokers significantly increases the risk of developing a range of dental health problems, including increased risk of caries, gingivitis, tooth loss, ulcer formation, oral cancers and PD.[55] In general, smokers are 4–20 times more likely to develop periodontitis compared with persons who never smoked and, amongst current smokers, 74.8% of their periodontitis was attributable to smoking.[56, 57] Smoking is a major preventable risk factor for PD and chronic destructive PD.

Smoking can adversely affect dental health by various mechanisms, such as defects in neutrophil function and host defences from nicotine leading to bacterial invasion and plaque formation, impairment of inflammatory and immune responses, increased alveolar bone loss, pocket formation and attachment loss, including adverse local and systemic effects (e.g. heart and lung disease).[58, 59] Smoking also reduces wound healing following local trauma and dental treatment.

Smokers are also exposed to various chemicals and heavy metals, such as cadmium and lead from cigarette smoking, which are associated with PD and may aggravate existing renal impairment.[60]

Smoking cessation can significantly reduce the risk of PD and increase the likelihood of tooth retention but it may take decades for this to happen.[61]

Sleep and dental pain

Oral pain that impacts on sleep is a common presentation to dentists. Other than oral pain, dentists may also be confronted with pain from orofacial and temperomandibular junction (TMJ) disorders. Pain is well known to disrupt numerous aspects of normal physical and psychological life, including work, social activities and sleep.[62, 63, 64]

Mind–body therapy

Dental anxiety

Dental anxiety is a common problem. High dental anxiety can be overwhelming for an individual and is strongly associated with poor oral health, particularly due to treatment avoidance. Studies of 272 adult private dental practice patients were assessed for anxiety, frequency of oral health care visits in the last 10 years and their preferred method to alleviate anxiety.[65]

Twenty-six participants (9.56%) scored high in dental anxiety. The study demonstrated that high anxiety was associated with infrequent oral health care visits and dental patients employ numerous strategies for reducing anxiety. They concluded that oral health care practitioners need to be aware of the patient's preferred technique for coping with anxiety and encourage them to use self-help techniques.

Mind–body techniques such as cognitive behaviour therapy (CBT), self-help techniques, relaxation and music therapy and exercise can be useful and effective for the management of panic and fear [see Chapter 4, anxiety].[66, 67, 68] Many of these techniques can also help address psychological symptoms associated with dental anxiety and fear.

Psychological interventions — general

A Cochrane systematic review identified 4 studies that assessed psychological interventions aimed at increasing compliance of oral hygiene in adult patients with PD.[69]

A total of 344 patients participated. Overall, whilst the quality of the studies were poor, there was evidence that psychological approaches improved self-efficacy beliefs in relation to flossing and improved behaviour patterns for oral hygiene related behaviours.

Brief relaxation and music distraction

A prospective RCT compared a brief relaxation method with music distraction and a control group.[70] Ninety patients with dental anxiety were randomised to either of the 3 groups. Both brief relaxation and music distraction reduced dental anxiety significantly. Brief relaxation was significantly superior to music distraction over the control group. Patients in the control group demonstrated no significant change in anxiety level.

The authors concluded brief relaxation was safe, economically sound and effective as a non-pharmacological approach to managing dental anxiety.

A trial of 44 adult subjects requiring surgery for root canal treatment procedure were randomised to a music group, which listened to selected sedative music using headphones throughout the root canal treatment procedure, or a control group where subjects wore headphones but without the music.[71] Heart rate, blood pressure and finger temperature were measured before the study and every 10 minutes until the end of the root canal treatment procedure. The level of anxiety experienced by the patient was measured before the study and at the end of the treatment procedure. The results revealed that there were no significant differences between the 2 groups for baseline data and procedure-related characteristics, except for gender. The music group showed a significant increase in finger temperature and a reduction in anxiety score over time compared with the control group. The authors concluded the findings:

> ... provide evidence for nurses and dentists that the use of soothing music for anxiety reduction in patients undergoing root canal treatment procedures is supported by research findings.[71]

Virtual image audio-visual eyeglass system

Virtual image, audio-visual (AV) eyeglasses may play a role in dental anxiety and pain. In a study of 27 patients, the participants completed a Dental Fear Survey and the Fear of Pain Questionnaire-III before dental treatment.[72] They were randomised to either watch and listen to a standard video using AV eyeglasses or not (control group). The AV eyeglass group demonstrated rescued anxiety and discomfort compared with control group. Patients showed a preference to use AV equipment compared to the traditional approach of no glasses and there was a significant reduction in treatment time in the first half of the dental procedure. Clinicians experienced no significant technical interference with their dental work by using the AV eyeglasses. The authors concluded AV virtual image eyeglasses may be beneficial in the reduction of fear, pain and procedure time for most dental patients.[72]

Hypnosis and dental anxiety

Pre-existing anxiety and cognitions about dental procedures can predict dental anxiety. Hypnosis may be helpful for some patients, but not all. A study found that patient characteristics such as hypnotisability, trait anxiety and negative cognitions can predict which people develop dental anxiety and who will be more responsive to hypnosis.[73] Rapid hypnotic induction techniques by oral health practitioners (dentists or dental nurses) can be useful for treating anxious patients prior to procedures.[74] Children may be more receptive to hypnosis. A double-blind, control trial of 29 children (ages 4–13) were randomised to both hypnosis group and a no hypnosis group before a local anaesthetic injection for a dental procedure.[75] Each subject was evaluated during utilisation of hypnosis before injection, and once without. Subjects were videotaped during the procedure and behaviour rated independently by 2 paediatric dentists, using the North Carolina Behaviour Rating Scale (NBRS). They found hypnosis significantly reduced pulse rate and crying, especially in the 4–6 year-old children.

Behavioural therapy for dental fear

Behaviour therapy may offer more benefit in reducing dental fear compared with hypnosis. In a study with 22 women (mean age of 31.8 years) who suffered dental fear and avoided dental care (median time of 9.5 years), participated in a clinical study and were randomly assigned to 1 of 2 groups; hypnotherapy (HT) versus behavioural treatment based on psychophysiological principles (PP).[76] Both therapies involved 8 sessions followed by standardised conventional dental test treatments. Pre- and post-treatment measures were dental fear, general fear, mood, and patient behaviour. PP group statistically significantly reduced dental fear and improved mood during dental situations compared with HT group. General fear levels insignificantly reduced. Overall 11 of the 22 patients completed the conventional dental treatment without complications, indicating that they were more relaxed during the treatment.

Relaxation oriented therapy (ROT) versus cognitively oriented therapy (COT)

A study of 112 adults that were found to be fearful of dental treatments reported that those who received COT by a trained psychologist prior to specialist care were more likely to complete the treatment program, but those who received ROT were more likely to experience significantly less generalised anxiety and fear, and dental fear during the procedure.[77] Dropouts were related to lower motivation (willingness to engage in dental treatment), and failed treatment was related to higher levels of general fear and anxiety. This study concluded that both COT and ROT interventions were effective in helping to reduce dental phobic reactions and to complete dental care, and that motivation was a significant predictor of treatment outcome.

An additional study compared ROT and COT with nitrous oxide sedation (NOS). Sixty-five patients with severe dental fear were randomly assigned to COT, ROT or NOS over 10 weekly sessions of individual therapy.[78] Overall there were low dropout rates. All patients who completed the therapy sessions completed dental treatment and anxiety scores on dental fear tests significantly reduced in all treatment groups. There were no major differences between each group or with the advent of any serious adverse events. Furthermore, on following up these participants at 1 year after initiating the trial with 62 patients, it was reported that 95% of the participants had attended dental treatment with continued favourable effects with respect to dental fear and general distress. The relaxation group established the greatest reductions on the dental fear measures.[79] All patients judged the 3 interventions namely, COT, ROT and NOS as beneficial for dental fear. Of the participants, 80% judged the treatment given in the year after the dental fear treatment as successful and all 3 treatment groups scored in the normative range for general distress both at the end of treatment and at follow-up.

In a further 5-year follow-up study of 43 patients, it was observed that the majority (81%) of the participants assessed the dental fear treatment they received 5 years previously to have been useful for dental fear and general psychological distress for participants in all 3 treatment groups.[80]

Diet

It is well established that nutritional intake plays a vital and significant role in oral and bone health. A number of reports have demonstrated that poor nutrition significantly affects teeth during development, exacerbates PD and dental diseases, craniofacial development (from *in utero*), risk of oral cancer and oral infections.[81, 82]

Dairy intake — calcium and vitamin D

Low dietary calcium intake is associated with reduced bone mass and increased risk of osteoporosis. Best sources of calcium foods include dairy products (milk, yoghurts and cheese), fish (sardines with bones), green leafy vegetables and fruits. The recommended dietary allowance for calcium is 800mg/day.[83] Vitamin D deficiency is associated with rickets in children, osteoporosis; osteomalacia (reduced mineralisation of bone) and is common in the elderly and dark skinned people. The best source of vitamin D is from sun exposure. (Refer to Chapter 30 on osteoporosis for more information on calcium and vitamin D.)

Early childhood caries (ECC)

ECC is preventable and affects very young children, especially those from low-income families and certain racial and ethnic minorities. Dental caries are due to a combination of factors, including colonisation of teeth with cariogenic bacteria, food types, frequency of exposure of these foods to the cariogenic bacteria, duration of breastfeeding, fluoride content in fluids and susceptible teeth, especially in very young children.

Data from the Third National Health and Nutrition Examination Survey (NHANES III) of 2- to 5-year-old children, found those consuming best dietary practices (uppermost tertile of the Healthy Eating Index [HEI]) were 44% less likely to exhibit severe ECC compared with children with the worst dietary practices (lowest tertile of the HEI).[84]

Sugars

Dental caries are more prevalent if sugars are consumed more frequently, particularly if retained in the mouth for long periods of time.[85] Sucrose forms glucan in the mouth that facilitates firm bacterial adhesion to teeth and limits diffusion of acid and buffers in the plaque.

Children should be encouraged to eat healthy snacks and foods, and discouraged from sugars and frequent consumption of juice, sugary drinks, snacks and sugary foods e.g. lollies, chocolates, toffees, lollipops. Children should be encouraged to brush their teeth immediately if consuming these foods.

Soft drinks

Five to 6 servings per week of soft drinks, particularly cola, are recognised as a risk factor and linked to low bone mineral density and osteoporosis according to a population study of over 2500 adults.[86] The harmful effects of soft drinks on general, dental and oral health are well confirmed.

Acidic diet and caries

It is well recognised that an acidic diet promotes caries. A study of 309 children's diets found that large consumption of high-acidic beverages (e.g. fruit juices), vinegar, fruit, vitamin C supplements with low consumption of water and milk is associated with increased risk in caries and erosion.[87] A recent Australian study investigated the erosive potential of beverages in schools.[88] This study found that the majority of the tested beverages sold from school canteens exhibited erosive potential.

Table 28.1 lists the acidity of common drinks. A pH less than 5.0 should generally be reduced or avoided. Water and milk are preferred drinks to maintain good oral health.

Table 28.1 Acidity of common drinks

Beverages	Acidity pH
Water	7.0
Milk	6.8
Flat mineral water	5.3
Soda water	5.1
Apricot yoghurt	5.1
Beer and/or wine	4.0
Sparkling mineral water	3.9
Orange juice	3.6
Apple juice	3.4
Diet coke	3.0
Ribena	2.8
Lemonade and Fanta®	2.7
Powerade	2.7
Coca cola® and Pepsi®	2.3
Vinegar	2.2
Lemon juice	2.0

Nutritional supplements

Vitamins

Vitamin D

Vitamin D has a pivotal role in bone metabolism, it controls intestinal calcium absorption plus its deposition into bone.[89] The main source of vitamin D is sunlight exposure (see Figure 28.1). Ninety percent of vitamin D is produced in the skin from sunshine exposure (UVB) with only 10% from dietary sources. Dietary sources include fatty fish (e.g. mackerel), cod liver oil, sun-exposed mushrooms and liver. The majority of women with osteoporosis have vitamin D deficiency and resulting bone loss.[90] The Geelong Vitamin D Study on postmenopausal women found that the majority of the participants were vitamin D deficient during winter.[91]

Vitamin D deficiency is likely to be the commonest nutritional deficiency in many countries, and may well be the most important one.[92–97] Risk factors for vitamin D deficiency include dark skin colour, dress codes (e.g. wearing veils), migrants, infants of migrant families, living in geographical prone areas, especially over winter (southern or northern latitude), institutionalisation, bed-bound, intellectual disability, prolonged and exclusive breastfeeding, restricted sun exposure,

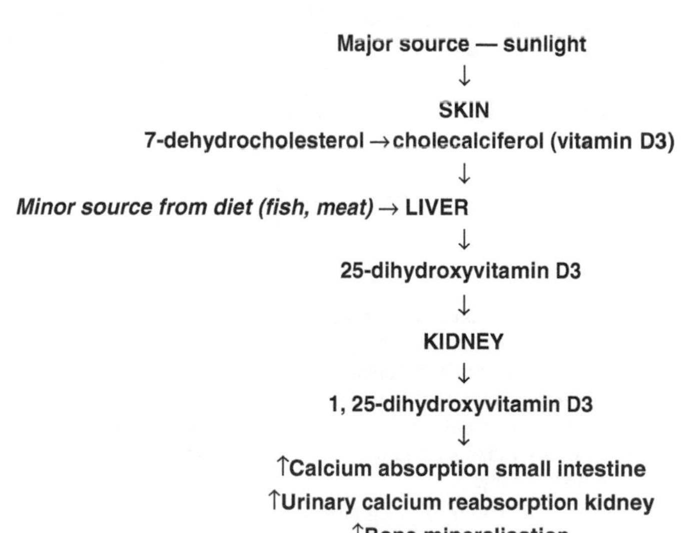

Figure 28.1 Major sources of sunlight
(Source: adapted from Nowson CA, Diamond TH, Psco JA, et. al. *Australian Family Physician*. 2004;33(3):133–8)

and certain medical conditions. Vitamin D deficiency has re-emerged as a public health issue particularly affecting infants and young children, potentially causing hypocalcemia, seizures, rickets, limb pain, tooth loss and poor dentition and risk of fracture.[98–104] Breastfed infants of mothers who were vitamin D deficient during pregnancy were at high risk of vitamin D deficiency.[105]

A position statement released recently by the Australian and New Zealand Bone and Mineral Society and Osteoporosis Australia and the Endocrine Society of Australia is summarised in Figure 28.2.[106]

Improved bone mineral density (BMD)

A large RCT of elderly people over a 5-year period demonstrated vitamin D combined with calcium supplementation has long-term benefit on BMD compared with calcium alone or control group, particularly in subjects with sub-optimal vitamin D levels.[107] Moreover, it is well documented that throughout the lifecycle the skeleton requires optimum development and maintenance of its integrity to prevent fracture. The data is promising for the use of combined calcium with vitamin D and the use of vitamin K.[108]

Periodontal disease (PD)

Numerous articles indicate vitamin D and calcium deficiency are associated with bone loss and increased inflammation, which are well recognised symptoms of PD. Whilst studies suggest calcium and vitamin D may benefit periodontal health and calcium deficiency may be a risk factor for periodontal disease, there are no RCTs done to date to test this hypothesis.[109]

Vitamin D and calcium enhances tooth retention

A placebo-controlled trial of 145 healthy subjects aged over 65 years were randomised over a 3-year period to calcium or vitamin D supplementation to assess bone loss from the hip. Furthermore, participants were further followed up for 2-years after discontinuation of study supplements and teeth were counted at 18 months and 5 years.[110] During the trial, subjects were less likely to lose 1 or more teeth (13%) whilst taking calcium and vitamin D supplements compared with a larger proportion of subjects (27%) whilst taking placebo. At the 2-year follow-up period, of those with total calcium intake >1000mg/day, 31 of 77 subjects (40%) lost 1 or more teeth compared with a larger proportion of 40 of 68 subjects (59%) who consumed less calcium.

Recommended dosage is calcium citrate 800mg/day or calcium carbonate 1000mg/day.

Vitamin B complex

Vitamin B may help wound healing post-surgery for PD. A randomised, double-blind, placebo-controlled trial of 30 patients with moderate to severe chronic periodontitis found that vitamin B complex at a dose of 50mg/day supplementation, in combination with surgery for 30 days following access flap surgery for PD, resulted in significantly better wound healing and clinical attachment levels up to 180 days compared with placebo and surgery.[111]

During the decades of the 1980s and 1990s several case reports of peripheral neuropathy associated with high-dose pyridoxine appeared in the scientific literature, where the consumption in most of the reported cases was of dosages that ranged from 1–5g per day.[112] Vitamin B6 is usually safe at intakes up to a maximum of 200mg/day in adults for short-term supplementation. However, vitamin B6 can cause neurological disorders, such as loss of sensation in legs and imbalance, when taken in high doses (50 mg or more per day) over a long period of time. Vitamin B6 toxicity can damage sensory nerves, leading to numbness in the hands and feet as well as difficulty

- Balance of evidence remains in favour of fracture prevention from combined calcium and vitamin D supplementation in elderly men and women.
- Adequate vitamin D status is essential for active calcium absorption in the gut and for bone development and remodelling.
- In adults with a baseline calcium intake of 500–900mg/day, increasing or supplementing this intake by a further 500–1000mg/day has a beneficial effect on bone mineral density.
- Calcium intake significantly above the recommended level is unlikely to achieve additional benefit for bone health.

Figure 28.2 Position statement: calcium and bone health

(Source: Australian and New Zealand Bone and Mineral Society and Osteoporosis Australia and the Endocrine Society of Australia, 2009)[106]

walking. Symptoms of a pyridoxine overdose may include poor coordination, peripheral neuropathy, staggering, numbness, decreased sensation to touch, temperature, and vibration and tiredness for up to 6 months. It is important to note though that there is a requisite to avoid overuse of single vitamin products (e.g. oral and injectable forms of vitamin B6) or concomitant use of multivitamin products that could lead to some patients routinely exceeding the upper limit for vitamins and hence risk severe toxicity.[113]

Vitamin C (ascorbate)

Low dietary intake of vitamin C is associated with increased risk of PD, particularly in past and present smokers.[114] Those with lowest vitamin C levels demonstrated greater clinical effects of PD. The effect appeared to be dose-responsive. For those taking 0–29mg/day of vitamin C the odds ratio (OR) for PD was 1.30 and for those taking 100–179mg/day the OR was 1.16, compared to those taking 180mg or more of vitamin C per day.

Multivitamins

Wound healing

The importance of nutritional intake for wound healing is well established.[115, 116] For example, the elderly are particularly prone to nutritional deficiencies due to various factors such as poor dentition, relying on dentures, difficulty chewing food, and being on various medications, and are therefore more likely to suffer chronic diseases. (See Chapter 2 for more information on nutritional assessment.) This makes the elderly more prone to poor wound healing with dental treatment.

Periodontal disease (PD)

In a 60 day, 2-cell, randomised, parallel clinical trial for PD patients, 63 patients were randomised to a vitamin tablet or placebo.[117] Clinical parameters assessed included gingival index (GI), bleeding index (BI), periodontal pocket depth (PD), and attachment levels (AL), all of which were recorded at baseline and at 60 days. After 60 days, the vitamin group demonstrated reduced clinical GI, BI, PD ($P < .0001$) but no significant changes for AL between both groups. However, further analysis of patients with PD > or = 4mm showed the vitamin group demonstrated clinically significant improvements in GI and PD compared with baseline, with no significant differences in BI and AL. The authors concluded 'multi-vitamin nutritional supplement might be a beneficial adjunct to the required established periodontal treatment'.[117]

A review of the literature to assess the effects of nutritional supplements (e.g. vitamin B-complex, vitamin C and dietary calcium) on general wound healing, periodontal disease status and response to periodontal therapy found that multivitamins may have a possible influencing factor on periodontal status and wound healing but more studies are required.[118]

Minerals

Magnesium

A cross-sectional epidemiological study of 4290 subjects (aged 20–80 years) recorded periodontal risk factors, serum magnesium and calcium levels, relating them to periodontal parameters.[119] Magnesium deficiency was found to be associated with PD. In a matched-pair study, 60 subjects using oral magnesium-containing drugs and 120 without were compared. Subjects aged over 40 years with higher serum magnesium and calcium was significantly associated with reduced probing depth ($p<0.001$), less attachment loss ($p = 0.006$), and an increased number of remaining teeth ($p = 0.005$). Subjects taking magnesium supplementation showed less attachment loss ($p<0.01$) and more remaining teeth than the control group. The authors concluded that these results suggest 'nutritional Mg supplementation may improve periodontal health'.[119]

Calcium

Whilst the association of low dietary calcium intake with periodontal disease is well recognised, a statistically significant association occurred for low total serum calcium and periodontal disease found in young females (20–39 years) with OR of 6.11 (95% CI: 2.36 to 15.84), after adjusting for tobacco use, gingival bleeding, and dietary calcium intake.[120] However, further studies are warranted to better define the role of calcium supplementation effect on risk of PD and tooth loss.

Fluoride

A number of studies confirm the value of oral ingestion and topical use of toothpastes, mouth rinses, varnishes and gels for their naturally occurring mineral fluoride; preventing dental caries and decay.

A Cochrane review of 25 studies involving 7747 children, found the effect of fluoride gel applied topically once or several times yearly by dental health practitioners led to, on average, a 21% reduction in dental caries, 'decayed, missing and filled tooth surfaces' compared with placebo.[121]

Similarly, a Cochrane review of 9 studies involving 2709 children found fluoride varnishes applied professionally 2–4 times a year substantially reduced tooth decay in children compared with no treatment controls.[122]

However, whilst Cochrane reviews found topical fluorides from supervised mouth rinses, varnishes and gels are helpful, they are not any more effective at reducing tooth decay in children and adolescents than using fluoride toothpaste alone.[123–126]

A number of systematic reviews have demonstrated that water fluoridation is associated with reduced dental caries and the number of teeth affected by caries in children.[127]

Fluoride added to the water supply, salt or milk as a public health measure has remained a controversial issue. There is evidence to suggest that there is a possible association between fluoride in drinking water during growth and development (5–10 years) and the incidence of osteosarcoma in boys aged 10–19 years.[128–134] A literature review (1970–2008) of all papers covering possible aetiological factors involved in the development of bone tumours in children and young adults found several associations have been reported with some consistency for osteosarcoma: the presence of hernias and Ewing sarcoma; high fluoride exposure and osteosarcoma; and parental farming and residence on a farm, younger age at puberty and family history of cancer for all bone tumours, especially osteosarcoma.[135] One study found higher levels of serum fluoride levels in 25 case patients with osteosarcoma compared with patients with other bone tumours, suggesting a role of fluoride in the disease.[136] One study also suggested a possible link between fluoride drinking and other tumours, such as brain tumours, T-cell system Hodgkin's disease, Non-Hodgkin lymphoma, multiple myeloma, melanoma of the skin and monocytic leukaemia, and concluded that the likelihood of fluoride being causal for cancer requires further assessment.[137]

However, an association with osteosarcoma risk has been disputed by authorities who have found, based on the research, that fluoridation of drinking water remains the most effective and socially equitable means of achieving community-wide exposure to the caries prevention, when consumed at a safe target range of 0.6–1.1mg/l, depending on the climate.[138–142]

A Cochrane review found that there is insufficient evidence to show that fluoride added to milk can prevent tooth decay.[143] Fluoride use for the prevention of osteoporosis and fractures remains controversial with a meta-analysis demonstrating no improvement, and a more recent study showing improvement in BMD in post-menopausal osteoporosis.[144, 145]

Potassium containing toothpastes — reduces tooth sensitivity

Dentine hypersensitivity is a common problem that causes sudden, sharp teeth pain and discomfort when exposed to touch, hot or cold foods. A Cochrane review of 6 studies found statistically significant effect of 6–8 weeks use of potassium nitrate toothpaste in improving dentine hypersensitivity although trials involved a small number of individuals for a conclusion to be generated.[146]

Zinc combined with herb blood root (*Sanguinaria candensis* extract)

Toothpaste and oral rinse

Sixty subjects with moderate levels of plaque and gingivitis were randomly assigned to a treatment group (combined use of toothpaste and oral rinse containing blood root extract and zinc chloride) and compared to placebo products in a 28-week clinical trial.[147] The treatment group significantly reduced non-invasive measures of plaque (21%), gingivitis (25%), bleeding on probing (43%) compared with placebo group. The product was well tolerated with 3 subjects of the 30 in the treatment group exhibiting minor soft-tissue irritations that resolved spontaneously without discontinuation of treatment.

Other nutritional supplements

Coenzyme Q_{10} (CoQ_{10})-PD

Topical application of CoQ_{10} to the periodontal pocket in 10 male patients suffering periodontitis led to significant improvements in symptoms and signs such as GI and bleeding on probing as a sole treatment or in combination with traditional non-surgical periodontal therapy, warranting more research.[148, 149]

Alpha-lipoic acid (burning mouth syndrome)

Burning mouth syndrome describes a group of symptoms of unknown cause that may include burning sensation of the lips, tongue, mouth, dryness and altered taste. A Cochrane review explored a number of therapies and found there was some evidence alpha-lipoic acid, coping strategies and anti-convulsants may help, but not analgesia, hormone therapies or antidepressants.[150]

Probiotics (caries prevention)

Probiotics may play an important role on oral health benefits. Studies report improvements in mouth flora associated with caries prevention, improved interspecies interactions and improved immuno-modulation effects.[151–55] Additional studies are warranted though.

Herbal medicines

Green tea extract (PD, caries prevention)

Green tea extract mouth rinses may play a role in the treatment of periodontal disease and prevention of dental caries as the green tea catechins can inhibit acid production in dental plaque bacteria.[156]

Blood root (*Sanguinaria candensis*)

When used in a toothpaste and oral rinse, blood root may reduce plaque, gingival inflammation and bleeding parameters for up to 6 months with no adverse effects.[157] However, blood root has produced mixed results in other studies, showing no benefit when used as a dentrifice.[158]

When combined with zinc as an oral rinse, there was demonstrable improvement in reducing plaque (21%), gingivitis (25%), and bleeding on probing (43%) compared with placebo group.[159] It is possible that the zinc component of the dentrifice plays the more important role here in view of the mixed results found in studies with the herb blood root.

Clove oil — analgesia

Clove oil has a long tradition of use in dental care, especially as a topical anaesthetic. In 1 study of 73 adult volunteers, topical agents applied to maxillary canine buccal mucosa were compared in efficacy for dental pain.[160] The 4 substances tested included homemade clove gel, benzocaine 20% gel, placebo that resembled clove, and a placebo resembling benzocaine.

After 5 minutes of application, each participant received 2 needle sticks and pain response was assessed using a 100mm visual analogue pain scale. Both clove and benzocaine gels equally significantly reduced mean pain scores compared with both placebos ($p = 0.005$). The authors concluded clove gel 'might possess a potential to replace benzocaine as a topical agent before needle insertion'.[160]

Eucalyptus extract chewing gum — gingivitis

A randomised placebo-controlled trial of healthy subjects with gingivitis found eucalyptus extract chewing gum could exhibit antibacterial properties and improve periodontal health over 12 weeks.[161] A high-concentration group ($n = 32$) using 0.6% eucalyptus extract chewing gum (90mg/day) was compared to a lower concentration group ($n = 32$) using 0.4% eucalyptus extract chewing gum (60mg/day) and to placebo group ($n = 33$) that used chewing gum without eucalyptus extract. Both eucalyptus chewing gum groups statistically reduced/improved plaque accumulation, improved gingival index, bleeding on probing, periodontal probing depth (PD) but not for clinical attachment level compared with placebo chewing gum.[161]

Table 28.2 summarises potential interactions and adverse effects that can occur during dental surgery if patients are taking complementary medicines and herbal medicines. [161, 163, 164]

Adverse effects of some herbal supplements that may cause rare oral manifestations are summarised in Table 28.3.

Table 28.2 Potential adverse herbal or complementary medicine effects on dental surgery

Effect during dental surgery	Herb or complementary medicine
↑ bleeding time	garlic, ginseng, gingko, glucosamine, high doses of fish oils
↑ sedating effect with anaesthetic	kava, hops, valerian, passionflower
Nutrient–herb–drug interaction(s)	↑ metabolism of many drugs used in the perioperative period (e.g. St John's wort); – bromelain, cayenne, chamomile, feverfew, dong quai, eleuthro/Seberian ginseng, garlic, ginkgo, ginger, ginseng and licorice interacting with aspirin; – aloe latex, ephedra, ginseng, rhubarb, cascara sagrada, licorice, and senna interacting with corticosteriods; – herbs acting on the gastrointestinal system such as slippery elm, altering the absorption of several orally administered drugs.

Physical therapies

Temperomandibular junction (TMJ) disorders

Pain and difficulty opening the oral cavity are features of TMJ disorder.

A systematic review of 12 studies that met inclusion criteria included 4 studies of therapeutic exercise interventions, 2 on acupuncture and 6 on electro-physical modalities to treat TMJ disorders.[165]

In general, postural exercises reduced pain and improved function and oral opening, manual therapy in combination with active exercises reduced pain and improved oral opening, and acupuncture reduced pain compared with no treatment. Also, muscular awareness relaxation therapy, biofeedback training and low-level laser therapy treatment significantly improved oral opening. In another study identified by the review, there were no significant differences in pain outcomes between acupuncture and sham.[165]

In another systematic review of 30 studies, active exercises and manual mobilisations, postural training in combination with other interventions, and mid-laser therapy may be more effective for TMJ disorder.[163] Relaxation techniques, biofeedback, electromyography training, and proprioceptive re-education were more effective than placebo treatment or occlusal splints. Combinations of active exercises, manual therapy, postural correction, and relaxation techniques were also effective for TMJ disorder. [166]

Splints and TMJ disorders

A Cochrane review of 12 RCTs demonstrated that there was no evidence of a statistically significant difference in the effectiveness of stabilisation splint (SS) therapy in reducing symptoms in patients with pain dysfunction syndrome compared with other active treatments such as acupuncture, bite plates, biofeedback, stress management, visual feedback, relaxation, jaw exercises and with no treatment.[167]

Table 28.3 Adverse oral manifestations of some herbs

Herb	Adverse manifestation
Feverfew	Aphthous ulcers, lip and tongue irritation and swelling
Feverfew and ginkgo	Gingival bleeding
Echinacea	Tongue numbness
St John's wort	Xerostomia
Yohimbe	Salivation
Kava	Oral and lingual dyskinesia

Occlusal adjustment for treating and preventing TMJ Disorders

Occlusal adjustment involves adjusting the teeth's biting surfaces with the aim to relieve symptoms of TMJ disorder. A Cochrane review of RCTs found no evidence for the use of occlusal adjustment in preventing or treating TMJ disorders.[168]

Acupuncture

TMJ dysfunction

A study of 60 case reports (50 females, 10 males; mean age of 40.6 years [range 14–68]) with TMJ dysfunction with an average pain score of 3.2 out of 5 explored the benefit of acupuncture for TMJ pain relief.[169] Each patient received acupuncture (mean of 3.4 treatments), lasting on average 12 minutes, by dentists over the TMJ and in the masticatory muscles, points on the neck, and additional relaxing points. There were significant reductions in mean pain scores with beneficial effects observed in 85% of cases and an average reduction in pain intensity by 75%.[169]

A review of the literature identified 6 RCTs that explored the efficacy of acupuncture in the treatment of craniomandibular dysfunction.[170] Whilst methodological flaws were found in most studies, the study concluded that acupuncture appeared to be suitable as a treatment for the management of TMJ dysfunction.

Xerosterma

A case report of 7 patients suffering xerostomia found that acupuncture was able to increase salivary flow and the ability to eat and speak, and improved sleep in all patients.[171]

In another study of 21 patients with severe xerostomia, 11 were treated with acupuncture and 10 received placebo acupuncture.[172] True acupuncture treatment significantly increased salivary flow rates during and after the acupuncture treatment over the observation year. Placebo acupuncture demonstrated some improvement of salivary flow rates only during treatment.

Gagging

Some people suffer pronounced gag reflex that severely limits their ability to accept dental care and clinicians' ability to provide the care. It compromises all aspects of dentistry, from diagnostic procedures to active treatment and can be distressing for all concerned.[173] Acupuncture may help reduce the gag reflex.

One study involved 21 dentists and 37 case reports (20 females and 17 males; mean age of 46.8 years) of patients who were unable to accept the impression-taking during dental care.[174] After acupuncture of the point CV-24, there was improvement up to 51–55% (mean 53%) for the 3 stages of impression-taking and up to 30 patients (81%) were able to accept the impression-taking. The authors concluded 'that acupuncture of point CV-24 is an effective method of controlling severe gag reflex during dental treatment including impression taking'.[174]

Bruxism

Abrasive wear and tear is common and is seen in a wide range of patients. Abrasion and attritive loss is commonly seen in individuals who suffer bruxism due to tooth grinding, which can also occur during sleep.[175, 176]

Occlusal splints and bruxism

A Cochrane review of 5 RCTs has reported that occlusal splints were of no benefit for treating sleep bruxism when compared to no treatment, although they may benefit by preventing tooth wear.[177]

Homeopathy and dentistry

A pilot study of 14 homeopathic dentists collected clinical and outcome data over a 6-month period of 726 individual patients (mean age of patients was 46.2 years) who received homeopathic treatment.[175] Of the followed-up 496 individual cases, positive outcome was demonstrated in 90.1% (negative in 1.8%; no change in 7.9%; outcome not recorded in 0.2%)

Strongly positive outcomes (scores of +2 or +3) were achieved most notably in the frequently treated conditions of pericoronitis, periodontal abscess, periodontal infection, reversible pulpitis, sensitive cementum, and toothache with decay.[178]

Conclusion

Based on current evidence, there are a number of holistic and lifestyle approaches that can help prevent and treat a number of oral health conditions.

It is important for dental practitioners to review the general health of the patient. Check for complementary medicines patients may be taking that may interfere with surgery, medication or other dental treatment. Also reinforce positive lifestyle factors for prevention of oral health problems and to help with dental care and recovery such as relaxation therapy, diet, sleep management, creating a healthy environment and avoiding toxins, such as smoking.

Table 28.4 summarises the level of evidence for lifestyle factors and complementary medicines that may be useful in dental health care.

Table 28.4 Levels of evidence for lifestyle and complementary medicines/therapies in the management of oral health disorders

Modality	Level I	Level II	Level IIIa	Level IIIb	Level IIIc	Level IV	Level V
Lifestyle							
Toothbrushing (powered)	x						
Chewing gum							
• Xylitol							
• Vitamin C			x				
• Eucalyptus			x				
Mouth rinses	x						
Tongue scraping	x						
Prudent sun exposure (vitamin D)						x	
Smoking cessation	x						
Environmental risks							
Mercury/cadmium						x	
Mind–body medicine							
Psychological interventions	x						
Brief relaxation and music distraction		x					

Virtual image audio-visual eyeglass system			x				
Hypnosis			x				
Behavioural therapy			x				
Relaxation and cognitive oriented therapy			x				
Nutritional influences							
High dairy/calcium intake						x	
Avoidance of sugar						x	
Avoidance of acid diet						x	
Dietary vitamin C						x	
Nutritional supplements							
Vitamins							
Vitamin D/calcium supp			x				
Vitamin B complex			x				
Multivitamin			x				
Minerals							
Calcium						x	
Magnesium			x				
Fluoride (topical)	x						
Fluoridation of water							
Zinc/blood root herb	x						
Other nutritional supplements							
Coenzyme Q10			x				
Alpha-lipoic acid	x						
Probiotics						x	
Herbal medicines							
Green tea extract mouth rinse					x		
Blood root herb		x(+/-)					
Clove oil top			x				
Physical therapies							
TMJ							
• therapeutic exercise, acupuncture, electrophysical modalities				x			
• splints			x				
• occlusal adjustment	x						
• acupuncture	x(-)						
Bruxism							
• occlusal splints	x(-)						
Xerosterma							
• acupuncture	x						
Gagging							
• acupuncture	x(-)						
Homeopathy					x		

Level I — from a systematic review of all relevant randomised controlled trials, meta–analyses.
Level II — from at least 1 properly designed randomised controlled clinical trial.
Level IIIa — from well-designed pseudo-randomised controlled trials (alternate allocation or some other method).
Level IIIb — from comparative studies (including systematic reviews of such studies) with concurrent controls and allocation not randomised, cohort studies, case-control studies, or interrupted time series with a parallel control group.
Level IIIc — from comparative studies with historical control, 2 or more single-arm studies or interrupted time series without a parallel control group.
Level IV — opinions of respected authorities based on clinical experience, descriptive studies or reports of expert committees.
Level V — represents minimal evidence that represents testimonials.

Clinical tips handout for patients — oral health

Refer to this link for details for prevention of dental caries:
http://www.dentalhealthweek.com.au/2008/bootcamp.htm

1 Lifestyle advice

- Maintain good general health with a healthy lifestyle.
- Ensure regular dental check-ups are maintained.

Toothbrushing

- Brush teeth 2–3 times daily after meals. Floss daily between all teeth.
- A powered toothbrush with a rotation oscillation action is preferable.
- Use fluoride toothpaste; avoid swallowing; children need supervision.

Sleep

- Restore normal sleep patterns. Early to bed, about 9–10 p.m. and awake with the sunrise. (See Chapter 22 for more advice.)

Sunshine

- Amount of exposure varies with local climate.
- At least 15 minutes of sunshine needed daily for vitamin D and melatonin production — especially before 10 a.m. and after 3 p.m. when the sun exposure is safest during summer; much more exposure is needed in winter, when supplementation with vitamin D may be needed.
- Ensure gradual, adequate skin exposure to sun; avoid excess clothing to maximise levels of vitamin D.
- Ensure direct exposure to about 10% of the body (hands, arms, face), without sunscreen and not through glass.
- More time in the sun is required for dark skinned people and people with vitamin D deficiency.
- Vitamin D is obtained in the diet from fatty fish, eggs, liver and fortified foods (some milks and margarines); diet alone is not a sufficient source of vitamin D.

2 Physical activity/exercise

- Exercise 30 minutes or more daily. If exercise is not regular, commence with 5 minutes daily and slowly build up to at least 30 minutes. Outdoor exercise in nature, fresh air and sunshine is ideal (e.g. brisk walking, light jogging, cycling, swimming, stretching.) The more time you spend outdoors the better.

3 Mind–body medicine

- Stress management program; for example, 6 x 40 minute sessions for patients to understand the nature of their symptoms, the symptoms' relationship to stress and the practice of regular relaxation exercises.
- Regular meditation practice of at least 10–20 minutes daily is helpful.
- Biofeedback and autogenic training is helpful.

Breathing

- Be aware of breathing from time to time. Notice if tendency to hold breath or over-breathe.
- Always aim to relax breath and the muscles around chest wall.

Rest and stress management

- Bruxism, or teeth-grinding, may occur as a result of nervous tension or difficulty sleeping. Relaxation plays an important role.
- Cognitive behavioural therapy and psychotherapy are extremely helpful to reduce any symptoms of dental fear, panic and anxiety; consider seeing a health professional to discuss any fears you have.
- It is not uncommon for people to feel uncomfortable or nervous about any dental procedure. Communicate with your dentist if you suffer any dental fears and anxiety before treatment. This can help you feel more relaxed about the dental treatment.
- In order to assist you, we recommend you relax before any dental procedure. You may have your own methods.
- Listen to your favourite music with an iPOD or CD during dental procedures. This may help you feel more relaxed during treatment.
- Consider massage therapy.
- Hypnosis may help.

Fun

- It is important to have fun in life. Joy can be found even in the simplest tasks, such as being with friends with a sense of humour funny movies/videos, comedy, hobbies, dancing, playing with pets and children.

4 Environment

- Avoid smoking, drugs, exposure to chemicals and heavy metals.

- Spend more time outdoors, with nature and fresh air.

5 Dietary changes

- Diet is most important for prevention of caries; water and milk are preferred drinks.
- Do not rush your meals; chew your food thoroughly as this aids digestion.
- If you wear dentures, grate or finely cut your food.
- Children should be encouraged to eat healthy snacks and foods, and discouraged from frequent consumption of juices, sugary drinks, snacks and sweet foods (e.g. lollies, chocolates, toffees, lollipops).
- Brush teeth immediately afterwards if consuming any of the abovementioned foods or drinks.
- Eat more fruit (at least 2 daily) and vegetables (at least 5 daily).
- Eat more nuts (e.g. walnuts, almonds, peanuts) and seeds (e.g. sesame, flax)
- Eat more legumes (e.g. soybeans, chickpeas, lentils, sprouts) and beans (e.g. alfalfa, mung beans).
- Eat more unprocessed carbohydrates with lower GI (e.g. wholegrain bread, wholemeal pasta, wholegrain rice).
- Increase fish intake, daily if possible, especially deep sea fish; canned fish is okay (mackerel, salmon, sardines, cod, tuna).
- Avoid large predatory fish such as shark and swordfish for children and pregnant women.
- Reduce red meat intake (preferably use red lean meat e.g. lamb, kangaroo). White meat is okay (e.g. free range organic chicken).
- Eat low-fat dairy (e.g. yoghurt, cheeses such as fetta and ricotta).
- For alternative sweeteners try honey (e.g. yellow box and stringy bark have the lowest GI), xylitol, or stevia drops.
- Drink more water (1–2 litres a day), teas (e.g. especially organic green, black and oolong tea) and vegetable juices.
- Chamomile tea may help you to relax. Drink 1 cup 30–60 minutes before meals.
- Reduce alcohol intake.
- Avoid high coffee consumption (e.g. >1 cup daily).
- Reduce salt intake.
- Avoid chemical additives — artificial sweeteners, preservatives, colourings and flavourings.
- Avoid hydrogenated fats, salt, fast foods, added sugar (such as in lollies, biscuits, cakes) and processed foods (e.g. white bread, white pasta, pastries).
- Avoid sugar, lollies, chocolate — brush teeth immediately after consumption of these foods.
- Avoid sugary soft drinks, especially cola.

6 Physical therapies

- While splints and occlusal adjustment are commonly prescribed by dentists — they may help alleviate pain from TMJ problems —there is little research to support this at this stage.
- Acupuncture may help reduce pain from TMJ problems.
- Occlusal splints worn at night may help reduce grinding of teeth.
- Dry mouth, and gagging during dental procedures may be alleviated with acupuncture treatment.

7 Supplements

Vitamins

Warning: Vitamin A — excessive intake of vitamin A, above 3000IU/day, may contribute to bone loss.

Vitamin D3

- Indication: correct vitamin D deficiency; improve bone density, prevent osteoporosis, fractures and falls; reduce muscle and whole body pain; reduces risk of tooth loss and poor dentition.
- Dosage: safe sunshine exposure of skin is the safest source of vitamin D.
  - Vitamin D (cholecalciferol 1000 international units).
  - Doctors should check blood levels and suggest supplementation if levels are low.
  - Adults: 400–1000IU/day for maintenance; 3000–5000IU/day for 1 month then 1000IU daily if vitamin D level below normal.
  - Children at risk: 200–400IU/day under medical supervision.
  - Pregnant and lactating women at risk: under medical supervision.
- Results: 3–6–12 months.
- Side-effects: very high doses can cause vitamin D toxicity; raised calcium levels in the blood.
- Contraindications: can increase aluminium and magnesium absorption; prolonged heparin therapy can increase resorption and reduce formation of

bone and hence more vitamin D and calcium are required; thiazide diuretics decrease urinary calcium and hence hypercalcaemia possible with vitamin D supplementation; high levels of vitamin D can reduce effectiveness of verapamil.

- The following drugs can decrease vitamin D levels: carbamazepine, cholestyramine, colestipol, phenobarbitol, phenytoin, rifampin, orlistat, stimulant laxatives, sunscreens.
- Corticosteroids increase the need for vitamin D; use vitamin D with caution in those with artery disease, hyperparathyroidism, lymphoma, renal disease and sarcoidosis.

Vitamin C

- Indication: maintain bone formation; tissue healing.
- Dosage: 500–1000mg/day.
- Results: >3 months.
- Side-effects: with high doses can cause nausea, heartburn, abdominal cramps and diarrhoea.
- Contraindications: can increase iron absorption. Use with caution if glucose-6-phosphate dehydrogenase deficiency.

Vitamin B group

- Indication: periodontal disease, post-surgical healing.
- Dosage: upper level of intake of vitamin B6 should not exceed 50mg/day.
- Results: uncertain.
- Side-effects: avoid overuse of single vitamin products (e.g. oral and injectable forms of vitamin B6) or concomitant use of multivitamin products could result in some patients routinely exceeding the upper limit for vitamins associated with severe toxicity. Toxicity in high doses of vitamin B6 includes peripheral neuropathy, such as tingling, burning and numbness of limbs.
- Contraindications: avoid in anaemia until assessed by a doctor.

Folate

- Indication: maintaining bone health when blood levels high in homocysteine.
- Dosage: 5mg/day.
- Results: uncertain.
- Side-effects: very mild and rare.
- Contraindications: avoid in anaemia until assessed by a doctor.

Vitamin B12

- Indication: maintaining bone health when blood levels high in homocysteine, especially in those with vitamin B12 deficiency such as vegans.
- Dosage: Between 600–1000mcg/day.
- Result: >3 months.
- Side-effects: does not cause side-effects even in large doses.
- Contraindications: concurrent use with vitamin C may decrease vitamin B12 absorption therefore best if taken at least 2 hours apart. Several drugs can reduce serum vitamin B12 levels. Excess alcohol intake can also decrease vitamin B12 absorption. Likely to be safe during pregnancy, although there is insufficient data.

Multivitamin

- Indication: wound healing, periodontitis.
- Dosage: 1 multivitamin (containing a mixture of multivitamin B, antioxidants, minerals and fish oils) daily.
- Result: 3 months.
- Side-effects: very mild and rare; gastrointestinal irritation can be avoided if taken after meals; avoid single vitamin B supplementation and high doses of vitamin B6 >50mg/day for prolonged periods of time. Vitamin B6 toxicity may cause neurological problems, such as tingling sensation, and balance problems that are often reversible but can be permanent.
- Contraindications: avoid any multivitamin with herbal ingredients and when vitamin A content is greater than 2000IU/day.

Minerals

Magnesium and calcium (best provided together)

- Indication: calcium and magnesium are necessary to support bone growth and increase bone density; more effective when combined with vitamin D and K.
- Dosage: magnesium — children: 65–120mg/day in divided doses; adults: 400–800mg/day including pregnant and lactating women.
  Calcium citrate — 800mg/day or calcium carbonate 1000mg/day in adults. Children 30–40mg/day.
- Results >1–2 years.
- Side-effects: oral magnesium can cause gastrointestinal irritation, nausea, vomiting, and diarrhoea. The dosage varies from person to person. Although rare, toxic levels can cause low blood pressure, thirst, heart arrhythmia, drowsiness and weakness. Calcium can

cause gastrointestinal irritation and constipation.
- Contraindications: patients with kidney disease.

Zinc

- Indication: may help maintain and improve bone density; oral zinc washes may help ulcers and gingivitis heal faster.
- Dosage: zinc sulfate; usual dosage in adult 5–10mg/day; can take up to 25mg/day. Zinc liquid 10mg/ml, 5–10mls for mouth washes twice daily.
- Side-effects: nausea, vomiting, metallic taste in mouth. Avoid long-term use and high dosage as this may cause copper deficiency, impair the immune system and cause anaemia.
- Contraindications: sideroblastic anaemia, above normal blood levels of zinc, severe kidney disease.

Alpha-lipoic acid

- Indication: may prevent nerve damage and can repair existing damage. Burning mouth syndrome.
- Dosage: 600–1200mg/day (oral).
- Side-effects: nausea and skin rashes have been reported.
- Contraindicated: must not be taken if thiamine deficient (e.g. alcoholic) unless thiamine supplementation is given.

Prevention of dental caries — additional tips

Refer to this link for details for prevention of dental caries:

http://www.dentalhealthweek.com.au/2008/bootcamp.htm

Probiotics

Probiotics such *Lactobacillus acidophilus*, *Lactobacillus plantarum*, *Bifidobacterium breve* and *Lactobacillus GG* found in yoghurt may help reduce caries.

Gum

Chewing xylitol (non-sugary) gum regularly may be help prevent dental caries.

Bad breath, oral infection and gingivitis

- If you suffer bad breath or an oral infection, consider warm salt water mouth rinses.
- Avoid any alcoholic mouth rinses.
- Eucalyptus chewing gum or green tea extract mouth rinses may help.
- Scraping the tongue with a tongue scraper or cleaner may help.
- Try probiotics such as *Lactobacillus plantarum*, *Bifidobacterium breve* and *Lactobacillus GG*.

Bruxism or tooth grinding

Try relaxation techniques and a warm bath before bed.

Mouth splints may help by relaxing muscles.

Other specific conditions

Burning mouth syndrome — try alpha-lipoic acid supplement.

Dental pain — try acupuncture; clove oil applied onto the painful gum may help.

Dry mouth — fish oil supplements; increase oils in diet; acupuncture may help.

Excess gagging — try acupuncture before dental treatment.

TMJ disorder — therapeutic mouth exercises, acupuncture, muscular awareness relaxation therapy, biofeedback training and low-level laser therapy may help. Splints may help by relaxing muscles.

Tooth sensitivity — gentle tooth brushing using potassium-containing toothpastes. Try warm saline water mouth rinses.

Warning: avoid the following herbs or supplements before any dental surgery:

↑ bleeding time — garlic, ginseng, gingko, glucosamine, high doses of fish oils

↑ sedating effect with anaesthetic: kava, hops, valerian, passionflower

herb–drug interactions: ↑ metabolism of drugs used in the perioperative period (e.g. St John's wort).

References

1 Kron, J. Holistic Dentistry. Journal of Complementary Medicine. 2007;6(1):42–7.
2 Australian Research Centre for Population Oral Health. Australian dentist labour force 2003. Aust Dent J 2006;51:(2):191–4.
3 Darby P. Dentists practising CAM. British Dental Journal 2002;193(5):244–5.
4 Watts TLP. Dentists practising CAM. British Dental Journal 2002;193(9):487.
5 Dailey YM, Humphris GM, Lennon MA. Reducing patients' state anxiety in general dental practice: a randomized controlled trial. J Dent Res 2002 May;81(5):319–22.
6 Beltran-Aguilar ED, Beltran-Neira RJ. Oral diseases and conditions throughout the lifespan. II. Systemic diseases. Gen Dent 2004;52(2):107–14.
7 Kinane DF, Marshall GJ. Periodontal manifestations of systemic disease. Aust Dent J 2001;46(1):2–12.
8 Beck JD, Offenbacher S. Systemic effects of periodontitis; epidemiology of periodontal disease and cardiovascular disease. J Periodontol 2005; 76(11 Suppl):2089–100.
9 Blaizot A, Vergnes JN, Nuwwareh S, et. al. Periodontal diseases and cardiovascular events: meta-analysis of observational studies. Int Dent J 2009;59(4):197–209.
10 Meurman JH, Sanz M, Janket SJ. Oral health, atherosclerosis and cardiovascular disease. Crit Rev Oral Biol Med 2004;15(6):403–13.
11 Pihlstrom BL, Michalowicz BS, Johnson NW. Periodontal diseases. Lancet 2005;366(9499): 1809–20.

12 Chiu B. Multiple infections in carotid atherosclerotic plaques. Am Heart J 1999;138:534–6.
13 Herring ME, Shah SK. Periodontal Disease and Control of Diabetes Mellitus. J Am Osteop Assoc 2006;106(7):416–21.
14 Kiran M, Arpak N, Unsal E,et. al. The effect of improved periodontal health on metabolic control in type 2 diabetes mellitus. J Clin Periodontol 2005 Mar;32(3):266–72.
15 Westfelt E, Rylander H, Blohmé G, et. al. The effect of periodontal therapy in diabetics. Results after 5 years. J Clin Periodontol. 1996 Feb;23(2):92–100.
16 Garcia R. Periodontal treatment associated with improved glycaemic control in type 2 diabetic patients. Evid Based Dent. 2007;8(1):13.
17 Skaleric U, Schara R, Medvescek M, et. al. Periodontal treatment by Arestin and its effects on glycemic control in type 1 diabetes patients. J Int Acad Periodontol 2004 Oct;6(4 Suppl):160–5.
18 Garcia RI, Nunn ME, Vokonas PS. Epidemiologic associations between periodontal disease and chronic obstructive pulmonary disease. Ann Periodontol 2001;6(1):71–7.
19 Wactawski-Wende J. Periodontal diseases and osteoporosis: association and mechanisms. Ann Periodontol 2001;6(1):197–208.
20 Robinson P, Deacon SA, Deery C, et. al. Manual versus powered toothbrushing for oral health. Cochrane Database of Systematic Reviews 2005, Issue 1. Art. No.: CD002281. doi: 10.1002/14651858.CD002281.pub2.
21 Stookey GK. The effect of saliva on dental caries. J Am Dent Assoc 2008 May;139:11S–17S.
22 Aksoy A, Duran N, Koksal F. In vitro and in vivo antimicrobial effects of mastic chewing gum against Streptococcus mutans and mutans streptococci. Arch Oral Biol. 2006 Jun;51(6):476–81. Epub 2005 Dec 15.
23 Takahashi K, Fukazawa M, Motohira H, et. al. A pilot study on antiplaque effects of mastic chewing gum in the oral cavity. J Periodontol. 2003 Apr;74(4):501–5.
24 Edgar WM. Sugar substitutes, chewing gum and dental caries-a review. Br Dent J 1998 Jan 10;184(1):29–32.
25 Gales MA, Nguyen TM. Sorbitol compared with xylitol in prevention of dental caries. Ann Pharmacother. 2000 Jan;34(1):98–100.
26 Mäkinen KK, Bennett CA, Hujoel PP, et. al. Xylitol chewing gums and caries rates: a 40-month cohort study. J Dent Res 1995 Dec;74(12):1904–13.
27 Van Loveren C. Sugar alcohols: what is the evidence for caries-preventive and caries-therapeutic effects? Caries Res 2004 May-Jun;38(3):286–93.
28 Mäkinen KK, Alanen P, Isokangas P, et. al. Thirty-nine-month xylitol chewing-gum programme in initially 8-year-old school children: a feasibility study focusing on mutans streptococci and lactobacilli. Int Dent J 2008 Feb;58(1):41–50.
29 Twetman S, Stecksén-Blicks C. Effect of xylitol-containing chewing gums on lactic acid production in dental plaque from caries active pre-school children. Oral Health Prev Dent 2003;1(3):195–9.
30 Lingstrom P, Fure S, Dinitzen B, et. al. The release of vitamin C from chewing gum and its effects on supragingival calculus formation. Eur J Oral Sci 2005 Feb;113(1):20–7.
31 Fedorowicz Z, Aljufairi H, Nasser M, et. al. Mouthrinses for the treatment of halitosis. Cochrane Database of Systematic Reviews 2008, Issue 4. Art. No.: CD006701. doi: 10.1002/14651858. CD006701.pub2.
32 Winn DN, Blot WJ, McLaughlin JK, et. al. Mouthwash Use and Oral Conditions in the Risk of Oral and Pharyngeal Cancer. Cancer Research 1991 June 1;51:3044–47.
33 Cole P, Rodu B, Mathisen A. Alcohol-containing mouthwash and oropharyngeal cancer: A review of the epidemiology. J Am Dent Assoc 2003 August 1;134(8):1079–87.
34 McCullough MJ, Farah CS. A review of the role of alcohol in oral carcinogenesis with particular reference to alcohol containing mouthwashes. Aust Dent J 2008;53(4):302–5.
35 La Vecchia C. Mouthwash and oral cancer risk: An update. Oral Oncology 2008 Oct 24. Epub ahead of print.
36 Walsh LJ. Are alcohol containing dental mouthrinses safe? A critical look at the evidence. Aust Dental Practice 2008;Nov/Dec:64–8.
37 Outhouse TL, Al-Alawi R, Fedorowicz Z, et. al. Tongue scraping for treating halitosis. Cochrane Database of Systematic Reviews 2006, Issue 2. Art. No.: CD005519. doi: 10.1002/14651858. CD005519.pub2.
38 Brand CA, Abi HY, Cough DE, et. al. Vitamin D deficiency: a study of community beliefs among dark skinned and veiled people. Intern J Rheumatic Dis 2008;11:15–23.
39 Diamond TH, Levy S, Smith A, et. al. High bone turnover in Muslim women with vitamin D deficiency. MJA 2002;177:139–41.
40 Australian Dental Association. Frequently Asked Questions. Amalgum Fillings. Online. Available: http://www.ada.org.au/faqs/faq, documentid, 26712. aspx (accessed 1 Sept 2009).
41 NHMRC. Dental Amalgam and Mercury in Dentistry - Report of an NHMRC Working Party. 1999. Online. Available: http://www.nhmrc.gov.a u/publications/synopses/d17syn.htm (accessed 1st September 2009).
42 DeRouen TA, Martin MD, Leroux BG, et. al. Neurobehavioural effects of dental amalgam in children: a randomized clinical trial. JAMA 2006;295(15):1784–92.
43 Bellinger DC, Trachtenberg F, Barregard L, et. al. Neuropsychological and renal effects of dental amalgam in children: a randomized clinical trial. JAMA 2006 Apr 19;295(15):1775–83.
44 Ye X, Qian H, Xu P, et. al. Nephrotoxicity, neurotoxicity, and mercury exposure among children with and without dental amalgam fillings. Int J Hyg Environ Health 2009 Jul;212(4):378–86.
45 Barregard L, Trachtenberg F, McKinlay S. Environ Health Perspect. Renal effects of dental amalgam in children: the New England children's amalgam trial. 2008 Mar;116(3):394–9.
46 Trachtenberg F, Barregard L, McKinlay S. The influence of urinary flow rate in children on excretion of markers used for assessment of renal damage: albumin, gamma-glutamyl transpeptidase, N-acetyl-beta-D -glucosaminidase, and alpha1-microglobulin. Pediatr Nephrol 2008;23(3): 445–56.
47 Mortada WL, Sobh MA, El-Defrawy MM, et. al. Mercury in dental restoration: is there a risk of nephrotoxicity? J Nephrol 2002 Mar-Apr;15(2):171–6.
48 Dental mercury use banned in Norway, Sweden and Denmark. Reuters, January 3, 2008. Online. Available: http://www.reuters.com/article/press Release/idUS108558+03-Jan-2008+PRN20080103 (accessed 1 September 2009)

49 Ministry of the Environment. Press release 21 December 2007. Minister of the Environment and International Development Erik Solheim: Bans mercury in products. http://www.regjeringen.no/en/dep/md/press-centre/Press-releases/2007/Bans-mercury-in-products.html?id = 495138 (accessed 1st September 2009)

50 Amendment of regulations of 1 June 2004 no 922 relating to restrictions on the use of chemicals and other products hazardous to health and the environment (Product regulations). Adopted by the Ministry of the Environment on 14 December 2007 pursuant to section 4 of the Product Control Act of 11 June 1979. Online. Available: http://www.regjeringen.no/Upload/MD/Vedlegg/Forskrifter/product_regulation_amendment_071214.pdf (accessed 1 September 2009)

51 Foods Standards Australia New Zealand (FSANZ). Online. Available: http://www.foodstandards.gov.au/foodmatters/mercuryinfish.cfm (accessed 1 Sept 2009)

52 US Food and Drug Administration; FDA; US Department of Health and Human Services. What You Need to Know About Mercury in Fish and Shellfish, Advice for Women Who Might Become Pregnant, Women Who are Pregnant, Nursing Mothers, and Young Children Online. Available: http://www.fda.gov/Food/ResourcesForYou/Consumers/ucm110591.htm (accessed 1 Sept 2009)

53 Chin G, Chong J, Kluczewska A, et. al. REVIEW. The environmental effects of dental amalgam. Australian Dental Journal 2000;45:(4):246–249.

54 Arora M, Weuve J, Schwartz J, et. al. Association of environmental cadmium exposure with periodontal disease in U.S. Adults. Environ Health Perspect 2009 May;117(5):739–44.

55 Albandar JM, Streckfus CF, Adesanya MR, et. al. Cigar, pipe, and cigarette smoking as risk factors for periodontal disease and tooth loss. J Periodontol 2000 Dec;71(12):1874–81.

56 Tomar SL, Asma S. Smoking-attributable periodontitis in the United States: findings from NHANES III. National Health and Nutrition Examination Survey. J Periodontol 2000 May;71(5):743–51.

57 Bergström J. Tobacco smoking and chronic destructive periodontal disease. Odontology 2004 Sep;92(1):1–8.

58 Obeid P, Bercy P. Effects of smoking on periodontal health: a review. Adv Ther 2000 Sep-Oct;17(5):230–7.

59 Barbour SE, Nakashima K, Zhang JB, et. al. Tobacco and smoking: environmental factors that modify the host response (immune system) and have an impact on periodontal health. Crit Rev Oral Biol Med 1997;8(4):437–60.

60 Mortada WI, Sobh MA, El-Defrawy MM. The exposure to cadmium, lead and mercury from smoking and its impact on renal integrity. Med Sci Monit 2004 Mar;10(3):CR112–6.

61 Krall EA, Dawson-Hughes B, Garvey AJ, et. al. Smoking, smoking cessation, and tooth loss. J Dent Res 1997 Oct;76(10):1653–9.

62 Brousseau M, Manzini C, Thie N, et. al. Understanding and managing the interaction between sleep and pain: an update for the dentist. J Can Dent Assoc 2003 Jul-Aug;69(7):437–42.

63 Bailey DR. Sleep disorders. Overview and relationship to orofacial pain. Dent Clin North Am 1997 Apr;41(2):189–209.

64 Lavigne GJ, Goulet JP, Zuconni M, et. al. Sleep disorders and the dental patient: an overview. Oral Surg Oral Med Oral Pathol Oral Radiol Endod 1999 Sep;88(3):257–72.

65 Biggs QM, Kelly KS, Toney JD. The effects of deep diaphragmatic breathing and focused attention on dental anxiety in a private practice setting. J Dent Hyg 2003 Spring;77(2):105–13.

66 Parslow R, Morgan AJ, Allen NB, et. al. Effectiveness of complementary and self-help treatments for anxiety in children and adolescents. Med J Aust 2008 Mar 17;188(6):355–9.

67 Royal Australian and New Zealand College of Psychiatrists Clinical Practice; Guidelines Team for Panic Disorder and Agoraphobia. Australian and New Zealand Journal of Psychiatry 2003;37:641–56.

68 Wipfli BM, Rethorst CD, Landers DM. The anxiolytic effects of exercise: a meta-analysis of randomized trials and dose-response analysis. J Sport Exerc Psychol 2008 Aug;30(4):392–410.

69 Renz A, Ide M, Newton T, et. al. Psychological interventions to improve adherence to oral hygiene instructions in adults with periodontal diseases. Cochrane Database of Systematic Reviews 2007, Issue 2. Art. No.: CD005097. doi: 10.1002/14651858.CD005097.pub2.

70 Lahmann C, Schoen R, Henningsen P, et. al. Brief relaxation versus music distraction in the treatment of dental anxiety: a randomized controlled clinical trial. J Am Dent Assoc 2008 Mar;139(3):317–24.

71 Lai HL, Hwang MJ, Chen CJ, et. al. Randomised controlled trial of music on state anxiety and physiological indices in patients undergoing root canal treatment. J Clin Nurs 2008 Oct;17(19):2654–60.

72 Frere CL, Crout R, Yorty J, et. al. Effects of audiovisual distraction during dental prophylaxis. J Am Dent Assoc 2001 Jul;132(7):1031–8.

73 DiClementi JD, Deffenbaugh J, Jackson D. Hypnotizability, absorption and negative cognitions as predictors of dental anxiety: two pilot studies. J Am Dent Assoc 2007 Sep;138(9):1242–50; quiz 1267-8.

74 Finkelstein S. Rapid hypnotic inductions and therapeutic suggestions in the dental setting. Int J Clin Exp Hypn 2003 Jan;51(1):77–85.

75 Gokli MA, Wood AJ, Mourino AP, et. al. Hypnosis as an adjunct to the administration of local anesthetic in pediatric patients. ASDC J Dent Child 1994;61(4):272–5.

76 Hammarstrand G, Berggren U, Hakeberg M. Psychophysiological therapy vs. hypnotherapy in the treatment of patients with dental phobia. Eur J Oral Sci 1995;103(6):399–404.

77 Berggren U, Hakeberg M, Carlsson SG. Relaxation vs. cognitively oriented therapies for dental fear. J Dent Res 2000 Sep;79(9):1645–51.

78 Willumsen T, Vassend O, Hoffart A. A comparison of cognitive therapy, applied relaxation, and nitrous oxide sedation in the treatment of dental fear. Acta Odontol Scand 2001 Oct;59(5):290–6.

79 Willumsen T, Vassend O, Hoffart A. One-year follow-up of patients treated for dental fear: effects of cognitive therapy, applied relaxation, and nitrous oxide sedation. Acta Odontol Scand 2001 Dec;59(6):335–40.

80 Willumsen T, Vassend O. Effects of cognitive therapy, applied relaxation and nitrous oxide sedation. A five-year follow-up study of patients treated for dental fear. Acta Odontol Scand 2003 Apr;61(2):93–9.

81 Moynihan P, Petersen PE. Diet, nutrition and the prevention of dental diseases. Public Health Nutr 2004 Feb;7(1A):201–26.

82 Sheiham A. Dietary effects on dental diseases. Public Health Nutr 2001 Apr;4(2B):569–91.

83 Gennari C. Calcium and vitamin D nutrition and bone disease of the elderly. Public Health Nutr 2001 Apr;4(2B):547–59.

84 Nunn ME, Braunstein NS, Krall Kaye EA, et. al. Healthy eating index is a predictor of early childhood caries. J Dent Res 2009 Apr;88(4):361–6.

85 Tinanoff N, Palmer CA. Dietary determinants of dental caries and dietary recommendations for preschool children. J Public Health Dent 2000 Summer;60(3):197–206; discussion 207–9.

86 Tucker KL, Morita K, Qiao N, et. al. Colas, but not other carbonated beverages, are associated with low bone mineral density in older women: The Framingham Osteoporosis Study. AJCN 2006;84:936–42.

87 Sullivan EA, Curzon ME. A comparison of acidic dietary factors in children with and without dental erosion. ASDC J Dent Child 2000;67(3):186–92.

88 Cochrane NJ, Cai F, Yuan Y, et. al. Erosive potential of beverages sold in Australian schools. Aust Dent J 2009;54(3):238–44.

89 Moyad MA. Vitamin D: a rapid review. Urol Nurs 2008;28(5):343–9.

90 Bischoff-Ferrari HA, Dietrich T, Orav EJ, et. al. Higher 25-hydroxyvitamin D concentrations are associated with better lower-extremity function in both active and non-active persons aged > or = 60 y. AJCN 2004;80:752–8.

91 Nowson CA, Margerison C. Vitamin D intake and vitamin D status of Australians. MJA 2002;177: 149–52.

92 Holick MF. Vitamin D deficiency. N Engl J Med 2007;357:266–81.

93 Van der Mei IA, Ponsonby AL, Engelsen O, et. al. The high prevalence of vitamin D insufficiency across Australian populations is only partly explained by season and latitude. Environ Health Perspect 2007;115(8):1132–9.

94 Guardia G, Parikh N, Eskridge T, et. al. Prevalence of vitamin D depletion among subjects seeking advice on osteoporosis: a five –year cross-sectional study with public health implications. Osteoporosis Int 2008;19(1):13–9.

95 Mart Kull Jr, Riina Kallikorm, Anu Tamm, et. al. Seasonal variance of 25-(OH) vitamin D in the general population of Estonia, a Northern European country. BMC Public Health 2009,9:22. doi:10.1186/1471-2458-9-22 http://www.biomedcentral.com/1471-2458/9/22.

96 John Livesey, et. al. Seasonal variation in vitamin D levels in the Canterbury, New Zealand population in relation to available UV radiation. The New Zealand Medical Journal 120(1262):1–13.

97 Weisber P, Kelley SS, Ruowei Li, et. al. Nutritional rickets among children in the United States: review of cases reported between 1986-2003. Am J Clin Nutr 2004;80(suppl):1697S–705S.

98 Munns C, Zacharin MR, et. al. Prevention and treatment of infant and childhood vitamin D deficiency in Australia and New Zealand: a consensus statement. MJA 2006;185:268–72.

99 Van der Meer IM, Karamali NS, Boeke JP, et. al. High prevalence of vitamin D deficiency in pregnant non-Western women in the Hague, Netherlands. Am J Clin Nutr 2006;84:350–53.

100 Bircan Erbas, Peter R Ebeling, Dianne Couch, et. al. Suburban clustering of vitamin D deficiency in Melbourne, Australia. Asia Pac J Clin Nutr 2008;17(1):63–7.

101 Terrence H Diamond, Sherel Levy, Angelina Smith, et. al. High bone turnover in Muslim women with vitamin D deficiency. MJA 2002 Aug 5;177: 139–41.

102 Grover SR, Morley M. Vitamin D deficiency in veiled or dark skinned pregnant women. MJA 2001;175:251–2.

103 Carmel Tohill, Anne Laverty. Sunshine, diet and mobility for healthy bones-an interventional study designed to implement these standards into the daily routine in an at risk population of adults with intellectual disability. Journal of Intellectual and Developmental Disability 2001;26(3):217–31.

104 Leif Mosekilde. Vitamin D and the elderly. Clinical Endocrinology 2005;62:265–81.

105 Thompson K, Morley R, Grover SR, et. al. Postnatal evaluation of vitamin D and bone health in women who were vitamin D-deficient in pregnancy, and in their infants. MJA 2004;181(9):486–88.

106 Kerrie M Sanders, Caryl A Nowson, Mark A Kotowicz, et. al. Position Statement. Calcium and bone health: position statement for the Australian and New Zealand Bone and Mineral Society, Osteoporosis Australia and the Endocrine Society of Australia. MJA 2009;190(6):316–320. Online. Available: http://www.mja.com.au/public/issues/190_06_160309/san10083_fm.html (accessed 1 Sept 2009).

107 Zhu K, Devine A, Dick IM, et. al. Effects of calium and vitamin S supplementation on hip bone mineral density and calcium-related analytes in elderly ambulatory Australian women: a 5-year randomized controlled trial. J Clin Endocrino Metabol 2007;93:743–49.

108 Lanham-New SA. Importance of calcium, vitamin D and vitamin K for osteoporosis prevention and treatment. Proc Nutr Soc 2008;67(2):163–76.

109 Hildebolt CF. Effect of vitamin D and calcium on periodontitis J Periodontol 2005;76:1576–87.

110 Krall EA, Wehler C, Garcia RI, et. al. Calcium and vitamin D supplements reduce tooth loss in the elderly. Am J Med 2001 Oct 15;111(6):452–6.

111 Neiva RF, Al-Shammari K, Nociti FH Jr, et. al. Effects of vitamin-B complex supplementation on periodontal wound healing. J Periodontol 2005;76(7):1084–91.

112 Head KA. Peripheral neuropathy: pathogenic mechanisms and alternative therapies. Altern Med Rev 2006;11(4):294–329.

113 Scott K, Zeris S, Kothari MJ. Elevated B6 levels and peripheral neuropathies. Electromyogr Clin Neurophysiol 2008;48(5):219–23.

114 Nishida M, Grossi SG, Dunford RG, et. al. Dietary vitamin C and the risk for periodontal disease. J Periodontol 2000 Aug;71(8):1215–23.

115 Anderson B. Nutrition and wound healing: the necessity of assessment. Br J Nurs 2005 Oct 27-Nov 9;14(19):S30, S32, S34 passim.

116 Casey G. Nurs Stand. Nutritional support in wound healing. 2003 Feb 19-25;17(23):55–8.

117 Munoz CA, Kiger RD, Stephens JA, et. al. Effects of a nutritional supplement on periodontal status. Compend Contin Educ Dent 2001;22(5): 425–8.

118 Neiva RF, Steigenga J, Al-Shammari KF, et. al. Effects of specific nutrients on periodontal disease onset, progression and treatment. J Clin Periodontol 2003 Jul;30(7):579–89.
119 Meisel P, Schwahn C, Luedemann J, et. al. J Dent Res. Magnesium deficiency is associated with periodontal disease. 2005 Oct;84(10):937–41.
120 Nishida M, Grossi SG, Dunford RG, et. al. Calcium and the risk for periodontal disease. J Periodontol 2000 Jul;71(7):1057–66.
121 Marinho VCC, Higgins JPT, Logan S, et. al. Fluoride gels for preventing dental caries in children and adolescents. Cochrane Database of Systematic Reviews 2002, Issue 2. Art. No.: CD002280. doi: 10.1002/14651858.CD002280.
122 Marinho VCC, Higgins JPT, Logan S, et. al. Fluoride varnishes for preventing dental caries in children and adolescents. Cochrane Database of Systematic Reviews 2002, Issue 3. Art. No.: CD002279. doi: 10.1002/14651858.CD002279.
123 Marinho VCC, Higgins JPT, Sheiham A, et. al. One topical fluoride (toothpastes, or mouthrinses, or gels, or varnishes) versus another for preventing dental caries in children and adolescents. Cochrane Database of Systematic Reviews 2004, Issue 1. Art. No.: CD002780. doi: 10.1002/14651858. CD002780.pub2.
124 Marinho VCC, Higgins JPT, Sheiham A, et. al. Combinations of topical fluoride (toothpastes, mouthrinses, gels, varnishes) versus single topical fluoride for preventing dental caries in children and adolescents. Cochrane Database of Systematic Reviews 2004, Issue 1. Art. No.: CD002781. doi: 10.1002/14651858.CD002781.pub2.
125 Marinho VCC, Higgins JPT, Logan S, et. al. Fluoride mouthrinses for preventing dental caries in children and adolescents. Cochrane Database of Systematic Reviews 2003, Issue 3. Art. No.: CD002284. doi: 10.1002/14651858. CD002284.
126 Marinho VCC, Higgins JPT, Logan S, et. al. Topical fluoride (toothpastes, mouthrinses, gels or varnishes) for preventing dental caries in children and adolescents. Cochrane Database of Systematic Reviews 2003, Issue 4. Art. No.: CD002782. doi: 10.1002/14651858.CD002782.
127 McDonagh MS, Whiting PF, Wilson PM, et. al. Systematic review of water fluoridation. BMJ 2000;321(7265):855–9.
128 Bassin EB. Association Between Fluoride in Drinking Water During Growth and Development and the Incidence of Ostosarcoma for Children and Adolescents. Doctoral Thesis, Harvard School of Dental Medicine 2001.
129 Cohn PD. A Brief Report On The Association Of Drinking Water Fluoridation And The Incidence of Osteosarcoma Among Young Males. New Jersey Department of Health Environ. Health Service 1992;1–17.
130 Gelberg KH, et. al. Fluoride Exposure and Childhood Osteosarcoma: A Case-Control Study. Am J Pub Hlth 1995;85:1678–1683.
131 Hoover RN, et. al. Time trends for bone and joint cancers and osteosarcomas in the Surveillance, Epidemiology and End Results (SEER) Program. National Cancer Institute. In: Review of Fluoride: Benefits and Risks Report of the Ad Hoc Committee on Fluoride of the Committee to Coordinate Environmental Health and Related Programs US Public Health Service 1991:F1–F7.
132 Moss ME, Kanarek MS, Anderson HA, et. al. Osteosarcoma, seasonality, and environmental factors in Wisconsin, 1979-1989. Arch Envir Health 1995;50:235–41.
133 Operskalski EA, et. al. A case-control study of osteosarcoma in young persons. Am J Epidemiol 1987;126:118–26.
134 Bassin EB, Wypij D, Davis RB, et. al. Age-specific fluoride exposure in drinking water and osteosarcoma (United States). Cancer Causes Control 2006 May;17(4):421–8.
135 Eyre R, Feltbower RG, Mubwandarikwa E, et. al. Epidemiology of bone tumours in children and young adults. Pediatr Blood Cancer. 2009 Jul 17. Epub ahead of print.
136 Sandhu R, Lal H, Kundu ZS, et. al. Serum Fluoride and Sialic Acid Levels in Osteosarcoma. Biol Trace Elem Res. 2009 Apr 24. Epub ahead of print.
137 Takahashi K, Akiniwa K, Narita K. Regression analysis of cancer incidence rates and water fluoride in the U.S.A. based on IACR/IARC (WHO) data (1978-1992). International Agency for Research on Cancer. J Epidemiol 2001 Jul;11(4):170–9.
138 Freni SC, Gaylor DW. International trends in the incidence of bone cancer are not related to drinking water fluoridation. Cancer 1992;70(3):611–8.
139 Mcguire SM, et. al. Is there a link between fluoridated water and osteosarcoma? Am Dent Assoc 1991;122:38–45.
140 Spencer AJ. Water fluoridation in Australia. Community Dental Health 1996;13(suppl 2): 27–37.
141 National Health and Medical Research Centre (NHMRC). Online. Available: www.nhmrc.gov.au/news/media/rel07/_files/fluoride_flyer.pdf (accessed 1 Sept 2009)
142 Yeung CA. A systematic review of the efficacy and safety of fluoridation. Evid Based Dent 2008;9(2): 39–43.
143 Yeung A, Hitchings JL, Macfarlane TV, et. al. Fluoridated milk for preventing dental caries. Cochrane Database of Systematic Reviews 2005, Issue 3. Art. No.: CD003876. doi: 10.1002/14651858.CD003876.pub2.
144 Haguenuaer D, Welch V, Shea B, et. al. Fluoride for the treatment of postmenopausal osteoporotic fractures: a meta-analysis. Osteoporosis Int 2000;11:727–738.
145 Pak CY, Sakhaee K, Zerwekh JE, et. al. Treatment of postmenopausal osteoporosis with slow-release of sodium fluoride. Final report of randomized controlled trial. Ann Int Med 1995;123:401–8.
146 Poulsen S, Errboe M, Lescay Mevil Y, et. al. Potassium containing toothpastes for dentine hypersensitivity. Cochrane Database of Systematic Reviews 2006, Issue 2. Art. No.: CD001476. doi: 10.1002/14651858.CD001476. pub2.
147 Harper DS, Mueller LJ, Fine JB, et. al. Clinical efficacy of a dentifrice and oral rinse containing sanguinaria extract and zinc chloride during 6 months of use. J Periodontol 1990;61(6):352–8.
148 Watts TL. Coenzyme Q10 and periodontal treatment: is there any beneficial effect? Br Dent J 1995;178(6):209–13.
149 Hanioka T, Tanaka M, Ojima M, et. al. Effect of topical application of coenzyme Q10 on adult periodontitis. Mol Aspects Med 1994;15(Suppl):s241–8.

150 Zakrzewska JM, Forssell H, Glenny A-M. Interventions for the treatment of burning mouth syndrome. Cochrane Database of Systematic Reviews 2004, Issue 4. Art. No.: CD002779. doi: 10.1002/14651858.CD002779.pub2.
151 Twetman S, Stecksén-Blicks C. Probiotics and oral health effects in children Int J Paediatr Dent 2008 Jan;18(1):3–10.
152 Caglar E, Kargul B, Tanboga I. Bacteriotherapy and probiotics' role on oral health. Oral Dis 2005 May;11(3):131–7.
153 de Vrese M, Schrezenmeir J. Probiotics, prebiotics, and synbiotics. Adv Biochem Eng Biotechnol 2008;111:1–66.
154 Meurman JH, Stamatova I. Probiotics: contributions to oral health. Oral Dis 2007 Sep;13(5):443–51.
155 Meurman JH. Probiotics: do they have a role in oral medicine and dentistry? Eur J Oral Sci 2005 Jun;113(3):188–96.
156 Hirasawa M, Takada K, Otake S. Inhibition of acid production in dental plaque bacteria by green tea catechins. Caries Res 2006;40(3):265–70.
157 Kuftinec MM, Mueller-Joseph LJ, Kopczyk RA. Sanguinaria toothpaste and oral rinse regimen clinical efficacy in short- and long-term trials. J Can Dent Assoc1990;56(7 suppl):31–3.
158 Cullinan MP, Powell RN, Faddy MJ, et. al. Efficacy of a dentifrice and oral rinse containing sanguinaria extract in conjunction with initial periodontal therapy. Aust Dent J 1997;42(1): 47–51.
159 Harper DS, Mueller LJ, Fine JB, et. al. Clinical efficacy of a dentifrice and oral rinse containing sanguinaria extract and zinc chloride during 6 months of use. J Periodontol 1990;61(6):352–8.
160 Alqareer A, Alyahya A, Andersson L. The effect of clove and benzocaine versus placebo as topical anesthetics J Dent 2006 Nov;34(10):747–50.
161 Nagata H, Inagaki Y, Tanaka M, et. al. Effect of eucalyptus extract chewing gum on periodontal health: a double-masked, randomized trial. J Periodontol. 2008 Aug;79(8):1378–85.
162 Izzo AA, Ernst E. Interactions between herbal medicines and prescribed drugs: a systematic review. Drugs. 2001;61(15):2163–75
163 Ang-Lee MK, Moss J, Yuan CS. Herbal medicines and perioperative care. JAMA. 2001 Jul 11;286(2):208–16
163 Abebe W. An overview of herbal supplement utilization with particular emphasis on possible interactions with dental drugs and oral manifestations. J Dent Hyg. 2003 Winter;77(1):37–46
165 McNeely ML, Armijo Olivo S, Magee DJ. A systematic review of the effectiveness of physical therapy interventions for temporomandibular disorders. Phys Ther 2006 May;86(5):710–25.
166 Medlicott MS, Harris SR. A systematic review of the effectiveness of exercise, manual therapy, electrotherapy, relaxation training, and biofeedback in the management of temporomandibular disorder. Phys Ther 2006 Jul;86(7):955–73.
167 Al-Ani MZ, Davies SJ, Gray RJM, et. al. Stabilisation splint therapy for temporomandibular pain dysfunction syndrome. Cochrane Database of Systematic Reviews 2004, Issue 1. Art. No.: CD002778. doi: 10.1002/14651858.CD002778. pub2.
168 Koh H, Robinson P. Occlusal adjustment for treating and preventing temporomandibular joint disorders. Cochrane Database of Systematic Reviews 2003, Issue 1. Art. No.: CD003812. doi: 10.1002/14651858.CD003812.
169 Rosted P, Bundgaard M, Pedersen AM. The use of acupuncture in the treatment of temporomandibular dysfunction--an audit. Acupunct Med 2006;24(1):16–22.
170 Fink M, Rosted P, Bernateck M, et. al. Acupuncture in the treatment of painful dysfunction of the temporomandibular joint -- a review of the literature. Forsch Komplementmed 2006 Apr;13(2):109–15.
171 Morganstein WM. Acupuncture in the treatment of xerostomia: clinical report. Gen Dent 2005 May-Jun;53(3):223–6.
172 Blom M, Dawidson I, Angmar-Månsson B. The effect of acupuncture on salivary flow rates in patients with xerostomia. Oral Surg Oral Med Oral Pathol 1992 Mar;73(3):293–8.
173 Dickinson CM, Fiske J. A review of gagging problems in dentistry: I. Aetiology and classification. Dent Update 2005 Jan-Feb;32(1):26–8, 31–2.
174 Rosted P, Bundgaard M, Fiske J, et. al. The use of acupuncture in controlling the gag reflex in patients requiring an upper alginate impression: an audit. Br Dent J 2006;201:721–5; 715.
175 Lavigne G, Kato T. Usual and unusual orofacial motor activities associated with tooth wear. Int J Prosthodont 2003;16(Suppl):80–2; discussion 89–90.
176 Barbour ME, Rees GD. The role of erosion, abrasion and attrition in tooth wear. J Clin Dent 2006;17(4):88–93.
177 Macedo CR, Silva AB, Machado MAC, et. al. Occlusal splints for treating sleep bruxism (tooth grinding). Cochrane Database of Systematic Reviews 2007, Issue 4. Art.No.:CD005514.doi:10.1002/14651858.CD005514. pub2.
178 Mathie RT, Farrer S. Outcomes from homeopathic prescribing in dental practice: a prospective, research-targeted, pilot study. Homeopathy 2007 Apr;96(2):74–81.

Chapter 29

Osteoarthritis

Introduction

Although diseases with the greatest consequent mortality (e.g. CVD, cancer) attract much of the public's attention, musculoskeletal or rheumatic diseases are the major cause of morbidity throughout the world, having a substantial influence on health and quality of life, but not mortality, and inflicting a vast burden of cost on health systems. Musculoskeletal disease is a major cause of disability and handicap, and arthritis is the most prevalent form of musculoskeletal disease.[1] Rheumatic diseases include more than 150 different conditions and syndromes with the common denominators being pain and inflammation. Five account for 90% of the cases — osteoarthritis (OA), rheumatoid arthritis (RA), fibromyalgia, systemic lupus erythematosus (SLE) and gout.[1–4]

Arthritis is a chronic disease affecting an estimated 43 million (20.8%) US adults and is the leading cause of disability in that country[3] with OA reported to be the most common joint disorder in the world.[4] In Western populations it is one of the most frequent causes of pain, loss of function and disability in adults. Radiographic evidence of OA occurs in the majority of people by 65 years of age and in about 80% of those aged over 75 years. In Australia in 2004, there were 3.4 million people (17% of the population) suffering from some form of arthritis, with 60% of these being females. Of this total, 1.39 million had OA and more than 438 000 had RA.[5] Table 29.1 summarises the symptoms of OA.

The associated worldwide trend in morbidity is significant because it often leads to a reduction in quality of life and related conditions such as fatigue, depression and insomnia. Attendant costs to the health care system are vast and current medications, while often effective, are frequently associated with significant side-effects.

Integrative management of osteoarthritis

The early 1990s saw an upsurge of complementary and alternative medicine (CAM) use, based on reports that recognised the extensive use of treatments outside the realm of conventional medicine.[6, 7] A recent review reported that patients with musculoskeletal conditions often employ CAM modalities[8] in one form or another. Collectively the evidence demonstrates that some CAM modalities show significant promise, as for example herbal medicines, nutritional supplements, acupuncture, and mind–body medicine.

International expert panels have developed useful patient-focused, evidence-based integrative consensus recommendations for the management of hip and knee osteoarthritis.[9, 10]

The evidence-based approaches identified by the panel for the optimal management of patients with OA hip or knee included a combination of non-pharmacological and pharmacological modalities of therapy.

These recommendations include those listed below.

- *Non-pharmacological modalities:* education and self-management; regular telephone contact; referral to a physical therapist; aerobic, muscle strengthening and water-based exercises; hydrotherapy; weight reduction; walking aids; knee braces; footwear and insoles; thermal modalities; transcutaneous electrical nerve stimulation; and acupuncture.
- *Pharmacological modalities:* acetaminophen; cyclooxygenase-2 (COX-2) non-selective and selective oral non-steroidal anti-inflammatory drugs (NSAIDs); topical NSAIDs and capsaicin; intra-articular injections of corticosteroids and hyaluronates; glucosamine and/or chondroitin sulfate for symptom relief; glucosamine sulfate, chondroitin sulfate and diacerein for possible structure-modifying effects; and the use of opioid analgesics for the treatment of refractory pain.
- *Surgical modalities* (if necessary): total joint replacements; unicompartmental knee replacement; osteotomy and joint preserving surgical procedures; joint lavage and arthroscopic debridement in knee OA; and joint fusion as a salvage procedure when joint replacement had failed.

Table 29.1 Symptoms of osteoarthritis

- Pain, stiffness, and limitation in full movement of the joint are typical.
  - The stiffness tends to be worse first thing in the morning but tends to dissipate after half an hour or so.
- Swelling and inflammation of an affected joint can sometimes occur.
  - Large joint swellings are unusual in OA.
- An affected joint tends to look a little larger than normal. This is due to overgrowth of the bone next to damaged cartilage.
- Deformities of joints due to OA are uncommon, but sometimes develop.
- Poor mobility if a knee or hip is badly affected.
- No symptoms may occur.
  - In some people who have an X-ray, changes that indicate some degree of OA may have no, or only very mild, symptoms.
  - The opposite can also be true; that is, a patient may have quite severe symptoms but with only minor changes seen on X-ray.

Environment

Despite popular belief arthritic pain has no seasonal variation and is not more common in winter according to a study of 1424 patients with osteoarthritis, rheumatoid arthritis or fibromyalgia followed up over 24 years.[11]

However, associated atmospheric change and cold temperatures did impact on pain severity according to a study of 200 patients with OA. The authors postulated that the changes in cold temperature may contribute to changes in viscosity of synovial fluid which indirectly affects inflammation.[12]

Mind–body medicine

The non-pharmacological management of OA has been recently reviewed.[13]

Multi-modal cognitive behavioural and/or mind–body therapies, in combination with educational and information components (such as patient education and/or self-management programs) may be appropriate adjunctive treatments in the management of OA.[14, 15] Cognitive behavioural therapy (CBT) has a positive effect on pain and other patient relevant outcomes in chronic pain management due to OA.[16, 17] The best effect of CBT has been documented when it was employed together with physical activity as part of a multi-modal treatment program.[18] Recent reviews have reported that there is limited evidence available for the role of hypnosis in the management of pain due to OA.[14, 15]

Mind–body medicine modalities are summarised in Table 29.2.

Physical activity/exercise

In primary care, physical activity is one of the foundations in the management of chronic musculoskeletal pain. Multiple research data supports the benefits of physical activity for alleviation of symptoms of OA; even vigorous exercise.[19] A Cochrane review concluded there were no significant differences in benefit between high intensity and low intensity aerobic exercise on participants with OA of the knee for functional status, gait, pain and aerobic capacity.[19] Both levels of exercise were beneficial. According to the review of non-pharmacological therapies for OA, exercise (aerobic, range-of-motion and strengthening) should be the leading intervention for OA patients, especially as obesity and being overweight are major risk factors for OA.[19] However, recently another Cochrane review concluded that aquatic exercise appeared to have some beneficial short-term effects for patients with hip and/or knee OA while no long-term effects had been reported.[20] Based on this data, it is possible to consider using aquatic exercise as the first part of a longer exercise program for OA patients.[21]

Both function and pain benefit from aerobic or strengthening activity for knee OA. This was confirmed in an RCT with older participants.[22] Older disabled persons with OA of the knee had modest improvements in measures of disability, physical performance, and pain from participating in either an aerobic or a resistance exercise program. These data suggest that exercise should be prescribed as part of the treatment for knee OA.

In a recent 18 month clinical study investigating additive effects of glucosamine or risedronate for the treatment of osteoarthritis of the knee combined with home exercise,[23] it was reported that there was improvement after 18 months in all groups using individual scales for evaluation of pain and function of the knee, however, with no significant differences observed between the groups. There were no additive effects of glucosamine or risedronate on the exercise therapy.[23]

Of interest, a large-scale study of 1279 middle-aged to elderly persons without knee OA (mean age 53.2 years; many of whom were classified as obese) who underwent both baseline and follow-up examinations after 9 years found that neither recreational walking, jogging, frequently working up a sweat, nor high activity levels relative to peers or even weight factors (Body Mass Index [BMI] above

Table 29.2 Mind–body medicine modalities reported to ameliorate symptoms of OA

Intervention	Actions †	Indications	Outcome measures(SS) †	Pain effect sizes and/ or quality grade
Meditation	MBSR programme versus waiting-list control — 8 sessions	Chronic low back pain	CPAQ SFe36 physical function	Moderate 32% attrition in intervention group, 6% attrition from control Included 3-month follow-up
Guided imagery	Guided imagery + PMR versus usual care • 12 sessions	OA	AIMS 2 pain Self-reported mobility	Low 4% attrition rate
Hypnosis	PMR versus hypnosis versus usual care • 8 sessions	OA	Pain VAS Pain medication (for hypnosis and relaxation groups compared with usual care)	Moderate 12% attrition • pain reduction most rapid in hypnosis group, study included 6 month follow up • no instructions for home practicePain medications decreased in hypnosis and relaxation groups
Tai chi	Tai chi versus meeting and telephone control • brief contact • 5 weeks contact • 12 weeks contact	OA	Satisfaction with health Arthritis self-efficacy Pain and functional measures Joint pain and stiffness, physical function (Korean Western Ontario and McMaster Universities [KWOMAC]) Joint tenderness, swollen joint count 50-foot walk Grip strength	Moderate 6–50% attrition rate in both groups
Yoga	Yoga + exercise or Yoga + relaxation + education versus self-care or wait-list • 8 sessions • 12 sessions	OA	Pain and physical function (Western Ontario and McMaster Universities [WOMAC])	Moderate overall 4–20% attrition rate in both groups

(Source: adapted and modified from Vitetta L, Cicuttini F, Sali A. Alternative therapies for musculoskeletal conditions. Best Pract Res Clin Rheumatol 2008:22(3):499–522)

† PMR = progressive muscle relaxation
AIMS 2 = arthritis impact measurement scales – 2
SS = statistically significant
CPAQ = chronic pain acceptance questionnaire
SF–36 = short form 36-item health survey
VAS = visual analogue scale

the median [7.7 kg/m2 for men and 25.7 kg/m2 for women]; mean BMI >30 kg/m^2 for both) did not protect against nor increased the risk of developing knee OA.[24]

Tai chi and yoga

A recent systematic review has reported that there was some encouraging evidence suggesting that tai chi may be effective for pain control in patients with knee OA.[25] However, the evidence was not persuasive for pain reduction or improvement of physical function. A prospective randomised control clinical trial of tai chi over a 12-week period demonstrated significant improvements in self-efficacy for arthritis symptoms (other than pain and function), total self-efficacy, tension levels and general health status, while pain and some lower limb functional scores showed moderate but not clinically significant improvements among older adults.[26]

A number of small studies have demonstrated that tai chi was effective for a number of people in different environments for the management of pain due to OA.[27–30] In 1 study these findings supported the practice of tai chi as beneficial for gait kinematics in elderly people with knee OA.[27] A longer-term application was suggested in order to substantiate the effect of tai chi as an alternative exercise in management of knee OA. A further study concluded that access to either hydrotherapy or tai chi classes could provide large and sustained improvements in physical function for many older, sedentary individuals with chronic hip or knee OA.[28] In a 12-week study of the efficacy of tai chi to improve physical function, the study results demonstrated that the tai chi group reported lower overall pain and better WOMAC (Western Ontario and McMaster Universities) Osteoarthritis Index gauge physical function than the attention control group at weeks 9 and 12.[29] All improvements disappeared after tai chi training ceased. In a study with older women with OA who were able to safely perform the 12 forms of sun-style tai chi exercise for 12 weeks, it was reported effective in improving arthritic symptoms, balance, and physical functioning.[30] A longitudinal study with a larger sample size was suggested as necessary to confirm the potential use of tai chi exercise in arthritis management.

In a case series study investigating yoga and strengthening exercises for people living with OA of the knee, the study found functional changes and improvement in quality of life in traditional exercise and a yoga based approach.[31] A single small study of the use of yoga for OA of the hands demonstrated improvements in pain and finger range of motion as compared to a control group.[32]

Nutritional influences

Diets

Obesity is a well-recognised risk factor for increased risk of OA, particularly of the knee and hip.[33] A recent study showed that a high BMI was associated with progression of loss of joint-space width associated with knee OA but not hip OA.[34] Dietary advice and intervention clearly have a place in musculoskeletal diseases and allow patients to experience some control over their own disease. Although there is no evidence for efficacy of trendy diets, a significant proportion of patients diagnosed with OA can benefit from excluding foods individually identified during the reintroduction phase of an elimination diet.[35] Also a proportion of patients who follow a vegetarian or Mediterranean-type diet will experience a significant benefit.

Extra-virgin olive oil contains oleocanthol which acts as a natural anti-inflammatory, and may be of benefit for arthritic joint pains.[36]

Obesity and high BMI are also associated with more severe disease in terms of the amount of pain experienced[37] and the need for joint replacement.[38, 39]

Dietary nutritional habits are an unavoidable widespread exposure for people for the development of chronic diseases that include musculoskeletal problems.[39, 40] The Mediterranean diet reflects the dietary patterns characteristic of several countries in the Mediterranean basin during the 1960s. Typically, the diet comprises abundant plant foods that includes fruits, vegetables, wholegrain cereals, beans, nuts and seeds; minimally processed, seasonally fresh and locally grown foods; fish and poultry; olive oil as the main source of lipid, with dairy products, red meat and wine in low to moderate amounts.[35, 40] Lifestyle changes that include adopting daily physical activity and smoking cessation together with changes in nutritional/dietary manipulations may lead to positive effects on musculoskeletal physiology with a consequent beneficial impact on the population health.

Early epidemiological studies have reported that diets rich in vitamins C and D slow progression of OA.[41]

Nutritional supplements

General

Dietary supplements, commonly referred to as natural medicine/compounds, and herbal medicines account for approximately $20 billion of annual sales in the US alone.[8]

A large number of dietary supplements are promoted to patients with osteoarthritis and as many as one-third of those patients have used a supplement to treat their condition.[8] These sales for complementary medicine products indicate that glucosamine-containing supplements are among the most commonly used products for osteoarthritis.[8] Glucosamine is available in multiple forms; the most common being glucosamine hydrochloride and glucosamine sulfate. Some marketed products contain a blend of these and many combine one of the forms with a variety of other ingredients.

Various nutritional products such as calcium and fish oils are commonly used for OA pain management. Given that nutrition is increasingly linked to a range of degenerative and developmental disorders, most supplements used for OA are promoted to reduce pain; for example, via their anti-inflammatory effects. Hence nutritional deficiencies and imbalances can result in metabolic and systemic disturbances that may increase susceptibility to joint disease.

Vitamins

Vitamin C and β-carotene

Perhaps the best study of vitamin C was the Framingham OA Cohort Study which demonstrated vitamin C intake was associated with reduced progression of arthritis in OA patients and lower incidence of knee pain.[42] Specifically, a significant threefold reduction in risk of OA progression was reported, which related predominantly to a reduced risk of cartilage loss. This was documented for both the middle and the highest tertile of vitamin C intake. Those with high ascorbate intake also had a significantly reduced risk of developing knee pain. A significant, though less consistent, reduction in risk of OA progression was also seen for beta-carotene.[42] Recently it has been reported that there was a beneficial effect with vitamin C intake on the reduction in bone size and the number of bone marrow lesions, both of which are important in the pathogenesis of knee OA.[43, 44]

Niacinamide

Small early trials have reported individual benefits with other vitamins. Namely, a double-blind control trial study of 72 OA patients treated with 3000mg/day in 6 divided doses of niacinamide over 12 weeks demonstrated improved pain scores, reduced global impact of OA, improved flexibility and reduced inflammatory markers (ESR) when compared to controls. Furthermore, the use of NSAIDs was reduced with use of niacinamide.[45]

Pantothenic acid

A small trial of 26 patients supplemented with 12.5mg/day pantothenic acid reported relief in severity of OA. However 3 patients reported the onset of general anaesthesia and *leg weakness* with the dosage, for which 12.5mg/day of pyridoxine was administered to elicit recovery.[46]

Folic acid and vitamin B12 cyanocobalamin

Folic acid (6400mcg) and cyanocobalamin (20mcg) consumed orally over a 2-month period demonstrated greater improvements in hand grip and number of tender joints when applied to 26 patients with OA of the hands when compared to NSAIDs.[47] All of these studies require follow-up with properly designed trials.

Antioxidants

A recent systematic review concluded that there is presently no convincing evidence that antioxidants such as selenium, vitamin A, vitamin C or the combination product selenium ACE is effective in the treatment of any type of arthritis.[48]

Vitamin D

Vitamin D emerges as a vitamin that could stimulate the synthesis of proteoglycan by articular chondrocytes.[49] This effect was explored within the Framingham OA Cohort Study.[50] In the 556 participants who had complete assessments, a significant threefold to fourfold increase in risk of progression of radiographically determined OA was seen in the middle and low tertiles of vitamin D intake and serum concentration.[48] Also, the Study of Osteoporotic Fractures Research Group showed that high serum concentrations of vitamin D protected against both incident and progressive hip OA.[51] In more recent results from 2 longitudinal cohort studies the Framingham Offspring cohort (715 subjects) and the Boston Osteoarthritis of the Knee Study (277 participants),[52] no association was found between baseline 25(OH)D concentration and radiographic deterioration of joint-space narrowing or cartilage loss. Though the evidence is contradictory for OA, the wide prevalence of vitamin D deficiency and the broad range of important roles played by vitamin D suggest that even OA patients should be encouraged to optimise their vitamin D status.[53, 54, 55]

Herbal medicines

A number of herbal supplements have been investigated for their efficacy in patients with OA (see Table 29.3, at the end of this section).[56–60]

Green tea extract (*Camellia sinensis*)

The anti-inflammatory and pharmacological properties of green tea extracts have been attributed to the high content of polyphenols/catechins, of which epigallocatechin-3-gallate (EGCG) predominates.[58, 61] The emerging molecular evidence thus far gives strong biological plausibility support to the *in vitro* observations that catechins extracted from green tea can exhibit both anti-inflammatory and chondro-protective effects and hence may be beneficial for the management of arthritis.[61]

Cat's claw (*Uncaria tomentosa, Uncaria guianensis*)

Extracts of cat's claw have been shown to possess antioxidant, anti-inflammatory and immuno-modulating properties.[57, 58] The most investigated of the active constituents in *Uncaria tomentosa* extract for immuno-modulating and anti-inflammatory effects are pentacyclic oxindole alkaloids, which are reported to induce an immune regulating factor.[58] In a recent review[57] the mechanism of cat's claw action was postulated to be through the inhibition of TNF-alpha. A small study has reported the safe and effective use of cat's claw in OA of the knee with *U guianensis* versus placebo.[62]

Other research groups have documented the safety and pharmacological profile of cat's claw.[57, 63, 64, 65] There is a requisite though for rigorously testing the effectiveness of the recommended doses, which are considered non-toxic, and there are no known contraindications or drug interactions noted at this stage. Until a full pharmacokinetic profile is investigated it would be prudent to avoid its use in women attempting pregnancy, during pregnancy and lactation.[57]

Devil's claw (*Harpogophytum procumbens*)

Harpogophytum procumbens has been shown to be effective for OA in 2 reviews.[65, 66] There is little evidence of efficacy for extracts containing less than 30mg/day of the active constituent, harpagoside, and that a correct dose is >50mg/day for OA of the knee and hip. Devil's claw exhibits cellular signalling modulating activities that down-regulate inflammatory markers.[67, 68, 69] A Cochrane review of five randomised clinical trials (RCTs) have reported on the effects of devil's claw in the treatment of OA.[70] Of these, 3 were placebo-controlled and 2 were compared to common pharmaceuticals (diacerhein and phenylbutazone). Three trials demonstrated significant positive results, while 2 studies that employed less than 30mg harpagoside recorded results that were less significant.[70] An aqueous extract of devil's claw (consisting of 60mg harpagoside) was found to be as effective as 12.5mg of rofecoxib for the treatment of acute non-specific lower-back pain in a double-blind pilot RCT.[70] Three other trials have also demonstrated efficacy in lower back pain, with 100mg of harpagoside, considered superior, when neurological deficits are present.[69, 70] A recent systematic review[71] has reported a prevalence of 3% of gastrointestinal complaints in 20 of 28 clinical trials investigated. A few reports of acute toxicity were found (e.g. gastrointestinal complaints, allergies) but there were no reports on chronic toxicity, perhaps due to the low doses utilised in most of the studies.[71]

Ginger (*Zingiber officinale*)

The fresh and/or dried roots of *Zingiber officinale* are reported to possess anti-inflammatory, antiseptic and carminative properties and has been used to treat inflammatory and rheumatic diseases.[72] The pungent phenolic constituent of ginger, 6-gingerol, has been shown to inhibit LPS-induced iNOS expression and production of NO in macrophages and to block peroxynitrite-induced oxidation and nitration reactions *in vitro*.[72–74] Cumulative laboratory animal data suggest that 6-gingerol is a potent inhibitor of NO synthesis and effective in inhibiting production of PGE2 and TNF-alpha and COX-2 expression in human synoviocytes by regulating NFκB activation and degradation of its inhibitor IkBa subunit.[72]

A recent RCT of a combined extract of the herbs *Zingiber officinale* and *Alpinia galanga*, comprising 255mg extracted from 2500–4000mg ginger and 500–1500mg galanga rhizome respectively, demonstrated a positive effect on knee OA.[75] Clinical trial participants in the ginger/galangal combined extract group experienced a 63% reduction in knee pain on standing versus 50% in the placebo group.[75] The highly purified and standardised extract had a statistically significant effect on reducing symptoms of OA of the knee with a high safety profile, and mild GI adverse events in the ginger extract group.[75] In a further cross-over RCT, in patients with OA, the ginger extract showed statistically significant efficacy in the first period of treatment before cross-over, however a significant difference was not observed in the study overall.[76]

Wintergreen (*Gaultheria yunnanensis*)

Topical natural products that include liniments, balms, creams, gels, oils, lotions, patches, ointments and other products that are applied to the skin are often sought with the intent to provide pain relief for mild arthritis pain that affects only a few joints, as well as to ease sore muscles, back pain and OA.[77,78] No clinical trials are currently available to evaluate these effects. However, *in vivo* studies have shown that a salicylate fraction isolated from wintergreen has analgesic and anti-inflammatory properties.[79] Caution, even with topical products, is required in patients receiving warfarin as adverse interactions and bleeding have been reported to be a risk with its use.[80]

Phytodolor

Phytodolor is a herbal proprietary product that includes aspen (*Populus tremula*), goldenrod (*Solidago virgaurea*) and golden ash (*Fraxinus excelsior*). Although most of the available literature is German, a recent systematic review of 6 RCTs which included the German studies concluded that Phytodolor reduced the pain associated with rheumatic disorders.[80] The dose administered was 30 drops TID for 3 of the trials and 40 drops TID for the remainder, with duration ranging from 2 to 4 weeks.

Boswellia and/or frankincense (*Boswellia serrata*)

Boswellia serrata (boswellia) is a popular Ayurvedic herb that is purported to exhibit effective analgesic, anti-inflammatory and anti-arthritic activity.[81–84] A recent RCT assessed the efficacy, safety and tolerability in 30 patients with OA of the knee over a 16-week period.[84] Patients receiving 333mg of boswellia extract containing 40% boswellic acid, 3 times daily, reported a significant decrease in knee pain and swelling, and an associated increase in function and range of movement. Adverse reactions of boswellia therapy were uncommon and included diarrhoea, epigastric pain, and nausea, all of which responded to simple symptomatic management.[84] A further RCT compared the same extract with valdecoxib, a non-steroidal anti-inflammatory drug in 66 patients with knee OA over 6 months. This study has a slower onset of action with pain relief persisting for 1 month after ceasing treatment, while valdecoxib acted faster but lasted only during therapy.[85]

White bark

There is a resurgence of interest in willow bark as a treatment for chronic pain syndromes associated with OA. While white willow (*Salix alba*) is the willow species most commonly used for medicinal purposes, crack willow (*Salix fragilis*), purple willow (*Salix purpurea*), and violet willow (*Salix daphnoides*) are all salicin-rich species and are available under the label of willow bark. RCTs of short duration have provided evidence of efficacy.[86]

Historically, Hippocrates was known to prescribe the bark and the leaves of the white willow bark to help relieve pain and fever.[86] In 1832, a German chemist produced salicylic acid from salicin, the active ingredient in willow bark. Acetyl salicylic acid was used to produce aspirin and is the more stable form, widely used internationally.[86]

Rosehip (rose haw)

Recent systematic searches of the literatures,[87,88] have demonstrated that rosehip powder or the seeds of the *Rosa canina* subspecies had a moderate effect in patients with OA. A study that enrolled 94 patients with OA of the hip or knee in a double-blind placebo-controlled (DBPC) cross-over trial,[89] reported that the 47 patients who were given 5g/day of the herbal remedy for a period of 3 months, resulted in a significant reduction in WOMAC pain ($P<0.014$) as compared to placebo, when testing after 3 weeks of treatment. Furthermore, the clinical data suggested that the herbal remedy not only alleviated symptoms but also reduced the consumption of 'rescue medication' for pain relief.

A recent meta-analysis of the literature identified 3 randomised control trials (RCTs) inclusive of 287 patients over a mean 3-month period and demonstrated rosehip powder significantly reduced OA pain compared with placebo, although long-term studies are required to assess its long-term efficacy and safety.[90]

Comfrey (*Symphytum officinale L*)

A recent randomised, double-blind, bi-centre, placebo-controlled clinical trial investigated the effect of a daily application of 6g (3 x 2g) of a commercially available preparation labelled as *Kytta-Salbe® f* over a 3-week period with patients suffering from painful OA of the knee.[91] The results documented suggested that the comfrey root extract ointment was significantly appropriate for the treatment of OA of the knee. Pain was reduced, mobility of the knee improved and quality of life increased.

French maritime pine bark extract

A randomised, double-blind, placebo-controlled trial of 100 patients with mild-moderate knee OA who were treated for 3 months with either 150mg French maritime pine bark extract once daily at meals or by placebo demonstrated reduction of symptoms in the treated group.[92] Patients on the herbal extract reported an improvement of WOMAC index, significant alleviation of pain and reduction of analgesia use compared with no effect with placebo. The pine bark extract was well tolerated and postulated to have anti-inflammatory actions.[92]

Capsaicin (*Capsicum frutescens*)

A recent systematic review has concluded that topically applied capsaicin has moderate to poor efficacy in the treatment of chronic musculoskeletal or neuropathic pain. Further, that it could be useful as an adjunct or sole therapy for a small number of patients who are unresponsive to, or intolerant of, other treatments.[93]

A summary of herbal medicines appears in Table 29.3.

Other supplements

Glucosamine

Even though the therapeutic effectiveness of glucosamine treatment on OA has been demonstrated by improved mobility and relief of pain in animal models as well as in RCTs[94] its effectiveness as a symptom and disease modifier for OA is still under debate. A recent meta-analysis concluded that the evidence for efficacy for improving symptoms in OA was conflicting and that glucosamine hydrocholoride was not effective.[95] A recent study reported that glucosamine sulfate was no better than placebo in reducing symptoms and progression of hip OA.[96]

A Cochrane review concluded that a specific type of glucosamine sulfate supplement (from Dona, Rotta Pharmaceuticals, Inc) was superior to placebo in the treatment of pain and functional impairment resulting from symptomatic OA.[97] Results for the non-Rotta preparation were not statistically significant. The review analysed data from 20 RCTs involving 2570 participants, of which 10 RCTs used the Rotta preparation. A second systematic review reviewed RCTs of at least 1 year's duration.[95] It was reported that glucosamine sulfate may be effective and safe in delaying the progression and improving the symptoms of knee OA. A previous Cochrane review of 16 RCTs had found that glucosamine was effective, however, these included smaller trials with less methodological rigor.[98]

A concern with most trials of glucosamine sulfate, glucosamine hydrochloride and chondroitin sulfate in the treatment of OA was weak research designs that had been employed.[99] The Glucosamine/Chondroitin Arthritis Intervention Trial (GAIT) was designed to address these inconsistencies and provide some clarity on the effectiveness of glucosamine (1500mg/day) and chondroitin (1200mg/day) for the treatment of knee pain in OA by employing a rigorous research design.[100] The GAIT found that glucosamine and chondroitin sulfate, alone or in combination, did not significantly reduce OA knee pain more than placebo.[100] A combination of glucosamine and chondroitin sulfate was found to be effective in a subgroup of patients with moderate-to-severe knee pain (79.2% versus 54.3 % for placebo).[100] The combined emerging data suggests that glucosamine has a structure-modifying effect. However, debate remains regarding this, largely in relation to methodological issues surrounding outcome measures used in the positive studies.

It has been reported that there is extensive heterogeneity among trials of glucosamine and that this is larger than would be expected by chance. Glucosamine hydrochloride does not appear to be effective.[101] Among trials with industry involvement, effect sizes were consistently reported to be higher. The potential explanations may include different glucosamine preparations, inadequate allocation concealment, and industry bias.[101]

Chondroitin sulfate (CS)

An RCT employing chondroitin sulfate (GS) on 40 patients with tibio-fibular OA of the knee, were allocated to receive 50 intramuscular injections (one injection twice weekly) for 25 weeks. CS had a significantly greater therapeutic effect on all symptoms evaluated.[102] No important local or systemic side-effects were noted.[102] Favourable effects have been reported in pain reduction and improvement in mobility when CS was given either intra-articularly or orally to elderly patients with joint degeneration.[103]

A double-blind RCT with 104 patients receiving oral chondroitin-4-sulfate and chondroitin-6-sulfate (CS4 and CS6) at a dose of 800mg/day or placebo for 1 year showed CS4 and CS6 had a beneficial effect, both in terms of clinical manifestations and anatomic progression, in patients with OA of the knee.[104] The main efficacy criterion was the Lequesne's functional index (LFI). Functional impairment was reduced by approximately 50%, with a significant improvement over placebo for all clinical criteria. Tolerance was excellent or good in more than 90% of cases. This study suggests that CS act as structure modulators as illustrated by improvement in the interarticular space visualised on x-rays of patients treated with CS4 and CS6.[104]

Table 29.3 Herbal medicines with demonstrated therapeutic anti-inflammatory and analgesic activity

Herbals/ botanicals	Actions	Indications	Dosages	Contraindications and cautions
Boswellia/ frankincense (*Boswellia serrata*)	Anti-inflammatory	OA	600–1200mg/ day extract standardised to 60% boswellic acids	Occasional mild diarrhoea or urticaria LD50 <2 g/kg
Devil's claw (*Harpogophytum procumbens*)	Anti-inflammatory Analgesic Chondro-protective Anti-rheumatic	OA	Liquid extract (1:2) 6–12 ml/day Trials indicate a need to use extracts with >50mg harpagoside for pain relief	High doses may increase effects of warfarin Theoretical interaction with anti-arrhythmic drugs — monitor use Not recommended in pregnancy May cause GI irritation Use with caution in patients with gastric and duodenal ulcers, gallstones and acute diarrhoea Suspend use 1 week before surgery LD_{50} <13.5 g/kg
Ginger (Zingiber officinale)	Anti-inflammatory Analgesic	OA	250mg QID	Theoretically may increase bleeding when high doses taken with anticoagulants and antiplatelet agents Caution advised in patients with gastric ulcers and reflux
Phytodolor	Anti-inflammatory Analgesic	OA	20 drops TID 1200mg/day in divided doses	None reported
Rosehip (rose haw)	Anti-inflammatory	OA	5g/day of powder orally administered Moderate efficacy reported	None reported
White willow bark (*Salix alba*)	Anti-inflammatory Analgesic	OA	Tincture (1:1) 1–2ml twice daily Trials for OA and lower back pain used preparations standardised to 240mg/day salicin in divided doses	High doses may theoretically increase effect of anticoagulants Avoid if salicylate sensitivity LD_{50} 28 ml/kg Requires thorough evaluation for renal, haematologic, and hepatic function

(Source: adapted and modified from Vitetta L, Cicuttini F, Sali A. Alternative therapies for musculoskeletal conditions. Best Pract Res Clin Rheumatol 2008:22(3):499–522)

A double-blind RCT of 42 patients with symptomatic OA of the knee examined the effect of 400mg CS twice daily for 1 year.[105] After 3 months, joint pain was significantly reduced in the CS group compared to the placebo group. This difference became more pronounced after 12 months. The increase in overall mobility capacity was significantly greater at 6 and 12 months in the CS group than in the placebo group. After 1 year, the mean width of the medial femoro-tibial joint was unchanged from baseline in the CS group, but had decreased significantly in the placebo group. Although no statistical comparison was presented for the change in joint-space width between the 2 groups, the finding suggests the possibility CS treatment may slow the progression of OA.[105] The proprietary chondroitin sulfate was studied in a further double-blind RCT of 85 patients with OA of the knee. Participants received Condrosulf® at a dose of 400mg twice daily or placebo for 6 months. Lequesne's index, spontaneous joint pain, and walking time all decreased progressively in the CS group, with a significant difference in favour of the CS group for each of these parameters.[106] In a double-blind RCT parallel group study using either CS 1g/day or placebo on 130 patients for 3 months followed by a 3-month post-treatment period, the CS group experienced greater but non-significant improvement than the placebo group at the treatment endpoint, as measured by the LFI. Improvement became significant in the completer population. In the intent-to-treat population, all variables tended toward greater improvement in the CS than the placebo group. One month after treatment, CS had a significantly higher persistent effect than placebo on the LFI, pain with activity, and other efficacy criteria. Adverse event rates did not differ significantly.[107]

To assess the clinical efficacy of CS in comparison with the NSAID diclofenac sodium, a multi-centre double-blind RCT, double-dummy study on 146 patients was conducted for 6 months.[108] Patients treated with diclofenac showed prompt reduction of clinical symptoms that reappeared, however, after the end of treatment. In the CS group, the therapeutic response appeared later but lasted up to 3 months after the end of treatment. It was concluded that CS had slow but gradually increasing clinical activity in OA, and these benefits lasted a long period after the end of treatment. Shortcomings in these studies were that they involved only a relatively small number of patients and no dose-finding investigations for CS could be found.

A double-blind prospective RCT study of 300 patients given a proprietary registered brand of chondroitin sulfate 800mg/day or placebo for 2 years investigated the structure-modulating properties of CS in gonarthrosis by measuring the modifications in minimum joint space width (JSW), mean thickness, and mean surface of the cartilage in internal femoro-tibial function.[109] There was a significant difference, with worsening of the arthritis in the placebo group compared to the CS group. In the group treated with CS, there were no significant variations in any radiological parameters, which remained remarkably stable. The statistical analysis revealed a significant difference in the CS group compared to the placebo group in regard to maintenance of the cartilage analysed, in both the intent-to-treat analysis and also in the per-protocol of analysis subjects who completed the study protocol. It was shown that CS was superior to placebo with regard to stabilisation of minimum JSW of the internal femoro-tibial articular space, the mean thickness, and the surface.[109] Hence there is sufficient controlled trial data to support the use of CS in symptomatic OA, having less side-effects than currently used NSAIDs. Chondroitin sulfates appear to have a role in prevention of disease progression. The requisite is that CS be further evaluated in studies of longer treatment duration, with larger numbers of patients, and using well-established measures of function and progression.

A recent meta-analysis reporting on a set of poor to moderate quality, largely heterogeneous (in methodology) trials that made interpretation of the data difficult, concluded that the results were unreliable. Further, the authors concluded that since large-scale, methodologically sound trials indicate that the symptomatic benefit of chondroitin is minimal or nonexistent, that chondroitin cannot be recommended.[110]

Despite these findings a recent well-performed long-term double-blind study of 622 patients with knee OA, randomised to 800mg of CS or placebo once daily for a 2-year period, demonstrated significant pain relief and radiological improvement by way of demonstrable reduction in minimum JSW loss on X-Rays in the CS group as compared with the placebo group.[111]

Collagen hydrolysate

Four open label and 3 double-blind trials have been reported in a review of the literature.[112] In a 24-week multi-country double-blind RCT on knee OA, 10g/day of collagen hydrosylate did not improve the WOMAC index.[113] Post-study analysis suggested that the hydrolysate could be more efficient in severe OA. A 60-day cross-over double-blind RCT on knee and hip OA compared 10g/day of collagen hydrolysate, gelatin, gelatin + glycin + calcium phosphate, or egg albumin[114] and found the gelatin preparations were not significantly different from each other and were superior to egg albumin in reducing pain as assessed by a patient questionnaire. According to the best evidence, efficacy for collagen hydrolysate is equivocal. However, a recent systematic review points to a growing body of evidence and provides a rationale for the use of collagen hydrolysate for patients with OA.[112]

Methylsulfonylmethane (MSM)

In a 12-week double-blind RCT on knee OA, 500mg of methylsulfonylmethane TID used alone, or in combination with 500mg of glucosamine HCl 3 times a day, significantly improved a Likert scale of pain and LFI.[115] The combination of both ingredients was not more efficacious than each ingredient used alone. In a further 12-week double-blind RCT on knee OA, 3g of methylsulfonylmethane given twice daily was more efficient than placebo in decreasing WOMAC pain and functional scores.[116] According to the best-evidence synthesis, MSM provides moderate evidence of efficacy for knee OA.[117]

S-Adenosyl Methionine (SAMe)

A practical amount of research evidence exists to support the use of SAMe for the treatment of pain associated with OA.[118] A meta-analysis of 11 RCTs comprising 1442 participants with an average age of 60.3 years from 2002, demonstrated that SAMe is as effective as NSAIDs in reducing the pain of OA, with significantly fewer side-effects.[119]

New Zealand green-lipped mussel (*Perna Canaliculus*)

The reported incidence of arthritis in coastal-dwelling Maoris is low, and it has been suggested that this is possibly due to their high consumption of green-lipped mussels.[120] However, results from clinical trials have been inconsistent, with a recent review concluding that there is little consistent and compelling evidence, to date, in the therapeutic use of freeze-dried green-lipped mussel powder products for RA and OA treatment but that further investigations are warranted.[120] Recently a study was conducted to validate the clinical efficacy and safety of Lyprinol (a patented extract from *Perna Canaliculus*), a 5-LOX inhibitor in patients with OA.[121] The results demonstrated that after a 4- and 8-week treatment period, 53% and 80% (respectively) of the trial participants experienced significant pain relief, and improvement of joint function. There was no reported adverse effect during the trial.

Lipids (avocado/soybean unsaponifiables)

Four double-blind RCTs and 1 systematic review have evaluated avocado/soybean unsaponifiables (ASUs) on knee and hip OA.[122–127] In two 3-month RCTs, 1 on OA of the knee only[123] and 1 on knee and hip OA,[125] 300mg once a day decreased NSAID intake. The efficacy of ASU at a dosage of 300mg/day and 600mg/day was consistently superior to that of placebo at all endpoints.[123] However, no statistical difference in any primary or secondary endpoints was detected between 300 and 600mg once a day.[123] In a 3-month RCT on knee and hip OA, 300mg once a day resulted in an improved LFI compared with placebo.[124] ASUs had a 2-month delayed onset of action as well as residual symptomatic effects 2 months after the end of treatment.[124] In a 2-year RCT on hip OA, 300mg once a day did not slow down narrowing of JSW.[125] In addition, none of the secondary endpoints LFI, visual analogue scale of pain, NSAID intake, and patients' and investigators' global assessments was statistically different from placebo after 1 year. However, a post-hoc analysis suggested that ASUs might decrease narrowing of JSW in patients with the most severe hip OA.[125]

Although ASUs might display medium-term symptom-modifying effects on knee and hip OA, their symptom-modifying effects in the long term (>1 year) have not been confirmed. Based on the best-evidence synthesis, ASUs is good for symptom-modifying effects in knee and hip OA with some evidence of absence of structure-modifying effects. A recent systematic review on ASUs recommended further investigation because 3 of the 4 rigorous RCTs suggest that ASUs is an effective symptomatic treatment, but the long-term study was largely negative.[126]

A Cochrane review identified 5 studies (4 different herbs) that met the criteria for the treatment of OA.[127] Two studies of ASU extracts showed beneficial effects on function, reduced pain, reduced requirement for NSAID medication and increased global evaluation. There were no serious side-effects reported. The reviewers concluded the evidence for

ASUs in the treatment of OA is convincing but evidence for the other herbal interventions is insufficient to either recommend or discourage their use.[128]

Fish oils/omega-3 (n-3) fatty acids

There are currently no RCTs on the effect of n-3 fatty acids in OA. However, there are suggestions that supplementation with long-chain n-3 PUFA may be beneficial for those with active/inflamed OA joints.[35] In a recent review, the authors reported that in a small unpublished trial carried out in Wales, OA patients supplemented with cod-liver oil showed reduced COX-2 expression and COX-2 protein levels and that the levels of inflammatory eicosanoids were reduced in some cases.[35]

Supplements for OA are summarised in Table 29.4.

Physical therapies

Hydrotherapy/water-based exercises

It is well known that hydrotherapy and water-based exercises can provide symptomatic relief of pain and improve joint flexibility for OA patients. A recent randomised study aimed to compare the outcomes between land-based and water-based exercise programs (1 hour sessions twice weekly) in 102 patients, 2 weeks after a total knee replacement, for up to 6 months and found equally significant improvements observed in both groups for joint pain, stiffness, flexibility and leg oedema.[128]

Acupuncture

Non-pharmacological treatments such as acupuncture are attractive because of their safety profile and the adverse events that have been well documented with the use of pharmaceuticals, especially when considering an elderly population.

Recent meta-analysis and systematic review concluded that acupuncture procedures that meet criteria for adequate treatment were significantly greater to sham acupuncture and to no additional intervention in improving pain and function in patients with chronic knee pain that was due to OA.[129, 130, 131] These recent studies confirm an earlier systematic review and meta-analysis that concluded that:

1. acupuncture is often used for treating and relieving chronic pain due to OA
2. the meta-analysis of 3 trials showed a significant effect of manual acupuncture compared with a sham acupuncture procedure
3. there were confirmed beneficial effects for ameliorating pain for peripheral joint OA.[130]

There is, however, due to the nature of the heterogeneity in the results, a requisite for further research to confirm these findings and provide more information on long-term effects.[131]

Magnetic therapies, TENS and low level laser therapy (LLLT)

Whilst research in the past showed magnetic therapy to be promising for the stimulation of cartilage growth in *in vitro* studies, a recent Cochrane review of 259 OA patients found small to moderate effects on outcomes for knee OA.[132] All outcomes were statistically significant with clinical benefit ranging from 13–23% greater with active treatment compared with placebo. The reviewers concluded that there was a significant need for further large-scale studies of pulsed electric stimulation with a focus on knee OA to establish the clinical relevance of this treatment for the management of OA.[132]

LLLT is a light source that generates extremely pure light, of a single wavelength. LLLT was introduced as an alternative non-invasive treatment for OA about 20 years ago, but its effectiveness is still controversial. A recent Cochrane review identified 7 trials of 184 patients randomised to laser and 161 patients to placebo laser.[133] Treatment duration ranged from 4 to 12 weeks. Pain was assessed by 4 trials. Three trials showed very positive effects on pain relief and 3 trials found no effect. Only 1 patient reported an erythema as a side-effect, and was then excluded for the rest of the study. Lower dosage of LLLT was found to be as effective as the higher dosage for reducing pain and improving knee range of motion.[133] In another trial with no scale-based pain outcome, significantly more patients reported pain relief (yes/no) with laser with an odds ratio of 0.05, (95% CI: 0.0 to 1.56). Of the 7 studies only 1 study found significant results for increased knee range of motion (WMD: -10.62 degrees, 95% CI: -14.07,-7.17). Other outcomes of joint tenderness and strength were not significant. The review concluded that there was an urgent need for further large-scale studies of laser therapy for OA. In particular, the application of laser therapy to the nerve as well as the joint was shown to be beneficial in 1 trial.[133]

Recently, a systematic review of physical treatments was conducted with meta-analysis of efficacy within 1–4 weeks and at follow up at 1–12 weeks after the end of treatment.[134]

Table 29.4 Supplements with demonstrated therapeutic anti-inflammatory and analgesic activity

Supplements	Actions	Indications	Dosages	Contraindications and Cautions
Glucosamine sulfate Glucosamine hydrochloride	Anti-inflammatory Chondro-protective	OA	1500mg/day usually in divided doses Most research has been conducted on glucosamine sulfate	Occasional mild digestive problems, headache, drowsiness and skin reactions Avoid in patients with shellfish allergy Avoid or caution with warfarin treatment
Chondroitin	Chondro-protective	OA	1200mg/day usually in divided doses	
Collagen hydrolysate	Chondro-protective	OA	10g/day	
Lipids (avocado/soybean unsaponifiables)	Chondro-protective	OA	300–600mg /day	
Methyl-sulfonylmethane	Chondro-protective	OA	500mg TID alone or in combination with glucosamine	
NZ green-lipped mussel	Anti-inflammatory	OA Results still remain inconclusive	1050–1150mg/day of freeze-dried powder	GI discomfort, gout, skin rashes and 1 case of granulomatous hepatitis have been reported in trials Contraindicated in people with shellfish allergies Theoretical caution with hypertension due to sodium content
SAMe	Anti-inflammatory	OA	A lower dose of 400mg/day may be used as a maintenance dose once a response occurs	Tricyclic and SSRI antidepressants as serotonin syndrome theoretically possible Thyroxine — monitor Betaine — monitor Extreme caution in bipolar disorder, schizophrenia, schizoaffective disorder and Parkinson's disease
Fish oils	Anti-inflammatory	OA	1–3g/day	Bleeding tendency in high dose (>10g/day) Avoid if seafood allergic

(Source: adapted and modified from Vitetta L, Cicuttini F, Sali A. Alternative therapies for musculoskeletal conditions. Best Pract Res Clin Rheumatol 2008:22(3):499–522)

The patient cohort had a mean age of 65.1 years and mean baseline pain of 62.9mm on a 100mm visual analogue scale. Within 4 weeks of the commencement of treatment manual acupuncture, static magnets and ultrasound therapies did not offer statistically significant short-term pain relief over placebo. Pulsed electromagnetic fields offered a small reduction in pain of –6.9mm. Transcutaneous electrical nerve stimulation (TENS), including interferential currents, electro-acupuncture and low LLLT, offered clinically relevant pain relieving effects of –18.8mm, –21.9mm and –17.7mm respectively, versus placebo control.[134]

Therapeutic touch

A single randomised control trial of 82 non-institutionalised patients with knee OA were randomised to therapeutic touch, or progressive muscle relaxation. The treatment group noted significant improvement in pain and distress compared with the muscle relaxation group who also had improvements in pain scores.[135] The differences in effectiveness existed between the therapeutic touch and progressive muscle relaxation groups. That is, the pain and distress scores were lower in the progressive muscle relaxation group. The differences approached significance for pain and were significant for distress.

Conclusion

There is an interaction between musculoskeletal disease and the affected individual's lifestyle and psychosocial circumstances.

Intervention programs often focus on only 1 or a few components in the management of musculoskeletal diseases. There is not 1 single format that can be advised to give an evidence-based approach to every patient. The requisite is therefore for an integrative approach to improve the quality of life for the patient, particularly with the aim to reduce pain and improve function of the joints. This approach may require a multi-team involvement to assist the patient meet their symptom management needs. The cornerstones for the treatment of musculoskeletal conditions hence require implementation of dietary and nutritional/ supplement interventions alongside physical activity (other manipulative or appropriate physical modalities), appropriate analgesia (nutritional, herbal or pharmaceutical), and patient education and engagement with a cognitive approach. Table 29.5 summarises the evidence for complementary medicine therapies.

Table 29.5 Levels of evidence for lifestyle and complementary medicines/therapies in the management of osteoarthritis

Modality	Level I	Level II	Level IIIa	Level IIIb	Level IIIc	Level IV	Level V
Lifestyle							
Diet and reduction in BMI					x		
Mind–body medicine							
CBT	x						
Hypnosis						x	
Physical activity/ exercise	x						
Tai chi		x					
Yoga				x			
Land and water-based exercises	x						
Nutritional supplements							
Beta-carotene					x		
Vitamin D				x			
Vitamin C					x		
Niacin					x		
Niacinamide vitamin B3					x		

Continued

Table 29.5 Levels of evidence for lifestyle and complementary medicines/therapies in the management of osteoarthritis—cont'd

Modality	Level I	Level II	Level IIIa	Level IIIb	Level IIIc	Level IV	Level V
Vitamin B12/folate					x		
Antioxidants (A, C, E, selenium)	x(-)						
Herbal medicine							
Catechins from green tea (*Camellia sinensis*)						x	
Cat's claw			x				
Harpogophytum procumbens	x						
Wintergreen (topical)						x	
Ginger (*Zingiber officinale*)		x(+/-)					
Capsicum spp. (topical)	x						
Phytodolor	x						
Boswellia serrata			x				
Willow bark			x				
Rosehip	x						
Comfrey (topical)		x					
Other supplements							
Glucosamine sulfate (rotta)	x*						
Chondroitin sulfate	x						
Collagen hydrolysate	x(+/-)	x					
Methylsulfonylmethane		x					
S-Adenosyl Methionine (SAME)		x					
New Zealand Green-lipped Mussels		x					
Lipids (avocado/soybean unsaponifiables)	x						
French maritime pine bark extract			x				
Omega-3 fatty acids						x	
Physical therapies							
Magnetic therapies	x						
Low Level Laser Therapy	x						
Acupuncture	x						
Therapeutic touch			x				

*Rotta glucosamine sulfate

Level I — from a systematic review of all relevant randomised controlled trials — meta-analyses.
Level II — from at least 1 properly designed randomised controlled clinical trial.
Level IIIa — from well-designed pseudo-randomised controlled trials (alternate allocation or some other method).
Level IIIb — from comparative studies (including systematic reviews of such studies) with concurrent controls and allocation not randomised, cohort studies, case-control studies, or interrupted time series with a parallel control group.
Level IIIc — from comparative studies with historical control, 2 or more single-arm studies or interrupted time series without a parallel control group.
Level IV — opinions of respected authorities based on clinical experience, descriptive studies or reports of expert committees.
Level V — represents minimal evidence that represents testimonials.

Clinical tips handout for patients — osteoarthritis

1 Lifestyle advice

Sleep

- Restore normal sleep patterns. Early to bed (about 9–10 p.m.) and awake with sunrise. (See Chapter 22 or more advice.)

Sunshine

- Amount of exposure varies with local climate.
- At least 15 minutes of sunshine needed daily for vitamin D and melatonin production — especially before 10 a.m. and after 3 p.m. when the sun exposure is safest during summer. Much more exposure is required in winter, when supplementation needs to be considered.
- Ensure gradual, adequate skin exposure to sun; avoid sunscreen and excess clothing to maximise levels of vitamin D.
- More time in the sun is required for dark skinned people.
- Direct exposure to about 10% of body (hands, arms, face), without sunscreen and not through glass.
- Vitamin D is obtained in the diet from fatty fish, eggs, liver and fortified foods (some milks and margarines). It is unlikely that adequate vitamin D concentrations can be obtained from diet alone.

2 Physical activity/exercise

- Exercise 30–60 minutes daily. If exercise is not regular, commence with 5 minutes daily and slowly build up to at least 30 minutes. Outdoor exercise with nature, fresh air and sunshine is ideal (e.g. brisk walking, light jogging, cycling, swimming, stretching, weight-bearing exercises). The more time you spend outdoors the better.
- Tai chi, qigong and yoga could be quite helpful.
- Splints may help to protect inflamed joints e.g. wrist splints when carrying shopping. Avoid prolonged use of splints as they can weaken muscles.

3 Mind–body medicine

- Stress management program — for example, six 40 minute sessions for patients to understand the nature of their symptoms, the symptoms' relationship to stress, and the practice of regular relaxation exercises.
- Regular meditation practice, at least 10–20 minutes daily.
- Psychological therapy and cognitive behaviour therapy may help to deal with difficult issues and stressors.

Breathing

- Be aware of breathing at all times. Notice if tendency to hold breath or over-breathe. Always aim to relax breath and the muscles around the chest wall.

Rest and stress management

Recurrent stress may cause a return of symptoms. Relaxation is important for a full and lasting recovery.

- Reduce workload and resolve conflicts. Contact family, friends, church or social groups for support.
- Listening to relaxation music helps.
- Relaxation massage therapy is helpful.
- Cognitive behavioural therapy and psychotherapy are extremely helpful.
- Hypnotherapy, biofeedback may be of help.

Focus on wellness, not just the disease.

Fun

- It is important to have fun in life.
- Joy can be found even in the simplest tasks, such as funny movies/videos, comedy, hobbies, dancing, playing with pets and children.

4 Environment

- Avoid smoking, environmental pollutants and chemicals — at work and in the home.

5 Dietary changes

- Do not rush your meals; relax before meals; chew your food thoroughly before swallowing as this aids digestion; develop regular relaxed eating patterns.
- Eat more vitamin C rich foods.
- Aim to lose weight if you or your health practitioner believes you are overweight.
- Vegetarian and Mediterranean diets are particularly useful for arthritis sufferers.
- Eat regular balanced healthy meals, ideally 3 small meals, and 2 snacks, each containing protein in order to avoid fluctuating blood sugar levels and provide amino acids for nerve transmitters such as tryptophan.

- Eat more fruit (>2/day) and vegetables (>5/day) — a variety of colours and those in season.
- Eat more nuts, seeds, beans, sprouts (e.g. alfalfa, mung beans, lentils).
- Increase fish intake (sardines, tuna, salmon, cod, mackerel) especially deep sea fish >3 servings per week.
- Reduce red meat intake — preferably eat lean red meat (e.g. lamb, kangaroo) and white meat (e.g. free range organic chicken).
- Eat wholegrains/cereals (variety): rice (brown, basmati, Mahatmi, Doongara), traditional rolled oats, buckwheat flour, wholegrain organic breads (rye bread, Essene, spelt, Kamut), brown pasta, couscous, millet, amaranth etc.
- Reduce dairy intake; consume low fat dairy products such as yoghurt and cheeses, unless there is a dairy intolerance.
- Drink more water (1–2 litres a day) and teas (especially green tea, black tea).
- Cold pressed olive oil — 4 teaspoons and 1 tablespoon flaxseed oil (uncooked) daily. Eat avocado.
- Dark chocolate — 100g/day unless not tolerated.
- Avoid hydrogenated fats, salt, fast foods, sugar (such as in soft drinks), lollies, biscuits, cakes and processed foods (e.g. white bread, white pasta, pastries).
- Avoid chemical additives — preservatives, colourings and flavourings.
- For sweetener try honey (e.g. manuka, yellow box and stringy bark have lowest GI).
- Avoid coffee.
- Avoid excessive high salicylate rich foods if they upset you (see Chapter 2).

6 Physical therapies

- Hydrotherapy is particularly useful.
- Acupuncture, electromagnetic therapy, low-level laser therapy and TENS may help relieve pain.
- Therapeutic touch such as reiki may help reduce pain.

7 Supplements

Fish oils

- Indication: may help reduce inflammatory joint pain; prevent heart disease.
- Dosage: 3–7g/day as tolerated and as indicated for high blood pressure (e.g. EPA 180/DHA 120mg).
- Results: 4–7 days.
- Side-effects: often well tolerated especially if taken with meals. Very mild and rare side-effects (e.g. gastrointestinal upset); allergic reactions (e.g. rash, breathing problems if allergic to seafood); blood thinning effects in very high doses > 10g/day (may need to stop fish oil supplements 2 weeks prior to surgery).
- Contraindications: sensitivity reaction to seafood; drug interactions; caution when taking high doses of fish oils >4g/day together with warfarin (your doctor will check your INR test).

Vitamins

Vitamin C

- Indication: may reduce OA pain; may help with gout.
- Dosage: 500–1000–1500mg/day or as tolerated.
- Results: unknown.
- Side-effects: usually well tolerated; gastrointestinal irritation (especially in high doses) such as nausea, heartburn, abdominal cramps, loose stools, diarrhoea. Reduce dosage if this occurs.
- Contraindications: avoid if you have renal impairment or kidney stones.

Vitamin D3 (cholecalciferol 25mg or 1000 international units)

Doctors should check blood levels and suggest supplementation if levels are low.

Sun exposure can help build up your vitamin D levels. Expose skin to sun adequately, but safely. Take with calcium supplements (e.g. Ca citrate).

- Indication: may help reduce pain of OA, leg pains; maintains healthy bone density, builds muscle strength and reduces falls in elderly, improves absorption of calcium and phosphate for healthy bones.
- Dosage: adult 1000mcg or more depending on blood levels. Children under 12 years, pregnant and lactating women: as professional prescribed.
- Results: 1–3 months.
- Side-effects: bone pain, excess calcium, gastrointestinal irritation, nausea, vomiting, and diarrhoea. The dosage varies from person to person.
- Contraindications: sensitivity to sulfites; avoid if you have high blood calcium levels (e.g. in cancer or kidney diseases).

Niacinamide/vitamin B3

Vitamin B3 includes niacin and niacinamide. Niacin is converted to niacinamide. Niacinamide is better tolerated than niacin. Best combined in a multi-B supplement.

- Indication: may help reduce pain of OA; pellagra, hyperlipidemia.
- Dosage: adult, 100–300mg/day to 3 times daily. Use with care in children, pregnant and lactating women.
- Results: 2–4 weeks.
- Side-effects: may cause liver impairment; gastrointestinal irritation, nausea, vomiting, and diarrhoea; flushing effect; in high doses can cause insulin resistance; dizziness, drowsiness, headaches.
- Contraindications: liver and kidney disease; diabetes, allergies, sensitivity to sulfites; avoid if you have high blood calcium levels (e.g. in cancer or kidney diseases).

Pantothenic acid/Vitamin B5

- Indication: may help reduce pain of OA; pantothenic deficiency; burning feet syndrome; dandruff. Best combined in a multi-B supplement.
- Dosage: adult, 5–10–12.5mg/day. Use with care in children, pregnant and lactating women. Avoid high doses. Safe to apply on joints as a topical cream.
- Results: 2–4 weeks.
- Side-effects: usually well tolerated; may cause pins and needles, paraesthesia and leg weakness (reversed with pyridoxine); gastrointestinal irritation, nausea, vomiting, and diarrhoea; dizziness, drowsiness, headaches.
- Contraindications: avoid taking with royal jelly which contains high amounts of pantothenic acid.

Folic acid and vitamin B12 cyanocobalamin

Folic acid (6400mcg) and cyanocobalamin (20mcg) consumed orally over a 2-month period demonstrated greater improvements in hand grip and number of tender joints.

Check with your health or medical practitioner. Best combined in a multi-B supplement.

Herbal medicines

Green tea (*Camellia sinensis*)

- Indication: may alleviate osteoarthritis pain and improve joint function and mobility. May improve mental alertness and energy.
- Dosage: 1–3 cups daily of infused green tea; avoid high doses in pregnancy, lactation and young children.
- Results: 2–7 days.
- Side-effects: usually well tolerated, however, in excess may develop symptoms related to caffeine intoxication that cause gastrointestinal irritation, reflux, heartburn, nausea, vomiting, abdominal discomfort and diarrhoea; dizziness, restlessness, agitation, headache, insomnia, tremor (like caffeine intoxication); liver impairment; allergic reaction.
- Contraindications: liver disease, caffeine sensitivity, anxiety disorder, high blood pressure, drug/amphetamine use; cardiac arrhythmias.

Devil's claw (*Harpogophytum procumbens*)

- Indication: may alleviate osteoarthritis pain and improve joint function and mobility; inflammatory back and joint pain; migraine.
- Dosage: 50–100mg harpagoside/day.
- Results: 2–7 days.
- Side-effects: Usually well tolerated. May cause gastrointestinal irritation, reflux, heartburn, nausea, vomiting, abdominal discomfort and diarrhoea; allergic reactions.
- Contraindications: avoid in pregnancy, lactation and young children. If taking blood thinners and warfarin avoid 1-2 weeks prior to surgery. Bleeding disorders.

Ginger (*Zingiber officinale*)

- Indication: may alleviate osteoarthritis pain and improve joint function and mobility; inflammatory back and joint pain; migraine; motion sickness, nausea of pregnancy and chemotherapy; low appetite.
- Dosage: 250mg 3–4 times daily in adults; 1g of dried powder as needed. Can use in pregnancy. Avoid high dosage in lactation and young children.
- Results: 2–7 days.
- Side-effects: usually well tolerated. May cause gastrointestinal irritation, reflux, heartburn, nausea, vomiting, abdominal discomfort and diarrhoea; allergic reactions.
- Contraindications: avoid with blood thinning medication; bleeding disorders.

Wintergreen (camphor/*gaultheria yunnanensis*), capsaicin topical, stinging nettle

May be combined with glucosamine and chondroitin, pantothenic acid (vitamin B5).

- Indication: may alleviate osteoarthritis pain and improve joint function and mobility; inflammatory back and joint pain; relieves pain; muscular pain; fibromyalgia. Capsaicin topical cream may also help neuropathic pain.
- Dosage: Topical use only. Camphor: 3–11% in low concentrations. Wintergreen liniment: 10% to 60% methyl salicylate. Capsaicin 0.025% to 0.075%. Topically 3–4 times daily.
- Results: 1–3 days.
- Side-effects: usually well tolerated. Avoid widespread use on skin; allergic reactions and dermatitis; tinnitus, confusion, salicylate-like reactions (see under Willow bark/*Salix alba*).
- Contraindications: avoid with blood thinning medication; bleeding disorders; children, pregnancy and lactation. Allergy to salicylates.

Boswellia/frankincense (*Boswellia serrata*)

- Indication: may alleviate osteoarthritis pain and improve joint function and mobility. Inflammatory back pain. Other forms of arthritis (e.g. rheumatoid arthritis, gout, spondylitis); inflammatory bowel disease; ulcerative colitis; asthma; dysmenorrhoea; pain.
- Dosage: 333mg 3 times daily in adults.
- Results: 2–7 days.
- Side-effects: usually well tolerated; may cause gastrointestinal irritation, reflux, heartburn, nausea, vomiting, abdominal discomfort and diarrhoea. Allergic reaction such as rash.
- Contraindications: avoid in pregnancy, lactation and young children.

Willow bark (*Salix alba*)

Willow bark has salycilate-like properties (anti-inflammatory).

- Indication: may alleviate osteoarthritis pain and improve joint function and mobility; inflammatory back pain; other forms of arthritis (e.g. rheumatoid arthritis, gout, spondylitis; headache; dysmenorrhoea; viral infections, pain.
- Dosage: 250mg salicin daily in adults.
- Results: 1–2 days.
- Side-effects: usually well tolerated; may cause gastrointestinal irritation, reflux, heartburn, nausea, vomiting, abdominal discomfort and diarrhoea. Salicylate toxicity (e.g. ringing in ears and confusion). Allergic reaction such as asthma, rash and anaphylaxis (rare). May cause kidney damage in high and prolonged use.
- Contraindications: avoid in children with fever (Reye's syndrome). Avoid if taking blood thinners (including garlic, gingko), aspirin and warfarin. Allergy or sensitivity to aspirin. Avoid if suffering allergic asthma or kidney disease. Avoid use at least 2 weeks prior to surgery due to blood thinning effects. Peptic ulcer.

Rosehip (rose haw) powder/tea

Fresh rose hips contains high concentrations of vitamin C.

- Indication: may alleviate osteoarthritis pain and improve joint function and mobility.
- Dosage: 5g/day orally in adults; 2.5mg tea infusion (hot water).
- Results: up to 1 week.
- Side-effects: usually well tolerated; may cause gastrointestinal irritation, nausea, vomiting, abdominal discomfort and diarrhoea.
- Contraindications: hemochromatosis and thalassemia; iron overload. Avoid in pregnancy, lactation and children. Avoid if taking warfarin.

Comfrey (*Symphytum officinale* L)

For topical use only.

- Indication: may alleviate OA pain and improve joint function and mobility.
- Dosage: 3–6g/day topically to arthritic joints; avoid extensive and prolonged use.
- Results: up to 1 week.
- Side-effects: may cause skin irritation and dermatitis.
- Contraindications: oral use as it has a history of causing liver damage. Avoid in pregnancy, lactation, children; if suffering liver disease; avoid applying to broken skin.

Other supplements

French maritime pine bark extract

- Indication: may alleviate OA pain and improve joint function and mobility. May also assist with hypertension, asthma and athletic performance.
- Dosage: 150–200mg/day with meals in adults; children >6 years of age 50–100mgs daily.
- Results: 1–2 weeks.
- Side-effects: usually well tolerated; may cause gastrointestinal irritation, nausea, vomiting, abdominal discomfort and diarrhoea; headache; dizziness.
- Contraindications: avoid in pregnancy, lactation.

Glucosamine sulfate (preferred)

Most forms of glucosamine are derived from shellfish; some are derived from bovine cartilage and others from corn starch suitable for vegetarians. Often glucosamine is combined with chondroitin sulfate.

- Indication: usually well tolerated; may alleviate osteoarthritis pain and improve joint function and mobility. May also improve degenerative changes on X-Ray findings if taken up to 2 years.
- Dosage: 1500mg 1–2 times daily in adults; evidence suggests topical use may help.
- Results: up to 4–6 weeks.
- Side-effects: allergic reaction such as skin reactions and asthma in those with seafood sensitivity. May cause gastrointestinal irritation, nausea, vomiting, abdominal discomfort and diarrhoea. May cause bleeding tendency. In rare situations, a severe allergic reaction can cause anaphylaxis. May aggravate asthma.
- Contraindications: known allergy to fish or shellfish. Avoid if taking warfarin as may cause increase in INR or if suffering from clotting disorders. Avoid in pregnancy, lactation and young children.

Chondroitin sulfate

- Chondroitin is derived from bovine (cow) cartilage.
- Indication: may alleviate osteoarthritis pain and improve joint function and mobility.
- Dosage: up to 1200mg/day in divided doses in adults.
- Results: up to 4–6 weeks.
- Side-effects: usually well tolerated; may cause gastrointestinal irritation, nausea, vomiting, abdominal discomfort and diarrhoea. May cause bleeding tendency in very high doses.
- Contraindications: avoid high doses of chondroitin if taking warfarin or suffer from a bleeding disorder; avoid in pregnancy, lactation and young children.

Collagen hydrolysate (gelatine)

This is a purified protein from animal collagen (e.g. pigs and cows); often found in food products.

- Indication: may alleviate joint pain and improve joint function and mobility; may assist with strengthening joints, hair and nails.
- Dosage: up to 10g/day in divided doses in adults.
- Results: up to 4–6 weeks.
- Side-effects: usually well tolerated; may cause gastrointestinal irritation, nausea, vomiting, abdominal discomfort and diarrhoea. Allergic skin reactions.
- Contraindications: Avoid if intolerance to cow or pig. Avoid in pregnancy, lactation and young children.

Methylsulfonylmethane (MSM)

This is a natural compound derived from green plants.

- Indication: may alleviate osteoarthritis pain and improve joint function and mobility; rheumatoid arthritis, tenosynovitis.
- Dosage: 1.5 to 6g/day in divided doses in adults.
- Results: up to 4–6 weeks.
- Side-effects: usually well tolerated; allergic reactions such as skin reactions and irritation. May cause gastrointestinal irritation, nausea, vomiting, abdominal discomfort and diarrhoea.
- Contraindications: young children, pregnancy and lactation.

S-Adenosyl Methionine (SAMe)

- Indication: may alleviate osteoarthritis pain; mild-moderate depression.
- Dosage: 400mg 2–3 times daily.
- Results: 3–7 days.
- Side-effects: very mild and rare.
- Contraindications: pregnancy, lactation, fertility, bipolar disorder, drug interaction; avoid use with other antidepressants.

New Zealand green-lipped mussel

Mollusc derived from mussel; rich in omega-3 fatty acids.

- Indication: may alleviate osteoarthritis pain and improve joint function and mobility; may also help rheumatoid arthritis, asthma.
- Dosage: 900–1200mg/day in divided doses in adults.
- Results: up to 4–6 weeks.
- Side-effects: usually well tolerated; allergic reaction such as skin reactions and asthma in those with seafood sensitivity. May cause gastrointestinal irritation, nausea, vomiting, abdominal discomfort and diarrhoea. May cause bleeding tendency. In rare situations, a severe allergic reaction can cause anaphylaxis. May aggravate asthma.
- Contraindications: known allergy to fish or shellfish. Avoid in pregnancy, lactation and young children.

Lipids (avocado/soybean unsaponifiables)

- Indication: may alleviate osteoarthritis pain and improve joint function and mobility; may help reduce cholesterol.
- Dosage: 300–600mg/day in divided doses in adults.
- Results: 1–2 weeks.
- Side-effects: usually well tolerated; may cause gastrointestinal irritation, nausea, vomiting, abdominal discomfort and diarrhoea.
- Contraindications: known allergy to avocado or soy. Avoid in pregnancy, lactation and young children.

References

1 Siebens HC. Musculoskeletal problems as comorbidities. Am J Phys Med Rehabil 2007;86: S69–S78.
2 Bergman S. Public health perspective-how to improve the musculoskeletal health of the population. Best Pract Res Clin Rheumatol 2007;21:191–204.
3 Centers for Disease Control and Prevention (CDC). Monitoring progress in arthritis management-United States and 25 states 2003. MMWR Morb Mortal Wkly Rep 2005;54:484–8.
4 Arden N, Nevitt MC. Osteoarthritis: epidemiology. Best Pract Res Clin Rheumatol 2006;20:3–25.
5 Arthritis Australia. Online. Available: http://arthritisaustralia.com.au/media/file/Access%20Economics%20Report%202001.pdf [accessed June 2008].
6 Eisenberg DM, Davis RB, Ettner SL, et. al. Trends in alternative medicine use in the United States 1990–1997: results of a follow-up national survey. JAMA 1998;280:1569–75.
7 MacLennan AH, Myers SP, Taylor AW. The continuing use of complementary and alternative medicine in South Australia costs and beliefs in 2004. Med J Aust. 2006;184:27–31.
8 Gregory PJ, Sperry M, Wilson AF. Dietary supplements for osteoarthritis. Am Fam Physician 2008;77(2):177–84.
9 Zhang W, Moskowitz RW, Nuki G, et. al. OARSI recommendations for the management of hip and knee osteoarthritis, part I: critical appraisal of existing treatment guidelines and systematic review of current research evidence. Osteoarthritis Cartilage 2007;15(9):981–1000.
10 Zhang W, Moskowitz RW, Nuki G, et. al. OARSI recommendations for the management of hip and knee osteoarthritis, Part II: OARSI evidence-based, expert consensus guidelines. Osteoarthritis Cartilage 2008;16(2):137–62.
11 Hawley DJ, Wolfe F, Lue FA, et. al. Seasonal symptom severity in patients with rheumatic diseases: a study of 1,424 patients. J Rheumatol 2001;28(8):1900–9.
12 McAlindon TM, Fomica, Schmid CH, Fletcher J. Changes in barometric pressure and ambient temperature influence osteoarthritis pain. Am J Med 2007;120(5):429–34.
13 Bremander A, Bergman S. Non-pharmacological management of musculoskeletal disease in primary care. Best Pract Res Clin Rheumatol 2008;22(3):563–77.
14 Morone NE, Greco CM. Mind-body interventions for chronic pain in older adults: a structured review. Pain Med 2007;8(4):359–75.
15 Astin JA. Mind-body therapies for the management of pain. Clin J Pain 2004;20:27–32.
16 Morley S, Eccleston C, Williams A. Systematic review and meta-analysis of randomised controlled trials of cognitive behaviour therapy and behaviour therapy for chronic pain in adults, excluding headache. Pain 1999; 80(1–2):1–13.
17 Linton SJ, Ryberg M. A cognitive-behavioral group intervention as prevention for persistent neck and back pain in a non-patient population: a randomised controlled trial. Pain 2001; 90(1–2):83–90.
18 Williams DA, Cary MA, Groner KH, et. al. Improving physical functional status in patients with fibromyalgia: a brief cognitive behavioral intervention. The Journal of Rheumatology 2002; 29(6):1280–86.
19 Brosseau L, MacLeay L, Robinson V, et. al. Intensity of exercise for the treatment of osteoarthritis. Cochrane Database Syst Rev 2003;(2):CD004259.
20 Bartels EM, Lund H, Hagen KB, et. al. Aquatic exercise for the treatment of knee and hip osteoarthritis. Cochrane Database Syst Rev 2007;(4):CD005523.
21 March LM, Stenmark J. Non-pharmacological approaches to managing arthritis. MJA 2001;175:S103–S107.
22 Ettinger WH Jr, Burns R, Messier SP, et. al. A randomised trial comparing aerobic exercises and resistance exercise with a health education program in older adults with knee osteoarthritis. The Fitness Arthritis and Seniors Trial (FAST) JAMA 1997;277(1):25–31.
23 Kawasaki T, Kurosawa H, Ikeda H, et. al. Additive effects of glucosamine or risedronate for the treatment of osteoarthritis of the knee combined with home exercise: a prospective randomised 18-month trial.J Bone Miner Metab 2008;26(3):279–87.
24 Felson DT, Niu J, Clancy M, et. al. Effect of recreational physical activities on the development of knee osteoarthritis in older adults of different weights: The Framingham Study. Arthritis Rheumatology 2007;57(1):6–12.
25 Lee MS, Pittler MH, Ernst E. Tai chi for osteoarthritis: a systematic review. Clin Rheumatol 2008;27(2):211–8.
26 Hartman CA, Manos TM, Winter C, et. al. Effects of tai chi training on function and quality of life indicators in older adults with osteoarthritis. J Am Geriatrics Society 2000;48(12):1553–59.
27 Shen CL, James CR, Chyu MC, et. al. Effects of tai chi on gait kinematics, physical function, and pain in elderly with knee osteoarthritis—a pilot study. Am J Chin Med 2008;36(2):219–32.
28 Fransen M, Nairn L, Winstanley J, et. al. Physical activity for osteoarthritis management: a randomised controlled clinical trial evaluating hydrotherapy or tai chi classes. Arthritis Rheum 2007;57(3):407–14.
29 Brismée JM, Paige RL, Chyu MC, et. al. Group and home-based tai chi in elderly subjects with knee osteoarthritis: a randomised controlled trial. Clin Rehabil 2007;21(2):99–111.
30 Song R, Lee EO, Lam P, et. al. Effects of tai chi exercise on pain, balance, muscle strength, and perceived difficulties in physical functioning in older women with osteoarthritis: a randomised clinical trial. J Rheumatol 2003;30(9):2039–44.
31 Bukowski EL, Conway A, Glentz LA, et. al. The effect of iyengar yoga and strengthening exercises for people living with osteoarthritis of the knee: a case series. Int Q Community Health Educ 2006–2007;26(3):287–305.

32 Garfinkel M, et. al. Evaluation of a yoga based regimen for treatment of osteoarthritis of the hands. J Rheumatol 1994;21(12):2341–3.

33 Reijman M, Pols HA, Bergink AP, et. al. Body mass index associated with onset and progression of osteoarthritis of the knee but not of the hip: the Rotterdam Study. Annals of the Rheum Dis 2007;66:158–62.

34 Marks R. Obesity profiles with knee osteoarthritis: correlation with pain, disability, disease progression. Obesity (Silver Spring Md) 2007; 15: 1867–74.

35 Rayman MP, Pattison DJ. Dietary manipulation in musculoskeletal conditions. Best Pract Res Clin Rheumatol 2008;22(3):535–61.

36 Beauchamp GK, Keast SJ. Phytochemistry Ibuprophen-like activity in extra-virgin olive oil. Nature 2005;437(7055):45–46.

37 Cooper C, Inskip H, Croft P, et. al. Individual risk factors for hip osteoarthritis: obesity, hip injury, and physical activity. Amer J Epid 1998;147:516–22.

38 Liu B, Balkwill A, Banks E, et. al. Relationship of height, weight and body mass index to the risk of hip and knee replacements in middle-aged women. Rheumatology (Oxford England) 2007;46:861–67.

39 Choi HK. Dietary risk factors for rheumatic diseases. Curr Opin Rheumatol 2005;17(2):141–6.

40 Rayman MP, Callaghan A. Nutrition and Arthritis. Blackwell Publishing, Oxford, 2006.

41 McAlindon TE, Felson DT, Zhang Y, et. al. Do antioxidant micronutrients protect against the development and progression of knee osteoarthritis? Arthritis and Rheumatism 1996; 39: 648–56.

42 Roemer FW, Guermazi A, Hunter DJ, et. al. The association of meniscal damage with joint effusion in persons without radiographic osteoarthritis: the Framingham and MOST osteoarthritis studies. Osteoarthritis Cartilage. 2008 Oct 17. Epub ahead of print.

43 Wang Y, Cicuttini FM, Vitetta L, et. al. What effect do dietary antioxidants have on the symptoms and structural progression of knee osteoarthritis over two years? Clin Exp Rheumatol 2006;24:213–14.

44 Wang Y, Hodge AM, Wluka AE, et. al. Effect of antioxidants on knee cartilage and bone in healthy, middle-aged subjects: a cross-sectional study. Arthritis Res Ther 2007;9(4):R66.

45 Jonas WB, Rapoza CP, Blair WF. The effect of niacinamide on osteoarthritis: a pilot study. Inflamm Res 1996; 45(7):330–34.

46 Annand J. Pantothenic acid and Osteoarthritis. Lancet 1963; 2:1168.

47 Flynn M, et. al. The effect of folate and cobalamin on osteoarthritic hands. J Am College of Nutr 1994;13(4).

48 Canter PH, Wider B, Ernst E. The antioxidant vitamins A, C, E and selenium in the treatment of arthritis: a systematic review of randomised clinical trials. Rheumatology (Oxford) 2007;46(8):1223–33.

49 McAlindon T, Felson DT. Nutrition: risk factors for osteoarthritis. Annals of the Rheumatic Diseases 1997;56:397–402.

50 McAlindon TE, Felson DT, Zhang Y, et. al. Relation of dietary intake and serum levels of vitamin D to progression of osteoarthritis of the knee among participants in the Framingham Study. Ann Int Med 1996;125:353–59.

51 Lane NE, Gore LR, Cummings SR, et. al. Serum vitamin D levels and incident changes of radiographic hip osteoarthritis: a longitudinal study. Study of Osteoporotic Fractures Research Group. Arthr Rheum 1999;42:854–60.

52 Felson DT, Niu J, Clancy M, et. al. Low levels of vitamin D and worsening of knee osteoarthritis: results of two longitudinal studies. Arthr Rheum 2007;56:129–36.

53 Zittermann A. Vitamin D in preventive medicine: are we ignoring the evidence? Br J Nutr 2003; 89: 552–72.

54 Hypponen E, Power C. Hypovitaminosis D in British adults at age 45 y: nationwide cohort study of dietary and lifestyle predictors. The American Journal of Clinical Nutrition 2007;85: 860–68.

55 Lementowski PW, Zelicof SB. Obesity and osteoarthritis. Am J Orthop 2008;37(3):148–51.

56 Vitetta L, Cicuttini F, Sali A. Alternative therapies for musculoskeletal conditions. Best Pract Res Clin Rheumatol 2008;22(3):499–522.

57 Hardin SR. Cat's claw: an Amazonian vine decreases inflammation in osteoarthritis. Complement Ther Clin Pract 2007;13(1):25–8.

58 Ahmed S, Anuntiyo J, Malemud CJ, et. al. Biological basis for the use of botanicals in osteoarthritis and rheumatoid arthritis: a review. Evid Based Complement Alternat Med. 2005;2:301–8.

59 Sharma RA, Steward WP, Gescher AJ. Pharmacokinetics and pharmacodynamics of curcumin. Adv Exp Med Biol. 2007;595:453–70.

60 Canter PH, Lee HS, Ernst E. A systematic review of randomised clinical trials of Tripterygium wilfordii for rheumatoid arthritis. Phytomedicine. 2006;13:371–7.

61 Curtis CL, Harwood JL, Dent CM, et. al. Biological basis for the benefit of nutraceutical supplementation in arthritis. Drug Discov Today 2004;9:165–72.

62 Piscoya J, Rodriguez Z, Bustamante SA, et. al. Efficacy and safety of freeze-dried cat's claw in osteoarthritis of the knee: mechanisms of action of the species Uncaria guianensis. Inflamm Res 2001;50(9):442–8.

63 Sandoval M, Okuhama NN, Zhang XJ, et. al. Anti-inflammatory and antioxidant activities of cat's claw (Uncaria tomentosa and Uncaria guianensis) are independent of their alkaloid content. Phytomedicine 2002;9:325–37.

64 Mur E, Hartig F, Eibl G, et. al. Randomised double-blind trial of an extract from the pentacyclic alkaloid-chemotype of Uncaria steoarth for the treatment of rheumatoid arthritis. J Rheumatol 2002;29:656–8.

65 Chrubasik JE, Roufogalis BD, Chrubasik S. Evidence of effectiveness of herbal antiinflammatory drugs in the treatment of painful osteoarthritis and chronic low back pain. Phytother Res. 2007;21:675–83.

66 Gagnier JJ, Chrubasik S, Manheimer E. Harpgophytum procumbens for osteoarthritis and low back pain: a systematic review. BMC Complement Altern Med 2004;4:13. Online. Available: http://www.biomedcentral.com/1472–688 2/4/13 (accessed 14 Oct 2009).

67 Fiebich BL, Heinrich M, Hiller KO, et. al. Inhibition of TNF-alpha synthesis in LPS-stimulated primary human monocytes by Harpagophytum extract SteiHap 69. Phytomed 2001;8:28–30.

68 Huang TH, Tran VH, Duke RK, et. al. Harpagoside suppresses lipopolysaccharide-induced Inos and COX-2 expression through inhibition of NF-kappa B activation. J Ethnopharmaco 2006;104:149–55.

69 Chrubasik S, Conradt C, Black A. The quality of clinical trials with Harpagophytum procumbens. Phytomed 2003;10:613–23.

70 Gagnier JJ, van Tulder MW, Berman B, et. al. Herbal medicine for low back pain: a Cochrane review. Spine 2007;32:82–92. Review.
71 Vlachojannis J, Roufogalis BD, Chrubasik S. Systematic review on the safety of Harpagophytum preparations for osteoarthritic and low back pain. Phytother Res 2008;22(2):149–52.
72 Ippoushi K, Azuma K, Ito H, et. al. (6)-Gingerol inhibits nitric oxide synthesis in activated J774.1 mouse macrophages and prevents peroxynitrite-induced oxidation and nitration reactions. Life Sci 2003;73:3427–37.
73 Thomson M, Al-Qattan KK, Al-Sawan SM, et. al. The use of ginger (Zingiber officinale Rosc.) as a potential anti-inflammatory and antithrombotic agent. Prostaglandins Leukot Ess Fatty Acids 2002;67:475–8.
74 Jolad SD, Lantz RC, Solyom AM, et. al. Fresh organically grown ginger (Zingiber officinale): composition and effects on LPS-induced PGE2 production. Phytochemistry 2004;65:1937–54.
75 Altman RD, Marcussen KC. Effects of a ginger extract on knee pain in patients with osteoarthritis. Arthritis Rheum 2001;44:2531–8.
76 Bliddal H, Rosetzsky A, Schlichting P, et. al. A randomised, placebo-controlled, cross-over study of ginger extracts and ibuprofen in osteoarthritis. Osteoarthritis Cartilage 2000;8:9–12.
77 Zhang B, Li JB, Zhang DM, et. al. Analgesic and anti-inflammatory activities of a fraction rich in gaultherin isolated from Gaultheria yunnanensis Biol Pharm Bull 2007;30(3):465–9.
78 Zhang B, He XL, Ding Y, et. al. Gaultherin, a natural salicylate derivative from Gaultheria yunnanensis: towards a better non-steroidal anti-inflammatory drug. Eur J Pharmacol 2006;530(1–2):166–71.
79 Chan TY. The risk of severe salicylate poisoning following the ingestion of topical medicaments or aspirin. Postgrad Med J 1996;72:109–12.
80 Ernst E, Chrubasik S. Phyto-anti-inflammatories. A systematic review of randomised, placebo-controlled, double-blind trials. Rheum Dis Clin Nort Am 2000;26:13–27.
81 Ammon HP. Boswellic acids in chronic inflammatory diseases. Planta Med 2006;72:1100–16.
82 Gayathri B, Manjula N, Vinaykumar KS, et. al. Pure compound from Boswellia serrata extract exhibits anti-inflammatory property in human PBMCs and mouse macrophages through inhibition of TNFalpha, IL-1beta, NO and MAP kinases. Int Immunopharmacol 2007;7(4):473–82.
83 Kimmatkar N, Thawani V, Hingorani L, et. al. Efficacy and tolerability of Boswellia serrata extract in treatment of osteoarthritis of knee—a randomised double-blind placebo controlled trial. Phytomedicine 2003;10:3–7.
84 Sontakke S, Thawani S, Pimpalkhute P, et. al. Open, randomised, controlled clinical trial of Boswellia serrata extract as compared to valdecoxib in osteoarthritis of knee. Indian J Pharmacol 2007;39:27–9.
85 Setty AR, Sigal LH. Herbal medications commonly used in the practice of rheumatology: mechanisms of action, efficacy, and side-effects. Semin Arthritis Rheum 2005;34:773–84.
86 Rinsema TJ. One hundred years of aspirin. Med Hist 1999;43(4):502–7.
87 Rossnagel K, Roll S, Willich SN. The clinical effectiveness of rosehip powder in patients with osteoarthritis. A systematic review. MMW Fortschr Med 2007;149:51–6.
88 Chrubasik C, Duke RK, Chrubasik S. The evidence for clinical efficacy of rose hip and seed: a systematic review. Phytother Res 2006;20:1–3.
89 Winther K, Apel K, Thamsborg G. A powder made from seeds and shells of a rose-hip subspecies (Rosa canina) reduces symptoms of knee and hip osteoarthritis: a randomised, double-blind, placebo-controlled clinical trial. Scand J Rheumatol 2005;34:302–8.
90 Christensen R, Bartels EM, Altman RD, et. al. Does the hip powder of Rosa canina (rosehip) reduce pain in osteoarthritis patients?--a meta-analysis of randomised controlled trials. Osteoarthritis Cartilage. 2008 Sep;16(9):965–72. Epub 2008 Apr 14.
91 Grube B, Grünwald J, Krug L, et. al. Efficacy of a comfrey root (Symphyti steoa. Radix) extract ointment in the treatment of patients with painful osteoarthritis of the knee: results of a double-blind, randomised, bicenter, placebo-controlled trial. Phytomedicine 2007;14(1):2–10.
92 Cisár P, Jány R, Waczulíková I, et. al. Effect of pine bark extract (Pycnogenol®) on symptoms of knee osteoarthritis. Phytotherapy Research. 2008;22: 1087–92.
93 Mason L, Moore RA, Derry S, et. al. Systematic review of topical capsaicin for the treatment of chronic pain. BMJ 2004;328:991.
94 Wang Y, Prentice LF, Vitetta L, et. al. The effect of nutritional supplements on osteoarthritis. Altern Med Rev 2004;9:275–96.
95 Poolsup N, Suthisisang C, Channark P, et. al. Glucosamine long-term treatment and the progression of knee osteoarthritis: systematic review of randomised controlled trials. Ann Pharmacother 2005;39:1080–7.
96 Rozendaal RM, Koes BW, van Osch GJ, et. al. Effect of glucosamine sulfate on hip osteoarthritis: a randomised trial. Ann Intern Med 2008;148(4): 268–77.
97 Towheed TE, Maxwell L, Anastassiades TP, et. al. Glucosamine therapy for treating osteoarthritis. Cochrane Database Syst Rev 2005;(2):CD002946.
98 Towheed TE, Anastassiades TP, Shea B, et. al. Glucosamine therapy for treating osteoarthritis. Cochrane Database Syst Rev 2001;(1):CD002946. Review.
99 Distler J, Anguelouch A. Evidence-based practice: review of clinical evidence on the efficacy of glucosamine and chondroitin in the treatment of osteoarthritis. J Am Acad Nurse Pract 2006;18: 487–93.
100 Reginster JY, Bruyere O, Neuprez A. Current role of glucosamine in the treatment of osteoarthritis. Rheumatology 2007;46:731–5.
101 Vlad SC, Lavalley MP, McAlindon TE, et. al. Glucosamine for pain in osteoarthritis: Why do trial results differ? Arthritis Rheum 2007;56:2267–77.
102 Clegg DO, Reda DJ, Harris CL, et. al. Glucosamine, chondroitin sulfate, and the two in combination for painful knee osteoarthritis. N Engl J Med 2006;354(8):795–808.
103 Oliviero U, Sorrentino GP, De Paola P, et. al. Effects of the treatment with Matrix on elderly people with chronic articular degeneration. Drugs Exp Clin Res 1991;17:45–51.
104 Conrozier T. Anti-arthrosis treatments: efficacy and tolerance of chondroitin sulfates (CS 4 and 6). Presse Med 1998;27:1862–1865.

105 Uebelhart D, Thonar EJ, Delmas PD, et. al. Effects of oral chondroitin sulfate on the progression of knee osteoarthritis: a pilot study. Osteoarthritis Cartilage 1998;6:39–46.
106 Bucsi L, Poor G. Efficacy and tolerability of oral chondroitin sulfate as a symptomatic slow-acting drug for osteoarthritis (SYSADOA) in the treatment of knee osteoarthritis. Osteoarthritis Cartilage 1998;6:31–36.
107 Mazieres B, Combe B, Phan Van A, et. al. Chondroitin sulfate in osteoarthritis of the knee: a prospective, double-blind, placebo controlled multicenter clinical study. J Rheumatol 2001;28:173–81.
108 Morreale P, Manopulo R, Galati M, et. al. Comparison of the osteoarthritisry efficacy of chondroitin sulfate and diclofenac sodium in patients with knee osteoarthritis. J Rheumatol 1996;23:1385–91.
109 Mathieu P. Radiological progression of internal femoro-tibial osteoarthritis in gonarthrosis. Chondro-protective effect of chondroitin sulfates ACS4-ACS6. Presse Med 2002;31:1386–90.
110 Reichenbach S, Sterchi R, Scherer M, et. al. Meta-analysis: chondroitin for osteoarthritis of the knee or hip. Ann Intern Med 2007;146:580–90.
111 Kahan A, Uebelhart D, De Vathaire F, et. al. Long-term effects of chondroitins 4 and 6 sulfate on knee osteoarthritis: The study on osteoarthritis progression prevention, a two-year, randomised, double-blind, placebo-controlled trial. Arthritis Rheum. 2009 Jan 29;60(2):524–33. Epub ahead of print.
112 Bello AE, Oesser S. Collagen hydrolysate for the treatment of osteoarthritis and other joint disorders: a review of the literature. Curr Med Res Opin 2006;22:2221–32.
113 Moskowitz RW. Role of collagen hydrolysate in bone and joint disease. Semin Arthritis Rheum 2000;30:87–99.
114 Adam M. Therapy for osteoarthritis: which effects have preparations of steoart? Therapiewoche 1991;38:2456–61.
115 Usha PR, Naidu MUR. Randomised, double-blind, parallel, placebo- controlled study of oral glucosamine, methylsulfonylmethane and their combination in osteoarthritis. Clinical Drug Investigation 2004;24:353–63.
116 Kim LS, Axelrod LJ, Howard P, et. al. Efficacy of methylsulfonylmethane (MSM) in osteoarthritis pain of the knee: a pilot clinical trial. Osteoarthritis Cartilage 2006;14:286–94.
117 Soeken K, Lee WL, Bausell RB, et. al. Safety and efficacy of S-adenosylmethionine (SAMe) for osteoarthritis. J Fam Practice 2002;5:425–30.
118 Tavoni A, Vitali C, et. al. Evaluation of S-adenosylmethionine in primary fibromyalgia. A double-blind cross-over study. Am J Med 1987;83:107–10.
119 Ameye LG, Chee WS. Osteoarthritis and nutrition. From nutraceuticals to functional foods: a systematic review of the scientific evidence. Arthritis Res Ther 2006;8:R127.
120 Cobb CS, Ernst E. Systematic review of a marine nutriceutical supplement in clinical trials for arthritis: the effectiveness of the New Zealand green-lipped mussel Perna canaliculus. Clin Rheumatol 2006;25:275–84.
121 Cho SH, Jung YB, Seong SC, et. al. Clinical efficacy and safety of Lyprinol, a patented extract from New Zealand green-lipped mussel (Perna Canaliculus) in patients with osteoarthritis of the hip and knee: a multicenter 2-month clinical trial. Eur Ann Allergy Clin Immunol 2003;35(6):212–6.
122 Appelboom T, Schuermans J, Verbruggen G, et. al. Symptoms modifying effect of avocado/soybean unsaponifiables (ASU) in knee osteoarthritis. A double-blind, prospective, placebo-controlled study. Scand J Rheumat 2001;30:242–7.
123 Blotman F, Maheu E, Wulwik A, et. al. Efficacy and safety of avocado/soybean unsaponifiables in the treatment of symptomatic osteoarthritis of the knee and hip. A prospective, multicenter, three-month, randomised, double-blind, placebo-controlled trial. Rev Rhum Engl Ed 1997;64:825–34.
124 Maheu E, Mazieres B, Valat JP, et. al. Symptomatic efficacy of avocado/soybean unsaponifiables in the treatment of osteoarthritis of the knee and hip: a prospective, randomised, double-blind, placebo-controlled, multicenter clinical trial with a six-month treatment period and a two-month followup demonstrating a persistent effect. Arthritis Rheum 1998;41:81–91.
125 Lequesne M, Maheu E, Cadet C, et. al. Structural effect of avocado/soybean unsaponifiables on joint space loss in osteoarthritis of the hip. Arthritis Rheum 2002;47:50–8.
126 Ernst E. Avocado-soybean unsaponifiables (ASU) for osteoarthritis — a systematic review. Clin Rheumatol 2003;22:285–8.
127 Little CV, Parsons T, Logan S. Herbal therapy for treating osteoarthritis. Cochrane Database of Systematic Reviews 2001 Issue 1. Art no CD002947
128 Harmer AR, Naylor JM, Crosbie J, et. al. Land-based versus water-based rehabilitation following total knee replacement: A randomised, single-blind trial. Arthritis Rheum. 2009 Jan 29;61(2):184–191. Epub ahead of print.
129 Manheimer E, Linde K, Lao L, et. al. Meta-analysis: acupuncture for osteoarthritis of the knee. Ann Int Med 2007;146:868–77.
130 White A, Foster NE, Cummings M, et. al. Acupuncture treatment for chronic knee pain: a systematic review. Rheumatology 2007;46: 384–90.
131 Kwon YD, Pittler MH, Ernst E. Acupuncture for peripheral joint osteoarthritis: a systematic review and meta-analysis. Rheumatology 2006;45: 1331–7.
132 Hulme J, Robinson V, DeBie R, et. al. Electromagnetic fields for the treatment of osteoarthritis. Cochrane Database Syst Rev 2002;(1):CD003523.
133 Brosseau L, Welch V, Wells G, et. al. Low level laser therapy (Classes I, II and III) for treating osteoarthritis. Cochrane Database Syst Rev. 2004;(3):CD002046.
134 Bjordal JM, Johnson MI, Lopes-Martins RA, et. al. Short-term efficacy of physical interventions in osteoarthritic knee pain. A systematic review and meta-analysis of randomised placebo-controlled trials. BMC Musculoskelet Disord 2007;8:51.
135 Eckes Peck SD. The effectiveness of therapeutic touch for decreasing pain in elders with degenerative arthritis. J Holist Nurs 1997;15:176–98.

Chapter 30

Osteoporosis

Introduction

Osteoporosis is a common skeletal condition that results in significant morbidity and mortality for men and women, with ever increasing health care costs.[1] Osteoporosis afflicts 75 million people in the US, Europe and Japan and results in more than 1.3 million fractures annually in the US alone.[1]

Osteoporosis is a metabolic bone disease, and the bones have a physiological appearance where matrix and mineral are both decreased. Fracture is a major morbidity of this disease.

In Australia, 1 in 2 women and 1 in 3 men over the age of 60 develop this disease. It is estimated that approximately 2 million Australians have osteoporosis, and this figure is expected to rise to 3 million by 2021.[1] It is predicted that by 2021, 1 in 3 hospital beds in Australia will be occupied by a woman with an osteoporotic fracture. Hip fracture is a serious consequence of osteoporosis.

Risk factors

There are numerous risk factors for osteoporosis, but only those related to lifestyle behavioural factors will be discussed.[2] The most important risk factors are:

- genetic factors — white or Asian ethnicity
- gender/hormones/ageing — female: premature menopause/amenorrhoea
- medical conditions (e.g. anorexia nervosa, malabsorption, coeliac disease, hyperthyroidism, kidney and liver disease)
- increased life stressors/depression
- decreased physical activity
- decreased weight-bearing exercises
- prudent nutrition — high animal protein; high sugar intake
- low body mass index; small body frame
- depleted vitamin D/sunlight exposure
- smoking
- medications (e.g. proton pump inhibitors; corticosteroids; thyroid drugs; chemotherapy; lithium).

Genetics

Although genes play a part in determining the risk of osteoporosis, the genetic contribution is not well understood. Two recent studies have reported gene variants associated with osteoporosis.[3,4] It is estimated that genes account for 25–45% of variation in a 5-year change in bone mineral density (BMD) in women and men.[5]

However, prospective 25-year follow up of a nationwide cohort of elderly Finnish twins has concluded that susceptibility to osteoporotic fractures in elderly Finns is not strongly influenced by genetic factors, especially in elderly women.[6]

Gender/hormones/ageing

It is estimated that 30% of 50-year-old women already have osteoporosis.[7] At age 65 years, 50% of women and 20% of men already have osteoporosis, and by age 75 years, 70% of men and women will have osteoporosis.[7] Women are reported to usually lose approximately 1–2% of cortical bone per year after the age of 40–50 years. Moreover, 3–7 times more bone is lost in the first 7–10 years after becoming menopausal.[8]

In men, osteoporosis begins 5–10 years later than in women.[9] Approximately 25% of men older than age 60 years will have an osteoporotic hip fracture. Mortality from fracture is higher in men.[9]

Using fracture as the benchmark for the risk of osteoporosis, risk for men in their lifetime is 13–25%, as compared to 50% in women.[10] Bone loss is increased by oestrogen or testosterone deficiency from any cause at any time.[11, 12]

Moreover, a recent literature review shows that the most successful and essential strategy for improving BMD in women with functional hypothalamic amenorrhea is to increase caloric intake such that body mass is increased and there is a resumption of menses.[13] However, the study also pointed out that further long-term studies to determine the persistence of this effect and to determine the size of this effect and other strategies on fracture risk are indeed warranted.

Lifestyle

Lifestyle risk factors for osteoporosis can impact growing bones in-utero resulting from maternal lifestyle and in early childhood. Epidemiological studies suggest there is a relationship of osteoporosis with birth weight, weight in infancy, hereditary, gender, diet, physical activity, sun exposure, endocrine status and smoking. Infants born to mothers who are vitamin D deficient are at risk of abnormal bone formation.[14]

The Mediterranean Osteoporosis Study has concluded that in both men and women lifestyle is important for bone health, and that there are a number of identifiable factors that can reverse the risk for osteoporosis.[15,16]

In men, the potentially *reversible* risk factors included low Body Mass Index (BMI), reduced physical activity, low exposure to sunlight, and low consumption of tea and alcohol and increased use of tobacco remained independent risk factors for 54% of hip fractures.[15]

In women, significant risk factors identified included low BMI, short fertile period, low physical activity, lack of sunlight exposure, low milk consumption, no consumption of tea, and a poor mental score.[14] No significant adverse effects for coffee or smoking were reported. Moderate consumption of spirits was a protective factor in young adulthood, with no other risk effects observed for overall alcohol consumption. A low BMI and milk consumption were significant risks only in the lowest 50% and 10% of the population, respectively. A late menarche, poor mental score, low BMI and physical activity, low exposure to sunlight, and a low consumption of calcium and tea remained independent risk factors, accounting for 70% of hip fractures.[14] Hence, approximately 50% of the hip fractures could be explained on the basis of potentially reversible risk factors. However, it should be noted that the use of risk factors to *predict* the occurrence of hip fractures had only a moderate sensitivity and specificity.

Recently, a study reported the 5-year risk of fracture among post-menopausal women of various ethnic backgrounds. The algorithm of 11 clinical factors included age, health status, weight, height, race/ethnicity, self-reported physical activity, history of fracture after age 54 years, parental hip fracture, current smoking, current corticosteroid use, and treated diabetes.[17]

Mind–body medicine

Stress and/or depression

There have been numerous reports that have investigated the association between depression and BMD. An early study has reported that women with depression have much lower BMD, and higher cortisol levels than controls.[18] A recent review has concluded, however, that while most studies support the data that depression is associated with an increased risk for both low BMD and fractures, variations in study design, sample compositions, and exposure measurements have made the causative role played by depression in osteoporosis difficult to conclude.[19]

Sunlight

Sunshine is the main source of vitamin D produced by the body in response to direct skin exposure to UVB. This means that no or minimal exposure to sun can contribute to vitamin D deficiency, with risk factors including: dress codes (e.g. wearing veils, migrants, infants of migrant families); dark skin colour; living in geographically prone areas, especially over winter (southern or northern latitude); institutionalisation; elderly; being bed-bound; intellectual disability; prolonged and exclusive breastfeeding; restricted sun exposure, and certain medical conditions.[20, 21] A study of 250 institutionalised patients following stroke demonstrated that regular sun exposure over 1 year increased vitamin D levels fourfold accompanied with a 3% increase in BMD, compared with the control group involving standard hospital care.[22]

Other than osteoporosis, osteomalacia and rickets, lack of sun exposure and vitamin D deficiency have been linked to many serious chronic diseases, including autoimmune diseases, infectious diseases, cardiovascular disease, hypertension, multiple sclerosis, depression, risk of infections, skin diseases, numerous cancers and diabetes.[23–47]

A recent review has proposed that sensible sun exposure can raise blood levels of 25(OH) D >30 ng/ml.[48] Vitamin D deficiency is the most significant contributor to osteoporosis, fractures and falls and is a major public health issue in some parts of the world. Supplementation of Vitamin D in the form of cholecalciferol is necessary to establish normal blood levels.[49]

Environment

Smoking

Smoking is a risk factor for osteoporosis. A meta-analysis of the literature demonstrates an association of BMD and increased lifetime risk of vertebral fractures by 13% in women and by 32% in men, and hip fracture 31% in women and 40% in men.[50] The effects were greatest in men and in the elderly, and were dose-dependent. BMD continued to significantly reduce over the time of continued smoking. Moreover, in an antioxidant vitamin supplement study it was reported that smoking had adverse effects on the skeleton.[51]

Physical activity/exercise

A Cochrane review has found that exercise is beneficial in the treatment of osteoporosis.[51] This benefit is demonstrated in all age groups, including post-menopausal women.[52, 53, 54] BMD can be improved by walking, weight-bearing and resistance exercises.[17, 55] It has also been reported that resistance and weight-bearing exercises can also improve muscle strength which can help reduce falls and osteoporotic fractures.[56, 57]

High intensity training

A recent review has reported that several studies with post-menopausal women demonstrate modest increases in bone mineral toward the normal that are observed in a healthy population in response to high-intensity training.[58] Physical activity continues to stimulate bone diameter increases throughout the lifespan. Therefore, these exercise-stimulated increases in bone diameter significantly decrease the risk of fractures by mechanically counteracting the thinning of bones and the increasing bone porosity and fragility.[17]

Vigorous walking

A recent study that investigated walking intensity in post-menopausal women demonstrated that exercise intensities about 115% of ventilator threshold or 74% of VO_2 max, or at walking speeds greater than 6.14 km/hr mechanical loading of 1.22 times their body weight was sufficient for increases in leg muscle mass and preservation of BMD in these post-menopausal women.[59] The study demonstrates vigorous speedy walking, not gentle amble walking, as helping to maintain BMD.

Athletic training

Moreover, young women who exercise athletically have higher bone mass than their sedentary counterparts, and this difference may be sustained in adulthood.[60] Hence, moderate physical activity during the years of peak bone acquisition may have lasting benefits for lumbar spine and proximal femoral BMD in post-menopausal women.[17]

Tai chi

Tai chi has been shown to be extremely effective in significantly reducing the risk of falls by improving balance.[61]

Nutritional influences

Diets

The metabolism associated with bone and muscle strength, and in particular for bone formation, requires calcium and phosphorus plus vitamins D, C, B and K, as well as the minerals boron, zinc, iron, fluoride, copper, magnesium, manganese, selenium, iodine, silicon and chromium.[62, 63]

Any disease that causes malabsorption of any of these nutrients can impact on BMD. For instance, a study of young children with coeliac disease, demonstrated improved BMD after 4 years on a strict gluten-free diet.[64]

Dairy intake

Of interest, a meta-analysis of 47 studies found little relationship between dietary calcium intake in childhood and bone health.[65] The review examined 37 studies that found no relationship between dairy or dietary calcium intake and measures of bone health. Only 9 studies demonstrated small positive effects on bone health from dairy foods, although 3 were confounded with milk-fortified vitamin D. These studies suggest vitamin D from safe sunshine exposure or supplementation may be the more significant source than dietary dairy intake alone. Also the study implies that once minimum calcium needs are met, extra calcium from dairy source is not required.

Caloric restriction and weight loss diets

Caloric restriction and weight loss diets may actually significantly reduce BMD according to a weight loss study of 50–60 year-old adults (BMI 23.5–29.9) which also demonstrated that the exercise group had no loss of BMD compared with control group.[66]

Western diets high in animal protein

An early study has reported that Western diets that consist of high levels of animal protein are acidic in character, and can lead to an acidic diet which then is believed to release alkaline salts of calcium from bone.[67]

A reduction in animal protein consumption has been proposed to decrease bone resorption and affect calcium balance in a favourable way. A high vegetable to animal ratio, with high dietary calcium intake, appears to protect against osteoporosis.[68]

Many factors are known to influence bone health. Protein can be both detrimental and beneficial to bone health and this depends on a variety of factors that include the amount of protein consumed in the diet, protein source, calcium intake, weight loss, and the acid/base balance of the overall diet.[69]

Alkaline diets

The notion that diets rich in vegetables, fruits and whole grains are more alkaline, and hence provide protection for bone health has not been supported by a recent randomised control trial (RCT).[70] The RCT of menopausal women has demonstrated that supplementation with a potassium citrate supplement over 2 years did not reduce bone turnover or increase BMD in healthy post-menopausal women. The results suggest that alkali provision does not explain any long-term benefit of fruit and vegetable intake on bone health.

Raw food vegetarian diet

A further study with participants consuming a long-term raw food vegetarian diet has concluded that this diet was associated with low bone mass at clinically important skeletal regions and was without evidence of increased bone turnover or impaired vitamin D status.[71]

Population diets

What may be of utmost importance is a population's eating pattern. Diets rich in fruit, vegetables, legumes and plant-based sources of calcium appear to play an important role in prevention of osteoporosis, together with maintaining adequate weight, not smoking, sun exposure and exercising.

Mediterranean diet

In Europe, there is a noticeable difference in the severity of osteoporosis, the lowest incidence being reported in the Mediterranean area.[72] The beneficial effect has been attributed mainly to a specific eating pattern. The Mediterranean diet has numerous food items that contain a complex array of naturally occurring bioactive molecules with anti-inflammatory and alkalinising properties that together may contribute to the bone-sparing effect that has been documented.[70]

DASH diet

The Dietary Approaches to Stop Hypertension (DASH), which is a diet rich in fruit and vegetables, has also been reported to reduce bone loss.[73] Moreover, the DASH diet has been demonstrated to reduce hypertension and has subsequently been shown to reduce coronary artery disease and stroke risk.

Tea

Older women who drink tea have a reported higher BMD than those who do not drink tea.[74] A Taiwanese study of 1037 people aged 30 years or more, found that those who drink green, black or oolong tea regularly over a decade have a higher BMD than those who drank tea occasionally.[75] A recent epidemiological study from the Middle East reported that habitual tea drinking did not impact on bone health, rather that multi-factorial factors (high education levels, being overweight, and being treated for HT) had positive effects on BMD in this population.[76]

However, a study that assessed risk factors for osteoporosis in Iranian women compared with Indian women has concluded that high habitual tea consumption (4–7 cups per day) was protective in both of these populations.[77]

A study of impaired hip structure, assessed by dual-energy X-ray absorptiometry areal BMD, which is an independent predictor for osteoporotic hip fracture, concluded that tea drinking was associated with preservation of hip structure in elderly women.[78] This study provides further evidence for the beneficial effects of daily tea consumption on the skeleton. Flavonoids in tea are thought to be responsible for their protective effects against the development of osteoporosis.[79]

Soft drinks

Five to 6 servings per week of soft drinks, particularly cola, are recognised as a risk factor and linked to low BMD according to a population study of over 2500 adults.[80]

Soy and soy isoflavones

A number of observational studies have suggested that populations with a high dietary soy intake have a lower incidence of osteoporosis and related fractures when compared to Western populations.[81]

Soy contains protein and also isoflavones (phytoestrogens), and has been reported to increase BMD.[82] The phytoestrogens have an affinity for oestrogen receptors and can behave similar to endogenous oestrogens. A meta-analysis of randomised controlled trials has shown that soy isoflavone intake inhibits bone resorption and can stimulate bone formation in menopausal women.[83] However, a recent RCT has reported that in apparently healthy early post-menopausal white European women the daily consumption of foods containing 110mg of soy isoflavone aglycone equivalents for 1 year did not prevent post-menopausal bone loss and did not affect bone turnover.[84]

Phytoestrogens act on both osteoblasts and osteoclasts through genomic and non-genomic pathways as evidenced through *in vitro* and *in vivo* studies.[85] Given that epidemiological studies and clinical trials suggest that soy isoflavones have beneficial effects on bone mineral density, bone turnover markers, and bone mechanical strength in post-menopausal women, the conflicting results make conclusions difficult to gauge. Differences in study design, oestrogen status of the body, metabolism of isoflavones among individuals in different population groups, and other dietary factors advocate that long-term safety and efficacy of soy isoflavone supplements in the prevention of osteoporosis remains to be demonstrated.

Dietary and supplemental omega-3 fatty acids (FAs)

An imbalance of omega-3 to omega-6 FAs is associated with lower BMD at the hip in both men and women.[86] Also an early study has reported that dietary omega-3 FAs can suppress production of osteoclast-activation.[87]

A small placebo-controlled trial using a combination of evening primrose oil and fish oil supplementation over a 3-year period increased spinal BMD.[88]

Reviews report that the available evidence demonstrates that increased daily intake of dietary n-3 FAs decreases the severity of autoimmune disorders, lessens the chance of developing cardiovascular disease, and protects against bone loss during post-menopause.[89]

A recent systematic review concludes that even though studies support the beneficial effects of n-3 FAs on bone health and osteoporosis, the dissimilar lipid metabolism in humans and animals, the various study designs, and controversies over the human clinical study outcomes make definite conclusions as to the efficacy of n-3 FAs in preventing osteoporosis difficult to interpret.[90]

Nutritional supplements

Vitamins

Vitamin D

Vitamin D has a pivotal role in bone metabolism, it controls intestinal calcium absorption plus its deposition into bone.[91] The main source of vitamin D is sunlight exposure (see Figure 30.1).[92] Ninety percent of vitamin D is produced in the skin from sunshine exposure (UVB) with only 10% from dietary sources. Dietary sources include fatty fish (e.g. mackerel), cod-liver oil, sun-exposed mushrooms and liver. The majority of women with osteoporosis have vitamin D deficiency and resulting bone loss.[93] The Geelong vitamin D study on post-menopausal women found that the majority of the participants were vitamin D deficient during winter.[94]

Vitamin D deficiency is likely to be the commonest nutritional deficiency in Australia and many other countries, and may well be the most important one.[95–100] As mentioned previously, risk factors for vitamin D deficiency include dark skin colour, dress codes (e.g. wearing veils, migrants, infants of migrant families), living in geographically prone areas especially over winter (southern or northern latitude), institutionalisation, being bed-bound, intellectual disability, elderly, prolonged and exclusive breastfeeding, restricted sun exposure, and certain medical conditions. Vitamin D deficiency has re-emerged as a major

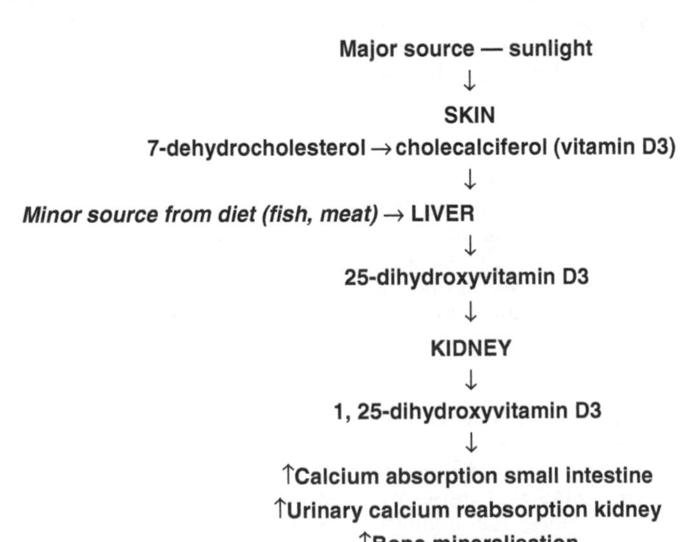

Figure 30.1 Major sources of sunlight

(Source: adapted from Nowson CA, Diamond TH, Psco JA, et. al. *Australian Family Physician*. 2004;33(3):133–8)

public health issue affecting at-risk groups such as the elderly, but also infants and young children potentially causing hypocalcemia, seizures, rickets, limb pain, tooth loss and poor dentition and risk of fracture.[101–107] Breastfed infants of mothers who were vitamin D deficient during pregnancy were at high risk of vitamin D deficiency.[108]

Vitamin D has a multiplicity of roles involving virtually every body system.

Supplementation with cholecalciferol, vitamin D3 is necessary when adequate sun exposure is difficult to ensure normal blood levels.

Improved Bone Mineral Density (BMD)

A large RCT of elderly people over a 5-year period demonstrated vitamin D combined with calcium supplementation has long-term benefit on BMD compared with calcium alone or control group, particularly in subjects with sub-optimal vitamin D levels.[109] Moreover, it is well documented that throughout the lifecycle the skeleton requires optimum development and maintenance of its integrity to prevent fracture. The data is promising for the use of combined calcium with vitamin D and the use of vitamin K.[110]

Reduction of fractures

A meta-analysis of randomised controlled studies found that vitamin D supplementation prevented hip and non-vertebral fractures in the elderly.[111] Of interest, in a study of osteoporotic women over 65 years of age with a history of previous hip fractures, calcium and vitamin D supplementation, up to 1 year, increased BMD, corrected secondary hyperparathyroidism, increased urinary excretion but did not reduce the risk of further fractures.[112]

Muscle strength and prevention of falls

Vitamin D3 supplementation can improve muscular strength and balance, which can help prevent falls and consequently fractures.[113,114] An Australian study that assessed the role of vitamin D on muscle strength in patients with previous fractures reported that muscle strength was most strongly associated with serum 25 hydroxy-vitamin D levels of >50 nmol/L.[115] The study concluded that there was a significant association between serum 25 hydroxy-vitamin D levels and left leg muscle strength. This association may also have benefits for BMD.

Reduction of pain

In a recent UK study that investigated the use of vitamin D and chronic widespread pain in a white middle-aged British population, it was reported that the current vitamin D status of the study population was associated with chronic widespread pain in women but not in men.[116] Follow-up studies were cited as needed to evaluate whether higher vitamin D intake could abrogate chronic widespread pain.

Doses of 700–800IU/day of vitamin D3 (cholecalciferol and ergocalciferol) were used in these studies. Vitamin D is contraindicated in hypercalcemia.

Traditionally, vitamin D3 is preferred over vitamin D2 which has a much shorter half-life than D3, and is also about one-third as potent. However, more recent research suggests that vitamin D2 is equally effective to vitamin D3 according to a double-blind randomised study of 68 healthy adults.[117] The subjects received either vitamin D2 (1000IU), vitamin D3 (1000IU), a combination of D2 plus D3 (500IU) or placebo over an 11-week period, in winter, which demonstrated mean blood levels significantly increased from baseline by 9ng/ml without any differences between groups and with no change in placebo. These findings suggest vitamin D2 and D3 supplements are equally effective in raising serum levels. Similarly a 6-week study of young children with hypovitaminosis D demonstrated equivalent outcomes in improved serum 25(OH)D3 concentration levels from supplementation with elemental calcium (50mg/kg/day) combined with either vitamin D2 (2000IU) daily, vitamin D2 (50 000IU) weekly, or vitamin D3 (2000IU) daily.[118]

The dosage of vitamin D3 will vary depending on the serum level. If the level is in the lower third of the usual range, or even lower, a dosage of 10–20,000IU/day is given for 1 week, and then 3000IU/day for 3 months when serum level needs to be retested.

Researchers found that a single high dose of vitamin D3 (100,000IU) every 3 months can also achieve normal serum levels in vitamin D deficient aged care residents without risks of side-effects.[119]

Another study demonstrated that a once-yearly intramuscular vitamin D3 injection (cholecalciferol 600 000IU) may be an effective method of raising serum levels and improving compliance, although this method cannot be recommended until larger long-term safety studies are performed to assess potential development of hypercaluria.

However, a recent study in JAMA shows a yearly oral dose of 500 000IU of cholecalciferol (alone) in elderly increased the risk of falls and fractures.[120]

If it is possible to increase sunlight exposure, then the dosage of oral vitamin D can be reduced. It is better to have the serum 25-hydroxyvitamin D in the upper half of the usual range because of the vital importance of this nutrient.

Toxicity, adverse reactions and interactions

Vitamin D toxicity is possible with very high doses of either 50–100 000IU/day or 10 000IU taken routinely for several months. Toxic levels cannot be obtained from excessive sun exposure.

Adverse reactions can only occur with very high doses.

Glucocorticoids inhibit vitamin D mediated calcium intestinal absorption. Vitamin D supplementation and possibly calcium is useful in patients taking glucocorticoids.

Ketoconazole can reduce the conversion of vitamin D to its active forms. Phenytoin valproate, rifampicin and isoniazide can increase breakdown of vitamin D.

Vitamin K

Vitamin K is essential for the activation of osteocalcin which is synthesised by osteoblasts, and it is important in reducing fracture risks and maintaining bone mineral density. Patients with osteopenia and fracture have significantly decreased levels of vitamin K. This fat-soluble vitamin comes in 2 forms, vitamin K1 and K2. Vitamin K1 is found in green leafy vegetables, whereas vitamin K2 is found in meat and fermented products such as natto (fermented soybeans) and cheese.[122, 123]

In a systematic and meta-analysis of RCTs investigating the efficacy of vitamin K in the prevention of fractures it was suggested that supplementation with vitamin K phytonadione (vitamin K1) and menaquinone-4 (vitamin K2) reduced bone loss and fracture incidence (up to 80% reduction in hip fractures).[124] In the case of menaquinone-4, there was a strong effect on incident fractures among Japanese patients.

A prospective randomised clinical study in osteoporotic patients using vitamin K2 found that it could maintain lumbar bone mineral density.[125] When given together with vitamin D3 it has an additive effect in reducing post-menopausal bone loss.[126] Another study over a 2-year period also demonstrated a synergistic effect of vitamin D3, calcium with vitamin K1 on BMD in 60-year-old healthy non-osteoporotic women.[127] Moreover, it has been recently proposed that there is an important role for vitamin K2 when used in combination with bisphosphonates or raloxifene in the prevention of fractures in post-menopausal women with osteoporosis with vitamin K deficiency.[128]

A recent RCT that employed a daily dose of 5mg of vitamin K1 supplementation for 2 to 4 years did not protect against age-related decline in BMD.[129] However, it was also documented that it may protect against fractures and cancers in post-menopausal women with osteopenia.

Interactions

Vitamin K is known to influence warfarin anticoagulation.

Vitamin C

Vitamin C is an important stimulus for osteoclast-derived proteins, and it is important in bone and collagen synthesis. In scurvy there is profound bone weakness.

A prospective study in a group of smokers with insufficient intake of vitamins C and E increased the risk of hip fracture, whereas a more adequate intake was protective.[51]

A recent study with high dose vitamin C has reported that it was associated with a better BMD and a lower 4-year bone loss in elderly men.[130] The total amount of vitamin C ingested (dietary + supplemental) was approximately 223mg/day.

Suggested dosages: 500–1000mcg calcium ascorbate, twice daily.

Adverse reactions and interactions

High doses of vitamin C can cause diarrhoea in some people, and should be avoided in people with severe renal impairment.

Vitamin C increases iron absorption and, hence, should to be used with caution in those with iron overload.

Aspirin can reduce the absorption and cellular uptake of ascorbate. Vitamin C enhances anti-tumour activity of cisplatin, cyclophosphamide, doxorubicin, etoposide, fluorouracil and tamoxifen. Vitamin C may reduce the activity of bortzomib and Velcade®. It may also interfere with several laboratory tests, and is best ceased beforehand.

Folate and B group vitamins

Elevated homocysteine levels have been linked to osteoporosis.[131,132] Folic acid, vitamin B6 and B12 can reduce homocysteine levels, and hence may have a role to play in maintaining bone health.[133,134] A Japanese study of 628 stroke patients (>65 years of age) with high baseline levels of homocysteine and lower levels of serum vitamin B12 compared with a healthy reference range were supplemented with folate (5mg/day) plus mecobalamin (vitamin B12 1500mg/day) or placebo.[135] After 2 years, the placebo group had significantly more hip fractures than the vitamin treatment group, BMD had not changed in both groups but, as expected, was significantly lower in the hemiplegic side for both groups. More studies are required.

Vitamin A

According to the Rancho Bernardo Study, Vitamin A above the recommended daily intake (2000–2800IU/day) is a significant risk factor for reducing bone mass in the elderly, who are at greater risk of vitamin A toxicity.[136] The BMD further reduced as the intake of vitamin A increased beyond this level. The authors recommended avoiding vitamin A above recommended daily intake levels in the elderly.

Minerals

Calcium

Calcium is required to support bone growth, bone healing and maintain bone strength.[137] It is controversial whether calcium supplementation can prevent or treat osteoporosis. It has been reported that in populations with extremely low calcium intake correlated with extremely low rates of bone fracture, and that others with high rates of calcium intake through the consumption of milk and milk products, had a higher rate of bone fracture.[65,138]

In post-menopausal women, neither milk nor a high calcium diet appears to reduce the risk of osteoporotic fracture.[51] Calcium supplementation does not prevent loss of bone matrix-calcium loss, nor vertebral or non-vertebral fractures.[139, 140]

A recent Cochrane review has documented that calcium supplements alone have a small positive effect on bone density.[141] The data show a trend toward a reduction in vertebral fractures, but it is unclear if calcium supplements reduce the incidence of non-vertebral fractures. In an RCT study with men, calcium at a dose of 1200mg/day was effective on BMD in a manner comparable with those found in post-menopausal women but at a dose of 600mg/day it was ineffective for treating BMD.[142] The study concluded that calcium supplements were of benefit on BMD in men. A further randomised control study of 930 elderly men and women over 80 years of age for a 4-year period demonstrated less fractures in those taking 1200mg of elemental calcium compared with the placebo group.[143] The benefit dissipated when calcium supplementation stopped. A similar study also demonstrated significantly reduced risk for all-site limb fractures for elderly taking calcium supplementation over a 5-year period compared with placebo.[144]

However, there is also a requisite to assess the incidence of cardiovascular events with calcium supplementation so that the balance of risk and benefit can be clearly ascertained. Cardiovascular risk with calcium supplements have been recently addressed in a study with post-menopausal women.[145] This study reported that calcium supplementation in healthy post-menopausal women was associated with increased trends in cardiovascular event rates. As previously discussed, this potentially detrimental effect should be balanced against the likely benefits of calcium on bone particularly in the elderly who are at higher risk of cardiovascular disease.

There is also evidence of an association between calcium intake and prostate cancer, a possible mechanism being the reduction of serum vitamin D by dietary calcium.[146, 147]

Calcium with vitamin D

Calcium appears to have a role when taken at a higher dose and in conjunction with vitamin D. A meta-analysis of 29 RCTs involving calcium and calcium plus vitamin D, supported the use of high dose calcium (1200mg or more), and vitamin D (800 IU or more), but outcomes varied depending on whether the rates of fracture or bone loss was used.[148] Patients with higher compliance of treatment had better outcomes.

A Cochrane review of 45 trials of older, post-menopausal women with osteoporosis, especially frail older people confined to institutions, demonstrated fewer hip fractures if given vitamin D with calcium, but not vitamin D alone.[149]

Historically, a further complication in calcium and vitamin D metabolism was the reporting of calcium and vitamin D malabsorption following Roux-en-Y gastric bypass surgery.[150] It was further reported that bone turnover was increased and hip bone density rapidly declined. This decline in hip BMD was strongly associated with patient weight loss itself. Adjustable gastric banding is now the most common procedure. However vigilance for nutritional deficiencies and bone loss in patients are required.

Recommended dosage is calcium citrate 800mg/day or calcium carbonate 1000mg/day.

The Position Statement released recently by the Australian and New Zealand Bone and Mineral Society, Osteoporosis Australia and the Endocrine Society of Australia is summarised in Figure 30.2.[151]

Sodium

Sodium causes an increase in renal calcium excretion.[152] In post-menopausal women and men, a higher salt intake has been reported to lead to greater rates of bone resorption.[153] In people who have a low calcium and high salt diet it is shown that they have lower BMD. If salt intake is kept below 2400mg/day, there is no negative impact on bone health. However, adequate intake of calcium or potassium can also neutralise the impact of sodium.[153]

- Balance of evidence remains in favour of fracture prevention from combined calcium and vitamin D supplementation in elderly men and women.
- Adequate vitamin D status is essential for active calcium absorption in the gut and for bone development and remodelling.
- In adults with a baseline calcium intake of 500–900mg/day, increasing or supplementing this intake by a further 500–1000mg/day has a beneficial effect on bone mineral density.
- Calcium intake significantly above the recommended level is unlikely to achieve additional benefit for bone health.

Figure 30.2 Position statement: calcium and vitamin D

(Source: Australian and New Zealand Bone and Mineral Society, Osteoporosis Australia and the Endocrine Society of Australia, 2009)149

Potassium

Potassium can influence calcium homeostasis especially urinary conservation and excretion of calcium. Low potassium diets increase urinary calcium losses and high potassium diets reduce it. Higher potassium intake, primarily from fruits and vegetables, has been associated with higher BMD, and less bone loss.[154] There are no controlled trials that have investigated potassium in osteoporosis.

Phosphorus

Phosphorus is the second most abundant mineral in bone. The calcium/phosphorus ratio should be 2.5:1. Excess phosphorus can cause osteoporosis by decreasing calcium absorption and generating acid in the body, leading to bone loss.[155] As phosphorus is common in usual diets, it is rare to have a deficiency.

Magnesium

Magnesium is the third most common mineral in bone. It can assist in calcium absorption, bone mineralisation and increases the dynamic strength of bone.[156]

Magnesium supplementation can increase BMD in post-menopausal women.[157, 158] The recommended dosage is 400–800mg/day.

Adverse reactions and interactions

Diarrhoea and gastric irritation can occur with higher doses of magnesium.

Magnesium supplementation can cause reduced absorption of aminoglycosides such as gentamicin and tetracycline antibiotics. Magnesium can decrease absorption of fluoroquinolones. There is increased magnesium loss with thiazide and loop diuretics. Magnesium may enhance hypertensive action of calcium channel blockers. It should be used with caution in those with renal failure, and heart block.

Manganese

Women with osteoporosis have been found to have decreased plasma levels of manganese, and an enhanced plasma response to an oral dose of manganese. There are no human studies that have investigated the role of manganese in the treatment of osteoporosis, but it is likely to be useful in combination with other nutrients.[159] A number of animal studies demonstrate manganese together with copper can have a favourable effect on bone density.[160]

Copper

Copper is needed for normal bone synthesis and a 2-year controlled study found that 3mg/day of copper reduced bone loss.[159–162]

Fluoride

Fluoride in osteoporosis and fracture rate remains controversial with an earlier meta-analysis showing no improvement, and a more recent study showing improvement in BMD.[163,164]

Strontium

Strontium ranelate appears to have comparable efficacy to that of alendronate in reducing the risk of vertebral fracture in post-menopausal women with a previous fracture.[165] A recent clinical trial has demonstrated that 2gm orally of strontium ranelate significantly decreased the relative risk of vertebral fractures by 45% in patients without prevalent vertebral fracture over 3 years, versus placebo. BMD was observed to linearly increase during the 3 years of treatment with strontium ranelate, in comparison with placebo. Further, strontium ranelate was well tolerated throughout the entire duration of the clinical trial.[166]

(Refer also to the pharmaceutical section, later this chapter.)

Table 30.1 The effect of pharmacological interventions on fracture risk when co-administered with calcium and vitamin D in post-menopausal women with osteoporosis

Pharmaceutical	Vertebral fracture	Non-vertebral fracture	Hip fracture
Alendronate	Yes	Yes	Yes
Ibandronate	Yes	Yes	No
Risedronate	Yes	Yes	Yes
Zoledronate	Yes	Yes	Yes
Raloxifene	Yes	No	No
Strontium ranelate	Yes	Yes	Yes
Teriparatide	Yes	Yes	No
PTH (1–84)	Yes	No	No

Yes: effectively evaluated
No: not effectively evaluated
(Source: adapted and modified from Compston J, Cooper A, Cooper C, et. al. Guidelines for the diagnosis and management of osteoporosis in post-menopausal women and men from the age of 50 years in the UK. Maturitas 2009 Jan 7)

Other mineral micronutrients (zinc, boron, silicon, chromium, selenium)

Additional trace micronutrients play a role in bone metabolism, but it is difficult to ascertain the role of these in the treatment of osteoporosis. Boron deficiency can result in deficiency of vitamin D, magnesium and calcium deficiency and can assist in increasing BMD although there are no RCTs demonstrating benefit on bone health.[167,168]

Studies using a combination of zinc, manganese, magnesium, copper and calcium have shown a reduction in spinal bone loss in post-menopausal women.[169–172]

Boron 3mg/day may have a positive effect on bone, but there are no controlled studies.[173]

Herbal medicines

A study of red clover isoflavone supplementation over a 1-year period demonstrated reduced loss of BMD of the lumbar spine compared with placebo, although more studies are required to support its use.[174] Isoflavones exert a mild oestrogenic effect which may explain its benefit on bone health. Further studies are warranted to replicate these findings.

The metabolism of bone occupies a complex balance between the deposition of matrix and mineralisation and resorption. It has been reported in a recent review that essential oils derived from herbs such as sage, rosemary, thyme and other herbs can inhibit osteoclast activity *in vitro* and *in vivo* and leading to an increase in BMD.[175] Also, that there are various herbal medicines from the traditional herbal formulae in Chinese and Ayurvedic medicine that have demonstrated effects in pharmacological models of osteoporosis, however, clinical studies of safety and efficacy are lacking and hence warranted.

Traditional Chinese medicine (TCM)

Two preliminary studies have found that the herbal formula Bushen Migu Ye[176] and Bushen Jiangu[177] may be useful in the treatment of osteoporosis.

Cannabinoids (*Cannabis sativa L*)

Recently, cannabinoid receptors have been described as having a positive effect on osteoblast differentiation. The presence of cannabinoid receptors in bone tissue indicates a more complex role in bone metabolism than previously thought.[178]

Pharmacological management of osteoporosis

The major pharmacological interventions are the bisphosphonates, strontium ranelate, raloxifene and parathyroid hormone peptides, as described in Table 30.1.[179]

These pharmacological interventions have been shown to reduce the risk of vertebral fracture when given with calcium and vitamin D supplements. Some of these drugs have been shown to also reduce the risk of non-vertebral fractures, and in some cases specifically at the hip.

Hormone replacement therapy

The use of combined low dose estradiol and progesterone can reduce risk of osteoporosis and rate of BMD loss.[180] Percutaneous estradiol and natural progesterone were assessed in a controlled clinical trial of 57 post-menopausal women and was found to reduce bone loss.[181]

DHEA/testosterone hormones also play a role in the treatment of osteoporosis.

Physical therapies

Whole-body vibration

As physical activity plays an important role in maintaining bone health, any therapies that mechanically stimulate bone and muscle may assist people with low bone density and osteoporosis. A review of the literature found whole-body vibration may play a role for maintaining or improving bone mass, especially in individuals who have limited physical activity.[182]

Conclusion

Health practitioners will frequently encounter patients with osteoporosis, a condition that is often asymptomatic until a fracture occurs.

An integrative approach for the prevention and treatment of osteoporosis is centred on a lifestyle approach that further suggests that the patient maintain an adequate dietary intake of calcium, vitamin D-adequate blood levels, together with lifestyle advice such as smoking cessation, safe sun exposure and daily physical activity that particularly includes weight-bearing exercises, in conjunction with pharmacotherapy where appropriate. Table 30.2 summarises the level of evidence for some CAM therapies for the management of osteoporosis.

Table 30.2 Levels of evidence for lifestyle and complementary medicines/therapies in the management of osteoporosis

Modality	Level I	Level II	Level IIIa	Level IIIb	Level IIIc	Level IV	Level V
Lifestyle			x				
Prudent sun exposure			x				
Mind–body medicine							
Stress and depression risk			x				
Physical activity	x		x				
Muscle strength training	x				x		
Tai chi						x	
Environment							
Smoking cessation	x						
Nutritional influences							
Mediterranean diet				x			
DASH diet				x			
Low BMI diet				x			
Soy/isoflavones				x			
Tea			x				
Nutritional supplements							
n-3 fatty acids				x			
Red clover isoflavones				x			
Vitamins							
• Vitamin D	x						
• Vitamin C			x				
• Vitamin K	x						
• B Group vitamins						x	

Continued

Table 30.2 Levels of evidence for lifestyle and complementary medicines/therapies in the management of osteoporosis—cont'd

Modality	Level I	Level II	Level IIIa	Level IIIb	Level IIIc	Level IV	Level V
Minerals							
• Calcium	X						
• Sodium						X	
• Potassium						X	
• Phosphorus						X	
• Magnesium			X				
• Manganese						X	
• Copper						X	
• Fluoride						X	
Herbal medicines							
Sage/rosemary/ thyme						X	
Cannabinoids						X	
Traditional Chinese herbal medicines						X	
Ayurvedic medicine herbs						X	
Pharmaceuticals*							
Alendronate		X					
Ibandronate		X					
Risedronate		X					
Zoledronate		X					
Raloxifene		X					
Strontium ranelate		X					
Teriparatide		X					
PTH (1–84)		X					
Hormone therapy							
Estradiol		X					
Progesterone		X					
DEA		X					
Testosterone		X					

*For the prevention of vertebral fractures (see Figure 30.2).

Level I — from a systematic review of all relevant randomised controlled trials, meta-analyses.

Level II — from at least 1 properly designed randomised controlled clinical trial.

Level IIIa — from well-designed pseudo-randomised controlled trials (alternate allocation or some other method).

Level IIIb — from comparative studies (including systematic reviews of such studies) with concurrent controls and allocation not randomised, cohort studies, case-control studies, or interrupted time series with a parallel control group.

Level IIIc — from comparative studies with historical control, 2 or more single-arm studies or interrupted time series without a parallel control group.

Level IV — opinions of respected authorities based on clinical experience, descriptive studies or reports of expert committees.

Level V — represents minimal evidence that represents testimonials.

Clinical tips handout for patients — osteoporosis

1 Lifestyle advice

Sleep

- Restore normal sleep patterns. Most adults require about 7 hours sleep a day. (See Chapter 22 for more advice.)

Sunshine

- Amount of exposure varies with local climate.
- At least 15 minutes of sunshine needed daily for vitamin D and melatonin production — especially before 10 a.m. and after 3 p.m. when the sun exposure is safest during summer. Much more exposure required in winter when supplementation needs to be considered.
- Ensure gradual, adequate skin exposure to sun; avoid sunscreen and excess clothing to maximise levels of vitamin D.
- More time in the sun is required for dark skinned people and people with vitamin D deficiency.
- Direct exposure to about 10% of the body (hands, arms, face), without sunscreen and not through glass.
- Vitamin D is obtained in the diet from fatty fish, eggs, liver and fortified foods (some milks and margarines); diet alone is not a sufficient source of vitamin D.

2 Physical activity/exercise

- Exercise 30–60 minutes daily. If exercise is not regular, commence with 5 minutes daily and slowly build up to at least 30 minutes.
- Outdoor exercise in nature, with fresh air and sunshine, is ideal (e.g. brisk walking, light jogging, cycling, swimming, stretching, resistance or weight bearing exercises). The more time you spend outdoors the better.
- Weight-bearing exercises are essential for building up bone and muscle.
- Tai chi can help with balance and build up strong muscles and bones.

3 Mind–body medicine

- Stress management program — for example, six 40 minute sessions for patients to understand the nature of their symptoms, the symptoms' relationship to stress, and the practice of regular relaxation exercises.
- Regular meditation practice at least 10–20 minutes daily, especially mindfulness meditation.

Breathing

- Be aware of breathing from time to time. Notice if tendency to hold breath or over-breathe.
- Snoring and irregular breathing during sleep needs to be reported and further investigated.
- Avoid exposure to polluted air as much as possible.

Rest and stress management

Recurrent stress may cause a return of symptoms. Relaxation is important for a full and lasting recovery.

- Reduce workload and resolve conflicts. Contact family, friends, church or social groups for support.
- Listening to relaxation music and daily baths may help.
- Relaxation massage therapy is helpful.
- Cognitive behavioural therapy and psychotherapy are extremely helpful to reduce any symptoms of depression and stress.

Fun

- It is important to have fun in life.
- Joy can be found even in the simplest tasks, such as funny movies/videos, comedy, hobbies, dancing, playing with pets and children.

4 Environment

- Don't smoke or, if already smoking, use whatever measures necessary to cease smoking.
- Avoid smoking, environmental pollutants and chemicals — at work and in the home.
- Walks in parks, office areas or around the home, with a view overlooking the garden or a park, can help with daily relaxation.

5 Dietary changes

- If overweight, aim to normalise and stabilise weight. Adopt calorie restriction and weight loss diet strategies, especially if not exercising.
- Eat regular healthy low-GI meals; ideally 3 small meals a day.
- A low-carbohydrate, high-protein diet (fish, legumes, nuts, seeds, cereals) and high vegetable oil plant-based diet is best.

- Eat more fruit, such as apples, prunes, guava fruit, avocado, olives and berries.
- Eat more vegetables with skin (for fibre), and use a variety of colours (e.g. carrots, brussel sprouts, broccoli, artichoke, okra, eggplant, yams) and use vegetables in season.
- Increase dietary fibre — oats, oat bran, barley, psyllium husks (1 tsp of psyllium husk twice daily). Pectin is a soluble fibre (polysaccharide) found in fruits.
- Eat more nuts (30–100g/day), especially walnuts and macadamia, and seeds (e.g. sunflower seeds, flaxseed).
- Eat more legumes (e.g. peas, beans, soy, chickpeas).
- Increase fish intake to 2–4 times weekly (daily if possible), especially deep sea fish. Canned fish is okay (mackerel, salmon, sardines, cod, tuna, salmon).
- Reduce red meat intake (preferably use red lean meat e.g. lamb, kangaroo) and white meat (e.g. free range organic chicken).
- Use cold-pressed olive oil and avocado.
- Eat more low-GI wholegrains/cereals (variety): traditional rolled oats and barley; rice (brown, basmati, Mahatmi, Dongara), buckwheat flour, wholegrain organic breads (rye bread, Essene, spelt, Kamut), brown pasta, millet, amaranth etc.
- Do not rush your meals, chewing your food thoroughly as this aids digestion.
- For sweetener try honey (e.g. yellow box and stringy bark have the lowest GI).
- Drink more water, 1–2 litres a day, and teas, especially organic green tea and black tea.
- Chamomile tea may help you to relax. Drink 1 cup 30–60 minutes before meals/bed.
- Minimise alcohol intake. Red wine is best; no more than 1–2 glasses daily.
- Avoid coffee.
- Avoid sugary soft drinks, especially cola.
- Avoid hydrogenated fats, salt, fast foods, added sugar such as lollies, biscuits, cakes, and processed foods (e.g. white bread, white pasta, pastries).
- Avoid high doses of vitamin A.
- Reduce salt intake.
- Avoid chemical additives — artificial sweeteners, preservatives, colourings and flavourings.

6 Physical therapies

- Whole-body vibration may play a role for maintaining or improving bone mass.

7 Supplements

Fish oils

- Indication: help improve bone density. Fish oils providing EPA 6.2g and DHA 3.4g/day have been used.
- Dosage: take with meals. Adult, 1g 1–2 capsules 1–2–3 x daily. Child, 500mg capsule 1–2 x daily; can be used in pregnancy or lactation as tolerated.
- Results: 1–2 years.
- Side-effects: often well tolerated especially if taken with meals. Very mild and rare side-effects; for example, gastrointestinal upset; allergic reactions (e.g. rash, breathing problems if allergic to seafood); blood thinning effects in very high doses > 10g/day (may need to stop fish oil supplements 2 weeks prior to surgery).
- Contraindications: allergic or sensitivity reaction to seafood; drug interactions; caution when taking high doses of fish oils >4g per day together with warfarin (your doctor will check your INR test).

Evening primrose oil

- Indication: help improve bone density; best combined with fish oils.
- Dosage: take with meals. Adult, 1–2 x 500mg–1g capsules 1–2 times daily. Child, 500mg capsule 1–2 x daily. Can be used in lactation as tolerated; avoid high doses in pregnancy.
- Results: 1–2 years.
- Side-effects: often well tolerated, especially if taken with meals. Very mild and rare side-effects; for example, gastrointestinal upset; allergic reactions (e.g. rash, breathing problems).
- Contraindications: avoid if you suffer epilepsy or seizures.

Vitamins

Warning: vitamin A. Excessive intake of vitamin A above 3000IU/day contributes to bone loss.

Vitamin D3

- Indication: correct vitamin D deficiency; improve bone density, prevent osteoporosis, fractures and falls; reduce muscle and whole body pain. Best combined with calcium (dietary and/or supplement).
- Dosage: safe sunshine exposure of skin is the safest source of vitamin D.
  - Doctors should check blood levels and suggest supplementation if levels are low.

- Adults: 400–1000IU/day, for maintenance; 3000–5000IU/day for 1 month then 1000IU/day if vitamin D level below normal.
- Children at risk: 200–400IU/day under medical supervision.
- Pregnant and lactating women at risk: under medical supervision.
- Results: 3–12 months.
- Side-effects: very high doses can cause vitamin D toxicity; raised calcium levels in the blood.
- Contraindications: hypercalcaemia; vitamin D3 can increase aluminium and magnesium absorption, prolonged heparin therapy can increase resorption and reduce formation of bone and hence more vitamin D and calcium required; thiazide diuretics decrease urinary calcium and hence hypercalcaemia possible with vitamin D supplementation; high levels of vitamin D can reduce effectiveness of verapamil.
- The following drugs can *decrease* vitamin D levels: carbamazepine, cholestyramine, colestipol, phenobarbitol, phenytoin, rifampin, orlistat, stimulant laxatives.
- Corticosteroids increase the need for vitamin D.
- Use vitamin D with caution in those with artery disease, hyperparathyroidism, lymphoma, renal disease and sarcoidosis.

Vitamin K

- Indication: correct vitamin K deficiency; improve bone density, prevent osteoporosis and fractures.
- Dosage: vitamin K1 and K2 best combined with calcium and vitamin D.
  - Adults, 200mcg/day — if on warfarin use low dose vitamin K, 50–150mcg/day under medical supervision.
  - Children, pregnant and lactating women at risk: under medical supervision.
- Results: 3–6 months.
- Side-effects: very high doses can cause vitamin K toxicity.
- Contraindications: can interact with Coenzyme Q_{10} by increasing its activity. Tiratricol, vitamin A and vitamin E antagonise vitamin K.
  Vitamin K antagonises warfarin. The following can deplete vitamin K levels: antibiotics, anticonvulsants, bile acid sequestrants, orlistat and rifampin.

Vitamin C

- Indication: maintain bone formation.
- Dosage: 500–1000mg/day.
- Results: >3 months.
- Side-effects: with high doses can cause nausea, heartburn, abdominal cramps and diarrhoea.
- Contraindications: can increase iron absorption. Avoid in hemochromatosis. Use with caution if glucose-6-phosphate dehydrogenase deficiency.

Folate

- Indication: maintaining bone health when blood levels high in homocysteine.
- Dosage: 5mgs/day.
- Results: uncertain.
- Side-effects: very mild and rare.
- Contraindications: avoid in anaemias until assessed by a doctor.

Vitamin B12

- Indication: maintaining bone health when blood levels high in homocysteine, especially in those with vitamin B12 deficiency.
- Dosage: between 600–1000mcg/day.
- Result: >3 months.
- Side-effects: does not cause side-effects, even in large doses.
- Contraindications: concurrent use with vitamin C may decrease vitamin B12 absorption therefore best if taken at least 2 hours apart. Several drugs can reduce serum vitamin B12 levels (e.g. metformin). Excess alcohol intake can also decrease vitamin B12 absorption. Likely to be safe during pregnancy, although there is insufficient data.

Minerals

Magnesium and calcium (best provided together)

- Indication: calcium and magnesium are necessary to support bone growth and increase bone density; more effective when combined with vitamin D and K.
- Dosage: magnesium: children up to 65–120mg/day in divided doses; adults, 400–800mg/day, including pregnant and lactating women.
- Calcium citrate: 800mg/day or calcium carbonate 1000mg/day in adults. Children 30–40mg/day.
- Results: >1–2 years.
- Side-effects: oral magnesium can cause gastrointestinal irritation, nausea, vomiting, and diarrhoea. The dosage varies from person to person. Although rare, toxic levels can cause low blood pressure, thirst, heart arrhythmia, drowsiness and weakness. Calcium can

cause gastrointestinal irritation and constipation.
- Contraindications: patients with kidney disease.

Copper

- Indication: reduce bone density loss and for bone synthesis.
- Should be combined with zinc, manganese and calcium.
- Dosage: adults, 3mg/day in; do not exceed 10mg/day; children, from 1mg–5mg/day. Safe in pregnancy and lactation.
- Side-effects: nausea, vomiting, liver and kidney damage with very high doses. Avoid long-term use and high dosage as this may cause copper toxicity, can reduce zinc absorption, cause anaemia, uraemia and cardiovascular collapse.
- Contraindications: decreases penicillamine absorption and at the same time decreases copper absorption. Ethambutol and zidovudine can decrease copper levels.

Zinc

- Indication: may help maintain and improve bone density.
- Dosage: zinc sulfate; usual dosage in adult 5–10mg, up to 25mg zinc sulfate daily.
- Side-effects: nausea, vomiting, metallic taste in mouth. Avoid long-term use and high dosage as this may cause copper deficiency, impair the immune system and cause anaemia.
- Contraindications: sideroblastic anaemia, above normal blood levels of zinc, severe kidney disease.

Other trace minerals that play a role in osteoporosis: boron, silicon, chromium, selenium, and manganese, combined with minerals discussed above.

References

1 South-Paul JE. Osteoporosis: part I. Evaluation and assessment. Am Fam Physician 2001;63(5): 897–904.
2 Adapted Sali A, Vitetta L. Management of Osteoporosis and Integrative Approach. Australian Doctor article In Press Jan 2009.
3 South-Paul JE. Osteoporosis: part II. Nonpharmacologic and pharmacologic treatment. Am Fam Physician 2001;63(6):1121–8.
4 Karasik D. Osteoporosis: an evolutionary perspective. Hum Genet 2008;124(4):349–56.
5 Shaffer JR, Kammerer CM, Bruder JM, et. al. Genetic influences on bone loss in the San Antonio Family Osteoporosis study. Osteoporos Int 2008 Apr 15. Epub ahead of print.
6 Kannus P, Palvanen M, Kaprio J, et. al. Genetic factors and osteoporotic fractures in elderly people: prospective 25 year follow up of a nationwide cohort of elderly Finnish twins. BMJ 1999;319:1334–7.
7 NIH Consensus Development Panel. Osteoporosis prevention, diagnosis and therapy. JAMA 2001;285:785–95.
8 Garnero P, et. al. Markers of bone resorption predict hip fracture in elderly women: the EPIDOS Prospective Study. J Bone Miner Res 1996;11:1531–8.
9 Campion JM, Maricic MJ. Osteoporosis in men. Am Fam Physician 2003;67(7):1521–6.
10 Looker AC, et. al. Prevalence of low femoral bone density in older U.S. adults from NHANES III. J Bone Miner Res 1997:12:1761–8.
11 Buchanan JR, et. al. Determinants of peak trabecular bone density in women: the role of androgens, estrogens, and exercise. J Bone Miner Res 1988;3:673–80.
12 Gasperino J. Androgenic regulation of bone mass in women. Clin Orthop 1995;311:278–86.
13 Vescovi JD, Jamal SA, De Souza MJ. Strategies to reverse bone loss in women with functional hypothalamic amenorrhea: a systematic review of the literature. Osteoporos Int 2008;19(4):465–78.
14 Thomson K, Morley R, Grover SR, et. al. Postnatal evaluation of vitamin D and bone health in women who were vitamin D-deficient in pregnancy, and in their infants. MJA 2004;181:486–8.
15 Kanis J, Johnell O, Gullberg B, et. al. Risk factors for hip fracture in men from southern Europe: the MEDOS study. Mediterranean Osteoporosis Study. Osteoporosis Int 1999;9(1):45–54.
16 Johnell O, Gullberg B, Kanis JA, et. al. Risk factors for hip fracture in European women: the MEDOS Study. Mediterranean Osteoporosis Study. J Bone Miner Res 1995;10(11):1802–15.
17 Robbins J, Aragaki AK, Kooperberg C, et. al. Factors associated with 5-year risk of hip fracture in post-menopausal women. JAMA 2007;298(20):2389–98.
18 Michelson D, Stratakis C, Hill L, et. al. Bone mineral density in women with depression. NEJM 1996;335:1176–81.
19 Mezuk B, Eaton WW, Golden SH. Depression and osteoporosis: epidemiology and potential mediating pathways. Osteoporos Int 2008;19(1):1–12.
20 Brand CA, Abi HY, Cough DE, et. al. Vitamin D deficiency: a study of community beliefs among dark skinned and veiled people. Intern J Rheumatic Dis 2008;11:15–23.
21 Diamond TH, Levy S, Smith A, et. al. High bone turnover in Muslim women with vitamin D deficiency. MJA 2002;177:139–41.
22 Sato Y, Metoki N, Iwamoto J, et. al. Amelioration of osteoporosis and hypovitaminosis D by sunlight exposure in stroke patients. Neurology 2003;61:338–42.
23 Holick MF. Vitamin D: a D-Lightful health perspective. Nutr Rev 2008;66:S182–94.
24 Daniel J Raiten, Mary Frances Piccano. Vitamin D and health in the 21st century: bone and beyond. Executive summary. Am J Clin Nutr 2004;80(suppl):1673S-7S.
25 Kristin K Deeb, Donald L Trump, Candace S Johnson. Vitamin D signaling pathways in cancer: potential for anticancer therapeutics. Nature Publishing Group 2007;7:684–700.
26 BM Van Amerongen, Dijkstra CD, Lips P, et. al. Multiple sclerosis and vitamin D: an update. European Journal of Clinical Nutrition 2004;58:1095–1109.
27 Miguel A. Hernán, Michael J. Olek, DO and Alberto Ascheri. Geographic variation of MS incidence in two prospective studies of US women. Neurology 1999;53:1711.

28 Munger KL, Zhang SM, O'Reilly E, et. al. Vitamin D intake and incidence of multiple sclerosis. Neurology 2004; 62: 60–5.
29 Armin Zitterman, Stefanie S Schleithoff, Reiner Koerfer. Putting cardiovascular diseases and vitamin D insufficiency into perspective. British Journal of Nutrition 2005;94:483–92.
30 Dobnig H, Pilz S, Sharnagl H, et. al. Independent association of low serum 25-hydroxyvitamin D and 1,25 dihydroxyvitamin D levels with all-cause and cardiovascular mortality. Arch Intern Med 2008;168:1340–49.
31 Bischoff-Ferrari HA, Giovannucci E, Willett WC, et. al. Estimation of optimal serum concentrations of 25-hydroxyvitamin D for multiple health outcomes. Am J Clin Nutr 2006;84:18–28.
32 Holick MF, Matsuoka LY, Wortsman J. Age, vitamin D, and solar ultraviolet. Lancet 1989;2:1104–05.
33 Heaney, RP. Functional indices of vitamin D status and ramifications of vitamin D deficiency. Am J Clin Nutr 2004;80:1706S–1709S.
34 Nnoaham KE, Clarke A. Low serum vitamin D levels and tuberculosis: a systematic review and meta-analysis. Int J Epidemiol 2008;37:113–19.
35 Lui PT, Stenger S, Li H, et. al. Toll-like receptor triggering of a vitamin D-mediated human antimicrobial response. Science 2006;311: 1770–73.
36 Adams JS, Liu PT, Chun R, et. al. Vitamin D in defense of the human immune response. Ann NY Acad Sci 2007;1117:94–105.
37 Guenther L, Van de Kerkhof PC, Snellman E, et. al. Efficacy and safety of a new combination of calcipotriol and betamethasone dipropionate (once or twice daily) compared to calcipotriol twice daily) in the treatment of psoriasis vulgaris:a randomized double-blind, vehicle-controlled clinical trial. Br J Dermatol 2002;147:316–23.
38 Forman JP, Giovannucci E, Holmes MD, et. al. Plasma 25-hydroxyvitamin D levels and risk of incident hypertension. Hypertension 2007;49:1063–9.
39 Wang TJ, Pencina MJ, Booth SL, et. al. Vitamin D deficiency and risk of cardiovascular disease. Circulation 2008;117:503–11.
40 Hsia J, Heiss G, Ren H, et. al. Calcium/vitamin D supplementation and cardiovascular events. Circulation 2007;115:846–54.
41 Garland CF, Garland FC. Do sunlight and vitamin D reduce the likelihood of colon cancer? Int J Epidemiol 1980;9:227–31.
42 Giovannucci E, Liu Y, Rimm EB, et. al. Prospective study of predictors of vitamin D status and cancer incidence and mortality in men. J Natl Cancer Inst 2006;98:451–9.
43 Garland CF, Gorham ED, Mohr SB, et. al. Vitamin D and prevention of breast cancer: Pooled analysis. J Steroid Biochem Mol Biol 2007;103:708–11.
44 Kumagai T, O'Kelly J, Said JW, et. al. Vitamin D2 analog 19-nor-1,25-dihydroxyvitamin D2: antitumor activity against leukemia, myeloma, and colon cancer cells. J Natl Cancer Inst 2003;95:896–905.
45 Lappe JM, Travers-Gustafson D, Davies KM, et. al. Vitamin D and calcium supplementation reduces cancer risk: results of a randomized trial. Am J Clin Nutr 2007;85:1586–91.
46 Hypponen E, Laara E, Reunanen A, et. al. Intake of vitamin D and risk of type 1 diabetes: a birth cohort study. Lancet 2001;358:1500–03.
47 Mathieu C, Gysemans C, Giulietti A, et. al. Vitamin D and diabetes. Diabetologia 2005;48:1247–57.
48 Holick MF. Vitamin D and sunlight: strategies for cancer prevention and other health benefits. Clin J Am Soc Nephrol 2008;3(5):1548–54.
49 Victorian Government Health Information. Low vitamin D in Victoria. Key health messages for doctors, nurses and allied health. Department of Health, State Government of Victoria. Online. Available: www.health.vic.gov.au/chiefhealthofficer/publications/low_vatamin_d_med.htm (accessed 31 August 1020)
50 Ward Kenneth D, Klesges Robert C. A meta-analysis of the effects of cigarette smoking on bone mineral density Calcified Tissue International; 2001;68:259–70.
51 Melhus H, Michaëlsson K, Holmberg L, et. al. Smoking, antioxidant vitamins and the risk of hip fracture. J Bone Miner Res 1999;14:129–35.
52 Bonaiuti D, Shea B, Iovine R, et. al. Exercise for preventing and treating osteoporosis in post-menopausal women. Cochrane Database Syst Rev 2002;(3):CD000333.
53 Hagberg JM, Zmuda JM, McCole SD, et. al. Moderate physical activity is associated with higher bone mineral density in post-menopausal women. J Am Geriatr Soc 2001;49:1411–17.
54 Wallace BA, Cumming RG. Systematic review of randomized trials of the effect of exercise on bone mass in pre- and post-menopausal women. Calcif Tissue Int 2000;67:10–18.
55 Kelley GA, Kelley KS, Tran ZV. Resistance training and bone mineral density in women: a meta-analysis of controlled trials. Am J Phys Med Rehabil 2001;80:65–77.
56 Raisz LG. Screening for osteoporosis. NEJM 2005;353:164–71.
57 Sinaki M, Itoi E, Wahner HW, et. al. Stronger back muscles reduce the incidence of vertebral fractures: a prospective 10 year follow-up of post-menopausal women. Bone 2002;30:836–41.
58 Borer KT. Physical activity in the prevention and amelioration of osteoporosis in women: interaction of mechanical, hormonal and dietary factors. Sports Med 2005;35(9):779–830.
59 Borer KT, Fogleman K, Gross M, et. al. Walking intensity for post-menopausal bone mineral preservation and accrual. Bone 2007;41(4): 713–21.
60 Rideout CA, McKay HA, Barr SI. Self-reported lifetime physical activity and areal bone mineral density in healthy post-menopausal women: the importance of teenage activity. Calcif Tissue Int 2006;79(4):214–22.
61 Wolf SL, Barnhart HX, Kutner NG, et. al. Reducing frailty and falls in older persons: an investigation of Tai Chi and computerized balance training. Atlanta FICSIT Group. Frailty and Injuries: Cooperative Studies of Intervention Techniques. J Am Geriatr Soc 1996;44:489–97.
62 Morgan KT. Nutritional determinants of bone health. J Nutr Elder 2008;27(1–2):3–27.
63 Yazdanpanah N, Zillikens M, Rivadeneira F, et. al. Effect of dietary B vitamins on BMD and risk of fracture in elderly men and women: The Rotterdam Study. Bone 2007;41: 987–94.
64 Kalayci AG, Kansu A, Girgin N, et. al. Bone mineral density and importance of a gluten-free diet in patients with celiac disease in childhood. Pediatrics 2001;108:E89.
65 Lanou AJ, Berkow SE, Barnard ND. Calcium, dairy products, and bone health in children and young adults: a re-evaluation of the evidence. Pediatrics 2005;115:736–43.

66 Villareal DT, Fontana L, Weiss EP, et. al. Bone mineral density response to caloric restriction-induced weight loss or exercise-induced weight loss: a randomized controlled trial. Arch Intern Med 2006;166:2502–10.

67 Bushinsky DA. Net calcium efflux from a live bone during chronic metabolic, but not respiratory, acidosis. Am J Physiol 1989;256:F836-F842.

68 Weikert C, Walter D, Hoffmann K, et. al. The relation between dietary protein, calcium, and bone health in women: results from the EPIC-Potsdam cohort. Ann Nutr Metab 2005;49:312–18.

69 Heaney RP, Layman DK. Amount and type of protein influences bone health. AJCN 2008;87(5):1567S-70S.

70 Macdonald HM, Black AJ, Aucott L, et. al. Effect of potassium citrate supplementation or increased fruit and vegetable intake on bone metabolism in healthy post-menopausal women: a randomized controlled trial. AJCN 2008;88(2):465–74.

71 Fontana L, Shew JL, Holloszy JO, et. al. Low bone mass in subjects on a long-term raw vegetarian diet. Arch Intern Med 2005;165(6):684–9.

72 Puel C, Coxam V, Davicco MJ. Mediterranean diet and osteoporosis prevention. Med Sci (Paris) 2007;23:756–60.

73 Fung T, Chiuve SE, McCullough ML, et. al. Adherence to a DASH-style diet and risk of coronary heart disease and stroke in women. Arch Intern Med 2008;168:713–20.

74 Hegart V, May HM, Khaw KT. Tea drinking and bone mineral density in older women. AJCN 2000;71:1003–1007.

75 Wu CH, Yang YC, Yao WJ, et. al. Epidemiological evidence of increased bone mineral density in habitual tea drinkers. Arch Intern Med 2002;162:1001–06.

76 Hamdi Kara I, Aydin S, Gemalmaz A, et. al. Habitual tea drinking and bone mineral density in post-menopausal Turkish women: investigation of prevalence of post-menopausal osteoporosis in Turkey (IPPOT Study). Int J Vitam Nutr Res 2007;77(6):389–97.

77 Keramat A, Patwardhan B, Larijani B, et. al. The assessment of osteoporosis risk factors in Iranian women compared with Indian women. BMC Musculoskelet Disord 2008;9:28.

78 Devine A, Hodgson JM, Dick IM, et. al. Tea drinking is associated with benefits on bone density in older women. AJCN 2007;86(4):1243–7.

79 Siddiqui IA, Afaq F, Adhami VM, et. al. Antioxidants of the beverage tea in promotion of human health. Antioxid Redox Signal 2004;6(3):571–82.

80 Tucker KL, Morita K, Qiao N, et. al. Colas, but not other carbonated beverages, are associated with low bone mineral density in older women: The Framingham Osteoporosis Study. AJCN 2006;84:936–42.

81 Zhang Y, Chen WF, Lai WP, et. al. Soy isoflavones and their bone protective effects. Inflammopharmacology 2008;16(5):213–5.

82 Potter SM, et. al. Soy protein and isoflavones: their effects on blood lipids and bone density in post-menopausal women. AJCN 1998;68(6 Suppl): 1375S-1379S.

83 Ma DF, Qin LQ, Wang PY, et. al. Soy isoflavone intake inhibits bone resorption and stimulates bone formation in menopausal women: meta-analysis of randomized controlled trials. Europ J Clin Nutr 2008;62:155–161.

84 Brink E, Coxam V, Robins S, et. al. PHYTOS Investigators. Long-term consumption of isoflavone-enriched foods does not affect bone mineral density, bone metabolism, or hormonal status in early post-menopausal women: a randomized, double-blind, placebo controlled study. AJCN 2008;87:761–70.

85 Atmaca A, Kleerekoper M, Bayraktar M, et. al. Soy isoflavones in the management of post-menopausal osteoporosis. Menopause 2008;15(4 Pt 1):748–57.

86 Simopoulos AP. Human requirement for omega-3 polyunsaturated fatty acids. Poult Sci 2000;79: 961–70.

87 Endres S, Ghorbani R, Kelley VE, et. al. The effect of dietary supplementation with n-3 polyunsaturated fatty acids on the synthesis of interleukin-1 and tumor necrosis factor by mononuclear cells. NEJM 1989;320:265–71.

88 Kruger MC, Coetzer H, de Winter R, et. al. Calcium, gamma-linolenic acid and eicosapentaenoic acid supplementation in senile osteoporosis. Aging 1998;10:385–94.

89 Fernandes G, Bhattacharya A, Rahman M, et. al. Effects of n-3 fatty acids on autoimmunity and osteoporosis. Front Biosci 2008;13:4015–20.

90 Salari P, Rezaie A, Larijani B, et. al. A systematic review of the impact of n-3 fatty acids in bone health and osteoporosis. Med Sci Monit 2008;14(3): RA37–RA44.

91 Moyad MA. Vitamin D: a rapid review. Urol Nurs 2008;28(5):343–9.

92 Nowson CA, Diamond TH, Psco JA, et. al. Australian Family Physician 2004;Vol 33(3):133–8.

93 Bischoff-Ferrari HA, Dietrich T, Orav EJ, et. al. Higher 25-hydroxyvitamin D concentrations are associated with better lower-extremity function in both active and non-active persons aged > or = 60 y. AJCN 2004;80:752–8.

94 Nowson CA, Margerison C. Vitamin D intake and vitamin D status of Australians. MJA 2002;177:149–52.

95 Holick MF. Vitamin D deficiency. N Engl J Med 2007;357:266–81.

96 Van der Mei IA, Ponsonby AL, Engelsen O, et. al. The high prevalence of vitamin D insufficiency across Australian populations is only partly explained by season and latitude. Environ Health Perspect 2007;115(8):1132–9.

97 Guardia G, Parikh N, Eskridge T, et. al. Prevalence of vitamin D depletion among subjects seeking advice on osteoporosis: a five –year cross-sectional study with public health implications. Osteoporosis Int 2008;19(1):13–9.

98 Mart Kull Jr, Riina Kallikorm, Anu Tamm, et. al. Seasonal variance of 25-(OH) vitamin D in the general population of Estonia, a Northern European country. BMC Public Health 2009, 9:22doi:10.1186/1471–2458-9–22. Online. Available: www.biomedcentral.com/1471–2458/9/22 (accessed 14 Oct 2009).

99 John Livesey, et. al. Seasonal variation in vitamin D levels in the Canterbury, New Zealand population in relation to available UV radiation. The New Zealand Medical Journal. Vol 120 No 1262:1–13.

100 Weisber P, Kelley SS, Ruowei Li, et. al. Nutritional rickets among children in the United States: review of cases reported between 1986–2003. Am J Clin Nutr 2004;80(suppl):1697S-705S

101 Munns C, Zacharin MR, et. al. Prevention and treatment of infant and childhood vitamin D deficiency in Australia and New Zealand: a consensus statement. MJA 2006;185:268–72.

102 Van der Meer IM, Karamali NS, Boeke JP, et. al. High prevalence of vitamin D deficiency in pregnant non-Western women in the Hague, Netherlands. Am J Clin Nutr 2006;84:350–3.
103 Bircan Erbas, Ebeling Peter R, Dianne Couch, et. al. Suburban clustering of vitamin D deficiency in Melbourne, Australia. Asia Pac J Clin Nutr 2008;17(1):63–7.
104 Diamond Terrence H, Sherel Levy, Angelina Smith, et. al. High bone turnover in Muslim women with vitamin D deficiency. MJA 2002 Aug 5;177: 139–141.
105 Grover SR, Morley M. Vitamin D deficiency in veiled or dark skinned pregnant women. MJA 2001;175:251–2.
106 Carmel Tohill, Anne Laverty. Sunshine, diet and mobility for healthy bones-an interventional study designed to implement these standards into the daily routine in an at risk population of adults with intellectual disability. Journal of Intellectual & Developmental Disability 2001;26(3):217–31.
107 Leif Mosekilde. Vitamin D and the elderly. Clinical Endocrinology 2005;62:265–81.
108 Thompson K, Morley R, Grover SR, et. al. Postnatal evaluation of vitamin D and bone health in women who were vitamin D-deficient in pregnancy, and in their infants. MJA 2004;181(9):486–8.
109 Zhu K, Devine A, Dick IM, et. al. Effects of calium and vitamin D supplementation on hip bone mineral density and calcium-related analytes in elderly ambulatory Australian women: a 5-year randomized controlled trial. J Clin Endocrino Metabol 2007;93:743–9.
110 Lanham-New SA. Importance of calcium, vitamin D and vitamin K for osteoporosis prevention and treatment. Proc Nutr Soc 2008;67(2):163–76.
111 Bischoff-Ferrari HA, et. al. Fracture prevention with vitamin D supplementation: a meta-analysis of randomized controlled trials. JAMA 2005;293: 2257–64.
112 Sosa M, Láinez P, Arbelo A, et. al. The effect of 25-dihydroxyvitamin D on the bone mineral metabolism of elderly women with hip fracture. Rheumatology 2000;39:1263–8.
113 Bischoff-Ferrari HA, Willett WC, Wong JB, et. al. Fracture prevention with vitamin D supplementation. A meta-analysis of randomized controlled trials. JAMA 2005;293:2257–64.
114 Jackson C, Gaugris S, Sen SS, et. al. The effect of cholecalciferol (vitamin D3) on the risk of fall and fracture: a meta-analysis. Q J Med 2007;1–8.
115 Inderjeeth CA, Glennon D, Petta A, et. al. Vitamin D and muscle strength in patients with previous fractures. NZ Med J 2007;120(1262):U2730.
116 Atherton K, Berry DJ, Parsons T, et. al. Vitamin D and chronic widespread pain in a white middle-aged British population: evidence from a cross-sectional population survey. Ann Rheum Dis 2008 Aug 12. Epub ahead of print.
117 Holick MF, et. al. Vitamin D2 is as effective as vitamin D3 in maintaining circulating concentrations of 25-hydroxyvitamin D. J Clin Endocrinol Metabol2008;93:677–81.
118 Gordon CM, LeBoff Williams A, Feldman HA, et. al. Treatment of hypovitaminosis D in infants and toddlers. J Clin Endocrin and Metabol 2008;93:2716–21.
119 Alison ER Wigg, Caroline Prest, Peter Slobodian, et. al. A system for improving vitamin D nutrition in residential care. Medical Journal of Australia 2006;185:195–98.
120 Terrence H Diamond, Kenneth W Ho, Peter G Rohl, et. al. Annual intramuscular injection of a megadose of cholecalciferol for treatment of vitamin D deficiency: efficacy and safety data. Medical Journal of Australia 2005;183:10–12.
121 Sanders KM, Stuart AL, Williamson EJ, et. al. Annual high-dose oral vitamin D and falls and fractures in older women. A randomised control trial. JAMA 2010;3030(18):1815–22.
122 Ikeda Y, Iki M, Morita A, et. al. Intake of fermented soybeans, natto, is associated with reduced bone loss in post-menopausal women: Japanese Population-Based Osteoporosis (JPOS) Study. J Nutr 2006 May;136(5):1323–8.
123 Garber AK, Binkley NC, Krueger DC, et. al. Comparison of phylloquinone bioavailability from food sources or a supplement in human subjects. J Nutr 1999 Jun;129(6):1201–3.
124 Cockayne S, Adamson J, Lanham-New S, et. al. Vitamin K and the prevention of fractures: systematic review and meta-analysis of randomized controlled trials. Arch Intern Med 2006;166(12):1256–61.
125 Shiraki M. (Vitamin K2) Nippon Rinsho 1998;56:1525–30.
126 Iwamoto J, Takeda T, Ichimura S. Effect of combined administration of vitamin D3 and vitamin K2 on bone mineral density of the lumbar spine in post-menopausal women with osteoporosis. J Orthoped Sci 2005;546–51.
127 Bolton-Smith C, McMurdo ME, Paterson CR, et. al. Two year randomized controlled trial of vitamin K (1) (phylloquinone) and vitamin D3 plus calcium on the bone health of older women. J Bone Miner Res 2007 Apr 22(4):509–19.
128 Iwamoto J, Takeda T, Sato Y. Role of vitamin K2 in the treatment of post-menopausal osteoporosis. Curr Drug Saf 2006;1(1):87–97.
129 Cheung AM, Tile L, Lee Y, et. al. Vitamin K supplementation in post-menopausal women with osteopenia (ECKO trial): a randomized controlled trial. PLoS Med 2008;5(10):e196.
130 Sahni S, Hannan MT, Gagnon D, et. al. High vitamin C intake is associated with lower 4-year bone loss in elderly men. J Nutr 2008;138(10):1931–8.
131 McLean R, et. al. Homocysteine is a predictive factor for hip fracture in older persons. New England Journal of Medicine 2004;352:2042–9.
132 McLean RR, Jacques PF, Selhub J, et. al. Homocysteine as a predictive factor for hip fracture in older persons. NEJM 2004;350:2042–49.
133 Homocysteine-lowering Trialists' Collaboration. Lowering blood homocysteine with folic acid-based supplements: meta-analysis of randomized trials. BMJ 1998;316:894–98.
134 Gjesdal CG, Vollset SE, Ueland PM, et. al. Plasma total homocysteine level and bone mineral density: the Hordaland Homocysteine Study. ArchIntern Med 2006;166:88–94.
135 Sato, et. al. Effect of folate and mecobalamin on hip fractures in patients with stroke: a randomized controlled trial. JAMA 2005;293:1082–88.
136 Promislow JH, Goodman-Gruen D, Slymen DJ, et. al. Retinol intake and bone mineral density in the elderly: the Rancho Bernardo Study. J Bone Min Res 2002;17:1349–58.
137 Morgan KT. Nutritional determinants of bone health. J Nutr Elder 2008;27:3–27.
138 Feskanich D, Willett WC, Stampfer MJ, et. al. Milk, dietary calcium, and bone fractures in women: a 12-year prospective study. Am J Public Health 1997;87:992–7.

139 Kreiger N, Gross A, Hunter G. Dietary factors and fracture in post-menopausal women: a case-controlled study. Int J Epidemiol 1992;21: 953–8.
140 Shea B, Wells G, Cranney A, et. al. Calcium supplementation on bone loss in post-menopausal women: Cochrane Database. Syst Rev (1) CD004526, 2004.
141 Shea B, Wells G, Cranney A, et. al. Osteoporosis Methodology Group; Osteoporosis Research Advisory Group. Calcium supplementation on bone loss in post-menopausal women. Cochrane Database Syst Rev 2004;(1):CD004526. Review. Update in: Cochrane Database Syst Rev 2006;(1):CD004526.
142 Reid IR, Ames R, Mason B, et. al. Randomized controlled trial of calcium supplementation in healthy, nonosteoporotic, older men. Arch Intern Med 2008;168(20):2276–82.
143 Bischoff-Ferrari HA, Rees JR, Grau MV, et. al. Effect of calcium supplementation on fracture risk: a double-blind randomized controlled trial. AJCN 2008;87:1945–51.
144 Prince RA, Devine A, Dhaliwal SS, et. al. Effects of calcium supplementation on clinical fracture and bone structure: results of a 5-year, double-blind, placebo-controlled trial in elderly women. Arch Int Med 2006;166:869–75.
145 Bolland MJ, Barber PA, Doughty RN, et. al. Vascular events in healthy older women receiving calcium supplementation: randomised controlled trial. BMJ 2008;336(7638):262–6.
146 Heaney R, McCarron DA, Dawson-Hughes B, et. al. Dietary changes favourably affect bone remodeling in older adults. J Am Diet Assoc 1999;99:1228–33.
147 Giovannucci E, Rimm EB, Wolk A, et. al. Calcium and fructose intake in relation to risk of prostate cancer. Cancer Res 1998;58:442–7.
148 Tang BM, Eslick GD, Nowson C, et. al. Use of calcium or calcium in combination with vitamin D supplementation to prevent fractures and bone loss in people aged 50 years and older: a meta-analysis. Lancet 2007;370:657–66.
149 Avenell A, Gillespie WJ, Gillespie LD, et. al. Vitamin D and vitamin D analogues for preventing fractures associated with involutional and post-menopausal osteoporosis. Cochrane Database of Systematic Reviews 2005, Issue 3. Art. No.: CD000227. doi: 10.1002/14651858.CD000227.pub2.
150 Fleischer J, Stein EM, Bessler M, et. al. The decline in hip bone density after gastric bypass surgery is associated with extent of weight loss. J Clin Endocrinol Metab 2008;93(10):3735–40.
151 Sanders Kerrie M, Nowson Caryl A, Kotowicz Mark A, et. al. Position Statement. Calcium and bone health: position statement for the Australian and New Zealand Bone and Mineral Society, Osteoporosis Australia and the Endocrine Society of Australia. MJA 2009; 190 (6): 316–20. Online. Available: http://www.mja.com.au/public/issues/190_06_160309/san10083_fm.html (accessed 14 Oct 2009).
152 Teucher B, Fairweather-Tait S. Dietary sodium as a risk factor for osteoporosis: where is the evidence? Proc Nutr Soc 2003;62:859–66.
153 Harrington M, Cashman KD. High salt intake appears to increase bone resorption in post-menopausal women, but high potassium intake ameliorates this adverse effect. Nutr Rev 2003;61:179–83.
154 Tucker KL, Hannan MT, Kiel DP. The acid-base hypothesis: diet and bone in the Frammingham Osteoporosis Study. Eur J Nutr 2001;40: 231–7.
155 Jüppner H. Novel regulators of phosphate homeostasis and bone metabolism. Ther Apher Dial 2007;11(Suppl 1):S3–S22.
156 Sojka JE, Weaver CM. Magnesium supplementation in osteoporosis. Nutr Rev 1995;53:71–4.
157 Mutlu M, Argun M, Kilic E, et. al. Magnesium, zinc and copper status in osteoporotic, osteopenic and normal post-menopausal women. J Int Med Res 2007;35(5):692–5.
158 Stendig-Lindberg G, Tepper R, Leichter I. Trabecular bone density in a two year controlled trial of peroral magnesium in osteoporosis. Magnes Res 1993;6:155–63.
159 Odabasi E, Turan M, Aydin A, et. al. Magnesium, zinc, copper, manganese, and selenium levels in post-menopausal women with osteoporosis. Can magnesium play a key role in osteoporosis? Ann Acad Med Sing 2008;37(7):564–7.
160 Rico H. Effects on bone loss of manganese alone or with copper supplement in ovariectomized rats A morphometric and densitomeric study. Eur J Obst Gynecol Reprod Biol 2002;90:97–101.
161 Eaton-Evans J, et. al. Copper supplementation and bone mineral density in middle-aged women. Proc Nutr Soc 1995;54:191A.
162 Palacios C. The role of nutrients in bone health, from A to Z. Crit Rev Food Sci Nutr 2006;46(8):621–8.
163 Haguenuaer D, Welch V, Shea B, et. al. Fluoride for the treatment of post-menopausal osteoporotic fractures: a meta-analysis. Osteoporosis Int 2000;11:727–38.
164 Pak CY, Sakhaee K, Zerwekh JE, et. al. Treatment of post-menopausal osteoporosis with slow-release of sodium fluoride. Final report of randomized controlled trial. Ann Int Med 1995;123:401–8.
165 Reginster JY, Meunier PJ, Roux C, et. al. Strontium ranelate: an anti-osteoporotic treatment demonstrated vertebral and nonvertebral antifracture efficacy over 5 years in post-menopausal osteoporotic women. International Osteoporosis Foundation Osteoporosis International 2006;17(Suppl 2): OC24.
166 Ortolani S, Vai S. Strontium ranelate: an increased bone quality leading to vertebral antifracture efficacy at all stages. Bone 2006;38(2 Suppl 1):19–22.
167 McCoy H, Kenney MA, Montgomery C, et. al. Relation of boron to the composition and mechanical properties of bone. Environ Health Perspect 1994;102(7):59–63.
168 Meacham SL, Taper LJ, Volpe SL. Effect of boron supplementation on blood and urinary calcium, magnesium, and phosphorus, urinary boron in athletic and sedentary women. AJCN 1995;61: 341–5.
169 Gur A. The role of trace minerals in the pathogenesis of post-menopausal osteoporosis and a new effect of calcitonin. J Bone Miner Metab 2002;20: 39–53.
170 Volte SL, et. al. The relationship between boron and magnesium status and bone mineral density in the human: a review. Magnes Res 1993;6:291–96.
171 Evans GW, et. al. Chromium picolinate decreases calcium excretion and increases dehydroepiandiosterone (DHEA) in post-menopausal women. FASEB J 1995;9:A449.

172 Tamaki J, Iki M. Evidence-based, best-practice guidelines for primary prevention of osteoporosis and osteoporotic fractures. Clin Calcium 2005;15(8):1312–8.

173 Nielsen FH. Studies on the relationship between boron and magnesium which possibly affects the formation and maintenance of bones. Mag Tr Elem 1990;9:61–9.

174 Charlotte Atkinson, Juliet E Compston, Nicholas E Day, Mitch Dowsett, Sheila A Bingham. The effects of phytoestrogen isoflavones on bone density in women: a double-blind, randomized, placebo-controlled trial. American Journal of Clinical Nutrition 2004;79:326–33.

175 Putnam SE, Scutt AM, Bicknell K, et. al. Natural products as alternative treatments for metabolic bone disorders and for maintenance of bone health. Phytother Res 2007;21(2):99–112.

176 Shen L, Du JY, Yang JY. Preliminary clinical study on prevention of bone loss in post-menopausal women with kidney invigoration. Zhongguo Zhong Xi Yi Jie He Za Zhi 1994;14(9):515–8.

177 Ding GZ, Zhang ZL, Zhou Y. Clinical study on effect of bushen jiangu capsule on post-menopausal Osteoporosis. Zhongguo Zhong Xi Yi Jie He Za Zhi 1995;15(7):392–4.

178 Bab I, Zimmer A, Melamed E. Cannabinoids and the skeleton: from marijuana to reversal of bone loss. Ann Med 2009;41(8):560–7.

179 Compston J, Cooper A, Cooper C, et. al. Guidelines for the diagnosis and management of osteoporosis in post-menopausal women and men from the age of 50 years in the UK. Maturitas 2009 Jan 7. Epub ahead of print.

180 Prestwood KM, Kenny AM, Kleppinger A, et. al. Ultralow-dose micronized 17beta-estradiol and bone density and bone metabolism in older women: a randomized controlled trial. JAMA 2003;290: 1042–8.

181 Riis BJ, Thomsen K, Strom, V, et. al. The effect of percutaneousestradiolandnaturalprogesteroneonpost-menopausal bone loss. Am J Obstet Gynecol 1987;156:61–5

182 Totosy de Zepetnek JO, Giangregorio LM, Craven BC. Whole-body vibration as potential intervention for people with low bone mineral density and osteoporosis: a review. J Rehab Res Dev 2009;46(4):529–42.

Chapter 31

Parkinson's disease

With contribution from Dr Lily Tomas

Introduction

Parkinson's disease (PD) is a degenerative neurological disorder that becomes more prevalent with age and is of unknown aetiology. It is characterised by a progressive degeneration of the nigrostriatal dopaminergic pathway subsequently leading to progressive tremor, bradykinesis, rigidity and postural instability. As such, the primary features of PD relate to a deficiency of dopamine, with the development of traditional pharmaceutical therapies being based around the replacement of this particular neurotransmitter. However, effective as these are, they do not address all features of the disease that may not be secondary to low dopamine.[1] This appears to be 1 of the prime reasons that complementary and alternative medicine (CAM) therapies are widely used by patients afflicted with this disease. Surveys throughout the world demonstrate that 40–76% patients with PD have used at least 1 CAM therapy since their original diagnosis.[2–5]

Incidence/prevalence in Australia

Patients using CAM are seeking to improve their motor symptoms (57.6%), for fatigue (19.6%), for pain relief (4.3%), for constipation (5.4%) or for no specific reason (13%).[2] The most common therapies used by Westerners include vitamins, herbs, massage and acupuncture. Users of CAM tend to be younger and have a younger age of onset of PD, and have a higher income and education level than non-users.[5] Patients with more severe motor dysfunction symptoms at onset are also more likely to use CAM.[4]

In 1998, the Parkinson's Disease Society (PDS) set up a working group to look at complementary therapies and PD. Their first initiative was to survey PDS members about their experiences of complementary therapies. Over 2000 people replied and the results are presented in Table 31.1.[6, 7]

Lifestyle

It has been suggested that there are several environmental, lifestyle, and physical attributes that appear to be precursors of PD.[8] In summary these include:

- constipation (as a result of reduced water intake)[9]
- adiposity
- years worked on a sugar or pineapple plantation and exposure to sugar cane processing
- years of exposure to pesticides.

Factors that showed an inverse association with PD included:

- coffee intake
- cigarette smoking.

Among dietary factors:

- carbohydrates increased the risk of PD
- the intake of polyunsaturated fats appeared to be protective
- total caloric intake, saturated and monounsaturated fats, protein, niacin, riboflavin, beta-carotene, vitamins A, B and C, dietary cholesterol, cobalamin, alpha-tocopherol and pantothenic acid showed no clear relation with clinical PD.

Mind–body medicine

Cognitive behavioural therapy (CBT)

There have been several studies demonstrating a benefit of CBT for those individuals suffering with PD. There is a strong comorbidity between PD and depression and for these patients there is a faster progression of physical symptoms, greater cognitive decline and poorer quality of life. It is important to note that depressed PD patients often differ from depressed non-PD patients and therefore CBT may need to be adapted to their individual needs.[10, 11]

One such study of individually tailored CBT demonstrated that PD patients with

Table 31.1 Complementary therapies utilised and reported effective, together with the percent benefits

CAM modality	Benefit described by those who reported a positive effect
Acupuncture/acupressure	Increased wellbeing (26%) Pain relief (10%)
Reflexology	Relaxation/stress relief (18%) Increased wellbeing (10%) General symptom improvement (10%)
Aromatherapy	Relaxation/stress relief (26%)
Relaxation	Relaxation/stress relief (29%)
Chiropractic	Improved stiffness/rigidity (19%) Pain relief (16%)
Massage/Shiatsu	Relaxation/stress relief (21%)
Healing	Increased wellbeing (19%) Relaxation/stress relief (17%)
Homeopathy	Relaxation/stress relief (10%)
Yoga	Stiffness/rigidity (26%) Improved wellbeing (9%)
Herbal medicines	Increased wellbeing (10%)

(Source: adapted and modified from Paccetti C, Mancini F, Agliera R et. al. Active music therapy in PD: an integrative method for motor and emotional rehabilitation. Psychosom Med 2000:62(3):386–93)

depression experienced a significant reduction in depressive symptoms and negative cognitions with a greater perception of social support over the course of treatment. These gains were maintained at 1 month follow-up. Larger randomised control trials (RCTs) are needed to further evaluate the efficacy of this intervention.[12] CBT has also been shown to be efficacious for carers of those with PD.[13]

Alexander technique (AT)

Alexander technique is a process of psycho–physical re-education. A systematic review of controlled clinical trials has shown that AT is effective in reducing disability of patients suffering with PD.[14] Earlier studies have also shown that AT may be effective for reducing depression for PD patients on drug therapy.[15, 16]

Imagery

One recent study has shown that the combination of motor imagery and real exercise practice was effective in the treatment of PD, particularly for reducing bradykinesia.[7, 17]

Music therapy

Available data shows that music therapy is effective on motor, affective and behavioural functioning in PD and ideally should be included in rehabilitation programmes.[18]

Repetitive transcranial magnetic stimulation (rTMS)

rTMS is a non-invasive brain stimulation technique that can produce lasting changes in excitability and activity in cortical regions underneath the stimulation coil (designated as a local effect), but also within functionally connected cortical or sub-cortical regions (designated as remote effects).[19] Moreover, although the results from a small efficacy study support the beneficial effects of rTMS on Parkinsonian symptoms, long-term studies with large numbers of participants should be conducted to assess the efficacy of the rTMS on PD.[20] A recent study has demonstrated that rTMS is significantly safe for use in PD patients.[21] However, a comprehensive screening schedule should include electroencephalogram

(EEG) before higher-frequency rTMS is applied.

Physical activity/exercise

A systematic review has stated that regardless of the strength of the evidence, the published literature that was reviewed reported that exercise resulted in improvements in postural stability and balance task performance in patients with PD.[22] It was also recognised that despite these improvements, the number and quality of the studies and the outcomes used were limited. The authors concluded that there is a need for longer term follow-up so as to establish the trajectory of change in PD patients and to determine if any gains are retained long term. The optimal delivery and content of physical activity interventions (i.e. dosing, component exercises) at different stages of the disease are not clear and require further study.

A recent RCT investigating changes in walking activity and endurance following rehabilitation for people with PD demonstrated that an interdisciplinary rehabilitation program can improve walking activity and endurance depending on baseline walking levels in people diagnosed with PD.[23]

Despite treatment with drugs or neurosurgery, people with PD are faced with progressively increasing mobility problems.[24] Recent meta-analyses have confirmed evidence to support exercise being beneficial with regard to physical functioning, health-related quality of life, strength, balance and gait speed for people with PD.[25, 26, 27] Tango dancing, in fact, has been shown to ameliorate some functional mobility deficits in those that are frail and elderly when compared to a general exercise programme.[28] A systematic review has also indicated that the effect of a physical treatment declines after the treatment has ended, suggesting the need for permanent treatment for patients with PD.[29]

A further study has demonstrated that the effects of aerobic exercise are more beneficial than qigong for people with advanced PD.[30]

There is currently insufficient evidence to support or refute the value of exercise in reducing falls or depression.[25] Those with PD are twice as likely to fall compared with the non-PD elderly. An Australian RCT is currently under way to investigate whether exercises focusing on balance, leg muscle strength and gait will benefit those with PD.[31]

Tai chi

The objective of a critical review was to assess the effectiveness of tai chi as a treatment option for PD.[32] The review concluded that the evidence was insufficient to suggest tai chi was an effective intervention for PD. Further research is hence required to investigate whether there are specific benefits of tai chi for people with PD, such as its potential effect on balance and on the frequency of falls.

Recently a pilot study has examined the effects of tai chi on balance, gait and mobility in people with PD.[33] This study reported that all tai chi participants reported satisfaction with the program and improvements in wellbeing. Furthermore, the tai chi program appeared to be an appropriate, a safe and effective form of exercise for some individuals with mild–moderately severe PD.[33]

Environment

Toxins

Health and disease are shaped for all individuals by interactions between their genes and environment, such is the phenomenon now known as epigenetics.[34, 35] In recent years, an increased emphasis has been placed on an integrating role of medicine in the prevention, early diagnosis and treatment of diseases that have been linked to environmental factors.[36]

A lack of heritability in idiopathic PD has implicated adulthood environmental factors in the aetiology of the disease. However, there is increasing evidence that exposure in the womb to a variety of environmental factors (such as exposure to pesticides, heavy metals and an iron-enriched diet) can either directly cause a reduction in the number of dopaminergic neurons, or cause an increased susceptibility to degeneration of these neurons with subsequent environmental insults or with aging alone.[37]

It should be noted that previous work in an electronics plant, use of chlorpyrifos products and exposure to fluorides are also associated with a significantly increased risk of developing PD. The association exists but is not as strong for previous work in a paper/lumber mill and exposure to cadmium.[38]

Repeated traumatic loss of consciousness is associated with increased risk of PD. Hypnotic, anxiolytic or anti-depressant drug use for more than 1 year and a family history of PD show significantly increased odds ratios for developing PD. Tobacco use is protective against developing PD.[39]

Recent evidence has demonstrated that cigarette smoking, alcohol use, fish intake and carbon monoxide intoxication are associated with reduced risk of PD.[36, 38] Consuming well-water and living/working on a farm are not associated with PD.[40]

Heavy metals

There have been a multitude of studies regarding the neurotoxic effects of certain heavy metals and their relationship to PD.[28] Several of these reports concern a village in Italy, Valcamonica, that was previously exposed to heavy metals, especially manganese. A high prevalence of PD was observed within the close vicinity (407/100 000) and it was determined that such Parkinsonian patients who had exposure to heavy metals developed a more severe neuropsychological phenotype, without detectable contribution from genetic factors.[41]

It is important to note, however, that manganese exposure can cause neuro-behavioural and neurological symptoms at concentrations much less than is currently considered to be the minimum *acceptable* level. The relationship appears to be dose-dependent, with adults presenting primarily with motor symptoms and children with dysfunctions in cognition and behaviour.[42] Preliminary studies show that manganese may be transported into the brain by either transferrin or non-transferrin-dependent mechanisms which may include calcium channels.[43]

Chronic occupational exposure to manganese or copper, individually, or dual combinations of lead, iron and copper have also been associated with PD.[44, 45]

Recently, PD has been characterised by elevated tissue iron (not currently connected with hemochromatosis) and mis-compartmentalisation of copper and zinc.[46] Zinc levels appear to be greater in PD independently from metal exposure whereas the perturbation of copper metabolism seem to be associated with exposure to environmental toxins or metals and could, indeed, be involved in the progression of the disease itself.[47]

Although brain uptake mechanisms for some metals have been identified, the efflux of metals from the brain has received little attention, preventing the integration of all processes that contribute to brain metal concentrations.[43]

As such new information comes to light, however, there has been steadily growing interest in how particular metal ions (especially zinc, copper and iron) are involved in neurobiological processes such as the regulation of synaptic transmission. Increasingly sophisticated medicinal chemistry approaches (that are correcting these metal imbalances without resulting in systemic disturbances of these essential minerals) are being investigated. Furthermore, this process shows great promise of being disease-modifying.[46]

Pesticides

There has been considerable research in the last decade as to the association between the neurotoxic effects of pesticides and the development of PD. Epidemiological evidence certainly suggests that exposure to pesticides may play a significant role in the aetiology of idiopathic PD.[35, 38, 40, 48] Indeed, most studies reveal that moderate pesticide exposure is linked to neurological symptoms and altered neuro-behavioural performance, reflecting cognitive and psychomotor dysfunction. There is less evidence that exposure is related to sensory/motor deficits or peripheral nerve conduction, but fewer studies have considered these outcomes. It is also possible that general malaise and mild cognitive dysfunction may be the most sensitive manifestation of symptoms of pesticide neurotoxicity.[49]

Many pesticides (organophosphates, carbamates, pyrethroids, organochlorines) target the nervous system of insect pests and, because of the similarity in brain biochemistry, such chemicals may also be neurotoxic to humans. Indeed, adverse effects on brain development can be severe and irreversible.[50] This may be of more concern in the case of developing brains that are particularly vulnerable to the adverse effects of neurotoxins.[50, 51]

There is strong human epidemiological evidence for persistent nervous system damage following acute intoxication with several pesticide groups such as organophosphates and certain fumigants.[52] Investigations are now concentrating on whether chronic low-level exposure to pesticides in adults, children or in-utero may also result in persistent nervous system damage.[51] There is evidence that exposure to the common agricultural pesticides such as maneb, paraquat and rotenone increases the risk of PD, particularly when exposure occurs at a younger age.[35, 53] Such an association suggests a causative role.[39] However, despite definitive evidence from animal and cell models that pesticides cause a neurodegenerative process leading to PD, human data are insufficient to support this claim for any specific pesticide primarily because of ethical challenges in exposure assessment.[53]

It is recommended that the residues of pesticides in food and other types of human exposures should be prevented with regards to those pesticide groups that are known to be neurotoxic. 'Whilst awaiting more definitive evidence, existing uncertainties should be considered in light of the need for precautionary action to protect brain development.'[50]

Nutritional influences

Diets

There has been much research attempting to elucidate the most beneficial diet in order to prevent and/or treat PD. Caloric restriction has been proposed to counteract neuronal loss and be associated with extended lifespan. Although there are mixed results, recent animal models with PD have not confirmed this association.[54, 55]

The dietary patterns of approximately 50 000 men and 80 000 women were followed for 16 years. During this time, 508 new cases of PD were diagnosed. It was found that a high intake of vegetables, fruit, legumes, whole grains, nuts, fish and poultry with a low intake of saturated fat and a moderate intake of alcohol was protective against PD. In comparison, a typical Western diet high in saturated/animal fats was directly associated with PD risk. Indeed, the benefits of a whole-food, plant-based diet with fish warrants further investigation.[56, 57]

Previous epidemiological studies have shown that consumption of diets rich in antioxidant and anti-inflammatory agents, such as those found in fruits and vegetables, may lower the risk of PD and other age-related neurodegenerative diseases. Further research suggests that the polyphenolic compounds found in fruits such as blueberries exert their positive effects through signal conduction and neuronal communication.[58]

Uric acid is a natural antioxidant and recent studies demonstrate that it may play a neuroprotective role in the pathogenesis of PD. Dietary manipulation of uric acid through increased consumption of purines (meat/crustaceans) may slow progression of the disease.[59] This finding was supported by several earlier studies which show that uric acid levels are lower in individuals with PD than controls. It should also be noted that plasma uric acid correlated strongly with serum ferritin in both patients and control groups.[60, 61]

As can be easily seen, correct levels of protein intake are currently debatable, with mixed results of studies showing positive benefits for both ketogenic and low-protein dietary regimes.[55, 62, 63] A further recent investigation demonstrated that low saturated fat/cholesterol, especially in the presence of high iron intake, may be associated with an increased risk of PD.[64]

The dietary patterns of approximately 58 000 men and 73 000 women from the American Cancer Society's Cancer Prevention Study II Nutrition Cohort were also followed for 9 years. It was found that dairy product consumption was positively associated with risk of PD, particularly in men. This is once again controversial and more studies are required to confirm these findings and explore possible underlying mechanisms.[65]

There have been multiple studies demonstrating the association between caffeine intake and PD. Results are mixed, with some studies showing a protective effect of caffeine and others with no effect.[66, 67, 68] A recent study showed that consumption of green tea was unrelated to risk of PD, however, black tea, a caffeine-containing beverage, showed an inverse association with risk of PD. Therefore, it was concluded that the ingredients of black tea other than caffeine appear to be responsible for this inverse association.[69]

Previous dietary exposure to food contaminants such as polychlorinated biphenyls (PCBs) and methyl mercury (MeHg) have also been positively associated with PD.[70]

Nutritional supplements

Vitamins and minerals

The nutraceutical treatment for PD is still in its infancy. For example, it has been postulated that imbalances in body metal levels could be a significant risk factor as the homeostasis of trace metals in the brain is important for brain function and also for the prevention of brain diseases.[71] Hair mineral analyses indicate significantly lower levels of iron in the hair of patients with PD compared with controls. Calcium and magnesium were slightly lower while zinc was higher in PD, but these differences were not significant.[72]

Atomic absorption spectrophotometer studies have correspondingly revealed a significant zinc deficiency combined with elevated iron and selenium in the CSF of patients with PD on L-dopa. This provided clear evidence of increased iron and selenium in the brain which could be correlated with decreased dopamine levels and increased oxidative stress in PD patients.[73]

Antioxidants

Vitamin E

A meta-analysis investigating the relationships between vitamin C, E and carotenoids and PD has demonstrated that dietary vitamin E may have a neuroprotective effect attenuating the risk of PD.[74]

B group vitamins

Vitamin B6

Adequate dietary vitamin B6 has also been shown to decrease the risk of PD, probably through its antioxidant effects rather than mechanisms related to homocysteine metabolism.[75]

Folate and vitamin B12

L-dopa treated PD patients have significantly lower serum folate and vitamin B12 than controls.[76] In fact, L-dopa treatment may represent an acquired cause of hyperhomocysteinaemia, as evidenced by studies in animals as well as PD patients.[77] PD patients with depression have significantly lower folate levels compared with non-depressed PD, and cognitively impaired PD patients have significantly lower vitamin B12 levels compared with non-cognitively impaired PD. Supplementation with cobalamin and folate is effective in reducing homocysteine, and this may have important implications in the management of PD patients who are at risk for vascular diseases, cognitive impairment or dementia. The effects of vitamin supplementation certainly warrant further attention and investigation given that elevated concentrations of total homocysteine in plasma (>12 micromol/l) is epidemiologically associated as a risk factor for several diseases of the central nervous system (CNS).[76]

A recent review has concluded that treatment with folate, B12, and B6 can improve cerebral function. Hence, preventive vitamin B supplementation and sufficient intake seem very important for secondary and primary prevention of neuropsychiatric disorders, especially in those individuals with a low intake or status of these vitamins.[78]

Vitamin D

Based upon several lines of evidence, vitamin D deficiency may also be a significant risk factor in the pathogenesis of PD.[79] Significantly more patients with PD have been found to have insufficient vitamin D compared with controls.[80] Furthermore, animal studies show that 1,25(OH)(2)D(3) may help to prevent dopaminergic neuron damage.[81]

More studies are warranted to assess the role of vitamin D deficiency in PD.

Zinc

Zinc has many critical functions in brain development and maintenance.[82] The CNS concentrates almost 10% total body zinc, a large proportion of which serves as zinc metalloproteins in neurons and glial cells. Ionic zinc exists in the synaptic vesicles, serving as an endogenous neuromodulator in synaptic neurotransmission. Dietary zinc deficiency significantly affects zinc homeostasis in the brain, causing deficiencies of neurotransmitters such as serotonin, gamma-butyric acid (GABA) and melatonin and brain dysfunctions such as cognitive impairment, olfactory dysfunction and depression.[83, 84] It is interesting to note that patients with PD often complain of these symptoms.[85]

PD is characterised by the loss of dopamine-producing cells which is believed to be caused by defects in mitochondrial oxidative phosphorylation and enhanced oxidative stress.[86–90] Zinc is required for the synthesis of superoxide dismutase (SOD), a powerful antioxidant. SOD is normally found in high concentrations in the substantia nigra where it protects neurons by scavenging free radicals.[91] PD patients show a significantly decreased zinc status compared with controls and zinc supplementation has been shown to significantly increase SOD in vitro.[85]

Zinc is also necessary for the synthesis of metallothionein, which has been shown to be neuroprotective against the nitric oxide synthase activation and peroxynitrite ion overproduction that may be involved in the aetiopathogenesis of PD.[86] Additional studies on the role of zinc in the development and treatment of PD are therefore warranted.[85]

Copper

Copper is a trace element whose role in the pathogenesis of PD has been widely discussed.[90,92] Low copper may result in incomplete CNS development whereas excess copper may be injurious. It may be involved in free radical production that results in mitochondrial damage, DNA breakage and neuronal injury.[93] Free copper is increased in the CSF and thus appears to be a good biomarker for PD.[91] Furthermore, a person who gradually accumulates copper will tend to experience a gradual reduction in zinc, with a subsequent increase in oxidative stress, which may eventually lead to PD.[82]

Iron

Iron accumulation in human and animal PD brains is beyond that observed in non-PD brains of a similar age.[71, 94, 95] For animal models, pre-treatment with iron chelators is neuro–protective.[96] Several case-control studies have described the association of high dietary iron and PD, but prospective data are lacking. In 1 study, total iron intake was not associated with an increased risk of PD but the risk was significantly increased among individuals with high nonheme iron and low Vitamin C.[97] A significantly decreased ferroxidase activity has also been found in patients with PD, confirming previous findings of iron deposition in this disorder.[91] At this time, there are only hypotheses as to the possible role of iron in the pathogenic processes of PD, including potential interactions between iron and other factors associated with PD.[94]

Magnesium

Magnesium deficiency has recently been shown to be involved in the pathogenesis of substantia nigra neuronal degeneration, hence contributing to the risk of PD.[36, 98, 99] Results from animal studies show that magnesium might protect dopaminergic neurons in the substantia nigra from degeneration. Thus, magnesium exerts both preventative and ameliorating effects with regards to neurite and neuron pathology in a PD model.[100, 101]

Other supplements

Coenzyme Q_{10} (CoQ_{10})

The concentration of CoQ_{10} has been reported recently to be in deficit in a number of brain regions (substantia nigra, cerebellum, cortex and striatum) from individuals with PD as compared to controls.[102] CoQ_{10} may therefore also be involved in the pathophysiology of PD.[103] A study that employed doses as high as 1200mg/day of CoQ_{10} in early PD showed that it was safe and well tolerated. Moreover, a recent nano-particular CoQ_{10} at a dosage of 300mg/day was safe and well tolerated and led to plasma levels similar to 1200mg/day of standard formulations. However, it did not improve primary or secondary outcome measures.[104] A large phase III clinical trial is currently under way to examine if high-dose CoQ_{10} will slow disease progression.[105]

Further, a new anti-parkinsonian agent has been tested in combination with CoQ_{10}; namely, GPI 1485 (a neuroimmunophilin ligand that binds FK-506-binding proteins) and the RCT study concluded that the combination may warrant further study in PD, even though the data are inconsistent.[106]

Omega-3 fatty acids

A recent nutrition review related to neurodegenerative diseases suggested that adequate omega-3 fatty acids in the diet will probably prevent most psychotic episodes and prove that neurodegenerative disorders with dementia are also to a large extent not only preventable but avoidable.[107] In addition, an RCT study has demonstrated that PD patients, with or without anti-depressants, show improvement in depressive symptoms when supplemented with omega-3 fish oils supplements.[108]

Levodopa (L-dopa)

L-dopa-induced dyskinesia (LID) is 1 of the major complications that occur in PD patients after prolonged treatment with L-dopa. Animal studies have demonstrated that combining L-dopa (a naturally occurring amino acid found in food and made from l–tyrosine in the human body) with a diet high in creatine (found in, for example, salmon, tuna, sashimi, sushi, lean red meat) could attenuate LID, possibly representing a novel way to control the motor complications associated with L-dopa therapy.[109]

Alpha-lipoic acid/acetyl L-carnitine

In a review of the *in vitro* and animal data, Beal has suggested that the considerable evidence that is available suggests that mitochondrial dysfunction may play a role in the pathogenesis of PD and that supplements such as alpha-lipoic acid and acetyl L-carntine may have a role in ameliorating symptoms by modulating cellular energy metabolism.[102] Moreover, anecdotal evidence has suggested that alpha-lipoic acid at a dose of 80mg/day and acetyl L-carnitine at 400mg/day in combination with a number of other antioxidant substances (e.g. CoQ_{10} + vitamin C + vitamin E) could be useful. However there are no clinical data to substantiate this notion.[111]

Herbal medicines

Curcumin and naringenin

The nutritional supplements, curcumin and naringenin, are phenolic antioxidant compounds that have also recently been shown to prevent significant loss of tyrosine-hydroxylase-positive cells, thereby increasing dopamine levels, in the substantia nigra of animals with induced PD.[112]

Gingko biloba

Gingko biloba is 1 of the most extensively studied herbal supplements for neurodegenerative conditions that has been reported to directly improve brain metabolism and increase brain blood flow. In a double-blind RCT *Gingko biloba* was reported to stabilise Alzheimer's disease and many of the participants demonstrated an improvement as noted in various standardised psychological tests.[113] A recent review suggests that *Gingko biloba* EGb 761 extracts exerts a combination of antioxidative, antiamyloidogenic and anti-apoptotic effects that are in tune with cognitive deficits, however, it may also have a metabolic role to play in PD.[114] Clinical trials are hence warranted.

Ayurvedic medicine

Ayurveda is a comprehensive natural health care system that originated in India more than 5000 years ago. Still being used in India as a primary health care system, it is now creating more interest worldwide.[115] PD or *paralysis agitans* and its pharmacological treatment was in fact described in this ancient medical system under the name Kampavata.[116]

Mucuna pruriens

Mucuna pruriens (MP) contains L-dopa and is the traditional herb used in Ayurveda to treat PD. It is interesting that PD existed before current environmental toxins, suggesting again that PD is of multi-factorial origin.[117, 118, 119]

The pharmaceutical preparation, HP-200, which contains MP has been shown to be effective in the treatment of PD. Indeed, it has been demonstrated, in animal models, to be more effective than conventional L-dopa.[120] MP possesses significantly higher anti-Parkinson activity compared with levadopa in the 6-hydroxydopamine lesioned rat model of PD.[121] Unlike synthetic levadopa treatment, MP cotyledon powder significantly restored the endogenous L-dopa, dopamine, noradrenaline and serotonin content in the *substantia nigra*. It should be noted that nicotine adenine dinucleotide and CoQ_{10} were also included in this powder.[121]

MP has been shown to possess anti-Parkinson and neuroprotective effects in animal models of PD. Its antioxidant activity was demonstrated by its ability to scavenge DPPH radicals, ABTS radicals and reactive oxygen species. Furthermore, MP inhibited the oxidation of lipids and deoxyribose sugar and exhibited divalent iron chelating activity. The results suggest that the neuroprotective and neurorestorative effects of MP may be related to its antioxidant activity, independent of the symptomatic effect. In addition, MP appears to be safe in the treatment of patients with PD.[122]

Traditional Chinese medicine (TCM)

The description and treatment of PD can also be found in the ancient Chinese medical system. When herbs-interposed moxibustion at Shenque acu-point CV8 was added to the routine Western medical therapy, the total effective rate was significantly better than in the control group.[123] Recent reviews of trials involving TCM, however, have concluded that larger, more well-designed RCTs need to be performed before any conclusion can be drawn regarding the efficacy of TCM for PD.[124, 125]

Physical therapies

Allied health care

Allied health care (e.g. occupational therapy, speech therapy, physiotherapy) is used by many patients with PD. Referral rates have been estimated to be 63% for physical therapy, 9% for occupational therapy and 14% for speech therapy. It is advisable to refer patients with PD to an allied health care professional with PD-specific expertise.[126]

Scientific evidence is beginning to emerge with specific interventions being increasingly integrated in rehabilitation programmes.[127] Recent Cochrane reviews, however, have revealed that there is insufficient evidence to support or refute the efficacy of OT, physiotherapy and speech therapy in PD. Larger placebo-controlled RCTs are needed to determine a consensus for 'best practice' regimens in these areas.[128, 129, 130]

Acupuncture

There is a plethora of studies, including meta-analyses, suggesting beneficial effects of acupuncture in the treatment of PD.[131–136] Acupuncture is safe and well tolerated in patients with PD.[134] Similar results have been obtained with electro-scalp acupuncture (ESA).[137] Tremor, rigidity and bradykinesia, in particular, have shown to be improved.[138] It has been found that ESA may possibly reduce the loss of dopamine transporters in the basal ganglia, delaying the progression of PD and alleviating clinical symptoms.[139] Larger, placebo-controlled RCTs with rigorous methods of randomisation are warranted.[132]

There have also been several studies combining traditional pharmaceutical therapies with acupuncture. It has been demonstrated that the combination can be synergistic and, furthermore, that the adverse effects of drugs may be reduced.[140, 141] The dose of medication required has also been shown to be reduced.[142]

Conclusion

PD is a progressive neurodegenerative disorder that affects neurophysiologic function, movement abilities, and quality of life.

Hence, an integrative approach to the management of PD can include a number of CAM modalities to improve quality of life. Furthermore these can also be integrated with other nutritional and lifestyle modification modalities (see Table 31.2).

Table 31.2 Levels of evidence for lifestyle and complementary medicines/therapies in the management of Parkinson's disease symptoms

Modality	Level I	Level II	Level IIIa	Level IIIb	Level IIIc	Level IV	Level V
Lifestyle modification							
Coffee intake				x			
Smoking				x			
Constipation (↓ water intake)				x			
Adiposity				x			
Mind–body medicine							
Cognitive behavioural therapy				x			
Alexander technique					x		
Imagery				x			
Music therapy				x			
Repetitive transcranial magnetic stimulation					x		
Physical activity/ exercise	x						
Tai chi				x			
Walking				x			
Tango dancing				x			
Environmental influences							
Heavy metals				x			
Occupational exposures					x		
Pesticides					x		
Diet							
Calorie restrictions						x	
Vegetarian diet				x			
Western diet				x			
Nutritional supplements							
(vitamins and minerals)							
Antioxidants (C, E. carotenoids)					x		
Vitamin D					x		
Vitamin B12					x		
Vitamin B6					x		
Folate					x		

Continued

Table 31.2 Levels of evidence for lifestyle and complementary medicines/therapies in the management of Parkinson's disease symptoms—Cont'd

Modality	Level I	Level II	Level IIIa	Level IIIb	Level IIIc	Level IV	Level V
Zinc					x		
Copper					x		
Iron					x		
Magnesium					x		
Other supplements							
Coenzyme Q_{10}		x					
Omega-3 fatty acids			x				
L-dopa					x		
Alpha–Lipoic Acid/ Acetyl L–Carnitine						x	
Herbal medicines							
Gingko biloba					x		
Ayurvedic medicine							
• *Mucuna pruriens*			x				
Traditional Chinese medicine					x		
Physical therapies							
Allied health					x		
Acupuncture	x						

Level I — from a systematic review of all relevant randomised controlled trials — meta-analyses.
Level II — from at least 1 properly designed randomised controlled clinical trial.
Level IIIa — from well-designed pseudo-randomised controlled trials (alternate allocation or some other method).
Level IIIb — from comparative studies (including systematic reviews of such studies) with concurrent controls and allocation not randomised, cohort studies, case-control studies, or interrupted time series with a parallel control group.
Level IIIc — from comparative studies with historical control, 2 or more single-arm studies or interrupted time series without a parallel control group.
Level IV — opinions of respected authorities based on clinical experience, descriptive studies or reports of expert committees.
Level V — represents minimal evidence that represents testimonials.

Clinical tips handout for patients — Parkinson's disease

1 Lifestyle advice

Sleep

- Herbal teas such as chamomile can be helpful in some cases.
- Magnesium (up to 350mg elemental twice daily) can be used to assist sleep at night (3 month trial).
- L-tryptophan (200mg bd) may be trialled for 1 month in the morning and 1 hour before bedtime.
- Melatonin (3–6mg) at bedtime may be trialled for 1 month (not with L-tryptophan).
- Herbal supplements including passionflower and valerian may be helpful in some cases.

Sunshine

- At least 15 minutes sunshine is needed daily for vitamin D production. More sun exposure is required in winter. Dark skinned people need more sun exposure.
- Sunscreen can block the conversion to vitamin D so sunscreen should be avoided during this specified time period.

2 Physical activity/exercise

- Regular exercise can improve physical functioning, quality of life, balance and gait speed.
- The practice of tai chi may also be beneficial.
- Dancing, such as tango dancing may be beneficial for those who are frail and elderly with PD.

3 Mind–body medicine

- Many Parkinson's patients also suffer with depression as a side-effect of their illness. Cognitive behavioural therapy, in particular, can be very useful.
- The Alexander technique is a process of psycho–physical education. It can help with reducing disability and depression in people with Parkinson's disease.
- Music therapy and visualisation may also be helpful.

4 Environment

- Manganese, lead, iron, copper and zinc imbalances have all been found to be possible contributing factors to PD.
- Patients with PD should ideally be tested for the presence of heavy metals. This can be done by testing plasma levels, hair mineral analysis or a comprehensive urinary element profile.
- Avoid pesticide residues in food wherever possible.

5 Dietary modification

- There are benefits from a whole-food, plant-based diet with fish and blueberries.
- If uric acid levels are high, decreased consumption of purines (meat/crustaceans) should be advised.
- Although controversial, dairy consumption may increase PD risk in men.
- Reduce caffeine intake and replace it with black tea.
- Increase creatine in the diet to possibly reduce L-dopa induced dyskinesia.

6 Physical therapies

- Acupuncture may be particularly beneficial for those with PD. The combination of pharmaceutical therapies and acupuncture may be synergistic and may also reduce the adverse effects of medications.

7 Supplementation

Supplements to reduce the risk of Parkinson's disease

Vitamin E

- Dosage: 200IU up to 500IU/day (mixed tocopherols).
- Side-effects: mild and rare.
- Contraindications: caution with warfarin and vitamin E at higher doses.

Vitamin B6

- Dosage: 20mg Pyridoxal-5-Phosphate (Activated B6).
- Side-effects: parasthesia in extremities, bone pain, muscle weakness at high doses. Reversible on cessation of supplement.
- Contraindications: caution with amiodarone, phenobarbitone, phenytoin.

Vitamin D3 (cholecalciferol)

- Indication: may help to prevent dopaminergic neuron damage.
- Dosage: depending upon serum levels of 25(OH)D3, between 1000–4000IU/day under medical supervision.
- Side-effects: mild and rare when used appropriately.
- Contraindications: hypersensitivity to vitamin D, systemic lupus erythematosus (SLE), hypercalcaemia. Caution in sarcoidosis and hyperparathyroidism. Possible interaction with calcium channel blockers and digitalis.

Magnesium
- Indication: may help to prevent substantia nigra neuronal degeneration.
- Dosage: if symptoms of deficiency are present (eyelid twitches, restless legs, feelings of tightness/cramps in legs/feet, palpitations, chocolate cravings), 350mg elemental magnesium twice daily for 3 months, then a smaller maintenance dose as dictated by return of symptoms.
- Side-effects: diarrhoea, gastric irritation.
- Contraindications: renal failure, heart block.

Supplements to treat PD

CoenzymeQ$_{10}$ (CoQ$_{10}$)
- Indication: to slow the progression of PD.
- Dosage: 150mg/day up to 2400mg/day.
- Results: 3 month trial.
- Side-effects: dizziness, nausea, abdominal discomfort, anorexia, diarrhoea.
- Contraindications: caution with warfarin.

Vitamin B12
- Indication: to improve cognition and reduce homocysteine (common side-effect of L–dopa treatment)
- Dosage: depending on levels, sublingual B12 1mg daily for 3 months or 10mg methylcobalamin I/M injection once weekly for 6 weeks. Ideal serum level 750–1500.
- Results: 6 weeks to 3 months.
- Side-effects: nil known.
- Contraindications: no known contraindication.

Folic acid
- Indication: to improve depression and reduce homocysteine in PD.
- Dosage: depending upon red cell levels, 1–5g/day.
- Results: 3 months trial.
- Side-effects: urticaria with allergy, nausea, flatulence, bitter taste in mouth, irritability, excitability.
- Contraindications: close supervision required if on anti-convulsants. Folate supplementation may mask vitamin B12 deficiency.

Tyrosine
- Indication: to naturally increase dopamine levels.
- Dosage: 500mg tds.
- Results: 3 months trial.
- Side-effects: migraines, gastrointestinal upset, fatigue, reflux, arthralgia, insomnia, nervousness.
- Contraindications: melanoma. Caution with manic conditions, hyperthyroidism, anti-depressants (MAOIs, SSRIs TCAs). Use only under medical supervision in combination with L-dopa.

EPA/DHA fish oils
- Indication: to improve depression in PD patients.
- Dosage: 2–4–9g/day.
- Results: 3 month trial.
- Side-effects: fishy burps, diarrhoea, gastrointestinal discomfort.
- Contraindications: caution with anticoagulants at very high doses. Doses >10g/day may cause bleeding tendency, avoid use 1-2 weeks prior to surgery.

Zinc
- Indication: to improve cognition, olfactory dysfunction and depression and reduce oxidative stress.
- Dosage: 35–45mg elemental zinc nocte.
- Results: 3 month trial; cease earlier if nausea occurs.
- Side-effects: nausea, vomiting, reduced copper after long-term use.
- Contraindications: high zinc levels, sideroblastic anaemia, severe kidney disease. Caution with amiloride.

Herbs

***Mucuna pruriens* (may not be available in Australia)**
- Indication: naturally contains L-dopa.
- Dosage: there is no rigorously proven effective dose, however 15 and 30g preparations have been used weekly.
- Results: good efficacy for controlling symptoms associated with PD.
- Side-effects: mild–moderate gastrointestinal complaints.
- Contraindications: not recommended for people prescribed L-dopa or monoamine oxidase inhibitors. Not to be used by pregnant or breastfeeding women.

Curcumin
- Indication: to increase dopamine levels in substantia nigra.
- Dosage: powdered extract 100–300mg/day.
- Results: 3 month trial.
- Side-effects: gastrointestinal upset.
- Contraindications: bile duct obstruction, breast cancer chemotherapy; cease 1 week prior to major surgery. Caution with warfarin.

References

1 Stoessl J. Potential therapeutic targets for PD. Expert Opin Ther Targets 2008;12(4):425–36.
2 Kim SR, Lee TY, Kim MS, et. al. Use of CAM by Korean patients with PD. Clin Neurol Neurosurg 2009;111(2):156–60.
3 Murphy SM, Rogers A, Hutchinson M, et. al. Counting the cost of CAM therapies in an Irish neurological clinic. Eur J Neurol 2008;15(12):1380–3.
4 Tan LC, Lau PN, Jamora RD, et. al. Use of complementary therapies in patients with PD in Singapore. Mov Disord 2006;21(1):86–9.
5 Rajendran PR, Thompson RE, Reich SG. The use of alternative therapies by patients with PD. Neurology 2001;57(5):790–4.
6 Parkinson's Disease Society. UK. Online. Available: www.parkinsons.org.uk/pdf/comptherapiesOct05.pdf. (accessed May 2009).
7 Paccetti C, Mancini F, Agliera R, et. al. Active music therapy in PD: an integrative method for motor and emotional rehabilitation. Psychosom Med 2000;62(3):386–93.
8 Abbott RD, Ross GW, White LR, et. al. Environmental, life-style, and physical precursors of clinical Parkinson's disease: recent findings from the Honolulu-Asia Aging Study. J Neurol 2003;250(Suppl 3):III30–9.
9 Ueki A, Otsuka M. Life style risks of Parkinson's disease: association between decreased water intake and constipation. J Neurol 2004;251(Suppl 7):vII18–23.
10 Dobkin RD, Menza M, Bienfait KL. CBT for the treatment of depression in PD: a promising nonpharmacological approach. Expert Rev Neurother 2008;8(1):27–35.
11 Cole K, Vaughan FL. The feasibility of using CBT for depression associated with PD: a literature review. Parkinsonism Relat Disord 2005;11(5):269–76.
12 Dobkin RD, Allen LA, Menza M. CBT for depression in PD: a pilot study. Mov Disord 2007;22(7):946–52.
13 Secker DL, Brown RG. CBT for carers of patients with PD: a preliminary RCT. J Neurol Neurosurg Psychiatry 2005;76(4):491–7.
14 Ernst E, Canter PH. The AT: a systematic review of controlled clinical trials. Forsch Komplementarmed Klass Nuturheilkd 2003;10(6):325–9.
15 C, Stallibrass. An evaluation of the AT for the management of disability in PD- a preliminary study. Clin Rehabil 1997;11(1):8–12.
16 Stallibrass C, Hampson M. The AT: its application in midwifery and the results of preliminary research into Parkinsons. Complement Ther Nurs Midwifery 2001;7(1):13–8.
17 Tamir R, Dickstein R, Huberman M. Integration of motor imagery and physical practice in group treatment applied to subjects with PD. Neurorehabil Neural Repair 2007;21(1):68–75.
18 Paccetti C, Aglieri R, Mancini F, et. al. Active music therapy and PD: methods. Funct Neurol 1998;13(1):57–67.
19 Helmich RC, Siebner HR, Bakker M, et. al. Repetitive transcranial magnetic stimulation to improve mood and motor function in Parkinson's Disease. J Neurol Sci 2006;248(1–2):84–96.
20 Derejko M, Niewiadomska M, Rakowicz M. The diagnostic and therapeutic application of transcranial magnetic stimulation. Neurol Neurochir Pol 2005;39(5):389–96.
21 Benninger DH, Lomarev M, Wassermann EM. Safety study of 50 Hz repetitive transcranial magnetic stimulation in patients with Parkinson's disease. Clin Neurophysiol 2009;120(4):809–15.
22 Dibble LE, Addison O, Papa E. The effects of exercise on balance in persons with Parkinson's disease: a systematic review across the disability spectrum. J Neurol Phys Ther 2009;33(1):14–26.
23 White DK, Wagenaar RC, Ellis TD, et. al. Changes in walking activity and endurance following rehabilitation for people with Parkinson disease. Arch Phys Med Rehabil 2009;90(1):43–50.
24 Keus SH, Munneke M, Nijkrake MJ, et. al. Physical therapy in PD: evolution and future challenges. Mov Disord 2009;24(1):1–14.
25 Goodwin VA, Richards SH, Taylor RS, et. al. The effectiveness of exercise interventions for people with PD: SR and meta-analysis. Mov Disord 2008;23(5):631–40.
26 Keus SH, Bloem BR, Hendriks EJ, et. al. Evidence-based analysis of physical therapy in PD with recommendations for practice and research. Mov Disord 2007;22(4):451–60.
27 Crizzle AM, Newhouse IJ. Is physical exercise beneficial for persons with PD? Clin J Sport Med 2006;16(5):422–5.
28 Hackney ME, Kantorovich S, Levin R, et. al. Effects of tango on functional mobility in PD: a preliminary study. J Neurol Phys Ther 2007;31(4):173–9.
29 Kwakkel G, de Goede CJ, van Wegen EE. Impact of physical therapy for PD: a critical review of the literature. Parkinsonism Relat Disord 2007;13 Suppl 3:S478–87.
30 Burini D, Farabollini B, Iacucci S, et. al. A RC cross-over trial of aerobic training vs Qigong in advanced PD. Eura Medicophys 2006;42(3):231–8.
31 Canning CG, Sherrington C, Lord SR, et. al. Exercise therapy for prevention of falls in people with PD: a protocol for a RCT and economic evaluation. BMC Neurology 2009;9:4.
32 Lee MS, Lam P, Ernst E. Effectiveness of tai chi for Parkinson's disease: a critical review. Parkinsonism Relat Disord 2008;14(8):589–94.
33 Hackney ME, Earhart GM. Tai Chi improves balance and mobility in people with Parkinson disease. Gait Posture 2008;28(3):456–60.
34 Edwards TM, Myers JP. Environmental exposures and gene regulation in disease aetiology. Cien Saude Colet 2008;13(1):269–81.
35 Brown TP, Rumsby PC, Capleton AC, et. al. Pesticides and PD-is there a link? Environ Health Perspect 2006;114(2):156–64.
36 Guzeva VI, Chukhlovina ML, Chuklovin BA. Environmental factors and Parkinsonian syndrome. Gig Sanit 2008;(2):60–62.
37 Barlow BK, Cory-Slechta DA, Richfield EK, et. al. The gestational environment and Parkinson's disease: evidence for neurodevelopmental origins of a neurodegenerative disorder. Reprod Toxicol 07;23(3):457–70.
38 Dhillon AS, Tarbutton GL, Levin JL, et. al. Pesticide/environmental exposures and PD in EastTtexas. J Agromedicine 2008;13(1):37–48.
39 Dick FD, De Palma G, Ahmadi A, et. al. Environmental risk factors for PD and parkinsonism: the Geoparkinson study. Occup Environ Med 2007;64(10):666–72.
40 Hancock DB, Martin ER, Mayhew GM, et. al. Pesticide exposure and risk of PD: a family-based case-control study. BMC Neurol 2008;8:6.

41 Luccini R, Albini E, Benedetti L, et. al. Neurological and neuropsychological features in PD patients exposed to neurotoxic metals. G Ital Med Lav Ergon 2007;29(3 Suppl):280–1.
42 Zoni S, Albini E, Luccini R. Neuropsychological testing for the assessment of manganese neurotoxicity: a review and a proposal. Am J Ind Med 2007;50(11):812–30.
43 RA, Yokel. Blood-brain barrier flux of aluminium, manganese, iron and other metals suspected to contribute to metal-induced neurodegenration. J Alzheimers Dis 2006;10(2–3):223–53.
44 Gorell JM, Johnson CC, Rybicki BA, et. al. Occupational exposure to Mn, Cu, Pb, Fe, Hg and Zn and the risk of PD. Neurotoxicology 1999;20 (2–3):239–47.
45 Coon S, Stark A, Peterson E, et. al. Whole-body lifetime occupational lead exposure and risk of PD. Environ Health Perpect 2006;114(12):1872–6.
46 Barnham KJ, Bush AI. Metals in Alzheimer's and PD. Curr Opin Chem Biol 2008;12(2):222–8.
47 Squitti R, Gorgone G, Binetti G, et. al. Metals and oxidative stress in PD from industrial areas with exposition to environmental toxins or metal pollution. G Ital Med Lav Ergon 2007;29(3 Suppl):294–6.
48 Li AA, Mink PJ, McIntosh LJ, et. al. Evaluation of epidemiologic and animal data associating pesticides with PD. J Occup Environ Med 2005;47(10):1059–87.
49 Kamel F, Hoppin JA. Association of pesticide exposure with neurologic dysfunction and disease. Environ Health Perspect 2004;112(9):950–8.
50 Bjorling-Poulson M, Anderson HR, Grandjean P. Potential developmental neurotoxicity of pesticides in Europe. Environ Health 2008;7:50.
51 Neurotoxicity of pesticides: a review. Costa LG, Giordano G, Guizzetti M et. al. Front Biosci 2008;13:1240–9.
52 Keifer MC, Firestone J. Neurotoxicity of pesticides 2007;12(1):17–25.
53 Costello S, Cockburn M, Bronstein J, et. al. PD and residential exposure to maneb and paraquat from agricultural applications in the central valley of Caifornia. Am J Epidemiol 2009;169(8):919–26.
54 Armentero MT, Levandis G, Bramanti P, et. al. Dietary restriction does not prevent nigrostriatal degeneration in the 6-hydroxydopamine model of PD. Exp Neurol 2008;212(2):548–51.
55 Barichella M, savardi C, Mauri A, et. al. Diet with LPP for renal patients increases daily energy expenditure and improves motor function in parkinsonian patients with motor fluctuations. Nutr Neurosci 2007;10(3–4):129–35.
56 Gao X, Chen H, Fung TT, et. al. Prospective study of dietary pattern and risk of PD. Am J Clin Nutr 07;86(5):1486–94.
57 de Luis Roman D, Aller R, castano O. Vegetarian diets: effects on health. Rev Clin Esp 2007;207(3):141–3.
58 Lau FC, Shukitt-Hale B, Joseph JA. Nutritional intervention in brain aging: reducing the effects of inflammation and oxidative stress. subcell Biochem 2007;42:299–318.
59 Schlesinger I, Schlesinger N. Uric acid in PD. Mov Discord 2008;23(12):1653–7.
60 Gao X, Chen H, Choi HK, et. al. Diet, urate and PD. Am J Epidemiol 2008;167(7):831–8.
61 Annanmaki T, Muuronen A, Murros K. Low plasma uric acid level in PD. Mov Disord 2007;22(8):1133–7.
62 Gasior M, Rogawski MA, Hartman AL. Neuroprotective and disease-modifing effects of the ketogenic diet. Behav Pharmacol 06;17(5–6):431–9.
63 Ma L, Zhang L, Gao XH, et. al. Dietary factors and smoking as risk factors for PD in a rural population in china: a nested case-control study. Acta Neurol Scand 2006;113(4):278–81.
64 Powers KM, Smith-weller T, Franklin GM, et. al. Dietary fats, cholesterol and iron as risk factors for PD. Parkinsonian Relat Disord 2009;15(1):47–52.
65 Chen H, O'Reilly E, McCullough ML, et. al. Consumption of dairy products and risk of PD. Am J Epidemiol 07;16599:998–1006.
66 Nakaso K, Ito S, Nakashima K. Caffeine activates the P13K/Akt pathway and prevents apoptotic cell death in a PD model of SH-SY5Y cells. Neuro Sci Lett 2008;432(2):146–50.
67 Facheris MF, Schneider NK, Lesnick TG et. al. Coffee, caffeine-related genes and PD: a case-control study. Mov Disord 2008;23(14):2033–40.
68 Tan EK, Chua E, Fook-Chong SM, et. al. Association between caffeine intake and risk of PD among fast and slow metabolisers. Pharmacogenet Genomics 2007;17(11):1001–5.
69 Tan LC, Koh WP, Yuan JM, et. al. Differential effects of black vs green tea on risk of PD in the Singapore Chinese Health Study. Am J Epidemiol 2008;167(5):553–60.
70 Petersen MS, Halling J, Bech S, et. al. Impact of dietary exposure to food contaminants on the risk of PD. Neurotoxicology 2008;2994:584–90.
71 A, Takeda. Essential trace metals and brain function. Yakugaku Zasshi 2004;124(9):577–85.
72 Forte G, Alimonte A, Violante N, et. al. Ca, Cu, Fe,mg, Si and Zn content of hair in PD. J Trace Elem Med Biol 2005;19(2–3):195–201.
73 Qureshi GA, Qureshi AA, Memon SA, et. al. Impact of Se, Cu and Zn in on/off PD patients on L-dopa therapy. J Neural Transm Suppl 2006;(71):229–36.
74 Etminan M, Gill SS, Samii A. Intake of Vit E,C and carotenoids and the risk of PD: a meta-analysis. Lancet Neurol 2005;4(6):362–5.
75 de Lau LM, Koudstaal PJ, Witteman JC, et. al. Dietary folate, Vitamin B12 and Vitamin B6 and the risk of PD. Neurology 2006;67(2):315–8.
76 Triantafyllou NI, Nikolau C, Boufidou F, et. al. Folate and Vit B12 levels in L-dopa treated PD patients: their relationship to clinical maifestations, mood and cognition. Parkinsonism Relat Disord 2008;14(4):321–5.
77 Lamberti P, Zoccolella S, Armenise E, et. al. Hyperhomocysteinaemia in L-dopa treated PD patients: effect of cobalamin and folate administration. Eur J Neurol 2005;12(5):365–8.
78 Herrmann W, Lorenzl S, Obeid R. Review of the role of hyperhomocysteinemia and vitamin B deficiency in neurological and psychiatric disorders--current evidence and preliminary recommendations. Fortschr Neurol Psychiatr 2007;75(9):515–27.
79 Newmark HL, Newmark J. Vit D and PD- a hypothesis. Mov Disord 2007;22(4):461–8.
80 Evatt ML, Delong MR, Khazai N, et. al. Prevalence of Vit D deficiency in patients with PD and Alzheimers. Arch Neurol 2008;65(10):1348–52.
81 Sanchez B, Relova JL, Gallego R, et. al. 1,25 Dihydroxyvitamin D3 administration to 6-hydroxydopamine-lesioned rats increases glial cell line-derived neurotrophic factor and partially restores tyrosine hydroxylase expression in SN and striatum. J Neurosci Res 2009;87(3):723–32.

82 Johnson S. Micronutrient accumulation and depletion in schizophrenia, epilepsy, autism and PD? Med Hypothese 2001;56(5):641–5.
83 Takeda A. Zinc homeostasis and functions of zinc in the brain. Biometals 2001;14(3–4):343–51.
84 Ciubotariu D, Nechifor M. Zinc involvements in the brain. Rev Med Chir Soc Med Nat Iasi 2007;111(4):981–5.
85 Forsleff L, Schauss AG, Bier ID, et. al. Evidence of functional zinc deficiency in PD. J Altern Comp Med 1999;5(1):57–64.
86 Ebadi M, Sharma SK, Ghafourifar P, et. al. Peroxynitrite in the pathogenesis of PD and the neuroprotective role of metallothioneins. Methods Enzymol 2005;396:276–98.
87 Henchcliffe C, Beal MF. Mitochondrial biology and ox stress in PD pathogenesis. Nat Clin Pract Neurol 2008;4(11):600–9.
88 Chen CM, Liu JL, Wu YR, et. al. Increased ox damage in peripheral blood correlates with severity of PD. Neurobiol Dis 2009;33(3): 429–35.
89 Mandel S, Packer L, Youdim, et. al. Proceedings from the '3rd International Conference on Mechanism of Action of Nutraceuticals.'. J Nutr Biochem 2005;16(9):513–20.
90 Chwiej J, Adamek D, Szczerbowska-Boruchowska M, et. al. Study of Cu chemical state inside single neurons from PD and control substantia nigra using the micro-XANES technigue. J Trace Elem Med Biol 2008;22(3):183–8.
91 Boll MC, Alcaraz-Zubeldia M, Montes S, et. al. A different marker profile in 4 neurodegenerative diseases. Free Cu, ferroxidase and SOD1 activities, lipid peroxidation and NO(x) content in the CSF. Neurochem Res 2008;33(9):1717–23.
92 Gaggelli E, Kozlowski H, Valensin D, et. al. Cu homeostasis and neurodegerative disorders (Alzheimers, prion, PD and ALS). Chem Rev 2006;106(6):1995–2044.
93 Desai V, Kaler SG. Role of copper in human neurological disorders. Am J Clin Nutr 2008;88(3):855S-8S.
94 Rhodes SL, Ritz B. Genetics of iron regulation and the possible role of iron in PD. Neurobiol Dis. 2008;32(2):183–95.
95 MB, Youdim. Brain iron deficiency and excess: cognitive impairment and neurodegeneration with involvement of striatum and hippocampus. Neurotox Res 2008;14(1):45–56.
96 Youdim MB, Grunblatt E, Mandel S. The copper chelator, D-peniccamine, does not attenuate MPTP induced dopamine depletion in mice. J Neural Transm 2007;114(2):205–9.
97 Logroscino g, Gao X, Chen H, et. al. Dietary iron intake and risk of PD. Am J Epidem 2008;168(12):1381–8.
98 Oyanagi K, Kawakami E, Kikuchi-Horie K, et. al. mg deficiency over generations in rats with special references to the pathogenesis of the P-dementia complex and ALS of Guam. Neuropathology 2006;2692):115–28.
99 K, Oyanagi. The nature of the P-dementia complex and ALS of Guam and Mg deficiency. Parkinsonism Relat Disord 2005;11 suppl 1:S17–23.
100 Hashimoto T, Nishi K, Nagasao J, et. al. Mg exerts both preventative and ameliorating effects in an in vivo rat PD model involving MPP+ toxicity in dopaminergic neurons. Brain Res 2008;1197: 143–51.
101 Tariq M, Khan HA, al Moutaery K, et. al. Effect of chronic administration ofmgSO4 on MPTP induced neurotoxicity in mice. Pharmacol Toxicol 1998;82(5):218–22.
102 Hargreaves IP, Lane A, Sleiman PM. The coenzyme Q10 status of the brain regions of Parkinson's disease patients. Neurosci Lett 2008;447(1):17–9.
103 Hargreaves IP, Lane A, Sleiman PM. The CoQ10 status of the brain regions of PD patients. Neurosci Lett 2008;447(1):17–9.
104 Storch A, Jost WH, Vieregge P, et. al. Randomized, double-blind, placebo-controlled trial on symptomatic effects of coenzyme Q(10) in Parkinson disease. German Coenzyme Q(10) Study Group. Arch Neurol 2007;64(7):938–44.
105 Henchcliffe C, Beal MF. Mitochondrial biology and ox stress in PD pathogenesis. Nat Clin Pract Neurol 2008;4(11):600–9.
106 A randomized clinical trial of coenzyme Q10 and GPI-1485 in early Parkinson disease. Investigators., The NINDS NET-PD. Neurology 2007;68(1): 20–8.
107 Are neurodegenerative disorder and psychotic manifestations avoidable brain dysfunctions with adequate dietary omega-3? LF, Saugstad. Nutr Health 2006;18(3):203–15.
108 Depression in PD: a double-blind, placebo-controled pilot study of omega-3 fatty acid supplementation. J Affect Disord 2008;111(2–3):351–9.
109 da Silva TM, Munhoz RP, Alvarez C, et. al. Oral creatine supplementation attenuates L-dopa induced dyskinesia in 6-hydroxydopamine lesioned rats. Valastro B, Dekundy A, Danysz W, et. al. Behav Brain Res 2009;197(1):90–6.
110 Beal MF. Bioenergetic approaches for neuroprotection in Parkinson's disease. Ann Neurol 2003;53 Suppl 3:S39–47.
111 Kidd PM. Parkinson's disease as multifactorial oxidative neurodegeneration: implications for integrative management. Altern Med Rev 2000;5(6):502–29.
112 Zbarsky V, datla KP, Parkar S, et. al. Neuroprotective properties of the natural phenolic antioxidants curcumin and naringenin but not quercetin and fisetin in a 6-OHDA model of PD. Free Radic Res 2005;39(10):1119–25.
113 Le Bars, P., Katz, M.M., Berman, N, et. al. Placebo Controlled, Double-blind Randomized Trial of an Extract of Gingko Biloba for Dementia. JAMA 278(16): 1327–32, 1997.
114 Ramassamy C. Emerging role of polyphenolic compounds in the treatment of neurodegenerative diseases: a review of their intracellular targets. Eur J Pharmacol 2006;545(1):51–64.
115 Sharma H, Chandola HM, Sing G, et. al. Utilization of Ayurveda in helath care: an approach for prevention, health promotion and treatment of disease. Part 2-Ayurveda in primary health care. J Altern Complement Med 2007;13(10); 1135–50.
116 Manyam BV. Paralysis agitans and levo-dpa in 'Ayurveda'-ancient Indian medical treatise. Mov Disord 1990;5(1):47–8.
117 Gourie-Devi M, Ramumg, Venkatarum BS. Treatment of PD in Ayurveda(ancient system of medicine): discussion peper. J R Soc Med 1991;84(8):491–2.
118 Manyam BV, Sanchez-Ramos JR. Traditional and complementary therapies in PD. Adv Neurol 1999;80:565–74.

119 Nader T, Rothenberg S, Averbach R, et. al. Improvements in chronic diseases with a comprehensive natural medine approach:a review and case series. Behav Med 2000;26(1):14–46.

120 Manyam BV, Dhanasekaran M, Hare TA. Effectv of antiparkinson drug HP-200 (Mucuna pruirns) on the central monoaminergic neurotransmitters. Phytother Res 2004;18(2):97–101.

121 Manyam BV, Dhanasekaran M, Hare TA. Neuroprotective effects of the anti-parkinson drug Mucuna pruriens. Phytother Res 2004;18(9):706–12.

122 Dhanasekaran M, Tharakan B, Manyam BV. Antiparkinson drug-Mucuna pruriens shows antioxidant and metal chelating activity. Phytother Res 2008;22(1):6–11.

123 Zhang JF, Sun GS, Zhao GH. Observation on therapeutic effect of herbs-partitioned moxibustion on PD of 54 cases. Zhongguo Zhen Jiu 2005;25(9):610–2.

124 Yang ZM, Tang XJ, Lao YR. Systematic evaluation on clinical literature related with treatment of PD with TCM. Zhongguo Zhong Xi Yi Jie He Za Zhi 2005;25(7):612–5.

125 Li Q, Zhao D, Bezard E. TCM for PD: a review of Chinese literature. Behav Pharmacol 2006;17(5–6):403–10.

126 Nijkrake MJ, Keus SH, Oostendorp RA, et. al. Allied health care in PD: referral,consulation and professional expertise. Mov Disord 2009;24(2):282–6.

127 Nijrake MJ, Keus SH, Kalf JG, et. al. Allied health acre interventions and complementary therapies in PD. Parkinsonism Relat Disord 2007;13 Suppl 3:S488–94.

128 Dixon L, Duncan D, Johnson P, et. al. OT for patients with PD. Cochrane database Syst Rev 2007;(3):CD002813.

129 Deane KH, Jones D, Playford Ed, et. al. Physio for patients with PD: a comparison of techniques. Cochrane Database Syst Rev 2001;(3):CD002817.

130 Deane KH, Whurr R, Playford ED, et. al. A comparison of speech and language therapy techniques for dysarthria in PD. Cochrane Database Syst Rev 2001;(2):CD002814.

131 Lee MS, Shin BC, Kong JC, et. al. Effectiveness of acupuncture for PD: a systematic review. Mov Disord 2008;23(11):1505–15.

132 Lam YC, Kum WF, Durairajan SS, et. al. Efficacy and safety of acupuncture for isiopathic PD: a systematic review. J Altern Complement Med 2008;14(6):663–71.

133 Cheng XR, Cheng K. Survey of studies on the mechanism of acupuncture and moxibustion treating diseases abroad. Zhongguo Zhen Jiu 2008;28(6):463–7.

134 Eng ML, Lyons KE, Greene MS, et. al. Open-label trial regarding the use of acupuncture and yin tui na in PD outpatients: a pilot study on efficacy, tolerabolity and QOL. J Altern Comp Med 2006;12(4):395–9.

135 Cristan A, Katz M, Cutrone E, et. al. Evaluation of acupuncture in the treatment of PD: a double-blind pilot study. Mov Disord 2005;20(9):1185–8.

136 Shulman LM, Wen X, weiner WJ, et. al. Acupuncture therapy for the symptoms of PD. Mov Disord 2002;17(4):799–802.

137 Wang X, Liang XB, Li FQ, et. al. Therapeutic strategies for PD: the ancient meets the future-TCM, electroacupuncture, gene therapy and stem cells. Neurochem Res 2008;33(10):1956–63.

138 Jiang XM, Huang Y, Zhuo Y, et. al. Therapeutic effect of ESA on PD. Nan Fang Yi Ke Da Xue Xue Bao 2006;26(1):114–6.

139 Huang Y, Jiang XM, Li DJ. Effects of ESA on cerebral dopamine transporter in patients with PD. Zhongguo Zhong Xi Yi Jie He Za Zhi 2006;26(4):303–7.

140 Chen XH, Li Y, Kui Y. Clinical observation on abdominal acupuncture plus Madopa for treatment of PD. Zhongguo Zhen Jiu 2007;27(8):562–4.

141 Chang XH, Zhang LZ, Li YJ. Observation on therapeutic effect of acupuncture combined with medicine on PD. Zhongguo Zhen Jiu 2008;28(9):645–7.

142 Ren XM. 50 cases of PD treated by acupuncture combined with Madopar. J Tradit Chin Med 2008;28(4):255–7.

Chapter 32

Pregnancy disorders

Introduction

Pregnancy is a special time in a woman's life that should be enjoyed with good health. Due to a surge of hormones and rapid physical changes by the body, a number of distressing symptoms may arise, especially if the woman is unprepared. Many women conceive without planning a pregnancy, so it is not always possible to be prepared for a pregnancy. Hence it is vital that women optimise their health as soon as they make the decision to plan a pregnancy.

Complementary and alternative medicines (CAMs) are frequently used in pregnancy, more than prescription medicines, according to Australian research.[1] These CAMs include massage (49%), vitamin and mineral supplements (30%) and yoga (18.4%) which are not likely to be harmful in pregnancy. The study highlighted more than three-quarters had used at least 1 complementary therapy 8 weeks prior to the study; one-third had used complementary medicine to alleviate a physical symptom such as headache, cough or cold with a 95% positive response to treatment compared with 6.8% of women on prescription medicine to treat a complaint.

Studies in the Netherlands found up to 36% of women were using herbs in pregnancy and up to 43% during breastfeeding.[2] The most commonly used herbs in pregnancy include red raspberry leaf, ginger, chamomile[3] and also echinacea and cranberry.[2] Less commonly used supplements were fish oil, herbal teas, blue cohosh, acidophilus, ombeshi plums, homeopathic drops, peppermint and St John's wort.

Symptoms of pregnancy

A number of problems can develop during pregnancy, including the following:[4]

- psychosocial and emotional stress
- high body temperature
- morning sickness [nausea and vomiting >50% of women]
- breasts changes
  - nipples may be tender and sensitive
  - some women describe their nipples to be irritatingly sensitive
  - breast may be sore and/or lumpy
  - nipples may deepen in colour
  - veins may become more noticeable and enlarged in the breast area
  - aereolas may darken
  - Montgomery's tubercles may increase
- increased cervical mucus
- fatigue
- frequent urination
- cramping
- spotting [in early pregnancy = 10% of normal pregnancies]
- constipation and wind
- changes in sense of smell
- nasal stuffiness/colds
- pimples/acne
- cravings/changes in taste
- heartburn
- varicose veins
- haemorrhoids
- back pain
- weight gain
- dental problems can worsen
- stretch marks and pigmentation of skin.

Lifestyle

Simple lifestyle strategies are not only useful for a pregnancy but also to optimise wellbeing for life. These include: rest, stress management, exercise, adequate sleep, fresh air, plenty of adequate sunshine and good dietary habits. Also, pregnant women should avoid illicit drugs, smoking, exposure to chemicals and alcohol.

Mind–body medicine

Sleep

A good nights sleep of up to 8 hours a night is essential in pregnancy and post-partum to help reduce fatigue, depression, mood disturbances and exhaustion. Recent evidence also suggests that a good nights sleep also contributes to shorter labour and an easier delivery.[5] Women who slept for less than 4–5 hours per night were more likely to have caesarean deliveries and experience longer labour times compared with women who were well rested.[5]

Psychosocial and psychological factors

Many women experience anxiety during pregnancy and fear of pain, especially with a vaginal delivery. Studies suggest that personality factors such as general anxiety, neuroticism, low self-esteem and vulnerability, and dissatisfaction with their partners, violence in the relationship, lack of social support and unemployment will contribute and amplify pregnancy related anxiety.[6, 7] Strategies such as increasing supports, meditation, counselling and cognitive behaviour therapy (CBT) should be aimed at reducing maternal anxiety and addressing issues with the partner. Even a telephone-based peer support line can make a significant difference in preventing postnatal depression among women at high risk.[8]

Duration between births

Women should be advised to avoid conceiving too quickly after giving birth to avoid subsequent birth complications. A large scale study of 89 000 women found shorter intervals between births (i.e. of less than 6 months between first and second pregnancy) was an independent risk factor for pre-term birth and neonatal death in the second pregnancy.[9]

Physical activity/exercise

It is clear that daily exercise benefits pregnant women both physically and emotionally but what is not certain is the level of intensity that is safe for pregnancy. A prospective study of 148 pregnant women examined whether vigorous exercise undertaken by recreational exercisers had any impact on infant birth weight and gestational age at birth.[10] The researchers found there were no differences between the different exercise groups in pregnancy outcome, and duration or frequency of vigorous exercise was not associated with any adverse outcome for the infant, such as mean birth weight.

Regular exercise maintains and improves fitness during pregnancy, including aerobic exercise. However, larger and better trials are needed before confident recommendations can be made about the benefits and risks, such as pre-term birth, of more vigorous exercise in pregnancy.[11]

Environmental factors

Pollution

Pollution is a public health issue and can cause adverse health outcomes in pregnancy. A large Australian study of 28 000 births recorded during the study period found exposure to low levels of air pollution from vehicle exhausts, particularly in the 1st trimester, resulted in more premature births before 37 weeks gestation, the risk increasing by 15–26%.[12] This association was strongest in winter and less in autumn compared with summer.

Smoking

Smoking should be completely avoided in pregnancy for its known adverse pregnancy outcomes that include intrauterine growth retardation, failure to thrive, low birth weight, premature death, fetal anomalies, and predisposition to asthma (maternal and child). Giving up smoking prior to pregnancy is preferred, although even ceasing early in the pregnancy (before 15 weeks gestation) can also be of benefit and reduce the risk of spontaneous pre-term birth and infants who are small for gestational age, according to a prospective cohort study.[13]

Smokers demonstrate lower levels of folate compared with non-smokers with similar dietary folate intake which may explain some of the negative pregnancy outcomes.[14] Passive smoking is also harmful.

Recent evidence suggests smoking during pregnancy also increased the risk of children developing behavioural problems and hyperkinetic disorder by threefold compared with non-smokers.[15]

Alcohol

The Australian new-draft alcohol guidelines state that for pregnant women and women planning pregnancy no drinking is the safest option.[16] A British study examining the effects of low–moderate prenatal alcohol exposure on pregnancy outcome found no convincing evidence of adverse effects.[17] Similar findings have been found by a Western Australian group, however, alcohol intake at higher levels, particularly heavy and binge drinking patterns, was associated with increased risk of pre-term birth even when drinking was ceased before the 2nd trimester.[18] Adverse effects of alcohol exposure on the fetus include fetal alcohol syndrome (1–3 % of live births), birth defects, neurodevelopmental disorders, miscarriage, still births, pre-term births and low birth weight.

Fetal alcohol exposure can be minimised through abstaining or reducing alcohol consumption or increasing effective contraception in females who engage in *risk* drinking.[19]

Animal studies suggest dietary zinc supplementation may play a role in preventing fetal alcohol syndrome due to prenatal ethanol exposure, although more studies are required.[20]

Maternal obesity

It is natural for a woman to gain on average up to 18kg during pregnancy without risking complications, although the recommended weight range is from 11.5 to 16kg.[21] The optimal birth weight for the infant is 3500–4500g. Women gaining weight at the lower end of the recommended range had a higher chance of low birth weight newborns weighing less than 3500g.

A study of 100 pregnant women were randomised to a program of dietary and lifestyle counselling that helped reduce excessive weight gain during pregnancy compared with the routine prenatal care group, who also had significantly more caesarean deliveries by 58.6% due to failure to progress (compared with lifestyle counselling group 25.0%, P = .02).[22]

Obesity is an independent risk factor for negative, adverse pregnancy outcome. It contributes to infertility, miscarriage, hypertension, increased deep vein thrombosis and pulmonary embolisms, pre-eclampsia, gestational diabetes, prematurity, congenital anomalies, fetal distress, still birth, longer labour, caesarean delivery, subsequent post-operative complications, and cardiovascular risk factors.[23–26]

A large scale cohort study of 54 000 pregnant women found the risk of fetal death (stillbirth) for obese women (Body Mass Index [BMI] >30) doubled by week 28 of gestation and quadrupled by week 40 compared to normal weight women.[27] They found that obesity was associated with placental dysfunction.

Nutritional influences

Diet

A number of studies have evaluated the role of diet in the prevention of gestational diabetes and pre-eclampsia. It is essential women maintain a healthy diet as nutritional needs are increased substantially during this time. Substantial epidemiological evidence documents diverse health benefits associated with diets high in fibre, fish and low in glycaemic index (GI).

Mediterranean diet

Of interest, the Mediterranean diet characterised by high intakes of fruit, vegetables, olive oil, fish, legumes, and cereals and low intakes of potatoes and sweets, is associated with reduced risk of Spina bifida in offspring compared with maternal intake not on Mediterranean diet.[28] The Mediterranean diet also correlated with higher levels of serum and RBC folate, serum vitamin B12 and lower plasma homocysteine.

Western diet

Maternal consumption of the Western diet (e.g. high in meat, pizza, legumes, and potatoes, and low in fruits) increases the risk of offspring with a cleft lip and/or cleft palate by approximately twofold.[29] The authors postulated low folate levels in the Western diet may account for this association and, therefore, recommend dietary and lifestyle profiles should be included in preconception screening programs.

Fish and heavy metal exposure in pregnancy

Fish is an important part of dietary intake. It contains a number of essential nutrients such as eicosopentaenoic acid (EPA) and docosohexaenoic acid (DHA), important for development of the fetal brain and retina, and is rich in iodine, iron, choline, selenium, and trace elements important for pregnancy and fetal growth. Also meta-analysis of the literature indicates maternal diet high in fish may reduce the risk of inflammatory conditions such as rheumatoid arthritis, atopy and asthma in the newborn, although more evidence is required.[30, 31]

Health benefits of fish may counterbalance any adverse effects of mercury exposure on the developing nervous system.[32] All fish contains some mercury in their flesh, mostly in the form of organic methyl mercury (MeHg), a known neurotoxin which can cause developmental delay, neurological problems and damage to the developing central nervous system (CNS). The quantity of MeHg present in fish varies depending on the dietary habits and age of the fish, and is particularly concentrated in the larger predatory fish at the top of the food chain.

Foods Standards Australia New Zealand (FSANZ) has useful advice on mercury in fish.[33] FSANZ found that most fish is safe for all population groups to eat 2–3 serves per week and recommends that pregnant women, women planning pregnancy and young children continue to consume a variety of fish as part of a healthy diet, but limit their consumption of the larger predatory fish such as shark, marlin, broadbill and swordfish (containing highest levels of MeHg) to no more than 1 serve per fortnight with no other fish to be consumed during that fortnight. For orange roughy (also sold as sea perch) and catfish, the FSANZ advice is to consume no more than 1 serve per week, with no other fish being consumed during that week.[33]

The FSANZ 'Advice on Fish Consumption' has been specifically developed for the Australian population and suggests that women in other countries check with their local authorities as mercury content of fish varies from country to country depending on the environmental exposure, patterns of fish consumption in the community and other food sources consumed containing mercury.

Nutritional risk factors in pregnancy

Recommended daily intakes (RDIs) are increased significantly during pregnancy and lactation due to extra demands by the pregnant mother and infant. The diet of the mother is of great importance to the fetus. Dietary guidelines are similar to those given to the general public with special attention to foods that provide good sources of iodine, calcium, iron, folate and dietary fibre.

The increased needs during pregnancy can vary from 12% for dietary fibre, 14% for vitamin A, 46% for vitamin B6, 50% for folate, 37% for zinc, 50% for iron, 46% for iodine, 30% for protein and 25% for essential fatty acids.[34, 35]

Teenage pregnancy requires special needs as a mother's body is still growing in many instances. The ideal weight gain for teenage pregnancy is 10kg; lower weight gain can lead to lower birth weight which can be associated with greater risk of developing type 2 diabetes and hypertension later in life, as well as a weight problem.[27]

Routine supplementation with iron, vitamin A, C and E are not recommended in pregnancy. [36]

Vegetarian mothers are at risk of deficiencies in protein, iron, vitamin B12, folate, calcium and zinc and should be screened early in pregnancy, if not beforehand, to minimise complications. Untreated vitamin B12 deficiency may lead to serious neurological consequences especially in exclusively breastfed babies. Vegan sources of omega-3 foods include soybeans, beans, linseed, walnuts, pecans and soy.

Vitamin D deficiency is common in dark skinned, veiled women and their breastfed offspring should also be screened with consideration to supplement with vitamin D.

Nutritional supplements

Fish oil for pregnancy and breastfeeding

Fish oils play an important role in pregnancy and in the development of the fetus and newborn. Pregnant women should be encouraged to eat at least 3 deep sea fish a week although there are real concerns with heavy metal toxicity in the larger predator fish (see section titled 'Fish and heavy metals').[37] A number of studies demonstrate fish oils can significantly reduce the risk of atopy, asthma (see Chapter 5 for asthma information) and other immune-mediated diseases by positively modulating inflammation and prostaglandin effects on the newborn child. In addition, the benefits of fish oils are carried through to breastfed babies. In bottle-fed babies, the benefits are through formulas enriched with fish oils.[38–42]

For instance, a population-based study of 533 pregnant women from 30 weeks gestation to birth were randomly assigned to receive 4 x 1g gelatin capsules/day of fish oil (2.7g n-3 PUFAs) or 4 x 1g similar-looking capsules/day with olive oil, or no oil capsules.[43] Over a 16-year follow-up of offspring, the risk of asthma was reduced by 63% and of allergic asthma by 87% in those pregnancies treated with fish oil compared with the olive oil group. This study supports a potential prophylactic role of fish oils late in pregnancy, reducing risk of asthma in the newborn.[43]

Women consuming fish oil supplements compared with olive oil capsules were also less likely to experience pre-term delivery and more likely to reach full term without any complications.[44] The high intake of fish oils might prolong pregnancy by shifting the balance of production of prostaglandins in parturition.

Fish oils play an important role in the development of the nervous system and augments cognitive function, IQ, vision and behaviour in offspring to mothers supplemented with fish oils during pregnancy and breastfeeding.[45–60]

However, a double-blind study randomised pregnant mothers to take 10ml of either cod-liver oil or corn oil from 18 weeks gestation until 3 months after delivery.[61] At 7 years of age, children were assessed and the researchers found higher maternal plasma phospholipid concentrations of alpha-linolenic acid (18:3n-3) and docosahexaenoic acid during pregnancy were correlated with enhanced cognitive function, such as sequential processing, but no significant effect was observed on global IQs or on BMI in the children.

Multi-nutrients and pregnancy

Micronutrients such as vitamins and minerals are necessary for the growing demands experienced by the pregnant mother and for the normal functioning, growth and development of the fetus. A Cochrane review of 9 trials including 15 378 women demonstrated multi-nutrient supplementation reduced the number of low birth weight and small-for-gestational-age babies and maternal anaemia, but close analyses of the data revealed no added benefit compared with iron/folic acid supplementation alone.[62] Further research is required to confirm the benefits of taking multi-nutrients during pregnancy.

A systematic review and meta-analysis of the use of prenatal supplementation with multivitamins found that they decreased the risk for paediatric brain tumour, neuroblastoma and leukaemia.[63]

Vitamin A deficiency

Vitamin A deficiency is common in developing countries such as Indonesia and Nepal due to poor nutritional intake where daily or weekly supplementation may be necessary as deficiency of vitamin A causes night-blindness, anaemia and other problems.[64] However, in women with adequate nutritional intake, vitamin A supplementation can cause toxicity, especially doses >10 000IU/day, and should be avoided. Toxic levels can cause miscarriage and birth defects. Note: beta-carotene intake is very safe.

Vitamin C deficiency

It is not clear if taking vitamin C supplementation in pregnancy is safe, because a Cochrane review found in a trial that vitamin C supplementation was linked with a moderate risk of pre-term birth, although more studies are required to confirm this adverse effect.[65] Vitamin C deficiency is linked with complications in pregnancy such as pre-eclampsia, anaemia and intrauterine growth retardation, and so women should be encouraged to eat foods rich in vitamin C such as fruit.

Vitamin D deficiency

Severe vitamin D deficiency can cause maternal osteomalacia and lead to significant morbidity in the mother and fetus. The prevalence of vitamin D deficiency in pregnant women is high and this can have serious health ramifications in the mother and child.[66, 67] Pregnant women who are deficient in vitamin D can lead to reduced weight gain and pelvic deformities that prevent normal delivery. For the fetus, vitamin D deficiency is linked with poor fetal growth, low birth weight, neonatal hypocalcemia with and without convulsions, neonatal rickets, defective tooth enamel, and pre-disposition to childhood rickets, particularly in breastfed, dark skinned children.[68, 69, 70] Deficiency is common in populations residing in geographically prone areas such as southern Australia (e.g. Melbourne) and in some high-risk communities such as migrants, women wearing veiled clothing, and people who spend more time indoors.[71] Ninety percent of the body's vitamin D is produced by the skin from sunlight (ultraviolet B light) exposure of non-covered skin without sunscreen, with only 10% coming from dietary sources. It is essential to restore vitamin D deficiency in mothers by advising safe sun exposure which is dependent on geographical areas and pigmentation of the skin (the darker the skin the more sun that is required), and supplement with cholecalciferol if needed, but this needs to be done cautiously to avoid vitamin D toxicity. Excessive vitamin D may cause hypercalcemia and fetal harm. Doses within RDI are safe. According to a Cochrane review of the literature, there is not enough evidence to date to evaluate the effects of vitamin D supplementation in pregnancy.[72] Vitamin D is excreted in milk in limited amounts, and with excessive use can cause toxicity in infants. If pharmacological supplementation is required, it is essential to monitor calcium levels in the infant and get maternal vitamin D checked regularly.

Folate deficiency

Folate is one of the most important nutrients for healthy fetal development. Pregnant women and the growing embryo require higher levels of folate for cell replication and growth. Rapidly dividing cells in the embryo fail to produce healthy DNA if folate levels are low. The recommended daily intake for folate is increased significantly by 50% in pregnancy. It is recommended that every woman planning a pregnancy should take 500mcg folate a few months prior to pregnancy and in the 1st trimester although recent studies indicate that folate supplementation in the 2nd trimester may help prevent pre-eclampsia.[73] Low folate levels are associated with increased risk of spontaneous abortion, anaemia, low birth weight and congenital malformations such as neural tube defects (NTD), oral clefts and cleft palate, and cardiovascular and urinary tract malformations.[74, 75] Overall, nutritional deficiency in the pregnant woman (not just folate deficiency) can increase the risk of orofacial cleft. Increasing intakes of vegetables, protein, fibre, fruit, ascorbic acid, iron, vitamin Bs and magnesium also reduce the risk of orofacial cleft.[76, 77]

Folate is essential for fetal brain and spinal cord development. A Cochrane review evaluated 4 trials of folate supplementation involving 6425 women. Peri-conceptional folate supplementation significantly reduced the incidence of NTD (relative risk 0.28, 95% confidence interval 0.13 to 0.58) without significant harmful effects such as miscarriage, ectopic pregnancy or stillbirth. The authors also found multivitamins were not associated with any additional beneficial preventative effects of NTDs even when given with folate.[78]

Medications interfering with folate

Maternal exposure to folate antagonist medication such as sulfamethoxazole-trimethoprim and anti-epileptic medication such as phenobarbital and sodium valproate may contribute to adverse pregnancy outcomes by affecting placental function, although more studies are required to confirm this finding and one needs to weigh the benefit to any potential risk.[79, 80] It is important to avoid any medication and herbal medicines that may harm the fetus in pregnancy unless there is a clear risk to the mother.

Anti-epileptic medication and folate

Pregnant women who require anti-epileptic medication, many of which antagonise folate action, are at increased risk of fetal abnormalities and birth defects such as NTDs.[81] Epileptic women in reproductive years should be advised to take folate peri-conceptually if on anti-epileptic medication that interferes with folate, although it is not clear what this dosage should be.

Women of child-bearing age prescribed, for example, sodium valproate should be warned about the potential risks of the drug, including teratogenesis, and should be strongly advised to ensure adequate contraception whilst taking this drug.[82, 83]

Minerals

Iron deficiency

The recommended daily intake for iron is increased significantly, by 50%, in pregnancy. Iron deficiency is linked with infertility, anaemia, increased risk of infection, fatigue, and behavioural and cognitive development problems.[84, 85, 86] It is possible that fetal oxygenation is compromised with iron deficiency.[85] While the benefits are clear for iron supplementation, if the mother demonstrates serum iron deficiency with or without anaemia, at this stage, there is not enough evidence to recommend routine iron supplementation in all pregnant women.[87]

Zinc deficiency

Zinc is an essential trace element and plays an important role in normal growth and development, protein synthesis and cellular integrity. Zinc deficiency can adversely effect pregnancy outcome, such as pre-term birth, intrauterine growth retardation, poor fetal bone growth and prolong labour.[88, 89] Zinc deficiency is common in low socioeconomic groups with poor nutritional intake and in third world countries. A trial of zinc supplements in HIV pregnant women improved infant mortality, birth weight and duration of pregnancy.[90] Its benefit was related to improving immune status.

Foods rich in zinc are found in pecans, wholegrains, lima beans, almonds, walnuts, hazelnuts, sardines and chicken. A Cochrane review of 17 randomised controlled trials (RCTs) involving over 9000 women and their babies demonstrated zinc supplementation resulted in a significant reduction in pre-term birth by 14%, reduced need for caesarean section and in 1 trial demonstrated reduced need for induction of labour, but did not reduce the risk of babies with low birth weight.[91] In a study held in Bangladesh, babies of women who took 30mg/day of elemental zinc during pregnancy were less likely to develop acute diarrhoea by 16%, dysentery by 64% and impetigo by 47%, compared with mothers on placebo.[92]

Iodine deficiency

Iodine is an essential trace element for the production of thyroid hormones T3 and T4. Studies indicate mild deficiency of iodine is common in pregnant women.[93] Sources of iodine include ocean fish, spinach, seaweed (such as kelp), garlic, watercress, citrus fruit, cereals, nuts (cashews), egg yolk and iodised salt. Researchers suggest pregnant women need to increase their intake of iodine and, if deficient, should consider supplementation from 100–200mcg/day.

A high frequency of iodine deficiency is known to occur in Australia, with almost 20% of pregnant women having a moderate to severe iodine deficiency. Mild deficiency occurred in almost 30% of women.[94]

Maternal iodine deficiency is known to cause neonatal cretinism. A suboptimal iodine intake by pregnant females without overt deficiency may compromise fetal development, even in the absence of cretinism, leading to developmental delays in the infant.[95]

It is possible to prevent cretinism with iodine supplementation pre-conception, and also if supplementation is given before the end of the 2nd trimester.[96]

Medical conditions associated with pregnancy or a complication of pregnancy

Gestational diabetes mellitus (GDM)

Between 1 to 14% of women develop GDM during pregnancy. Dietary advice is essential to help reduce the incidence of diabetes in pregnancy and subsequently in life. GDM can cause significant health problems, such as a very large baby, and increase the risk of negative and adverse pregnancy outcomes, such as an increased risk of induced birth and caesarean section, prematurity and increased infant morbidity and mortality. GDM is also associated with an increased risk of diabetes for mother and child later in life.

Depression as a risk factor for GDM

Among low-income pregnant women, those with diabetes (pre-existing of gestational) were twice as likely to suffer peri-natal depression and more likely to have post-partum depression after adjustment for other confounding factors, according to a retrospective cohort study.[97]

Lifestyle and GDM

Lifestyle risk factors play a role in the development of diabetes in any person and these include stress management, sunshine for vitamin D, dietary factors, exercise and sleep strategies. (See Chapter 13 for diabetes and Chapter 22 for sleep.)

Exercise and GDM

An analysis of 21 765 women as part of the Nurses Health study II found that women who perform regular exercise, especially brisk walking 30 minutes daily, before pregnancy have a significantly reduced risk of developing GDM, by up to 34%, when compared with women who did the least amount of exercise.[98]

Diet and GDM

Diet factors play a significant role in the control of diabetes, with wholegrain carbohydrates and low GI diets being particularly helpful.

Low GI diet and GDM

A low GI diet can effectively halve the need to use insulin compared with a high GI diet, according to a recent randomised study.[99]

A Cochrane review identified 3 trials including 107 women.[100] Two trials assessed low versus high GI diets for pregnant women. Women on low GI diets, had less large-for-gestational-age infants and lower maternal fasting glucose levels. The other trial assessed high fibre versus control diet but the trial did not report on the outcomes. The reviewers concluded based on these findings that whilst 'a low glycaemic index diet was seen to be beneficial for some outcomes for both mother and child, results from the review were inconclusive'.[100]

Weight gain and GDM

Women of reproductive age should be encouraged to maintain a normal healthy weight as weight gain and maternal obesity is associated with increased risk for diabetes, adverse pregnancy and neonatal outcome.[101] See the maternal obesity section earlier in this chapter.

Cinnamon and GDM

Cinnamon has been reported to enhance insulin sensitivity. (See Chapter 13 for diabetes information.)

Nutrients and GDM

Nutrients in GDM may be of some help, such as fish oil and chromium supplementation, to improve insulin sensitivity, although great care is required, especially with high doses, as there are no adequate studies in pregnancy. (See Chapter 13 for diabetes information.)

Pre-eclampsia (PE)

PE is a serious condition affecting pregnant women and occurs in about 2–8% of women, characterised by high blood pressure, with or without proteinuria.

Exploring diet and lifestyle are essential to lower the risk of developing PE, particularly increasing nutrient rich foods for antioxidants, vitamin E, calcium and magnesium as deficiency of these nutrients can predispose to PE. This is commonly seen in under-nourished, low socio-economic communities. A diet high in sugar and fat, cigarette smoking and low physical activity are known risk factors for PE. Stress is a contributor to PE-like hypertension. It is likely other lifestyle risk factors may also play a role in PE and strategies such as stress management, dietary changes (increasing vegetables, high fish intake), exercise and sleep restoration should assist in the management of PE (see Chapter 19 on hypertension). Calcium and magnesium appear to be particularly effective and may play an important role as therapeutic agents for PE. PE can cause serious morbidity and can lead to death in pregnant women, who should be monitored closely, including for onset and progression of chronic kidney disease.[102]

Stress and PE

Work stress is a significant predictor and risk factor for developing PE.[103] In a trial on pregnant normotensive women, heart rate increased and mean arterial blood pressure rose by more than 2.9mmHg, and in some up to 10mmHg on work days.[104] Higher blood pressures occurred in women experiencing greater job stress.

Fibre and PE

High dietary fibre plays an important role in the prevention of PE. A study of over 1500 pregnant women found that women consuming more than 21.2g/day of fibre were associated with reduced risk of PE by up to 70% and mean concentrations of triglycerides was higher and high density lipoprotein (HDL) cholesterol was lower compared with women consuming less than 11.9g of fibre daily.[105]

Salt and PE

Whilst a low salt diet is recommended for the prevention of hypertension, there is currently insufficient evidence to advise reduction of dietary salt during pregnancy for the prevention of PE and its complications.[106]

Antioxidants and PE

Findings from a Cochrane review could not recommend the use of antioxidants for the prevention of PE[107] although another Cochrane review found women taking vitamin supplements 'may be less likely to develop pre-eclampsia and more likely to have a multiple pregnancy'.[108]

Vitamins C and E and PE

Inadequate dietary intake of vitamin E during pregnancy is associated with PE and low birth weight. A Cochrane review found in trials that pregnant women supplemented with vitamin E in combination with other supplements compared with placebo were at reduced risk of developing clinical PE, however, the data was too few to recommend supplementation in pregnancy at this stage.[109]

One double-blind RCT of 283 women at risk of PE (previous history of PE or placental blood flow abnormalities) were assigned to 1000mg/day of vitamin C and 400IU/day of vitamin E or placebo at 16-22 weeks gestation.[110] Vitamin supplementation correlated with a significant 21% reduction in plasma markers reflecting endothelial and placental function. Plasma ascorbic acid increased 32% on average, and the α-tocopherol level increased by 54%. PE developed in 17% of placebo recipients but in only 8% of women given vitamins. Furthermore, small-for-gestational-age infants were less frequent, although less significant in the vitamin-supplemented group. Subsequent research demonstrated similar findings.[111, 112]

Another study found 1000mg of vitamin C or 400IU of vitamin E did not reduce the risk of PE compared with placebo, however, the synthetic form of vitamin E was used in this study.[113] Women should be encouraged to eat foods high in vitamin E found in vegetable oils, nuts, cereals and some leafy green vegetables.

However, a recent study warns against peri-conception use of vitamin E supplements with high dietary vitamin E intake above 14.9mg/day as it increased the risk of congenital heart defects (CHDs) in offspring by nine fold.[114]

Folate and PE

A prospective cohort study of 2951 women at 12–20 weeks gestation found supplementation with multivitamins containing folic acid in the 2nd trimester reduced the risk of developing PE.[73]

Mineral supplementation for PE

Calcium and PE

In a review of the literature of RCTs found calcium supplementation to play an important role in the prevention of PE and pre-term delivery more than any other supplement.[115]

A randomised placebo-controlled study of 524 healthy first-time pregnant women whose mean dietary calcium was less than RDI, found 2g of elemental calcium supplementation daily during pregnancy was associated with a significant reduced risk of PE by 69% and pre-term delivery by 49% compared with placebo.[116, 117]

Furthermore, a Cochrane review of the literature of 12 good quality trials supports the findings that calcium may play an important role in the prevention of PE, the authors concluding that calcium supplementation could 'almost halve the risk of PE, and reduce the rare occurrence of the composite outcome death or serious morbidity'.[118]

Magnesium and PE

According to a Cochrane review magnesium supplementation during pregnancy may be able to reduce PE and fetal growth retardation.[119] In a large scale international trial from 33 different countries 10 141 pregnant women were randomised to magnesium sulfate or placebo. The trial was cut short due to the positive conclusive findings demonstrating magnesium sulfate led to a significant 58% reduction of PE and 45% reduction in maternal death compared with placebo.[120]

Herbs for PE

Garlic and PE

Meta-analyses have demonstrated that garlic is a valid therapeutic treatment for hypertension, but its role in PE is not so clear. (See Chapter 19 for hypertension information.) A Cochrane review identified 1 study of 100 pregnant women that showed dried garlic capsules did not prevent PE compared with placebo and demonstrated no significant differences in side-effects except women on garlic reported odour.[121]

Hyperemesis gravidarum (HG)

Nausea and vomiting

Nausea and vomiting may occur in the early stages of pregnancy and can be quite intense and disabling for the mother. In some mothers, nausea and vomiting persist throughout the whole pregnancy. HG occurs in 0.5–2% of pregnant women, although up to 85% of women will experience some level of nausea. When symptoms are severe, some women require hospitalisation and intravenous fluid therapy to avoid dehydration.

Many trials have compared the use of vitamin B6 and ginger with anti-emetic medication. A Cochrane review of the literature found anti-emetic medication to reduce the frequency of nausea but there is little research that explores adverse fetal outcome from this medication and it can cause side-effects such as drowsiness in the mother. The reviewers found evidence for ginger, acupressure (of pericardium P6) and vitamin B6 in reducing severity of nausea and vomiting.[122]

Vitamin B6 and nausea

Vitamin B6 needs to be used with caution as high doses (more than 50mgs/day) and prolonged use have been associated with neurotoxicity such as peripheral neuropathy (e.g. tingling, burning and numbness of limbs), and should be stopped immediately should these symptoms develop.[123, 124] Vitamin B6 should be used cautiously for therapeutic purposes and not used routinely, although a trial did suggest it may protect against tooth decay in pregnant women.[125, 126]

Ginger (*zingiber officinale*) and nausea

Ginger is a popular remedy used by pregnant women for the treatment of nausea in pregnancy. A Cochrane review of 6 RCTs involving 675 pregnant women assessed the evidence for efficacy and safety of ginger therapy for nausea and vomiting in early pregnancy.[127] The authors concluded that ginger may be an effective treatment choice for nausea and vomiting associated with early pregnancy but further studies with larger numbers of women are required to confirm the promising preliminary data for the safety of this therapy. Four of the 6 RCTs showed superiority of ginger over placebo and 2 of them showed equivalence to vitamin B6 in relieving the severity and episodes of nausea and vomiting.[128]

Acupuncture, acupressure and nausea

A Cochrane review identified 26 trials of 3347 participants suffering nausea and vomiting and found significant reduction in the risk of nausea and need for anti-emetic medication with acupuncture point stimulation (pericardium 6) compared with sham acupuncture.[129] There were minimal side-effects with this method. This treatment should be considered for pregnant women suffering severe nausea.

Gingivitis

Topical or systemic folate may play a role in relieving gingivitis in pregnancy.[130]

Cramps

Calcium and magnesium can provide effective treatment for pregnancy-induced leg cramps.[131, 132, 133]

Ectopic pregnancy

Ectopic pregnancy occurs in 1–2% of pregnancies and is a leading cause of pregnancy-related deaths in the 1st trimester. Whilst traditional Chinese herbal medicines are used in China to treat ectopic pregnancy, most of the trials are of poor quality.[134] Surgery is highly recommended for the treatment of any ectopic pregnancy, and to exclude any predisposing factors to ectopic pregnancy, such as fallopian tube disorders.

Miscarriage

Lifestyle and miscarriage

A large UK population case-control study identified risk factors for 1st trimester miscarriage and found lifestyle factors and stress play an important role in increasing the risk of miscarriage.[135] The findings of this case-control population-based study are summarised in Table 32.1.[18,135]

Stress and miscarriage

Stress is a risk factor for miscarriage, particularly with stressful and traumatic events. Stress may contribute to hormonal imbalance such as lowered progesterone and raised cortisol levels through neuroendocrine pathways.

Caffeine and miscarriage

Furthermore, a recent study suggests caffeine consumption of at least 2 cups daily (200mg or more) increases the risk of miscarriage by up to 40% compared with women with no intake of caffeine.[136]

Table 32.1 Lifestyle and behavioural risk and protective factors for miscarriage

Increase risk of miscarriage	Protective factors for miscarriage	No association with miscarriage
High maternal age Previous miscarriage Termination and infertility assisted conception Low pre-pregnancy Body Mass Index Regular or high alcohol consumption Feeling stressed (including trend with number of stressful or traumatic events) High paternal age Changing partner Nutrient deficiencies (e.g. iodine,folate) Poor diet Illness (e.g. coeliac disease)	Previous live birth Nausea Vitamin supplementation Eating fresh fruits and vegetables daily	Low caffeine consumption (1 cup daily) Smoking Moderate or occasional alcohol consumption Educational level Socioeconomic circumstances Working during pregnancy

(Source: Maconochie N, Doyle P, Prior S, Simmons R. Risk factors for first trimester miscarriage — results from a UK-population-based case-control study. BJOG 2007;114(2))

Nutritional factors and miscarriage

A Cochrane review of the literature found research to date indicates that pregnant women taking a daily multivitamin supplementation prior to or early in pregnancy does not reduce the risk of miscarriage or stillbirth.[137] It is likely that supplements used did not contain enough of the nutrients that can be protective. The quality of the nutrients is also important. The amount of nutrients and the type of nutrient, especially whether they were synthetic or natural, may have been an important factor in this study, which could explain this unexpected result.

Despite these findings, numerous studies have demonstrated the association between increased homocysteine and spontaneous miscarriage.[138, 139] Folic acid and vitamin B6 and B12 take part in the metabolism of homocysteine.

Coeliac disease is associated with damaged intestinal mucosa leading to a malnourished state caused by the malabsorption of macro and micronutrients. Miscarriages are more frequently observed in those with coeliac disease.[140] Therefore coeliac disease must be considered in the pre-conceptional screening and treatment of patients with reproductive disorders.

Iodine deficiency is a risk factor for growth and development of up to 800 million people living in iodine deficient environments throughout the world. The effects on growth and development, called the Iodine Deficiency Disorders, includes miscarriages.[94, 95, 96] Poor diet or diets that are vitamin deficient such as folate have been associated with an increased risk of women losing their baby early in pregnancy.[141]

Sperm and miscarriage

Older sperm are also risk factors for miscarriage. [143]

Congenital heart defect (CHD) in newborn

Saturated fats, riboflavin and nicotinamide and newborn CHD

Fatty acids play an important role in embryonic development, and B-vitamins riboflavin and nicotinamide play a role as co-enzymes in lipid metabolism. Vitamin B deficiency is linked with increased incidence of CHD.[144] A study demonstrated that maternal diets low in dietary riboflavin (<1.20mg/d) and nicotinamide (<13.5mg/d) increased the risk of a child with CHDs by twofold, especially in mothers who did not take multivitamins, and particularly those on high saturated fatty diets.[145] These findings were independent of dietary folate intake.

Vitamin E increases risk of newborn CHD

High vitamin E dietary intake and supplements have been associated with CHD in offspring (see under heading above, 'Vitamins C and E and PE').[114]

Pre-term birth, low birth weight, fetal failure to thrive

Stress and pre-term birth (PTB)

Epidemiological evidence suggests that maternal psychosocial stress, strenuous physical activity and fasting are independent risk factors for PTB and low birth weight.[146]

Depression, anxiety, stress and PTB

Depression and anxiety are risk factors for pre-term labour. Screening of pregnant women for depression may be useful as antenatal depression is significantly associated with almost twice the risk of pre-term delivery (before 37 weeks) compared with non-depressed women, according to a cohort study of 791 women assessed at 10 weeks gestation and followed up during pregnancy.[147] Severe depression increased the risk by up to 2.2 times compared with women not suffering antenatal depression. The authors concluded that their findings show that pregnant women with depressive symptoms are a risk factor for PTB and exacerbated by stressful events, low educational level, and a history of fertility and obesity. It is likely excess cortisol produced in response to stress may play a role, although other factors may also contribute.

A study of 634 pregnant women revealed that depression was positively associated with underweight women (pre-pregnancy BMI below 19) and together with anxiety correlated with a higher incidence of pre-term delivery.[148] Anxiety also correlated with vaginal bleeding. These findings indicate that depression and anxiety are associated with spontaneous pre-term labour.

Yoga reduces risk of PTB, PE, intrauterine growth retardation

A study demonstrated yoga consisting of gentle, daily physical postures, meditation and breathing improves pregnancy outcome, significantly reduces risk of PE, intrauterine growth retardation, pre-term labour and low birth weight newborns.[149] No significant adverse events were reported in the yoga group. Yoga helps with relaxation, postural and stretching exercise so may have benefits in other areas of pregnancy, such as anxiety, headaches and back pain.

Sex in pregnancy

Contrary to popular belief, having sex in pregnancy does not induce labour.

Exercise reduces risk of PTB

Vigorous exercise in pregnancy, such as swimming, cycling and aerobics, reduces risk of pre-term birth by 20% when engaged in the 1st trimester and by 50% in the 2nd trimester.[150]

Poor dental hygiene and PTB

A meta-analysis of RCTs concluded periodontal disease treatment with scaling and/or root planning during pregnancy may significantly reduce PTB or low birth weight infant incidence, but not spontaneous abortion or stillbirth.[151]

Maternal periodontitis and PTB

It is known that a number of diseases including cardiovascular diseases, respiratory diseases, diabetes mellitus and osteoporosis are linked to periodontitis. A number of studies have found that maternal periodontitis can lead to adverse pregnancy outcomes including pre-term, low birth weight or small-for-gestational-age babies.[152, 153]

It is important that a thorough dental examination is carried out either prior to pregnancy or once pregnancy has been confirmed.

Smoking and PTB

Numerous studies have investigated the influence of smoking on the outcome of pregnancy. A large US study found that small fetal size at 10–19 weeks is associated with tobacco use in pregnancy, early pre-term births and low birth weight plus poor fetal growth.[154] This finding is supported by another study.[155]

An Australian study concluded that smoking by indigenous and non-indigenous mothers led to growth restriction in full-term births.[156]

Mothers who are able to quit smoking early in pregnancy reduced the risk of having a pre-term or low birth weight baby to nearly that of mothers who did not smoke.[157]

A systematic review and meta-analysis investigated the role of environmental tobacco smoke and has shown that this too can lead to fetal failure to thrive.[158]

There is a clear dose-related impact of smoking on risk of spontaneous pre-term labour and should be avoided in pregnancy.[159] The highest risk occurred in women who smoked more than 10 cigarettes daily.

Diet and PTB

Fish reduces risk of PTB

A study of over 8700 pregnant women demonstrated that eating as little as 15g/day of fish significantly reduced the risk of pre-term delivery or having a low birth weight baby compared with women not eating any fish.[160] Pregnant women who did not eat fish increased their risk of pre-term delivery or having a low birth weight baby by up to 3.5 times compared with fish eaters.

In another study researchers found a significant reduction of 90% of pre-term delivery among healthy women on fruit, vegetables, wholegrains and low cholesterol diet substituted with fatty fish, vegetable oils, nuts and nut butter in place of meat, butter, cream and fatty dairy foods.[161] This has enormous health implications and reinforces the important role of women of child-bearing age to be on a healthy low cholesterol diet.

Caffeine effects and PTB

Studies consistently demonstrate the adverse effects of maternal caffeine consumption on fetal development.[162–165] A large prospective observational study of over 2600 low-risk pregnant women showed maternal consumption of caffeine from 100mg/day to over 300mg/day (1–3 cups/day) at any stage throughout the pregnancy was associated with a significant risk of fetal growth restriction.[166] An intake of 200mg/day of caffeine was associated with a significant reduction of birth weight by 60–70g, and consumption of caffeine >100mg/day with each trimester led to drops in birth weight by 34–59g in the 1st trimester, 24–74g in the 2nd and 66–89g in the 3rd trimester. Caffeine is rapidly absorbed and crosses the placenta freely. Cytochrome P450 1A2, the principal enzyme involved in caffeine metabolism, is absent in the placenta and the fetus.

A recent study confirms these findings and demonstrated that the equivalent of only 1 dose of caffeine (just 2 cups of coffee) ingested during pregnancy may be enough to affect fetal heart development.[167] The authors strongly advise pregnant women should not consume coffee.

Another study found that coffee consumption during pregnancy was associated with miscarriage, in particular if more than 3 cups of coffee were consumed per day.[168]

Fish oil supplements protect against PTB

Long chain polyunsaturated fatty acids are essential for infant growth and development. Maternal intake of 500mg DHA-rich tuna fish oil supplements taken daily during lactation improved cognitive development and reduced risk of developmental delay in pre-term babies when assessed at 18 months.[169] The main side-effect was a 'fishy burp taste'.

Magnesium protective for PTB

Magnesium is a promising nutrient not only for PE treatment but also in the prevention of pre-term labour and birth. An analysis of trials involving over 2600 pregnant women found oral magnesium treatment in early pregnancy was associated with reduced risk of pre-term birth, a lower frequency of low birth weight and less small-for-gestational age infants compared with placebo.[170] Furthermore, the women treated with magnesium required less hospitalisation during pregnancy and less risk of antepartum haemorrhage compared with placebo treated women. However, the Cochrane review noted the poor quality trials are likely to have resulted in a biasness favouring magnesium supplementation and concluded at this stage that there is 'not enough high quality evidence to show that dietary magnesium supplementation during pregnancy is beneficial'.[170]

A recent Cochrane review of 5 trials involving 6145 babies demonstrated giving intravenous magnesium sulfate to women at risk of pre-term birth significantly reduced the risk of cerebral palsy and the overall mortality of the infant.[171] Side-effects included nausea, vomiting, headaches and palpitations. Epidemiological and scientific studies suggest that magnesium sulfate before birth may be neuroprotective for the fetus.

Placental disruption

Multivitamins and folate

A large population-based study of 280 127 deliveries recorded over a 5-year period demonstrated that women who took any supplement during pregnancy had a 26% reduced risk of developing placental disruption, folate supplement reduced the risk by 19% and a multivitamin supplement was associated with a 28% reduction compared with no supplementation.[172] Combining folate with multivitamins reduced the risk of placental abruption by a further 32%.

Failure to thrive

Poor nutrition and failure to thrive

Birth weight is a key determinant of natal mortality, morbidity, subsequent growth and development, as well as early onset of adulthood diseases.[173]

Poor nutrition is especially common in developing countries where fetal failure to thrive is a common problem. [64, 65, 66, 174] The role of diet and specific nutrients in avoiding failure to thrive are discussed earlier in this chapter.

Premature rupture of membranes (PROM)

Occupational fatigue and PROM

A large-scale study of 2929 pregnant women at 22 to 24 weeks gestation were enrolled in a multi-centre (10 sites) as part of the Pre-term

Prediction Study, which identified a high volume of working hours and occupational fatigue as significant risk factors for PROM. This was particularly evident in nulliparous compared with multiparous women.[175]

Frequency of meals and PROM

Poor nutritional status is a risk factor to developing PROM. Pregnant women who eat only once daily had a slightly increased risk of having a pre-term birth and a significant risk of developing PROM compared with women who ate 3 times daily.[176]

Vitamin C and E and PROM

Vitamin C is required for the synthesis of collagen and plays an important role in the maintenance of chorioamniotic membranes. Low dietary vitamin C intake before conception and during 2nd trimester is a risk factor for PROM and pre-term delivery.[177]

A randomised double-blind trial of 109 pregnant women found daily supplementation with 100mg of vitamin C reduced the risk of PROM up to 20 weeks gestation compared with placebo.[178] Pregnant women should be encouraged to ingest a diet high in vitamin C rich foods such as red sweet peppers, kale, parsley, fruit, and tomatoes. Where there is a strong history of recurring PROM, supplementation with vitamin C may be warranted.

Vitamin E is a lipid-soluble antioxidant that inhibits membrane-damaging effects of reactive oxygen species-induced lipid peroxidation. It is hypothesised that dietary vitamins C and E in low doses may prevent damage by reactive oxygen species that can impair fetal membrane integrity and reduce mid-gestation levels of vitamin C associated with PROM.[179]

Fish oils and PROM

A randomised trial of fish oils in high-risk pregnancies found there may be a potential role for its use in the prevention of PROM although more studies are warranted.[180]

Genital tract infections

Pre-term labour can be caused by maternal genital infection in 30–50% of cases and lead to serious complications in the newborn. Clearing infections in the vagina can reduce the rate of pre-term births. Studies explored the use of probiotics, such as *Lactobacillus* preparations and yoghurts containing live cultures, either orally or vaginally, by women diagnosed with bacterial vaginosis in early pregnancy. A Cochrane review concluded that whilst probiotics reduced risk of genital infection by 81%, there was insufficient data to firmly conclude in the few trials that probiotics can prevent pre-term labour or its complications.[181] Another Cochrane review did find that probiotics are particularly useful for the prevention of severe necrotising enterocolitis in pre-term during enteral feeding by the infant.[182]

Pelvic and back pain in pregnancy

Back and pelvic pain are common symptoms of pregnancy aggravated by the weight of the growing newborn and then carrying after the baby is born. Management strategies include: exercise, rest, heat or cooling compresses, a supportive belt, using pillows during sleep and sitting, massage, acupuncture, chiropractic, relaxation, yoga and Reiki, and if necessary the use of medication such as paracetamol.

A Cochrane review was undertaken of 8 studies (1305 participants) that examined the effects of adding various pregnancy-specific exercises, physiotherapy, acupuncture and pillows to usual prenatal care.[183] Women who were not instructed to do exercise, stretching or have acupuncture and just received usual prenatal care reported more use of analgesics, physical modalities and sacroiliac belts.

Exercise helps back pain

The abovementioned Cochrane review found strengthening exercises, stabilising exercises, sitting pelvic tilt exercises and water gymnastics reduced pain intensity and back pain-related sick leave in pregnant women more than usual prenatal care alone.[183]

Acupuncture helps pelvic and back pain

The Cochrane reviewers found that acupuncture relieved pelvic pain, particularly relief from evening pain, more than exercises, and in 1 study was more effective than physiotherapy in reducing the intensity of pain. Acupuncture relieved intensity of pain by up to 60% compared to 14% of those receiving usual prenatal care.[183]

A systematic review of the literature that included 3 RCTs found statistically significant reduction in pain using acupuncture compared with control, particularly the combination of acupuncture and standard treatment with physiotherapy, for women suffering mixed pelvic and back pain in pregnancy.[184] No serious adverse events were reported across all trials with only minor adverse events, such as local pain, bruising, sweating and nausea.[184]

Stretching helps pelvic and back pain

According to the Cochrane review, stretching exercises resulted in total pain relief by up to 60% compared with usual care (11%).[183]

Labour and labour pain

Mind–body factors and labour

Ten percent of women experience fear of labour. Feeling fear without counselling was associated with a negative birth experience.[185] Counselling helped women have a more positive experience with childbirth but, of interest, it was associated with a higher risk of having a caesarean section.

More research is required to explore non-drug and surgical interventions for the safe delivery of the newborn as interventions such as caesarean sections carry a high risk to both mothers and newborns and whilst epidurals are effective in reducing pain they come at a high risk, resulting in higher chances of instrumental delivery.[186]

Music and labour

Music plays an important role in the management of anxiety (see Chapter 4 on anxiety) and for pain relief. A systematic review of the literature identified 51 studies involving 3663 patients experiencing acute or chronic pain (not pregnant) and found music reduced pain by up to 50%, and reduced the need for morphine-like analgesics.[187] It would appear calm, gentle, soothing music may play a role in helping reduce pain and anxiety during labour, as gentle music poses little risk or harm to the mother, although research is required to confirm this.

Yoga and labour

Practising regular yoga during pregnancy is associated with improved birth outcomes, improved maternal comfort and reduced labour pain.[188–191] Also, yoga practise was associated with higher incidence of vaginal birth rate and less need for caesarean section.

Acupuncture, acupressure, hypnosis, massage, relaxation, aromatherapy and labour

A Cochrane literature review explored trials using non-drug approaches such as acupuncture, mind-body techniques, massage, reflexology, herbal medicines, homoeopathy, hypnosis and music for pain management during labour.[192] They identified 14 trials including 1448 pregnant women:

- 3 trials acupuncture (n = 496)
- 2 acupressure (n = 172)
- 1 audio-analgesia (n = 24), 'sea sounds'
- 1 aromatherapy (n = 22)
- 5 hypnosis (n = 729), including self-hypnosis
- 1 massage (n = 60)
- 1 relaxation (n = 34).

The authors concluded that acupuncture and self-hypnosis reduced the need for pain relief and led to women feeling more satisfied with their pain during labour compared with controls, plus requiring less analgesia and the need for an epidural. However, the other studies were of too poor a quality to comment.

Water births and labour

A Cochrane review of 8 trials including 2939 women found statistically significant reduction in pain and the use of epidural/spinal/paracervical analgesia/anaesthesia amongst women allocated to water immersion during the first stage of labour compared to those not allocated to water immersion.[193] Also, women were less likely to require analgesia and there were no adverse outcomes on labour duration, operative delivery or neonatal outcomes, although more research is still warranted.

Pelvic floor exercises and labour

A study of 120 healthy nulliparous women who engaged in a series of weekly pelvic floor training sessions over 12 weeks in the second half of the pregnancy, experienced better childbirth than women in the control group who experienced longer active pushing in the second stage of labour.[194]

Homeopathy and labour

There is no evidence to support the use of homeopathy in inducing labour, based on 2 trials.[195]

Heat packs and labour

A heat pack heated with warm water to 45–59 degrees can be quite soothing and reduce pain and severity of trauma to perineum during second stage of labour.[196]

Breech

External cephalic version (ECV) and breech

ECV is often overlooked as a suitable option for breech presentation in favour of caesarean section.[197]

Moxibustion and breech

Moxibustion is a method used in Chinese medicine that involves the burning of a herb close to the skin. In breech, traditional Chinese medicine (TCM) practitioners apply moxibustion near the little toe. A Cochrane review identified 3 trials of 597 women, but only 1 trial reported relevant outcome measures.[198] This study demonstrated that moxibustion reduced the need for ECV or the use of oxytocin before and during labour for women who had vaginal deliveries. Whilst the authors concluded the research to date is not convincing, it would appear a very simple, non-harmful approach to trial if needed.

Labour pain

Perineal massage and labour

A Cochrane review of 3 good quality trials involving 2434 women comparing digital perineal massage with control demonstrated a clear benefit using perineal massage during pregnancy as little as once or twice weekly from 35 weeks gestation.[199] Antenatal perineal massage significantly reduced the incidence of perineal trauma requiring suturing (episiotomy) especially in women without previous vaginal birth. In women with a history of previous vaginal birth they reported significant reduction of pain at 3 months post-partum.[199] As such, women should be encouraged to undertake perineal massage, which can be done by the woman or her partner.

Perineal pain after labour

Cooling packs

Perineal tears following labour can cause much pain and discomfort for the mother and it is common practice after labour to apply ice or cold packs onto tears or cuts. [200] A review of the literature demonstrates that ice packs provide pain relief up to 72 hours following birth but women preferred gel pads (ease of use) when compared with ice packs or no treatment. There were no differences in level of bruising or oedema in each group.[200]

Ultrasound

There is little evidence to evaluate the use of ultrasound in treating perineal pain following childbirth.[201]

Antenatal and postnatal depression

Antenatal depression (AND) is common, affecting from 7.4% in the 1st trimester up to 12.8% in the 2nd trimester. Psychosocial and psychological support is vital for the wellbeing of the mother and child during and following pregnancy, especially for the prevention of post-partum depression.

A Cochrane review found too few trials to confidently make any recommendations for other therapies, such as massage therapy or depression-specific acupuncture, for the treatment of antenatal depression.[202]

Postnatal depression (PND) affects up to 15% of mothers. It is vital that PND is detected and treated early. Mothers require guidance and emotional and physical support, especially in the first few months following birth. It is a time when they experience poor sleep, may experience pain, illness, problems with lactation, have difficulty cooking, lack exercise and sunshine and all these factors can contribute to fatigue, exhaustion and depression. There is a traditional North American Indian saying: 'it takes a whole village to bring up a child'. The level of support in smaller communities, extended families, villages and so forth, can play a vital role in supporting the mother, especially a first-time mother who needs guidance and assistance within the first year following birth. There are many cultures where women become more supportive to new mothers and provide assistance with cooking and cleaning.

A meta-analyses of the literature identified 9 studies (n = 956) that found psychosocial interventions such as peer support or non-directive counselling, cognitive behavioural therapy (CBT), interpersonal psychotherapy, and psychodynamic therapy significantly reduced evidence of depression within the first year after delivery, compared to usual care in women with PND.[203] Professional counselling reduced rates of PND by 40%, while support from other mothers reduced the risk by up to 50%. Research consistently supports the value of psychological and psychosocial support in reducing the incidence of PND.[204]

Infants of mothers with PND are more likely to experience cognitive and psychomotor developmental delays, although the mechanism is not clear.[205]

Lifestyle and AND/PND

There is clear evidence that lifestyle factors, such as diet, exercise, sunshine, sleep and stress management, play an important role in the management of depression. (See Chapter 12 for more information on depression.)

Psychosocial and psychological support and AND/PND

Antidepressant use in pregnancy should be avoided as much as possible, because of adverse effects on the fetus, and should be weighed against the risk and harm to the mother.[206–209] Counselling is not only recommended for treatment of depression but can help reduce risk of developing depression.

Sleep and PND

Two-thirds of clinically significant depression symptoms in pregnancy occur in mothers reporting an infant with a sleep problem. An Australian study of mothers with infants 6–12 months of age found that sleep deprivation was a factor in PND.[210] If the infant had a sleep problem, the mother was twice as likely to have PND. The same group showed that by improving the mother's sleep, this improved the PND.[211]

In another study, this group is investigated for behavioural intervention for sleep problems on maternal depression.[212] They concluded that sleep intervention in infancy resulted in sustained positive effects on maternal depression.

Fish oils and PND

It is well recognised that a diet high in fish and omega-3 supplementation may help with depression. (See Chapter 12 for more information on depression.) A small pilot study found omega-3 supplementation may help women with PND.[213] A review of the literature found 3 trials of omega-3 fatty acids versus placebo for perinatal depression show conflicting results.[214] It is likely women with lower levels of omega-3 fatty acids during pregnancy are more likely to develop depression than those with higher levels.

Iron and PND

An increased risk of PND occurs in women who have suffered post-partum anaemia such as that due to blood loss. Iron can help prevent the onset of PND.[215]

Herbal medicine

Safety of herbs in pregnancy

There is little research that supports the safety and use of many herbs in pregnancy, except for a few such as ginger, and one needs to rely on traditional evidence. For instance, the herb liquorice is known to inhibit cortisol metabolism and increase blood pressure, and may increase the risk of pre-term pregnancy.[216] Traditionally liquorice was used to induce abortions.

One study looked at the use and safety of echinacea in pregnant women compared with control for the treatment of upper respiratory tract infections.[217] There was no increase in congenital malformations in the echinacea group versus the placebo group.

Red raspberry leaf tea is widely used by pregnant women to tonify the uterus during pregnancy and shorten the labour but to date there is no convincing research to demonstrate this.

The Medicines Control Agency report titled 'The Safety of Herbal Medicinal Products' warns that many herbs have pharmacologically active ingredients that may act unpredictably when ingested in high concentrations and quantities.

The following should be avoided in pregnancy:[218]

- liquorice — estrogenic activity and reputed abortifacient[219, 220, 221]
- aloes — cathartic, reputed abortifacient
- chamomile — may stimulate the uterus in large quantities, reputed abortifacient
- feverfew — reputed abortifacient
- ginseng — has estrogenic effect
- St John's wort — slight uterine activity in vitro
- gingko — birth defects.

Lactation

The herbs listed below may affect breast milk production, although there has been very little scientific research to test their safety in the mother and baby, or their efficacy during breastfeeding. They can be ingested or consumed as teas by the mother, and were traditionally used to promote milk production during breastfeeding:

- alfalfa
- bitter melon
- blessed thistle
- chaste tree berry
- caraway
- celery root
- fennel seed
- fenugreek
- goat's rue
- raspberry.

During lactation mothers should be encouraged to rest, reduce stress levels, drink adequate fluids and eat small frequent protein meals.

Herbs traditionally used to reduce milk production during breastfeeding:

- castor bean
- jasmine flower
- sage
- cabbage leaf applied to breast for engorgement.

Breastfeeding

An early study on breastfeeding and cognitive function has suggested that a longer duration of breastfeeding benefits cognitive development.[222] This was confirmed by a subsequent meta-analysis.[223]

A recent study, that is the largest randomised trial ever conducted in the area of human lactation, provides significantly strong evidence that prolonged and exclusive breastfeeding improves children's cognitive development.[224]

What has been reported to be of further importance is maternal intake of very-long-chain n-3 polyunsaturated fatty acids (PUFAs) during pregnancy and lactation, which may have significant favourable effects for later mental development of children.[225] Additional studies have confirmed these results.[226, 227]

Lactational amenorrhoea — family planning

Lactational amenorrhea method (LAM) is a contraceptive method where the mother uses breastfeeding also for contraception. It has a failure rate of 0.9 to 1.2% and in other studies up to 2.45%, so cannot be relied on solely but together with other methods, such as the use of condoms, it can be a very effective natural method of contraception.[228]

Conclusion

Pregnancy is a natural state and due to physical, emotional and hormonal changes throughout the pregnancy with the growth of the fetus, this can pose a number of different health challenges for the woman at any stage. Pregnancy for some women can cause a myriad of distressing symptoms. This chapter covers some of the common pregnancy-related complaints.

It is vital women are fit and healthy before entering pregnancy. For example, it is vital women eat well to maintain a healthy weight, avoid gestational diabetes and constipation, exercise regularly to help develop a good strong posture to support their back during the pregnancy, practise regular stress management strategies and increase their supports from friends and family for emotional wellbeing. A pregnancy multivitamin that contains 500mcg of folate taken once daily commenced at least 3 months ahead of a planned pregnancy can be useful for the prevention of a number of pregnancy-related diseases, such as neural tube defect. Consuming alcohol, smoking and drug intake should be avoided during the planning and pregnancy period. Pregnancies also occur unplanned, so efforts for good health and positive lifestyle and behavioural changes need to occur as soon as possible during the pregnancy.

This chapter has covered a whole range of conditions and health problems that may occur in pregnancy that can be treated or symptomatically managed using a range of evidence-based complementary medicines and therapies together with lifestyle changes, such as exercise, diet and stress management. Pregnancy itself is not a disease and so in this chapter (unlike other chapters) we have not prepared a table of evidence for lifestyle and complementary medicine/therapies in the management of pregnancy. Because we have covered a number of different disease and symptom states throughout the chapter, not just 1 or 2 diseases (as covered in other chapters), such a table might be quite confusing.

So, in summary, healthy lifestyle and behavioural changes before, during and after pregnancy can positively impact on the mother's and child's wellbeing.

Clinical tips handout for patients — pregnancy

1 Lifestyle advice

Sleep

- Ensure at least 7–8 hours sleep. During third trimester naps may be necessary during the day but avoid unless completely necessary as it may lead to sleep disturbance. (See Chapter 22 for more advice.)

Sunshine

- Amount of exposure varies with local climate.
- At least 15 minutes of sunshine needed daily for vitamin D and melatonin production — especially before 10 a.m. and after 3 p.m. when the sun exposure is safest during summer; much more exposure in winter when supplementation with vitamin D needs to be considered.
- Ensure gradual adequate skin exposure to sun; avoid sunscreen and excess clothing to maximise levels of vitamin D.
- More time in the sun is required for dark skinned people.
- Direct exposure to about 10% of body (hands, arms, face), without sunscreen and not through glass.
- Vitamin D is obtained in the diet from fatty fish, eggs, liver and fortified foods (some milks and margarines); it is unlikely that adequate vitamin D concentrations can be obtained from diet alone.

2 Physical activity/exercise

- Exercise 30–60 minutes daily.
- If exercise is not regular, commence with 5 minutes daily and slowly build up to at least 30 minutes. Outdoor exercise with nature, fresh air (avoid polluted air) and sunshine is ideal (e.g. brisk walking, light jogging, cycling, swimming, stretching, resistance or weight bearing exercises).
- Weight bearing or resistance exercises are essential for building up bone and muscle.
- Yoga can decrease stress during pregnancy and improve labour management.
- Tai chi can help with balance and build up strong muscles and bones.
- Stretching exercises can help pregnancy and labour.

3 Mind–body medicine

- Stress management program — for example, six 40 minute sessions for patients to understand the nature of their symptoms, the symptoms' relationship to stress, and the practice of regular relaxation exercises.
- Regular meditation practice at least 10–20 minutes daily.

Breathing

- Be aware of breathing from time to time. Notice if tendency to hold breath or over-breathe.

Rest and stress management

- Increased stress can occur during pregnancy.
- Reduce workload and resolve conflicts.
- Accept support and help from friends, family members, neighbours, especially in the first 3–6 months following labour.
- Listening to relaxation music and daily baths help.
- Massage therapy is most useful in pregnancy and during labour.
- Avoid overworking whilst pregnant, especially if you are feeling fatigued.
- Cognitive behavioural therapy and psychotherapy are extremely helpful to reduce any symptoms of depression.
- Counselling can help reduce the risk of developing depression especially after difficult pregnancies or birth.

Fun

- It is important to have fun in life. Joy can be found even in the simplest tasks, such as being with friends with a sense of humour, funny movies/videos, comedy, hobbies, dancing, playing with pets and children.

4 Environment

- Try to minimise exposure to pollution and chemicals, especially during the 1st trimester.
- Office or home environment is enhanced with a view overlooking garden or park.
- Avoid smoking — it can lead to a number of problems for the baby and pregnancy outcome and must be completely avoided.

5 Dietary changes

- Best if not overweight before and during pregnancy.
- Avoid excess weight gain as this can be associated with problems for the mother and also baby.

- Avoid calorie restriction and weight loss diets especially if not exercising.
- Do not rush your meals; chewing your food thoroughly aids digestion.
- Small frequent meals may be preferred during pregnancy.
- Eat more fruit and vegetables — variety of colour and those in season. Can be raw or steamed.
- Use cold pressed olive oil and avocado.
- Increase intake of nuts (e.g. walnuts, peanuts, almonds).
- Eat more seeds and legumes (e.g. beans, soy, lentils, chickpeas).
- Eat more vegetable protein compared to animal protein.
- Use unprocessed carbohydrates with lower GI — wholegrains/cereals (variety) such as wholegrain bread, wholemeal pasta and low GI rice (brown, basmati, mahatma, doongara), traditional rolled oats with cinnamon, buckwheat flour, organic breads best (e.g. rye, Essene, spelt, Kamut), couscous, millet, amaranth etc.
- Constipation can be a problem so wheat bran and oat bran may be added to breakfast.
- Increase fish intake, at least 3 times weekly, especially deep sea fish. Canned is okay (mackerel, salmon, sardines, cod, tuna). Avoid fish with a high content of mercury and other pollutants.
  - Limit to 1 serve (150g) per fortnight of billfish (swordfish, broadbill and marlin) and shark (flake), with no other fish eaten during that fortnight.
  - Limit to 1 serve (150g) per week of orange roughy (deep sea perch) or catfish, with no other fish eaten during that week.
- Reduce red meat intake (preferably use red lean meat e.g. lamb, kangaroo) and use white meat (e.g. free range organic chicken).
- Consume low-fat dairy products, such as yoghurt and hard cheeses.
- For sweetener try honey (e.g. yellow box and stringy bark have the lowest GI).
- Drink more water (about 1–2 litres a day), and vegetable juices.
- Drink more teas, low caffeine is best (e.g. organic green, black, oolong tea).
  - Chamomile tea may help you to relax (do not exceed more than 1 cup daily).
  - Peppermint and ginger teas can aid digestion (1 cup before meals may help).
- Avoid drinks with high caffeine (e.g. no more than 1 cup of coffee per day, not strong).
- Avoid sugary soft drinks, especially cola.
- Avoid hydrogenated fats, salt, fast foods, added sugar such as lollies, biscuits, cakes, and processed foods (e.g. white bread, white pasta, pastries).
- Avoid alcohol during pregnancy. If drinking alcohol do not exceed 1 glass per day.
- Avoid high salt intake.
- Avoid chemical additives — artificial sweeteners, preservatives, colourings and flavourings.

Avoid the following foods as they may contain the harmful bacteria *Listeria*, which can cause increased risk of miscarriage, stillbirth or premature labour in pregnancy, and is destroyed only with cooking:

- soft cheeses, such as brie, camembert, fetta, blue vein and ricotta
- paté, quiches and delicatessen meats such as ham and salami
- raw seafood such as oysters and sashimi or smoked seafood such as salmon (canned varieties are safe)
- unpasteurised foods
- soft-serve ice-cream.

Refer to the website for Foods Standards Australia New Zealand for more information:

http://www.foodstandards.gov.au/_srcfiles/Listeria.pdf

Nutrition

Good nutrition during pregnancy is vital for the developing baby and its mother. Normal weight gain during pregnancy is around 10–16kg.

Due to increased nutrient demands by the body, it is advisable to *increase* the foods rich in the following nutrients:

- calcium: dairy foods, such as milk, hard cheeses (e.g. cheddar, tasty) and yoghurt, and calcium-fortified soymilk
- iron: red meats, dried fruits and leafy green vegetables
- folic acid (folate): asparagus, broccoli, brussel sprouts, cabbage, cauliflower, chick peas, dried beans, leeks, lentils, parsley, peas, spinach, wholegrain bread.

Warnings

- Liver should be avoided due to its high vitamin A content. Paté is also a risk factor for Listeria exposure.
- Vitamin A supplements are not recommended for pregnant women as

excessive intake of vitamin A may cause birth deformities.

Heartburn symptoms

Try small frequent meals and avoid eating late at night, especially before bed. Avoid bending, lifting or lying down after meals, and excessive consumption of tea or coffee. Use large pillows to sleep on and raise your bed-head by a few inches.

Nausea and vomiting symptoms

- Eat small frequent snacks and meals. Suck on sour food such as a lemon. Relax and have plenty of fresh air. Try drinks containing ginger.
- Avoid large, spicy, fried, strong-smelling foods.
- Avoid dehydration by drinking small sips of fluids frequently, such as ginger, peppermint or red raspberry leaf tea and water.
  - Fresh ginger tea: steep a few peeled slices of fresh ginger root in 2 cups of hot water.
  - Red raspberry leaf tea: steep 1 tablespoon of red raspberry leaf in a pot of hot water. Drink up to 4 cups daily. Can interfere with iron, calcium and magnesium absorption and therefore best to consume at separate times to supplements.
- Try acupuncture or acupressure to pericardium 6, located on the wrists (2 finger-breadths from the distal crease line on the wrist). Apply gentle pressure to this point. Should alleviate nausea immediately.

6 Physical therapies

- Physiotherapy, acupressure and acupuncture may help with back and pelvic pain, headaches and nausea of pregnancy.
- A thorough dental examination and treatment of conditions such as periodontal disease can positively impact upon pregnancy outcome.

Labour

- Perineal massage once or twice weekly from 35 weeks can reduce risk of tear during vaginal birth.
- Standing and squatting may help with pain and progression of labour.
- Water birth, topical heat or cooling packs and acupuncture may help with labour pain.

7 Supplements

Fish oils

- Indication: can help prevent allergy problems in baby and improve IQ in child. May be helpful to mother.
- Dosage: take with meals. Adult: 1g 1–2 capsules 1–3 x daily; can be used in pregnancy or lactation as tolerated.
- Results: during pregnancy and post pregnancy.
- Side-effects: often well tolerated, especially if taken with meals. Very mild and rare side-effects (e.g. gastrointestinal upset); allergic reactions (e.g. rash, breathing problems) if allergic to seafood; blood thinning effects in very high doses > 10g/day (may need to stop fish oil supplements 2 weeks prior to surgery).
- Contraindications: sensitivity reaction to seafood; drug interactions; caution when taking high doses of fish oils >4g/day together with warfarin (your doctor will check your INR test).

Multivitamins and minerals

- Indication can help prevent folic acid, zinc, magnesium, copper, selenium, iron and calcium depletion.
- Dosage: best to use a multivitamin and mineral supplement that has been especially designed for pregnant women and take as directed.
- Results: during pregnancy plus post pregnancy.
- Side-effects: should be safe when special formula designed for pregnant women is used.
- Contraindications: should be safe to use if a pregnancy formula.

Vitamins

Do not take vitamin A supplements as excessive intake of vitamin A above 3000IU/day can contribute to genetic problems in the baby.

Do not take vitamin E supplements in early pregnancy as it is linked to heart problems in the baby.

Vitamin B6, B12

- Indication: nausea, vegetarianism.
- Dosage: Vitamin B6: upper level of intake should not exceed 50mg/day; may use twice this dose for short periods only if severe nausea or 25mg 8 hourly.
  - Vitamin B12: between 600–1000mcg daily.
  - Results: B6: within 1 hour if it works.

- B12: variable depending on whether deficiency or not.
- Side-effects: Vitamin B6: avoid use of multiple single-vitamin products (e.g. oral and injectable forms of vitamin B6) or concomitant use of multivitamin products could result in some patients exceeding the upper limit for toxicity. Toxicity from high doses of vitamin B6 (> 50mg/day) includes peripheral neuropathy, such as tingling, burning and numbness of limbs.
- Vitamin B12: generally minimal side-effects.

Contraindicated: vitamin B6 in high dosage (>50mgs/day) especially with long-term use.

Vitamin D3

Indication: correct vitamin D deficiency; osteomalacia. In fetus deficiency linked to low birth weight, neonatal hypocalcaemia and rickets plus defective tooth enamel.

- Dosage: safe sunshine exposure of skin is the safest source of vitamin D.
  - Vitamin D (cholecalciferol 1000 international units).
  - Doctors should check blood levels and suggest supplementation if levels are low.
  - Adults: 400–1000IU/day -for maintenance; 3000–5000IU daily for 1 month then 1000IU daily if vitamin D level below normal, ensure repeat blood measurement.
  - Children at risk: 200–400IU daily under medical supervision.
  - Pregnant and lactating women at risk: under medical supervision.
- Results: 6–12 months.
- Side-effects: Very high doses can cause vitamin D toxicity; raised calcium levels in the blood.
- Contraindications: Can increase aluminum and magnesium absorption, prolonged heparin therapy can increase resorption and reduce formation of bone and hence more vitamin D and calcium required, thiazide diuretics decrease urinary calcium and hence hypercalcaemia possible with vitamin D supplementation, high levels of vitamin D can reduce effectiveness of verapamil.

Vitamin C

- Indication: may reduce risk of pre-eclampsia with vitamin E; may prevent premature rupture of membranes; only take if high risk.
  - Dosage: 500–1000mg/day.
- Results: 6–9 months.
- Side-effects: with high doses can cause nausea, heartburn, abdominal cramps and diarrhoea.
- Contraindications: can increase iron absorption. Use with caution if glucose-6-phosphate dehydrogenase deficiency.

Vitamin E

- Indication: may reduce risk of pre-eclampsia with vitamin C; only take if high risk of pre-eclampsia.
- Dosage: 200IU/day.
- Results: 6–9 months.
- Side-effects: doses below 1500IU/day are very unlikely to result in haemorrhage. Rarely can cause diarrhoea, flatulence, nausea, heart palpitations.
- Contraindications: use with caution if bleeding disorder or if taking with blood thinning medication. Avoid using high doses in periconception period.

Folate

- Indication: prevention of abnormal fetal development; NTD; cleft palate; medications that affect folate levels (eg. anti-epileptics).
- Dosage: 500–1000mcg/day.
- Results: 3 months pre-conception and first 3 months during pregnancy for fetal development.
- Side-effects: very mild and rare.
- Contraindications: avoid in anaemias until assessed by a doctor.

Minerals

Iron

- Indication: use only for iron deficiency.
- Dosage: 50–100mg of elemental iron 3 times daily.
- Results: can vary and therefore must measure at regular intervals.
- Side-effects: during pregnancy oral iron can cause gastrointestinal irritation, abdominal pain, constipation or diarrhoea, nausea and vomiting. Doses less than 45mg/day rarely cause problems. Best to take iron with vitamin C-rich meals as this reduces side-effects. Can combine with vitamin C to increase iron absorption.
- Contraindications: ensure that excess iron is not taken as this can have adverse outcomes to pregnancy. Iron can interfere with absorption of zinc and calcium and therefore best if taken at separate times.

Magnesium and calcium (best provided together)

- Indication: cramps; to support bone growth and increase bone density; more effective when combined with vitamins D and K; pre-eclampsia.
- Dosage: magnesium: 400–800mg/day including pregnant and lactating women.
  - Calcium citrate: 800mg/day or calcium carbonate 1000mg/day in adults.
- Results: >1–2 days for cramps.
- Side-effects: oral magnesium can cause gastrointestinal irritation, nausea, vomiting, and diarrhoea. The dosage varies from person to person. Although rare, toxic levels can cause low blood pressure, thirst, heart arrhythmia, drowsiness and weakness. Calcium can cause gastrointestinal irritation and constipation.
- Contraindications: patients with kidney disease and diarrhoea.

Copper

- Indication: reduce bone density loss and for bone synthesis. Should be combined with zinc, manganese and calcium.
- Dosage: 3mg/day in adults; do not exceed 10mg/day. Safe in pregnancy and lactation. Children: from 1–5mg/day.
- Side-effects: nausea, vomiting, liver and kidney damage with very high doses. Avoid long-term use and high dosage as this may cause copper toxicity; can reduce zinc absorption; may cause anaemia, uraemia and cardiovascular collapse.
- Contraindications: decreases penicillamine absorption and at the same time decreases copper absorption. Ethambutol and zidovudine can decrease copper levels.

Zinc

- Indication: deficiency can lead to pre-term birth, fetal growth retardation and can prolong labour.
- Dosage: elemental zinc 25–50mg daily if deficiency. Recommended dietary intake is 11mg/day.
- Side-effects: nausea, vomiting, metallic taste in mouth. Avoid long-term use and high dosage as this may cause copper deficiency, impair the immune system and cause anaemia. Absorption may be impaired by calcium, iron and folate — separate doses by 2 hours.
- Contraindications: sideroblastic anaemia, above normal blood levels of zinc, severe kidney disease.

Iodine

- Indication: mild deficiency is common in pregnancy. It plays a critical role in neuropsycho–intellectual development of the newborn.
- Dosage: 220mcg/day.
- Side-effects: over consumption can lead to hypothyroidism or hyperthyroidism and post-partum thyroiditis. High doses can lead to a brassy taste in mouth, increased salivation, gastric irritations plus skin lesions. Soy can inhibit iodine absorption and T3 plus T4 production.
- Contraindications: if thyroid problems exist use with caution.

Herbs

Ginger

- Indication: nausea.
- Dosage: 1–2g of dried ginger daily has been used safely.
- Side-effects: nausea, vomiting, heartburn and bloating plus stomach irritation. Theoretical risk of bleeding increased with warfarin and anti-platelet drugs.
- Contraindications: use with caution if heartburn or gastric ulcers present.

References

1 Skouteris H, Wertheim EH, Rallis S, et. al. Use of complementary and alternative medicines by a sample of Australian women during pregnancy. ANZJ Obstet Gynecol 2008;48:384–90.

2 Hedvig N and Gro CH. Use of herbal drugs in pregnancy: a survey among 400 Norwegian women. Pharmacoepidemiology and Drug Safety 2004;13:371–80.

3 Forster DA, Denning A, Wills G. Herbal medicine use during pregnancy in a group of Australian women. BMC Pregnancy and Childbirth 2006;6:21.

4 Murtagh J. General Practice.mcgraw–Hill, Australia, 4th Ed. ISBN: 0074717790 EAN: 9780074717790.

5 Lee KA, Gay CL. Sleep in late pregnancy predicts length of labour and type of delivery. Ame J Obstet Gynecol 2004;191:2041–46.

6 Saisto T, Salmela-Aro K, Nurmi JE, et. al. Psychosocial characteristics of women and their partners fearing vaginal childbirth. BJOGl 2001;108:492–98.

7 Heather J Rowe, Maggie Kirkman, E Annarella Hardiman, et. al. Considering abortion: a 12-month audit of records of women contacting a Pregnancy Advisory Service. MJA 2009;190(2):69–72.

8 Dennis C-L, Hodnett E, Reisman Heather M, et. al. Effect of peer support on prevention of postnatal depression among high risk women: multisite randomised controlled trial. Published 15 January 2009, doi:10.1136/bmj.a3064 Cite this as: BMJ 2009;338:a3064.

9 Smith GCS, Pell JP, Dobbie R. Interpregnancy interval and risk of pre-term birth and neonatal death: retrospective cohort study. BMJ 2003;327:313–16.

10 Duncombe D, Skouteris H, Eleanor H, et. al. Vigorous exercise and birth outcomes in a sample of recreational exercisers: A prospective study across pregnancy. ANZ J Obstet Gynaecol 2006;46: 288–92.
11 Kramer MS, McDonald SW. Aerobic exercise for women during pregnancy. Cochrane Database of Systematic Reviews 2006, Issue 3. Art. No.: CD000180. doi: 10.1002/14651858.CD000180. pub2.
12 Hansen C, Neller A, Williams G, et. al. Maternal exposure to low levels of ambient air pollution and pre-term birth in Brisbane, Australia. BJOG 2006;113:935–41.
13 McCowan Lesley ME, Dekker Gustaaf A, Eliza Chan, et. al. Spontaneous pre-term birth and small for gestational age infants in women who stop smoking early in pregnancy: prospective cohort study. Published 26 March 2009, doi:10.1136/bmj. b1081. Cite this as: BMJ 2009;338:b1081.
14 McDonald SD, Perkins SL, Jodouin CA, et. al. Folate levels in pregnant women who smoke: an important gene/environment interaction. Am J Obstet Gynecol 2002 Sep;187(3):620–5. PubMed PMID: 12237638.
15 Linnet KM, Wisborg K, Obel C, et. al. Smoking during pregnancy and the risk for hyperkinetic disorder in offspring. Pediatrics 2005 Aug;116(2):462–7.
16 Elliott EJ, Bower C. Alcohol and pregnancy: the pivotal role of the obstetrician. Aust NZ J Obstet Gynecol 2008;48:236–9. Online. Avaialble: www.nhmrc.gov.au/guidelines/_files/draft_australian_alcohol_guidelines.pdf (accessed April 2010).
17 Henderson J, Gray R, Brocklehurst P. Systematic review of effects of low/moderate prenatal alcohol exposure on pregnancy outcome. BJOG 2007;114:243–52.
18 O'Leary CM, Nassar N, Kurinczuk JJ, et. al. The effect of maternal alcohol consumption on fetal growth and pre-term birth. BJOG 2009;116: 390–400.
19 Mengel MB, Searight HR, Cook K. Clinical review preventing alcohol/exposed pregnancies. Amer Board Fam Med 2006;19:494–505.
20 Summers Brooke L, Rofe Allan M. Peter Coyle Dietary Zinc Supplementation Throughout Pregnancy Protects Against Fetal Dysmorphology and Improves Postnatal Survival After Prenatal Ethanol Exposure in Mice. Alcoholism: Clinical and Experimental Research. Published Online: Jan 12 2009 doi: 10.1111/j.1530–0277.2008.00873.x.
21 Thorsdottir I, Torfadottir JE, Birgisdottir BE, et. al. Weight gain in women of normal weight before pregnancy: complications in pregnancy or delivery and birth outcome. Obstet Gynecol 2002;99:799–806.
22 Asbee Shelly M, Jenkins Todd R, Butler Jennifer R, et. al. Preventing Excessive Weight Gain During Pregnancy Through Dietary and Lifestyle Counseling: A Randomised Controlled Trial. Obstetrics and Gynecology 2009 February;113(2-1):305–312. doi: 10.1097/AOG.0b013e318195baef.
23 Cedergren MI. Maternal morbid obesity and the risk of adverse pregnancy outcome. Obstet Gynecol 2004;103:219–24.
24 Vahratian A, et. al. Maternal prepregnancy overweight and obesity and the patter of labour progression in term nulliparous women. Obstet Gynecol 2004;104:943–51.
25 van der Steeg JW, Steures P, Eijkemans MJ, et. al. Obesity affects spontaneous pregnancy chances in subfertile, ovulatory women. Hum Reprod 2008 Feb;23(2):324–8.
26 Leddy MA, Power ML, Schulkin J. The impact of maternal obesity on maternal and fetal health. Rev Obstet Gynacol 2008;1:170–78.
27 Nohr EA, Bech BH, Davies MJ, et. al. Prepregnancy Obesity and Fetal Death: A Study Within the Danish National Birth Cohort. Obstet Gynecol 2005;106:250–59.
28 Vujkovic M, Steegers EA, Looman CW, et. al. The maternal Mediterranean dietary pattern is associated with a reduced risk of spina bifida in the offspring. British Journal of Obstetrics and Gynecology 2009;116(3): 408–15.
29 Vujkovic Marijana, Ocke Marga C, van der Spek Peter J, et. al. Maternal Western Dietary Patterns and the Risk of Developing a Cleft Lip With or Without a Cleft Palate. Obstetrics and Gynecology August 2007;110:378–384. © 2007 by The American College of Obstetricians and Gynecologists.
30 Woods RK, Thien FC, Abramson MJ. Dietary marine fatty acids (fish oil) for asthma. Cochrane Database Syst Rev 2000;(4):CD001283.
31 Dunstan JA, Mori TA, Barden A, et. al. Fish oil supplementation in pregnancy modifies neonatal allergen-specific immune responses and clinical outcomes in infants at high risk of atopy: a randomised,controlled trial. J Allergy Clin Immunol 2003 Dec;112(6):1178–84.
32 Myers GJ, Davidson PW, Strain JJ. Nutrient and methyl mercury exposure from consuming fish. J Nutr 2007;137(12):2805–8.
33 Foods Standards Australia New Zealand. Online. Available: www.foodstandards.gov.au/foodmatters/mercuryinfish.cfm (accessed January 2009).
34 Stanton R. Complete Book of Food and Nutrition. Simon and Schuster, Sydney, 2007.
35 Shabert JK. In Krause's Food and Nutrition and Diet Therapy (11th edn). Saunders, Philadelphia, 2004:182–213, Chapter 7.
36 Royal Australian and New Zealand College of Obstetricians and Gynaecologists (RANZCOG). Online. Available: http://www.ranzcog.edu.au/publications/statements/C-obs25.pdf (accessed February 2009).
37 Williams C, Birch EE, Emmett PM, et. al. Stereoacuity at age 3.5 y in children born full-term is associated with prenatal and postnatal dietary factors: a report from a population-based cohort study. AJCN 2001;73(2):316–322.
38 Dunstan JA, Prescott SL. Does fish oil supplementation in pregnancy reduce the risk of allergic disease in infants? Curr Opin Allergy Clin Immunol 2005;5(3):215–21.
39 Auestad N, Scott DT, Janowsky JS, et. al. Visual, cognitive, and language assessments at 39 months: a follow-up study of children fed formulas containing long-chain polyunsaturated fatty acids to 1 year of age. Pediatrics 2003;112(3 Pt 1):e177–83.
40 Helland IB, Saugstad OD, Smith L, et. al. Similar effects on infants of n-3 and n-6 fatty acids supplementation to pregnant and lactating women. Pediatrics 2001;108(5):E82.
41 Helland IB, Smith L, Saarem K, et. al. Maternal supplementation with very-long-chain n-3 fatty acids during pregnancy and lactation augments children's IQ at 4 years of age. Pediatrics 2003;111(1): e39–e44.

42 Dunstan JA, Roper J, Mitoulas L, et. al. The effect of supplementation with fish oil during pregnancy on breast milk immunoglobulin A, soluble CD14, cytokine levels and fatty acid composition. Clin Exp Allergy 2004;34(8):1237–42.
43 Olsen SF, Østerdal ML, Salvig JD, et. al. Fish oil intake compared with olive oil intake in late pregnancy and asthma in the offspring: 16 y of registry-based follow-up from a randomised controlled trial. ALCN 2008;88(1):167–75.
44 Olsen SF, Sørensen JD, Secher NJ, et. al. Randomised controlled trial of effect of fish-oil supplementation on pregnancy duration. Lancet 1992;339(8800):1003–7.
45 Martinez M. Tissue levels of polyunsaturated fatty acids during early human development. J Pediatr 1992;120(4 pt 2):S129–S138.
46 Harris WS, Connor WE, Lindsey S. Will dietary omega-3 fatty acids change the composition of human milk? AJCN 1984;40(4):780–785.
47 Helland IB, Saarem K, Saugstad OD, et. al. Fatty acid composition in maternal milk and plasma during supplementation with cod liver oil. Eur J Clin Nutr 1998;52(11):839–845.
48 Bakker EC, Ghys AJ, Kester AD, et. al. Long-chain polyunsaturated fatty acids at birth and cognitive function at 7 y of age. Eur J Clin Nutr 2003;57(1):89–95.
49 Ghys A, Bakker E, Hornstra G, et. al. Red blood cell and plasma phospholipid arachidonic and docosahexaenoic acid levels at birth and cognitive development at 4 years of age. Early Hum Dev 2002;69(1–2):83–90.
50 Innis SM, Gilley J, Werker J. Are human milk long-chain polyunsaturated fatty acids related to visual and neural development in breast-fed term infants? J Pediatr 2001;139(4):532–538.
51 Smuts CM, Huang M, Mundy D, et. al. A randomised trial of docosahexaenoic acid supplementation during the third trimester of pregnancy. Obstet Gynecol2003;101(3):469–479.
52 Malcolm CA, McCulloch DL, Montgomery C, et. al. Maternal docosahexaenoic acid supplementation during pregnancy and visual evoked potential development in term infants: a double blind, prospective, randomised trial. Arch Dis Child Fetal Neonatal Ed 2003;88(5):F383–F390.
53 Colombo J, Kannass KN, Shaddy DJ, et. al. Maternal DHA and the development of attention in infancy and toddlerhood. Child Dev 2004;75(4):1254–1267.
54 Lauritzen L, Jorgensen MH, Olsen SF, et. al. Maternal fish oil supplementation in lactation: effect on developmental outcome in breast-fed infants. Reprod Nutr De 2005;45(5):535–547.
55 Jensen CL, Voigt RG, Prager TC, et. al. Effects of maternal docosahexaenoic acid intake on visual function and neurodevelopment in breastfed term infants. AJCN 2005;82(1):125–132.
56 Dunstan JA, Simmer K, Dixon G, et. al. Cognitive assessment at 2(1/2) years after fish oil supplementation in pregnancy: a randomised controlled trial. Arch Dis Child Fetal Neonatal Ed 2008;93(1):F45–F50.
57 Helland IB, Smith L, Saarem K, et. al. Maternal supplementation with very-long-chain n-3 fatty acids during pregnancy and lactation augments children's IQ at 4 years of age. Pediatrics 2003;111(1).
58 Innis SM, Friessen RW. Essential n-3 fatty acids inpregnant women and early visual acuity maturation in term infants. Am J Clin Nutr 2008;87(3):548–557.
59 Eilander A, Hundscheid DC, Osendarp SJ, et. al. Effects of n-3 long chain polyunsaturated fatty acid supplementation on visual and cognitive development throughout childhood: a review of human studies. Prostaglandins Leukot Essent Fatty Acids 2007;76(4):189–203.
60 Decsi T, Koletzko B. N-3 fatty acids and pregnancy outcomes. Curr Opin Clin Nutr Metab Care 2005;8(2):161–6.
61 Helland IB, Smith L, Blomén B, et. al. Effect of supplementing pregnant and lactating mothers with n-3 very-long-chain fatty acids on children's IQ and body mass index at 7 years of age. Pediatrics 2008;122(2):e472–9.
62 Haider BA, Bhutta ZA. Multiple micronutrient supplementation for women during pregnancy. Cochrane Database of Systematic Reviews 2006, Issue 4. Art. No.: CD004905. doi: 10.1002/14651858.CD004905.pub2.
63 Goh YI, Bollano E, Einarson TR, et. al. Prenatal multivitamin supplementation and rates of pediatric cancers: a meta–analysis. Clin Pharmacol Ther 2007;81:685–691.
64 van den Broek N, Kulier R, Gülmezoglu AM, et. al. Vitamin A supplementation during pregnancy. Cochrane Database of Systematic Reviews 2002, Issue 4. Art. No.: CD001996. doi: 10.1002/14651858.CD001996.
65 Rumbold A, Crowther CA. Vitamin C supplementation in pregnancy. Cochrane Database of Systematic Reviews 2005, Issue 1. Art. No.: CD004072. doi: 10.1002/14651858.CD004072.pub2.
66 Hollis BW, Wagner CL. Editorial. Vitamin D deficiency during pregnancy: an ongoing epidemic. AJCN 2006;84:273.
67 Van der Meer IM, Karamali NS, Boeke JP, et. al. High prevalence of vitamin D deficiency in pregnant non-Western women in the Hague, Netherlands. Am J Clin Nutr 2006;84:350–353.
68 Munns C, Zacharin MR, et. al. Prevention and treatment of infant and childhood vitamin D deficiency in Australia and New Zealand: a consensus statement. MJA 2006;185:268–272.
69 Weisber P, Kelley SS, Ruowei Li, et. al. Nutritional rickets among children in the United States:review of cases reported between 1986–2003. Am J Clin Nutr 2004;80(suppl):1697S–705S.
70 Pettifor JM. Nutritional rickets: deficiency of vitamin D, calcium, or both? Am J Clin Nutr 2004;80(suppl):1725S-9S.
71 Nozza JM, Rodda CP. Vitamin D deficiency in mothers of infants with rickets. MJA 2001;175: 253–55.
72 Mahomed K, Gulmezoglu AM. Vitamin D supplementation in pregnancy. Cochrane Database of Systematic Reviews 1999, Issue 1. Art. No.: CD000228. doi: 10.1002/14651858. CD000228.
73 Wen SW, Chen XK, Rodger M, et. al. Folic acid supplementation in early second trimester and the risk of preeclampsia. Am J Obstet Gynecol 2008;198(1):45.e1–e7.
74 Mills GL, Johansson A, Nordmark A, et. al. Plasma foalte levels and risk of spontaneous abortion. JAMA 2002;288:1867–73.
75 Hernández-Díaz S, Werler MM, Walker AM, et. al. Folic acid antagonists during pregnancy and the risk of birth defects. NEJM 2000;343:1608–14.

76 Krapels IP, van Rooij IA, Ocké MC, et. al. Maternal dietary B vitamin intake, other than folate, and the association with orofacial cleft in the offspring. Eur J Nutr 2004;43(1):7–14. Epub 2004 Jan 6.
77 Krapels IP, van Rooij IA, Ocké MC, et. al. Maternal nutritional status and the risk for orofacial cleft offspring in humans. Nutr 2004;134(11):3106–13.
78 Lumley J, Watson L, Watson M, et. al. Periconceptional supplementation with folate and/or multivitamins for preventing neural tube defects. Cochrane Database of Systematic Reviews 2001, Issue 3. Art. No.: CD001056. doi: 10.1002/14651858.CD001056.
79 Wen SW, Zhou J, Yang Q, et. al. Maternal exposure to folic acid antagonists and placenta-mediated adverse pregnancy outcomes. CMAJ 2009;179: 1263–8.
80 Wen SW, Walker M. Risk of fetal exposure to folic acid antagonists. J Obstet Gynaecol Can 2004;26:475–80.
81 Lagrange AH. Folic acid supplementation for women with epilepsy who might become pregnant nature clinical practice neurology. Nature Clinical Practice Neurology 2009;5(1):16–7.
82 Vajda FJ, O'Brien TJ, Hitchcock A, et. al. Critical relationship between sodium valproate dose and human teratogenicity: results of the Australian register of anti-epileptic drugs in pregnancy. J Clin Neurosci 2004 Nov;11(8):854–83.
83 Whitehall J, Smith J. Valproate and babies. Aust NZ J Psychiatry 2008;42:837.
84 Chavarro JE, Rich-Edwards JW, et. al. Iron intake and risk of ovulatory infertility. Obstet Gynecol 2006;108:1145–52.
85 Lozoff B, De Andraca I, Castillo M, et. al. Behavioural and developmental effects of preventing iron-deficiency anemia in healthy full-term infants. Pediatrics 2003;112 (4):846–854.
86 Eden AN. Iron deficiency and impaired cognition in toddlers: an underestimated and undertreated problem. Paediatr Drugs 2005;7(6):347–52.
87 Peña-Rosas JP, Viteri FE. Effects of routine oral iron supplementation with or without folic acid for women during pregnancy. Cochrane Database of Systematic Reviews 2006, Issue 3. Art. No.: CD004736. doi: 10.1002/14651858.CD004736.pub2.
88 Favier M, Hininger-Favier I. Zinc and pregnancy. Gynecol Obstet Fertil 2005;33(4):253–8.
89 Merialdi M, et. al. Randomised controlled trial of prenatal zinc supplementation and fetal bone growth. AJCN 2004;79:826–30.
90 Fawzi WW, Villamor E, Msamanga GI, et. al. Improves infant mortality, birth weight and duration of pregnancy in HIV mums:Trial of zinc supplements in relation to pregnancy outcomes, hematologic indicators, and T cell counts among HIV-1-infected women in Tanzania. Am J Clin Nutr 2005;81:161–7.
91 Mahomed K, Bhutta Z, Middleton P. Zinc supplementation for improving pregnancy and infant outcome. Cochrane Database of Systematic Reviews 2007, Issue 2. Art. No.: CD000230. doi: 10.1002/14651858.CD000230.pub3.
92 Osendarp SJ, van Raaij JM, Darmstadt GL, et. al. Zinc supplementation during pregnancy and effects on growth and morbidity in low birth weight infants: a randomised placebo controlled trial. Lancet 2001;357:1080–85.
93 Travers CA. et. al. Iodine status in pregnant women and their newborns: are our babies at risk of iodine deficiency? MJA 2006;184:617–20.
94 Gunton JE, Hams G, Fiegert M, et. al. Iodine deficiency in ambulatory participants at a Sydney teaching hospital: is Australia truly iodine replete. MJA 1999;171(9):467–70.
95 Glinoer D. Feto-maternal repercussions of iodine deficiency in pregnancy. Ann Endocrinol 2003;64(1):37–44.
96 Xue-Yi C, Jiang XM, Dou ZH, et. al. Timing of vulnerability of the brain to iodine deficiency in endemic cretinism. NEJM 1994;331(26):1739–44.
97 Kozhimannil KB, Pereira MA, Harlow BL. Association between diabetes and perinatal depression among low-income mothers. JAMA 2009 Feb 25;301(8):842–7.
98 Zhang C, Solomon CG, Manson JE, et. al. A prospective study of pregravid physical activity and sedentary behaviours in relation to the risk for gestational diabetes mellitus. Arch Intern Med 2006 Mar 13;166(5):543–8.
99 Moses Robert G, Barker Megan, Winter Meagan, et. al. Gestational diabetes; can a low glycemic index diet reduce the need for insulin? A randomised trial. Diabetes Care Publish Ahead of Print published online ahead of print March 11, 2009. doi: 10.2337/dc09–0007.
100 Tieu J, Crowther CA, Middleton P. Dietary advice in pregnancy for preventing gestational diabetes mellitus. Cochrane Database of Systematic Reviews 2008, Issue 2. Art. No.: CD006674. doi: 10.1002/14651858.CD006674.pub2.
101 Ray JG, Vermeulen MJ, Shapiro JL, et. al. Maternal and neonatal outcomes in pregestational and gestational diabetes mellitus, and the influence of maternal obesity and weight gain: the DEPOSIT study. Diabetes Endocrine Pregnancy Outcome Study in Toronto. QJM 2001;94:347–56.
102 Hamano T. Women with a history of preeclampsia should be monitored for the onset and progression of chronic kidney disease. J Nutr 2007;137: 2805–08.
103 Marcoux S, Bérubé S, Brisson C, et. al. Job strain and pregnancy-induced hypertension. Epidemiology 1999;10:376–82.
104 Walker SP, Permezel M, Brennecke SP, et. al. Blood pressure in late pregnancy and work outside the home. Obstetrics and Gynecology 2001;97:361–5.
105 Qui C, Coughlin KB, Frederick IO, et. al. Dietary fibre intake in early pregnancy and risk of subsequent preeclampsia. Am JHypertension 2008;21:903–9.
106. Duley L, Henderson-Smart D, Meher S. Altered dietary salt for preventing pre-eclampsia, and its complications. Cochrane Database of Systematic Reviews 2005, Issue 4. Art. No.: CD005548. doi: 10.1002/14651858.CD005548.
107 Rumbold A, Duley L, Crowther CA, et. al. Antioxidants for preventing pre-eclampsia. Cochrane Database of Systematic Reviews 2008, Issue 1. Art. No.: CD004227. doi: 10.1002/14651858. CD004227.pub3.
108 Rumbold A, Middleton P, Crowther CA. Vitamin supplementation for preventing miscarriage. Cochrane Database of Systematic Reviews 2005, Issue 2. Art. No.: CD004073. doi: 10.1002/14651858.CD004073.pub2.
109 Rumbold A, Crowther CA. Vitamin E supplementation in pregnancy. Cochrane Database of Systematic Reviews 2005, Issue 2. Art. No.: CD004069. doi: 10.1002/14651858.CD004069. pub2.

110 Chappell Lucy C, Seed Paul T, Briley Annette L, et. al. Effect of Antioxidants on the Occurrence of Pre-Eclampsia in Women at Increased Risk: A Randomised Trial. Obstetrical Gynecological Survey 2000;55:129–30.

111 Chappell Lucy C, Seed Paul T, et. al. Vitamin C and E supplementation in women at risk of preeclampsia is associated with changes in indices of oxidative stress and placental function. Am J Obstet Gynecol 2002;187:777–84.

112 Beazley D, Ahokas R, Livingston J, et. al. Vitamin C and E supplementation in women at high risk for preeclampsia: A double-blind, placebo-controlled trial. American Journal of Obstetrics and Gynecology 2002;192:520–21.

113 Poston L, Briley AL, Seed PT, et. al. Vitamin C and vitamin E in pregnant women at risk for pre-eclampsia (VIP trial): randomised placebo-controlled trial. Lancet 2006;367:1145–54.

114 Smedts HPM, de Vries JH, Rakhshandehroo M, et. al. High maternal vitamin E intake by diet or supplements is associated with congenital heart defects in the offspring. British Journal of Obstetrics and Gynaecology 2009;16(3):416–423.

115 Villar J, Merialdi M, Gulmezoglu AM. Nutritional interventions during pregnancy for the prevention or treatment of maternal morbidity and pre-term delivery: An overview of randomised controlled trials. J Nutr 2003;133:1606S–1625S.

116 Kumar A, Shukla DK, et. al. Calcium supplementation for the prevention of pre-eclampsia, Int J Gynaecol Obstet 2008;104(1): 32–6.

117 Villar J, Abdel-Aleem H, Merialdi M, et. al. World Health Organization randomised trial of calcium supplementation among low calcium intake pregnant women. Am J Obstet Gynecol 2006;194:639–49.

118 Hofmeyr GJ, Atallah AN, Duley L. Calcium supplementation during pregnancy for preventing hypertensive disorders and related problems. Cochrane Database of Systematic Reviews 2006, Issue 3. Art. No.: CD001059. doi: 10.1002/14651858.CD001059.pub2.

119 Makrides M, Crowther CA. Magnesium supplementation in pregnancy. Cochrane Database of Systematic Reviews 2001, Issue 4. Art. No.: CD000937. doi: 10.1002/14651858.CD000937.

120 Altman D, Carroli G, Duley L, et. al. Do women with pre-eclampsia, and their babies, benefit from magnesium sulphate? The Magpie Trial: a randomised placebo-controlled trial. Lancet 2002;359:1877–90.

121 Meher S, Duley L. Garlic for preventing pre-eclampsia and its complications. Cochrane Database of Systematic Reviews 2006, Issue 3. Art. No.: CD006065. doi: 10.1002/14651858.CD006065.

122 Jewell D, Young G. Interventions for nausea and vomiting in early pregnancy. Cochrane Database of Systematic Reviews 2003, Issue 4. Art. No.: CD000145. doi: 10.1002/14651858.CD000145.

123 Renwick AG. Toxicology of micronutrients: Adverse effects and uncertainty. J Nutr 2006;136:493S–501S.

124 Australian Adverse Drug Reactions Bulletin 2008 August;27;(4).

125 Thaver D, Saeed MA, Bhutta ZA. Pyridoxine (vitamin B6) supplementation in pregnancy. Cochrane Database of Systematic Reviews 2006, Issue 2. Art. No.: CD000179. doi: 10.1002/14651858.CD000179.pub2.

126 Thaver D, Saeed MA, Bhutta ZA. Pyridoxine (vitamin B6) supplementation in pregnancy. Cochrane Database of Systematic Reviews 2006, Issue 2. Art. No.: CD000179. doi: 10.1002/14651858.CD000179.pub2.

127 Jewell D, Young G. Interventions for nausea and vomiting in early pregnancy. The Cochrane Database of Systematic Reviews 2003, Issue 4. Art. No.: CD000145. doi: 10.1002/14651858.CD000145.

128 Barrelli F, Capasso R, et. al. Effectiveness and safety of ginger in the treatment of pregnancy-induced nausea and vomiting. Obstet Gynecol 2005;105(4):849–56.

129 Lee A, Done ML. Stimulation of the wrist acupuncture point P6 for preventing postoperative nausea and vomiting. Cochrane Database of Systematic Reviews 2004, Issue 3. Art. No.: CD003281. doi: 10.1002/14651858.CD003281.pub2.

130 Pack AR, Thomson ME. Effects of topical and systemic folic acid supplementation on gingivitis in pregnancy. J Clin Periodontol 1980;7:402–14.

131 Dahle LO, Berg G, Hammar M, et. al. The effect of oral magnesium substitution on pregnancy-induced leg cramps. Am J Obstet Gynecol 1995;173:175–80.

132 Young GL, Jewell D. Interventions for leg cramps in pregnancy. Cochrane Database Syst Rev 2002;(1):CD000121.

133 Hammar M, Larsson L, Tegler L. Calcium treatment of leg cramps in pregnancy. Effect on clinical symptoms and total serum and ionized serum calcium concentrations. Acta Obstet Gynecol Scand 1981;60:345–7.

134 Dengfeng W, Taixiang W, Lina Hu, et. al.Chinese herbal medicines in the treatment of ectopic pregnancy. Cochrane Database of Systematic Reviews 2007, Issue 4. Art. No.: CD006224. doi:10.1002/14651858.CD006224.pub2.

135 Maconochie N, Doyle P, Prior S, et. al. Risk factors for first trimester miscarriage--results from a UK-population-based case-control study. BJOG 2007;114(2):170–86.

136 Weng X, Odouli R, Li DK. Maternal caffeine consumption during pregnancy and the risk of miscarriage: a prospective cohort study. Am J Obstet Gynecol 2008;198(3):279.e1–e8.

137 Rumbold A, Middleton P, Crowther CA. Vitamin supplementation for preventing miscarriage. Cochrane Database of Systematic Reviews 2005, Issue 2. Art. No.: CD004073. doi: 10.1002/14651858.CD004073.pub2.

138 de la Calle N, Usandizaga R, Sancha M, et. al. Homocysteine, folic acid and B-group vitamins in obstetrics and gynaecology. Eur J Obstet Gynecol Reprod Biol 2003;107(2):125–34.

139 Nelen WL, Blom HJ, Thomas CM, et. al. Methylenetetrahydrofolate reductase polymorphism affects the change in homocysteine and folate concentrations resulting from low dose folic acid supplementation in women with unexplained recurrent miscarriages. J Nutr 1998;128(8): 1336–41.

140 Rostami K. Coeliac disease and reproductive disorders: a neglected association. Eur J Obstet Gynecol Reprod Biol 2001;96(2):146–9.

141 Hetzel BS. Story of iodine deficiency: an international challenge in nutrition. Oxford University Press, New York, 1989.

142 George L, Mills JL, Johansson AL, et. al. Plasma folate levels and risk of spontaneous abortion. JAMA 2002;288:1867–73.

143 Slama R, Bouyer J, Windham G, et. al. Influence of paternal age on the risk of spontaneous abortion. Am J Epidemiol 2005;161:816–23.
144 Verkleij-Hagoort AC, de Vries JH, et. al. Dietary intake of B-vitamins in mothers born a child with a congenital heart defect. Eur J Nutr 2006;45(8): 478–86.
145 Smedts HP, Rakhshandehroo M, Verkleij-Hagoort AC, et. al. Maternal intake of fat, riboflavin and nicotinamide and the risk of having offspring with congenital heart defects. Eur J Nutr 2008;47(7): 357–65.
146 Hobel C, Culhune J. Role of psychosocial and nutritional stress on poor pregnancy outcome. J Nutr 2003;133:1790S-1717S.
147 Li D, Liu L, Odouli R. Presence of depressive symptoms during early pregnancy and the risk of pre-term delivery: a prospective cohort study. Hum Reprod. 2009 Jan;24(1):146–53. Epub 2008 Oct 23. PubMed PMID: 18948314.
148 Dayan J. Creveuil, C Herlicoviez M, et. al. Role of Anxiety and Depression in the Onset of Spontaneous Pre-term Labour. Am J Epidemiol 2002:155(4): 293–301.
149 Narendran S, Nagarathna R, Narendran V, et. al. Swami Vivekananda Yoga Anusandhana Samsthana (sVYASA), Vivekananda Yoga. Research Foundation, Bangalore, India. 'Efficacy of yoga on pregnancy outcome.J Altern Complement Med 2005;11(2):237–44.
150 Evenson KR, Siega-Riz AM, Savitz DA, et. al. Vigorous Leisure Activity and Pregnancy Outcome. Epidemiology 2002;13:653–59.
151 Polyzos Nikolaos P, Polyzos Ilias P, Mauri Davide, et. al. Effect of periodontal disease treatment during pregnancy on pre-term birth incidence: a metaanalysis of randomised trials. American Journal of Obstetrics and Gynecology 2009 March;225–32.
152 Marakoglu I, Gursoy UK, Marakoglu K, et. al. Periodontitis as a risk factor for pre-term low birth weight. Yonsei Med J 2008;49(2):200–3.
153 Pitiphat J, Joshipura KJ, Gillman MW, et. al. Maternal periodontitis and adverse pregnancy outcomes. Community Dent Oral Epidemiol 2008;36:3–11.
154 Mercer BM, Merlino AA, Milluzzi CJ, et. al. Small fetal size before 20 weeks' gestation: associations with maternal tobacco use, early pre-term birth, and low birth weight. Am J Obstet Gynecol 2008;198(6):673.e1–e7.
155 Suzuki K, Tanaka T, Kondo N, et. al. Is maternal smoking during early pregnancy a risk factor for all low birth weight infants? J Epidemiol 2008;18: 89–96.
156 Wills R, Coory MD. Effect of smoking among Indigenous and non-Indigenous mothers on pre-term birth and full-term low birth weight. MJA 2008;189(9):490–4.
157 Jaddoe VWV, Troe E, Hofman A, et. al. Active and passive smoking during pregnancy and the risks of low birth weight and pre-term birth: the generation R study. Paed Perinat Epidem 2008;20:162–71.
158 Leonardi-Bee J, Smyth A, Britton J, et. al. Environmental tobacco smoke and fetal health: systematic review and meta-analysis. Arch Dis Child Fetal Neonatal Ed 2008;93(5):F351–61.
159 Kyrklund-Blomberg Nina B, Cnattingius Sven. Pre-term birth and maternal smoking: Risks related to gestational age and onset of delivery. Am J Obstet Gynecol 1998;179(4):1051–55.
160 Olsen SF, Secher NJ. Low consumption of seafood in early pregnancy as a risk factor for pre-term delivery: prospective cohort study. BMJ 2002;324:447–50.
161 Khoury J, Henriksen T, Christophersen B, et. al. Effect of a cholesterol-lowering diet on maternal, cord, and neonatal lipids, and pregnancy outcome: a randomised clinical trial. Am J Obstet Gynecol 2005;193:1292–301.
162 Cook Derek G, Peacock Janet L, Feyerabend Colin, et. al. Relation of caffeine intake and blood caffeine concentrations during pregnancy to fetal growth: prospective population based study. BMJ 1996 313:1358–62.
163 Bodil Hammer Bech, Carsten Obel, et. al. Effect of reducing caffeine intake on birth weight and length of gestation: randomised controlled trial. BMJ 2007;334:409.
164 Clausson B, Granath F, Ekbom A, et. al. Effect of caffeine exposure during pregnancy on birth weight and gestational age. Am J Epidemiol 2002;155:429–36.
165 Bracken MB, Triche EW, Belanger K, et. al. Association of maternal caffeine consumption with decrements in fetal growth. Am J Epidemiol 2002;155:429–36.
166 CARE Study Group. Maternal caffeine intake during pregnancy and risk of fetal growth restriction: a large prospective observational study. BMJ 2008;337:a2332.
167 Wendler CC, Busovsky-McNeal B, Ghatpande S, et. al. Embryonic caffeine exposure induces adverse effects in adulthood . FASEB J 2008 as doi:10.1096/ fj.08–124941.
168 Bech BH, Nohr EA, Vaeth M, et. al. Coffee and fetal death: a cohort study with prospective data. Am J Epidmiol 2005;162:983–990.
169 McPhee, A. JAMA 2009;301:175–182.
170 Makrides M, Crowther CA. Magnesium supplementation in pregnancy. Cochrane Database of Systematic Reviews 2001, Issue 4. Art. No.: CD000937. doi: 10.1002/14651858.CD000937.
171 Doyle LW, Crowther CA, Middleton P, et. al. Magnesium sulphate for women at risk of pre-term birth for neuroprotection of the fetus. Cochrane Database of Systematic Reviews 2007, Issue 3. Art. No.: CD004661. doi: 10.1002/14651858. CD004661.pub2.
172 Nilsen RM, Vollset SE, Rasmussen SA, et. al. Folic acid and Multivitamin Supplement Use and Risk of Placental Abruption: A Population-based Registry Study. Am J Epidemiol 2008. Epub ahead of print.
173 Elizabeth KE, Krishnan V, Zachariah P. Auxologic, biochemical and clinical (ABC) profile of low birth weight babies – a two-year prospective study. Trop Med 2007;53(6):374–82.
174 Elizabeth KE, Krishnan V, Vijayakumar T. Umbilical cord blood nutrients in low birth weight babies in relation to birth weight and gestational age. Indian J Med Res 2008;128(2):128–33.
175 Newman RB, Goldenberg RL, Moawad AH, et. al. Occupational fatigue and pre-term premature rupture of membranes. National Institute of Child Health and Human Development Maternal-Fetal Medicine, Units Network. Am J Obstet Gynecol 2001 Feb;184(3):438–46.
176 Siega-Riz AM, Herrmann TS, Savitz DA, et. al. Frequency of eating during pregnancy and its effect on pre-term delivery. Am J Epidemiol 2001;153:647–52.
177 Siega-Riz AM, Promislow JH, Savitz DA, et. al. Vitamin C and the risk of pre-term delivery. Am J Obstet Gynecol 2003;189(2):519–25.

178 Casanueva E, Ripoll C, Tolentoin M, et. al. Vitamin C supplementation to prevent premature rupture of the chorioamnionic membranes: a randomised trial. ACJN. 2005;81:859–64.

179 Woods JR Jr, Plessinger MA, Miller RK. Vitamins C and E: missing links in preventing pre-term premature rupture of membranes? Am J Obstet Gynecol. 2001 Jul;185(1):5–10.

180 Olsen SF, Secher NJ, Tabor A, et. al. Randomised clinical trials of fish oil supplementation in high risk pregnancies. Fish Oil Trials In Pregnancy (FOTIP) Team. BJOG 2000;107:382–95.

181 Othman M, Neilson JP, Alfirevic Z. Probiotics for preventing pre-term labour. Cochrane Database of Systematic Reviews 2007, Issue 1. Art. No.: CD005941. doi: 10.1002/14651858.CD005941.pub2.

182 AlFaleh KM, Bassler D. Probiotics for prevention of necrotizing enterocolitis in pre-term infants. Cochrane Database of Systematic Reviews 2008, Issue 1. Art. No.: CD005496. doi: 10.1002/14651858.CD005496.pub2.

183 Pennick V, Young G. Interventions for preventing and treating pelvic and back pain in pregnancy. Cochrane Database of Systematic Reviews 2007, Issue 2. Art. No.: CD001139. doi: 10.1002/14651858.CD001139.pub2.

184 Carolyn E, Manheimer, E, Pirotta, M, White A. Acupuncture for pelvic and back pain in pregnancy: a systematic review. American Journal of Obstetrics and Gynecology 2008;March;254–59.

185 Waldenström U, Hildingsson I, Ryding EL. Antenatal fear of childbirth and its association with subsequent caesarean section and experience of childbirth. BJOG 2006;113:638–46.

186 Anim-Somuah M, Smyth R, Howell C. Epidural versus non-epidural or no analgesia in labour. Cochrane Database of Systematic Reviews 2005, Issue 4. Art. No.: CD000331. doi: 10.1002/14651858.CD000331.pub2.

187 Cepeda MS, Carr DB, Lau J, et. al. Music for pain relief. Cochrane Database of Systematic Reviews 2006, Issue 2. Art. No.: CD004843. doi:10.1002/14651858. CD004843.pub2.

188 Chuntharapat S, Petpichetchian W, Hatthakit U. Yoga during pregnancy: effects on maternal comfort, labour pain and birth outcomes. Complement Ther Clin Pract 2008;14:105–15.

189 Narendran S, Nagarathna R, Narendran V, et. al. Efficacy of yoga on pregnancy outcome. J Altern Complement Med 2005;11:237–44.

190 Chuntharapat S, Petpichetchian W, Hatthakit U. Yoga during pregnancy: effects on maternal comfort, labour pain and birth outcomes. Complement Ther Clin Pract 2008;14:105–15.

191 Narendran S, Nagarathna R, Narendran V, et. al. Efficacy of yoga on pregnancy outcome. J Altern Complement Med 2005;11:237–44.

192 Smith CA, Collins CT, Cyna AM, et. al. Complementary and alternative therapies for pain management in labour. Cochrane Database of Systematic Reviews 2006, Issue 4. Art. No.: CD003521. doi: 10.1002/14651858.CD003521.pub2.

193 Cluett ER, Nikodem VC, McCandlish RE, et. al. Immersion in water in pregnancy, labour and birth. Cochrane Database of Systematic Reviews 2002, Issue 2. Art. No.: CD000111. doi: 10.1002/14651858.CD000111.pub2.

194 Salvesen KA, Mørkved S. Randomised controlled trial of pelvic floor muscle training during pregnancy. BMJ 2004;329:378–80.

195 Smith CA. Homoeopathy for induction of labour. Cochrane Database of Systematic Reviews 2003, Issue 4. Art. No.: CD003399. doi: 10.1002/14651858.CD003399.

196 Dahlen HG, Homer CS, Cooke M, et. al. Perineal outcomes and maternal comfort related to the application of perineal warm packs in the second stage of labour: a randomised controlled trial. Birth 2007;34(4):282–90.

197 Raynes-Greenow CH, Roberts CL, Barratt A, et. al. Pregnant women's preferences and knowledge of term breech management, in an Australian setting. Midwifery 2004;20:181–87.

198 Coyle ME, Smith CA, Peat B. Cephalic version by moxibustion for breech presentation. Cochrane Database of Systematic Reviews 2005, Issue 2. Art. No.: CD003928. doi: 10.1002/14651858. CD003928.pub2.

199 Beckmann MM, Garrett AJ. Antenatal perineal massage for reducing perineal trauma. Cochrane Database of Systematic Reviews 2006, Issue 1. Art. No.: CD005123. doi: 10.1002/14651858.CD005123.pub2.

200 East CE, Begg L, Henshall NE, et. al. Local cooling for relieving pain from perineal trauma sustained during childbirth. Cochrane Database of Systematic Reviews 2007, Issue 4. Art. No.: CD006304. doi: 10.1002/14651858. CD006304.pub2.

201 Hay-Smith J. Therapeutic ultrasound for post-partum perineal pain and dyspareunia. Cochrane Database of Systematic Reviews 1998, Issue 3. Art. No.: CD000495. doi: 10.1002/14651858. CD000495.

202 Dennis CL, Allen K. Interventions (other than pharmacological, psychosocial or psychological) for treating antenatal depression. Cochrane Database of Systematic Reviews 2008, Issue 4. Art. No.: CD006795. doi: 10.1002/14651858.CD006795. pub2.

203 Dennis CL. Review: Psychosocial and psychological interventions reduce post-partum depressive symptoms. Evidence-Based Mental Health 2008;11:79.

204 Morrell CJ, Slade P, Warner R, et. al. Clinical effectiveness of health visitor training in psychologically informed approaches for depression in postnatal women: pragmatic cluster randomised trial in primary care. BMJ 2009;338:a3045.

205 Cornish AM, McMahon CA, Ungerer JA, et. al. Postnatal depression and infant cognitive and motor development in the second postnatal year: The impact of depression chronicity and infant gender. Infant Behav Dev 2005;28:407–17.

206 Cowley D. Antidepressants in Pregnancy: The Ongoing Story. Journal Watch Psychiatry December 29, 2006. http://psychiatry.jwatch.org/cgi/content/full/2006/1229/4 (accessed February 2009).

207 ACOG Committee on Obstetric Practice. ACOG Committee Opinion No. 354: Treatment with selective serotonin reuptake inhibitors during pregnancy. Obstet Gynecol 2006;108:1601–3.

208 Levinson-Castiel R, Merlob P, Linder N, et. al. Neonatal abstinence syndrome after in utero exposure to selective serotonin reuptake inhibitors in term infants. Arch Pediatr Adolesc Med 2006;160:173–6.

209 Chun-Fai-Chan B, Koren G, Fayez I, et. al. Pregnancy outcome of women exposed to bupropion during pregnancy: a prospective comparative study. Am J Obstet Gynecol 2005;192:932–6.

210 Hiscock H, Wake M. Infant sleep problems and postnatal depression: a community-based study. Pediatrics. 2001;107(6):1317–22.

211 Hiscock H, Wake M. Randomised controlled trial of behavioural infant sleep intervention to improve infant sleep and maternal mood. BMJ 2002;324(7345):1062–5.

212 Hiscock H, Bayer JK, Hampton A, et. al. Long-term mother and child mental health effects of a population-based infant sleep intervention: cluster-randomised, controlled trial. Pediatrics 2008;122(3):e621–7.

213 Freeman MP, et. al. Randomised dose-ranging pilot trial of omega-3 fatty acids for post-partum depression. Acta Psychiatr Scand 2006;113(1): 31–5.

214 M. Freeman. Complementary and alternative medicine for perinatal depression. Journal of Affective Disorders 112(1):1–10.

215 Allen L. Multiple micronutrients in pregnancy and lactation: an overview. AJCN 2005;81:1206s–1212s.

216 Strandberg TE, Anderson S, Järvenpää AL, McKeigue PM. Premature birth and liquorice consumption during pregnancy. American Journal Epidemiology 2002;156(9):803–5

217 Gallo M, et. al. Pregnancy outcome following gestational exposure to echinacea: a prospective controlled study. Arch Intern Med 2000;160:3141–43.

218 Medicines Control Agency Report. Online. Available: http://www.mhra.gov.uk/index.htm (accessed February 2009).

219 Järvenpää AL, Vanhanen H, McKeigue PM. Birth Outcome in Relation to Licorice Consumption during Pregnancy. Am J Epidemiol 2001;153:1085–8.

220 Strandberg TE, Andersson S, Järvenpää AL, et. al. Pre-term Birth and Licorice Consumption during Pregnancy. Am J Epidemiol 2002;156:803–5.

221 Hughes J, Sellick S, King R, et. al. Pre-termbirth and licorice consumption during pregnancy. Am J Epidemiol 2003;158:190–4.

222 Angelsen NK, Vik T, Jacobsen G, et. al. Breast feeding and cognitive development at age 1 and 5 years. Arch Dis Child 2001;85(3):183–8.

223 Anderson JW, Johnstone BM, Remley DT. Breast-feeding and cognitive development: a meta-analysis. AJCN 1999;70(4):525–35.

224 Kramer MS, Aboud F, Mironova E, et. al. Breastfeeding and child cognitive development: new evidence from a large randomised trial. Arch Gen Psychiatry 2008;65(5):578–84.

225 Helland IB, Smith L, Saarem K, et. al. Maternal supplementation with very-long-chain n-3 fatty acids during pregnancy and lactation augments children's IQ at 4 years of age. Pediatrics 2003;111(1):e39–e44.

226 Gustafsson PA, Duchen K, Birberg U, et. al. Breastfeeding, very long polyunsaturated fatty acids (PUFA) and IQ at 6 1/2 years of age. Acta Paediatr 2004;93(10):1280–87.

227 Lauritzen L, Hoppe C, Straarup EM, et. al. Maternal fish oil supplementation in lactation and growth during the first 2.5 years of life. Pediatr Res 2005;58 (2):235–42.

228 Van der Wijden C, Brown J, Kleijnen J. Lactational amenorrhea for family planning. Cochrane Database of Systematic Reviews 2003, Issue 4. Art. No.: CD001329. doi: 10.1002/14651858.CD001329. Online. Available: www.cochrane.org/reviews/en/ab0 01329.html (accessed January 2009).

Chapter 33

Premenstrual syndrome

With contribution from Dr Gillian Singleton

Introduction

A great majority of women will experience premenstrual symptoms at some time in their lives. Some women, however, experience more severe and troublesome symptoms that can impact daily living. This condition is defined as premenstrual syndrome (PMS). PMS can affect up to 90% of women of childbearing age with 2–10% of women experiencing severe, incapacitating symptoms. PMS is characterised by the cyclical recurrence of broad and varied symptoms which are in the luteal phase of the menstrual cycle, and which remit at the onset of menstruation or in the days following.[1–5] These symptoms include emotional, behavioural and physical symptoms (which are outlined in more detail in Table 33.1).[6,7] Some women predominantly experience mood, cyclical mastalgia or dysmenorrhoea symptoms during the luteal phase.

Premenstrual dysphoric disorder (PMDD)

When premenstrual symptoms are dominated by severe disturbances of mood and behaviour that are associated with major disruption to daily activities and relationships, the condition is known as premenstrual dysphoric disorder (PMDD).[3] PMDD affects around 3–5% of women of reproductive age.[5, 8, 9]

Some studies have found an association between the luteal phase and exacerbations of psychiatric disorders, including obsessive-compulsive disorder, schizophrenia, increased alcohol consumption in alcoholism, and increased incidence of suicide attempts. This postulates serotonin dysregulation as a possible causative factor.[10]

The DSM IV diagnostic criteria for PMDD include at least 5 of 11 symptoms occurring in the week prior to menstruation for the majority of months of the previous year, which remit in the post-menstrual week.[11] These symptoms markedly interfere with daily activities and interpersonal relationships.

Table 33.2 lists the common symptoms of PMDD.

Dysmenorrhoea

Primary dysmenorrhoea is defined as the occurrence of painful menstrual cramps, in the absence of pelvic pathology, and occurs in up to 80% of young women, with over 50% of these individuals experiencing limitations to their daily activities, such as work and schooling.[12] Primary dysmenorrhoea is hypothesised to be caused by uterine contractions in response to prostaglandin, leukotriene and vasopressin release.

This condition needs to be differentiated from secondary dysmenorrhoea where the pain is caused by an underlying disease process. Causes of secondary dysmenorrhoea include endometriosis, adenomyosis, post-surgical adhesions, endometrial fibroid tumours, pelvic inflammatory disease, psychosomatic disorders, depression, inflammatory bowel disease, diverticulitis, bladder problems and urogenital cancers. It is obviously important to exclude these secondary causes of pelvic pain prior to treatment.

Cyclical mastalgia

Breast pain or mastalgia is a common symptom experienced by women especially in the premenstrual phase. Overall, 92% of patients with cyclical mastalgia and 64% with non-cyclical mastalgia can obtain relief of their pain with the use of available therapies.[13]

Aetiology of premenstrual symptoms

Several hypotheses have been postulated as to the exacerbating factors for and causation of symptoms of PMS, PMDD, cyclical mastalgia and dysmenorrhoea. These include:

- excess or deficiency of progesterone
- abnormal secretion of oestrogen
- abnormality of endogenous opiates
- excess or deficiency of cortisone, androgens or prolactin
- excess anti-diuretic hormone from posterior pituitary gland

Table 33.1 Common symptom of PMS

Psychological	Irritability, anger, depressed mood, tearfulness, anxiety, tension, mood swings, difficulties with concentration and memory, confusion, restlessness, decreased self-esteem, tension, feelings of being overwhelmed, of loneliness and hopelessness
Behavioural	Insomnia, changes in libido, food cravings or overeating
Physical	Fatigue, dizziness, headaches, mastalgia, back pain, abdominal pain and bloating, weight gain, constipation, fluid retention (up to 1kg of weight), nausea, myalgias and arthralgias

Table 33.2 Common symptoms of PMDD using DSM IV criteria

Depressive symptoms	Markedly depressed mood, feelings of hopelessness, self-deprecation Affective lability. Suddenly feeling sad or tearful, with increased sensitivity to personal rejection Decreased interest in usual activitiesLethargy, fatigue, marked lack of energy Accompanying depressive symptoms there is always the danger for suicidal ideation and risk-taking behaviours Marked changes in appetite and cravings for certain foodsInsomnia or hypersomnia
Anxiety symptoms	Marked anxiety, and tension Persistent or marked irritability, anger, and subsequent increased interpersonal conflicts Feeling overwhelmed or out of control
Cognitive symptoms	Subjective sense of having difficulty concentrating
Physical symptoms	Breast tenderness or swelling, headaches, joint or muscular pain, weight gain, bloating

- excess or deficiency of prostaglandins
- psychological, social or genetic factors.

Pharmaceutical and hormone therapies

A number of pharmaceuticals and hormone therapies are used successfully for the management and alleviation of symptoms of PMS, PMDD, cyclical mastalgia and dysmenorrhoea but it is not within the scope of this chapter to cover these therapies. Pharmaceutical and hormone treatment include:

- prostaglandin inhibitors (e.g. non-steroidal anti-inflammatory medication)
- analgesics
- hormonal therapies — oestrogen, and/or progestogen treatment (e.g. IUD, oral contraceptive pill, minipill, depo provera) and testosterone
- antidepressants and anti-anxiolytic agents such as selective serotonin reuptake inhibitors
- antidiuretics and anti-diuretic hormone inhibitors
- anti-androgens.

Role of complementary medicine and integrative therapies in PMS

Treatment goals for PMS, PMDD, cyclical mastalgia and dysmenorrhoea are determined by the severity of the symptomatology, with the aim to ameliorate or eliminate symptoms and reduce the impact of symptoms on activities of daily living and interpersonal relationships.

The use of complementary medicine is popular amongst women with PMS, PMDD and dysmenorrhoea and plays an important role in management of symptoms.[14] While mainstream medical treatment for PMS is commonly used, a large scale survey of medical and nurse practitioners, including gynaecologists, indicated that at least 90% reported recommending at least 1 complementary therapy, primarily for pain management for women with PMS.[15] Chiropractic, acupuncture, massage, and behavioural medicine techniques such as meditation and relaxation training were cited as the most commonly recommended.

A 2003 systematic review[16] identified 33 randomised control trials (RCTs) for complementary medicine use in PMS, 13 of which were for dysmenorrhoea. There is an increasing body of evidence supporting the use of complementary therapies and lifestyle interventions in the management of PMS symptoms. To date a number of therapeutic interventions including calcium supplementation, vitex agnus castus, stress reduction, cognitive behavioural therapy (CBT) and relaxation therapy and exercise have been shown to be beneficial. The authors' conclude that preliminary studies indicate a role for further research on magnesium, vitamin B1 and B6, low-fat diet, fish oil supplementation for dysmenorrhoea, St John's wort and L-tryptophan supplementation for PMDD.[16]

Another review of the literature for treatment of PMS and PMDD identified a number of useful non-pharmacological treatments with some evidence for efficacy including cognitive behavioural relaxation therapy, aerobic exercise, as well as calcium, magnesium, vitamin B6, L-tryptophan supplementation and a complex carbohydrate drink. [17]

This chapter will outline in more detail potential lifestyle and non-pharmaceutical approaches which may assist PMS symptoms, including the evidence on efficacy and safety for these approaches.

General lifestyle interventions

Lifestyle interventions such as dietary changes, sodium and caffeine restriction, regular daily exercise, and stress reduction can improve quality of life (QOL) and significantly reduce symptoms of PMS, including mood and pain symptoms, experienced by women. Patient education and supportive strategies, such as use of a symptom diary, can help in diagnosing, understanding and managing the disorders. It is clear that women need reassurance and education about effective treatment options available to them.

Symptom diary and management

The PMS Symptom Management Program (PMS-SMP) includes non-pharmacological strategies incorporating self-monitoring, emphasis on personal choice, self-regulation, and self/environmental modification, with peer support and professional guidance. A study designed to establish the effectiveness of this program randomised 91 women with severe PMS to early treatment groups (n = 40) or waiting treatment groups (n = 51) over an 18-month period.[18] The PMS-SMP was effective in reducing PMS severity by 75%, premenstrual depression, and general distress by 30–54%, as well as increasing wellbeing and self-esteem in women experiencing severe PMS compared with antidepressant drug treatments that report a 40–52% reduction in PMS severity in studies. The improvement was maintained in the long-term follow-up.[18]

Addressing attitude to menstruation and rest

An area rarely addressed in the literature is the importance of assessing the woman's attitude towards menstruation. A woman's attitude and perception can be influenced by her family member's or her peer's previous experiences with menarche and menstruation on the background of her own level of knowledge about this stage of her life. Negative experience of peers and female role models with menarche and menstruation can obviously influence a young woman's perception of what to expect with her own menses. Alternatively, if menarche comes unexpectedly, she may respond negatively or positively, depending on her own life skills and her level of communication with her family members and peers.

There are a multitude of negative terms which have been used in many societies to describe menarche; conversely there are cultures where menarche is celebrated and viewed as a positive entrance into womanhood. An example of this is Ayurveda, which is an ancient Asian tradition of medicine that is over 2000 years old. Ayurvedic tradition views menstruation as an opportunity for a woman's body to 'purify', rather than as a problem. They encourage respect for menstruation and aim to facilitate it and employ methods to experience greater comfort. The tradition promotes women to stay at home as much as possible during menstruation as the woman's body undergoes changes. There any many traditional cultures with similar beliefs which advise women to rest during menstruation.

Minimising sexual activity during the premenstrual phase may help reduce pelvic pain.

Mind–body medicine

Cognitive and behavioural interventions

Improving knowledge, supportive therapy, addressing dysfunctional thinking and encouragement of behavioural changes can significantly impact on women's perception of PMS and menstruation and on their ability to better manage their symptoms appropriately. Educating women about the biological changes in their bodies has been reported to facilitate an increased sense of control and relief of symptoms.[19]

There has been evidence of an increased placebo-response rate demonstrated in symptomatic improvement from formal psychological interventions such as relaxation therapy and CBT in some studies.[20] These interventions include keeping a symptom diary to help identify when behavioural and psychological changes are necessary, having adequate rest and exercise, and making healthy dietary changes.[21]

A number of studies have supported the role of CBT in managing PMS, particularly for pain and dysphoric symptoms. A study of 84 women with PMS, examined the efficacy of enhanced coping skills training that included cognitive restructuring, reducing negative emotions, effective problem-solving assertiveness and relaxation training, in direct comparison with hormone treatment with Duphaston, a synthetic progestogen.[22] The group of women randomised to coping skills training obtained substantial relief of affective and cognitive symptoms when compared to women in the hormone therapy group; this relief was particularly noted in women with severe PMS symptoms. These symptomatic benefits persisted at the 3-month follow-up following intervention.[22]

A 2005 Cochrane systematic review of 14 RCTs looking at management strategies for chronic pelvic pain, demonstrated that 'counselling supported by ultrasound scanning was associated with reduced pain and improvement in mood'.[23]

A 2007 Cochrane systematic review of the effectiveness of behavioural therapies in management of dysmenorrhoea included 5 RCTs. The results of this review demonstrated that there is some evidence for the use of behavioural interventions such as relaxation techniques and pain management training in reducing symptoms to cause fewer restrictions in daily activities.[24]

Another study aimed to modify dysfunctional thinking as a means of impacting on negative premenstrual symptoms.[25] The CBT group involved cognitive restructuring and assertion training. A comparison group called 'information-focused therapy' (IFT) were presented with information only on relaxation training, nutritional and vitamin guidelines, dietary and lifestyle recommendations, and assertion training, and did not address belief restructuring. Both groups equally displayed amelioration of anxiety, depression, negative thoughts and physical changes in women with PMS.

A 2009 systematic review of studies that investigated the use of CBT for PMS or PMDD identified 3 RCTs comparing CBT with pharmacotherapy and a number of case studies.[26] The researchers highlighted the benefits of applying mindfulness and acceptance-based CBT interventions to individuals with PMS/PMDD and suggested more methodologically rigorous research be done in this area.

Psychosocial support

It is important that the impacts of PMS/PMDD on a woman's life and relationships are dealt with on a social level. The involvement of partners, friends, family, teachers and employers in the education process is important to allow them to understand the woman who is experiencing severe symptoms that may impact on her ability to function in her normal daily activities, and that she may benefit from empathy, social support and possibly financial assistance.

Counselling may also be required to address sexual, fertility and relationship consequences in women affected by chronic pelvic pain, dysmenorrhoea, mood changes, lowered libido and dyspareunia.

Stress reduction, relaxation therapies and massage

A number of studies have demonstrated that women can gain symptomatic benefit from the use of relaxation therapies and massage.

A 2004 study of 114 women divided them into high and low symptom severity PMS groups and compared these groups on stress and QOL variables. The results revealed that women with severe PMS symptoms had significantly more stress and poorer QOL than women with low symptom scores.[27]

A 5-month study published in *Obstetrics and Gynecology*, examined the effects of the relaxation response on PMS symptoms in 46 women who were randomly assigned to 1 of 3 groups: a charting group who kept a daily diary of symptoms experienced, a reading group who read leisure material twice daily in combination with charting symptoms, and a relaxation response group who elicited a relaxation response twice daily as well as charting symptoms.[28] The relaxation response group showed significant improvement (58.0%), in comparison to the reading groups (27.2%) and the charting group (17.0%) of reduction in physical and emotional symptoms. The authors conclude that 'regular relaxation response is an effective treatment for physical and emotional premenstrual symptoms, and is most effective in women with severe symptoms'.[28]

Another trial had 24 women with PMDD randomly assigned to either a massage therapy or a relaxation therapy group (Progressive Muscle relaxation therapy).[29] The massage therapy group demonstrated reduction in pain, anxiety and depressed mood immediately after the massage sessions, especially in women treated weekly for 5 weeks, who also experienced reduced fluid retention and overall menstrual distress. The relaxation group also demonstrated improved symptoms but not to the same degree of benefit from massage therapy. While the findings demonstrate massage therapy may be an effective short-term treatment for severe symptoms of PMS, no long-term changes were observed in the massage therapy group.

Sleep

Sleep disturbances are common in women with severe symptoms of PMS, PMDD and dysmenorrhoea. Variations in core temperature, metabolic rate and hormones throughout the menstrual cycle may contribute to changes in sleep patterns and quality of sleep particularly in the luteal phase and menstruation.[30] Women experiencing negative mood changes in the premenstrual period also demonstrate significantly less delta wave sleep during both menstrual cycle phases in comparison with asymptomatic subjects.[31] Evidence also indicates that variations in other circadian rhythms, such as melatonin and cortisol, may also be affected in the luteal phase of the menstrual cycle which may negatively impact sleep patterns.

A study of 68 nurses under 40 years of age completed a survey evaluating sleep, menstrual function and pregnancy outcomes. Fifty-three percent of the women noted menstrual changes when working shift work and the findings suggest that sleep disturbances may lead to menstrual irregularities, and changes in menstrual function.[32] Another study also demonstrated how disruption of circadian rhythms as seen in women working night shifts are more likely to report menstrual irregularities, longer menstrual cycles, abnormalities of reproductive function and mood changes than non-shift workers.[33] The authors also concluded there was accumulating evidence 'that circadian disruption increases the risk of breast cancer in women, possibly due to altered light exposure and reduced melatonin secretion'.[33]

A regular structured sleep schedule is therefore recommended, especially during the luteal phase, to minimise premenstrual symptoms.

Sunshine and vitamin D

It is likely that regular exposure to sunshine plays an important role in regulating hormones and sleep patterns, by affecting melatonin circadian rhythms, which is known to affect the menstrual cycle.

The primary source of vitamin D is sunshine exposure which is best combined with regular exercise and may play a role in normalising menstrual cycles.

In a very small study of women suffering polycystic ovarian disease, they received 50 000IU of vitamin D weekly or biweekly, and this helped to normalise their menstrual cycles in over 50% of patients.[34] Whilst the exact underlying mechanism is unclear, it would appear more research is warranted in this area as vitamin D deficiency is common, particularly in cooler climates, in dark skinned women and women with certain dress codes (e.g. veils), and vitamin D may play an important hormone regulatory effect. It is also documented that vitamin D plays an important role in mood regulation, amelioration of depression, myalgias, back pain and in the management of migraine headaches and thus may reduce some of the symptoms experienced with PMS, PMDD and dysmenorrhoea (see chapters on depression, headaches and migraines and musculoskeletal medicine for more references).[35–38]

Interestingly, a number of controlled studies of active bright light therapy in the late luteal phase significantly reduced depression and pre-menstrual tension scores in women with PMDD, compared to baseline, while placebo dim red light treatment did not.[39, 40] These results suggest that bright light therapy can be an effective treatment for depression in the luteal phase, although exposure to daily sunshine and/or vitamin D supplementation (especially if sunshine exposure is not possible), may obviously be more feasible and convenient.

Physical activity/exercise

A number of studies demonstrate that exercise has a positive impact on symptoms of PMS, PMDD and dysmenorrhoea.

A prospective study examined the relationship between exercise participation and menstrual pain, physical symptoms, and negative mood in 21 sedentary women and 20 women who participated in regular exercise for 2 complete menstrual cycles.[41] All women experienced pain during menses compared to the follicular and luteal phases. The findings demonstrated that exercise participants reported less pain than sedentary women during menses, however there was no reported difference in pain experienced in the follicular and luteal phases between the groups. The sedentary group also reported greater symptoms of anxiety during menses. Likewise, another study demonstrated moderate exercise training without major weight, hormonal or menstrual cycle alteration significantly reduced premenstrual and menstrual symptoms including circulatory symptom problems, psychic tension, irritable behaviour, belligerence, and other personality alterations.[42]

A preliminary study of middle-aged women demonstrated that women with PMS who practised regular aerobic exercise reported fewer symptoms than the control subjects.[43]

In a prospective, controlled 6-month trial of exercise training, 2 groups of women, 1 previously sedentary, were commenced on a 6-month conditioning exercise program of increased running or marathon training, and were compared with a control group of women who were not actively involved in an exercise training program but were normally active.[44] Over the 6-month period of the study the first 2 groups demonstrated a reduction in PMS symptoms including fluid retention, depression and anxiety symptoms compared with the control group of women. The control group demonstrated no change in PMS symptomatology. This study demonstrates the direct positive effects of conditioning exercise on PMS. There was no documented hormonal, menstrual cycle, or weight changes in either groups.[44]

Nutritional influences

Diet

A growing body of evidence supports the use of dietary change in managing premenstrual symptoms. Individuals with diets rich in omega-3 fatty acids, calcium and vitamin D and low in animal fats, salt and caffeine are believed to have a reduced incidence of troublesome premenstrual symptoms. The following section outlines the evidence basis for suggesting these dietary changes in patients who experience such symptoms.

Fish

A diet with high content of omega-3 fatty acids as found in oily fish (salmon, trout and mackerel) and in some plant foods, such as raw, fresh nuts and seeds (e.g. walnuts, linseeds, flaxseeds) can contribute to anti-inflammatory effects within the body by raising the series-one and series-three prostaglandins. Conversely, diets high in saturated animal fats usually cause a rise in the series-two prostaglandin levels contributing to increased muscle contractions and inflammation which can lead to uterine contraction pain with menstruation.

A 1995 study of a group of Danish women, which analysed dietary intake of omega-3 and omega-6 fatty acids and correlated results with severity of menstrual pain, demonstrated that a higher ratio of dietary omega-3 to omega-6 fatty acids correlates with reduced menstrual pain.[45]

(Refer to nutritional supplements section later in this chapter for further information regarding omega-3 fatty acid supplementation.)

Vegetarian plant-based diet

A study of 33 women over 4 menstrual cycles was conducted in which the women adhered solely to a plant-based vegetarian diet for 2 menstrual cycles then returned to their normal diets and took a placebo supplement for a further 2 cycles. This study demonstrated that a low-fat, plant-based vegetarian diet of grains, vegetables, legumes and fruits, significantly reduced the duration (from 3.9 to 2.7 days) of pain and reduced associated premenstrual symptoms such as fluid retention and behavioural changes when the diet cycles were compared to the placebo cycles on a normal diet.[46] Several reasons were postulated for its benefit. The plant-based dietary factors were found to raise serum sex-hormone binding globulin (SHBG) by 19% in the diet phase compared to the supplement phase. SHBG binds and inactivates estrogens. It is hypothesised that estrogenic stimulation of the endometrium is then reduced which in turn may limit proliferation of tissues which produce prostaglandins. Another possible reason for symptomatic benefit is that vegetarian diets are generally lower in total fat and that the ratio of omega-3 to omega-6 fatty acids is increased compared to diets rich in animal fats, which results in reduced fluid retention and reduced dysmenorrhoea.

Calcium and vitamin D dietary intake

A case-controlled study within the prospective Nurses Health Study II cohort of women aged 27–44 years free from PMS at baseline were followed up over a 10-year period and assessed for dietary intake of calcium and vitamin D by using a food frequency questionnaire to correlate with development of PMS.[47]

After adjustment for age, parity, smoking status, and other risk factors, women with the highest vitamin D intake (median, 706IU/day) experienced a 40% reduction in the development of PMS symptoms when compared with those in the lowest intake group (median, 112IU/day). Similarly, women with the highest intake of dietary calcium food sources, such as skim or low-fat milk, were also inversely related to PMS, with a 30% risk reduction of developing PMS compared with women with a low intake (median, 529mg/day).[47] Further large-scale clinical trials are warranted to confirm these findings.

(Refer to nutritional supplements section later in this chapter for further information on calcium supplementation.)

Salt restriction

Restricting salt intake may help to minimise abdominal bloating, fluid retention, breast swelling and tenderness. There is a paucity of studies into this intervention. However, in light of the broader health benefits the provision of this advice to patients is obviously worthwhile.

Caffeine restriction

Caffeine is thought to increase premenstrual irritability, insomnia and the incidence of dysmenorrhoea and other premenstrual symptomatology.

A 1985 study investigated the possible association between severity of premenstrual symptoms and consumption of caffeine. The study concluded that consumption of caffeine-containing beverages was strongly associated with PMS symptoms. A dose-dependant relationship was found in women with severe premenstrual symptoms.[48]

Nutritional supplements

Vitamins

Vitamins B6 and B1

There is an increasing body of evidence supporting the use of vitamins B6 and B1 in PMS.

A 2001 Cochrane review, identified 1 small randomised placebo-controlled trial of vitamin B6 which showed that it was more effective at reducing pain than both placebo and a combined formula of magnesium and vitamin B6.[49]

A 2009 systematic review of 10 RCTs of herbs and nutrients suggests that chasteberry herb and vitamin B6 may be effective for PMS, although there was stronger evidence for the use of calcium. The review concluded that vitamin B6 supplementation in doses of 50–100mg/day are likely to be of benefit in reducing premenstrual symptoms.[50]

It should be noted, however, that these doses are far in excess of the recommended daily intake (RDI) of this vitamin and that there is a risk of toxicity if daily doses of 50mg are exceeded. Several cases have been reported to the Australian Adverse Drug Reaction Advisory Committee (ADRAC) in recent years reporting neuropathy which can present with paresthesia, nerve shooting pains, hyperaesthesia and muscle fasciculation in patients taking more than 50mg of vitamin B6/day and thus excessive doses for prolonged periods of time should obviously be avoided.[51] Patients should be warned to stop taking vitamin B6 if they should develop unexplained neurological symptoms suggestive of peripheral neuropathy, such as tingling, burning and numbness of limbs.

One large trial identified by the 2001 Cochrane review demonstrated that 100mgs/day of vitamin B1 to be more effective than placebo in reducing dysmenorrhoea. Vitamin B1 (thiamine) is generally well tolerated, however its absorption may be impaired by concomitant intake of antibiotics, iron and tannins and thus intake of these substances should be separated by 2 hours.[11, 49]

Vitamin E

There is conflicting evidence on the potential role of vitamin E in the management of dysmenorrhea.

The 2001 Cochrane review, referred to previously, identified 1 small trial comparing a combination of vitamin E (taken daily) and ibuprofen (taken during menses) versus ibuprofen (taken during menses) alone that showed no difference in pain relief between the 2 treatments. It should be noted that there was no placebo group in this study.

In a more recent placebo-controlled trial published in the *British Journal of Obstetrics and Gynecology* in 2005, 278 teenage girls with primary dysmenorrhoea were randomised to either vitamin E supplements or placebo.[52] Both groups were permitted to consume 200mgs of ibuprofen 8-hourly for pain as needed. The vitamin E group were instructed to take vitamin E 200mgs twice daily for 5 days (two days before and 3 days after the beginning of menstruation) over 4 consecutive menstrual periods. A symptomatic questionnaire was used to establish the severity and duration of the pain, and also to measure blood loss. The vitamin E group demonstrated significantly less pain, of shorter duration, requiring less consumption of ibuprofen (4.3%) compared with the placebo group (89.4%) for pain. They also noted significant reduction in menstrual blood loss, without any significant side-effects. The mechanism of action for vitamin E is not clear, but is thought to be due to the inhibition of prostaglandin synthesis, which is implicated as a cause of uterine contraction pain.

Minerals

Magnesium

A number of small trials support the use of magnesium in patients with dysmenorrhea and premenstrual mood changes. The results of these studies suggest that further, larger-scale research is warranted.

A 2001 Cochrane review identified 3 small trials that compared the effects of magnesium and placebo for pain relief in women with dysmenorrhoea.[49] Overall the trials showed magnesium to be more effective than placebo for pain relief and the women required less concomitant analgesic medication with its use. There were minimal adverse effects reported. The author's conclude that 'magnesium is a promising treatment for dysmenorrhoea', but it was uncertain from the trials which dose or regime of treatment should be used.[49]

A 1991 small double-blinded randomised placebo-controlled trial examined the effects of supplementation of 360mg/day of magnesium on premenstrual mood changes. Results demonstrated that magnesium supplementation lessened mood symptoms in women with previous PMS compared to placebo.[53]

Calcium

There exists some good evidence to justify the recommendation for use of calcium in PMS. A 2009 systematic review of RCTs found good quality evidence for the use of calcium in PMS.[50]

According to a large case-control study published in *Archives of Internal Medicine 2005*,[54] individuals in the highest quintile of dietary intake of calcium and vitamin D had the risk of PMS reduced by 30%, compared to those with the lowest level of intake. Individuals who ingested 4 or more servings of low-fat milk per day had a 46% reduction in risk compared with women who drank milk once a day. In light of the many health benefits of increased calcium and vitamin D intake including reduced risk of osteoporosis, researchers suggest recommending increased intake of foods rich in these nutrients, even for younger women.

A large study of 466 women reported in *The American Journal of Obstetrics and Gynaecology*[55] showed that 1200mg calcium carbonate versus a placebo taken over 3 months produced a significant reduction in pain and discomfort, fluid retention, mood disorders, and food cravings (48% effective compared to 30% with placebo) in the premenstrual phase.

Calcium may cause constipation and flatulence and should not be co-administered with zinc, magnesium or caffeine. Calcium is best combined with magnesium and vitamin D. Calcium can also interact with calcium channel blockers and cardiac glycosides; high-dose supplementation should be avoided with these medications.[56]

Zinc

Zinc may play a role in the alleviation of dysmenorrhoea, however the current evidence for this is weak. An analysis of 5 case studies of women using up to 30mg of zinc once to 3 times a day for 1 to 4 days immediately prior to menses was able to prevent dysmenorrhoea although the researchers recommended additional study.[57] Whilst no side-effects were recorded in the case studies, it is uncertain if high dose zinc may impact on pregnancy. So, women should be warned to avoid pregnancy if taking high doses of zinc for PMT. The author postulated that zinc, like the non-steroidal anti-inflammatory drugs used to treat cramping, reduces the production of prostaglandins or zinc improves micro-vessel circulation to help prevent cramping and pain.[58]

It should be noted that zinc supplementation can cause gastrointestinal side-effects and that concomitant administration with calcium, coffee, folate and iron may impair zinc absorption and thus doses should be separated in time during the day (e.g. separate with different meals during the day).

Omega-3 fatty acids

Dietary supplementation with omega-3 fatty acids may have a beneficial effect on symptoms of dysmenorrhoea.

In a 4-month double-blinded randomised placebo-controlled trial, 42 teenage girls with dysmenorrhoea were randomised to either fish oil (720mgs DHA and 1080mgs EPA) plus 1.5mg of vitamin E supplements or placebo for 2 months, then the treatment groups switched treatments for a further 2 months.[58] After 2 months of the fish oil/vitamin E treatment, there was a marked reduction in symptoms and requirement for analgesia, compared with no changes demonstrated in the placebo groups. Of interest, the dietary intake of fish for most of the girls in the study was extremely low.

Tryptophan

Tryptophan is an amino acid which is naturally found in dairy products, seafood, red and white meat, nuts, seeds and soy products and is a precursor to niacin and serotonin. Serotonin depletion has been hypothesised to play a role in premenstrual dysphoria. This hypothesis has been examined in a number of small studies. One such study examined the effects of acute tryptophan depletion on 16 women with PMS. Tryptophan depletion was associated with a significant worsening of premenstrual mood symptoms which correlated with a reduction in tryptophan levels relative to other amino acids suggesting a role for this serotonin precursor.[59]

A number of small studies have demonstrated a positive effect of tryptophan supplementation on premenstrual dysphoria symptoms. In 1 randomised placebo-controlled trial of 71 patients with premenstrual dysphoric disorder, patients were treated with either 6g/day of L-tryptophan or placebo from day 17 to day 23 of the menstrual cycle over 3 consecutive cycles. There was a statistically significant improvement in dysphoria, irritability, tension and mood swings in the tryptophan group compared to the placebo group.[60]

Another double-blinded cross-over small study of 12 women with PMS examined the effects of a carbohydrate-rich beverage known to increase serum tryptophan levels compared to 2 other iso-caloric beverages in the luteal phases over 3 menstrual cycles preceded by a 1-month placebo cycle. Symptoms of depression, anger, confusion and carbohydrate cravings were reduced significantly when the experimental carbohydrate beverage was consumed compared to the iso-caloric beverages which did not impact serum tryptophan levels. Interestingly, the ability of the women to perform memory word recognition tasks was improved after consumption of the experimental beverage compared to placebo.[61]

More comprehensive research is obviously required in this area, however this collection of small studies bears significant promise for the use of L-tryptophan in the treatment of premenstrual dysphoria in the future.

There is a risk of significant interactions if tryptophan is taken with antidepressants and lithium. Side-effects include dry mouth, nausea, headaches and tremors. In 1989 the FDA in the United States reported an association between the consumption of a particular Japanese manufactured L-tryptophan and fatalities from eosinophilia myalgia syndrome.[62] This disorder is thought to have been related to a contaminant which arose in the process of creating L-tryptophan from genetically modified bacteria by the manufacturer.

Herbal medicine

There are a number of herbs which have a good evidence basis for use in PMS, in particular chasteberry (*vitex agnus castus*), discussed in more detail below. A number of herbs have been implicated for the treatment of PMS, such as dong quai (*Angelica sinensis*), cramp bark (*Viburnum opulus*), black cohosh and wild yam (*Dioscorea villosa)* but little research evidence is currently available.

Red clover (Isoflavones)

Isoflavones are a subgroup of phytoestrogens that have a weak anti-oestrogenic effect on oestrogen receptor sites in pre-menopausal women. A double-blind RCT of either placebo, 40mg or 80mg of isoflavones in 18 women demonstrated that 9 of the 12 women on treatment had a worthwhile improvement in their cyclical mastalgia symptoms, compared to only 2 of 6 on placebo.[63] Pain reduced by 13% for placebo, 44% for 40mg of isoflavone per day and 31% for 80mg/day.

Chasteberry (*vitex agnus castus*)

Perhaps the best researched herb for PMS to date, is *vitex agnus castus* (VAC). Its use dates back to Hippocrates. A trial was published in *Archives of Gynecology and Obstetrics* of 50 women with PMS who were treated with 20mgs/day of Ze440 (VAC extract) over 3 menstrual cycles.[64] The patients were studied over 8 menstrual cycles, 2 baseline, 3 treatment and 3 post-treatment. Symptoms reduced by 42.5% in the group during the treatment phase and interestingly symptoms remained 21.7 % below baseline symptoms in the 3 cycles post-treatment cessation. The main criticism of this study is that it was not blinded or placebo controlled.

A randomised, placebo-controlled trial of 170 women, published in the *British Medical Journal* (2001), concluded that a specific extract of VAC Ze440 (180mgs) was 'an effective and well-tolerated treatment for the relief of symptoms' of PMS.[65] Women selected for the trial were diagnosed with the PMS on the basis of DSM II R criteria and took either the placebo or VAC treatment for 3 months. Compared with placebo, the VAC group demonstrated statistically significant improvement (52% response rate compared to the placebo response of 24%) of PMS symptoms including irritability, mood alteration, anger, headache and breast fullness. Abdominal bloating was the only measured symptom which did not have a significant response to VAC.

A 2007 review which examined the results of 2 non-randomised and 3 randomised controlled studies (two with placebo and 1 with fluoxetine) for a total of 1991 women concluded that VAC was 'safe, effective and efficient in the treatment of cyclical mastalgia'.[66]

A 2003 randomised trial of 41 women compared fluoxetine (a selective serotonin reuptake inhibitor [SSRI]) with a VAC extract (20–40mg/day) for the treatment of PMDD.[67] Patients' symptoms improved equally for Fluoxetine (68.4%) — this group demonstrated a significant reduction, particularly in psychological symptoms — and VAC (57.9%) which demonstrated a significant effect in relieving mainly physical symptoms. Unfortunately, there was no placebo arm in this study, so these findings need to be interpreted with caution.

It is not clear how VAC works. VAC extracts have been shown in some studies to have a dopaminergic effect and to reduce excessive levels of serum prolactin. It is generally well tolerated and side-effects are infrequent.

St John's wort (*Hypericum perforatum*)

Animal studies have demonstrated that *Hypericum* inhibits the reuptake of serotonin, noradrenaline and dopamine and upregulates serotonin receptors and thus may play a role in ameliorating premenstrual dysphoria symptoms.[68]

A 2008 Cochrane review demonstrated that there is a role for St Johns wort in the management of depression and that results for St Johns wort were comparable to antidepressants with less side-effects experienced.[69] Unfortunately, there is a paucity of large, randomised, placebo-controlled trials into the potential use for *Hypericum* in management of premenstrual dysphoric symptoms.

A small, prospective, uncontrolled, observational pilot study of 19 women with PMS had participants take 300mg of St Johns wort over 2 menstrual cycles. Response rates were recorded through self-reporting on the Hospital Anxiety and Depression scale and Social Adjustment scale. Results demonstrated a significant reduction in all-outcome measures with an overall improvement of 51% compared to baseline symptoms. Two-thirds of the women reported at least a 50% reduction in symptom severity with good compliance and tolerability demonstrated.[70]

Further large-scale, randomised placebo-controlled trials are obviously required into this area. It should be noted that St Johns wort is known to interact with a number of medications including antidepressants, anticonvulsants and the oral contraceptive pill. Side-effects include gastrointestinal symptoms, photosensitivity and skin reactions. Interestingly, the incidence of side-effects is thought to be tenfold lower than for SSRIs.[66]

Essence of fennel

An RCT demonstrated that both essence of fennel 2% given orally 4 hourly and mefanamic acid given 6 hourly were effective for pain relief in women with moderate to severe dysmenorrhoea, when compared with placebo.[71]

Evening primrose oil (EPO)

Despite widespread popularity for its use in PMS, a systematic review[72] of EPO for the treatment of PMS demonstrated to be ineffective. This review commented on the poor design of the majority of the studies which had been included. The 2 most well-constructed studies included in this review were randomised cross-over or placebo-controlled, however they were small, including a total of only 76 patients. A more recent review of treatments for cyclical mastalgia found a possible role for EPO 1–3g/day, together with reducing saturated fats in the diet.[13]

Traditional Chinese medicine (TCM)

A 2009 Cochrane review into the use of TCM in management of premenstrual symptoms examined 2 large RCTs including 549 women. One of these studies was well designed and demonstrated that Jingqianping granules caused a statistically significant reduction in premenstrual symptoms. The reviewers noted, however, that the researchers provided the formula for the granules themselves and thus recommended that further trials occur to ensure that these results are reproducible.[73]

Physical therapies

Low-level heat therapy

Continuous low-level topical heat therapy using an abdominal patch for 12 hours was as effective as ibuprofen for the treatment of dysmenorrhoea, according to a randomised placebo and active controlled study published in *Obstetrics and Gynecology* in 2001.[74] Therefore, topical heat packs can help alleviate dysmenorrhoea.

Transcutaneous electrical nerve stimulation (TENS) and acupuncture

A recent Cochrane review of 9 RCTs identified 7 involving TENS, 1 acupuncture, and 1 for both treatments.[75] The author's findings concluded that overall high frequency TENS was shown to be more effective for pain relief than placebo TENS, with insufficient evidence for low-frequency TENS.

Acupuncture

Systematic reviews of research into the use of acupuncture have been positive for a number of pain conditions including back pain, fibromyalgia and headaches. Unfortunately more evidence is required to prove benefits in premenstrual pain including dysmenorrhoea and mastalgia. A 2003 systematic review of controlled trials into the use of acupuncture and acupressure for dysmenorrhoea included 4 studies, only 2 of which were patient blinded. These studies demonstrated promising results for reduction of symptoms in patients experiencing dysmenorrhoea, however the author concluded that more comprehensive research is required.[76]

Spinal manipulation

A 2004 Cochrane review concluded there is no evidence that spinal manipulation is more effective than sham manipulation in the treatment of primary and secondary dysmenorrhoea.[77] Five RCTs were included in this review. Interestingly, however, when the results were compared to control groups who had no treatment the author's concluded that sham or true manipulative techniques were 'possibly more effective'. There was no difference noted in adverse effects when the sham and true manipulation groups were compared.[78]

Conclusion

PMS and its often associated conditions of cyclical mastalgia, dysmenorrhoea and PMDD are extremely common conditions which impact the lives of many women in our society. There is a significant amount of evidence for the use of integrative therapies and lifestyle management of these symptoms as has been discussed in this chapter.

In summary, the use of cognitive and behavioural interventions such as symptom diaries, cognitive restructuring, the use of mindfulness and acceptance-based approaches, coping skills training and relaxation techniques have been shown to be effective. Stress reduction strategies have also been shown to be beneficial as has an emphasis on good sleep hygiene. Regular exercise regimes and sun exposure with normalisation of vitamin D levels have been shown to be of benefit as have dietary interventions. Dietary recommendations which have an evidence basis include increasing intake of omega-3 fatty acids, calcium, vitamin D, vegetarian plant-based diets and minimising saturated fats, caffeine and salt.

Nutritional supplementation and the use of herbal medications are popular with women. There is an increasing body of evidence for the use of vitamins B1, B6, magnesium, calcium and omega-3 fatty acids in women with predominant physical premenstrual symptoms and tryptophan for women with predominant dysphoria symptoms. Red clover, essence of fennel and *vitex agnus castus* have demonstrated beneficial effects in the management of physical symptoms and St John's wort may have a role for women with predominant mood symptoms, however more research is clearly needed in regard to this particular herb. There is a potential role for evening primrose oil in the treatment of cyclical mastalgia and TCM for treatment of premenstrual symptoms although more research is required.

Regarding physical therapies, there is a role for heat therapy and TENS in management of dysmenorrhoea and a potential role for acupuncture and acupressure. The role of spinal manipulation is not supported by evidence, however more research is required to further elucidate whether this therapy may be an effective treatment.

Table 33.3 is a summary of the levels of evidence for the various forms of integrative therapies outlined in this chapter.

Table 33.3 Levels of evidence for lifestyle and complementary medicines/therapies in the management of premenstrual syndrome

Modality	Level I	Level II	Level IIIa	Level IIIb	Level IIIc	Level IV	Level V
Lifestyle							
PMS-stress management program		x					
Exercise				x		x	
Light therapy/ sunshine		x					
Sleep hygiene					x		
Mind–body medicine							
Cognitive behaviour therapy	x						
Relaxation therapy	x						
Family and social support							x
Nutrition/diet							
Salt restriction							x
Caffeine restriction				x			
Plant based vegetarian diet				x			
Fish				x			
HIgh calcium diet				x			
High vitamin D diet				x			
Nutritional supplements							
Fish oil		x					
Tryptophan		x					
Vitamin supplements							
Vitamin B1		x					
Vitamin B6	x						
Vitamin E		x					
Vitamin D				x			
Mineral supplements							
Magnesium	x*						
Calcium	x						
Zinc						x	
Herbal medicines							
Red clover		x*					
Vitex agnus castus	x						
St John's wort					x		
Evening primrose oil (mastalgia only)	x						
Traditional Chinese medicine		x					
Essence of fennel					x		

Continued

Table 33.3 Levels of evidence for lifestyle and complementary medicines/therapies in the management of premenstrual syndrome—cont'd

Modality	Level I	Level II	Level IIIa	Level IIIb	Level IIIc	Level IV	Level V
Physical therapies							
Heat therapy		x					
High frequency TENS		x					
Acupuncture/ acupressure		x*					
Spinal manipulation							x

* Caution is advocated in interpreting these results as conclusive–as further evidence is required.

Level I — from a systematic review of all relevant randomised controlled trials — meta-analyses.

Level II — from at least 1 properly designed randomised controlled clinical trial.

Level IIIa — from well-designed pseudo-randomised controlled trials (alternate allocation or some other method).

Level IIIb — from comparative studies (including systematic reviews of such studies) with concurrent controls and allocation not randomised, cohort studies, case-control studies, or interrupted time series with a parallel control group.

Level IIIc — from comparative studies with historical control, 2 or more single-arm studies or interrupted time series without a parallel control group.

Level IV — opinions of respected authorities based on clinical experience, descriptive studies or reports of expert committees.

Level V — represents minimal evidence that represents testimonials.

Clinical tips handout for patients — premenstrual symptoms

1 Lifestyle advice

Sleep

- Restore normal sleep patterns. Early to bed about 9–10 p.m. and awakening upon sunrise. Early morning sun exposure can be useful in regulating sleep patterns. (See Chapter 22 for more advice.)

Sunshine

- At least 15 minutes of sunshine needed daily for vitamin D and melatonin production — especially before 10 a.m. and after 3 p.m. when sun exposure is safest in summer.
- Ensure adequate skin exposure to sun. During the exposure period avoid sunscreen and excess clothing to maximise levels of vitamin D.
- More time in the sun is required for dark skinned people.
- Individuals living in cooler climates may need to consider vitamin D supplementation in the cooler months if adequate sun exposure is not possible.

2 Physical activity/exercise

- Yoga may be of help; other examples: qigong and tai chi.
- See this free website for a video demonstrating yoga postures that may help with menstrual pain: http://thephj.com/videos/article/menstral_pain_relief_with_yoga/
- Exercise at least 30–60 minutes daily. If exercise is not regular, commence with 5 minutes daily and slowly build up to at least 30 minutes. Outdoor exercise in nature, with fresh air and sunshine, is ideal (e.g. brisk walking, light jogging, cycling, swimming, stretching, weight bearing exercises).
- The more time you spend outdoors the better, especially in natural park-like settings.

4 Mind–body medicine

- Understanding your condition is very important as is an understanding of what factors may exacerbate and what you can do to minimise or relieve your symptoms. Maintaining a positive attitude towards your menses is beneficial.
- Some women find keeping a menstrual symptom diary useful. Stress reduction, relaxation strategies, particularly meditation and mindfulness, and acceptance-based cognitive approaches have also been found to be beneficial.

5 Dietary changes

- Eat regular, balanced healthy meals, ideally 3 small meals, and 2 snacks, each containing protein in order to avoid fluctuating blood sugar levels and provide amino acids for nerve transmitters such as tryptophan.
- Eat more fruit (>2/day) and vegetables (>5/day) — a variety of colours and those in season.
- Eat more nuts, seeds and legumes (e.g. beans, lentils) and sprouts (e.g. alfalfa, mung beans).
- Eat wholegrains/cereals (variety): rice (brown, basmati, Mahatmi, Doongara), traditional rolled oats, buckwheat flour, wholegrain organic breads (rye bread, Essene, spelt, Kamut), brown pasta, couscous, millet, amaranth etc.
- A vegetarian plant-based diet has been shown to reduce premenstrual symptoms.
- Increase fish intake (sardines, tuna, salmon, cod, mackerel) especially deep sea fish >3 servings per week. This has been shown to reduce menstrual pain symptoms.
- Increase intake of calcium-containing foods as these have also been shown to reduce premenstrual symptoms. Examples of these foods include nuts, low-fat dairy products (e.g. Greek feta), fish with bones (particularly salmon and sardines), tofu, broccoli and bok choy.
- Avoid saturated fats, particularly animal fats.
- Minimise caffeine intake as this is thought to cause menstrual pain and premenstrual irritability.
- Minimise salt intake as this is thought to contribute to fluid retention, abdominal bloating and breast tenderness.

6 Physical therapies

- Local heat such as heat packs during menstruation has been shown to reduce pain.
- TENS treatment has demonstrated usefulness for reduction of period pain symptoms.
- Acupuncture/acupressure may also be useful in reducing period pain.

7 Supplements

Vitamins

Vitamin D3

- Indication: may help PMS
- Dosage: safe sunshine exposure of skin is the safest source of vitamin D.
  - Doctors should check blood levels and suggest supplementation if levels are low.
  - Adults: 400–1000IU/day, for maintenance; 3000–5000IU/day for 1 month then 1000IU/day if vitamin D level below normal.
  - Children at risk: 200–400IU/day under medical supervision
  - Pregnant and lactating women at risk: under medical supervision.
- Results: 3–12 months
- Side-effects: very high doses can cause vitamin D toxicity; raised calcium levels in the blood.
- Contraindications: hypercalcemia; vitamin D3 can increase aluminium and magnesium absorption, prolonged heparin therapy can increase resorption and reduce formation of bone and hence more vitamin D and calcium required; thiazide diuretics decrease urinary calcium and hence hypercalcaemia possible with vitamin D supplementation; high levels of vitamin D can reduce effectiveness of verapamil.

  The following drugs can decrease vitamin D levels: carbamazepine, cholestyramine, colestipol, phenobarbitol, phenytoin, rifampin, orlistat, stimulant laxatives. Corticosteroids increase the need for vitamin D.

  Use vitamin D with caution in those with artery disease, hyperparathyroidism, lymphoma, renal disease and sarcoidosis.

Vitamin B1 and B6

- Indication: premenstrual syndrome and period pain.
- Dosage: upper level of intake of vitamin B6 should not exceed 50mg/day.
  - Vitamin B1: 100mg/day.
- Results: reduced premenstrual symptoms.
- Side-effects: overuse of single vitamin products; avoid use of multiple single-vitamin products (e.g. oral and injectable forms of vitamin B6) or concomitant use of multivitamin products could result in some patients routinely exceeding the upper limit for vitamins associated with severe toxicity. Toxicity symptoms in high doses of vitamin B6 include tingling, burning and numbness of limbs.
- Contraindications: avoid in anaemias until assessed by a doctor.
- Interactions: absorption may be impaired by being taken with iron supplements, antibiotics and tannins (found in tea) thus these substances should be separated from vitamin B intake by 2 hours.

Vitamin E (natural)

- Indication: period pain.
- Dosage: 200mg twice daily 2 days prior to menstruation. Continue for 5 days.
- Results: reduced period pain and reduced menstrual blood loss.
- Side-effects: rare in these doses. May cause nausea, diarrhoea and flatulence.
- Contraindications: avoid doses > 1000IU/day 1 week prior to surgery.

Minerals

Magnesium

- Indication: period pain and premenstrual depressed mood.
- Dosage: 360mg/day from day 15 of cycle to the onset of period.
- Results: 1–2 menstrual cycles
- Side-effects: oral magnesium can cause gastrointestinal irritation, nausea, vomiting, and diarrhoea. Although rare, toxic levels can cause low blood pressure, thirst, heart arrhythmia, drowsiness and weakness.
- Contraindications: patients with kidney disease.
- Interactions: may interfere with the absorption of some antibiotics and anti-arrhythmic medications.

Calcium

- Indication: period pain, premenstrual fluid retention, mood disorders and food cravings.
- Dosage: 1200mgs/day.
- Results: 1–2 menstrual cycles.
- Side-effects: constipation and flatulence.
- Contraindications: in individuals with chronic renal disease, unless medically supervised, and hyperparathyroidism.
- Interactions: some blood pressure and heart medications. Check with your doctor.

Zinc

- Indication: period pain (although research is not convincing).
- Dosage: 30mg 1–3 times daily commencing 1 to 4 days prior to onset of period.

- Side-effects: gastric irritation, nausea, vomiting, metallic taste in mouth. Avoid long-term use and high dosage as this may cause copper deficiency, impair the immune system and cause anaemia.
- Contraindication: sideroblastic anaemia; above normal blood levels of zinc; severe kidney disease. Avoid high doses in pregnancy.
- Interactions: calcium, folate and iron supplements and coffee may impair absorption of zinc, therefore separate ingestion of these.

Fish oils

- Indication: period pain.
- Dosage: fish oils providing EPA 6.2g and DHA 3.4g/day have been used. Take with meals. Adult: 1g x 1–2 capsules 1–3 times daily.
- Results: 2–3 menstrual cycles.
- Side-effects: often well tolerated especially if taken with meals. Very mild and rare side-effects; for example, gastrointestinal upset; burping with fishy smells; allergic reactions (e.g. rash, breathing problems); avoid if allergic to seafood; blood thinning effects in very high doses > 10g daily (may need to stop fish oil supplements 2 weeks prior to surgery).
- Contraindications: sensitivity reaction to seafood; drug interactions; caution when taking high doses of fish oils >4g/day together with warfarin (your doctor will check your INR test).

Tryptophan

- Indication: premenstrual depressed mood.
- Dosage: up to 6g/day.
- Results : 1 menstrual cycle.
- Side-effects: nausea, headaches, dry mouth, tremors.
- Contraindications: antidepressants and lithium. Concomitant use should be avoided.

Herbal medicine

Red clover

- Indication: premenstrual breast pain.
- Dosage: 40–80mg/day.
- Results: 1-2 menstrual cycles.
- Side-effects: no adverse effects reported at these dosages.
- Interactions: should be used in caution with patients who take anticoagulants and there is a theoretical risk of interaction with synthetic oestrogens.
- Contraindications: individuals with oestrogen-sensitive tumours (e.g. breast cancer).

Chasteberry *(Vitex agnus castus)*

- Indications: premenstrual syndrome.
- Dosage: 20mg Ze440 (chasteberry) extract daily.
- Results: 2–3 menstrual cycles.
- Side-effects: rare. Skin rash, nausea, gastrointestinal disturbances and headaches.
- Interactions: use with caution when taken with oral contraceptive pill. Consult your doctor.
- Contraindications: pregnancy; individuals with oestrogen-sensitive tumours (e.g. breast cancer).

Evening primrose oil

- Indication: mastalgia, breast discomfort, atopic eczema, psoriasis.
- Dosage: 2-4 g/day.
- Side effects: usually well tolerated; may increase bleeding time so be careful when using with other anticoagulants.
- Contraindications: avoid if you suffer seizures or epilepsy.

St John's wort

- Indication: premenstrual depressed mood.
- Dosage: 300–900mg/day.
- Results: 1–3 weeks.
- Side-effects: very mild and rare, include: photosensitivity skin rash; digestion disturbance; dizziness; fatigue; dry mouth.
- Contraindications: pregnancy; lactation.
- Drug interaction: avoid use with most pharmaceutical medications such as the oral contraceptive pill, other antidepressants, epileptic medication — check with your doctor.

References

1. Collier J, ed. SSRIs for premenstrual dysphoric disorder. *Drug and Therapeutics Bulletin* 2002;40(9):70–2.
2. ACOG Practice Bulletin. Clinical management guidelines for obstetrician-gynecologists. Number 15, April 2000. Premenstrual syndrome. Obstet Gynecol 2000;95:1–9.
3. Frackiewicz EJ, Shiovitz TM. Evaluation and management of premenstrual syndrome and premenstrual dysphoric disorder. J Am Pharm Assoc (Wash). 2001 May-Jun;41(3):437–47.
4. Zaafrane F, Faleh R, Melki W, et. al. An overview of premenstrual syndrome.J Gynecol Obstet Biol Reprod (Paris). 2007 Nov;36(7):642–52.
5. Pernol M, Benson, R. Benson and Pernoll's handbook of obstetrics and gynaecologymcgraw Hill Publishing 2001 pp725–726.

6 Wyatt K, Dimmock PW, O'Brien PM. Premenstrual syndrome. In: Barton S, ed. Clinical evidence. 4th issue. London: BMJ Publishing Group, 2000: 1121–33.
7 Moline ML, Zendell SM. Evaluating and managing premenstrual syndrome. Medscape Womens Health 2000;5:1–16.
8 Dell DL. Premenstrual syndrome, premenstrual dysphoric disorder, and premenstrual exacerbation of another disorder. Clinical obstetrics and gynecology 2004;47(3):568–75.
9 Steiner M, Born L. Diagnosis and treatment of premenstrual dysphoric disorder: an update. Int Clin Psychopharmacol 2000;15(suppl 3):S5–17.
10 Limosin F, Ades J. Psychiatric and psychological aspects of premenstrual syndrome Encephale. 2001 Nov-Dec;27(6):501–8
11 *Diagnostic and Statistical Manual of Mental Disorders, Fourth Edition DSM-IV.* American Psychiatric Association. Diagnostic and statistical manual of mental disorders. 4th ed. Washington, D.C.: American Psychiatric Association, 1994: 717–8.
12 Hillen TI, Grbavac SL, Johnston PJ, et. al. Primary dysmenorrhea in young Western Australian women: prevalence, impact, and knowledge of treatment. J Adolesc Health. 1999 Jul;25(1):40–5.
13 Millet AV, Dirbas FM. Clinical management of breast pain: a review. Obstet Gynecol Surv. 2002 Jul;57(7):451–61.
14 Girman, A, Lee, R, Kligler, B. An integrative medicine approach to premenstrual syndrome [Editorial]. American Journal of Obstetrics and Gynecology 2003;188(5, part 2):S56–S65.
15 Gordon NP, Sobel DS, Tarazona EZ. Use of and interest in alternative therapies among adult primary care clinicians and adult members in a large health maintenance organization. West J Med. 1998 Sep;169(3):153–61.
16 Fugh-Berman A, Kronenberg, F. Complementary and alternative medicine (CAM) in reproductive-age women: a review of randomised controlled trials. Reprod Toxicol. 2003 Mar-Apr;17(2):137–52.
17 Rapkin A. A review of treatment of premenstrual syndrome and premenstrual dysphoric disorder. Psychoneuroendocrinology. 2003 Aug;28 Suppl 3:39–53
18 Taylor D. Effectiveness of professional-peer group treatment: Symptom management for women with PMS. Nurs Health 1999;22:496–511.
19 ACOG Practice Bulletin. Clinical management guidelines for obstetrician-gynecologists. Number 15, April 2000. Premenstrual syndrome. Obstet Gynecol 2000;95:1–9.
20 Blake F, Salkovskis P, Gath D, Day A, Garrod A. Cognitive therapy for premenstrual syndrome: a controlled trial. J Psychosom Res 1998;45:307–18.
21 Kessel B. Premenstrual syndrome. Advances in diagnosis and treatment. Obstet Gynecol Clin North Am 2000;27:625–39.
22 Morse CA. et. al. A comparison of hormone therapy, coping skills training, and relaxation for the relief of premenstrual syndrome. J Behav Med. 1991 Oct;14(5):469–89.
23 Stones W, Cheong YC, Howard FM. Interventions for treating chronic pelvic pain in women. *Cochrane Database of Systematic Reviews* 2005, Issue 2. Art. No.: CD000387. DOI: 10.1002/14651858.CD000387.
24 Proctor ML, Murphy PA, Pattison HM, Suckling J, Farquhar CM. Behavioural interventions for primary and secondary dysmenorrhoea. *Cochrane Database of Systematic Reviews* 2007, Issue 3. Art. No.: CD002248. DOI: 10.1002/14651858.CD002248.pub3.
25 Christensen AP, Oei TP. The efficacy of cognitive behaviour therapy in treating premenstrual dysphoric changes. J Affect Disord. 1995 Jan 11;33(1):57–63.
26 Lustyk MK, Gerrish WG, Shaver S, Keys SL. Cognitive-behavioural therapy for premenstrual syndrome and premenstrual dysphoric disorder: a systematic review. Arch Womens Ment Health. 2009 Feb 27. [Epub ahead of print].
27 Lustyk MK, Widman L, Paschane A, Ecker E. Stress, quality of life and physical activity in women with varying degrees of premenstrual symptomatology. Women Health. 2004;39(3):35–44.
28 Goodale IL, Domar AD, Benson H. Alleviation of premenstrual syndrome symptoms with the relaxation response. Obstet Gynecol 1990 Apr;75(4):649–55
29 Hernandez-Reif M, Martinez A, Field T, Quintero O, Hart S, Burman I. Premenstrual symptoms are relieved by massage therapy. J Psychosom Obstet Gynaecol. 2000 Mar;21(1):9–15. PubMed PMID: 10907210.
30 Driver HS, Dijk DJ, Werth E, et. al. Sleep and the sleep electroencephalogram across the menstrual cycle in young healthy women. Journal of Clinical Endocrinology and Metabolism, Vol 81, 728–735.
31 Lee KA, Shaver JF, Giblin EC, Woods NF. Sleep patterns related to menstrual cycle phase and premenstrual affective symptoms. Sleep. 1990 Oct;13(5):403–9.
32 Labyak S, Lava S, Turek F, Zee P. Effects of shiftwork on sleep and menstrual function in nurses. Health Care For Women International, Volume 23, Numbers 6-7, 1 September 2002, pp. 703–714(12)
33 Baker FC, Driver HS. Circadian rhythms, sleep, and the menstrual cycle. Sleep Med. 2007 Sep;8(6): 613–22.
34 Thys-Jacobs S, Donovan D, Papadopoulos A, et. al. Vitamin D and calcium dysregulation in the polycystic ovarian syndrome. Steroids 1999;64(6):430–5.
35 Lansdowne AT, Provost SC. Vitamin D3 enhances mood in healthy subjects during winter. Psychopharmacology (Berl). 1998:135(4):319–23.
36 Gloth FM III, Alam W, Hollis B. Vitamin D vs broad spectrum phototherapy in the treatment of seasonal affective disorder. J Nutr Health Aging 1999; 3(1):5–7.
37 Al Faraj S, Al Mutairi K. Vitamin D deficiency and chronic low back pain in Saudi Arabia. Spine. 2003;28(2):177–9.
38 Thys-Jacobs S. Vitamin D and calcium in menstrual migraine. Headache 1994 Oct;34(9):544–6
39 Lam RW, Carter D, Misri S, et. al. A controlled study of light therapy in women with late luteal phase dysphoric disorder. Psychiatry Res 1999 Jun 30;86(3):185–92.
40 Parry BL, Berga SL, Mostofi N, et. al. Plasma melatonin circadian rhythms during the menstrual cycle and after light therapy in premenstrual dysphoric disorder and normal control subjects. J Biol Rhythms. 1997 Feb;12(1):47–64.
41 Hightower M. Effects of Exercise Participation on Menstrual Pain and Symptoms. Women and Health 1998;26(4):15–27.
42 Prior JC, Vigna Y, Alojada N. Conditioning exercise decreases premenstrual symptoms European Journal of Applied Physiology 1986;55(4): 349–355.
43 Steege JF, Blumenthal JA. The effects of aerobic exercise on premenstrual symptoms in middle-aged women: a preliminary study. J Psychosom Res 1993;37:127–33.

44 Prior JC, Vigna Y, Sciarretta D, et. al. Conditioning exercise decreases premenstrual symptoms: a prospective, controlled 6-month trial. Fertil Steril 1987 Mar;47(3):402–8.

45 Deutsh B. Menstrual pain in Danish women correlated with low n-3 polyunsaturated fatty acid intake Eur J Clin Nutr 1995; 49:508–16.

46 Barnard ND, Scialli AR, Hurlock D, Bertron P. Diet and sex-hormone binding globulin, dysmenorrhea, and premenstrual symptoms. Obstet Gynecol. 2000 Feb;95(2):245–50. PubMed PMID: 10674588.

47 Bertone-Johnson ER, Hankinson SE, Bendich A, et. al. Calcium and vitamin D intake and risk of incident premenstrual syndrome. Arch Intern Med 2005;165(11):1246–52.

48 Rossignol AM. Caffeine-containing beverages and premenstrual syndrome in young women. Am J Public Health. 1985 Nov;75(11):1335–7.

49 Proctor ML, Murphy PA. Herbal and dietary therapies for primary and secondary dysmenorrhoea. Cochrane Database Systematic Rev 2001;(3):CD002124.

50 Whelan AM, Jurgens TM, Naylor H. Herbs, vitamins and minerals in the treatment of premenstrual syndrome: a systematic review. Canadian J Clin Pharmacol 2009 Fall;16(3):e407–29. Epub 2009 Oct 29

51 High-dose vitamin B6 may cause peripheral neuropathy. ADRAC bulletin Volume 27, Number 4, August 2008 http://www.tga.gov.au/adr/aadrb/aadr0808.htm

52 Ziaei S, Zakeri M, Kazemnejad A. A randomised controlled trial of vitamin E in the treatment of primary dysmenorrhoea. British Journal of Obstetrics and Gynecology. 2005 Apr;112(4):466–9.

53 Facchinetti MD, Borella P, Sances G, et. al. Oral magnesium successfully relieves premenstrual mood changes Obstetrics and Gynecology Vol 78 n 2 1991 pp 177–181.

54 Bertone-Johnson ER, Hankinson SE, Bendich A, et. al. Calcium and Vitamin D intake and risk of incident premenstrual syndrome Archives of Internal Medicine 2005;165:1246–52.

55 Thys-Jacobs S, Starkey P, Bernstein D, et. al. Calcium carbonate and the premenstrual syndrome: effects on premenstrual and menstrual symptoms. *American Journal of Obstetrics and Gynaecology*, 1998; 179:444–452.

56 Braun L, Cohen M. Herbs and Natural supplements an evidence based guide 2nd edn. Elsevier Australia 2007 pp198–99.

57 Eby GA. Zinc treatment prevents dysmenorrhea. Medical Hypotheses Volume 69, Issue 2, 2007, Pages 297–301 doi:10.1016/j.mehy.2006.12.009.

58 Harel Z, Biro FM, Kottenhahn RK, et. al. Supplementation with omega-3 fatty acids in the management of dysmenorrhoea in adolescents. *American Journal of Obstetrics and Gynaecology* 1996;174(4): 1335–1338.

59 Menkes DB, Coates DC, Fawcett JP. Acute tryptophan depletion aggravates premenstrual syndrome J Psychiatry Neurosci. 1994 Mar;19(2):114–9.

60 Sayegh R, Schiff I, Wurtman J, Spiers P, McDermott J, Wurtman R. The effect of a carbohydrate-rich beverage on mood, appetite, and cognitive function in women with premenstrual syndrome. Obstet Gynecol 1995 Oct;86(4 Pt 1):520–8.

61 Sayegh R, Schiff I, Wurtman J, et. al. The effect of a carbohydrate-rich beverage on mood, appetite and cognitive function in women with premenstrual syndrome. J Affect Disord. 1994 Sep;32(1): 37–44.

62 FDA/DFSAN information paper on L-tryptophan Feb 2001 http://www.cfsan.fda.gov/~dms/ds-tryp1.html

63 Ingram DM, Hickling C, West L, et. al. A double-blind randomised controlled trial of isoflavones in the treatment of cyclical mastalgia. Breast. 2002 Apr;11(2):170–4.

64 Berger D, Schaffner W, Schrader E, et. al. Efficacy of Vitex agnus castus L. extract Ze 440 in patients with pre-menstrual syndrome (PMS). Archives of Gynecology and Obstetrics. 264(3): 150–3, 2000 Nov.

65 Schellenberg R. Treatment for the Premenstrual Syndrome With Agnus Castus Fruit: Prospective, Randomised, Placebo Controlled Study, British Medical Journal 2001, 322;134–7.

66 Carmichael AR. Can Vitex Agnus Castus be used for the treatment of cyclical mastalgia? What is the current evidence? eCAM 2008:5(3)247–50.

67 Atmaca M, Kumru S, Tezcan E. Fluoxetine versus Vitex Agnus Castus Extract in the Treatment of Premestrual Disphoric Disorder, Human Psychopharmacology 2003 Apr; 18(3) 191–5.

68 Braun L, Cohen M. Herbs and natural supplements. An evidence based guide 2nd edn. Elsevier 2007 pp 551–553.

69 Linde K, Berner MM, Kriston L. St John's wort for major depression. Cochrane Database of Systematic Reviews 2008, Issue 4. Art. No.: CD000448. DOI: 0.1002/14651858.CD000448.pub3

70 Stevinson C, Ernst E. A pilot study of Hypericum perforatum for the treatment of premenstrual syndrome. Altern Complement Med. 2004 Dec;10(6):925–32.

71 Namavar Jahromi B, Tartifizadeh A, Khabnadideh S. Comparison of fennel and mefenamic acid for the treatment of primary dysmenorrhea. Int J Gynaecol Obstet. 2003 Feb;80(2):153–7.

72 Budeiri D, Li Wan Po A, Dornan JC. Is evening primrose oil of value in the treatment of premenstrual syndrome? Control Clin Trials 1996;17:60–8.

73 Jing Z, Yang X, Ismail KM, Chen X, Wu T. Chinese herbal medicine for premenstrual syndrome. Cochrane Database Syst Rev. 2009 Jan 21;(1):CD006414. Review. PubMed PMID: 19160284.

74 Akin MD, Weingand KW, Hengehold DA, et. al. Continuous low-level topical heat in the treatment of dysmenorrhea. Obstet Gynecol. 2001 Mar;97(3):343–9.

75 Proctor ML, Smith CA, Farquhar CM, Stones RW. Transcutaneous electrical nerve stimulation and acupuncture for primary dysmenorrhoea (Cochrane Review) *The Cochrane Library, Issue 3, 2005*.

76 White AR. A review of controlled trials of acupuncture for women's reproductive health care. J Fam Plann Reprod Health Care. 2003 Oct;29(4):233–6.

77 Proctor ML, Hing W, Johnson TC, Murphy PA. Spinal manipulation for primary and secondary dysmenorrhoea. The Cochrane library 2004. Issue 1.

Chapter 34

Prostate disease and cancer

Introduction

Clinicians encounter in clinical practice 3 common diseases of the prostate, namely, benign prostatic hypertrophy (BPH), prostate cancer and prostatitis (inflammation of the prostate).

Benign prostatic hypertrophy (BPH)

BPH is a common, often worrisome condition that affects ageing men.[1] Approximately 60% of men in the Baltimore Longitudinal Study of Ageing[2] demonstrated some degree of clinical BPH by age 60.[3] Autopsy studies have confirmed microscopic evidence of BPH in 40% of men aged 50–60 years, and 90% of men aged 80 to 90 years.[3] The profound impact of this condition spans all ethnic/racial groups, and African American and Latino men are affected to at least a similar degree as white European American men.[3] BPH has been found to have an effect on quality of life (QOL) similar to that of other chronic diseases such as diabetes mellitus, hypertension, and heart disease.[4–7] Also, depressive mood is more likely to occur in men with BPH.[8] Despite the high prevalence of BPH, its specific cause is unknown, but the evidence suggests a multi-factorial process comparable to that of other chronic diseases, perhaps such as cardiovascular disease.[9, 10, 11] The risk factors for BPH include high blood pressure, low levels of high-density lipoprotein cholesterol, increased weight gain (associated with waist-to-hip ratio increases), and peripheral arterial disease.[10–15]

Prostate cancer

Early estimates from autopsy data have reported that in Western countries, approximately 30–40% of all men will develop microscopic prostate cancer during their lifetime.[16, 17] However, as the growth of most prostate cancers is slow, the risk of developing overt clinical disease in the US has been reported to be approximately 8–10% (lifetime risk), and the risk of actually dying from prostate cancer is approximately 3%, whereas the autopsy-based prevalence is 80% by the age of 80 years. Furthermore, epidemiological data from the US suggests that for a 50 year-old man with a life expectancy of a further 25 years, there is a 40–45% lifetime risk of having microscopic cancer.[17, 18]

In recent years, the veritable epidemic of prostate cancer has probably resulted from the widespread use of prostate-specific antigen (PSA) testing which allows the earlier diagnosis in men who have not yet developed symptoms. As an example, it is estimated that in 2005 in the USA there will be approximately 235 000 new diagnoses of prostate cancer and 29 000 deaths.[17, 18, 19]

In Australia, prostate cancer is the underlying cause of 4.3% of all male deaths registered in 2004.[20] The median age of death from prostate cancer is 80.4 years. Prostate cancer is primarily a disease of men over the age of 50 years, and the trend towards an ageing worldwide population is likely to lead to an increased incidence of cases of prostate cancer. In 2004 in Australia there were 15,759 new cases and 2,792 deaths from prostate cancer (~18%).[20] Approximately 11% of men in Australia will develop prostate cancer in their lifetime.[21]

Prostatitis

Prostatitis is the most common reason why men see a urologist with 1 in 2 men experiencing this condition in their lifetime. Prostatitis can be acute or chronic, bacterial, non-bacterial or inflammatory, plus non-inflammatory.[22] More than 90% of symptomatic patients have chronic prostatitis and/or chronic pelvic pain syndrome. Very little is known about the aetiology of chronic abacterial prostatitis. It is possible that this form of prostatitis may be some form of autoimmune disease.

Bacterial prostatitis is treated using conventional approaches. The other forms of prostatitis are best managed using an integrative approach, as with other chronic medical problems.

Risk factors for prostate cancer

Alcohol

High alcohol consumers such as those that drink more than 10 drinks per day have triple the risk for development of prostate cancer.[23] Another study reported that men who drank 4 glasses of red wine, 4 times weekly, had 50% *reduction* in relative risk of prostate cancer.[24] This study reported that middle-aged men showed a relative risk reduction of 6% for each additional glass of red wine consumed per week.[24] This study also demonstrated that consumption of alcohol above this level may increase risk of prostate cancer.

Meat and dairy

Studies have shown an association between circulating blood levels of some insulin-like growth factors (IGFs) and their binding proteins and the subsequent risk for prostate cancer.[25] A recent study has investigated individual patient data from 12 prospective studies.[26] This study investigated prostate cancer risk with relevance to IGFs, and their binding proteins. The study reported that men with high blood levels of IGF-1 were up to 40% more likely to develop prostate cancer than those with low levels. The conclusion was that high circulating IGF-I concentrations were associated with a moderately increased risk for prostate cancer.[25] However, there were limitations with the study and these included that IGF-1 concentrations were measured in only 1 sample for each participant, and the laboratory methods to measure IGFs differed in each study. Not all patients had disease stage or grade information, and the diagnosis of prostate cancer could have varied among the studies.

Occupational exposure

Herbicides and pesticides are 2 common xenobiotics (chemicals and toxins that are foreign to the body) that can increase prostate cancer risk by causing DNA damage and altering hormone metabolism. Over 60 studies have investigated the relationship between farming and prostate cancer, and have generally shown an elevated risk for farmers.[27]

Endocrine disrupters — substances that mimic natural hormones — are xenobiotics that also increase prostate cancer risk, but also disrupt hormone metabolism. Endocrine disrupters include polychlorinated, biphenyls or PCBs (used to make plastic), ink, electrical and electronic equipment, and plasticizers (substances used to make plastic food-wrap more pliable). Dairy and beef products contain fat which can be contaminated with toxic pesticide and hormone residues which can act as endocrine disruptors.[28, 29]

Lifestyle

Benign prostatic hyperplasia and prostate cancer

Lifestyle modifications have received minimal attention in the medical literature, however, a limited number of studies seem to suggest a consistent beneficial impact of lifestyle interventions that can prevent BPH or cancer and that lifestyle interventions may diminish the progression of existing disease.[30] The incidence of clinical prostate disease is around 30 times higher in Western men than in Eastern men of similar age.[30] Recently, it was reported that excess Body Mass Index (BMI) has been associated with adverse outcomes in prostate cancer, and hyperinsulinaemia is a candidate mediator of increased risk.[31] The study concluded that elevated BMI levels and a high plasma concentration of C-peptide both predisposed men who had been previously diagnosed with prostate cancer to an increased likelihood of dying of their disease.[31] Furthermore, that in those patients with both factors, the survival outcome from the disease was with the lowest probability.

Prostate cancer

There is strong edpimiological evidence that links the development of prostate cancer to a Western type lifestyle.[22] Furthermore, that there are specific components of the Western diet such as low fibre/high meat/ high saturated fat consumptions that may have clinical significance in the late stages of tumour growth, promotion and disease progression.

A small study that investigated a plant based diet in combination with a mindfulness based stress reduction program reported significant reduction in the rate of PSA increase and slowed the rate of tumour progression in patients with biochemically proven recurrent prostate cancer.[32] A recent and more robust study investigated lifestyle in patients with prostate cancer.[33] Participation was in The Prostate Cancer Lifestyle Trial, a 1-year randomised controlled clinical trial that consisted of 93 patients with early-stage prostate cancer (Gleason score <7, PSA 4–10 ng/mL) who were undergoing active surveillance. The study reported that lifestyle and dietary changes could be important in delaying or even avoiding conventional treatment.

Mind–body medicine

Lifestyle changes and stress reduction

Psychosocial interventions can improve quality of life (QOL) and significantly improve survival in patients diagnosed with prostate cancer.[34] A pilot study that enrolled prostate cancer patients into a mindfulness based stress reduction program reported enhanced QOL and decreased stress symptoms and also resulted in beneficial changes in hypothalamic-pituitary-adrenal (HPA) axis functioning.[35] The study demonstrated that mental relaxation, stress management, ways to develop self-esteem and spirituality, imagery techniques and problem solving improved prognosis with the active group living twice as long as the men in the control group.[35] The effects of comprehensive lifestyle changes from multiple Ornish research reports[36–41] has demonstrated that patients with prostate cancer participating in the Prostate Cancer Lifestyle Trial gain significant quality of life benefits. A study investigating a reduction in PSA levels demonstrated inhibition of the human cell line–LNCaP cell growth, and fewer prostate cancer-related clinical events at the end of 1 year compared with control participants.[36] The *in vitro* growth of the prostate cancer cells was inhibited 8 times more than in the control group using the serum from these patients. Another aspect of the Ornish study found that needle biopsy of prostate in the experimental group had significant changes in their prostate cancer genes and also increase in telomerase activity.[36] Hence an enhanced understanding of the molecular response to comprehensive lifestyle changes by prostate cancer cells is further warranted.[37, 38]

The Ornish study of early stage prostate cancer patients,[39] for instance, that randomised 93 men with prostate cancer (PSA 4–10ng/mL, cancer Gleeson scores < 7.0) to an intervention group versus a control group (no expectation of dietary or lifestyle changes), and observed over 1 year reported overall disease improvement. During the study time, the intervention group made vigorous lifestyle changes, namely, adhered to a vegan diet, daily moderate aerobic exercise and stress management techniques, weekly group support and daily supplementation of fish oil (3g/day), vitamin E (400IU/day), selenium (200mcg/day) and vitamin C (2g/day). The growth of prostate cancer cells were inhibited by 70% in the intervention group compared with 9% in the control. None of the patients in the intervention group required further conventional treatment and overall PSA dropped by 4%, compared with 6 patients in the control group requiring further conventional treatment and demonstrating an average increase of PSA of 6%. Diet and lifestyle changes may be the primary contributing factors, but it is hard to separate this benefit from the concomitant use of supplements.[39] A further study with a plant-based diet, high in fibre and low in saturated fat, combined with a stress management technique (mindfulness-based stress reduction) was able to decrease the rate of PSA increase and may slow the rate of tumour progression in cases of biochemically recurrent prostate cancer.[40] An additional recent study by this group further highlights the importance that plant based nutrition may have on slowing progression or preventing the development of prostate cancer.[41] This study suggested that a very-low-fat vegan diet increased intake of protective dietary factors and that it simultaneously may decrease intake of pathogenic dietary factors.

Nutrients and risk of prostate cancer

A recent observational study has highlighted serious concerns with the high use of multivitamins in men, increasing the risk of advanced prostate cancer.[42] The study enrolled 295 344 men aged 50–71 years who were cancer free over 1995–1996. Over a 5-year follow-up, 10 241 men were diagnosed with prostate cancer. The study demonstrated a 32% increase risk of advanced prostate cancer and a 98% increase risk of fatal prostate cancer among men ingesting multivitamins more than 7 times per week! This association was strongest in men with a family history of prostate cancer or those who took individual micronutrients such as selenium, beta-carotene or zinc. Unfortunately, they did not detail the exact quantities of multivitamins taken by those surveyed. The researchers acknowledge limitations of this study include its lack of information regarding duration of multivitamin use, information which may have helped to determine whether associations were limited to long-time users and that small case numbers limited their ability to investigate 3-way interactions among multivitamin use, single supplement use, and family history of prostate cancer. Furthermore, the authors speculate that the adverse effect of multivitamin supplements in combination with supplemental zinc on prostate cancer risk could be due to non-essential, potentially harmful trace elements contained in zinc supplements, such as cadmium, a known carcinogen.

The authors did acknowledge that previous research demonstrated a positive association of multivitamin and mineral use amongst men (with PSA<3) leading to a marked reduction in prostate cancer risk, even up to 52% compared with placebo.

Prostatitis

Stress reduction is beneficial, as it may be a factor leading to this disorder. Quality of life, in general, is very poor in these patients, as a consequence of their illness and hence they can benefit from stress reduction, as well as relaxation techniques.[43]

As with the management of other chronic illness, improvement in diet, especially by reducing pro-inflammatory foods and increasing anti-inflammatory foods, inclusion of a probiotic and regular exercise may be helpful.

Physical activity/exercise

A recent study demonstrated that men who were more active had less lower urinary tract symptoms.[15] More intense exercise, such as running and participating in sport activity, can significantly reduce the symptoms of BPH. In the Health Professionals Follow-up Study, after adjusting for age, race, ethnicity, alcohol intake, diet and smoking, it was found that men who were more active were also less likely to have BPH symptoms or surgery for the condition.[15]

Biologically plausible mechanisms exist to explain the protective effect of physical activity on the development of prostate cancer; the epidemiological data supporting this hypothesis is still incomplete.[44] It is relevant to know whether exercise is indoors or outdoors, the latter providing an opportunity for increased vitamin D production through sun exposure.

Exercise can improve immunity, and reduce stress and depression, increase exposure to sunlight, all of which could increase protection against prostate cancer. Some evidence indicates that physical activity cannot only decrease the chance of prostate cancer, but may slow its progression.[45] Resistance exercise in men receiving androgen deprivation therapy for prostate cancer reduces fatigue and improves QOL, and muscular fitness.[46]

Exercise is protective against BPH and prostate cancer. Men walking 2 to 3 hours per week have 25% lower risk of BPH. Exercise has been found to be protective and in 1 study in men younger than 60, found those that exercised were 4 times less likely to develop prostate cancer.[47]

Pelvic floor exercises for urinary incontinence following prostatectomy

Loss of urine following prostate surgery is a common occurrence. Most men report gradual improvement over several months after surgery, however, some men can remain incontinent.

The loss of urine should be evaluated by a clinician as it can have complicated sequelae.

Conservative treatment can be useful for some men. Incontinence can be of the urgent or stress related types.

Pelvic floor exercises and re-education of patients may help prevent and reduce the incidence of urinary incontinence after prostate surgery.[48] A recent randomised prospective study investigating the benefit of implementing pelvic floor muscle exercises 30 days prior to surgery demonstrated efficacy.[49] The study concluded that preoperative pelvic floor muscle exercises could improve early continence and quality of life outcomes in men following radical prostatectomy for prostate cancer.

Nutritional influences

Vegetables, legumes, soy and fruit

Diet plays an important role in the development of prostate disease.[50] There is now a significant amount of research that strongly suggests that nutrition is closely linked with prostate health.[30, 50–55] A diet rich in fruit, vegetables and fish and low in meat is likely to protect against BPH and prostate cancer.[51–55] High meat, fat and possibly milk intake[51, 52] and polyunsaturated fatty acids[53–55] are also risk factors. According to a recent study of 6000 men over 30 years of age, high consumption of fatty fish, such as salmon, herring and mackerel was reported to be associated with a 50% reduced risk of prostate cancer.[56] Men who ate no fish had a 2–3 fold higher risk of developing prostate cancer than men who ate moderate or high amounts. These benefits are further established in a recent epidemiological review that reported that the benefits were due to high omega-3 fatty acids contained in fatty fish[57] which proved to inhibit the growth of prostate cancer cells in previous *in vitro* studies, albeit the exact mechanisms remain unclear.

In those countries where legumes and soy are the main protein source consumed in large amounts, BPH and the reported prostate cancer incidence is very low.[58] It has been reported and hypothesised that soy is rich in isoflavones which actively concentrates in the prostate gland, regulates activity of androgens and oestrogens by acting on oestrogen receptors, and the isoflavonoids, genestein and diadzein are known to inhibit the enzyme 5-alpha-reductase.[50, 58–60] This then prevents the development of BPH, and may explain the lower rates of prostate cancer in Asian countries. In BPH, there is an increase in dihydrotestosterone (DHT) and DHT receptors. The conversion of testosterone to DHT is mediated by 5-alpha-reductase. This enzyme inhibition can prevent the development of BPH.

Broccoli and cruciferous vegetables

Epidemiological studies suggest men who consume at least 1 portion of cruciferous vegetables (such as broccoli, cauliflower, cabbage and brussel sprouts) per week are at lower risk of the incidence of prostate cancer.[52, 61] Diets rich in broccoli may reduce the risk of prostate cancer according to a 12-month study that randomised men to either a broccoli-rich or a pea-rich diet.[62] The researchers quantified and interpreted changes in global gene expression patterns in the human prostate gland by biopsy before, during and after the 12-month diet and biopsies of the prostate were taken. Whilst the underlying mechanism for this observation is still not clear, the authors postulated that consuming broccoli interacts with GSTM1 genotype to result in complex changes to signalling pathways associated with inflammation and carcinogenesis in the prostate. It was proposed that these changes may be mediated through the chemical interaction of isothiocyanates with signalling peptides in the plasma. The report describes broccoli interacting with oncogenic signalling pathways in the prostate.[62]

Fish, omega-3 fatty acids

The type of fat in the diet plays a role in prostate cancer risk. Oily fish may help to reduce the risk of prostate cancer as omega-3 fatty acids appear to have inhibitory effects on tumour cells whereas omega-6 fatty acids (those contained in margarines rather than gamma-linolenic acid contained in evening primrose and borage seed oil) may have stimulatory effects. Omega-3 fatty acids can influence 5-alpha-reductase activity. Canola products increase the rate of prostate cancer and it is thought to be due to the instability with heat of alpha linolenic acid in canola. Also, omega-3 fatty acids found in fish are protective most probably due to their anti-inflammatory action through their influence on prostaglandins and leukotrienes.[63]

A small study examined the effects on men with dietary changes rich in plant-based foods and fish and its effect on QOL and PSA over 3 months.[64] The intervention group significantly reduced the consumption of saturated fats, dairy foods and animal proteins, and increased consumption of vegetable proteins. The researchers concluded that men with an increasing PSA level after primary treatment were able to make a change to a prostate-healthy diet, accompanied by increases in QOL. No significant difference was found in the log PSA slope between the 2 groups; however, the PSA doubling time increased substantially in the intervention group compared with that in the controls.[64] Further studies are required with larger samples.

Dairy products

A large study found the risk of BPH was significantly lower in men with a high intake of total vegetables, dark yellow vegetables, other vegetables, tofu and red meat and a greater risk with increasing intake of high-fat dairy products.[65] It is thought that a high intake of calcium foods and dairy products is associated with an increased risk of prostate cancer by lowering concentrations of 1,25-dihydroxyvitamin D(3),[66, 67] 1,25(OH_2D3), a hormone thought to protect against prostate cancer. The Physicians' Health Study, a cohort of male US physicians in an 11-year follow-up study, documented 1012 incident cases of prostate cancer among 20 885 men. After adjustment for baseline age, BMI, smoking, exercise, and randomised treatment compared with men consuming less than or equal to 1–2/day servings of dairy products, those consuming >2.5 servings had an increase relative risk of prostate cancer by 34%.[66] Men consuming >600mg/day of calcium had a 32% higher risk of prostate cancer. Of interest, at baseline, men who consumed >600mg Ca/day from skim milk had lower plasma 1,25(OH_2D3) concentrations than did those consuming less than or equal to 150mg Ca/day, which explains the lack of protection towards developing prostate cancer. However, a recent large meta-analyses has concluded that the case-control analyses using calcium as the exposure of interest demonstrated no association with increased risk of prostate cancer in the review.[68] Dietary intake of vitamin D also was not related to prostate cancer risk. Moreover, the data from observational studies did not support an association between dairy product use and an increased risk of prostate cancer.[68]

Soy milk

Drinking soy milk (several glasses per day) lowered risk of prostate cancer by 70% in 1 study.[50, 69] Soy contains cancer-fighting substances called isoflavones, especially genistein which inhibits prostate cancer growth. Soy can inhibit oestrogen, cell growth, block activity of 5-alpha-reductase and tyrosine-specific protein kinase, plus reduce angiogenesis.

Phytoestrogens have been shown to cause prominent prostate cancer apoptosis in a human study.[70] The major difference between Asian and US diets is the consumption of soy-based food stuffs. Soy protein powder decreases serum testosterone levels in healthy men and acts as an estrogen receptor (ER)-beta agonist, possibly inducing a biological effect to reduce the risk for prostate cancer development.[71] This, however, needs to be carefully verified.

In general, there is support for the intake of legumes and yellow-orange plus cruciferous vegetables being inversely related to the risk of prostate cancer.[72] Decreased prostate cancer risk has been found in Seventh-Day Adventists who have high intakes of lycopenes, lentils and peas.[69] In general, multiple servings of fruit have also been shown to be inversely related to progression of prostate cancer.[51]

Pomegranate juice

Pomegranate juice is a major source of phytochemicals, and when consumed by men with a rising PSA after surgery or radiotherapy for their prostate cancer, it caused a statistically significant prolongation of PSA doubling with time.[73] Approximately 2 x 30mls of pomegranate juice was consumed daily over the 2-year period of the trial. The serum of the men taking pomegranate also influenced *in vitro* prostate cancer cell proliferation and apoptosis, as well as oxidative stress.[73]

Special foods and teas

Green tea (*Camellia sinensis*)

Tea produced from the leaves of the plant *Camellia sinensis* along with water, is the most widely consumed beverage in the world.[74] Alterations in the manufacturing process result in black, green, and oolong tea, which account for approximately 75%, 23%, and 2% of the global production, respectively. Even though each of these non-herbal teas is derived from the same source, different processing techniques render them chemically different from each other.[74]

Green tea has been reported in numerous recent reviews to be of benefit in preventing prostate diseases.[75–80] According to a recent study[79] with 404 men living in Southeast China, it was reported that compared to non-green tea drinkers, the risk of prostate cancer was 62% lower in all tea drinkers. Those who drank more than 3 cups daily reduced their risk by 63% and 88% for those who had consumed green tea for more than 40 years and 91% lower for those who consumed more than 1.5kg of tea leaves yearly.[80] Green tea suppresses prostate cancer cells *in vitro*.

Lycopene

Based largely on the scientific evidence from epidemiologic, *in vitro*, animal and human clinical trials data, it is evident that lycopene, a non-provitamin A carotenoid, is a promising agent for the chemo-prevention of prostate cancer.[81, 82] Lycopene is a natural plant compound found predominantly in tomatoes.

In the Health Professionals Follow-up study that followed just over 47 000 middle-aged male practitioners since 1986, a significant difference was reported in prostate cancer incidence in men with a high dietary intake of lycopene with a relative risk reduced to 0.84, even after adjusting for other risk factors such as smoking and other dietary factors.[83] The main source of lycopene in the study was from tomato sauce. Men who ate the most sauce had the highest lycopene levels and lower prostate cancer rates. Another study found that men who consumed tomato sauce-based pasta dishes for 3 weeks before radical prostatectomy, had increased lycopene levels in blood and prostate, reduction in serum PSA levels and damage to prostate cancer cells.[83] Recently the US Food and Drug Administration stated that lycopene was not associated with a reduced risk of prostate, lung, colorectal, breast, cervical or endometrial cancer.[84] The role of lycopene in the area of prostate cancer prevention subsequent to this study was defended by an expert commentary.[85]

Garlic (*Allium sativum*)

Animal and *in vitro* studies provide evidence of an anti-carcinogenic effect of active ingredients in garlic.[86, 87] A significant protective effect has also been noted in men with a consumption of >10g/day of allium vegetables.[88] After adjusting for age and intake for other foods, high consumption of garlic and scallions were associated with the greatest protective effects.[88]

Pumpkin seeds (*Curcurbita pepo*)

A German multi centre study with 2245 patients diagnosed with BPH (Stage I to II) investigated the therapeutic use and safety of a pumpkin seed extract.[89] Urinary symptoms were recorded by the International-Prostate-Symptom-Score according to the American Urological Association, the influence on quality of life has been recorded by a QOL index. Patients were treated for 12 weeks with

1–2 capsules per day containing 500mg of a pumpkin seed extract (15–25:1). The prostate symptom score decreased by 47.4% and QOL improved by 46.1% during therapy.

An early double-blind, placebo-controlled study of 3 months duration in 53 patients with BPH demonstrated that a daily intake of 4800mg of *Cucurbita pepo* (pumpkin seed) combined with the herb *Serenoa repens* (saw palmetto) showed significant improvement in objective and subjective parameters such as micturition time, frequency, dysuria, urinary flow (6.7 to 9.7 ml) as well as a reduction in residual volume by 32%. No side-effects were noted.[90]

A more recent double-blind, placebo-controlled study of 12 months duration in 47 patients with BPH demonstrated that a daily intake of 4800mg of *Cucurbita pepo* (pumpkin seed oil at a dose of 320mg/day) combined with the herb *Serenoa repens* (saw palmetto oil at a dose of 320mg/day) when compared with placebo or the 2 oils given singly. The study showed significant improvement in the international prostate symptom score (both oils singly or in combination), quality of life (both oils singly or in combination), serum prostate specific antigen (oil combination alone), prostate volume (no improvement) and maximal urinary flow rate improvement with both oils.[91]

Turmeric (*Curcumin*)

Curcumin is known to be a COX-2 inhibitor and can induce apoptosis of prostate cancer cells, as well as enhancing cytotoxicity of chemotherapeutic agents, and conferring radio-sensitising effects on prostate cancer cells.[92] *Curcumin* can induce apoptosis in both androgen-dependent and androgen-independent prostate cancer cells by inhibiting tyrosine kinase activity of epidermal growth factor receptor, and depletes this protein.[93] *Curcumin* may be a novel modality by which one can interfere with the signal transduction pathways of the prostate cancer cell and prevent it from progressing to its hormone refractory state.

Nutritional supplements

Prostate cancer

Vitamin E

Vitamin E, even in small doses, offers protection against prostate cancer.[94, 95] In the Alpha-Tocopherol Beta-Carotene Cancer Prevention Study, a large placebo-controlled trial involving 29 133 men (smokers aged 50–69 years), it was reported that there was a 32% decrease in prostate cancer incidence and mortality from prostate cancer by 41% among those males who received vitamin E (alpha-tocopherol at a 50mg dose per day).[95, 96] Natural vitamin E (d-alpha-tocopherol) and mixed tocopherols (alpha, beta and gamma tocopherol) may confer additional protection. It is possible that vitamin E combined with selenium may offer more protection.[96] Vitamin E inhibits human prostate cancer cell growth via modulating the cell cycle regulatory machinery.[97] Sources of vitamin E include wheat germ, canola oil, nuts, spinach and egg yolk.

However, a recent long-term RCT trial study utilising individual supplements of 400IU of vitamin E every other day and 500mg of vitamin C daily has reported that neither vitamin E nor C supplementation reduced the risk of prostate or total cancer.[98]

A recent randomised placebo controlled trial of 35,533 men from 427 participating sites in the United States, Canada, and Puerto Rico (Selenium and Vitamin E Cancer Prevention Trial [SELECT]) found that neither oral selenium (200 microgram/day from L-selenomethionine) nor vitamin E (400 IU/day of all rac-alpha-tocopheryl acetate) alone or in combination did not prevent prostate cancer in this population of relatively healthy men compared with placebo.[99]

Furthermore, it is best to avoid high doses of vitamin E greater than 400IU/day as some research suggests it may increase all-cause mortality, although there are mixed findings in a number of different studies and warrants further research.[100, 101]

Vitamin D

Experimental evidence suggests that vitamin D may reduce the risk of cancer through the regulation of cellular proliferation and differentiation as well as inhibition of angiogenesis.[102] These anti-cancer properties have been attributed primarily to 1,25-dihydroxyvitamin D, the hormonal form of vitamin D.[102, 103, 104] Moreover, numerous studies have reported the inverse association between ultraviolet solar exposure and mortality rates for prostate cancer.[104] Analysis of the serum from 250 000 participants found that low vitamin D was a risk factor for prostate cancer.[105] *In vitro* studies show that vitamin D can inhibit proliferation and also promotes differentiation in human prostate cancer cells.[106] Receptors for vitamin D exist on human prostate cancer cells. Prostate cancer patients who have the highest levels of vitamin D mainly from sun exposure have a better prognosis.[106]

Selenium

The prevention of prostate cancer with nutritional supplements came to prominence in 1996 when the Nutritional Prevention of Cancer Trial reported a 65% reduction in prostate cancer incidence in men receiving selenium supplementation.[107]

Non-experimental epidemiological studies suggest that individuals with a higher selenium status are at decreased risk of cancer, and that includes cancer of the prostate.[108–110] A US study reported that men with high selenium levels have a lower risk of prostate cancer.[109] In a double-blind cancer prevention trial of 974 men, 400mcg of selenium per day reduced the incidence of prostate cancer by 63%.[110] In a similar study involving over 10 000 people, selenium supplements of 200mcg/day reduced the risk of prostate cancer by two-thirds.[111] *In vitro* experiments using human prostate cancer cells showed that selenium caused apoptosis and in animal experiments it retarded hormone refractory prostate cancer.[112, 113]

The National Cancer Institute in cooperation with the Southwest Oncology Group has begun one of the largest prostate cancer prevention studies, the Selenium and Vitamin E Chemoprevention Trial (SELECT).[114] In reviewing all of the available evidence comprehensively for the study, the authors concluded that there was promising evidence in support of these antioxidant compounds in the primary prevention of prostate cancer.[114]

Zinc

Despite theories that zinc may benefit the prostate by inhibiting 5 alpha-reductase,[115] the Health Professionals Follow-up Study[116] did not confirm this hypothesis. In this study, men who took low doses of zinc were compared to men who took more than 100mg of supplemental zinc a day and men who took supplemental zinc for more than 10 years; the latter 2 groups doubled their risk of prostate cancer. Chronic oversupply of zinc should be avoided as it could play a role in prostate carcinogenesis. Zinc obtained from food was not linked to an increased risk.[117]

Nutritional supplements, prostatitis and BPH

Zinc and magnesium are depleted in prostatic fluid of patients with prostatitis and BPH.[118, 119, 120] Preliminary studies indicate that zinc and magnesium supplementation with appropriate doses may be of some value.[120, 121]

Herbal medicine

Prostatitis

A study that investigated the safety and efficacy of saw palmetto versus finasteride in men with category III prostatitis or chronic pelvic pain syndrome in a 1 year prospective trial reported no efficacy for the herb.[122] Long-term efficacy was reported for finasteride only. A multi-centre trial using saw palmetto (*Serenoa repens*) showed a positive response.[123] A recent multi-centre trial reported that a mixture of *Serenoa repens* plus selenium and lycopene was effective in ameliorating the symptoms associated with chronic prostatitis/chronic pelvic pain.[124] A placebo-controlled trial using quercetin found a response rate of 82%.[125] Saw palmetto and quercetin have an anti-inflammatory action and this may explain their mechanism of action.[126–129]

Benign prostatic hypertrophy

Saw palmetto (*Serenoa repens*)

The plant saw palmetto has been used for hundreds of years in traditional medicine, particularly for male genitourinary conditions such as libido, impotence and problems of micturition. Clinical studies have confirmed its use in the treatment for BPH.[129]

The exact mechanism of action of saw palmetto is not known. *Serenoa repens* extracts are rich in fatty acids, especially its principle ingredient beta-sitosterol a weak inhibitor of 5-alpha-reductase and anti-inflammatory effects on the prostate. Beta-sitosterol is also found in soy products as well as other herbs that have been used to treat diseases of the prostate, including pygeum bark, stinging nettle root and pumpkin seed extract.[129] It is a weak inhibitor of 5-alpha-reductase and may decrease DHT receptors as well as having an anti-inflammatory effect on the prostate. Finasteride is a more powerful inhibitor of 5-alpha-reductase. The mechanism of action of the sterols on the prostate remains unknown. Saw palmetto does not reduce the size of the gland.[130]

A systematic review of 18 clinical trials involved nearly 3000 men with mild to moderate BPH, and included 16 double-blind trials with a mean duration period study of 9 weeks.[131] It was concluded that saw palmetto improved urinary flow and was well tolerated with minimal and infrequent adverse effects, notably upper digestive upset and minimal withdrawal rates of 9% when compared with 7% for placebo. Compared with placebo, saw palmetto improved urinary symptom scores, symptoms, and flow measures.

The Cochrane reviewers reported that the weighted mean difference (WMD) for the urinary symptom score was −1.41 points (scale range 0–19), (95% confidence interval [CI] = −2.52, −0.30, n = 1 study) and the risk ratio (RR) for self-rated improvement was 1.76 (95% CI = 1.21, 2.54, n = 6 studies). The WMD for nocturia was −0.76 times per evening (95% CI = −1.22, -0.32; n = 10 studies). The WMD for peak urine flow was 1.86 ml/sec (95%CI = 0.60, 3.12, n = 9 studies). Compared with finasteride, saw palmetto produced similar improvements in urinary symptom scores (WMD = 0.37 IPSS points [scale range 0–35], 95% CI = −0.45, 1.19, n = 2 studies) and peak urine flow (WMD = −0.74 ml/sec, 95% CI = −1.66, 0.18, n = 2 studies). Adverse effects due to saw palmetto were mild and infrequent. Withdrawal rates in men assigned to placebo, saw palmetto or finasteride were 7%, 9%, and 11%, respectively. The authors' concluded the evidence suggests that *Serenoa repens* provides mild to moderate improvement in urinary symptoms and flow measures. Also, that *Serenoa repens* produced similar improvement in urinary symptoms and flow compared to finasteride and was associated with fewer adverse treatment events. The long-term effectiveness, safety and ability to prevent BPH complications are not as yet known.[131]

In a 6-month double-blind randomised control trial (RCT) 1098 men with mild to moderate BPH were randomised to saw palmetto extract 320mgs/day or finasteride 5mgs/day.[132] The results concluded that saw palmetto and finasteride were equally effective in the management of BPH; both relieved symptoms in two-thirds of patients with less side-effects in the saw palmetto group. The study used the International Prostate Symptom Score (IPSS) as a primary end-point and found reduction by 39% in the finasteride group compared with 37% in the saw palmetto group. Quality of life improved by 41% in the finasteride compared with 38% in the saw palmetto group. Prostate volume reduced by 18% in finasteride compared with 6% in the saw palmetto group. PSA levels reduced by 41% in finasteride group with no changes in the saw palmetto group; an advantage as it allows for continued monitoring for prostate cancer. Sexual function, libido and potency were adversely affected in the finasteride group by 4.4% compared with the saw palmetto group by 1.1%.[132]

A large double-blind randomised study compared finasteride, tamsulosin and perimixon (a lipido-sterolic extract of *Serenoa repens*)[133] evaluation of male sexual function in patients with lower urinary tract symptoms (LUTS) associated with BPH treated with a phytotherapeutic agent (Permixon). After 6-months, when compared to pre-treatment data, the study demonstrated that there was a slight negative impact on sexual disorders, especially ejaculation disorders in the Tamsulosin and Finasteride treated patients compared with a slight improvement on sexual function with Permixon therapy.[133]

A US study comparing saw palmetto and placebo found no statistical significance between the 2 groups in urinary flow rate, prostate size, residual volume after voiding, quality of life, or serum PSA levels during the 1-year study. The incidence of side-effects was also similar in the 2 groups.[134]

Curcumin

Numerous herbal medicine compounds (i.e. curcumin) for the chemo-prevention of prostate cancer have been investigated.[135–138] Currently, there are no clinical trials investigating the efficacy of curcumin for the prevention or treatment of prostate diseases.

African plum tree *(Pygeum africanum extract)*

A recent updated Cochrane review of 18 RCTs involving 1562 men taking *Pygeum africanum extract* from African plum tree versus placebo found twice as likely improvements in overall urinary symptoms. *Pygeum africanum* extract may be a useful treatment option for men with lower urinary symptoms consistent with BPH.[139,140] Additional placebo-controlled studies are warranted.

Stinging nettle (*Urticae radix* and *diocia*)

A recent review has documented the clinical evidence of effectiveness for stinging nettle in the treatment of BPH, based on many open studies and a small number of randomised controlled studies.[141–144] The data indicate that a proprietary methanolic extract is effective in improving BPH complaints.[144] Overall the studies have reported improvements of prostate size, nocturia, frequency of micturition, urine flow and residual urine.[139] Moreover, the risk for adverse events during stinging nettle treatment was reported to be very low, as was its toxicity. However, pre-clinical safety data are yet to be completed.[141, 142]

In most studies, stinging nettle has been combined with saw palmetto or *pygeum*.[140, 141, 142] A combination of 300mg of *Urtica dioica* root extract combined with 25mg of *Pygeum africanum* bark extract demonstrated improvement in QOL and reduced BPH symptoms.[142] Results of studies using combinations with saw palmetto have demonstrated a response equal to finasteride, an alpha blocker.[143–146] The mechanism action of stinging nettle is not clear but it is a potent antioxidant and also has anti-inflammatory activity.[147, 148]

Red clover (*Trifolium pretense*)

A small study of 20 men with BPH were treated with 60mg of red clover daily for 1 year. The study noted a statistically significant reduction of PSA by 33%.[149] Also, the mean prostate volume had decreased slightly from 49.3 cm^3 to 44.3 cm^3 after 12 months ($P < 0.097$). Sexual hormone levels did not change throughout the study period. The authors also noted a significant increase in levels of all 3 liver transaminases after 3 months to the high normal range.[149] This is a concern and raises the issue of potential herb–drug interactions as red clover affected the hepatic metabolism and may affect drugs metabolised by the liver (e.g. anaesthetics).

Prostate cancer

PC SPES and PC PLUS

PC stands for prostate cancer and SPES is Latin for hope. PC SPES is a product composed of 8 herbs but was removed from the market in the US because of impurities. PC SPES has been replaced by a new product with the same herbs without impurities, PC PLUS (called prostasol). PC SPES was shown to be useful in the treatment of both hormone-sensitive and hormone-insensitive prostate cancers. The herbs in this product have several actions, including inhibition of angiogeneses, stimulation of immunity, inducing an oestrogenic effect and inhibiting 5-alpha-reductase.[150]

Potential side-effects include fluid retention and thrombosis, as with oestrogen therapy.

Amazonian plant extract

An orally active Amazonian plant extract (BIRM) inhibits prostate cancer growth and metastasis.[151] This study evaluated the anti-tumour activity of a simple Ecuadorian oral solution: an extract of an Amazonian plant extract, that was characterised *in vitro* and *in vivo* using established prostate cancer (CaP) cell lines and a tumour model in 4 human and 1 rat CaP cell lines. The plant extract appears to exert anti-tumour compounds with potent anti-proliferative activity *in vitro* and *in vivo* against prostate cancer cells.[151] More research is warranted though.

Physical therapies

Acupuncture

Prostatitis

A meta- analysis from China[152] has concluded that acupuncture therapy was significantly effective for the treatment of chronic prostatitis. This result was further reinforced in a recently clinical trial.[153] This trial reported that acupuncture appeared to be safe and a potentially effective treatment in improving the symptoms and quality of life of men clinically diagnosed with chronic prostatitis and chronic pelvic pain syndrome.

Prostate cancer

A recent systematic review on the management of hot flushes in men diagnosed with prostate cancer has alluded to the possibility that acupuncture may assist in managing hot flushes.[154] The review concluded though that recommendation was difficult given that there were no robust RCTs. An additional systematic review consisted of 6 studies. One study was an RCT clinical trial that compared the effects of manual acupuncture with that of acupuncture plus electro-acupuncture. The other 5 studies of this review were uncontrolled observational studies and hence the evidence was limited.[155] The review concluded that the overall evidence was weak and acupuncture could not be recommended as an effective treatment for hot flushes in patients with prostate cancer.

Conclusion

Health care professionals should educate patients about the potential positive effects of simple lifestyle changes on BPH and prevention of prostate cancer. Some of the potential lifestyle and CAM factors that may positively affect the prostate are summarised in Table 34.1. Preliminary data continue to support the importance of lifestyle changes for men who are trying to prevent BPH and for men already diagnosed with the condition or for the prevention and treatment of prostate cancer. Clinicians must incorporate lifestyle modification advice (such as diet, exercise, sunshine exposure for vitamin D and stress management) into standard medical consultations, and future management guidelines should be adopted similar to what has been done for cardiovascular disease. This can improve educational efforts and help reduce the burden of prostate diseases.

A great deal of the evidence relating to prostate cancer is at a preliminary stage. However, the Ornish studies[36, 37, 38] are strongly suggestive that an integrative approach is likely to be beneficial. This is especially appropriate in those patients that are treated conservatively. The Ornish approach can be offered as an addition to established therapies.

Lifestyle changes go further than disease-specific concerns and can potentially improve overall health and wellbeing (both emotionally and physically), plus significantly reduce the risk for chronic disease development.

Table 34.1 Levels of evidence for lifestyle and complementary medicines/therapies in the management of prostate cancer (a), benign prostatic hypertrophy (b), and prostatitis (c)

Modality	Level I	Level II	Level IIIa	Level IIIb	Level IIIc	Level IV	Level V
Lifestyle behaviour modification							
Stress reduction + diet + exercise (a), (b)		x (a), (b)					
Mind–body medicine							
Mindfulness-based stress reduction (a)		x					
Physical activity/ exercise							
Physical activity/ exercise (a), (b)			x(a)	x(b)			
Pelvic floor exercise (a)		x					
Nutritional influences							
Vegetables and fruit in the diet (a, b)				x(a, b)			
Legumes, soy (a)							
Alcohol (a)		x					
Green tea (a)						x	
Fish/fish oils (a)				x			
Broccoli (a)		x					
Lycopene (a), (c)		x (a), (c)					
Garlic (a)			x				
Pumpkin seeds (b)					x		
Supplements							
Vitamin E (a)		x (+/-)					
Selenium (a), (c)		x					
Vitamin D (a)						x	
Zinc (c)					x		
Quercetin (a), (c)		x (c)				x (a)	

Continued

Table 34.1 Levels of evidence for lifestyle and complementary medicines/therapies in the management of prostate cancer (a), benign prostatic hypertrophy (b), and prostatitis (c)—cont'd

Modality	Level I	Level II	Level IIIa	Level IIIb	Level IIIc	Level IV	Level V
Herbal medicines							
Saw palmetto (b), (c)	x (b)	x (c)					
African plum tree (b)	x						
Red clover (b)					x		
Stinging nettle (b)				x			
PC SPES PLUS(a)			x				
Physical therapies							
Acupuncture							
• Prostatitis	x						
• Prostate cancer (hot flushes)				x			

Level I - from a systematic review of all relevant randomised controlled trials - meta-analyses.
Level II - from at least 1 properly designed randomised controlled clinical trial.
Level IIIa - from well-designed pseudo-randomised controlled trials (alternate allocation or some other method).
Level IIIb - from comparative studies (including systematic reviews of such studies) with concurrent controls and allocation not randomised, cohort studies, case-control studies, or interrupted time series with a parallel control group.
Level IIIc - from comparative studies with historical control, 2 or more single-arm studies or interrupted time series without a parallel control group.
Level IV - opinions of respected authorities based on clinical experience, descriptive studies or reports of expert committees.
Level V - represents minimal evidence that represents testimonials.

Clinical tips handout for patients — prostate disease

1 Lifestyle advice

Sleep

- Restore normal sleep patterns. Early to bed (about 9–10 p.m.) and awake upon sunrise. (See Chapter 22 for more advice.)

Sunshine

- Amount of exposure varies with local climate.
- At least 15 minutes of sunshine needed daily for vitamin D and melatonin production — especially before 10 a.m. and after 3 p.m. when the sun exposure is safest during summer. Much more exposure is required in winter, when supplementation needs to be considered.
- Ensure gradual adequate skin exposure to sun; avoid sunscreen and excess clothing to maximise levels of vitamin D.
- More time in the sun is required for dark skinned people.
- Direct exposure to about 10% of body (hands, arms, face), without sunscreen and not through glass.
- Vitamin D is obtained in the diet from fatty fish, eggs, liver and fortified foods (some milks and margarines); it is unlikely that adequate vitamin D concentrations can be obtained from diet alone.

2 Physical activity/exercise

- Exercise 30 minutes or more daily. If exercise is not regular, commence with 5 minutes daily and slowly build up to at least 30 minutes. Outdoor exercise in nature, fresh air and sunshine is ideal (e.g. brisk walking, light jogging, cycling, swimming, stretching.) The more time you spend outdoors the better.
- Pelvic floor exercises can help prevent incontinence after prostate surgery. Speak with your doctor/health practitioner for more advice and instructions on how to do pelvic floor exercises, particularly when practised before and after surgery.

3 Mind–body medicine

- Stress management program — for example, six 40 minute sessions for patients to understand the nature of their symptoms, the symptoms' relationship to stress, and the practice of regular relaxation exercises.
- Regular meditation practice, at least 10–20 minutes daily.

Breathing

- Be aware of breathing at all times. Notice if tendency to hold breath or over-breathe. Always aim to relax breath and the muscles around the chest wall.

Rest and stress management

Recurrent stress may cause a return of symptoms. Relaxation is important for a full and lasting recovery.

- Reduce workload and resolve conflicts. Contact family, friends, church, social or other groups for support.
- Listening to relaxation music and daily baths help.
- Other examples for stress management: yoga, counselling, meditation, personal growth, psychotherapy, tai chi, massage therapy.

Fun

- It is important to have fun in life. Joy can be found even in the simplest tasks, such as being with friends with a sense of humour, funny movies/videos, comedy, hobbies, dancing, playing with pets and children.

4 Environment

- Don't smoke and avoid smoking environments.
- Avoid environmental pollutants and chemicals — at work and in the home.
- Ensure office or home has a view overlooking garden or park.

5 Dietary changes

- Eat more fruit (>2/day) and vegetables (>5/day) — variety of colours and those in season.
- Eat more nuts; for example, walnuts, hazelnuts, almonds, peanuts; seeds, beans, sprouts (e.g. alfalfa, mung bean, lentils).
- Increase intake of legumes (soy 60 grams per day, beans, lentils, chickpeas), soy, tomatoes, broccoli, garlic, pumpkin seeds.
- Increase fish intake, especially deep sea fish, at least 3 times per week. Canned is okay (mackerel, salmon, sardines, cod, tuna, salmon).
- Reduce red meat intake — preferably use red lean meat (e.g. lamb, kangaroo) and white meat (e.g. free range organic chicken fillets).
- Use cold pressed olive oil and avocado.
- Use only dark chocolate (25–50g daily) unless not tolerated.
- Eat a variety of wholegrains/cereals (best if not toasted). Cooked traditional

rolled oats for breakfast are particularly helpful, as is rice (brown, basmati, Mahatma, Dongara), buckwheat flour, wholegrain organic breads (rye bread, Essene, spelt, Kamut) — when toasting make hot and crisp, not brown, to avoid acrylamide — brown pasta, couscous, millet, amaranth, etc.
- Use turmeric spice in cooking.
- Pomegranate juice 30mls 2 x daily may help prostate cancer.
- Increase dietary intake of lycopene-rich foods such as tomato sauces and fresh tomatoes, or a supplement of lycopene 4–10mg/day.
- Reduce dairy intake. Use low-fat dairy products, such as low-fat yoghurt, unless there is a dairy intolerance. Soy (organic) milk is an alternative and is protective.
- Drink more water 1–2 litres a day and teas, especially green tea, chamomile, peppermint and black teas (best if organic).
- Avoid artificial sweeteners — replace with honey (e.g. manuka, yellow box and stringy bark have lowest GI).
- Avoid hydrogenated fats, salt, fast foods, sugar such as soft drinks, lollies, biscuits, cakes and processed foods (e.g. white bread, white pasta, pastries).
- Minimise alcohol intake to no more than 1–2 glasses daily.
- Avoid chemical additives — preservatives, colourings and flavourings.

6 Physical therapies

- Acupuncture may be beneficial for prostate and back pain management in those patients diagnosed with prostatitis.

7 Nutritional supplements

Vitamin E (natural gamma tocopherol)

- Indication: may help reduce spread of prostate cancer.
- Dosage: 50–200IU/day.
- Results: uncertain.
- Side-effects: very mild and rare; nausea, vomiting, diarrhoea, sensitivity reactions; avoid high doses >400IU/day as some research suggest it may increase risk of all-cause mortality.
- Contraindications: avoid high doses before surgery; pharmaceutical medication such as warfarin especially with vitamin K deficiency, impaired coagulation, hemorrhagic stroke.

Vitamin D3 (cholecalciferol)

- Indication: may help reduce spread of prostate cancer. Natural source is from the sun.
- Dosage: 1000IU/day; your doctor should check your blood levels to determine correct dosage to avoid toxicity.
- Results: uncertain.
- Side-effects: very mild and rare; nausea, vomiting, diarrhoea, sensitivity reactions.
- Contraindications: avoid if you suffer high calcium levels, systemic lupus erythematosis, sarcoidosis and hyperparathyroidism as these conditions can impact on calcium levels; pharmaceutical medication such as lipid lowering drugs; calcium channel blockers for hypertension.

Selenium (sodium selenite, organic selenium found in yeast)

- Indication: may help reduce spread of prostate cancer.
- Dosage: 50–100mg/day; do not exceed >600mg/day (health professional supervision required to avoid toxicity).
- Results: uncertain.
- Side-effects: very mild and rare; nausea, vomiting, rash, sensitivity reactions, toxicity in high doses; nail changes, irritability, fatigue.
- Contraindications: pregnancy, lactation, children <12 years of age.

Zinc sulfate or gluconate; elemental zinc

- Indication: benign prostatic hypertrophy.
- Dosage: up to 25mg elemental zinc daily in adults.
- Results: uncertain.
- Side-effects: avoid high doses and long-term use as this increases the risk of prostate cancer; dry mouth, metallic taste on tongue, nausea, vomiting, diarrhoea; may cause copper deficiency in high doses; avoid in advanced prostate cancer.
- Contraindications: avoid in iron deficiency until assessed by a doctor.

Herbal supplements

African plum tree *(Pygeum africanum* extract)

- Indications: BPH.
- Dosage: 75–200mg/day of a standardised extract. 100mg/day serves as the mode dose.
- Results: minimum of 30 days for improvement in overall urinary symptoms in men with low grade benign prostatic hypertrophy. It should be noted that a dose given as 50mg/TDS or 100mg/day are considered equally efficacious and safe for up to 2 months of continuous use.
- Side-effects: although more clinical trials are necessary, mild gastrointestinal upset has been reported.

- Contraindications: no contraindications are known, however as with all herbal medicines, herb–drug interactions surveillance is always necessary.

Red clover (*Trifolium pretense*)

- Indications: elevated PSA with no malignancy and secondary to BPH.
- Dosage: 60mg/day.
- Results: significant reduction in PSA levels (33%) after 1 year, with no change in hormonal levels.
- Side-effects: elevated liver enzymes, in particular liver transaminases.
- Contraindications: there is a potential for significant herb–drug interactions, such as with anaesthetics.

Saw palmetto (*Serenoa repens*)

- Indication: mild–moderate benign prostatic hypertrophy.
- Dosage: 1–1.6mg 1–2 x daily.
- Results: 1–4 weeks.
- Side-effects: very mild and rare. Includes headache, nausea, vomiting, digestion disturbance, aggravation of urinary problems, and sensitivity to herb; gynecomastia.
- Contraindications: pregnancy, lactation, children, fertility, drug interaction; avoid use with pharmaceutical medication such as anticoagulants (warfarin, aspirin, non-steroidal medication), oral contraceptive pill, androgens, estrogens, and immune stimulants. Check with your doctor.

Stinging nettle (*Urticae radix*)

- Indication: mild–moderate benign prostatic hypertrophy.
- Dosage: extract of stinging nettle 120mg plus a specific extract of saw palmetto 160mg twice daily.
- Results: 1–4 weeks.
- Side-effects: very mild and rare. Includes headache, nausea, vomiting, digestion disturbance, allergic skin reactions (orally and topically), sensitivity to herb, lower blood pressure, lower glucose levels in diabetics, drowsiness.
- Contraindications: fertility, pregnancy and lactation; children; people with kidney disease as stinging nettle is a diuretic; avoid use with pharmaceutical medication such as anti-hypertensives and warfarin, as stinging nettle contains vitamin K. Check with your doctor.

Turmeric (Curcumin)

- Indication: may help prevent and reduce spread of prostate cancer.
- Dosage: 500mg of turmeric 4 times daily; add turmeric to cooking.
- Results: uncertain.
- Side-effects: very mild and rare; gastrointestinal upset (e.g. nausea, stomach pains, vomiting, diarrhoea); sensitivity reactions; blood clotting problems; rash when applied topically to skin.
- Contraindications: pregnancy and lactation; children; pharmaceutical medication such as anticoagulant and anti-platelet drugs (e.g. aspirin, warfarin, clopidogrel); discontinue turmeric at least 2 weeks before elective surgical procedures.

References

1 Nickel JC. Inflammation and benign prostatic hyperplasia. Urol Clin North Am 2008;35(1):109–15.
2 Arrighi HM, Metter EJ, Guess HA, et. al. Natural history of benign prostatic hyperplasia and risk of prostatectomy: the Baltimore Longitudinal Aging Study. Urology 1991;38(suppl 1):4–8.
3 Sarma AV, Wei JT, Jacobson DJ, et. al. Comparison of lower urinary tract symptom severity and associated bother between community dwelling black and white men: the Olmsted County Study of Urinary Symptoms and Health Status and the Flint Men's Health Study. Urology 2003;61:1086–1091.
4 Berry SJ, Coffey DS, Walsh PC, et. al. The development of human benign prostatic hyperplasia with age. J Urol 1984;132:474–79.
5 Kupelian V, Wei JT, O'Leary MP, et. al. Prevalence of lower urinary tract symptoms and effect on quality of life in a racially and ethnically diverse random sample: the Boston Area Community Health (BACH) Survey. Arch Intern Med 2006;166:2381–87.
6 Parsons JK, Carter HB, Partin AW, et. al. Metabolic factors associated with benign prostatic hyperplasia. J Clin Endocrinol Metab 2006;91: 2562–68.
7 Michel MC, Heemann U, Schumacher H, et. al. Association of hypertension with symptoms of benign prostatic hyperplasia. J Urol 2004;172:1390–93.
8 Clifford GM, Farmer RD. Drug or symptom-induced depression in men treated with beta1-blockers for benign prostatic hyperplasia? A nested case control study. Pharmacoepidemiol Drug Saf 2002;11:55–61.
9 Morton MS, Turkes A, Denis L, et. al. Can dietary factors influence prostatic disease? BJU Int 1999;84:549–54.
10 Moyad MA. Lifestyle changes to prevent BPH: Heart healthy prostate healthy. Urol Nurs 2003;23:439–41.
11 Gibbons EP, Colen J, Nelson JB, et. al. Correlation between risk factors for vascular disease and the American Urological Association Symptom Score. BJU Int 2007;99:97–100.
12 Parsons JK. Modifiable risk factors for benign prostatic hyperplasia and lower urinary tract symptoms: new approaches to old problems. J Urol 2007;178:395–401.
13 Lee S, Min HG, Choi SH, et. al. Central obesity as a risk factor for prostatic hyperplasia. Obesity (Silver Spring) 2006;14:172–79.
14 Dahle SE, Chokkalingam AP, Gao YT, et. al. Body size and serum levels of insulin and leptin in relation to the risk of benign prostatic hyperplasia. J Urol 2002;168:599–604.
15 Platz EA, Kawachi I, Rimm EB, et. al. Physical activity and benign prostatic hyperplasia. Arch Intern Med 1998;158:2349–56.

16 Damber JE, Aus G. Prostate cancer. Lancet 2008;371:1710–21.
17 Jemal A, Siegel R, Ward E, et. al. Cancer statistics, 2007. CA Cancer J Clin 2007;57(1):43–66.
18 Connolly D, Black A, Gavin A, et. al. Baseline prostate-specific antigen level and risk of prostate cancer and prostate-specific mortality: diagnosis is dependent on the intensity of investigation. Cancer Epidem Biomarkers Prev 2008;17(2):271–8.
19 Klotz L. Active surveillance for favorable risk prostate cancer: rationale, risks, and results. Urol Oncol 2007;25(6):505–9.
20 Australian Institute of Health and Welfare (AIHW). Cancer survival and prevalence in Australia: cancers diagnosed from 1982 to 2004. Online. Available: www.aihw.gov.au/publications/can/cspia-cdf-82–04/cspia-cdf-82–04.pdf (accessed March 2010).
21 Prostate Cancer Foundation of Australia. Online. Available: www.prostate.org.au/articleLive/pages/Prostate-Cancer-Statistics.html (accessed March 2010).
22 Krieger JN, Nyberg L Jr, Nickel JC. NIH consensus definition and classification of prostatitis. JAMA 1999;282(3):236–7.
23 Putnam SD, Cerhan JR, Parker AS, et. al. Lifestyle and anthropometric risk factors for prostate cancer in a cohort of Iowa men. Ann Epidemiol 2000;10(6):361–9.
24 Schoonen WM, Salinas CA, Kiemeney LA, et. al. Alcohol consumption and risk of prostate cancer in middle-aged men. Int J Cancer 2005;113(1):133–40.
25 Stattin P, Bylund A, Rinaldi S, et. al. Plasma insulin-like growth factor-I, insulin-like growth factor-binding proteins, and prostate cancer risk: a prospective study. JNCI 2000;92(23):1910–7.
26 Roddam AW, Allen NE, Appleby P, et. al. Insulin-like growth factors, their binding proteins, and prostate cancer risk: analysis of individual patient data from 12 prospective studies. Ann Intern Med 2008;149(7):461–71.
27 Parent M, Siemiatycki J. Occupation and prostate cancer. Epidemiological Reviews 2001;23:138–43.
28 Simone CB. Cancer and nutrition, a ten-point plan to reduce your risk of getting cancer. Avery Publishing Group, Inc, Garden City Park, NJ, 1994:148.
29 Robbins J. Diet for a new America, how your food choices affect your health, happiness and the future of life on Earth. Stillpoint Pubish, Walpole, NH, 1987:315, 331, 343.
30 Moyad MA, Lowe FC. Educating patients about lifestyle modifications for prostate health. Am J Med 2008;121(8 Suppl 2):S34–S42.
31 Ma J, Li H, Giovannucci E, et. al. Prediagnostic body-mass index, plasma C-peptide concentration, and prostate cancer-specific mortality in men with prostate cancer: a long-term survival analysis. Lancet Oncol 2008;9(11):1039–47.
32 Saxe GA, Hébert JR, Carmody JF, et. al. Can diet in conjunction with stress reduction affect the rate of increase in prostate specific antigen after biochemical recurrence of prostate cancer? J Urol 2001;166(6):2202–7.
33 Frattaroli J, Weidner G, Dnistrian AM, et. al. Clinical events in prostate cancer lifestyle trial: results from two years of follow-up. Urology 2008;72(6):1319–23.
34 Ramachandra P, Booth S, Pieters T, et. al. A brief self-administered psychological intervention to improve well-being in patients with cancer: results from a feasibility study. Psychooncology 2009;18(12):1323–6.
35 Carlson LE, Speca M, Patel KD, et. al. Mindfulness-based stress reduction in relation to quality of life, mood, symptoms of stress and levels of cortisol, dehydroepiandrosterone sulfate (DHEAS) and melatonin in breast and prostate cancer outpatients. Psychoneuroendocrinology 2004;29(4):448–74.
36 Ornish D, Weidner G, Fair WR, et. al. Intensive lifestyle changes may affect the progression of prostate cancer. J Urol 2005;174:1065–70.
37 Ornish D, Magbanua MJ, Weidner G, et. al. Changes in prostate gene expression in men undergoing an intensive nutrition and lifestyle intervention. PNAS 2008;105(24):8369–74.
38 Ornish D, Lin J, Daubenmier J, et. al. Increased telomerase activity and comprehensive lifestyle changes: a pilot study. Lancet Oncol 2008; 9(11):1048–57.
39 Daubenmier JJ, Weidner G, Marlin R, et. al. Lifestyle and health-related quality of life of men with prostate cancer managed with active surveillance. Urology 2006;67(1):125–30.
40 Dewell A, Weidner G, Sumner MD, et. al. Relationship of dietary protein and soy isoflavones to serum IGF-1 and IGF binding proteins in the Prostate Cancer Lifestyle Trial. Nutr Cancer 2007;58(1):35–42.
41 Dewell A, Weidner G, Sumner MD, et. al. A very-low-fat vegan diet increases intake of protective dietary factors and decreases intake of pathogenic dietary factors. J Am Diet Assoc 2008;108(2):347–56.
42 Lawson KA et. al. Multivitamin Use and Risk of Prostate Cancer in the National Institutes of Health-AARP Diet and Health Study. J National Cancer Inst 2007;99:754–64.
43 McNaughton Collins M, Pontari MA, O'Leary MP, et. al. Chronic Prostatitis Collaborative Research Network. Quality of life is impaired in men with chronic prostatitis: the Chronic Prostatitis Collaborative Research Network. J Gen Intern Med 2001;16(10):656–62.
44 Lee IM, Sesso HD, Chen JJ, et. al. Does physical activity play a role in the prevention of prostate cancer? Epidemiology Reviews 2001;23:132–37.
45 Giovannucci E, Liu Y, Leitzmann MF, et. al. A prospective study of physical activity, and incident and fatal prostate cancer. Arc Int Med 2005;165:1005–10.
46 Segal RJ, Reid RD, Courneya KS, et. al. Resistance exercise in men receiving androgen deprivation therapy for prostate cancer. J Cli Onc 2003;21:1653–59.
47 Lagiou A, Samoli E, Georgila C, et. al. Occupational physical activity in relation with prostate cancer and benign prostatic hyperplasia. Eur J Cancer Prev 2008;17(4):336–9.
48 Van Kampen M, De Weerdt W, Van Poppel H, et. al. Effect of pelvic-floor re-education on duration and degree of incontinence after radical prostatectomy: a randomised controlled trial. Lancet 2000;355:98–102.
49 Centemero A, Rigatti L, Giraudo D, et. al. Preoperative Pelvic Floor Muscle Exercise for Early Continence After Radical Prostatectomy: A Randomised Controlled Study. Eur Urol 2010 Mar 1.
50 Aldercreutz H, Mazur W. Phytoestrogens and Western diseases. Ann Med 1997;29(2):95–120.
51 Kolonel LN, Hankin JH, Whittemore AS, et. al. Vegetables, fruits, legumes and prostate cancer: a multi-ethnic case-controlled study. Cancer Epidemiol Biomarkers Prev 2000;9:795–804.
52 Cheung E, Wadhera P, Dorff T, et. al. Diet and prostate cancer risk reduction. Expert Rev Anticancer Ther 2008;8(1):43–50.

53 Stacewicz-Sapuntzakis M, Borthakur G, et. al. Correlations of dietary patterns with prostate health. Mol Nutr Food Res 2008;52(1):114–30.

54 Schulman C, Ekane S, Zlotta A. Nutrition and Prostate Cancer: Evidence or suspicion? Urology 2001;58:318–34.

55 Key TJ, Fraser GE, Thorogood M, et. al. Mortality in vegetarians and non-vegetarians: a collaborative analysis of 8300 deaths among 76,000 men and women in five prospective studies. Public Health Nutr 1998;1(1):33–41.

56 Terry P, Lichtenstein P, Feychting M, et. al. Fatty fish consumption and risk of prostate cancer. Lancet 2001;357:1764–6.

57 Terry PD, Rohan TE, Wolk A. Intakes of fish and marine fatty acids and the risks of cancers of the breast and prostate and of other hormone-related cancers: a review of the epidemiologic evidence. Am J Clin Nutr 2003;77(3):532–43.

58 Sarkar FH, Li Y. Soy isoflavones and cancer prevention. Cancer Invest 2003;21(5):744–57.

59 Morton MS, Chan PS, Cheng C, et. al. Lignans and isoflavonoids in plasma and prostatic fluid in men: samples from Portugal, Hong Kong, and the United Kingdom. Prostrate 1997;32:122–28.

60 Guy L, Védrine N, Urpi-Sarda M, et. al. Orally administered isoflavones are present as glucuronides in the human prostate. Nutr Cancer 2008;60(4):461–8.

61 Kirsh VA, Peters U, Mayne ST, et. al.Prostate, Lung, Colorectal and Ovarian Cancer Screening Trial. Prospective study of fruit and vegetable intake and risk of prostate cancer. JNCI 2007;99(15):1200–9.

62 Traka M, Gasper AV, Melchini A, et. al. Broccoli consumption interacts with GSTM1 to perturb oncogenic signaling pathways in the prostate. PLoS ONE 2008;3(7):e2568.

63 Good for the heart but not for the prostate? The alpha-linolenic acid dilemma. Harv Mens Health Watch 2002;6(6):1–3.

64 Carmody J, Olendzki B, Reed G, et. al. A Dietary Intervention for Recurrent Prostate Cancer After Definitive Primary Treatment: Results of a Randomized Pilot Trial. Urology 2008; 72(6):1324–8.

65 Ambrosini GL, de Klerk NH, Mackerras D, et. al. Dietary patterns and surgically treated benign prostatic hyperplasia: a case control study in Western Australia. BJU Intern 2008;101:853–860.

66 Giovannucci E et. al. Calcium and fructose intake in relation to risk of prostate cancer. Cancer Res 1998;58:442–7.

67 Chan JM, Stampfer MJ, Ma J, et. al. Dairy products, calcium, and prostate cancer risk in the Physicians' Health Study. Am J Clin Nutr 2002;76(2): 490–1.

68 Huncharek M, Muscat J, Kupelnick B. Dairy products, dietary calcium and vitamin D intake as risk factors for prostate cancer: a meta-analysis of 26,769 cases from 45 observational studies. Nutr Cancer 2008;60(4):421–41.

69 Jacobsen BK, Nutsen SF, Fraser GE. Does high soy milk intake reduce prostate cancer incidence? The Adventist's Health Study (United States). Cancer Causes Contr 1998;9:553–7.

70 Stevens FO. Phytoestrogens and prostate cancer: possible preventive role. Medical Journal of Australia 1997;1671:38–40.

71 Goodin S, Shen F, Shih WJ, et. al. Clinical and biological activity of soy protein powder supplementation in healthy male volunteers. Cancer Epidemiol Biomarkers Prev 2007;16(4):829–33.

72 Mills PK et. al. Cohort study of diet, lifestyle, and prostate cancer in Adventists men. Cancer 1989;64:598–604.

73 Pantuck AJ et. al. Phase 2 study of pomegranate juice for men with rising prostate-specific antigen following surgery or radiation for prostate cancer. Clin Cancer Res 2006;12:4018–25.

74 Syed DN, Suh Y, Afaq F, et. al. Dietary agents for chemoprevention of prostate cancer. Cancer Lett 2008;265(2):167–76.

75 Carlson JR, Bauer BA, A. Vincent, P, et. al. Reading the tea leaves: anticarcinogenic properties of epigallocatechin-3-gallate, Mayo Clin Proc 2007; 82:725–32.

76 Adhami VM, Mukhtar H. Anti-oxidants from green tea and pomegranate for chemoprevention of prostate cancer. Mol Biotechnol 2007;37(1):52–7.

77 Fleshner N, Zlotta AR. Prostate cancer prevention: past, present, and future. Cancer 2007;110(9): 1889–99.

78 Adhami VM, Mukhtar H. Polyphenols from green tea and pomegranate for prevention of prostate cancer. Free Radic Res 2006;40(10):1095–104.

79 Lee AH, Fraser ML, Meng X, et. al. Protective effects of green tea against prostate cancer. Expert Rev Anticancer Ther 2006;6(4):507–13.

80 Jian L, Ping Xie L, Lee AH, et. al. Protective effect of green tea against prostate cancer: A case-control study in southeast China. Inter J Cancer 2004;108:130–35.

81 Dahan K, Fennal M, Kumar NB. Lycopene in the prevention of prostate cancer. J Soc Integr Oncol 2008;6(1):29–36.

82 Chen L, Stacewicz-Sapuntzakis M, Duncan C, et. al. Oxidative DNA damage in prostate cancer patients consuming tomato sauce-based entres as a whole-food intervention. JNCI 2001;93:1872–9.

83 Giovanucci E, Rimm EB, Liu Y, et. al. A prospective study of tomato products, lycopene, and prostate cancer risk. JNCI 2002;94(5):391–8.

84 Peters U, Leitzmann MF, Chatterjee N, et. al. Serum lycopene, other carotenoids and prostate cancer risk: a nested case-control study in prostate, lung, colorectal, and ovarian cancer screening trial. Cancer Epidem Biomark Prev 2007;16:962–8.

85 Giovannucci E. Editorial. Lycopene and Prostate. JNCI 2007;99:1060–62.

86 Fleischauer AT, Arab L. Garlic and cancer: a critical review of the epidemiologic literature. J Nutr 2001;131(3s):1032S-40S.

87 Devrim E, Durak I. Is garlic a promising food for benign prostatic hyperplasia and prostate cancer? Mol Nutr Food Res 2007;51(11):1319–23.

88 Hsing AW, Chokkalingam AP, Gao YT, et. al. Allium vegetables and risk of prostate cancer: a population-based study. JNCI 2002;94:1648–51.

89 Schiebel-Schlosser G, Friederich M. Phytotherapy of BPH with pumpkin seeds - A multicentric clinical trial. Zeitschrift fur Phytotherapie [Germany] 1998;19(2):71–76.

90 Carbin BE, Larsson B, Lindahl O. Treatment of benign prostatic hyperplasia with phytosterols. Br J Urol 1990;66(6):639–41.

91 Hong H, Kim CS, Maeng S. Effects of pumpkin seed oil and saw palmetto oil in Korean men with symptomatic benign prostatic hyperplasia. Nutr Res Pract 2009 Winter;3(4):323–7.

92 Anand P, Sundaram C, Jhurani S, et. al. Curcumin and cancer: an "old-age" disease with an "age-old" solution. Cancer Lett 2008;267(1):133–64.

93 Dorai T, Gehani N, Katz A. Therapeutic potential of curcumin in human prostate cancer. II. Curcumin inhibits tyrosine kinase activity of epidermal growth factor receptor and depletes the protein. Mol Urol 2000 Spring;4(1):1–6.

94 The Alpha-Tocopherol, Beta-Carotene Cancer Prevention Study Group. The effect of vitamin E and beta-carotene on the incidence of lung cancer and other cancers in male smokers. NEJM 1994;330:1029–35.

95 Heinonen OP, Albanes D, Virtamo J, et. al. Prostate cancer and supplementation with alpha-tocopherol and beta-carotene: incidence and mortality in a controlled trial. JNCI 1998;90:440–6.

96 Helzlsouer KJ, Huang HY, Alberg AJ, et. al. Association between alpha-tocopherol, gamma-tocopherol, selenium, and subsequent prostate cancer. JNCI 2000;92:2018–23.

97 Ni J, Chen M, Zhang Y, et. al. Vitamin E succinate inhibits human prostate cancer cell growth via modulating cell cycle regulatory machinery. Bio Phys Res Commun 2003;300:357–63.

98 Gaziano JM, Glynn RJ, Christen WG, et. al. Vitamins E and C in the prevention of prostate and total cancer in men: the Physicians' Health Study II randomized controlled trial. JAMA 2009;301(1):52–62.

99 Lippman SM, Klein EA, Goodman PJ, et. al. Effect of selenium and vitamin E on risk of prostate cancer and other cancers: the Selenium and Vitamin E Cancer Prevention Trial (SELECT) 2009;301(1): 39–51.

100 Miller ER 3rd, Pastor-Barriuso R, Dalal D, et. al. Meta-analysis: high-dosage vitamin E supplementation may increase all-cause mortality. Ann Intern Med 2005;142(1):37–46;

101 Bjelakovic G Nikolova D, Gluud LL, Simonetti RG, et. al. Mortalitly in randomized trials of antioxidant supplements for primary and secondary prevention. Systematic review and meta-analysis. JAMA 2007;297:842–857.

102 Ali MM, Vaidya V. Vitamin D and cancer. J Cancer Res Ther 2007;3(4):225–30.

103 Luscombe CJ, Fryer AA, French ME, et. al. Exposure to ultraviolet radiation: association with susceptibility and age at presentation with prostate cancer. Lancet 2001;358:641–42.

104 Donkena KV, Karnes RJ, Young CY. Vitamins and prostate cancer risk. Molecules 2010;15(3):1762–83.

105 Corder EH, Friedman GD, Vogelman JH, et. al. Vitamin D and prostate cancer: a prediagnositic study with stored sera. Cancer Epidemiol Biomark Prev 1993;2:467.

106 Robsahm TE, Tretli S, Dahlback A, et. al. Vitamin D3 from sunlight may improve the prognosis of breast, colon and prostate cancer. Cancer Causes Control 2004;15:149–58.

107 Clark LC, Combs GF Jr, Turnbull BW, et. al. Nutritional Prevention of Cancer Study Group. Effects of selenium supplementation for cancer prevention in patients with carcinoma of the skin: a randomized controlled trial. JAMA 1996;276(24):1957–63.

108 Platz EA, Helzlsouer KJ. Selenium, zinc, and prostate cancer. Epidemiological Reviews 2001;23:93–101.

109 Willett WC, Polk BF, Morris JS, et. al. Prediagnostic serum selenium and risk of cancer. Lancet 1983;2:130–4.

110 Reid ME, Duffield-Lillico AJ, Slate E, et. al. The nutritional prevention of cancer: 400mcg per day selenium treatment. Nutr Cancer 2008;60(2):155–63.

111 Clark LC, Dalkin B, Krongrad A, et. al. Decreased incidence of prostate cancer with selenium supplementation: results of a double-blind cancer prevention trial. Br J Urol 1998;81(5):730–4.

112 Ghosh J. Rapid induction of apoptosis in prostate cancer cells by selenium: reversal by metabolites of arachidonate 5-lipoxygenase. Biochem Biophys Res Commun 2004;315(3):624–35.

113 Corcoran NM, Najdovska M, Costello AJ. Inorganic selenium retards progression of experimental hormone refractory prostate cancer. J Urol 2004;171: 907–10.

114 Pak RW, Lanteri VJ, Scheuch JR, et. al. Review of vitamin E and selenium in the prevention of prostate cancer: implications of the selenium and vitamin E chemoprevention trial. Integr Cancer Ther 2002 Dec;1(4):338–44.

115 Leake A, Chisholm GD, Habib FK. The effect of zinc on the 5 alpha-reduction of testosterone by the hyperplastic human prostate gland. J Steroid Bioch 1984;20:651–5.

116 Leitzmann MF, Stampfer MJ, Wu K, et. al. Zinc supplement use and risk of prostate cancer. JNCI 2003;95(13):1004–7.

117 Gonzalez A, Peters U, Lampe JW, et. al. Zinc intake from supplements and diet and prostate cancer. Nutr Cancer 2009;61(2):206–15.

118 Gómez Y, Arocha F, Espinoza F, et. al.(Zinc levels in prostatic fluid of patients with prostate pathologies) Invest Clin 2007;48(3):287–94.

119 Edorh AP, Tachev K, Hadou T, et. al. Magnesium content in seminal fluid as an indicator of chronic prostatitis. Cell Mol Biol (Noisy-le-grand) 2003;49 Online Pub:OL419–23.

120 Dutkiewicz S. Zinc and magnesium serum levels in patients with benign prostatic hyperplasia (BPH) before and after prazosin therapy. Mater Med Pol 1995;27(1):15–7.

121 Sapota A, Daragó A, Taczalski J, et. al. Disturbed homeostasis of zinc and other essential elements in the prostate gland dependent on the character of pathological lesions. Biometals 2009 Jul 23.

122 Kaplan SA, Volpe MA, Te AE. A prospective, 1-year trial using saw palmetto versus finasteride in the treatment of category III prostatitis/chronic pelvic pain syndrome. J Urol 2004;171(1):284–8.

123 Lopatkin NA, Apolikhin OI, Sivkov AV, et. al. (Results of a multicenter trial of serenoa repens extract (permixon) in patients with chronic abacterial prostatitis) Urologiia 2007;(5):3–7.

124 Morgia G, Mucciardi G, Galì A, et. al. Treatment of Chronic Prostatitis/Chronic Pelvic Pain Syndrome Category IIIA with Serenoa repens plus Selenium and Lycopene (Profluss(R)) versus S. repens Alone: An Italian Randomized Multicenter-Controlled Study. Urol Int 2010 Mar 24.

125 Shoskes DA, Zeitlin SI, Shahed A, et. al. Quercetin in men with category III chronic prostatitis: a preliminary prospective, double-blind, placebo-controlled trial. Urology 1999;54(6):960–3.

126 Hsieh TC, Wu JM. Targeting CWR22Rv1 prostate cancer cell proliferation and gene expression by combinations of the phytochemicals EGCG, genistein and quercetin. Anticancer research 2009;29(10):4025–32.

127 Jung YH, Heo J, Lee YJ, et. al. Quercetin enhances TRAIL-induced apoptosis in prostate cancer cells via increased protein stability of death receptor 5. Life Sci 2010;86(9–10):351–7.

128 Yuan H, Young CY, Tian Y, et. al. Suppression of the androgen receptor function by quercetin through protein-protein interactions of Sp1, c-Jun, and the androgen receptor in human prostate cancer cells. Mol Cell Biochem 2010 Feb 11.
129 Abe M, Ito Y, Oyunzul L, et. al. Pharmacologically relevant receptor binding characteristics and 5alpha-reductase inhibitory activity of free Fatty acids contained in saw palmetto extract. Biol Pharm Bull 2009;32(4):646–50.
130 Marks LS, Hess DL, Dorey FJ, et. al. Tissue effects of saw palmetto and finasteride: use of biopsy cores for in situ quantification of prostatic androgens. Urology 2001;57(5):999–1005.
131 Wilt TJ, Ishani A, Stark G, et. al. Saw Palmetto extracts for treatment of Benign Prostrate Hyperplasia: a systematic review. JAMA 1998;280(18):1604–09.
132 Carraro J, Raynaud J, Koch G. Comparison of Phytotherapy (Permixon) with Finasteride in the Treatment of BPH: A Randomized International Study of 1,098 Patients. Prostate 1996;29:231–40.
133 Zlotta AR, Teillac P, Raynaud JP, et. al. Evaluation of male sexual function in patients with Lower Urinary Tract Symptoms (LUTS) associated with Benign Prostatic Hyperplasia (BPH) treated with a phytotherapeutic agent (Permixon), Tamsulosin or Finasteride. Eur Urol 2005;48(2):269–76.
134 Bent S, Kane C, Shinohara K, et. al. Saw palmetto for benign prostatic hyperplasia. NEJM 2006;354(6):557–66.
135 Von Löw EC, Perabo FG, Siener R, et. al. Review. Facts and fiction of phytotherapy for prostate cancer: a critical assessment of preclinical and clinical data. In Vivo 2007;21(2):189–204.
136 Hour TC, Chen J, Huang CY, et. al. Curcumin enhances cytotoxicity of chemotherapeutic agents in prostate cancer cells by inducing p21 (WAF1/CIPI) and C/EBPbeta expressions and suppressing NF-kappa B activation. Prostate 2002;51:211–8.
137 Chendil D, Ranga RS, Meigooni D, et. al. Curcumin confers radiosensitising effect in prostate cancer cell lines PC-3. Oncogene 2004;23:1599–1607.
138 Dorai T, Gehani N, Katz A. Therapeutic potential of curcumin in human prostate cancer. II. Curcumin inhibits tyrosine kinase activity of the epidermal growth factor and depletes the protein. Mol Urol 2000;4:1–6.
139 Wilt T, Ishani A, Mac Donald R, et. al. Pygeum africanum for benign prostatic hyperplasia. Cochrane Database Systematic Review 2002;(1):CD001044.
140 Levin RM, Das AK. A scientific basis for the therapeutic effects of Pygeum africanum and Serenoa repens. Urol Res 2000;28(3):201–9.
141 Chrubasik JE, Roufogalis BD, Wagner H, et. al. A comprehensive review on the stinging nettle effect and efficacy profiles. Part II: urticae radix. Phytomedicine 2007;14(7–8):568–79.
142 Krzeski T, Kazón M, Borkowski A, et. al. Combined extracts of Urtica dioica and Pygeum africanum in the treatment of benign prostatic hyperplasia: double-blind comparison of two doses. Clin Ther 1993;15(6):1011–20.
143 Sökeland J. Combined sabal and urtica extract compared with finasteride in men with benign prostatic hyperplasia: analysis of prostate volume and therapeutic outcome. BJU Int 2000;86(4):439–42.
144 Popa G, Hägele-Kaddour H, Walther C. (Benign prostate syndrome: urinary tract symptoms can be eased with phytotherapy) MMW Fortschr Med 2005 Aug 18;147(33–34):42.
145 Schneider HJ, Honold E, Masuhr T. (Treatment of benign prostatic hyperplasia. Results of a treatment study with the phytogenic combination of Sabal extract WS 1473 and Urtica extract WS 1031 in urologic specialty practices) Fortschr Med 1995;113(3):37–40.
146 Bondarenko B, Walther C, Funk P, et. al. Long-term efficacy and safety of PRO 160/120 (a combination of sabal and urtica extract) in patients with lower urinary tract symptoms (LUTS). Phytomedicine 2003;10 Suppl 4:53–5.
147 Gülçin I, Küfrevioglu OI, Oktay M, et. al. Antioxidant, antimicrobial, antiulcer and analgesic activities of nettle (Urtica dioica L.). J Ethnopharmacol 2004;90(2–3):205–15.
148 Riehemann K, Behnke B, Schulze-Osthoff K. Plant extracts from stinging nettle (Urtica dioica), an antirheumatic remedy, inhibit the proinflammatory transcription factor NF-kappaB. EBS Lett 1999;442(1):89–94.
149 Engelhardt PF, Riedl CR. Effects of one-year treatment with isoflavone extract from red clover on prostate, liver function, sexual function, and quality of life in men with elevated PSA levels and negative prostate biopsy findings. Urology 2008;71(2):185–90.
150 Hsieh TC, Wu JM. Mechanism of action of herbal supplement PC-SPES: elucidation of effects of individual herbs of PC-SPES on proliferation and prostate specific gene expression in androgen-dependent LNCaP cells. Int J Oncol 2002;20(3):583–8.
151 Dandekar DS, Lokeshwar VB, Cevallos-Arellano E, et. al. An orally active Amazonian plant extract (BIRM) inhibits prostate cancer growth and metastasis. Cancer Chemother Pharmacol 2003;52(1):59–66.
152 Wang CY, Han RF. [Acupuncture for chronic prostatitis: a meta-analysis] Zhonghua Nan Ke Xue 2008;14(9):853–6.
153 Tugcu V, Tas S, Eren G, et. al. Effectiveness of Acupuncture in Patients with Category IIIB Chronic Pelvic Pain Syndrome: A Report of 97 Patients. Pain Med 2010 Jan 22.
154 Frisk J. Managing hot flushes in men after prostate cancer--a systematic review. Maturitas 2010;65(1):15–22.
155 Lee MS, Kim KH, Shin BC, et. al. Acupuncture for treating hot flushes in men with prostate cancer: a systematic review. Support Care Cancer 2009;17(7):763–70.

Chapter 35

Renal disease

Introduction

Chronic Kidney disease

Chronic kidney disease has increased in prevalence in the US by 20–25% from the 1988–1994 period of the National Health and Nutrition Examination Survey[1,2] and affects an estimated 31 million people in that country.[1]

Kidney diseases can be divided into glomerular diseases and tubulointerstitial disorders. The former tend to be immunologically mediated and the latter are most often due to toxins and/or infective insults. Some common kidney diseases include:

- nephritic/nephrotic syndromes
- acute renal failure
- azotemia
- pyelonephritis
- uremia
- acquired renal cystic disease
- polycystic kidney disease.

Kidney disease is defined as any one of several chronic conditions that are caused by damage to the cells of the kidney. It is a major cause of disease and death in the US and important causative factors have been identified (see Table 35.1).

Since chronic kidney disease cannot be cured, treatment focuses on slowing the progression and avoiding complete kidney failure.

Diabetes is the single leading cause of kidney failure in the US. Nephropathy is a condition that affects one-third or more of people who have had type 1 (juvenile) diabetes for at least 20 years. About 20–40% of people with type 2 (adult onset) diabetes also have kidney disease.[3]

A recent descriptive study from Germany has found that use of complementary and alternative medicines (CAMs) is common among renal patients.[4] This is consistent with other reports that have indicated that the consumption of complementary medicine products, including herbs, herbal teas, or nutritional supplements such as vitamins or minerals, has increased in the last decade.[5]

A high rate of complementary medicine product use has been documented for a number of different patient populations with chronic diseases, such as liver-transplant recipients,[6] HIV-positive patients,[7] patients with epilepsy,[8] and patients with diabetes,[9] and clinicians are often inadequately informed about CAM consumption by their patients.[10]

The prevalence and patterns of CAM utilisation among renal patients with chronic kidney diseases was recently investigated.[11] The study revealed the following facts.

- An important finding, which is consistent with current thinking, was that patients reported that only a minority of clinicians had taken an active interest in consumption of CAMs.
- Fifty-seven percent of dialysis patients and 49% of transplant patients reported to be regular CAM consumers.
- CAM consumption was positively associated with female gender and negatively with diabetes as comorbidity.
- Forty-one different CAM products had been named, with mineral supplements and vitamins ranking first.
- Numerous renal patients had regularly consumed herbal teas and citrus juices (50% and 35%, respectively).
- Of concern was that approximately 40% of the documented CAM/health food consumption had potential risks for patients because of constituents that either accumulate in renal failure or interact with pharmaceutical medications.
- Approximately 50% of dialysis patients and 73% of transplant patients used to inform their physicians about CAM consumption.
- Patient awareness of the interaction risks linked to CAM was especially low in dialysis patients when compared to transplant patients (39% versus 78%) and increased when clinicians had routinely questioned patients about their CAM consumption.[11]

In addition, CAM products (e.g. herbal products, functional foods such as probiotics) and physical therapies (e.g. acupuncture) have been used in other non-chronic associated kidney diseases.[12]

Table 35.1 Key and other factors associated with kidney disease

Factor
Age
Obesity*
Diabetes*
High blood pressure*
Heart disease*
Urinary tract system blockages
Medication: overuse or adverse reactions
Illicit drug abuse
Inflammation and/or disease processes
Family history of kidney failure*
Low birth weight
Trauma and/or accident
Environmental toxins

*Key factors

Lifestyle and other risk factors

Age

Kidney function is reduced in older people; that is, greater risk with increasing age.[13]

Obesity

Obesity is strongly associated with several major health risk factors.[14] These include type 2 diabetes mellitus (T2DM), hypertension and heart disease, which have significant causal correlations to chronic kidney disease.[15] Moreover, studies have reported that Body Mass Index (BMI) was associated with an increased risk of the development of end-stage renal disease.[16, 17]

Diabetes

Approximately 40% of new incident dialysis patients have been diagnosed with diabetes which today is considered the most important and increasing risk factor for kidney disease.[18, 19] T2DM (see Chapter 13 on diabetes) is the number 1 cause of kidney failure, responsible for more than 1 of every 3 new cases.[18]

High blood pressure (hypertension)

Hypertension is the second most common cause of kidney failure.[20] High blood pressure puts more stress on blood vessels throughout the body, including the nephrons. Normal blood pressure is defined as less than 130/85 — and this is the considered target for persons diagnosed with diabetes, heart disease, or chronic kidney disease. Weight control, physical activity (see later in this chapter), and medications can control blood pressure — and can assist in preventing or slowing the progress from kidney disease to kidney failure.

Urinary tract system blockages

Scarring from infections or a malformed lower urinary tract system as a result of a birth defect can force urine backflow, damaging the kidneys.[21] Blood clots or plaques of cholesterol that block the kidney's blood vessels can reduce blood flow to the kidneys and also cause damage. Repeated kidney stones can block the flow of urine from the kidneys and is an additional cause of obstruction that can damage the kidneys.

Overuse of medications

A number of pharmaceutical drugs are known to cause renal failure as a side-effect.

Continued use of analgesic medications containing ibuprofen, naproxen, or acetaminophen have been linked to interstitial nephritis, that can lead to kidney failure.[22] A US study suggested that ordinary use of analgesics (e.g. 1 pill per day) was not harmful in men who were not at risk for kidney disease.[23] However, concomitant use of NSAIDs and dehydration (e.g. severe diarrhoea) can predispose to renal impairment and failure, especially in the elderly. Allergic reactions to, or side-effects of, antibiotics such as penicillin and vancomycin may also cause nephritis and lead to kidney damage.[24] Note that adverse reactions can also occur with complementary medicines (CMs) (e.g. herbs and high-dose vitamins).

Illicit drug abuse

The illicit use of drugs involves millions of people worldwide and is associated with a variety of medical complications. Use of certain non-prescription drugs, such as heroin or cocaine, can damage the kidneys, and may lead to kidney failure and the need for dialysis.[25, 26]

Inflammation and/or diseases

Certain illnesses, like glomerulonephritis, can damage the kidneys and lead to chronic kidney disease.[27] Moreover, persons at increased risk of kidney disease include those diagnosed with systemic lupus erythematosus, sickle cell anaemia, cancer, HIV/AIDS, hepatitis C, and congestive heart failure.[28–32]

Family history — surrogate marker for risk of future nephropathy

Persons are at an increased risk if they have 1 or more family members who have chronic kidney disease, are on dialysis, or have had a kidney transplant.[33] Diabetes and high blood pressure can also have familial trends and present with risks for chronic kidney disease (see previous sections in this chapter).

Low birth weight

A recent systematic review has concluded that existing scientific data indicates that low birth weight is associated with subsequent risk of chronic kidney disease.[34] Further well-designed population-based studies are required, though, in order to accurately assess birth weight and kidney function and important cofounders, such as maternal and socioeconomic factors.

Trauma and/or accident

Accidents/injuries,[35] surgical procedures, and radio-contrast dyes used to monitor blood flow to the heart and other organs are a risk for developing contrast nephropathy due to reduced blood flow to the kidneys, causing acute kidney failure.[36]

Environmental toxins

The kidneys can be the target of numerous xenobiotic toxicants, including environmental chemicals.[37] The kidney's anatomical, physiological, and biochemical features make it particularly susceptible to many environmental compounds. Factors contributing to the sensitivity of the kidneys include: large blood flow; the presence of a variety of xenobiotic transporters and metabolising enzymes; and concentration of solutes during urine production.[36]

Glomerulonephritis is the most common cause of end-stage renal failure in most countries, and is exacerbated and may be causal by exposure to chemicals present in the workplace, the home and in the public environment. The most common nephrotoxic chemicals are hydrocarbons, present in organic solvents, glues, fuels, paints and motor exhausts. Exposure is common among painters, printers, cabinet makers, fitters and mechanics, electricians, and in the manufacturing industry.[38, 39] Other compounds with nephrotoxicity potential include lead, mercury, cadmium and some pharmaceuticals (e.g. gentamycin).[40–43]

A recent study has demonstrated that contact with cadmium and lead increases the risk for chronic kidney disease.[44] Given that these substances are widely distributed in populations at large, this study provides novel evidence of an increased risk with environmental exposure to both metals.

Mind–body medicine

Research shows that regular use of stress management techniques (e.g. cognitive behavioural therapies) can significantly influence those chronic disease conditions that can have adverse health effects on kidney function such as cardiovascular disease (CVD), T2DM and hypertension (see Chapters 10, 13 and 19, respectively).

Furthermore, the psychosocial assessment of the patient with end-stage renal disease is critically important because there is growing evidence that the psychosocial status of the patient significantly impacts medical outcomes and the objective of medical therapy is to maximise a patient's sense of wellbeing and their quality of life (QOL), in particular for those patients that are receiving chronic peritoneal dialysis.

Muscular relaxation

Progressive muscle relaxation training was investigated in 46 patients who had been treated with dialysis.[45] The study demonstrated that progressive muscle relaxation training for dialysis patients helped decrease state- and trait-anxiety levels and had a positive impact on the QOL of these patients.

Cognitive behavioural therapy (CBT)

Three small trials have reported benefit with CBT for patients undergoing haemodialysis.[46, 47, 48] The first study assessed the influence of CBT on chronic haemodialysis patients' ability for self-care and to achieve fluid intake-related behavioural objectives.[44]

The participants were 10 patients participating in a 4-week base-line phase, a 6-week intervention phase and a 4-week follow-up phase. The results showed that the average achievement of the fluid intake objective in the intervention phase was 65%. Fifty percent of participants achieved their objectives at least 75% of the time without individualised reinforcement. Hence, it was concluded that CBT was effective in helping patients change their fluid intake behaviours.

In a further study with an RCT design, enhancing adherence to haemodialysis fluid restrictions was investigated in a group of 56 participants receiving haemodialysis from 4 renal outpatient settings.[46] The study showed that applying group-based CBT (4 weeks duration) was feasible and effective in enhancing adherence to haemodialysis fluid restrictions.

Another study, with a nurse-delivered haemodialysis patient education program incorporating CBT compared to a standard patient education program on patients' salt intake and weight gain, found that both programs were shown to be effective, but CBT had a longer effect (12 weeks versus 8 weeks).[47]

Patients with end-stage renal disease often are diagnosed with *depression*[49] and *sleep disorders*[50] which have been linked to increased mortality. A recent randomised controlled pilot trial with 24 peritoneal dialysis patients reported that CBT may be effective for improving the quality of sleep and decreasing fatigue and inflammatory cytokine levels in these patients. CBT was concluded to be an effective non-pharmacological therapy for peritoneal dialysis patients with sleep disturbances.[51]

It should be noted though that there are few data to support the role of CBT, social support group interventions, and electroconvulsive therapy for treatment of sleep disturbances and depression in patients with chronic kidney disease. Larger randomised, controlled clinical trials aimed at the treatment of these conditions in patients with end-stage renal disease are very much warranted.

Educational interventions

There is increasing evidence that educational interventions aimed at empowering patients are successful in chronic disease management.

A systematic review of randomised clinical trials was recently conducted from studies that included patients diagnosed with any of the following stages of chronic kidney disease such as early pre-dialysis and dialysis.[52] Twenty-two studies were identified involving a wide range of multi-component interventions with variable aims and outcomes depending on the area of kidney disease care. Eighteen studies provided significant results for analysis. The majority of studies aimed to improve diet and/or fluid concordance in dialysis patients and involved short- and medium-term follow-up. A single major long-term study was a 20-year follow-up of a pre-dialysis educational intervention that showed increased survival rates. This review concluded that multi-component structured educational interventions were effective in pre-dialysis and dialysis care, but the quality of many studies was suboptimal.[52] Further, effectively framed and developed educational interventions for implementation and evaluation are required. The study also concluded that this strategy could lead to possible prevention or delay in the progression of kidney disease.

Physical activity/exercise

Exercise can help keep people strong, flexible and better prepared to handle life stressors and illnesses.[53] This is important for patients with kidney disease because, for example, independent of the course of kidney disease, physical fitness decreases continuously with the progression of chronic renal disease.[54] Hence, people with kidney disease, both early and late stage, can benefit from participation in appropriate physical activity programs[55] given that life expectancy in haemodialysis patients is reduced fourfold on average versus healthy age-matched individuals.[56]

End-stage renal disease patients present many cardiovascular complications and suffer from impaired exercise capacity. A number of studies have investigated exercise programs for patients with renal disease and found beneficial morphological, functional and psychosocial effects in end-stage renal disease patients on haemodialysis.[57, 58, 59]

One study noted that intense exercise training improved left ventricular systolic function at rest in haemodialysis patients. Moreover, it was reported that both intense and moderate physical training led to enhanced cardiac performance during supine sub-maximal exercise.[55] An additional study compared the effects of 3 modes of exercise training on aerobic capacity and aimed to identify the most favourable, efficient and preferable to patients on haemodialysis with regard to functional improvements and participation rate in the programs.[56] Fifty-eight volunteer participants were screened for low-risk status and selected from the dialysis population. The 48 patients who completed the study protocol were randomly assigned either to 1 of the 3 training groups or to a control group. These results showed that intense exercise training on non-dialysis days was the most effective way of training, whereas exercise during haemodialysis was also effective and preferable.[56] An additional study by the same research group showed that haemodialysis patients can adhere to long-term physical training programs on the non-dialysis days, as well as during haemodialysis, with considerable improvements in physical fitness and health. Also, although training out of haemodialysis seemed to result in better outcomes, the dropout rate was higher.[57]

A more recent study investigated a total of 50 patients with chronic kidney disease (stage 5) on haemodialysis and 35 healthy individuals who served as controls. The 50 chronic kidney disease patients were divided into 2 groups — the haemodialysis group consisted of 31 patients who received usual care without any physical activity during the haemodialysis sessions, while the haemodialysis/physical activity group included 19 patients who followed a program of physical exercise for 6 months.[60] The study established that exercise training during haemodialysis exerted a beneficial effect on the levels of the vasoactive eicosanoid hormone-like substances in patients on haemodialysis.[60]

A recent single centre prospective study whose objective was to examine the relationship between visceral and somatic protein stores and physical activity in individuals with end-stage renal disease showed that the association between somatic protein and visceral protein stores is weak in patients with chronic kidney disease. Whereas increased levels of physical activity and total daily protein intake were associated with higher lean body mass in patients with chronic kidney disease, higher adiposity was associated with higher C-reactive protein and lower albumin values.[61]

Furthermore, an additional study with the objective of determining whether 24 weeks resistance training during haemodialysis could improve exercise capacity, muscle strength, physical functioning and health-related QOL compared to a low-intensity aerobic program was investigated in 27 patients recruited from 2 haemodialysis clinics.[62] It was concluded that resistance training during haemodialysis significantly improved patient's physical functioning.

A recent review presented empirical evidence that intradialytic exercise can mitigate primary independent risk factors for early mortality in end-stage renal disease, hence, reducing the progression of skeletal muscle wasting, improving systemic inflammation, cardiovascular function and dialysis adequacy.[63] The review concludes that intradialytic cycling and/or progressive resistance training can alleviate primary independent risk factors for early mortality in end-stage renal disease.

Clinical trials have further supported the benefits gained with resistance training exercise by end-stage renal disease patients on haemodialysis.[64, 65] The first study which was a single-blinded, randomised, placebo-controlled trial of an exercise intervention in haemodialysis patients administered erythropoietin. The intervention consisted of progressive resisted isotonic quadriceps and hamstrings exercises and training on a cycle ergometer 3 times weekly for 12 weeks. The results showed that the exercise program improved physical impairment measures, but had no effect on symptoms or health-related QOL.[62] The second randomised study was designed to determine whether anabolic steroid administration and resistance exercise training combined induced anabolic effects among patients who were receiving maintenance haemodialysis.[63] This study found that patients who exercised increased their strength in a training-specific fashion, and exercise was associated with a significant improvement in self-reported physical functioning as compared with non-exercising groups. Nandrolone decanoate and resistance exercise combined produced anabolic effects among patients who were on haemodialysis.

Moreover it should be noted that as of 2008 there have been over 50 reports, including several randomised controlled trials (RCTs) that have evaluated the effects of intradialytic exercise in end-stage kidney disease.[61]

Nutritional influences

Diets and nutritional practices have significant multiple health-related risk factors with ramifications that, if prolonged, can lead to kidney disease.[66] An example of such a multiple health-related risk factor is obesity and its related risks (see Chapters 10, cardiovascular disease; 13, diabetes; and 19, hypertension).

Weight loss management of obese patients is crucial.[14, 15, 16]

Mediterranean diet

Traditional diets among Mediterranean cultures (Mediterranean diet) are characterised by the abundance of natural whole foods, especially fruits and vegetables, along with olive oil, fish, and nuts. The diet includes moderate amounts of wine and is low in saturated fat.[67]

A study reported that adhering to a Mediterranean diet provides for a healthier and nutritional hypolipidemic approach in renal transplant recipients.[68] This study reported that this diet led to a significant reduction in total cholesterol levels by 10%, triglycerides by 6.5%, low-density lipoprotein-cholesterol (LDL-cholesterol) by 10.4% and the ratio of LDL-cholesterol to high-density lipoprotein-cholesterol (HDL-cholesterol) decreased by 10%, while HDL-cholesterol levels remained unchanged. This provided a reduction instead of an increase in the number of participants with hypercholesterolemia, permitting the selection of individual candidates for further pharmacological treatment by carefully evaluating risk–benefit costs. Recently it was reported that the Mediterranean diet was found to be ideal for post-transplantation patients without serious pathologic dyslipidemia.[69] Moreover, it was concluded that in the case of patients with substantial dyslipidemia, appropriate pharmacologic treatment lowering proatherosclerotic lipid levels should be used in combination with the Mediterranean diet.

A further benefit that has been attributed to the Mediterranean diet for patients with kidney disease is that the diet, being rich in seafood and vegetables, was associated with less interdialytic weight gain compared with a diet rich in protein and carbohydrates.[70]

Given that T2DM is a risk factor for developing kidney disease, recently it has been reported that adherence to a Mediterranean diet may delay the use of antihyperglycemic drug therapy in patients with newly diagnosed T2DM, thereby extending an additional benefit to the kidneys.[71]

Dietary Approaches to Stop Hypertension (DASH) diet

The association between obesity, hypertension and nephrolithiasis has been recently reviewed.[72] The review concluded that adopting a lower sodium diet with increased fruits and vegetables and low-fat dairy products (e.g. as stipulated in the Dietary Approaches to Stop Hypertension [DASH] diet) may be useful for the prevention of both kidney stones and hypertension. It was also suggested that in those patients in whom dietary modification and weight loss was ineffective, thiazide diuretics are likely to improve blood pressure control and decrease calciuria.

Diet plays an important role in the pathogenesis of kidney stones. A recent report has prospectively examined the relationship between a DASH-style diet and incident kidney stones in the Health Professionals Follow-up Study (n = 45 821 men; 18-year follow-up), Nurses Health Study I (n = 94 108 older women; 18-year follow-up), and Nurses Health Study II (n = 101 837 younger women; 14-year follow-up). Consumption of a DASH-style diet was found to be associated with a marked decrease in kidney stone risk.[73]

It is interesting to note that the DASH diet has been reported to not increase albumin excretion rates despite a 3% increase in energy from the consumed protein.[74]

Protein diet

Low protein diets are commonly prescribed for patients with idiopathic calcium nephrolithiasis.

A recent Cochrane review of 10 studies from over 40 studies with a total of 2000 patients were analysed, of which 1002 had received reduced protein intake and 998 a higher protein intake.[75] The review concluded that studies investigating protein intake reductions in patients with chronic kidney disease reduced the occurrence of renal death by 32% as compared with those studies with patients on higher or on unrestricted protein intake. Also, the study concluded that the optimal level of protein intake could not be confirmed from these data. An earlier Cochrane review investigating protein intake in children with chronic renal failure found that reducing protein intake did not appear to have a significant impact in delaying the progression to end-stage kidney disease in children.[76]

A recent study compared the effect of very low protein diet supplemented with keto-analogs of essential amino acids (dose of 0.35g/kg/day), low protein diet (dose of 0.60g/kg/day), and free diet on blood pressure in patients with chronic kidney disease stages 4 and 5.[77] It was shown that in moderate to advanced chronic kidney disease, a very low protein diet had antihypertensive effects that were likely due to a reduction of salt intake, type of proteins, and keto-analog supplementation, independent of actual protein intake.

Results of several case-control studies suggest that high consumption of meat (all meat, red meat, or processed meat) is associated with an increased risk of renal cell cancer. Recently a pooled analysis of 13 prospective studies was conducted that included 530 469 women and 244 483 men and had follow-up times of up to 7–20 years to examine associations between meat, fat, and protein intakes and the risk of renal cell cancer.[78] The study concluded that consumption of fat and protein or their subtypes, such as red meat, processed meat, poultry and seafood, were not associated with risk of renal cell cancer.

In a prospective, stratified, multi-centre randomised trial, 191 children aged 2–18 years, who were diagnosed with chronic renal failure from 25 paediatric nephrology centres across Europe, were included in the study. This study was designed to determine whether a low-protein diet could slow disease progression.[79] Patients were divided into 3 groups according to their primary renal disease, and then stratified based on whether their disease was progressive or non-progressive. There was random assignment to the control and diet groups. Protein intake in the diet group was 0.8 to 1.1g/kg/day, with adjustments made for age. There were no protein intake restrictions in the control group. The study continued in all patients for 2 years, and 112 of the participants agreed to continue for an additional year. There were realistic rates of compliance (66%), and no statistically significant differences in the decline of creatinine clearance were found. Furthermore no adverse effects were reported, including no adverse effects on growth from a protein-restricted diet. This study suggests that there is little value in protein restriction in paediatric chronic renal failure.

Vegetarian diet and fluid intake

A diet that is reduced in saturated fat and cholesterol, and that emphasises fruits, vegetables and low-fat dairy products, dietary and soluble fibre, whole grains and protein from plant sources is advantageous for health.[80]

A recent epidemiological case-control study has highlighted the importance of the role of specific foods or nutrients on cancer development, in particular renal cell cancer.[81] This study has reported a significant direct trend in risk for bread (highest versus the lowest intake quintile), and a modest excess of risk was observed for pasta and rice, and milk and yoghurt. Poultry, processed meat and vegetables were inversely associated with renal cell cancer risk. No relation was found for coffee and tea, soups, eggs, red meat, fish, cheese, pulses, potatoes, fruits, desserts and sugars. The results of this study provide additional clues on dietary correlates for renal cell cancer and in particular indicate that a diet rich in refined cereals and poor in vegetables may have an adverse role on renal cell cancer. It is interesting to note that subsequent to this, a study tested whether an underlying intolerance of bread ingredients was responsible for the adverse influence of bread on renal cell cancer.[82] This study reported that serum levels of IgG against *Saccharomyces cerevisiae* may well predict survival in patients with metastatic renal cell cancer. The data reported in this study suggested that it was not cereals but baker's yeast, the critical component of bread, that may cause immune deviation and impaired immune surveillance in predisposed patients with renal cell cancer.

Approximately 80% of kidney stones contain calcium, and the majority of calcium stones consist primarily of calcium oxalate.[83] Small increases in urinary oxalate can have a major effect on calcium oxalate crystal formation and higher levels of urinary oxalate are a major risk factor for the formation of calcium oxalate kidney stones.[79]

An RCT investigated nephrolithiasis by randomly assigning 99 participants who had calcium oxalate stones for the first time to a low animal protein, high fibre diet that contained approximately 56–64g/day of protein, 75mg/day of purine (primarily from animal protein and legumes), one-quarter cup of wheat bran supplement, and fruits and vegetables.[84] After adjustment for possible confounders of age, gender, education and baseline protein and fluid consumption the study showed that the relative risk of a recurrent stone in the intervention group was 5.6 compared with the control group. It was concluded that following a low animal protein, high fibre, high fluid diet had no advantage over advice to increase fluid intake alone.

Dietary oxalate and kidney stone risk is centred on the contribution of oxalate intake to urinary oxalate excretion. A recent study that investigated the intake of oxalate and the risk for nephrolithiasis found that the relative risks for participants who consumed 8 or more servings of spinach per month compared with fewer than 1 serving per month were 1.30 for men and 1.34 for older women.[85]

Foods high in oxalic acids include rhubarb, spinach, beans, eggplant, garlic, cauliflower, broccoli and carrots. Fluids high in oxalic acids include cranberry juice, orange juice, black tea and cocoa. Reducing the intake of these foods and/or fluids in patients with renal impairment and/or those with a tendency to oxalate calcium may help.[86]

For secondary prevention of nephrolithiasis a recent Cochrane review that determined efficacy and safety of diet, fluid, or supplement interventions found that high fluid intake decreased risk of recurrent nephrolithiasis. The review also found that reduced soft drink intake lowered risk in patients with high baseline soft drink consumption.[87] (See also 'Water intake' later this chapter.)

Along a related trend of enquiry, a prospective study that examined the relationship between fructose intake and incident kidney stones in the Nurses Health Study I (93 730 older women), the Nurses Health Study II (101 824 younger women), and the Health Professionals Follow-up Study (45 984 men) concluded that the multivariate relative risks of kidney stones significantly increased for participants in the highest compared to the lowest quintile of total-fructose intake for all 3 study groups. Moreover, free-fructose intake was also associated with increased risk. Non-fructose carbohydrates were not associated with increased risk in any cohort. The study clearly suggested that fructose intake was an independent risk associated with incident kidney stones.[88]

A small study with 10 patients investigated dietary sodium supplementation in stone-forming patients with hypocitraturia.[89] The results demonstrated that dietary sodium supplementation increased voided urine volume and decreased the relative risk super-saturation ratio for calcium oxalate stones in patients with a history of hypocitraturic calcium oxalate nephrolithiasis.

An early study investigated a vegetarian soy diet and its effects on hyperlipidemia in a prospective cross-over trial of 20 participants, aged 17–71 years (mean age 41 years) with nephrotic syndrome.[90] Following a 2-month baseline period in which the patients consumed their usual diets, the participants were changed to the vegetarian soy diet for 2 months, after which they resumed their usual diet for a further 2-month washout period. The vegetarian soy diet was rich in monounsaturated and polyunsaturated fatty acids and fibre, low in fat and protein, and free of cholesterol.

During the 2-month vegetarian/soy diet period, serum concentrations of total cholesterol, LDL-cholesterol, HDL-cholesterol, and apolipoproteins *a* and *b* were significantly lower than they were during the baseline period — although still not within normal limits. There was also a significant decrease in urinary protein excretion during the soy diet period. All values returned toward baseline levels during the washout period, but remained lower than the pre-diet values. The study concluded that the decreases were similar to the result of a 6-week treatment regimen with 40mg/day of a statin drug (lovastatin). It was also concluded that further studies were needed to confirm these effects and to evaluate patient compliance to more long-term dietary restriction.

Additional studies have investigated the beneficial effects of soy diets on patients with T2DM and nephropathy.[91, 92] These studies have found that isolated soy protein consumption improved several markers (i.e. decreased albumin excretion, improvement of LDL:HDL ratios) that may be beneficial for T2DM patients with nephropathy.

Given that changes in dietary protein consumption have important roles in the prevention and management of several forms of kidney disease, a recent review has hypothesised that perhaps by substituting soy protein for animal protein, this could decrease hyperfiltration in diabetic patients and, hence, may significantly reduce urine albumin excretion and improve renal function.[93]

Recently it was shown in a large prospective cohort study (375 851 participants recruited in EPIC centres of 8 countries) that total consumption of fruits and vegetables was not related to risk of renal cell cancer.[94]

Alcohol

An early review has reported that alcohol over-consumption has multiple effects on kidney function as well as on water, electrolyte and acid-base homeostasis.[95] Increased blood pressure was demonstrated in men above 80g and in women above 40g ethanol consumption daily. In contrast, young adults consuming only 10–20g/day had lower blood pressure than the abstinent group, indicating a J-curve relationship. This is consistent with a decreased risk for coronary heart disease associated with regular consumption of small alcohol amounts. In fact, a large prospective cohort study (US Physicians Health Study) has reported that in apparently healthy men, alcohol consumption was not associated with an increased risk of renal dysfunction. Instead, the data suggested an inverse relationship between moderate alcohol consumption and the risk of renal dysfunction.[96] The study reported that men who had 7 or more drinks of wine per week had a 30% lower risk of raised creatinine levels.[96]

Further investigations into the relationships between wine consumption and kidney disease have been limited. A recent review has reported that there is convincing evidence of a beneficial effect of controlled wine consumption in patients with renal disease.[97] The evidence is built around the fact that long-term alcohol abuse has been associated with many renal alterations in humans. In experimental studies wine polyphenols enhance kidney antioxidant defences, exert protective effects against renal ischemia/reperfusion injury, and inhibit apoptosis of mesangial cells. Controlled clinical trials are, however, needed to confirm the hypothesis.

The mechanisms responsible for the association between alcohol over-consumption and post-infectious glomerulonephritis remain unclear. Moreover, the severe alcohol abuse that was reported to predispose to acute renal failure appeared to be associated with general catabolic effects.[89]

Water intake

A report from the University of Sydney presented at the Australian and New Zealand Nephrology meeting in 2005, detailed a study that people who drank approximately 3 litres of water per day halved their risk for chronic kidney disease.[98] This report needs to be verified with further studies. The study also reported that those individuals who had a higher intake of fibre (42.3g/day) also appeared to have a reduced risk for chronic kidney disease with a reduction in risk by 34%.

Coffee

It is an established fact that caffeine has a diuretic effect. Various studies have demonstrated that in healthy volunteers the acute administration of caffeine, or drinks containing it, causes a short-term increase in diuresis with a concomitant excretion of substances such as sodium, potassium, chlorides, magnesium, and calcium.[99, 100, 101]

Whether caffeine reduces or increases the risk for kidney stones is contentious. In the most recent study from 2004, Massey and Sutton[102] demonstrated that caffeine consumption at a dose of 6mg/kg of lean mass after 14 hours of fasting in 39 volunteers caused an increase in the excretion of calcium, magnesium and citrate, with an increase in the Tiselius index for calcium oxalate stones formation from 2.4 to 3.1 in those participants with a history of calcium lithiasis and from 1.7 to 2.5 in those participants without this history. In general, the consumption of coffee seemed to increase, albeit modestly, the risk of forming calcium oxalate stones. A report in a less recent study demonstrated that the administration of caffeine in healthy young women caused an increased urinary loss of calcium and magnesium, with a significant reduction in the reabsorption percentage after its consumption whereas other parameters, such as creatinine clearance, were not modified.[103]

Studies on the effects of caffeine in participating patients with nephropathy or chronic renal failure, and in those on dialysis, are scarce and therefore no conclusive information can be provided. It should be noted though that studies on patient populations have shown that the consumption of caffeine during dialysis might become a useful semi-pharmacologic option for the prevention and treatment of symptomatic intradialytic hypotension.[102, 103] Also it is now a strong consensus that chronic caffeine consumption does not contribute to restless leg syndrome, one of the most frequently observed disturbances of patients on haemodialysis.[106, 107]

Hence, from a detailed review of the current literature there are significant conflicting opinions and research data regarding the extremes of the diuretic, prolithiasic and toxic effects of caffeine.[101]

Food allergy

Early studies have reported on sensitisation to usual foods and idiopathic nephritic syndrome.[106, 107] These reports point to a significant contribution for the role of food hypersensitivity to idiopathic nephritic syndrome. An oligoantigenic diet has been proposed to be useful.

Nutritional supplements

Vitamins and minerals

There is limited evidence for the use of multivitamin/mineral preparations for kidney disease. Given that a decline in renal function is related directly to cardiovascular mortality, the administration of vitamins and or minerals that could benefit cardiovascular health may also be useful for maintaining kidney function.[110]

Folate

A cross-over RCT of 23 children/teenagers with chronic renal failure, aged 7–17 years, was conducted, whereby each participant received 8 weeks of 5mg/m^2 folic acid per day and 8 weeks of placebo, separated by a washout period of 8 weeks.[111] There was a significant decrease in homocysteine levels during the folic acid phase from 10.3 mol/L to 8.6 mol/L with an insignificant rise in LDL lag times during the folic acid period. Based on a significantly improved flow mediated vessel diameter in the folic acid group, the study concluded that an 8-week regimen of folic acid could improve endothelial function. Because of the inconclusive folic acid supplementation studies in adults, the authors have speculated that this positive finding might be related to timing of treatment, in that atherosclerosis in children is at an earlier stage of its natural history.[111] Although folic acid is extremely safe, studies with clinically relevant outcomes are required before folate supplementation can be recommended for routine use in children with chronic renal failure.

Vitamin D

Single vitamin studies have concentrated on reducing the risk for adverse events such as in those patients with chronic kidney disease who have significant abnormalities of bone remodelling and mineral homeostasis and are at increased risk of fracture. A recent systematic study reviewed the scientific evidence of RCTs that reported the use of bisphosphonates, vitamin D sterols, calcitonin, and hormone replacement therapy to treat bone disease following kidney transplantation.[112] The review found that treatment with a bisphosphonate or vitamin D sterol or calcitonin after kidney transplantation may protect against immunosuppression-induced reductions in bone mineral density and prevent fracture.

Vitamin C

The role of vitamin C in kidney oxalate urolithiasis remains a risk according to recent studies,[113] particularly in those predisposed to forming kidney stones.[114] A recent double-blind cross-over RCT investigated the effects of 2 different vitamin C formulations and found that vitamin C with metabolites (ester-C) significantly reduced urine oxalate levels compared to ascorbic acid.[115] This study requires further evaluation with respect to inhibiting oxalate kidney stone formation.

Vitamin E/B6/B12

The Antioxidant Therapy In Chronic Renal Insufficiency (ATIC) Study showed that a multi-step treatment strategy improved carotid intima-media thickness, endothelial function, and microalbuminuria in patients with stages 2–4 chronic kidney disease. Recently an RCT[116] investigated a sequential treatment consisting of pravastatin 40mg/day; after 6 months, vitamin E 300mg/day; and after another 6 months, homocysteine-lowering therapy (folic acid, 5mg/day; pyridoxine, 100mg/day; and vitamin B12, 1mg/day, all in 1 tablet) were added and continued for another year. This regimen was compared to placebo. It was concluded that analysis of separate treatment effects suggested that vitamin E significantly decreased plasma concentrations of asymmetric dimethylarginine (ADMA) — an endogenous inhibitor of nitric oxide synthase (linked to greater CVD risk in patients with chronic kidney failure). Levels were reduced by 4% in the treatment group compared with the placebo group.

A study that investigated dietary supplementation of red grape juice, a source of polyphenols, and vitamin E on neutrophil NADPH-oxidase activity and other cardiovascular risk factors in haemodialysis patients found that the regular ingestion of concentrated red grape juice by haemodialysis patients reduced neutrophil NADPH-oxidase activity and plasma concentrations of oxidised LDL and inflammatory biomarkers to a greater extent than does that of vitamin E.[117] This effect of red grape juice consumption may favour a reduction in cardiovascular risk and assist kidney function. The re-regulation of cellular metabolism by polyphenolic compounds may constitute a biologically plausible rescue mechanism of metabolism in patients with chronic kidney disease. Moreover, it has also been recently shown that gamma tocopherol and DHA were well-tolerated and reduced selected biomarkers of inflammation in haemodialysis patients thereby reducing the risk of cardiovascular complications in this patient population.[118] Larger trials are required though for further evaluation. Also, on assessing clinical trials utilising vitamin E it is important to distinguish if the supplement and/or compound being investigated is alpha tocopherol or mixed alpha and gamma tocopherols or gamma tocopherol alone.

Magnesium

Magnesium is an essential mineral for optimal metabolic function. Studies that have demonstrated the promising effectiveness include results such as lowering the risk of metabolic syndrome and improving glucose and insulin metabolism,[119] which may have an intimate association with the development of progressive renal failure. Furthermore, because the kidneys have a very large capacity for magnesium excretion, hypermagnesemia usually occurs in the setting of renal insufficiency as well as excessive magnesium intake. It has been documented that body excretion of magnesium can be enhanced by use of saline diuresis, furosemide, or dialysis, depending on the clinical situation.[120] Magnesium has been implicated in diverse consequences, both beneficial and deleterious, in patients with chronic renal failure and dialysis.[121] Hence, there is a requisite for prudent supplementation with magnesium for renal patients.

A recent review has reported that there is biologically plausible data available for the role of magnesium in end-stage renal disease and its possible favourable therapeutic application in these patients.[122] The benefit of magnesium supplementation has been recently reported in a study with haemodialysis patients.[123] Although further studies are required this study reported that magnesium could play an important protective role in the progression of atherosclerosis by protecting carotid intima media thickness in patients on dialysis.

A recent pilot study and an RCT have investigated magnesium for the control of serum phosphate.[124, 125] The pilot study, investigating outpatients on haemodialysis, concluded that magnesium carbonate was generally well tolerated and was effective in controlling serum phosphorus while reducing elemental calcium ingestion. The RCT used 46 stable haemodialysis patients who were randomly allocated to receive either magnesium carbonate (n = 25) or calcium carbonate (n = 21) for 6 months. The study showed that magnesium carbonate administered for a period of 6 months was an effective and inexpensive agent to control serum phosphate levels in haemodialysis patients. It was further concluded that the administration of magnesium carbonate in combination with a low dialysate magnesium concentration avoided the risk of severe hypermagnesemia.[125]

Dietary factors have also been investigated as risks for the development of kidney stones. A large prospective cohort study reported that the association between calcium intake and kidney stone formation varied with age. Magnesium intake decreased and total vitamin C intake seemed to increase the risk of symptomatic nephrolithiasis.[126] Given that age and body size affect the relationship between diet and kidney stones, dietary recommendations for stone prevention should be customised to the individual patient.

A recent double-blind, RCT studied 20 normo-calciuric participants randomised to either placebo or potassium-magnesium citrate (42 mEq potassium, 21 mEq magnesium, 63 mEq citrate/day) before and during 5 weeks of strict bed rest.[127]

The study showed that provision of alkali as a combination of potassium–magnesium citrate was an effective countermeasure for the increased risk of renal stone disease associated with immobilisation. Also, the study reported that despite an observed increase in urine calcium concentration, the relative saturation of calcium oxalate decreased due to citrate chelation of calcium. Moreover, the concentration of non-dissociated uric acid decreased due to the significant increase in urine pH.

Other supplements

L-arginine (amino acid supplement)

The same research group conducted a second cross-over RCT of 21 children/teenagers aged 7–17 years with chronic renal failure and previously documented endothelial dysfunction to determine the effect of dietary supplementation with oral L-arginine on the response of the endothelium to shear stress.[128] Each child was given a 4-week regimen of 2.5 g/m^2 or 5 g/m^2 of oral L-arginine 3 times/day, and then a regimen of placebo after a 4-week washout period. A significant rise in levels of plasma L-arginine after the treatment phase was recorded, however, there was no significant improvement in endothelial function and, therefore, dietary supplementation with L-arginine was deemed not useful in the treatment of children with chronic renal failure.[128]

Omega-3 fatty acids (fish oils)

A significant body of research exists on the therapeutic use of omega-3 fatty acids for adults suffering from immunoglobulin A (IgA) nephropathy.[129] Recently omega-3 supplementation was reported to be significantly associated with the improvement of both renal vascular function and tubule function.[130]

A meta-analysis conducted in 1997 of 5 RCTs (n = 202) with fish oil reported that although the mean difference was not statistically significant there was a 75% probability of at least a small beneficial effect of supplementation with omega-3 fatty acids.[131] Also, a sub-analysis on 3 of the studies indicated that omega-3 treatment may be more beneficial to more highly proteinuric patients. There was considerable heterogeneity among the 5 studies, including severity of disease, dosing, treatment duration, and length of follow-up, hence additional longer-term research with larger sample sizes is necessary.

The largest study that was included in the meta-analysis was a multi-centre double-blind RCT of 106 adults with IgA nephropathy.[132] The test group (n = 55) received 12g/day of fish oil for 2 years, and the control group (n = 51) received placebo. There was a significant difference between the 2 groups with respect to the primary end point, a 50% or more increase in serum creatinine. The study concluded that 2 years of fish oil may significantly slow the rate of decline in renal function. No adverse events were reported, however, some participants in the treatment group complained of an unpleasant aftertaste after consuming the fish oil capsules. The same research group conducted a further study to assess the long-term outcome of the patients enrolled in this trial, with a mean follow-up time of 6.4 years.[133] After the study, the placebo group had been un-blinded and was free to take fish oil. Seventeen patients from the original study switched to fish oil. In the long-term follow-up study, the study found that patients in the original treatment group were still at significantly less risk of reaching the primary end point than the patients in the original placebo group — including those who had switched to fish oil after the trial's completion. Hence, commencing fish oil therapy early appears to offer patients the best clinical outcome.

Since the initial meta-analysis was published, 2 additional trials have been conducted.[132, 133] One of these RCTs compared the effect of low-dose versus high-dose omega-3 fatty acid consumption in 73 patients with severe IgA nephropathy.[134] For 2 years, the low-dose group (n = 37) received 1.88g of eicosapentanoic acid (EPA) and 1.47g of docosahexanoic acid (DHA) daily. The high-dose group (n = 36) received 3.76g of EPA and 2.94g of DHA daily. Using a 50% or more increase in serum creatinine as the primary end point, the study demonstrated that both dosage regimens were similarly effective in slowing the rate of decline in renal function. Additional research is required to determine the optimal dosage of fish oil to be prescribed, however, on current evidence fish oil supplementation is effective.

A second and more recent RCT with 28 adults diagnosed with IgA nephropathy assessed the effect of a low-dose regimen of omega-3 fatty acids.[135] The test group (n = 14) received 0.85 g of EPA and 0.57 g of DHA twice/day for 4 years. Although the study indicated that the control group of participants (n = 14) was treated symptomatically, no treatment was specified. In both groups, hypertension was treated with angiotensin-converting enzyme inhibitors, beta blockers, and/or calcium channel blockers. At the end of the study, significantly fewer participants in the test group had a 50% or more increase in their serum creatinine than in the control group. No adverse events were reported. The study suggested that the effect of fish oil may be dose dependent — with higher doses being more beneficial at preventing decline in renal function.

Recent studies indicate that the effect of a purified preparation of omega-3 fatty acids on proteinuria in patients with IgA nephropathy was dose dependent and was associated with a dose-dependent effect of the FAs on plasma phospholipid EPA and DHA levels.[136]

A recent meta-analysis[137] that consisted of 17 trials with 626 participants investigated participants in the trials with a single underlying diagnosis such as IgA nephropathy (n = 5), diabetes (n = 7), or lupus nephritis (n = 1). The dose of omega-3 long-chain polyunsaturated fatty acids (LCPUFAs) ranged from 0.7 to 5.1g/day, and the median follow-up was 9 months. The study concluded that omega-3 LCPUFAs supplementation reduced urine protein excretion but not the decline in glomerular filtration rate.[137]

A recent RCT investigating the combined treatment of proteinuric IgA nephropathy with renin-angiotensin system blockers and polyunsaturated fatty acids (PUFAs) reported efficacy with PUFAs.[138] This study tested the effect of a 6-month course of PUFA (3g/day) in a group of 30 patients with biopsy-proven IgA neuropathy and proteinuria already treated with renin-angiotensin system blockers randomised to receive PUFA supplementation or to continue their standard therapy. The study reported reduction of proteinuria was 72.9% in the PUFA group and 11.3% in the renin-angiotensin system blockers group. A reduction of ≥ 50% of baseline proteinuria was achieved in 80% of PUFA patients and 20% of renin-angiotensin system blockers patients. Erythrocyturia was significantly lower in the PUFA group. No significant changes in renal function, blood pressure and triglycerides were observed.

When taken in recommended doses, fish oils have been reported to be extremely safe for adults.[139] It should also be noted that oral daily amounts exceeding 10g of fish oil or 3g of DHA plus EPA may lead to an increased risk of bleeding. Based on the known safety and efficacy data that currently exists, there is promising evidence to warrant the inclusion of fish oil supplementation in the treatment of adult IgA nephropathy. Potential use in children warrants further investigations though.

Probiotics

The prophylactic and therapeutic use of probiotic micro-organisms is a wide and contentious area of research.

A pilot study has assessed the effect of probiotics on oxaluria in 6 adults with idiopathic calcium oxalate urolithiasis and hyperoxaluria.[140] The 6 patients received a daily dose of 8×10^{11} colony-forming units (CFU) of a freeze-dried lactic acid bacteria preparation for 4 weeks. There was a significant reduction in 24-hour oxalate excretion in all 6 patients compared to baseline. The mean reduction in oxaluria was 30g/day. The reduced levels persisted for at least 1 month after treatment was ceased.

Clinical trials increasingly provide a plausible biological and scientific basis for the use of probiotics in medicinal practice including urology. A recent review concluded that dietary measures and novel probiotic therapy are promising adjuncts for preventing recurrent nephrolithiasis.[141]

Integrative medicine approaches for treating urinary tract infections (UTIs) have included the use of probiotics and cranberry juice.[142, 143] (For more information on cranberry juice see the next section).

Several clinical trials with varying outcomes have investigated the effect of direct administration of probiotics as suppositories for the prevention of UTIs.

An early study investigated infection recurrence in 41 adult women with acute lower UTIs. The participants were randomly treated for 3 days with pharmaceuticals and showed an infection eradication rate of 100% with norfloxacin and in 95% with trimethoprim/sulfamethoxazole. UTI recurred in 29% of patients treated with norfloxacin and in 41% of those treated with trimethoprim/sulfamethoxazole. Post drug therapy randomisation to vaginal administration of suppositories (*L. rhamnosus* GR-1 and *L. fermentum* B-24) or placebo (skim-milk suppositories) resulted in a recurrence rate of UTI of only 21%, while in patients given the placebo the recurrence rate was 47%.[144]

A later study[145] by this same research group investigated the effects of suppositories containing the same *Lactobacillus* species as the previous study versus suppositories containing *Lactobacillus* growth factor (to enhance growth of already existing *Lactobacilli*). Fifty-five women (mean age 34; ≥4 UTIs in past 12 months) were randomly selected to *Lactobacillus* or growth factor suppositories once weekly for 12 months. At the end of 12 months both groups exhibited a 73% lower incidence of UTIs than in the 12 months prior to study onset with 1.6 per patient and 1.3 per patient in the *Lactobacillus* and growth factor groups, respectively.

In a small pilot study, 9 women with recurrent UTIs (≥2 in the past 12 months) used a *L. crispatus* vaginal suppository every other night for 1 year. Infection rates were significantly reduced from 5.0±1.6 in the year prior to treatment to 1.3±1.2 during the year of treatment.[146]

Some studies with probiotic suppositories for UTI prevention have not reported a benefit.[147] In an RCT, 47 women (≥3 UTIs in the previous 12 months) who were assigned to *L. rhamnosus* or *L. casei* or placebo suppositories twice weekly for 26 weeks reported no significant difference on the incidence of monthly UTI between the treatment and placebo groups.

In another RCT, 30 women with a median UTI incidence of 3 in the previous 12 months were randomised to receive *L. crispatus* suppositories or placebo suppositories once daily for 5 days and followed for 6 months.[148] The study showed that *L. crispatus* CTV-05 can be given as a vaginal suppository with minimal side-effects to healthy women with a history of recurrent UTI. No severe negative effects were reported, although 7 women in the treatment group only experienced asymptomatic pyuria.

In a small study of 10 adult women, *L. rhamnosus* GR-1 and *L. fermentum* RC-14 was orally administered twice daily for 14 days and resulted in bacterial recovery from vaginal tissue within 1 week of commencing supplementation.[149] In 6 cases of asymptomatic or intermediate bacterial vaginosis it was reported to be resolved within 1 week of therapy.

In addition, oral probiotic supplements have been shown to benefit paediatric populations. In a multi-centre RCT in 12 neonatal intensive care units, 585 pre-term newborns were randomised to oral *L. rhamnosus* GG (n = 295) or placebo (n = 290) once daily until discharge. Incidence of UTIs in the *Lactobacillus* group was 3.4% compared to 5.8% in the placebo group — clinically relevant, however not statistically significant.[150] A cautionary note should be added when supplementing neonates with probiotics, as they appear to carry a higher risk of serious complications such as sepsis.

In a case report, a girl of 6 years of age with no urinary tract anatomical abnormalities experienced 3 consecutive UTIs — once a month for 3 months.[151] The patient was treated with increasingly potent antibiotic regimens — the last 2 which spread to the kidneys. After the third episode and antibiotic treatment, urine was negative for *E. coli* but faeces was positive for a uropathogenic strain of *E. coli*. The patient was commenced on *L. acidophilus* DDS-1 twice daily for 1 month, followed by once daily for 5 months. After 2 months, the stool was negative for the pathogenic strain of *E. coli*. During probiotic treatment the patient had no UTI recurrence. It is of interest that when the probiotics were ceased the patient experienced a UTI within 2 weeks — caused by *Klebsiella pneumoniae*.[151]

Recent reviews have reported that despite enhanced cure rates in some studies and the evidence from the available studies that suggests that probiotics can be beneficial for preventing recurrent UTIs in women with a good safety profile,[152] concerns about product stability and limited documentation of strain-specific effects prevent strong recommendations being made for the use of *Lactobacillus*-containing probiotics in the treatment of bacterial vaginosis.[153, 154] The results of studies employing *Lactobacilli* for the prophylaxis of UTI remain contentious due largely to the small sample sizes investigated in the clinical trials, however this should not be misinterpreted as no evidence.

It should be noted that the best management approach to preventing recurrent UTIs, other than appropriate hygiene, is to support the immune system (see Chapter 20).

Cranberry (*Vaccinium macrocarpon*)

A US survey of 117 caregivers of children being treated at a paediatric nephrology clinic reported that 29% of the parents administered cranberry products to their children for therapeutic purposes.[155] Recurrent UTI was reported by 15% of the survey parents as a problem, and the use of cranberry products was 65% among children with recurrent UTI versus 23% among children with other renal problems.

A recent meta-analysis[156] of 10 trials using the Cochrane criteria for inclusion summarised the cranberry trials. Of the 10 trials, 5 were cross-over and 5 were parallel group studies. Cranberry juice was used in 7 trials, while tablets were used in 4 (one trial used both). The conclusions reached were that cranberry juice significantly reduced the incidence of UTIs over a 12-month period. It seems to be most effective in women with recurrent infections than for the elderly (both genders); individuals with neurogenic bladder do not appear to derive much benefit from cranberry juice.

Recent additional systematic reviews report on clinical trials investigating the use of cranberry for UTIs.[157, 158] The findings of the first Cochrane collaboration supported the potential use of cranberry products in the prophylaxis of recurrent UTIs in young and middle-aged women. However, the authors also noted that the heterogeneity of clinical study designs and the lack of consensus regarding the dosage regimen and formulation to use cranberry products made recommendations difficult to advise.[157]

At the same time, in a further review for the Cochrane collaboration, the benefit of prophylactic antibiotics for the prevention of recurrent UTI in children remained unclear because of the underpowered and sub-optimally designed trials.[158] However, the review concluded that the studies suggested that any benefit was likely to be small, and clinical significance may be limited. The trials of complementary interventions (vitamin A, probiotics, cranberry, nasturtium and horseradish) generally gave favourable results but were not conclusive. Hence, it was further concluded that children and their families who utilise these supplements should be aware that further infections are possible despite their use.[158]

Herbal medicines

Herbal *Western* medicines have a long historical use for the treatment of pathologies of the kidneys and the urinary tract.[159] Examples of herbal medicines with traditional use in uncomplicated UTIs are:

- *Arctostaphylos uva ursi* (Bearberry) — an historical use as an urinary antiseptic, diuretic and astringent
- *Echinacea purpurea* — an historical use and verified through numerous clinical trials as anti-bacterial
- *Solidago virgaurea* (Golden rod) — an historical use as an anti-inflammatory that can be found in products that are currently available to the public.

However, clinical trials as to their efficacy and safety are largely absent.

It is important to note that herbal medicines that can help with CVD, T2DM and hypertension may also indirectly assist with renal function (see Chapters 10, 13 and 19, respectively).

Traditional Chinese medicine (TCM)

Often many of the RCTs on TCMs have been conducted in China and the results are not readily available to clinicians in Western countries. We have identified a number of RCTs and a meta-analysis that have evaluated TCMs of herbal extracts in children with nephrotic syndrome.[160–163] *Tripterygium wilfordii* glycosides have been demonstrated to have immunosuppressive and anti-inflammatory effects.[158]

In the first RCT the study analysed the response of 80 children between the ages of 1 and 13 to *Tripterygium wilfordii* glycosides plus prednisone (n = 39) versus the control treatment of cyclophosphamide plus prednisone (n = 41) for the treatment of relapsing primary nephrotic syndrome. Gradual reduction in prednisone doses were administered to both groups over 12–18 months. The TCM group was given 1mg/kg of *Tripterygium wilfordii* glycosides orally 2–3 times/day over a period of 3 months. Also, cyclophosphamide (10mg/kg/day) was given to the control group by intermittent intravenous pulse over 3–6 months. After a follow-up period of 3–7 years (mean 4.9 years). No significant difference between the relapse rates in the 2 groups was reported. The study concluded that a combination of prednisone and *Tripterygium wilfordii* glycosides is as effective as prednisone plus cyclophosphamide, although methodologically these were not equivalent. Less adverse events (i.e. GI upset, alopecia) were reported by the investigational group than in the control group.

The second RCT tested the efficacy of an oral liquid preparation of a combination of 10 Chinese medicinal plants (*Chai-Ling-Tang*) on 69 children between 5–12 years of age with steroid-dependent nephrotic syndrome.[159] The test group (n = 37) was given decreasing doses of prednisone until they had protein-free urine for 3 weeks. This group was also given consistent doses of *Chai-Ling-Tang* for 1.5 years. The control group (n = 32) was treated with tapering doses of prednisone, along with 2.5mg/kg/day of cyclophosphamide for 8 weeks. Both groups were followed-up for at least 2 years. The results showed that with respect to relapse rate, time to absence of proteinuria, amount of prednisone intake, and side-effects there was no improvement in the comparative treatment group. There was, though, a trend to improvement in these measures for the TCM arm of the study. Furthermore, it was suggested that the TCM could serve as a substitute for patients who do not respond to or have severe adverse events from taking cyclophosphamide. Further research on the TCM efficacy and safety are warranted.

The third RCT investigated whether *tiaojining*, a combination product of 6 principle Chinese medicinal herbs, reduced the risk of infection in 660 children with nephrotic syndrome.[160] The participating children ranged from 1–13 years of age. The experimental group was treated with *tiaojining* 3 times/day plus baseline treatment (prednisone) for 8 weeks. The control group received prednisone alone for 8 weeks. The study concluded that *tiaojining* was effective in the prophylaxis of infection in nephritic children. No adverse events were reported. As methodological quality was weak, further clinical studies are needed.

A systematic review of 14 RCTs (n = 524) was conducted to determine the effect of *Radix astragali* combined with conventional treatment for nephrotic syndrome, including prednisone and cyclophosphamide, on nephrotic adults.[161] The meta-analysis showed that *Radix astragali* could enhance the therapeutic effect of the conventional therapies and also reduce the recurrence of primary nephrotic syndrome. Also, compared with the participants who received only conventional treatment, those receiving the investigational product/treatment had reduced 24-hour proteinuria, increased plasma levels of albumin, and reduced levels of total cholesterol. Only 1 of the included articles indicated that there were no adverse events reported. Therefore, additional studies are required to fully understand possible adverse outcomes. Dosage varied among the trials investigated from 1–4g of dried root orally 3 times/day, or a full dropper of tincture orally 2 or 3 times/day.

A systematic review of 18 randomised and quasi-randomised trials (n = 1322) was conducted to evaluate the use of rhubarb (*Rheum rhabarbarum*) in chronic renal failure patients.[164] The included trials assessed rhubarb versus conventional medicine, as well as rhubarb versus TCM herbs. Rhubarb was found to be significantly more effective in treating chronic renal failure than conventional medicine alone. There was no significant difference between the efficacy of rhubarb and that of other traditional Chinese herbs in the treatment of chronic renal failure. The review concluded that rhubarb was effective in reducing the symptoms of chronic renal failure. The small participant numbers made it difficult to conclude whether rhubarb can slow or stop the long-term progression of the disease. Half the included articles reported that no adverse effects were found.[162]

It was concluded that rhubarb was likely to be safe when used for short periods (i.e. less than 8 days) and in low doses, but cramps and diarrhoea have been reported. Chronic use of rhubarb can lead to numerous adverse effects, including electrolyte depletion, oedema, colic, atonic colon, and hyperaldosteronism. Rhubarb leaves contain oxalic acid and are considered toxic if ingested. Patients with renal disorders should be monitored closely when using rhubarb, due to potential electrolyte disturbances.[165] Dosing information for children is unavailable.

TCM in the treatment of chronic renal failure was studied in 248 adult participants aged 20–65 years.[166] For 12 months, the TCM group (n = 120) was given conventional drugs (including prednisone and furosemide) in combination with 5 decoctions of traditional Chinese herbs to treat the primary disease. These herbs were specifically targeted to supplement the kidneys, as per by TCM assumptions, to invigorate blood flow. Patients were dosed and treated individually, based on their specific characteristics. Patients in the control group (n = 128) were treated with only conventional medicine for the 12-month period. Although both groups improved, significant differences were found in improved symptoms and in creatinine clearance between the 2 groups. Adverse events were not documented in this study, and safety was unknown. The study findings require further detailed research.

In a small trial, 40 patients with chronic renal failure were randomly divided into 2 groups. The trial investigated *Baoyuan Qiangshen* II tablet (TCM) group and essential amino acid added capoten group. The study reported improved kidney function.[167] Additional clinical studies by the same research group from China further investigated the *Baoyuan Qiangshen* II tablet preparation. Sixty patients with chronic renal failure were divided into 2 groups randomly; the tested group treated with *Baoyuan Qiangshen* II tablet combined with Lotensin and the control group treated with an essential amino acid combined with Lotensin.[168] It was concluded that the test treatment was significantly better than the control and that it could significantly alleviate tubular interstitial injury thereby improving renal function and enhancing the effective rate in treating chronic renal failure.

Physical therapies

Vibrational massage therapy

An early study that evaluated the use of vibrational massage therapy after extracorporeal shockwave lithotripsy in 103 adults with lower caliceal stones showed benefit.[169] The test group (n = 51) received shockwave lithotripsy and 20–25 minute sessions of vibrational massage therapy in 2-day intervals for 2 weeks, whereas the control group (n = 52) received shockwave lithotripsy alone. The results showed that the stone-free rates in the test and control groups were 80% and 60%, respectively. There was a significantly higher rate of stone recurrence in the control group than in the experimental group. The mean time to calculus recurrence was 16 months in the test group versus 11.4 months in the control group. There were more reports of renal colic in the control group. Additional complications, such as pyelonephritis and fever, were reported equally in both groups. Additional studies for further efficacy are warranted.

Tai chi

Tai chi is a potent intervention that improves balance, upper- and lower-body muscular strength and endurance, and upper- and lower-body flexibility. A study has found that tai chi exercise programs support current public health initiatives to reduce disability from chronic health conditions and enhance physical function in older adults.[170] Moreover, a recent review has reported that tai chi exercises may reduce blood pressure and serve as a practical, non-pharmacologic adjunct to conventional hypertension management.[171] This cumulative data strongly supports the use of tai chi for patients diagnosed with end-stage kidney disease.

A pilot study evaluated the effect of a tai chi based exercise training program on the QOL in a group of 9 patients on peritoneal dialysis.[172] The major finding of this study was that 3 months of tai chi exercise training significantly improved the mental health dimension score in 6 patients on peritoneal dialysis.

Acupuncture

Acupuncture is a complex therapeutic modality that has been used to treat a variety of diseases and pathological conditions. Acupuncture has become increasingly popular as a therapy for pain and several chronic disorders, including kidney disease, that are difficult to manage with conventional treatments. Acupuncture and acupuncture-like somatic nerve stimulation have been reported in different kidney diseases and several complications related to them.[173]

An extensive portion of the recent scientific literature that has been published on acupuncture for the treatment of renal diseases has originated from China, such as RCTs and reviews.[174–179] The studies have comprised RCTs on early interventions to treat kidney problems as well as to ameliorate symptoms associated with kidney diseases. A review of the literature between 1982 and 2007 has concluded that acupuncture and moxibustion can increase human immunity, reduce urinary protein, improve renal function, antagonise the side-effects of glucocorticoid hormones and that medication combined with acupuncture-moxibustion has the advantages of convenience, lower costs, safety and with no adverse effects.[177]

A randomised trial to evaluate the effect of acupuncture compared to a conventional analgesic in the treatment of 38 adult males with renal colic from urolithiasis was found to be effective.[180] The severity of renal colic was assessed before treatment and 30 minutes following treatment. The mean pain scores were not significantly different between groups prior to treatment. The experimental group (n = 22) received acupuncture treatment, and the active control group (n = 16) received an intramuscular injection of avafortan (analgesic/antispasmodic). There was no significant difference in the reduction in mean pain score between the 2 groups. However, acupuncture had a significantly faster analgesic onset. There were no adverse effects with the acupuncture group.

An RCT was recently completed that investigated the efficacy of acupuncture in 68 adults with uremic pruritis.[181] Patients in the test group (n = 34) were treated with acupuncture in 30-minute sessions twice a week for 4 weeks while receiving haemodialysis. For comparisons the control group (n = 34) was treated with 4mg of Chlor-Trimeton 3 times daily and a topical dermatitis ointment 3 times daily for 2 weeks along with haemodialysis. Patients were then observed for the alleviation of pruritus. The effective rate was 95% in the acupuncture group, significantly higher than the effective rate of 70.6% in the control group. Sixteen patients in the acupuncture group maintained this improvement for 3 months and 18 patients for 1 month. Conversely, in the control group, all cases experienced recurrence of uremic pruritus immediately once treatment was ceased.[181] Given that safety data for acupuncture is high, some clinicians may want to consider including acupuncture for patients with uremic pruritus.

Acupressure

An additional RCT study investigated the effects of acupressure in 60 adults with uremic pruritus.[182] Acupressure is part of TCM and involves pressing and/or massaging various acupuncture points on the body. The treatment group (n = 30) received acupressure in 15–20 minute sessions 3 times per week for 5 weeks either immediately before or after dialysis. Conversely the control group (n = 30) did not receive any treatment other than dialysis. Frequency, intensity, and localisation of pruritus as well as its effects on the patient's QOL were used to assess the efficacy of acupressure on pruritus. There were significant differences in mean pruritus scores between the 2 groups after 6 weeks, 12 weeks, and 18 weeks — with the acupressure group having significantly lower scores. The report concluded that acupressure was thought to be even safer than acupuncture, as it avoids needle insertion. Acupressure is a further modality for clinicians to consider for patients with pruritus.

A double-blinded RCT has reported that adult patients receiving acupressure along with conventional care returned a better quality of sleep and QOL than those not receiving any acupressure.[183] Ninety-eight patients experiencing sleep disturbances were randomly assigned to an acupressure group (n = 35), a placebo group (n = 32), or a control group (n = 31). The acupressure group received acupoint massage during haemodialysis 3 times a week for 4 weeks. The placebo group received sham acupressure, which involved massage on non-acupoints which were of similar frequency and duration as the acupressure group, whereas the control group received only standard care. Data was collected at baseline and at 1 week post-treatment. After treatment, sleep quality and QOL scores were significantly more improved in the acupressure group than in the control group. Interestingly, sham acupressure also had similar improvements.[183]

A further RCT assessed the effect of a combined acupressure/massage regimen on fatigue and depression in 58 end-stage renal disease patients receiving haemodialysis.[184] Patients were randomly assigned to either the acupressure group (n = 28) or the control group (n = 30). The acupressure group received 12 minutes of acupressure plus 3 minutes of lower limb massage 3 times a week during dialysis for 4 weeks. The control group received only routine care during dialysis. After the 4-week study period, there were significant differences in the perceived fatigue and feelings of depression (for depression this was borderline significant) between the 2 groups. This study shows promise, though further studies are warranted.

Aromatherapy

The effects of aromatherapy combined with massage was investigated in a small trial of 29 patients aged 26–65 years with uremic pruritis.[185] The test group (n = 13) received aromatherapy with massage 3 times per week for 1 month, along with haemodialysis. Lavender oil and tea tree oil were used in the aromatherapy group. The control group (n = 16) received only haemodialysis during the study period. Frequency, severity, and location of pruritus were assessed and pre-test scores were not significantly different between the groups. Following the treatment period the pruritus scores were significantly lower in the test group versus the control group.

Homeopathy

A small double-blinded RCT[186] assessed the effect of individualised homeopathic treatments on 28 adults (19 completed the study) with uremic pruritus who were on haemodialysis. Those in the test group received a homeopathic treatment, whereas those in the control group were given a placebo. The study had a 60-day follow-up period after starting treatment. In total, 40 homeopathic medications were prescribed, with each patient in the test group receiving more than 1 throughout the course of the study. Although there was a significant decrease in pruritus scores in the treatment group, the difference in post-treatment scores was not significant between the 2 groups at the end of the study.[186] The study methodology was weak.

Conclusion

This chapter has reviewed the best evidence that was available for the therapeutic management of patients with kidney disease. Patients with kidney disease may have additional health problems and therefore the integrative care approach of these patients, as with any other chronic disease, is multi-factorial.

Advantageous nutritional practices and sensible supplement use by patients with kidney disease can assist with management issues, as is the case, for example, with those patients undergoing haemodialysis.

Exercise-based rehabilitation programs benefit patients after myocardial infarction, bypass surgery, chronic lung disease, rheumatologic disorders, and stroke and other neurological conditions. Hence, exercise training may improve the functional capacity of patients with kidney diseases, thereby offering them a better QOL. Adoption of routine counselling and encouragement for physical activity has the potential to improve outcomes, improve physical functioning, and optimise QOL and overall health of those patients who may be undergoing dialysis.

As a final thought, a recent systematic review has investigated health-related QOL factors as predictors of mortality in end-stage renal disease.[187] This study overwhelmingly concluded that health-related QOL factors predict mortality in end-stage renal disease. The physical domains and nutritional biomarkers are those factors that were most closely associated with the highest health-related QOL.

Table 35.2 Levels of evidence for lifestyle and complementary medicines/therapies in the management of renal diseases

Modality	Level I	Level II	Level IIIa	Level IIIb	Level IIIc	Level IV	Level V
Lifestyle modification							
Age				x			
Obesity	x						
T2DM	x						
Hypertension/ cardiovascular disease	x						
Urinary tract system blockages				x			
Overuse of medications				x			
Illicit drug use				x			
Inflammation/diseases				x			
Family history	x						
Low birth weight				x			
Trauma/accidents				x			
Environmental toxins			x				
Mind–body medicine							
Cognitive behavioural therapy				x			
Educational interventions	x						
Muscular relaxation					x		
Physical activity/exercise							
General exercise		x					
Resistance exercise				x			
Nutritional influences							
Weight management diet (obese)				x			

Continued

Table 35.2 Levels of evidence for lifestyle and complementary medicines/therapies in the management of renal diseases—cont'd

Modality	Level I	Level II	Level IIIa	Level IIIb	Level IIIc	Level IV	Level V
Mediterranean diet			x				
DASH diet			x				
Protein diet (low)	x						
Soy protein			x				
Vegetarian diet			x				
Alcohol			x				
Caffeine					x		
Food allergy					x		
Vitamins, minerals and nutritional supplements							
Folate		x					
B6 plus B12 in combination					x		
Vitamin E		x					
Vitamin C + metabolites (ester-C)				x			
Vitamin D	x						
Magnesium				x			
L-arginine				x(-)			
Omega-3 fatty acids	x						
Probiotics	x						
Cranberry juice/tablets	x						
Red grape juice						x	
Herbal medicines							
Arctostaphylos uva ursi						x	
Echinacea purpurea						x	
Solidago virgaurea						x	
Radix astragali	x						
Chinese herbal medicine							
Tripterygium wilfordII				x			
Chai-Ling-Tang				x			
Tiaojining				x			
Rheum rhabarbarum	x						
Baoyuan Qiangshen II				x			
Physical therapies							
Vibrational massage therapy				x			
Tai chi				x			
Acupuncture			x				
Acupressure			x				
Natural therapies							
Aromatherapy				x			
Homeopathy			x				

Level I — from a systematic review of all relevant randomised controlled trials — meta-analyses.
Level II — from at least 1 properly designed randomised controlled clinical trial.
Level IIIa — from well-designed pseudo-randomised controlled trials (alternate allocation or some other method).
Level IIIb — from comparative studies (including systematic reviews of such studies) with concurrent controls and allocation not randomised, cohort studies, case-control studies, or interrupted time series with a parallel control group.
Level IIIc — from comparative studies with historical control, 2 or more single-arm studies or interrupted time series without a parallel control group.
Level IV — opinions of respected authorities based on clinical experience, descriptive studies or reports of expert committees.
Level V — represents minimal evidence that represents testimonials.

Clinical tips handout for patients — renal disease

1 Lifestyle advice

Sleep

- Restore normal sleep patterns. Most adults require about 7 hours sleep. (See Chapter 22 for more advice.)

Sunshine

- Eye protection should be worn in the form of sunglasses at all times when exposed to the sun for prolonged periods of time.
- Amount of exposure varies with local climate.
- At least 15 minutes of sunshine needed daily for vitamin D and melatonin production — especially before 10 a.m. and after 3 p.m. when the sun exposure is safest during summer. Much more exposure is required in winter, when supplementation needs to be considered.
- Ensure gradual adequate skin exposure to sun; avoid sunscreen and excess clothing to maximise levels of vitamin D.
- More time in the sun is required for dark skinned people.
- Direct exposure to about 10% of body (hands, arms, face), without sunscreen and not through glass.
- Vitamin D is obtained in the diet from fatty fish, eggs, liver and fortified foods (some milks and margarines); however, it is unlikely that adequate vitamin D concentrations can be obtained from diet alone.

2 Physical activity/exercise

- Exercise for 30 minutes or more daily. If exercise is not regular, commence with 5 minutes daily and slowly build up to at least 30 minutes. Outdoor exercise with nature, fresh air and sunshine is ideal (e.g. brisk walking, light jogging, cycling, swimming, stretching). Weight bearing exercises or resistance exercise are beneficial. The more time you spend outdoors the better.
- Tai chi can improve quality of life in patients on dialysis.

3 Mind–body medicine

- Stress management programs are important for life-stressor management; for example, six 40 minute sessions for patients to understand the nature of their symptoms, the symptoms' relationship to stress and the practice of regular relaxation exercises.
- Regular meditation practice at least 10–20 minutes daily.

Breathing

- Be aware of breathing from time to time. Notice if tendency to hold breath or over-breathe. Always aim to relax the breath and the muscles around the chest wall.

Rest and stress management

- Recurrent stress may cause a return of symptoms. Relaxation is important for a healthy lifestyle.
- Reduce workload and resolve conflicts. Contact family, friends, church, social or other groups for support.
- Listening to relaxation music and daily baths help.
- Massage therapy helps.
- Exercise aids in stress reduction.
- Cognitive behaviour therapy and psychotherapy are extremely helpful.

Fun

- It is important to have fun in life. Joy can be found even in the simplest tasks, such as being with friends with a sense of humour funny movies/videos, comedy, hobbies, dancing, playing with pets and children.
- Try to maintain an 'easy-going approach to life'; avoid feeling time-pressured or rushed.

4 Environment

- Reduce your exposure to chemicals wherever possible, including household cleaning agents, paints and solvents, petrochemical fumes, passive smoking, over-medication with pharmaceutical drugs (review with your doctor), drinking water bottles exposed to the sun, etc.
- Investigate whether there are any sources of mould in your environment and remove them wherever possible.
- Reduce your exposure to electromagnetic radiation wherever possible. Carry your mobile phone away from the body rather than in your pocket. Turn off home appliances at the power point when not in use.

5 Dietary changes

- Eat regular healthy low GI meals, ideally 3 small meals, and 2 snacks per day; each containing protein in order to avoid fluctuating blood sugar levels and provide amino acids for nerve transmitters, such as tryptophan.

- Eat more fruit and vegetables — variety of colours and those in season.
- Increase dietary fibre.
- Eat more nuts; for example, walnuts, peanuts; seeds, beans (e.g. soy), sprouts (e.g. alfa, mung bean, lentils).
- Increase fish intake — canned is okay (mackerel, salmon, sardines, cod, tuna, salmon), and especially deep sea fish — daily if possible.
- Reduce red meat intake — preferably eat lean red meat (e.g. lamb, kangaroo) and white meat (e.g. free range organic chicken). Substitute soy for red meat.
- Use cold pressed olive oil and avocado.
- Use only dark chocolate — preferably 85% or more of cocoa.
- Eat low GI wholegrains/cereals (variety): rice (brown, basmati, Mahatmi, Doongara), traditional rolled oats, buckwheat flour, wholegrain organic breads (rye bread, Essene, spelt, Kamut), brown pasta, millet, amaranth etc.
- Reduce dairy intake: low-fat dairy products such as yoghurt and occasionally cheeses, unless there is a dairy intolerance.
- Drink more water 1–3 litres a day.
- Drink teas (e.g. especially organic green tea, black tea) plus vegetable juices.
- Moderate levels of caffeine can help diabetes control. Avoid high dosage as it can cause restlessness and agitation.
- Avoid hydrogenated fats, salt, fast foods, sugar (such as in soft drinks), lollies, biscuits, cakes and processed foods (e.g. white bread, white pasta, pastries).
- Minimise alcohol intake to no more than 1–2 glasses daily (non-sweet) as it is a brain depressant and can disturb sleep.
- Avoid chemical additives — preservatives, colourings and flavourings.
- Avoid artificial sweeteners. For sweetener try honey (e.g. manuka, yellow box and stringy bark have lowest GI).

6 Physical therapies

The following physical therapies may help (see text for further detail):

- muscular relaxation
- vibrational massage therapy
- tai chi
- acupuncture
- acupressure.

Aromatherapy may help relieve uremic pruritis (itchy skin) from kidney disease.

7 Supplements

Fish oils

- Indication: anti-inflammatory action; may help IgA nephropathy, proteinuria, renal impairment; hypertension and diabetes; cardiovascular disease.
- Dosage: Take with meals. Adult: 2–4g (1g containing EPA 180/DHA 120mg) daily.
  - Child: 1–2 x 500mg capsule twice daily (500–1000mg/day EPA and DHA); can be used in pregnancy or lactation as tolerated.
- Results: 1–4 days.
- Side-effects: often well tolerated especially if taken with meals. Very mild and rare side-effects (e.g. gastrointestinal upset); allergic reactions (e.g. rash, breathing problems if allergic to seafood); blood thinning effects in very high doses > 10g daily (may need to stop fish oil supplements 2 weeks prior to surgery).
- Contraindications: sensitivity reaction to seafood; drug interactions; caution when taking high doses of fish oils >4g/day together with warfarin (your doctor will check your INR test).

Vitamins and minerals

Folate

- Indication: elevated blood levels of homocysteine.
- Dosage: 0.5–1mg/day as in a multivitamin and mineral supplement.
- Results: uncertain.
- Side-effects: very mild and rare.
- Contraindications: avoid in anaemias until assessed by a doctor.

Vitamin B group, especially B6 and B12

- Indication: elevated blood levels of homocysteine; metformin can reduce vitamin B12.
- Dosage: upper level of intake of vitamin B6 should not exceed 50mg/day.
- Results: uncertain.
- Side-effects: avoid overuse of single vitamin products (e.g. oral and injectable forms of vitamin B6) or concomitant use of multivitamin products could result in some patients routinely exceeding the upper limit for vitamins associated with severe toxicity. Toxicity in high doses of vitamin B6 includes peripheral neuropathy, such as tingling, burning and numbness of limbs.
- Contraindications: avoid in anaemias until assessed by a doctor.

Vitamin D3 (cholecalciferol 1000IU)

Doctors should check blood levels and suggest supplementation if levels are low.

Natural vitamin E

- Indication: may improve renal function in chronic kidney disease; can help reduce platelet aggregation.
- Dosage: 200–500–1000IU daily (D-alpha-tocopherol or mixed isomers).
- Side-effects: doses below 1500IU/day are very unlikely to result in haemorrhage, diarrhoea, flatulence, nausea, heart palpitations.
- Contraindications: use with caution if bleeding disorder or if taking with blood thinning medication. If using very high dose, reduce dose before surgery.

Magnesium carbonate

- Indication: Must use only under medical supervision. Improves insulin sensitivity and hence glucose level. May be useful for patients with T2DM and nephropathy. Hypertension. May help phosphate control in hemodialysis
- Dosage: children, up to 65–120mg/day in divided doses. Adults, 350mg/day including pregnant and lactating women.
- Results: 2–3 days.
- Side-effects: oral magnesium especially at a dose greater than 400mg/day can cause gastrointestinal irritation, nausea, vomiting and diarrhoea. The dosage varies from person to person. Although rare, toxic levels can cause low blood pressure, thirst, heart arrhythmia, drowsiness and weakness.
- Contraindications: patients with kidney failure and heart block.

Probiotics

- Indications: UTIs; bacterial vaginosis; following a course of antibiotics; vaginal suppositories can help prevent recurrent UTIs.
- Dosage: oral; depending upon condition, different probiotics may be required. Generalised treatment dose before breakfast:
  - *Lactoballus fermentum* 2 billion CFU (combined multistrain is preferred)
  - *Lactobacillus rhamnosus* 12 billion CFU
  - *Lactobacillus acidophilus* 4 billion CFU
  - *Lactobacillus casei* 2 billion CFU
  - *Bifidobacterium bifidum* 1 billion CFU
  - *Bifidobacterium longum* 1 billion CFU.
- Results: few days to a few weeks depending on condition.
- Side-effects: gastrointestinal disturbance if wrong probiotic.
- Contraindications: true cow's milk allergy if contained in product.

Note: for recurrent UTIs see Chapter 20.

Cranberry

- Indications: for prevention of urinary tract infections can be taken as juice or dried extract
- Dosage: 350–900 ml/day or 5–30ml/day of unsweetened 100% cranberry juice.
- Results: maintenance of prevention for UTIs.
- Side-effects: patients with diabetes or glucose intolerance may want to drink sugar-free cranberry juice to avoid a high sugar intake. High doses of cranberry may cause stomach distress and diarrhoea. Some commercially available products are high in calories.
- Contraindications: interacts with warfarin. Cranberry juice has a moderately high concentration of oxalate, a common component of kidney stones, and should be limited in persons with a history of nephrolithiasis (kidney oxalate stones).

Herbal medicines

Note: When consuming herbal medicines always consult your doctor.

Although there is a paucity of clinical trials the following herbal medicines have been documented to have historical use in kidney diseases associated with low grade UTIs. Employing these may be of benefit. Check with manufacturers for administration dose, results and contraindications. The following herbs have a traditional use for UTIs:

- *Arctostaphylos uva ursi* (bearberry).
- *Echinacea purpurea*
- *Solidago virgaurea.* (golden rod).

Chinese herbal medicines

The following have been investigated mainly in China for nephrotic syndrome and nephritic syndrome or chronic renal failure. Caution is hence advocated with their use (consult your doctor).

- *Tripterygium wilfordii*
- *Chai-Ling-Tang*
- *Tiaojining*
- *Rheum rhabarbarum* (rhubarb)
- *Baoyuan Qiangshen II.*
- *Radix astragalus*

References

1 US Renal Data System. USRDS 2008 Annual Report: Atlas of Chronic Kidney Disease and End-Stage Renal Disease in the United States. Bethesda, MD: National Institute of Diabetes and Digestive and Kidney Diseases, National Institutes of Health; 2008. http://www.usrds.org/default.asp (accessed June 2009)

2 Coresh J, Selvin E, Stevens LA, et. al. Prevalence of chronic kidney disease in the United States. JAMA 2007;298(17):2038-2047.
3 Rabkin R. Diabetic nephropathy. Clin Cornerstone. 2003;5(2):1-11.
4 Nowack R, Ballé C, Birnkammer F, et. al. Complementary and alternative medications consumed by renal patients in southern Germany. J Ren Nutr 2009;19(3):211-9.
5 Tindle HA, Davis RB, Phillips RS, Eisenberg DM: Trends in use of complementary and alternative medicine by US adults:1997-2002. Altern Ther Health Med 2005;11:42-49.
6 Neff GW, O'Brien C, Montalbano M, et al: Consumption of dietary supplements in a liver transplant population. Liver Transplant 2004;10:881-885.
7 Liu JP, Manheimer E, Yang M: Herbal medicines for treating HIV infection and AIDS. Cochrane Database Syst Rev 3. CD003937, 2005.
8 Chen LC, Chen YF,Yang LL, Chou MH, Lin MF: Drug utilization pattern of antiepileptic drugs and traditional Chinese medicines in a general hospital in Taiwan—a pharmaco-epidemiologic study. J Clin Pharm Ther 2000;25:125-129.
9 Yeh GY, Eisenberg MM, Davis RB, Phillips RS: Use of complementary and alternative medicine among persons with diabetes mellitus: results of a national survey. Am J Pub Health 2000;92:1648-1652.
10 Tilburt JC, Miller FG. Responding to medical pluralism in practice: a principled ethical approach. J Am Board Fam Med 2007;20(5):489-94.
11 Burrowes JD; van Houten G: Use of alternative medicine by patients with stage 5 chronic kidney disease. Adv Chronic Kidney Dis 2005;12:312-325.
12 Markell MS. Potential benefits of complementary medicine modalities in patients with chronic kidney disease. Adv Chronic Kidney Dis 2005;12(3):292-9.
13 Zhou XJ, Rakheja D, Yu X, et. al. The aging kidney. Kidney Int 2008;74(6):710-20.
14 Mokdad AH, Ford ES, Bowman BA, et. al. Prevalence of obesity, diabetes, and obesity-related health risk factors, 2001. JAMA 2003;289(1):76-9.
15 Poirier P, Giles TD, Bray GA, et. al. Obesity and cardiovascular disease: pathophysiology, evaluation, and effect of weight loss: an update of the 1997 American Heart Association scientific statement on obesity and heart disease from the Obesity Committee of the Council on Nutrition, Physical Activity, and Metabolism. Circulation 2006;113(6):898-918.
16 Iseki K, Ikemiya Y, Kinjo K, et. al. Body mass index and the risk of development of end-stage renal disease in a screened cohort. Kidney Int 2004;65(5):1870-6.
17 Hsu CY, McCulloch CE, Iribarren C, et. al. Body mass index and risk for end-stage renal disease. Ann Intern Med. 2006;144(1):21-28.
18 Wild S, Roglic G, Green A, et. al. Global prevalence of diabetes: estimates for the year 2000 and projections for 2030. Diabetes Care 2004;27(5):1047-1053.
19 Yach D, Stuckler D, Brownell KD. Epidemiologic and economic consequences of the global epidemics of obesity and diabetes. Nat Med 2006;12(1):62-66.
20 Hajjar I, Kotchen TA. Trends in prevalence, awareness, treatment, and control of hypertension in the United States, 1988-2000. JAMA 2003;290(2):199-206.
21 Abuelo JG. Normotensive ischemic acute renal failure. NEJM 2007;357(8):797-805.
22 House AA, Silva Oliveira S, Ronco C. Anti-inflammatory drugs and the kidney. Int J Artif Organs 2007;30(12):1042-6.
23 Rexrode KM, Buring JE, Glynn RJ, et. al. Analgesic use and renal function in men. JAMA 2001;286(3):315-21.
24 Pallotta KE, Manley HJ. Vancomycin use in patients requiring hemodialysis: a literature review. Semin Dial 2008;21(1):63-70.
25 Goldstein RA, DesLauriers C, Burda A, Johnson-Arbor K. Cocaine: history, social implications, and toxicity: a review. Semin Diagn Pathol 2009;26(1):10-7.
26 Dettmeyer RB, Preuss J, Wollersen H, Madea B. Heroin-associated nephropathy. Expert Opin Drug Saf 2005;4(1):19-28.
27 Abdullah A, Khanam A, Biswas S, et. al. Medical causes and histological pattern of glomerulonephritis. Mymensingh Med J 2008;17(1):38-41.
28 Szczech LA. Renal disease: the effects of HIV and antiretroviral therapy and the implications for early antiretroviral therapy initiation. Curr Opin HIV AIDS 2009;4(3):167-70.
29 Rehermann B. Hepatitis C virus versus innate and adaptive immune responses: a tale of coevolution and coexistence. J Clin Invest 2009;119(7):1745-54.
30 Mackelaite L, Alsauskas ZC, Ranganna K. Renal failure in patients with cirrhosis. Med Clin North Am 2009;93(4):855-69,
31 Tsaras G, Owusu-Ansah A, Boateng FO, Amoateng-Adjepong Y. Complications associated with sickle cell trait: a brief narrative review. Am J Med 2009;122(6):507-12.
32 Hage FG, Venkataraman R, Zoghbi GJ, Perry GJ, DeMattos AM, Iskandrian AE. The scope of coronary heart disease in patients with chronic kidney disease. J Am Coll Cardiol 2009;53:2129-40.
33 Satko SG, Sedor JR, Iyengar SK, Freedman BI. Familial clustering of chronic kidney disease. Semin Dial 2007;20(3):229-36.
34 White SL, Perkovic V, Cass A, et. al. Is low birth weight an antecedent of CKD in later life? A systematic review of observational studies. Am J Kidney Dis 2009;54(2):248-61.
35 Yuan F, Hou FF, Wu Q, Chen PY, Xie D, Zhang X. Natural history and impact on outcomes of acute kidney injury in patients with road traffic injury. Clin Nephrol 2009;71(6):669-79.
36 Cox CD, Tsikouris JP. Preventing contrast nephropathy: what is the best strategy? A review of the literature J Clin Pharmacol 2004;44(4):327-37.
37 Van Vleet TR, Schnellmann RG. Toxic nephropathy: environmental chemicals. Semin Nephrol 2003;23(5):500-8.
38 Meyer BR, Fischbein A, Rosenman K, et. al. Increased urinary enzyme excretion in workers exposed to nephrotoxic chemicals. Am J Med 1984;76(6):989-98.
39 Goyer RA. Environmentally related diseases of the urinary tract. Med Clin North Am 1990;74(2):377-89.
40 Anders MW. Chemical toxicology of reactive intermediates formed by the glutathione-dependent bioactivation of halogen-containing compounds. Chem ResToxicol 2008;21(1):145-59.
41 Lock EA, Reed CJ. Trichloroethylene: mechanisms of renal toxicity and renal cancer and relevance to risk assessment. Toxicol Sci 2006;91(2):313-31.

42 Jakubowski M. Influence of occupational exposure to organic solvents on kidney function. Int J Occup Med Environ Health 2005;18(1):5-14.
43 Perazella MA. Renal vulnerability to drug toxicity. Clin J Am Soc Nephrol 2009;4(7):1275-83.
44 Navas-Acien A, Tellez-Plaza M, Guallar E, et. al. Blood Cadmium and Lead and Chronic Kidney Disease in US Adults: A Joint Analysis. Am J Epidemiol 2009 Aug 21 (Epub ahead of print)
45 Yildirim YK, Fadiloglu C. The effect of progressive muscle relaxation training on anxiety levels and quality of life in dialysis patients. EDTNA ERCA J 2006;32(2):86-8.
46 Sagawa M, Oka M, Chaboyer W. The utility of cognitive behavioural therapy on chronic haemodialysis patients' fluid intake: a preliminary examination. Int J Nurs Stud 2003;40(4):367-73.
47 Nozaki C, Oka M, Chaboyer W. The effects of a cognitive behavioural therapy programme for self-care on haemodialysis patients. Int J Nurs Pract 2005;11(5):228-36.
48 Sharp J, Wild MR, Gumley AI, Deighan CJ. A cognitive behavioral group approach to enhance adherence to hemodialysis fluid restrictions: a randomized controlled trial. Am J Kidney Dis 2005;45(6):1046-57.
49 Cukor D, Peterson RA, Cohen SD, Kimmel PL. Depression in end-stage renal disease hemodialysis patients. Nat Clin Pract Nephrol 2006;2(12):678-87.
50 Hanly P. Sleep disorders and end-stage renal disease. Curr Opin Pulm Med 2008;14(6):543-50.
51 Chen HY, Chiang CK, Wang HH, et. al. Cognitive-behavioral therapy for sleep disturbance in patients undergoing peritoneal dialysis: a pilot randomized controlled trial. Am J Kidney Dis 2008;52:314-23.
51 Mason J, Khunti K, Stone M, et. al. Educational interventions in kidney disease care: a systematic review of randomized trials. Am J Kidney Dis 2008;51(6):933-51.
52 Pomeroy J, Soderberg AM, Franks PW. Gene-Lifestyle Interactions and Their Consequences on Human Health. Med Sport Sci 2009;54:110-135.
54 Fuhrmann I, Krause R. Principles of exercising in patients with chronic kidney disease, on dialysis and for kidney transplant recipients. Clin Nephrol 2004;61 Suppl 1:S14-25.
55 Fassett RG, Robertson IK, Geraghty, DP, et. al. Physical Activity Levels in Chronic Kidney Disease Patients Entering the LORD Trial. Medicine and Science in Sports and Exercise 2009;41:985-991.
56 U.S. Renal Data System. U.S. Renal Data System, USRDS 2007 Annual Data Report: Atlas of End-Stage Renal Disease in the United States, National Institutes of Health, National Institute of Diabetes and Digestive and Kidney Diseases. Bethesda, MD, 2007.
57 Deligiannis A, Kouidi E, Tassoulas E, et. al. Cardiac effects of exercise rehabilitation in hemodialysis patients. Int J Cardiol 1999;70(3):253-66.
58 Konstantinidou E, Koukouvou G, Kouidi E, et. al. Exercise training in patients with end-stage renal disease on hemodialysis:comparison of three rehabilitation programs. J Rehabil Med 2002;34(1):40-5.
59 Kouidi E, Grekas D, Deligiannis A, Tourkantonis A. Outcomes of long-term exercise training in dialysis patients: comparison of two training programs. Clin Nephrol 2004;61 Suppl 1:S31-8.
60 Karamouzis I, Grekas D, Karamouzis M, Kallaras K, et. al. Physical training in patients on hemodialysis has a beneficial effect on the levels of eicosanoid hormone-like substances. Hormones (Athens) 2009;8(2):129-37.
61 Majchrzak KM, Pupim LB, Sundell M, Ikizler TA. Body composition and physical activity in end-stage renal disease. J Ren Nutr 2007;17(3):196-204.
62 Segura-Orti E, Kouidi E, Lison JF. Effect of resistance exercise during hemodialysis on physical function andquality of life: randomized controlled trial. Clin Nephrol 2009;71(5):527-37.
63 Cheema BS. Review article: Tackling the survival issue in end-stage renal disease: time to get physical on haemodialysis. Nephrology 2008;13:560-9.
64 DePaul V, Moreland J, Eager T, Clase CM. The effectiveness of aerobic and muscle strength training in patients receiving hemodialysis and EPO: a randomized controlled trial. Am J Kidney Dis 2002;40(6):1219-29.
65 Moinuddin I, Leehey DJ. A comparison of aerobic exercise and resistance training in patients with and without chronic kidney disease. Adv Chronic Kidney Dis 2008;15(1):83-96.
66 Reisin E, Jack AV. Obesity and hypertension: mechanisms, cardio-renal consequences, and therapeutic approaches. Med Clin North Am. 2009;93(3):733-51.
67 Curtis BM, O'Keefe JH Jr. Understanding the Mediterranean diet. Could this be the new 'gold standard' for heart disease prevention? Postgrad Med 2002;112:35-38.
68 Barbagallo CM, Cefalù AB, Gallo S, et. al. Effects of Mediterranean diet on lipid levels and cardiovascular risk in renal transplant recipients. Nephron. 1999;82(3):199-204.
69 Stachowska E, Gutowska I, Strzelczak A, et. al. The use of neural networks in evaluation of the direction and dynamics of changes in lipid parameters in kidney transplant patients on the Mediterranean diet. J Ren Nutr 2006;16(2):150-9.
70 Ozdemir FN, Akçay A, Elsurer R, et. al. Interdialytic weight gain is less with the Mediterranean type of diet in hemodialysis patients. J Ren Nutr 2005;15(4):371-6.
71 Esposito K, Maiorino MI, Ciotola M, et. al. Effects of a Mediterranean-style diet on the need for antihyperglycemic drug therapy in patients with newly diagnosed type 2 diabetes. Ann Intern Med 2009;151:306-314.
72 Obligado SH, Goldfarb DS. The association of nephrolithiasis with hypertension and obesity: a review. Am J Hypertens 2008;21(3):257-64.
73 Taylor EN, Fung TT, Curhan GC. DASH-Style Diet Associates with Reduced Risk for Kidney Stones. J Am Soc Nephrol. 2009 Aug 13. (Epub ahead of print)
74 Jacobs DR Jr, Gross MD, Steffen L, et. al. The effects of dietary patterns on urinary albumin excretion: results of the Dietary Approaches to Stop Hypertension (DASH) Trial. Am J Kidney Dis 2009;53(4):638-46.
75 Fouque D, Laville M. Low protein diets for chronic kidney disease in non diabetic adults. Cochrane Database Syst Rev 2009 Jul 8;(3):CD001892.
76 Chaturvedi S, Jones C. Protein restriction for children with chronic renal failure. Cochrane Database Syst Rev 2007 Oct 17;(4):CD006863.
77 Bellizzi V, Di Iorio BR, De Nicola L, et. al. Very low protein diet supplemented with ketoanalogs improves blood pressure control in chronic kidney disease. Kidney Int 2007;71(3):245-51.
78 Lee JE, Spiegelman D, Hunter DJ, et. al. Fat, protein, and meat consumption and renal cell cancer risk: a pooled analysis of 13 prospective studies. JNCI 2008;100(23):1695-706.

79 Wingen AM, Fabian-Bach C, Schaefer F, Mehls O: Randomised multicentre study of a low-protein diet on the progression of chronic renal failure in children: European Study Group of Nutritional Treatment of Chronic Renal Failure in Childhood, *Lancet* 1997;349(9059):1117-23.

80 Khan NA, Hemmelgarn B, Herman RJ, et al Canadian Hypertension Education Program. The 2009 Canadian Hypertension Education Program recommendations for the management of hypertension: Part 2-therapy. Can J Cardiol 2009;25(5):287-98.

81 Bravi F, Bosetti C, Scotti L,et. al. Food groups and renal cell carcinoma: a case-control study from Italy. Int J Cancer 2007;120(3):681-5.

82 Ramoner R, Rahm A, Gander H, et. al. Serum antibodies against Saccharomyces cerevisiae: a new prognostic indicator in metastatic renal-cell carcinoma. Cancer Immunol Immunother 2008;57(8):1207-14.

83 Coe FL, Parks JH, Asplin JR: The pathogenesis and treatment of kidney stones. NEJM 1992;327: 1141-1152.

84 Hiatt RA, Ettinger B, Caan B, et. al. Randomized controlled trial of a low animal protein, high fibre diet in the prevention of recurrent calcium oxalate kidney stones. Am J Epidemiol 1996;144(1): 25-33.

85 Taylor EN, Curhan GC. Oxalate intake and the risk for nephrolithiasis. J Am Soc Nephrol 2007;18(7):2198-204.

86 Oxalic Acid and Food. Online Available: www.oxalicacidinfo.com (accessed 3 september 2010).

87 Fink HA, Akornor JW, Garimella PS, Diet, Fluid, or Supplements for Secondary Prevention of Nephrolithiasis: A Systematic Review and Meta-Analysis of Randomized Trials. Eur Urol 2009 Mar 13. (Epub ahead of print)

88 Taylor EN, Curhan GC. Fructose consumption and the risk of kidney stones. Kidney Int 2008;73(2): 207-12.

89 Stoller ML, Chi T, Eisner BH, et. al. Changes in urinary stone risk factors in hypocitraturic calcium oxalate stone formers treated with dietary sodium supplementation. J Urol 2009;181(3): 1140-4.

90 D'Amico G, Gentile MG, Manna G, et al: Effect of vegetarian soy diet on hyperlipidaemia in nephritic syndrome. Lancet 1992;339(8802):1131-34.

91 Azadbakht L, Shakerhosseini R, Atabak S, et. al. Beneficiary effect of dietary soy protein on lowering plasma levels of lipid and improving kidney function in type II diabetes with nephropathy. Eur J Clin Nutr 2003;57(10):1292-4.

92 Teixeira SR, Tappenden KA, Carson L, et. al. Isolated soy protein consumption reduces urinary albumin excretion and improves the serum lipid profile in men with type 2 diabetes mellitus and nephropathy. J Nutr 2004;134(8):1874-80.

93 Anderson JW. Beneficial effects of soy protein consumption for renal function. Asia Pac J Clin Nutr 2008;17 Suppl 1:324-8.

94 Weikert S, Boeing H, Pischon T, et. al. Fruits and vegetables and renal cell carcinoma: findings from the European prospective investigation into cancer and nutrition (EPIC). Int J Cancer 2006;118(12):3133-9.

95 Vamvakas S, Teschner M, Bahner U, Heidland A. Alcohol abuse: potential role in electrolyte disturbances and kidney diseases. Clin Nephrol 1998;49(4):205-13.

96 Schaeffner ES, Kurth T, de Jong PE, et. al. Alcohol consumption and the risk of renal dysfunction in apparently healthy men. Arch Intern Med 2005;165(9):1048-53.

97 Presti RL, Carollo C, Caimi G. Wine consumption and renal diseases: new perspectives. Nutrition 2007;23(7-8):598-602.

98 Water consumption and chronic kidney disease. Australian and New Zealand Society of Nephrology Proceedings 2005. Reported in Australian Doctor 9th September 2005.

99 Massey LK, Wise KJ: The effect of dietary caffeine on urinary excretion of calcium, magnesium, sodium and potassium in healthy young females. Nutr Res 1984;4:43-50.

100 Armstrong LE. Caffeine, body fluid-electrolyte balance, and exercise performance. Int J Sport Nutr Exerc Metab 2002;12(2):189-206.

101 Bolignano D, Coppolino G, Barillà A, et. al. Caffeine and the kidney: what evidence right now? J Ren Nutr 2007;17(4):225-34.

102 Massey LK, Sutton RA. Acute caffeine effects on urine composition and calcium kidney stone risk in calcium stone formers. J Urol 2004;172(2):555-558.

103 Bergman EA, Massey LK, Wise KJ, Sherrard DJ. Effects of dietary caffeine on renal handling of minerals in adult women. Life Sci 1990;47(6): 557-564.

104 Perazella MA: Pharmacologic options available to treat symptomatic intradialytic hypotension. Am J Kidney Dis 2001;38:S26-S36.

105 Sulowicz W, Radziszewski A: Pathogenesis and treatment of dialysis hypotension. Kidney Int Suppl (104):S36-S39, 2006

106 Gigli GL, Adorati M, Dolso P, et al: Restless legs syndrome in end-stage renal disease. Sleep Med 2004;5(3):309-315.

107 Lui SL, Ng F, Lo WK: Factors associated with sleep disorders in Chinese patients on continuous ambulatory peritoneal dialysis. Perit Dial Int 2002;22(6):677-682.

108 Lagrue G, Laurent J, Rostoker G. Food allergy and idiopathic nephrotic syndrome. Kidney Int Suppl 1989;27:S147-51.

109 Laurent J, Wierzbicki N, Rostoker G, et. al. (Idiopathic nephrotic syndrome and food hypersensitivity. Value of an exclusion diet) Arch Fr Pediatr 1988;45(10):815-9.

110 Patel TV, Singh AK. Role of vitamin D in chronic kidney disease. Semin Nephrol 2009;29:113-21.

111 Bennett-Richards K, Kattenhorn M, Donald A, et al: Does oral folic acid lower total homocysteine levels and improve endothelial function in children with chronic renal failure? Circulation 2002;105(15):1810-15.

112 Palmer SC, McGregor DO, Strippoli GF. Interventions for preventing bone disease in kidney transplant recipients. Cochrane Database Syst Rev. 2007 Jul 18;(3):CD005015.

113 Massey LK, Liebman M, Kynast-Gales SA. Ascorbate increases human oxaluria and kidney stone risk. J Nutr 2005;135(7):1673-7.

114 Chai W, Liebman M, Kynast-Gales S, Massey L. Oxalate absorption and endogenous oxalate synthesis from ascorbate in calcium oxalate stone formers and non-stone formers. Am J Kidney Dis 2004;44(6):1060-9.

115 Moyad MA, Combs MA, Crowley DC, et. al. Vitamin C with metabolites reduce oxalate levels compared to ascorbic acid: a preliminary and novel clinical urologic finding. Urol Nurs 2009;29:95-102.

116 Nanayakkara PW, Kiefte-de Jong JC, et. al. Randomized placebo-controlled trial assessing a treatment strategy consisting of pravastatin, vitamin E, and homocysteine lowering on plasma asymmetricdimethylarginine concentration in mild to moderate CKD. Am J Kidney Dis 2009;53:41-50.
117 Castilla P, Dávalos A, Teruel JL, et. al. Comparative effects of dietary supplementation with red grape juice and vitamin E on production of superoxide by circulating neutrophil NADPH oxidase in hemodialysis patients. AJCN 2008;87(4):1053-61.
118 Himmelfarb J, Phinney S, Ikizler TA, et. al. Gamma-tocopherol and docosahexaenoic acid decrease inflammation in dialysis patients. J Ren Nutr 2007;17(5):296-304.
119 Guerrera MP, Volpe SL, Mao JJ. Therapeutic uses of magnesium. Am Fam Physician 2009;80(2):157-62.
120 Musso CG. Magnesium metabolism in health and disease. Int Urol Nephrol. 2009;41(2):357-62.
121 Navarro-Gonzalez JF, Mora-Fernandez C, Garcia-Perez J. Clinical implications of disordered magnesium homeostasis in chronic renal failure and dialysis. Semin Dial 2009;22(1):37-44.
122 Tzanakis IP, Oreopoulos DG. Beneficial effects of magnesium in chronic renal failure: a foe no longer. Int Urol Nephrol 2009;41(2):363-71.
123 Turgut F, Kanbay M, Metin MR, et. al. Magnesium supplementation helps to improve carotid intima media thickness in patients on hemodialysis. Int Urol Nephrol 2008;40(4):1075-82.
124 Spiegel DM, Farmer B, Smits G, Chonchol M. Magnesium carbonate is an effective phosphate binder for chronic hemodialysis patients: a pilot study. J Ren Nutr 2007;17(6):416-22.
125 Tzanakis IP, Papadaki AN, Wei M, et. al. Magnesium carbonate for phosphate control in patients on hemodialysis. A randomized controlled trial. Int Urol Nephrol 2008;40(1):193-201.
126 Taylor EN, Stampfer MJ, Curhan GC. Dietary factors and the risk of incident kidney stones in men: new insights after 14 years of follow-up. J Am Soc Nephrol 2004;15(12):3225-32.
127 Zerwekh JE, Odvina CV, Wuermser LA, Pak CY. Reduction of renal stone risk by potassium-magnesium citrate during 5 weeks of bed rest. J Urol 2007;177(6):2179-84.
128 Bennett-Richards KJ, Kattenhorn M, Donald AE, et. al. Oral L-arginine does not improve endothelial dysfunction in children with chronic renal failure, Kidney Int 2002;62(4):1372-78.
129 Donadio JV, Grande JP. The role of fish oil/omega-3 fatty acids in the treatment of IgA nephropathy. Semin Nephrol 2004;24(3):225-43.
130 Sulikowska B, Niewęgłowski T, Manitius J, et. al. Effect of 12-month therapy with omega-3 polyunsaturated acids on glomerular filtration response to dopamine in IgA nephropathy. Am J Nephrol 2004;24(5):474-82.
131 Dillon JJ. Fish oil therapy for IgA nephropathy: Efficacy and interstudy variability. J Am Soc Nephrol 1997;8(11):1739-44.
132 Donadio JV, Bergstralh EJ, Offord KP, et. al. A controlled trial of fish oil in IgA nephropathy. NEJM 1994;331(18):1194-99.
133 Donadio JV, Grande JP, Bergstralh EJ, et. al. The long-term outcome of patients with IgA nephropathy treated with fish oil in a controlled trial. J Am Soc Nephrol 1999;10(8):1772-77.
134 Donadio JV, Larson TS, Bergstralh EJ, Grande JP: A randomized trial of high-dose compared with low-dose omega-3 fatty acids in severe IgA nephropathy. J Am Soc Nephrol 2001;12:791-99.
135 Alexopoulos E, Stangou M, Pantzaki A, et. al. Treatment of severe IgA nephropathy with omega-3 fatty acids: The effect of a 'very low dose' regimen, Ren Fail 2004;26(4):453-59.
136 Hogg RJ, Fitzgibbons L, Atkins C, et. al. Efficacy of omega-3 fatty acids in children and adults with IgA nephropathy is dosage- and size-dependent. Clin J Am Soc Nephrol 2006;1(6):1167-72.
137 Miller ER 3rd, Juraschek SP, Appel LJ, et. al. The effect of n-3 long-chain polyunsaturated fatty acid supplementation on urine protein excretion and kidney function: meta-analysis of clinical trials. AJCN 2009;89(6):1937-45.
138 Ferraro PM, Ferraccioli GF, Gambaro G, et. al. Combined treatment with renin-angiotensin system blockers and polyunsaturated fatty acids in proteinuric IgA nephropathy: a randomized controlled trial. Nephrol Dial Transplant 2009;24(1):156-60.
139 http://www.nrv.gov.au/nutrients/fat.htm (Accessed August 2009)
140 Campieri C, Campieri M, Bertuzzi V, et al: Reduction of oxaluria after an oral course of lactic acid bacteria at high concentration. Kidney Int 2001;60(3):1097-105.
141 Tracy CR, Pearle MS. Update on the medical management of stone disease. Curr Opin Urol 2009;19(2):200-4.
142 Guay DR. Cranberry and urinary tract infections. Drugs 2009;69(7):775-807.
143 Minocha A. Probiotics for preventive health. Nutr Clin Pract 2009;24(2):227-41.
144 Reid G, Bruce AW, Taylor M. Influence of three day antimicrobial therapy and Lactobacillus vaginal suppositories on recurrence of urinary tract infections. Clin Ther 1992;14:11-16.
145 Reid G, Bruce AW, Taylor M. Instillation of Lactobacillus and stimulation of indigenous organisms to prevent recurrence of urinary tract infections. Microecol Ther 1995;23:32-45.
146 Uehara S, Monden K, Nomoto K, et. al. A pilot study evaluating the safety and effectiveness of Lactobacillus vaginal suppositories in patients with recurrent urinary tract infection. Int J Antimicrob Agents 2006;28:S30-S34.
147 Baerheim A, Larsen E, Digranes A. Vaginal application of Lactobacilli in the prophylaxis of recurrent lower urinary tract infection in women. Scand J Prim Health Care 1994;12:239-243.
148 Czaja CA, Stapleton AE, Yarova-Yarovaya Y, Stamm WE. Phase I trial of a Lactobacillus crispatus vaginal suppository for prevention of recurrent urinary tract infection in women. Infect Dis Obstet Gynecol 2007;2007:35387.
149 Reid G, Bruce AW, Fraser N, et. al. Oral probiotics can resolve urogenital infections. FEMS Immunol Med Microbiol 2001;30:49-52.
150 Dani C, Biadaioli R, Bertini G, et. al. Probiotics feeding in prevention of urinary tract infection, bacterial sepsis and necrotizing enterocolitis in preterm infants. A prospective double-blind study. Biol Neonate 2002;82:103-108.
151 Gerasimov SV. Probiotic prophylaxis in pediatric recurrent urinary tract infections. Clin Pediatr (Phila) 2004;43:95-98.

152 Falagas ME, Betsi GI, Tokas T, Athanasiou S. Probiotics for prevention of recurrent urinary tract infections in women: a review of the evidence from microbiological and clinical studies. Drugs 2006;66(9):1253-61.
153 Barrons R, Tassone D. Use of Lactobacillus probiotics for bacterial genitourinary infections in women: a review. Clin Ther 2008;30: 453-468.
154 Abad CL, Safdar N. The role of lactobacillus probiotics in the treatment or prevention of urogenital infections--a systematic review. J Chemother 2009;21(3):243-52.
155 Scazzocchio F, Cometa MF, Tomassini L, Palmery M. Antibacterial activity of *Hydrastis Canadensis* extract and its major isolated alkaloids. Planta Med 2001;67:561-564.
156 Jepson RG, Craig JC. Cranberries for preventing urinary tract infections. Cochrane Database Syst Rev 2008;1:CD001321.
157 Guay DR. Cranberry and urinary tract infections. Drugs 2009;69(7):775-807.
158 Williams G, Craig JC. Prevention of recurrent urinary tract infection in children. Curr Opin Infect Dis 2009;22(1):72-6.
159 Touwaide A, De Santo NG, Aliotta G. The origins of Western herbal medicines for kidney diseases. Adv Chronic Kidney Dis 2005;12(3): 251-60.
160 Li RH, Peng ZP, Wei YL, Liu CH. Clinical observation on Chinese medicinal herbs combined with prednisone for reducing the risks of infection in children with nephrotic syndrome. Information J Chinese Medicine 2000;7(10):60-61.
161 Liu XY. Therapeutic effect of chai-ling-tang (sairei-to) on the steroid-dependent nephrotic syndrome in children. Am J Chin Med 1995;23(3/4):255-60.
162 Wang YP, Liu AM, Dai YW, Yang C, Tang HF. The treatment of relapsing primary nephrotic syndrome in children, J Zhejiang University Science 2005;6(7):682-85.
163 Fan J, Liu L, Li Z, Su B, Guan J. A meta-analysis of Radix Astragali for primary nephrotic syndrome in adults. Zhong yao xin yao yu lin chuang yao li 2003;14:62-66.
164 Li Z, Qing P, Ji L, su B, He L, Fan J. Systematic review of rhubarb for chronic renal failure. Chin J Evid-Based Med 2004;4:468-73.
165 Wojcikowski K, Johnson DW, Gobe G. Herbs or natural substances as complementary therapies for chronic kidney disease: ideas for future studies. J Lab Clin Med 2006;147(4):160-6.
166 Zhang M, Zhang D, Zhang W, Liu S: Treatment of chronic renal failure by supplementing the kidney and invigorating blood flow J Tradit Chin Med 2004;24(4):247-51.
167 Zhu PJ, Zhou X, Wei XJ. (Effect of boayuan qiangshen II tablet on plasma and urine superoxide dismutase and malondialdehyde in patients with chronic renal failure) Zhongguo Zhong Xi Yi Jie He Za Zhi 1997;17(11):649-52.
168 Zhu P, Wei X, Zhao W. (Effect of Baoyuan Qiangshen capsule no. II on tubular interstitial injury in chronic renal failure patients) Zhongguo Zhong Xi Yi Jie He Za Zhi 1999;19(12):721-4.
169 Kosar A, Ozturk A, Serel TA, Akkus S, Unal OS: Effect of vibration massage therapy after extracorporeal shockwave lithotripsy in patients with lower caliceal stones, J Endourol 1999;13(10):705-07.
170 Taylor-Piliae RE, Haskell WL, et. al. Improvement in balance, strength, and flexibility after 12 weeks of Tai chi exercise in ethnic Chinese adults with cardiovascular disease risk factors. Altern Ther Health Med 2006;12(2):50-8.
171 Yeh GY, Wang C, Wayne PM, Phillips RS. The effect of tai chi exercise on blood pressure: a systematic review. Prev Cardiol 2008 Spring;11:82-9.
172 Mustata S, Cooper L, Langrick N, et. al. The effect of a Tai Chi exercise program on quality of life in patients on peritoneal dialysis: a pilot study. Perit Dial Int 2005;25(3):291-4.
173 Garcia GE, Ma SX, Feng L. Acupuncture and kidney disease. Adv Chronic Kidney Dis 2005;12(3):282-91.
174 Song YH. (Observation on therapeutic effects of combined acupuncture and medicine therapy and simple medication on renal hypertension of chronic kidney disease) Zhongguo Zhen Jiu 2007;27(9):641-4.
175 Zhang ZL, Ji XQ, Zhang P, Zhang XH, Meng ZJ, Yang XJ. (Randomized and controlled study on needling method of harmonizing spleen-stomach for early intervention of diabetic nephropathies and the mechanism of protecting kidney). Zhongguo Zhen Jiu 2007;27(12):875-80.
176 Lin Q, Hu YL, Han CW, Li Y. (Eye acupuncture for treatment of renal and ureteral colic). Zhongguo Zhen Jiu 2007;27(9):663-4.
177 Chu Q, Wang L, Liu GZ. (Effect of acupuncture on hemorheology in patients with diabetic nephropathy). Zhen Ci Yan Jiu 2007;32(5):335-7.
178 Tian FS, Yang WG, Song HL, et. al. (Randomized controlled study on acupuncture for treatment of diabetic paralytic squint). Zhongguo Zhen Jiu 2008;28(2):84-6.
179 Wan RJ, Li YH. (Survey of acupuncture and moxibustion for clinical treatment of renal diseases). Zhongguo Zhen Jiu 2009;29(4):342-4.
180 Lee YH, Lee WC, Chen MT, et. al. Acupuncture in the treatment of renal colic. J Urol 1992;147: 16-18.
181 Gao H, Zhang W, Wang Y. Acupuncture treatment for 34 cases of uremic cutaneous pruritus, J Tradit Chin Med 2002;22(1):29-30.
182 Jedras M, Bataa O, Gellert R, et. al. Acupressure in the treatment of uremic pruritus. Dial Transplant 2003;32(1):8-10.
183 Tsay SL, Rong JR, Lin PF. Acupoints massage in improving the quality of sleep and quality of life in patients with end-stage renal disease. J Adv Nurs 2003;42(2):134-42.
184 Cho YC, Tsay SL. The effect of acupressure with massage on fatigue and depression in patients with end-stage renal disease. J Nurs Res 2004;12(1): 51-59.
185 Ro YJ, Ha HC, Kim CG, Yeom HA. The effects of aromatherapy on pruritus in patients undergoing hemodialysis. Dermatol Nurs 2002;14(4):231-34.
186 Cavalcanti AM, Rocha LM, Carillo R Jr, et. al. Effects of homeopathic treatment on pruritus of haemodialysis patients: A randomised placebo-controlled double-blind trial. Homeopathy 2003;92(4):177-81.
187 Spiegel BM, Melmed G, Robbins S, Esrailian E. Biomarkers and health-related quality of life in end-stage renal disease: a systematic review. Clin J Am Soc Nephrol 2008;3(6):1759-68.

Chapter 36

Rheumatoid arthritis

With contribution from Greg de Jong

Introduction

Affecting between 0.5–1.% of the population, rheumatoid arthritis is an autoimmune disorder that progressively destroys articular joint function through excessive inflammation of synovial tissue and other local structures.[1] This process can be rapid enough that when left untreated 20–30% of people can be seriously afflicted such that they become permanently work disabled as a result of the disease process within 2 years.[2] However widespread systemic influences are also prevalent, so much so that mortality amongst rheumatoid arthritis sufferers is 1.5–1.6 times greater than the general population.[3]

Traditionally, diagnosis of rheumatoid arthritis is based on the American Rheumatism Association criteria which states that 4 of the following 7 criteria should be met:

1 morning stiffness in and around the joints lasting at least 1 hour before maximal improvement
2 three joint areas with simultaneous swelling out of 14 possible areas (proximal inter-phalangeal [PIP] joint, metacarpal-phalangeal [MCP] joint, wrist, elbow, knee, ankle, and metatarsal phalangeal [MTP] joint; right or left)
4 arthritis of hand joints (PIP, MCP, wrist)
5 presence of rheumatoid nodules
6 positive serum rheumatoid factor
7 radiographic changes consistent with rheumatoid arthritis in posterior hand and/or wrist (must include erosion or bone decalcification localised in or adjacent to involved joint — not simply osteoarthritic changes).[4]

Early identification of rheumatoid arthritis is considered critical as prompt intervention provides a window of opportunity to limit progressive damage from the disease process.[5] Significantly one-third of patients with rheumatoid arthritis already have bone and joint damage prior to diagnosis and it has been identified that a delay in initiating treatment, (with Disease Modifying Anti-Rheumatic Drugs DMAR), of as little as 3 months can have significant impact on the amount of observable X-ray damage identified 5 years later.[6] (Examples of DMAR: Methotrexate, leflunomide, sulfasalazin, gold, hydroxychloroquinine, etanercept, inflixima, adalimumab.) This has led to growing interest in the use of anti-cyclic citrullinated protein antibody markers as an indication of the early presence and, potentially, a prediction of the development of rheumatoid arthritis amongst both healthy people and those with undifferentiated arthritis.[7, 8] Disease progression indicators include early low functional scores, low economic status, early multiple joint involvement, high erythrocyte sedimentation rates, high C-reactive protein measures, early X-ray changes and/or a positive rheumatoid factor.[2]

Individuals with rheumatoid arthritis commonly use complementary and alternative medicines (CAM). Reasons given include: the inadequacy of conventional treatment to meet the needs of the patient (disease remission, decrease pain, return of function and so on); concern regarding side-effects; a desire to reduce the stress of a disease; patients consider CAM as safer and 'natural'; and/or that they have been influenced by advertising claims.[9] Interestingly, a US study identified that the likelihood of using CAM therapies for a number of musculoskeletal conditions including rheumatoid arthritis increased with the degree of scepticism of the user of mainstream medical approaches.[10]

Noting this, and given the asserted importance of early treatment for rheumatoid arthritis (with DMAR drugs) in order to reduce the long-term effects of the disease process, it is therefore important that a balance of evidence-based information is provided to the patient, both for CAM and mainstream medicine, if the individual is to achieve an optimal integrative approach to therapy.

Lifestyle factors

Genes

Genetic factors are estimated to comprise 50–60% of the incidence of rheumatoid arthritis.[1] Growing evidence suggests an interactive link between genetic susceptibility (e.g. HLA-DR genetic profile) and environmental triggers (e.g. smoking) that lead to the eventual immunological assault of the disease.[11, 12]

Smoking

The immune system is influenced by smoking on many levels — the induction of an inflammatory response, suppression of immune responses, cytokine imbalance, induction of apoptosis and the formation of anti-DNA antibodies as a result of DNA damage.[13] Unsurprisingly therefore, a strong association is present between tobacco use and extra-articular manifestations of rheumatoid arthritis, including cardiovascular events, although not to the extent of radiographic changes.[14]

In a subset of rheumatoid arthritis patients the presence of an HLA-DR shared epitone gene also interacts with smoking leading to immune system dysregulation and the formation of autoantibodies to citrullinated peptides significant to the disease process.[11, 12] Significantly this immune system response as a result of gene-smoking interaction may be initiated years before symptomatic presentation of rheumatoid arthritis.[11] Smokers who have the HLA-DR gene are also at higher risk (7.5) of rheumatoid factor seropositive rheumatoid arthritis than non–smokers with the gene (2.8), or smokers without the gene (2.4) as compared with non-smokers/no gene (1.0).[15]

It has therefore been suggested that smoking cessation counselling should be mandatory for all rheumatoid arthritis patients and their relatives.[16]

Nutritional influences

Diets

A review of dietary factors considered to diminish the risks of rheumatoid arthritis indicate that foods high in olive oil, oil-rich fish, fruit, vegetables and betacryptoxanthins (found in red fruit and vegetables) were protective for rheumatoid arthritis.[17, 18] A review of trials on red meat, coffee and alcohol demonstrated mixed results and no firm conclusions could be made as to their influence on rheumatoid arthritis.[17] However, these conclusions differ to a further study of diet and risk which indicated that although consumption of high-fat fish (> or = 8g of fat/100g fish) appear to provide a risk reduction, medium-fat fish (3–7g/100g fish) was actually associated with increased risk of rheumatoid arthritis. A prospective study by the Mayo Clinic suggested that cauliflower, broccoli and other cruciferous vegetables and fruit were protective of rheumatoid arthritis.[19] However, a further study indicated that fruit, coffee, olive oil and meat intake showed no association with rheumatoid arthritis risk reduction, nor did intake of vitamins A, E, C, D, zinc, selenium or iron.[20] A review of studies into the relationship between obesity and rheumatoid arthritis presently suggests obesity may lead to less changes on radiography and better survival rates, although this needs to be confirmed.[21] Hence, the implications of diet on the risk of rheumatoid arthritis is, presently, contradictory.

Vegetarian and vegan diets have been advocated for rheumatoid arthritis patients. A 13-month trial in which a period of fasting was followed by a vegetarian diet indicated that pain diminished but physical function and morning stiffness did not change in the active group.[22] A vegan diet free of gluten provided benefit for 40.5% of the active group who completed 1 year of the diet plan. Notably, however, only 25 of 38 patients in the active vegan group were able to comply with 9 months or more of the program, suggesting compliance is a problem.[23]

Studies of Mediterranean (Cretan) diets, suggests they may be of benefit in reducing the pain of rheumatoid arthritis when committed to over a 12-week period.[24, 25] A UK pilot study trialled a pragmatic approach to the Mediterranean diet by providing community-based intervention that included hands-on cooking classes. As a result a change in dietary patterns was noticed with an increase in fruit, vegetable and legume consumption and improvements in monounsaturated: polyunsaturated fats ratios. Significant improvements were observed for pain and morning stiffness scores at 6 months.[25]

Studies of food allergies and/or intolerances suggest the possibility of an involvement in rheumatoid arthritis. Rheumatoid arthritis patients have been found to have increased immunoglobulin M (IgM) activity to cow's milk (alpha-lactalbumin, casein), cereals, hen's eggs (ovalbumin), cod fish and pork meat within their intestinal fluid.[26] It was postulated that such activity amongst other examples of cross-reactive food antibodies may ultimately lead to autoimmune responses in the joint via hypersensitivity reactions to circulating immune complexes.[26] Consistent with this, small trials of an elemental diet indicate the potential for improvement in rheumatoid arthritis patients.[27–29]. A review of allergens in 1 trial indicated that grains, milk, beef and eggs were common culprits.[27]

It must be highlighted that a Cochrane review (2009) concluded that the effects of diet remain uncertain due to the nature of the identified trials and the risk of bias. The review raised further concerns that all of the above diets (Mediterranean, fasting, vegan, vegetarian, elemental) risked both non-compliance and weight loss within patient groups and there was the potential for adverse effects as a result.[30]

Sleep

Sleep disturbances appear to be common amongst patients with rheumatoid arthritis. Amongst arthritis sufferers in general 60% of patients experience problems with sleep,[31] including 72% of patients above 55 years of age.[32] The problem also exists amongst children with juvenile rheumatoid arthritis.[33] Despite this sleep difficulties are seldom addressed with rheumatoid arthritis sufferers.[31] Sleep disturbances include longer times to fall asleep, repetitive night waking and early morning waking with subsequent day tiredness and fatigue.[34]

Mind–body medicine

Adjustment to the pain and disability that result from rheumatoid arthritis require psychological and emotional resilience. Capacity to initiate active coping strategies has been identified as critical in maintaining psychological wellbeing.[35, 36] As a result various mind–body medicine approaches have been advocated to aid coping with rheumatoid arthritis.

Cognitive behavioural therapies (CBTs) and education

CBT approaches may provide additional benefit to depressive symptoms in rheumatoid arthritis receiving routine medical management up to 18 months after an 8-week program.[37] However, a study of CBT comparing CBT to a standard education program for newly diagnosed arthritis patients found there was no difference on health status between the 2 approaches over 6 months.[38]

A Cochrane review (2003) indicated that patient education was of small benefit to rheumatoid arthritis in the short term, improving disability, joint count, depression and psychological status, yet there was little evidence that gains were maintained over the long term.[39] However studies continue to mount suggestive of benefits from arthritis education programmes subsequent to this review. Disease specific programs appear to be more valuable than generalised chronic self help programs.[40] Internet[41] and modular delivered behavioural arthritis programs[42] may be viable means of delivering information compared to standardised approaches.

Small studies indicate several mind-body medicines have the potential of influencing aspects of rheumatoid arthritis. Stress management programs decrease pain and psychological functioning by improving self-efficacy, coping strategies and overcoming feelings of helplessness.[43] Brief motivational training by telephone has also been demonstrated to assist in cognitive and emotional coping.[44] Tentative evidence suggests that private verbal or written emotional disclosure may be effective in the intermediate term to maintain psychological functioning, noting in the short term they may cause an increase in emotionality.[45–47]. However, results are mixed, and a further study of private emotional disclosure and, in particular, emotional disclosure in the presence of a clinician, was of no significant benefit.[48]

Meditation and/or relaxation

A study comparing cognitive behavioural therapies, emotional regulation and mindfulness meditation delivered in small group environments identified that rheumatoid arthritis patients who suffered with recurrent depression had greater benefit from meditation in terms of positive and negative effect and physician ratings of joint pain, whereas CBTs provided greater gains in pain control.[49] Positive effects of mindfulness-based stress reduction may be beneficial in aiding psychological distress and wellbeing as compared to controls, however, gains may take up to 6 months to be achieved.[50] The use of Benson's Relaxation Technique has shown benefit in a small study of 8 weeks as compared to controls in reducing anxiety, depression and feelings of wellbeing.[51] These early studies suggest that meditation and/or relaxation may have potential in improving the wellbeing of rheumatoid arthritis patients.

Physical activity/exercise

Comprehensive multidisciplinary approaches to rehabilitation often involve a combination of therapeutic and general exercise, occupational therapy and the use of orthotic splints. Such programs should be introduced as early as possible and concurrent with pharmacological intervention.[52] However, due to a paucity of trials in this area little is known as to the extent of effectiveness other than by inference from evidence for the individual therapies themselves within a program.[53]

Aerobic exercise

A review of reconditioning programs has established that dynamic and aerobic activity individualised to the patient's level of disability is more beneficial than rest in patients with rheumatoid arthritis, and the activities do not aggravate inflammation nor cause joint damage. The goal of such programs should be to avoid functional decline.[54] There is strong evidence from a systematic review suggesting that exercise, whether of low or high intensity, is effective in improving disease and functional Balneotherapy (hydrotherapy and spatherapy) measures in patients with rheumatoid arthritis.[55]

Balneotherapy (hydrotherapy and spatherapy)

Noting that methodological flaws and poor study structure in trials of balneotherapy are prevalent (spa therapy, hydrotherapy), present evidence is suggestive that it is of benefit for the patient with rheumatoid arthritis.[56]

Tai chi

A Cochrane review (2004) of tai chi for rheumatoid arthritis indicated statistically significant benefits were obtained with measures of lower extremity range of motion improving. This form of exercise does not appear to exacerbate symptoms of rheumatoid arthritis, however the review did not identify improvements in most other outcomes of disease activity.[57] While subsequent small trials continue to be suggestive of benefits to pain, fatigue and function scores as compared to no intervention,[58, 59] tai chi does not appear to provide additional benefit when compared to physically active controls or stretching and an exercise program.[60]

Yoga

Evidence for benefit from yoga is minimal. Results from a preliminary trial of 8 (12 sessions) weeks of yoga are suggestive of benefit but longer trials are required.[61] Similarly, a small Indian trial demonstrated potential benefits of yoga for increasing grip strength.[62]

Nutritional supplements

A New Zealand review of micronutrient adequacy of the diets of patients with rheumatoid arthritis demonstrated that only 23% achieved adequate calcium intake (as compared to recommended dietary intake [RDI]), 29% adequate vitamin E, 10% adequate zinc and only 6% adequate selenium.[63] Only 46% reached adequate RDI for folic acid, with a significant reduction noted in the subgroup of patients taking methotrexate. Protein intake and iron were adequate, and unrelated to the presence or absence of anemia.[63] A US dietary review suggested that rheumatoid arthritis patients consumed excess total fat but insufficient polyunsaturated fat and fibre, with inadequacies in pyridoxine, zinc and magnesium compared to the RDI, and copper and folate when compared to the typical American diet.[64]

Omega-3 (fish oils)

High-level evidence now exists for the symptomatic benefit achieved from fish oils and, given the increased risk of cardiovascular events in rheumatoid arthritis patients, they should be recommended to all patients.[65] The anti-inflammatory effects of fish oils result from their influence on eicosanoid pathways leading to less pro-inflammatory cytokines, as well as an inhibition of T-lymphocytes and catabolic enzymes.[66] A meta-analysis of 3–4 months use of fish oils amongst rheumatoid arthritis patients demonstrated reductions in joint pain intensity, morning stiffness, number of painful/tender joints and a reduction in the consumption of non-steroidal anti-inflammatory drugs (NSAIDs).[67] Animal models are also suggestive of the potential for omega-3 oils to slow the disease process and reduce disease severity.[68]

Gamma linoleic acid (omega-6, evening primrose oil, borage)

A Cochrane review (2000) indicated that evidence existed for the potential benefit of gamma linoleic acid (GLA) in the treatment of rheumatoid arthritis with improvements in pain, morning stiffness and joint tenderness noted.[69] Like fish oils, GLA down regulates the pro-inflammatory pathways active in rheumatoid arthritis,[70] however, it is not thought to alter the disease process.[71] Indeed, although patients are often able to reduce or even stop their NSAID with GLA usage,[70] symptoms often return within 3 months once supplementation is ceased.[71] Dosages of up to 2.8g/day have been trialled with success.[71]

Antioxidants

A cohort study of older women examining the relationship between antioxidant and micronutrient intake and the risk of rheumatoid arthritis noted an inverse relationship between intake of vitamin C, vitamin E and betacryptoxanthin (found in red fruit and vegetables) and the presence of rheumatoid arthritis.[72] However, a systematic review of randomised clinical trials (RCTs) relating to the use of antioxidant vitamins (2007) indicated that evidence was lacking as to the benefits of supplementation.[73]

In the abovementioned review, 4 trials of vitamin E suggested that vitamin E was superior to placebo but equivalent to diclofenac in treating rheumatoid arthritis, however, methodology of the trials was weak.[73] However, a large trial of near to 40 000 healthy female patients concluded that there was no evidence that the use of 600IU vitamin E supplementation prevented the development of rheumatoid arthritis during a 10-year follow up as compared to a no supplement control group.[74]

A subsequent trial in 2008 in which a pilot group of rheumatoid patients consumed 20g of an antioxidant rich spread per day (10 weeks) suggested improvements in the number of swollen joints and general health, although no change in laboratory markers was noted.[75]

Vitamin D

It has been established that vitamin D3 has a significant role in the maintenance of immune homeostasis including the regulation of normal immune tolerance to self.[76] This is relevant to rheumatoid arthritis and may explain both latitude and seasonal variations in rheumatoid arthritis activity as a consequence of the essential sunlight–vitamin D interaction.[77] Furthermore, preliminary evidence suggests the potential that a subgroup of rheumatoid arthritis patients may be influenced by the presence of a vitamin D gene polymorphism that contributes to their illness.[78] Vitamin D intake also appears to be inversely proportional to the risk of developing rheumatoid arthritis as established by a Women's Health Study of 29 368 women aged between 55–69 years. In this study the results were significant in regard to total dietary and supplementary intake of vitamin D with both reducing the risk of developing rheumatoid arthritis.[79]

It has therefore been argued that a careful balance must be achieved between the risk of sun exposure and sun neglect in patients as vitamin D deficiency is an important risk factor (e.g. for autoimmune diseases and rheumatoid arthritis) and that vitamin D supplementation should be considered.[80]

Zinc

A review of the risk of developing rheumatoid arthritis established that the use of supplemental zinc has a protective effect.[72] Plasma zinc levels have been found to be low in patients with rheumatoid arthritis and correlate with bio-humoral and clinical markers of the disease.[81] However, there appears to be little present evidence to suggest whether zinc supplementation is of benefit in rheumatoid arthritis or not.

Iron

Iron deficiency appears common amongst patients with rheumatoid arthritis, estimated at 33–60%. A systemic review of anaemia in rheumatoid arthritis suggested patients with anaemia usually had more severe disease and that the treatment of the anaemia assisted in the successful treatment of the overall disease process.[82] It should, however, be noted, that iron is linked to acceleration of reactive oxygen species in the inflammatory process[83] and that a haemochromatosis-linked arthritis exists,[84] such that definitive clinical measures and care need be taken in the use of iron supplements in the patient with rheumatoid arthritis.

Glucosamine

Despite widespread research and usage in osteoarthritis, there are few studies that evaluate the effectiveness of glucosamine specifically upon rheumatoid arthritis. Two small Japanese studies provided conflicting evidence; glucosamine is either effective in providing symptomatic but not anti-rheumatic effects,[85] or it is ineffective (along with chondroitin and quercetin) on all disease parameters of rheumatoid arthritis.[86]

Herbal medicines

An evaluation of the benefits of herbal medicine on rheumatoid arthritis is made difficult by the recommendation of numerous herbs, most with low levels of supportive evidence based on single, often methodologically flawed, trials.[87]

Two trials using 1200mg/day of curcumin both demonstrated improvements in pain, morning stiffness and swelling.[88, 89] Single trials have also suggested that pomegranate extract,[90] garlic,[91] ginger,[92] bromelain,[93] cat's claw,[94] and boswellia[95] may be effective, although confident recommendation requires to be justified by further trials.

A systematic review of Ayurvedic medicinal approaches to rheumatoid arthritis found a paucity of evidence and that existing trials failed to demonstrate any effect.[96]

Several Chinese herbal medicines have been studied for their potential benefit for rheumatoid arthritis patients, however, evidence is generally lacking. The most commonly studied TCM herb, *Tripterygium wilfordli* (thundergod vine), has been demonstrated to have beneficial effects according to a systematic review of randomised trials, however, the authors noted that a risk–benefit analysis suggested that due to concern for serious side-effects (renal, cardiac, haematopoietic and reproductive complications) the herb could not be recommended for use.[97]

Homeopathy

Three small trials comparing the benefit of homeopathy whilst on standard medical care to placebo controls demonstrated no benefit to the active group as compared to controls.[98, 99, 100] On this evidence homeopathy cannot presently be recommended for rheumatoid arthritis.

Physical therapies

Little evidence exists as to the efficacy of massage and manipulation in rheumatoid arthritis, other than a short trial of massage on the juvenile forms of the disease.[101]

Acupuncture

A Cochrane review (2005) identified only 2 low-quality trials of acupuncture in rheumatoid arthritis, 1 of which demonstrated no benefit as compared to sham treatment. The second trial, involving electric stimulation through the needles, was suggestive of benefit for pain about the knee.[102] Two systematic reviews in 2008 provided slightly different interpretations of the data available. While a Korean review concluded that there was presently no evidence to advocate the use of acupuncture,[103] a US review suggested that the evidence was conflicting with some active controlled trials demonstrating favourable results for acupuncture groups, including changes in erythrocyte sedimentation rate (ESR) and C-reactive protein (CRP) measures.[104]

Electrical modalities and/or heat therapy

A series of Cochrane reviews have established the following facts.

- Paraffin wax baths provide benefit for patients with symptoms in the hands including range of motion, pinch grip, pain and stiffness (4 weeks treatment).[105]
- There are no significant effects from heat or ice application.[105]
- Low-level laser therapy may provide short-term benefits, but modality parameters (e.g. wavelength, treatment length etc.) need to be more clearly defined.[106]
- Limited evidence suggests the benefit of sub-aquatic ultrasound to the hands of rheumatoid sufferers.[107]
- Transcutaneous electrical nerve stimulation (TENS) may assist with rheumatoid arthritis but the benefits could relate to the type of TENS used. AL-TENS (i.e. acupuncture-like TENS) may reduce rest pain and increase grip strength, C-TENS (i.e. conventional TENS) may reduce joint tenderness. As results are conflicting, further study is required before definitive comment may be made.[108]
- Weak evidence suggests electrical stimulation may aid pinch strength and muscle endurance.[109]
- Patients prefer to use resting splints, particularly if padded, although no benefit was noted in pain, grip strength or number of swollen joints. The use of extra depth shoes, in particular, when combined with semi-rigid insoles, may provide pain relief.[110]

Conclusion

The use of an integrated approach to the management of rheumatoid arthritis would appear advantageous, particularly where treatments with proven efficacy (fish oils, evening primrose oils) may be used to reduce symptoms and, potentially, reduce the use of medications with side-effects (e.g. non-steroidal anti-inflammatory drugs). However, a note of caution would appear appropriate: given the demonstrated importance of the use of Disease Modifying Anti-Rheumatic Drugs (DMAR) as early as possible to prevent future deterioration, a careful balance between pharmacological and non-pharmacological interventions must be achieved in order that an over-emphasis on CAM in itself is not of detriment to the patient. Therefore, until and unless CAM therapies are proven to have a disease-modifying affect rather than symptoms minimisation alone, they should remain an adjunct to, rather than a replacement for, conventional care. Table 36.1 summarises the evidence for complementary medicine/therapies.

Table 36.1 Levels of evidence for lifestyle and complementary medicines/therapies in the management of rheumatoid arthritis

Modality	Level I	Level II	Level IIIa	Level IIIb	Level IIIc	Level IV	Level V
Lifestyle non-modifiable							
Genes				x			
Lifestyle modifiable							
Smoking					x		
Sleep					x		
Mind–body Medicine							
Cognitive behavioural therapy				x			
Patient education	x						
Mindfulness-based stress reduction				x			
Physical activity/ exercise	x						
Aerobic and/or dynamic activity	x						
Tai chi	x						
Nutritional influences	x						
Mediterranean diet				x			
Vegetarian diet				x			
Nutritional supplements							
Omega-3 fatty acids	x						
Omega-6 fatty acids	x						
Antioxidants (E, C, beta-cryptoxanthin)	x						
Vitamin D				x			
Zinc	x				x		
Iron					x		
Glucosamine					x(-)		
Herbal medicines							
Tripterygium wilfordli	x						
Curcumin				x			
Pomegranate					x		
Garlic					x		
Ginger					x		
Bromelain					x		
Cat's Claw					x		
Boswellia					x		
Ayurvedic medicine	x						
Traditional Chinese medicine	x						

Continued

Table 36.1 Levels of evidence for lifestyle and complementary medicines/therapies in the management of rheumatoid arthritis—cont'd

Modality	Level I	Level II	Level IIIa	Level IIIb	Level IIIc	Level IV	Level V
Homeopathy					x(-)		
Physical therapies (overall)					x		
Acupuncture	x(+/-)						
Electrical modalities and/or heat therapy	x						

Level I — from a systematic review of all relevant randomised controlled trials — meta-analyses.
Level II — from at least 1 properly designed randomised controlled clinical trial.
Level IIIa — from well-designed pseudo-randomised controlled trials (alternate allocation or some other method).
Level IIIb — from comparative studies (including systematic reviews of such studies) with concurrent controls and allocation not randomised, cohort studies, case-control studies, or interrupted time series with a parallel control group.
Level IIIc — from comparative studies with historical control, 2 or more single-arm studies or interrupted time series without a parallel control group.
Level IV — opinions of respected authorities based on clinical experience, descriptive studies or reports of expert committees.
Level V — represents minimal evidence that represents testimonials.

Clinical tips handout for patients — rheumatoid arthritis

1 Lifestyle

Sleep

- Restore normal sleep patterns. Wake with the sun and go to sleep between 9–10p.m.

Sunshine

- Amount of exposure varies with local climate.
- At least 15 minutes of sunshine needed daily for vitamin D and melatonin production — especially before 10 a.m. and after 3 p.m. when the sun exposure is safest during summer; much more exposure in winter when supplementation needs to be considered.
- Ensure gradual adequate skin exposure to sun; avoid sunscreen and excess clothing to maximise levels of vitamin D.
- More time in the sun is required for dark-skinned people.
- Direct exposure to about 10% of body (hands, arms, face), without sunscreen and not through glass.

2 Physical activity/exercise

- Exercise 30–60 minutes daily within the limits of functional disability. If exercise is not regular, commence with 5 minutes at a time and slowly build up increment length towards 30 minutes. Exercising several short manageable sessions per day that total 30 minutes while increasing increment time is also beneficial. Outdoor exercise with nature, fresh air and sunshine is ideal.
- Yoga and tai chi may be helpful approaches as long as postural programs are assessed for risk. Some positions (e.g. inverted postures) may not be appropriate, and indeed dangerous, so monitoring by a qualified instructor is essential.
- Hand exercises in a wax bath or warm water may assist with maintaining hand function.

3 Mind–body medicine

- Stress management programs may be helpful including journaling and/or verbal disclosure of emotions. The use of a counsellor does not appear to provide additional benefit.
- Meditation and/or relaxation, at least 10–20 minutes per day, can be helpful

Education

- Participate in an arthritis self-management program to increase your knowledge of the disease and available coping strategies.

Community

- Actively engage in your community in order to increase your support networks.

Fun

- Enjoy life! Find ways to make life as pleasurable as possible. Seek joy in the simple aspects of life.

4 Environment

- Quit smoking through whatever means are available. Support is often essential as smoking cessation over the long term is a challenge.

5 Dietary changes

- Consider undertaking a food elimination and re-introduction regime, under medical or health practitioner supervision, to establish if you have any food intolerances and/or allergies that affect your rheumatoid arthritis (e.g. grain, milk, beef, eggs). This is preferable to strict long-term elemental, vegan or vegetarian diets as it may not be as limiting once food reintroduction is complete.
- Eat regular balanced healthy meals; ideally 3 main meals and 2 snacks per day, each containing protein.
- Increase fish intake (sardines, tuna, salmon, cod, mackerel), especially deep sea fish. Eat > 3 fish meals per week.
- Two small serves of red meat per week should be consumed to ensure adequate iron levels.
- Consume high quantities of fruit (>2/day) and vegetables (>5/day) (in particular red varieties).
- Use extra virgin cold pressed olive oil and avocado in dressings.
- Cook with garlic, ginger and plenty of fresh herbs and spices (e.g. turmeric).
- Nuts, seeds, bean sprouts (e.g. alfalfa, mung beans, lentils).
- Enjoy dark chocolate.
- Reduce dairy intake but consume full-fat varieties to increase vitamin D intake from fat-soluble sources.
- Drink 1–2 litres of water per day.
- Short-term fasting may be of benefit during symptom exacerbation.
- Avoid hydrogenated fats, salt, fast foods, sugar (such as in soft drinks), lollies, biscuits, cakes and other processed foods (e.g. white breads, white pasta, pastries).

- Moderate coffee and alcohol consumption only; 1–2 serves per day. Assess whether either affect your symptoms.
- Avoid chemical additives — preservatives, colourings, flavourings.
- For sweeteners try honey (e.g. manuka, yellow box and stringy bark).

6 Physical therapies

- Acupuncture may be effective in reducing symptoms of rheumatoid arthritis. Trial on a short term basis for benefit.
- The use of gentle heat may provide symptomatic relief.
- Wax baths may be an effective treatment for arthritis in the hands.
- Therapeutic laser, ultrasound and TENS may be worth a trial for symptomatic relief.
- Foot orthotics and hand splinting may be of benefit.
- Hydrotheraphy and spa baths can help.

7 Supplements

Omega-3 (fish oils)

- Indications: may provide an anti-inflammatory effect and reduce the symptoms of rheumatoid arthritis allowing a reduction in the use of pain killers.
- Dosage: 4–9g/day maximum (depending on dietary intake of fish) during exacerbations or beginning treatment; 2–4/g maintenance dosage.
- Contraindications: care should be taken at higher dosage (> 10g/day) if you have a clotting disorder or are using a blood thinning drug (e.g. Coumadin, warfarin) and you may need to stop fish oils 1–2 weeks prior to surgery.

Evening primrose oil

- Indications: may provide an anti-inflammatory effect and reduce the symptoms of rheumatoid arthritis allowing a reduction in the use of pain killers.
- Dosage: 3g/day.
- Contraindications: care should be taken at higher dosage if you have a clotting disorder or are using a blood thinning drug (e.g. Coumadin). Patients with schizophrenia should take caution due to interactions with some medications. Avoid if you suffer seizures of epilepsy.

Vitamins and minerals

- A broad-based multivitamin with high anti-oxidant value is recommended.

Vitamin D3 (cholecalciferol)

- Indications: recommendation based on clinical tests performed by your doctor.
- Dosage: studies suggest may begin with supplementation up to 50 000IU/week (7500IU/day) until levels normalised, after which 1000IU maintenance dosage.
- Contraindications: some people may be sensitive to vitamin D supplementation.
  - Potentially vitamin D may reduce the effectiveness of calcium channel blockers and therefore need to be used under medical supervision (patients with cardiac conditions).
  - Patients with systemic lupus erythmatosis, hypercalcemia, sarcoidosis, hyperparathyroidism and patients taking digitalis should take care with high doses and, therefore, require medical supervision.

Zinc

- Indications: zinc levels are often low in rheumatoid arthritis patients.
- Dosage: 20–50mg/day.
- Contraindications: needs to be balanced with copper intake (ratio 10:1). Take separate to iron, NSAIDs, coffee, calcium by 2 hours.

Iron

- Indications: supplement if clinically anaemic according to pathology results only (must be established not to have hemochromatosis; approximately 1 in 400).
- Dosage: up to 35mg 1–2/day.
- Contraindications: careful balance may be required as excessive iron may be pro-inflammatory.

Herbal supplements

Curcumin

- Indications: may have an anti-inflammatory affect allowing a reduction in the use of pain killers such as NSAIDs.
- Dosage: 1200mg/day recommended.
- Contraindications: may increase the risk of bleeding in high doses. Contraindicted in cases of bile duct obstruction. May negatively affect chemotherapy in breast cancers so should not be used. Suspend use 1 week prior to major surgery.

Herbs such as garlic, ginger, pomegranate extract, boswellia, bromelain and cat's claw may be of benefit.

References

1 Kobayashi S, Momohara S, Kamatani, et. al. Molecular aspects of rheumatoid arthritis: role of the environment. FEBS J 2008 Sep;275(18):4456–62.
2. Rindfleisch JA, Muller D. Diagnosis and management of rheumatoid arthritis. Am Fam Physician 2005 Sep 15; 17(6):1037–47.
3 Sokka T, Aberson B, Pincus T. Mortality in rheumatoid arthritis: 2008 update. Clin Exp Rheumatol 2008 Sep-Oct;26(5 suppl 51):s35–s61.
4 Arnett FC, Edworthy SM, Bloch DA, et. al. The American Rheumatism Association 1987 revised criteria for the classification of rheumatoid arthritis. Arthritis Rheum 1988;31:315–24.
5 Quinn MA Cox S. The evidence for early intervention Rheum. Dis Clin North America 2005 Nov;31(4):575–89.
6 O'Dell J Drug. Therapy: Therapeutic Strategies for Rheumatoid Arthritis. N Engl J Med 2004;350:2591–602.
7 Mimori T. Clinical significance of anti-CCP antibodies in rheumatoid arthritis. Intern Med 2005 Nov;44(11):1122–6.
8 Avouac J, Gossec L, Dougados M. Diagnostic and predictive value of anti-cyclic citrullinated protein antibodies in rheumatoid arthritis: a systematic review. Ann Rheum Dis 2006 Jul;65(7):845–51.
9 Vitetta L, Cicuttini F, Sali A. Alternative therapies for musculoskeletal conditions. Best Prac Res Clin Rheumatol 2008 Jun;22(3):499–522.
10 Callahan LF, Freburger JK, Mielenz TJ, et. al. Medical scepticism and the use of complementary and alternative care providers by patients followed by rheumatologists. J Clin Rheumatol 2008Jun;14(3):143–7.
11 Klareskog L, Alfredsson L, Rantapaa-Dahlqvist S, et. al. What precedes development of rheumatoid arthritis. Ann Rheum Dis 2004 Nov;63 (Suppl 2): ii28–ii31.
12 Klareskog L, Padyukov L, Lorentzen J, et. al. Mechanisms of disease: Genetic susceptibility and environmental triggers in the development of rheumatoid arthritis. Nat Clin Pract Rheumatol 2006 Aug;2(8):425–33.
13 Harel-Meir M, Sherer Y, Shoenfield Y. Tobacco smoking and autoimmune rheumatic disease. Nat Clin Pract Rheumatol 2007 Dec;3(12):707–15.
14 Vittecoq O, Lequerre T, Goeb V, et. al. Smoking and inflammatory diseases. Best Pract Res Clin Rheumatol 2008 Oct;22(5):923–35.
15 Padyukov L, Silva C, Stolt P, et. al. A gene environment interaction between smoking and shared epitope genes in HLA-Dr provides a high risk of seropositive rheumatoid arthritis. Arthritis Rheum 2004 Oct;50(10):3085–92.
16 Klareskog L, Padyukov L, Alfredsson L. Smoking as a trigger for inflammatory rheumatic disease. Curr Opion Rheumatol 2007 Jan;19(1):49–54.
17 Pattison DJ, Harrison RA, Symmons DP. The role of diet in susceptibility to rheumatoid arthritis: a systematic review. J Rheumatol 2004 Jul;31(7):1310–9.
18 Pattison DJ, Symmons DP, Yound A. Does diet have a role in the aetiology of rheumatoid arthritis. Proc Nutr Soc 2004 Feb;63(1):137–43.
19 Cerhan JR, et. al. Antioxidant micronutrients and risk of rheumatoid arthritis in cohort of older women. Am J Epidemiol 2003;157:345–54.
20 Pedersen M, Stripp C, Klarlund M. Diet and the risk of rheumatoid arthritis in a prospective cohort. J Rheumatol 2005 Jul;32(7):1249–52.
21 Magliano M. Obesity and arthritis. Menopause Int 2008 Dec 14(4):149–54.
22 Muller H, de Toldedo FW, Resch KL. Fasting followed by vegetarian diet in patienst with rheumatoid arthritis. Scand J Rheumatol 2001;30(1):1–10.
23 Hafstrom I, Ringertz B, Spangberg A, et. al. A vegan diet free of gluten improves the signs and symptoms of rheumatoid arthritis: the effects on arthritis correlates with a reduction in antibodies to food allergens. Rheumatology(Oxford) 2001 Oct;40(10):1175–9.
24 Skoldstam L, et. al. An experimental study of a Mediterranean diet for patients with rheumatoid arthritis. Scan J Rheumatol 2003;62:208–14.
25 McKellar G, Morrison E, McEntegart A, et. al. A pilot study of a Mediterranean-type diet intervention in female patients with rheumatoid arthritis living in areas of social deprivation in Glasgow. AnnRheum Dis 2007;66(9):1239–43.
26 Hyatum M, Kanerud L, Hallergren R, et. al. The gut-joint axis: cross reactive food antibodies in rheumatoid arthritis. Gut 2006 Sep;55(9): 1240–7.
27 Hicklin JA, et. al. The effect of diet in rheumatoid arthritis. Clin Allergy 1980;10:463
28 Darlington LR, Ramsay NW. Diets for rheumatoid arthritis. Lancet 1991;338:1209
29 Podas T, Nightingale JM, Oldham R, et. al. Is rheumatoid arthritis a disease that starts in the intestines? A pilot study comparing an elemental diet with oral prednisone. Postgrad Med J 2007 Feb;83(976):128–31.
30 Hagen KB, Byfuglien MGjeitung, Falzon L, et. al. Dietary Interventions for Rheumatoid Arthritis Cochrane Database of Systematic Reviews 2009, Issue 1, Art. No.:CD006400
31 Davis GC. Improved sleep may reduce arthritis pain. Holistic Nurs Prac 2003May-June;17(3):128–35.
32 Abad VC, Sarinas PS, Guilleminault C. Sleep and rheumatologic diseases. Sleep Med Rev 2008 Jun 12(3):211–28.
33 Labyak SE, Bourguignon C, Docherty S. Sleep quality in children with juvenile arthritis. Holistic Nurs Prac 2003 Jul-Aug 17(4):193–200.
34 Bourguignon C, Labyak SE, Taibi D. Investigating sleep in disturbances in adults with rheumatoid arthritis. Holistic Nurs Prac 2003 Sep-Oct, 17(5):241–9.
35 Treharne GY, Lyons AC, Booth DA, et. al. Psychological wellbeing across 1 year with rheumatoid arthritis: coping resources as buffers of perceived stress. Br J Health Psychol 2007 Sep;12 (Pt 3):323–45.
36 Curtis R, Groarke A, Coughlan R, et. al. Psychological stress as a predictor of psychological adjustment in patients with rheumatoid arthritis. Patientt Educ Couns 2005 Nov;59(2):192–8.
37 Sharpe L, Sensky T, Timberlake N, et. al. Long term efficacy of a cognitive behavioural treatment from a randomised controlled trial for patients recently diagnosed with rheumatoid arthritis. Rheumatology 2003;42(3):435–41.
38 Freeman K, Hammond A, Lincoln NB. Use of cognitive behavioural arthritis education programmes in newly diagnosed rheumatoid arthritis. Clin Rehabil 2002 Dec;16(8):828–36.
39 Riemsma RP, Kirwan JR, Taal E, et. al. Patient education for adults with rheumatoid arthritis. Cochrane Database of Systematic Reviews 2003. Issue 2.Art.No.: CD003688

40 Lorig K, Ritter PL, Plant K A. disease specific self-help program compared with a generalised chronic disease self-help program for arthritis patients. Arthritis Rheum 2005 Dec 15;53(6):950–7.
41 Lorig K, Ritter PL, Laurent DD, et. al. The Internet-based arthritis self-management program: a one year randomised trial for patients with arthritis or fibromyalgia. Arthritis Rheum 2008 Jul 15:59(7):1009–17.
42 Hammond A, Bryan J, Hardy A. Effects of a modular behavioural arthritis education programme: a pragmatic parallel group randomised controlled trial. Rheumatology (Oxford) 2008 Nov;47(11):1712–8.
43 Rhee SH, Parker JC, Smarr KL, et. al. Stress Management in rheumatoid arthritis: what is the underlying mechanism? Arth Care Res 200;13(6):435–42.
44 Rau J, Ehlebracht-Konig I, Petermann F. Impact of motivational intervention on coping with chronic pain: results of a controlled efficacy study. Schmertz 2008 Oct;22(5):575–78., 590–5.
45 Wetherell MA, Byrne-Davis L, Dieppe P, et. al. Effects of emotional disclosure on psychological and physiological outcomes in patients with rheumatoid arthritis: an exploratory home-based study. J Health Psych 2005;10(2):277–85.
46 Van Middendorp H, Sorbi MJ, van Doornen LJ, et. al. Feasibility and induced cognitive emotional change of an emotional disclosure intervention adapted for home application. Patient Educ Couns 2007 May;66(2):177–87.
47 Kelley JE, Lumley MA, Leisen JC. Health effects of emotional disclosure in rheumatoid arthritis patients. Health Psychol 1997 Jul;16(4):331–4.
48 Keefe FJ, Anderson T, Lumley M, et. al. A randomized controlled trial of emotional disclosure in rheumatoid arthritis: can clinician assistance enhance the effects? Pain 2008 Jul;137(1):164–72.
49 Zautra AJ, Davis MC, Reich JW, et. al. Comparison of cognitive behavioural and mindfulness meditation interventions on adaptation to rheumatoid arthritis for patients with and without history of recurrent depression. J Consult Clin Psychol 2008 Jun;76(3):408–421.
50 Pradhan EK, Baumgarten M, Langenberg P, et. al. Effect of Mindfulness-Based Stress Reduction in rheumatoid arthritis patients. Arth Rheum 2007;57(7):1134–42.
51 Bagheri-Nesami M, Mohseni-Bandpei MA, Shayesteh-Azar M, et. al. The effect of Benson relaxation Technique on rheumatoid arthritis patients: extended report. Int J Nurs Pract 2006 Aug;12(4):214–9.
52 Arioloi G, Maddali Bongi S, Pappone N. The rehabilitative approach in rheumatoid arthritis. Rheumatismo 2008 Oct-Dec;60(4):242–8.
53 Hammond A. Rehabilitation in rheumatoid arthritis: a critical review. Musculoskeletal Care;2004:2(3):135–51.
54 Mayoux Benhamou MA. Reconditioning in patients with rheumatoid arthritis. Ann Readapt Med Phys 2007 Jul;50(6):382–5, 377–81.
55 Metsios GS, Stavropolou-Kalinpglou A, Veldhuijzen van Zanten JJ. Rheumatoid arthritis, cardiovascular disease and physical exercise: a systematic review. Rheumatology (Oxford) 2008 (Mar);47(3):239–48.
56 Verhagen AP, Bierma-Zeinstra SM, Cardosos JR, et. al. Balneotherapy for rheumatoid arthritis Cochrane Data Base of Systematic Reviews, 2003;(4):CD000518
57 Han A, Robinson V, Judd M, et. al. Tai chi for treating rheumatoid arthritis Cochrane Data Base of Systematic Reviews 2004(3):CD004849
58 Lee KY, Jeong Oy. The effect of Tai Chi movement in patients with rheumatoid arthritis. Taehan Kanho Hakhoe Chi 2006 Apr;36(2):278–85.
59 Wang C. Tai chi improves pain and functional status in adults with rheumatoid arthritis: results of a single-blinded randomised controlled trial. Med Sport Sci 2008;52:218–219.
60 Lee MS, Pittler MH, Ernst E. Tai chi for rheumatoid arthritis: systematic review. Rheumatology (Oxford) 2007 Nov;46(11):1648–51.
61 Badsha H, Cahabra V, Leibman C, et. al. The benefits of yoga for rheumatoid arthritis: results of a preliminary, structured 8 week programme. Rheumatol Int 209 Jan 31. Epub ahead of print.
62 Dash M, Telles S. Improvement in hand grip strength in normal volunteers and rheumatoid arthritis patients following yoga training Indian. J Physiol Pharmacol 2001 Jul;45(3):355–60.
63 Stone J, Doube A, Dudson D, et. al. Inadequate calcium, folic acid, vitamin E, zinc and selenium intake in rheumatoid arthritis patients: results of a dietary survey. Semin Arthritis Rheum 1997 Dec;27(3):180–5.
64 Krener JM, Bigaouette J. Nutrient intake of patients with rheumatoid arthritis is deficient in pyridoxine, zinc, copper and magnesium. J Rheumatol 1996 Jun 23(6):990–4.
65 Proudman SM, Cleland LG, James MJ. Dietary omega-3 fats for treatment of inflammatory joint disease: efficacy and utility. Rheum Dis Clin North Am 2008 May;34(2):469–79.
66 Sales C, Oliviero F, Spinella P. Fish oil supplementation in rheumatoid arthritis. Reumatismo 2008 Jul-Sep;60(3):174–9.
67 Goldberg RJ, Katz J. A meta-analysis of the analgesic effects of omega-3 polyunsaturated fatty acid supplementation for inflammatory joint pain. Pain 2007 May;129(1–2.):210–213.
68 Calder PC. Session 3: Joint Nutrition Society and Irish Nutrition and Dietetic Institute Symposium on Nutrition and autoimmune disease; PUFA, inflammatory processes and rheumatoid arthritis. Proc Nutr Soc 2008 Nov;67(4):409–418.
69 Little CV, Parsons T. Herbal therapy for treating rheumatoid arthritis Cochrane Data Base of Systematic Reviews Issue 4 CD002948
70 Belch JJ, Hill A. Evening Primrose oil and borage oil in rheumatologic conditions. Am J Clin Nutr 71(1) (Suppl) 2000;352–6.S
71 Zurier RB, et. al. Gamma linoleic acid treatment of rheumatoid arthritis: a randomised placebo controlled trial. Arthritis Rheum1996;39(11), 1808–17.
72 Cerhan JR, Saag KG, Merlino LA, et. al. Antioxidant micronutrients and risk of rheumatoid arthritis in a cohort of older women. Am J Epidemiol 2003 Feb 15;157(4):345–54.
73 Canter PH, Wider B, Ernst E. The antioxidant vitamins A,C,E and selenium in the treatment of arthritis: a systematic review of randomised clinical trials. Rheumatology (Oxford):2007 Aug;46(8): 123–33.

74 Karlson EW, Shadick NA, Cook NR, et. al. Vitamin E in the primaty prevention of rheumatoid arthritis: the Women's Health Study. Arthritis Rheum 2008 Nov 15;59(11):1589–95.

75 Van Vught PM, Rijken PJ, Rietveld AG, et. al. Antioxidant intervention in rheumatoid arthritis: results of an open pilot study. Clin Rheumatol 2008 Jun;27(6):771–5.

76 Szodoray P, nakken G, Gaal J. The complex role of vitamin D in autoimmune diseases. Scand J Immunol 2008 Sep;68(3):261–9.

77 Cutolo M, Otsa F, Uprus M. Vitamin D in rheumatoid arthritis. Autoimmun Rev 2007 Nov;7(1):59–64.

78 Rass P, Pakozdi A, Lakatos P. Vitamin D receptor gene polymorphism in rheumatoid arthritis and associated osteoporosis. Rheumatol Int 2006 Sep;26(11):964–71.

79 Merlino LA, Curtis J, Mikuls TR. Vitamin D intake is inversely associated with rheumatoid arthritis: results from the Iowa Women's Health Study. Arthritis Rheum 2004 Jan;50(1):72–7.

80 Holick MF. Sunlight and vitamin D for bone health and prevention of autoimmune diseases, cancer and cardiovascular disease. Am J Clin Nutr 2004 Dec;80(6 Suppl):1678S-88S

81 Milanino R, Frigo A, Bambara Lm, et. al. Copper and zinc status in rheumatoid arthritis: studies of plasma, erythrocytes, and urine, and their relationship to disease activity markers and pharmacological treatment. Clin Exp Rheumatol 1993 May-Jun;11(2):271–81.

82 Wilson A, Yu HT, Goodnough LT, et. al. Prevalence and outcomes of anemia in rheumatoid arthritis: a systematic review of the literature. Am J Med 2004 Apr 5;116(Suppl 7a):50S-57S

83 Morris CJ, Earl JR, Trenam CW. Reactive oxygen specias and iron – a dangerous partnership in inflammation. Int J Biochem Cell Biol 1995 Feb;27(2):109–22.

84 Axford JS. Rheumatic manifestations of haemochromatosis. Baillieres Clin Rheumatol 1991 Aug;5(2):351–65.

85 Nakamura H, Masuko K, Yudoh K, et. al. Effects of glucosamine administration on patients with rheumatoid arthritis. Rheumatol Int 2007 Jan;27(3):213–18.

86 Matsuno H, Nakamura H, Katayama K, et. al. Effects of oral administration of glucosamine-quercetin-glucoside on the synovial fluid properties in patients with osteoarthritis and rheumatoid arthritis. Biosci Biotechnol Biochem 2009 Feb;73(2):288–92.

87 Soeken KL, Miller SA, Ernst E. Herbal medicines for the treatment of rheumatoid arthritis: a systematic review. Rheumatology (Oxford) 2003 May;42(5):652–9.

88 Deodhar SD, Srimal RC. Preliminary study on antirheumatic activity of curcumin (diferuloymethane). Indian J Med Res 1980 71 632–4.

89 Chopra A, et. al. Randomized double blind trial of an ayurvedic plant derived formulation for treatment of rheumatoid arthritis. J Rheumatol 2000 27(6) 1365–72.

90 Shukla M, Gupta K, Rasheed Z. Consumption of hydrolysable tannins-rich promegranate extract suppresses inflammation and joint damage in rheumatoid arthritis. Nutrition 2008 Jul-Aug; 24(7–8.):733–43.

91 Denisov LN, Adrianova IV, Timofeeva SS. Garlic effectiveness in rheumatoid arthritis. Ter Arkh 1999;71(8):55–8.

92 Srivastava KV, Mustafa T. Ginger (Zingiber officinale) in rheumatism and musculoskeletal disorders. Med Hypothesis 1992;39(4):342–8.

93 Cohen A, Goldman J. Bromelain therapy in rheumatoid arthritis. Pennsylvania Med J 1964;67:27–30.

94 Mur E, et. al. Randomised double blind trial of an extract from the penta-cyclic alkaloid-chemotype of uncaria tomentose for the treatment of rheumatoid arthritis. J Rheumatol 2002;27(6):1365–72.

95 Sander O, Herborn G, Rau R. Is H15(Resin extract of Boswellia serrata, "incense") a useful supplement to established drug therapy of chronic polyarthritis? Results of a double blind pilot study. Z Rheumatol 1998 Feb;57(1):11–6.

96 Park J, Ernst E. Ayurvedic medicine for rheumatoid arthritis: a systematic review. Semin Arthritis Rheum 2005 Apr;34(5):705–13.

97 Canter PH, Lee Hs, Ernst E. A systematic review of randomised clinical trials of Tripterygium wilforii for rheumatoid arthritis. Phyomedicine 2006 May;13 (5):371–7.

98 Andrade LE, Ferraz MB, Atra E, et. al. A randomised controlled to evaluate the effectiveness of homeopathy in rheumatoid arthritis. Scand J Rheumatol 1991;20(3):204–208.

99 Gibson RG, Gibson SL, MacNeil AD. Homeopathic therapy in rheumatoid arthritis: evaluation by double blind clinical therapeutic trial. Br J Clin Pharmacol 1980 May;9(5):453–9.

100 Fisher P, Scott Dl. A randomised trial of homeopathy in rheumatoid arthritis. Rheumatology (Oxford) 2001 Sep;40(9):1052–5.

101 Field T, Hernandez-Reif M, Seligman S. Juvenile rheumatoid arthritis: benefits from massage therapy. J Paediatr Psychol 1997 Oct;22(5):607–17.

102 Casimiro L, Barnsley L, Brosseau L, et. al. Acupuncture and electroacupuncture for the treatment of rheumatoid arthritis Cochrane Database of Systematic Reviews 2005 Issue 4 CD003788.

103 Lee MS, Shin BC. Ernst Acupuncture for rheumatoid arthritis: a systematic review. Rheumatology (Oxford) 2008 Dec;47(12):1747–53.

104 Wang C, de Pablo P, Chen X. Acupuncture for pain relief in patients with rheumatoid arthritis: a systematic review. Arthritis Rheum 2008 Sep 15:59(9):1249–56.

105 Welch V, Brosseau L, Cosimiro I, et. al. Thermotherapy for treating rheumatoid arthritis Cochrane Database of Systematic Reviews 2002 Issue 2 CD002826.

106 Brosseau L, Robinson V, Wells G, et. al. Low level laser therapy (Classes I,II,III) for treating rheumatoid arthritis Cochrane Database of Systematic Reviews 2000 Issue 2 CD002049.

107 Casimiro L, Brosseau L, Welch V. Therapeutic ultrasound for the treatment of rheumatoid arthritis Cochrane Database of Systematic Reviews 2002 Issue 3 CD003787.

108 Brosseau L, Judd MG, Marchand S, et. al. Transcutaneous electrical nerve stimulation (TENS) for the treatment of rheumatoid arthritis in the hand. Cochrane Database of Systematic Reviews 2003 Issue 3 CD004377.

109 Pelland L, Brosseau L, Casimiro L. Electrical stimulation for the treatment of rheumatoid arthritis. Cochrane Database of Systematic Reviews2002 Issue 2 CD003687.

110 Ergan m, Brosseau L, Farmer, et. al. Splints and orthosis for treating rheumatoid arthritis. Cochrane Database of Systematic Reviews 2001 Issue 4 CD004018.Table 36.1 Levels of evidence for lifestyle and complementary medicines/therapies in the management of rheumatoid arthritis

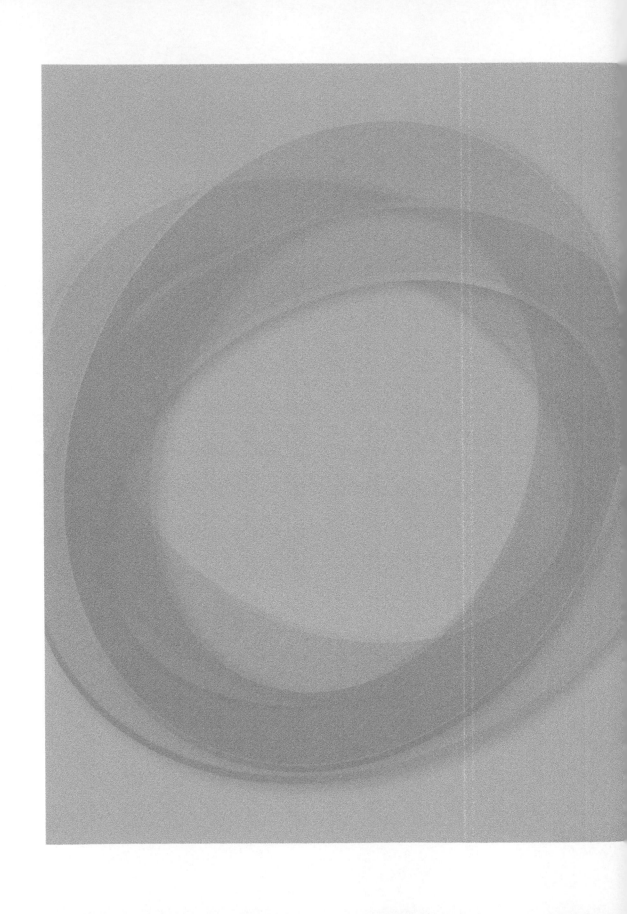

Part 3

Precaution when practising complementary medicine

Chapter 37

Herb–nutrient–drug interactions

With contribution from Dr Antigone Kouris-Blazos

Introduction

In the United States, approximately 1 in 4 persons prescribed pharmaceutical medications also consume a dietary supplement.[1, 2] Dietary supplements that include herbs, vitamin and/or mineral preparations, and other dietary supplements such as glucosamine and fish oils, may augment or antagonise the actions of prescription and non-prescription drugs. This is because supplements have demonstrated pharmacologic actions that may then go on to produce therapeutic outcomes.[3] Moreover, supplements that do not have a documented pharmacologic action can also significantly affect the absorption, metabolism, and disposition of other pharmaceutical products. Health professionals usually question the nutritional adequacy and safety of a patient's diet, however the nutritional impact of medications is often overlooked. Pharmaceuticals have both beneficial and adverse effects, although there is a strong focus on the benefits. Furthermore, drug–drug interactions are generally integral to decision-making yet the impact of drug–food and drug–nutrient interactions are rarely acknowledged or, mostly, deemed clinically insignificant.

Some vitamin–mineral–herbal supplements require separation from medications by about 2–4 hours to avoid potential problems with absorption or interactions. See the medications in Table 37.1 for more specific advice in relation to this rule.

Key points regarding herb-nutrient-drug interactions

Examine food habits or metabolic changes carefully in any patient who unexpectedly gains or loses weight while taking drugs.

Grapefruit juice, Seville orange juice and pomegranate juice inhibit cytochrome p450 (CYP450) and 3A4/5 in the liver and gut for up to 72 hours and can therefore increase serum concentration of some drugs (e.g statins, antidepressants, beta blockers, calcium channel blockers, hormone replacement therapy [HRT], warfarin, anticonvulsants, antipsychotics) into toxic ranges.

As a general rule separate vitamin–mineral–herbal supplements from medications by about 2–4 hours as they may increase or decrease each others absorption in the gut and/or affect metabolism, thus increasing risks of toxicity or insufficiency.

Types of herb–drug interactions

There are 2 types of interactions that occur between natural products and pharmaceuticals.

1. Pharmacodynamic interactions occur when the intrinsic action of a nutritional or dietary supplement augments or antagonises the activity of a pharmaceutical product.
2. Pharmacokinetic interactions are those that result from changes in metabolism, excretion, or (less frequently) absorption of the active aspect of the dietary or nutritional supplement or the drug, resulting in a more pronounced or alternatively reduced pharmacologic activity of the drug.

The evidence documenting dietary supplement–drug interactions varies extensively. There is at present no process for the systematic evaluation of dietary/nutritional supplement products for possible interactions with prescription medications. As a result of this deficit, there is an incomplete knowledge of the interactions that may occur. The information is largely researched from many different sources including animal studies, human case reports, case series, historical contraindications, and the extrapolation from basic pharmacology data, or from clinical trials. Many of the recommendations associated with herb–drug interactions are based on speculation rather than research.[4] According to a recent study,

Table 37.1 Common herbs and nutrients and their interactions with medications

Drugs	Interactions
Central nervous system and sedating medication	
Herb	**Effect**
St John's wort	SSRIs and any other medication with serotoninergic effect (e.g. tramadol) Warn patients not to initiate St John's wort when receiving SSRI medication — may cause serotonin syndrome Patients should discuss use of St John's wort with their GP and their pharmacist Any drug metabolised by CYP450 3A4/5, 2C9, 1A2 or eliminated by PGP (e.g. oral contraceptive pill [OCP], benzodiazepines, tricyclic antidepressants, anti-epileptics, HIV inhibitors, cyclosporine and immunosuppressants, digoxin, theophylline) All medications should be checked prior to initiating St John's wort. Can cause break-through bleeding and pregnancy in women taking OCP Patients should be cautioned to discuss St John's wort at the time of initiating any new medication
Kava kava Valerian Passiflora	Avoid with alcohol, benzodiazepines, barbiturates, psychoactive medication, narcotic opioids such as codeine, pethidine and oxycodone, and anti-anxiolytics as may potentiate sedating effect
Anticoagulant medications[a]	
Nutrient or herb	**Effects on anticoagulant**
St John's wort	Reduced serum levels of warfarin and reduces INR. Monitor INR carefully
Gingko biloba	Does not interact with warfarin and/or aspirin directly. Has anti-platelet activity. Does not significantly affect clotting status of warfarin. In combination with NSAIDS such as aspirin can cause severe bleeding (e.g. intra-cranial haemorrhage)
Ginger	May affect clotting status and potentiate effect of warfarin
Garlic	Has intrinsic anti-platelet activity. No serious haemorrhagic risk for monitored patients on warfarin, but care must still be taken Large doses of garlic may potentiate warfarin and aspirin effect
Asian ginseng *(Panax ginseng)*	No effect on warfarin
American ginseng *(Panax quinquefolius)*	Decreases serum warfarin levels
Siberian ginseng *(Eleutherococcus senticosus)*	Has not been studied, however contains constituents that inhibit platelet aggregation
Devil's claw *(Harpagophytum procumbens)*	Potentiates anticoagulant effects
Glucosamine	Potentiates warfarin effect and increases INR
Fish oils	3–6g daily does not affect coagulation status in patients on warfarin. Caution is still needed due to their anti-platelet effect, especially at higher doses and stop use 2 weeks before surgery

Continued

Table 37.1 Some common herbs and nutrients and their interactions with medications—cont'd

Drugs	Interactions
Vitamin E	Enhances anti-platelet effect of aspirin. No clear increased risk of bleeding in patients on warfarin
Cranberry juice, Seville oranges, pomegranate juice	Patients taking warfarin used to be advised not to drink cranberry juice due to reports of increased incidence of bruising and possible increase of INR due to inhibition of P450. Recent reviews fail to confirm this effect Conclusion: interaction may occur with more than 250ml cranberry juice daily or cranberry supplements with warfarin Grapefruit juice, Seville orange juice and pomegranate juice inhibit CYP450 3A4/5 for up to 72 hours and can therefore increase serum concentration of some drugs into toxic ranges
Papaya	May increase INR
Red clover (*Trifolium pratense*)	Due to its coumarin content, red clover may increase the risk of bleeding. Avoid use with warfarin and 2 weeks prior to surgery
Saw palmetto (*Serenoa repens*)	May increase risk of bleeding. Avoid use with warfarin and 2 weeks prior to surgery
Cardiovascular medications[(b)]	
Herb	**Effect**
St John's wort[(c)]	Decreases serum levels of verapamil, statins and digoxin
Ginseng[(c)]	Increases digoxin levels
Licorice	Increases urinary excretion of potassium and reduces serum potassium. Can increase blood pressure. Avoid with antihypertensive medication, potassium depleting medication such as thiazide diuretics, corticosteroids such as prednisolone, corticosteroid inhalants and cortisol, digoxin
Hawthorn	May interact adversely with Digoxin. May potentiate blood pressure lowering effects, thereby requiring modified drug doses
Fibre and gastrointestinal tract (GIT) supplements	
Supplement	**Effect**
Psyllium (dietary fibre)[(d)]	Decreases serum concentrations of carbamazepine Decreases absorption of lithium
Slippery elm bark	May reduce absorption of any medication as it coats the lining of the GIT
Diabetes medications	
Nutrient and/or herb	**Effect on diabetes medication**
Hawthorn	No interaction found
Chromium, psyllium, ginseng, fenugreek, gymnema, bitter melon	All have hypoglycaemic effects in patients with diabetes, which may be unpredictable. No specific changes in hypoglycaemic doses are needed unless blood sugar level changes occur
HIV medications	
Nutrient and/or herb	**Effect on HIV medication**
Garlic and vitamin C	Reduce serum antiretroviral medications

Continued

Table 37.1 Some common herbs and nutrients and their interactions with medications—cont'd

Drugs	Interactions
Milk thistle, echinacea species and goldenseal	No clinically relevant effect
St John's wort	Risk of dangerous interaction. Discourage use of herb
Ginkgo	Possible drug failure
Hormonal medications	
Nutrient and/or herb	**Effect on hormonal medication**
Ginseng	Can exert weak estrogenic effect Potentiates effect of oestrogen
Saw palmetto (*Serenoa repens*)	May exert anti-estrogenic effect Anti-androgenic effect due to 5 alpha-reducatse inhibitor effect — potentiates finasteride effect which is a more powerful inhibitor
Soy	Can exert weak estrogenic effect Potentiates effect of oestrogen
Red clover (*Trifolium pratense*)	Can exert weak estrogenic effect Potentiates effect of oestrogen
Vitex agnus castus	May potentiate progesterone effect
High dose iodine/kelp/seaweed	Thyroxine medication High dose of iodine may reduce effectiveness of medication or stimulate and/or block thyroxine production by the thyroid gland

(a) All patients on warfarin should be monitored closely with the introduction of any complementary medicine such as garlic, fish oils, ginseng and ginkgo.
(b) Given the serious consequences associated with small changes in the coagulation status, patients on warfarin should be carefully monitored when: 1) initiating or stopping any nutritional or herbal supplement 2) commencing new bottles of the same product in case of product variation.
(c) Monitor serum digoxin levels in patients taking St John's wort and ginseng.
(d) Separate psyllium by several hours to allow the absorption of drugs to occur more effectively.

overall the risk of actual harm from a herb–drug interaction is low.[5] According to the authors the 5 most common natural products with a potential to affect medications include garlic, St John's wort, ginkgo, valerian and kava. These herbal medicines accounted for 68% of the potential clinically significant interactions in the survey. The 4 most common prescription medicines affected by supplements are antithrombotics, such as warfarin, antidepressants, sedatives and anti-diabetic agents.

Types of nutrient–drug interactions

Pharmaceuticals can affect and be affected by nutrition.

1 Pharmaceuticals can influence nutrient absorption, metabolism, distribution or elimination. They can affect physiological changes such as fluid or electrolyte disturbances, which in turn may increase essential micronutrient requirements or altered nutritional status.
2 Specific nutrients, foods or beverages may interact with drugs to affect drug absorption, metabolism, distribution or elimination, which in turn may alter drug response pharmacokinetic interactions. They can also enhance or reduce the pharmacological effect — pharmacodynamic interactions.

Drugs can also affect many nutritional factors such as appetite, taste acuity and gastrointestinal function. Food habits or metabolic changes should be examined carefully in any patient who unexpectedly gains or loses weight or has altered bowel motions while taking drugs.

As a general rule, it is advisable to separate vitamin and/or mineral supplements from medications by about 2–4 hours to reduce any potential interactions. However, where the drug affects metabolism or excretion of a nutrient such a simple rule may not apply.

Even though a patient's diet may be supplying a moderate amount of vitamins and/or minerals, they may be tipped into nutritional insufficiency or deficiency due to their medications. If these deficiencies are not corrected through diet (and supplements if indicated) they may further complicate the management of the condition or create new health problems.

Nutrient supplementation may not necessarily be needed in combination with a nutrient-depleting pharmaceutical. Clinical symptoms of nutrient deficiency and/or insufficiency combined with laboratory data are needed to verify changes in nutritional status. A nutrient dense diet, however, makes an important contribution to the health of medicated patients and reduces the risk of nutritional disorders or altered drug efficacy. Health professionals need to be knowledgeable and vigilant of nutrition-related clinical symptoms that may be caused by pharmaceuticals.

Figure 37.1 lists the top 12 nutrient-depleting drugs (see also Appendix 2).[6, 7]

Nutrient absorption

Pharmaceuticals can affect the absorption of nutrients via:

- drug induced hyper or hypo peristalsis
- binding to the nutrient in the lumen of the intestine
- interfering with absorption of the nutrient (e.g. by decreased bile acid availability)
- damage to the intestinal mucosa causing malabsorption; for example, reduced cell mitosis resulting in loss of enzyme activity (e.g. lactase) or altered gut permeability, or altered gut bacterial flora, or altered carrier proteins (e.g. fructose carrier protein which can lead to fructose malabsorption)
- altering gut pH; for example, some nutrients are pH sensitive for absorption and increased pH will decrease their absorption — this is especially true for folate, Fe, Mg, Ca and Zn
- bacterial overgrowth e.g. as gut pH increases gut microflora survive further up the gastrointestinal (GI) tract and access nutrients before the host, resulting in reduced availability of nutrients for absorption by the host.

Nutrient metabolism

Altered cellular metabolism can result from the pharmaceutical:

- inducing enzyme systems; for example, induction of hepatic microsomal enzymes such as the cytochrome P450 can increase the turnover of nutrients (clearing effect)
- inhibiting enzyme systems through which the vitamins are converted to their active forms; for example, drugs binding to dihydrofolate reductase can cause a folate deficiency (inactivating effect).

Nutrient excretion

Drugs can cause nutrient deficiencies via increased urinary and/or faecal excretion — this is especially true for several minerals such as potassium, calcium, zinc, magnesium and sodium. Some drugs can also decrease nutrient urinary excretion increasing the risk of dangerously high serum levels, such as the potassium sparing diuretics.

Patient populations and specific pharmaceuticals

Proton pump inhibitors (PPI) and histamine receptor antagonists (HRA)

These drugs almost completely shut down the stomach's ability to produce hydrochloric acid and, as a result, affect absorption of Ca, Fe, Mg, Zn, Se, vitamins B1, B12, C, D, E, and folate, and thus a multivitamin is usually recommended with these drugs. They can alter taste and impair appetite and can cause anaemia through reduced absorption of these nutrients. PPI, but not HRA, are linked to increased risk of bone fractures — PPIs are thus contraindicated in patients with osteoporosis. If prescribing Mg/Ca supplements, magnesium hydroxide and calcium carbonate supplements require stomach acid for digestion — citrate versions are preferable. Antacids containing magnesium hydroxide (e.g. Mylanta®) can block absorption of PPI and HRA so their consumption must be separated by 2–4 hours. PPI and HRA may not be tolerated by patients with fructose intolerance and/or irritable bowel syndrome. Low stomach acidity can increase risk of small intestinal bowel overgrowth so a probiotic food or supplement may also be useful. (See Appendix 2 for references.)

Antacid medication

Antacids neutralise stomach acid and their high levels of calcium can interfere with the absorption of Fe, Zn, Cr, Cu, vitamins A, B1, B12, folate, D, E, K. They can also impair appetite and alter taste. Aluminium in some antacids (e.g. Mylanta®) can bind dietary phosphates and this can further lead to calcium depletion and cause osteomalacia. Ca/Mg citrate, vitamin C supplements, citrus juices and milk can increase aluminium absorption so should be separated from drug consumption by at least 2 hours. Fe/Zn/fibre supplements and foods high in oxalates (e.g. tea, wheat germ) and phytates (e.g. bran, oats) can reduce absorption of antacids. Long-term use of antacids can increase serum magnesium levels. Elderly patients should not take antacids at meal times or with other dietary supplements. (See Appendix 2 for references.)

Psychiatric medications

St John's wort is today most widely known as a herbal treatment for depression. St John's wort has been documented to be one of the most common natural products with a potential for interaction.[5, 8]

St John's wort pharmacodynamic action may have an effect on serotonin levels even though this is not probably its inherent mechanism of action in the treatment of depression. It has been associated with serotonin syndrome due to raised serotonin levels in patients also receiving a selective serotonin reuptake inhibitor (SSRI).[9] It has been reported that St John's wort should gradually be reduced when an SSRI is initiated.[10]

Similarly, patients should be cautioned not to initiate St John's wort use when receiving SSRI medications.

St John's wort pharmacokinetic interactions have been extensively demonstrated to decrease serum levels of psychiatric medications metabolised by the CYP450 enzyme system.[11, 12, 13] Also, although changes in serum levels of benzodiazepines and tricyclic antidepressants with the use of St John's wort have been reported, these changes may not result in a significant clinical effect.[12–15]

Oral contraceptive pill (OCP)

As St John's wort can induce the enzyme cytochrome P450, it can potentially affect the levels of any drugs that are metabolised by this pathway, such as anti-epileptics and the oral contraceptives. There have been reported cases of break-through bleeding in women taking the OCP and St John's wort increasing the risk of pregnancy.[16] However, a recent study has reported that a low dose of St John's wort extract Ze117 which was reported to have a low hyperforin content, did not interact with the pharmacokinetics of the hormonal components of the low-dose oral contraceptive.[17]

Anticoagulant medication

Warfarin

There have been documented case reports on interactions between the anticoagulant warfarin and St John's wort, *Ginkgo biloba* (gingko), garlic, and ginseng.[18, 19]

Studies have demonstrated that St John's wort increases the metabolism of warfarin, leading to significantly reduced serum levels of the drug.[20–23] However, the clinical response to the combination has not been quantified.

Care must be taken with patients on warfarin starting any complementary medicine. INR

1. Proton pump inhibitors and histamine receptor antagonists (Ca, Fe, Mg, Zn, Se, vitamins B1, B12, C, D, folate)
2. Loop and thiazide diuretics (Mg, K, Zn, CoQ10 vitamins B1, B12, B6, folate)
3. Corticosteroids (protein, Mg, Ca, Zn, Cr, Se, phosphorus, vitamins A, B6, C, D, K, folate)
4. Bile acid sequestrants (fat, Mg, Ca, Fe, Zn, Cr, vitamins A, B12, D, E, K, folate)
5. Some antibiotics (vitamins B1, B2, B5, B6, K and folate)
6. Oestrogens (Mg, Zn, Ca, vitamins B6, B12, folate, D)
7. Anticonvulsants (carnitine, Ca, vitamins A, biotin, B12, folate, D, E, K)
8. Benzodiazepines (carnitine, Ca, vitamins A, biotin, B2, B6, B12, folate, D, K)
9. Aspirin (Ca, Fe, K, Zn, vitamins B12, folate, C)
10. Colchicine (Fat, Na, K, carotene, vitamin B12)
11. Laxatives (fluid, K, Ca, Mg, Zn, phosphorus, vitamins A, D, E, K)
12. Antacids (Fe, Zn, Cr, Cu, vitamins A, B1, B12, folate, D, E, K)

Figure 37.1 Top nutrient-depleting drugs*

*Consider recommending foods high in these nutrients; if blood tests suggest deficiency then a supplement may be needed (see Chapter 2, Nutritional assessment and therapies).

should be checked within 2 weeks of starting the complementary medicine.

Ginkgo biloba extracts from the ginkgo leaves contains flavonoid glycosides and terpenoids (ginkgolides, bilobalides). It has many alleged nootropic properties, and is mainly used as a memory and concentration enhancer and as an anti-vertigo agent.[24] Animal and *in vitro* data suggest that *Ginkgo biloba* extracts may modulate CYP3A4 enzyme system activity.[25] *Ginkgo biloba* does not interact with warfarin or aspirin but has been demonstrated to have anti-platelet activity.[26, 27] A randomised cross-over study to assess the pharmacokinetics and pharmacodynamics of warfarin with ginkgo and ginger demonstrated that at recommended dosage these herbs do not significantly affect clotting status of warfarin in healthy subjects.[26] However, in combination with non-steroidal anti-inflammatory drugs (NSAIDs), such as aspirin, ginkgo has been reported to cause severe bleeding, including intracranial bleeding.[28–30]

Animal studies, and some early investigational studies in humans, have suggested possible cardiovascular benefits of garlic. Garlic has intrinsic anti-platelet activity.[31] However, a recent clinical trial has demonstrated that garlic is safe and poses no serious haemorrhagic risk for monitored patients prescribed warfarin.[32] Further, a recent review of the literature concluded that there is no evidence that supports the concern of perioperative bleeding in users of garlic.[33] Nevertheless, care must be taken when prescribed with warfarin.

A low-level of evidence clinical study found no effect of Asian ginseng *(Panax ginseng)* in combination with warfarin.[30] American ginseng *(Panax quinquefolius)*, a separate plant, decreases warfarin serum levels in humans, resulting in less anticoagulation.[30] Further, another study has reported that American ginseng significantly reduced peak plasma warfarin level and warfarin INR.[34] Siberian ginseng *(Eleutherococcus senticosus)* has not been studied; however, it contains a constituent that inhibits platelet aggregation. A recent review concludes that there is no evidence linking the use of ginseng to perioperative bleeding.[33] Specifically, patients receiving American ginseng should be monitored when changing products or even bottles of the same product.[35, 36]

Putative antioxidants such as vitamin E and essential fatty acids from fish oil are often cited in scientific reviews of nutritional supplement–drug interactions.[37, 38] In a small clinical study of 16 patients, fish oils (3–6g/day) were reported to not affect the coagulation status in patients who were receiving warfarin.[39] Nevertheless, caution is needed due to anti-platelet effects of fish oils. A recent expert opinion on fish oils has surmised that the benefits of triglyceride lowering with omega-3 fatty acids more than outweighs any theoretical risks for increased bleeding.[40]

In vitro studies demonstrate enhancement of the anti-platelet effect of aspirin by vitamin E and therefore it has been suggested that it may have an effect on bleeding time.[41] However, clinical trials with and without warfarin and vitamin E have demonstrated no clear increased risk of bleeding even though high doses of vitamin E were used and could have antagonised vitamin K levels.[42–44]

Cranberry juice contains polyphenolic and phytochemical compounds with possible benefits to the cardiovascular system, immune system and as an anti-cancer agent.[45–49] In 2004 the Committee on Safety of Medicines — the UK agency dealing with drug safety — advised patients taking warfarin not to drink cranberry juice because adverse effects such as increased incidence of bruising were reported from case reports, possibly resulting from the presence of salicylic acid native to polyphenol-rich plants such as the cranberry. It may also increase INR by inhibiting the CYP450 enzyme-reducing metabolism of warfarin. However, recent reviews of case reports and pilot studies have failed to confirm this effect, collectively indicating no significant interaction between daily consumption of 250 mL of cranberry juice and warfarin.[50, 51, 52] A controlled study demonstrated no effect on coagulation.[50]

Given that warfarin has a narrow therapeutic index and the serious consequences associated with small changes, the anticoagulation status in patients taking dietary supplements containing blood thinning herbs or vitamins (see Table 37.2 at the end of this chapter) should be carefully monitored whenever they initiate or stop taking any nutritional supplement. Moreover, patients on warfarin should also be monitored when they commence new bottles of the same product in case of product variations, and until the effect in the individual patient is known.

Also, patients should avoid major changes to diet to keep vitamin K intake around 65–80ug/day. A high intake of vitamin K rich foods, even for a single day, will alter plasma coagulation for several days afterward. Variation in vitamin K should not exceed 250–500ug/day. (See food sources for vitamin K in Appendix 1.)

Aspirin

Aspirin can reduce the absorption of B12, folate, vitamin C, Fe, Zn, Ca and increase the risk of gastrointestinal bleeding and anaemia with chronic use, primarily at high doses. Aspirin can also reduce appetite. A high intake of omega-3 EPA/DHA (>3000mg/day) from fish oil or flaxseed oil (>30g/day) or evening primrose oil (>1g/d) or vitamin E (>100IU) with aspirin may increase risk of haemorrhagic stroke. Other blood thinning herbs and/or foods that have the potential to increase the blood thinning effects of aspirin (and warfarin or clopidogrel) if taken at high supplemental doses include: *Aloe vera*, carnitine, chamomile, chondroitin, cinnamon, CoQ_{10}, cranberry, devil's claw, dong quai, feverfew, garlic, ginger, gingko, ginseng, glucosamine, goji, grape seed extract, green tea, krill oil, policosanol, saw palmetto, turmeric and willow bark. (See Appendix 2 for references.)

For a list of herbs and foods that may interact with anticoagulant medication, see Table 37.2.

Cardiovascular medication

Loop and thiazide diuretics increase the excretion of K, Mg, Zn, vitamins B1, B12, B6, folate and impair appetite. High K foods and/or supplements are frequently prescribed; however, long-term use (more than 6 months) might lead to Mg deficiency which in turn can increase loss of K and B1. It is probably prudent to check red blood cell magnesium along with serum potassium and prescribe a magnesium supplement if low (e.g. magnesium orotate/chelate/ citrate are better absorbed). B1 deficiency can aggravate congestive heart failure, oedema, muscle pain, poor appetite, mental confusion and risk of falls. Thiazide diuretics can increase blood levels of calcium by decreasing excretion and, indirectly, by affecting vitamin D metabolism, therefore calcium and vitamin D supplements should be used with caution.

Ace inhibitors and angiotensin II antagonists attach to zinc and can cause zinc deficiency, which in turn may account for some of the drug side-effects (impaired appetite, altered taste, skin numbness and/or tingling). Garlic, hawthorn, olive leaf and fish oil supplements may increase the antihypertensive effects of the drugs requiring adjustment of medication dose. K supplements and high K foods are contraindicated due to increased risk of hyperkalaemia. These drugs contain magnesium so high-dose Mg supplements (>300mg/day) should be used with caution to avoid excessive intake. (See Appendix 2 for references.)

Of all the supplements used by patients who have cardiac disease, St John's wort (used to treat mood disorders) is associated with the most interactions. It can decrease serum concentrations of drugs including most calcium channel blockers and statins.[53, 54, 55] Blood pressure and lipid levels, respectively, should be monitored closely if a patient is taking 1 of these drugs concomitantly with St John's wort.

The mechanisms of St John's wort on the pharmacokinetics of other drugs is due to induction of cytochrome P450 (CYP450) isoenzymes CYP3A4, CYP2C9, and CYP1A2, and of the transport protein P-glycoprotein, leading to decreased concentration of medications.[56] In 1 study, St John's wort was reported to have decreased digoxin blood levels by 25%. The most likely mechanism was by inducing P-glycoprotein and the clearance of digoxin.[57, 58]

Ginseng which is a commonly used herb[5] has been reported to cause an increase in digoxin serum levels in a case report of 1 patient.[59] At present digoxin levels should be monitored in patients taking Siberian ginseng or St John's wort (or any supplement for that matter, since digoxin has a narrow therapeutic window).

Laxative medication

Laxatives can cause steatorrhoea with chronic use which is associated with reduced absorption of fat soluble vitamins (A, D, E, K) and increased excretion of K and Mg. Milk/Ca/ Mg medication are not recommended within 2 hours of the laxative. It may be prudent to recommend a multivitamin with chronic use of laxatives

Psyllium commonly used as a dietary fibre is not absorbed by the small intestine. The purely mechanical action of psyllium mucilage absorbs excess water while stimulating normal bowel elimination. Although its main use has been as a laxative, it is more appropriately termed a true dietary fibre. With other related bulk-forming laxatives, these dietary supplements are often not considered to be medications by many patients. However, they can slow or diminish absorption of many pharmaceutical drugs.[60]

Psyllium has been reported to reduce the concentration of carbamazepine absorption and its serum levels.[61] In addition, a case report has demonstrated that psyllium decreased the absorption of lithium.[62]

Hence, this data tends to indicate that bulk laxatives such as psyllium may need to be separated by several hours to allow absorption of drugs to occur more effectively.

Diabetes medication

Metformin/pioglitazone/sulfonylureas can decrease absorption of vitamin B12 and folate. Magnesium supplements can increase

Table 37.2 Potential blood thinning foods and herbs

Potential blood thinning foods and herbs which may interact with blood thinning medication and theoretically should be avoided at least 1–2 weeks prior to and 1 week after surgery
Alfalfa supplements (or supplements containing alfalfa)
Aloe vera
Andrographis
Angelica root (contains coumarin-like substances and may interact with warfarin)
Anise
Aspirin/salicylates
Barley grass powder or juice
Beef liver (is high in vitamin A and K which can interact with warfarin)
Bilberry (high doses)
Bitter orange
Black cohosh
Borage oil
Bromelain enzyme supplements
Canola oil (>1 tablespoon)
Carnitine supplements
Celery seed supplements (contains coumarin-like substances and may interact with warfarin)
Cinnamon supplements
Chamomile tea (contains coumarin-like substances and may interact with warfarin)
Chondroitin
CoQ_{10}
Coleus
Corn silk (contains coumarin-like substances and may interact with warfarin)
Cranberry (>1 cup juice) or supplements
Dandelion
Danshen
Devils claw
Dong quai (contains coumarin-like substances and may interact with warfarin)
Evening primrose oil
Feverfew supplements
Flaxseed oil (>1/2 tablespoon)
Fenugreek supplements (contains coumarin-like substances and may interact with warfarin)
Fish oil *(>10 gram EPA + DHA daily)*
Garlic *(>4g/day)* fresh or supplements
Ginger *(>10g/day)* fresh or supplements
Ginkgo supplements
Ginseng supplements
Glucosamine
Goji berry juice, tea or supplements
Grapefruit (affects liver enzymes)
Grapefruit seed extract supplements
Green lipped mussel supplements
Grape seed supplements
Guarana
Guggul
Guar gum
Herbal teas (some) — goldenseal, meadow sweet, chamomile
Horse chestnut (contains coumarin like substances and may interact with warfarin)
Horseradish
Inositol supplements
Ipriflavone/isoflavones supplements
Kiwis (>2)
Krill oil
Licorice (contains coumarin like substances and may interact with warfarin)
Linseed oil (>1/2 tablespoon)
Papain enzymes (from Papaya; e.g. in meat tenderiser)
Meadowsweet
Milk thistle
Oligomeric proanthocyanidins (OPCs)
Passionflower (contains coumarin-like substances and may interact with warfarin)
Pau d'arco (high doses)
Phosphatidyl serine supplements
Phytoestrogen supplements
Policosanol
Pomegranate juice (affects liver enzymes)
Quinine
Red clover (contains coumarin-like substances and may interact with warfarin)
Red rice yeast extract
Reishi
Royal jelly
Rosemary supplements
Saw palmetto
St John's wort
Turmeric supplements
Vitamin E supplements (>250IU)
Wheat grass powder or juice
White willow/willow bark
Woodruff sweet (contains coumarin-like substances and may interact with warfarin)

(Source: EBSCO Publishing. Online. Available: http://healthlibrary.epnet.com/GetContent.aspx?token=1edc3d6e-4fec-4b20-baca-795e48830daa [accessed 4 Sept 2010]; Braun L, Cohen M. Herbs and Natural Supplements: an evidence-based guide (2nd edn). Elsevier, Sydney, 2007; Health Notes Online. Available: http://www.pccnaturalmarkets.com/health/2411003/ [accessed 4 Sept 2010]) absorption of pioglitazone and sulfonylureas these drugs can also reduce appetite and alter taste. K/Mg citrate supplements may reduce their therapeutic effect. Short-term studies have not found glucosamine supplements to have an adverse effect on blood glucose levels in diabetics. Sulfonylureas can affect thyroid function (and cause weight gain) by reducing the uptake of iodine by the thyroid. (See Appendix 2 for references.)

Currently nutrient-herb–drug interactions are not well documented in patients being treated for type 2 diabetes mellitus (T2DM). However, a number of supplements have been reported to have intrinsic effects on serum glucose. In a recent randomised controlled trial (RCT) to demonstrate a hypotensive effect of hawthorn in patients with diabetes taking medication, it was reported that no herb–drug interaction was found.[63]

Chromium and psyllium also have been reported to have hypoglycaemic effects.[64, 65, 66] Also ginseng, fenugreek and *Gymnema sylvestre* have demonstrated *in vivo* hypoglycaemic activity and in patients with diabetes this effect might be additive when combined with oral hypoglycaemics or insulin.[67, 68, 69]

Recently it has been reported that bitter melon (*Momordica charantia*) has a similar affect to rosiglitazone.[70] The cumulative evidence demonstrates that bitter melon and fenugreek may be useful for the treatment of T2DM.[71]

Patients taking supplements containing vitamin E, Mg, Cr, CoQ_{10}, lipoic acid, inositol or foods/supplements with *Aloe vera* juice, bitter melon, cinnamon, fenugreek, garlic, ginger, gymnema, ginseng, bilberry, guggul, gingko, milk thistle, guar, green tea, olive leaf extract, psyllium and turmeric may need closer monitoring of their blood glucose levels. These supplements may, therefore be useful in the pre-diabetic patient.

The effect of these supplements may be unpredictable in T2DM, and hypoglycaemic medication may need to be altered if blood glucose changes occur.[2]

Thyroxine (T4)

Thyroxine does not cause nutrient deficiencies, however, its absorption is reduced by food and mineral supplements. Thyroxine should be taken on an empty stomach, ideally 1 hour before food or 2 hours after food. Meals high in fibre and/or soy should also be separated from thyroxine by several hours. Any supplements or fortified foods (e.g. Anlene milk) containing minerals, especially Ca, Fe, Zn, chromium and Se, should be taken with a gap of 4 hours from taking thyroxine. Secretion of TSH, production of T4 by the thyroid and conversion of endogenous or exogenous T4 to T3 in the thyroid, liver and other tissues requires an adequate intake of I, Fe, Se, Zn, Mg, omega-3 fatty acids, vitamin A and tyrosine. Correcting deficiencies of these nutrients may have an additive effect on thyroid function that may result in a need for a reduced dose of thyroxine. This may be desirable since thyroxine therapy can have side-effects (e.g. potentiates glucose intolerance). Mild iodine deficiency has re-emerged in Australia over the last 10–15 years, with 43% of the population having inadequate iodine intakes. (See also Chapter 32, pregnancy disorders.) Good food sources of iodine include kelp/seaweed, fish and iodised salt. Iodine deficiency can be detected by way of several fasting urinary iodine tests (iodine/creatine ratio). If iodine deficiency is identified, a low dose iodine supplement (100mcg/day) approaching the RDI of 150mcg/day may be necessary with a concomitant reduction in thyroxine dose. High dose iodine supplements should be avoided as they can block thyroid hormone synthesis and create an underactive state. A T4:T3 ratio >3 may suggest selenium deficiency. However, since both I and Se deficiencies can co-exist, iodine deficiency must be corrected first to enable the thyroid to respond to selenium supplementation. Foods and/or supplements that may have an additive effect on thyroid function include low dose iodine/kelp/seaweed, Fe, tyrosine, withania and brahmi. Foods and/or supplements that may reduce thyroid function or the effects of thyroxine include high dose iodine/kelp/seaweed, isoflavones, lemon balm, bugleweed, red rice yeast extract, SAMe, carnitine, and celery seed. Goitrogenic foods include raw broccoli, cauliflower, cabbage, garlic, onion, linseed, rapeseed, lima beans, soy, peanuts, swede, sweet potato, and millet; they usually reduce utilisation of iodine by the thyroid by blocking the uptake of iodine, particularly when dietary iodine intake is low, potentially reducing thyroid production. This may be a useful effect in patients with hyperthyroidism. However, if iodine intake is adequate in patients with hypothyroidism, these foods will have a minor effect on thyroid production and will probably not cause problems. (See Appendix 2 for references.)

HIV medication

Herbal medicines are widely used by HIV patients. Several herbal medicines have been shown to interact with antiretroviral drugs, which might lead to drug failure.[68] *Echinacea purpurea* (echinacea), garlic, ginkgo, milk thistle, and St John's wort have the potential to cause significant interactions with antiretroviral medication.

Most antiretrovirals are metabolised via the CYP3A4 and P-glycoprotein systems. Dietary supplements that induce these systems may decrease serum levels of the antiretroviral drugs.

St John's wort is the herbal supplement with the most evidence of an effect on these enzyme systems.[72] Some degree of clinical research has demonstrated reductions in antiretroviral serum concentrations in patients who have taken garlic and vitamin C.[73, 74] Other herbal products such as milk thistle, echinacea species, and goldenseal inhibit CYP450 enzymes in vitro, but do not appear to give rise to a clinically relevant effect.[72–76]

The effectiveness of HIV therapy should be monitored in patients taking these supplements, particularly St John's wort. Because of the risk of dangerous interactions, patients prescribed antiretrovirals should be discouraged from using St John's wort.[2]

Anticonvulsant medications

An extensive early review has reported that there are numerous plant products that demonstrate anticonvulsant activity.[77] Even though there may not be an unequivocal and overwhelming scientific literature for herbal medicines interacting with anticonvulsant medications, there is strong biological plausibility for significant interactions between some herbal medicines (e.g. kava, valerian) and anticonvulsant medications. The Epilepsy Society of Southern New York in the US has cautioned that certain herbs, supplements and alternative medicines can cause or worsen seizures and may interact with pharmaceutical medications (see the table on the website).[78] Moreover, many herbal medicines from Traditional Chinese medicine (TCM) cultures, for example, have been documented to treat seizures and may have sedative effects, and can interact with other herbal medicines and supplements, as well as prescription medications.[79, 80, 81]

Sedatives

The 5 most common natural products with a potential for interaction with pharmaceuticals included garlic, valerian, kava, ginkgo, and St John's wort, and that these herbal medicines accounted for 68% of the potential clinically significant interactions in the survey.[82] The study concluded that the 4 most common classes of prescription medications with a potential for interaction with herbal medicines included sedatives, antithrombotic medications, antidepressant agents, and anti-diabetic agents.

A study on the action of Kava in neurotransmission concluded that kava pyrones exhibited a profile of cellular actions that show a large overlap with several mood stabilisers, especially lamotrigine.[83]

Immunosuppressant medication

A systematic review has concluded that St John's wort interacts with cyclosporine, causing a decrease of cyclosporine blood levels and leading in several cases to transplant rejection.[84] An animal study has demonstrated that the immunosuppressive methotrexate has significant interactions with the eastern Asia herb of the root extract of kudzu (*Pueraria lobata*).[85] The co-administration of the herb with methotrexate significantly decreased the elimination of the drug and resulted in markedly increased exposure of methotrexate to the rats. Other herbs and/or nutrients that have the potential to stimulate the immune system and possibly counter the effects of immunosuppressants and corticosteroids include alfalfa, astragalus, andrographis, baical skullcap, echinacea, ginseng, goldenseal, withania, licorice root, and/or the mineral zinc.

Summary

A recent US report shows that approximately 66% of patients do not tell their medical practitioners about their nutritional/dietary supplement use.[86] Patients may not consider nutritional supplements to be legitimate drugs or to carry adverse risks.[87] Therefore, all patients should be asked about their use of dietary supplements irrespective of the type of supplement consumed. Clinicians should question their patients openly about their vitamins, herbs, other supplements, teas, tinctures, or natural products that they are consuming. All of these supplements should be treated as other drugs and recorded in the patient record.

References

1 Kaufman DW, Kelly JP, Rosenberg L, et. al. Recent patterns of medication use in the ambulatory adult population of the United States: the Slone survey. JAMA 2002;287:337–44.

2 Gardiner P, Graham RE, Legedza AT, et. al. Factors associated with dietary supplement use among prescription medication users. Arch Intern Med 2006;166:1968–74.

3 Dietary Supplement Health and Education Act of 1994. Pub L No 103–417. Online. Available: www.fda.gov/opacom/laws/dshea.html#sec3 (accessed 15 April 2008).

4 Gardiner P, Phillips R, Shaughnessy AF. Herbal and dietary supplement--drug interactions in patients with chronic illnesses. Am Fam Physician 2008;77(1):73–8.

5 Sood A, Sood R, Brinker FJ, et. al. Potential for interactions between dietary supplements and prescription medications. Am J Med 2008;121(3):207–11.
6 Hamilton Smith C, Bidlack WR. Dietary concerns associated with the use of medications. J Am Diet Assoc 1984;84(8):901–14.
7 Wahlqvist ML. Nutrition and health problems related to substance abuse and medications. Food and Nutrition, Allen and Unwin, 1997.
8 Zhou S, Chan E, Pan SQ, et. al. Pharmacokinetic interactions of drugs with St John's wort. J Psychopharmacol 2004;18(2):262–76.
9 Hammerness P, Basch E, Ulbricht C, et. al., for the Natural Standard Research Collaboration. St John's wort: a systematic review of adverse effects and drug interactions for the consultation psychiatrist. Psychosomatics 2003;44:271–82.
10 Singh YN. Potential for interaction of kava and St. John's wort with drugs. J Ethnopharmacol 2005;100:108–13.
11 Izzo AA. Drug interactions with St. John's wort (Hypericum perforatum): a review of the clinical evidence. Int J Clin Pharmacol Ther 2004;42: 139–48.
12 Markowitz JS, DeVane CL. The emerging recognition of herb-drug interactions with a focus on St. John's wort (Hypericum perforatum). Psychopharmacol Bull 2001;35:53–64.
13 Peng CC, Glassman PA, Trilli LE, et. al. Incidence and severity of potential drug-dietary supplement interactions in primary care patients: an exploratory study of 2 outpatient practices. Arch Intern Med 2004;164(6):630–6.
14 Izzo AA, Ernst E. Interactions between herbal medicines and prescribed drugs: a systematic review. Drugs 2001;61:2163–75.
15 Roots I. Interaction of a herbal extract from St. John's wort with amitriptyline and its metabolites. Clin Pharmacol Ther 2000;67:69.
16 Hall SD, Wang Z, Huang SM, et. al. The interaction between St John's wort and an oral contraceptive. Clin Pharmacol Ther 2003;74(6):525–35.
17 Will-Shahab L, Bauer S, Kunter U, et. al. St John's wort extract (Ze 117) does not alter the pharmacokinetics of a low-dose oral contraceptive. Eur J Clin Pharmacol 2009;65(3):287–94.
18 Vaes LP, Chyka PA. Interactions of warfarin with garlic, ginger, ginkgo, or ginseng: nature of the evidence. Ann Pharmacot 2000;34:1478–82.
19 Hu Z, Yang X, Ho PC, et. al. Herb-drug interactions: a literature review. Drugs 2005;65:1239–82.
20 Jiang X, Williams KM, Liauw WS, et. al. Effect of St John's wort and ginseng on the pharmacokinetics and pharmacodynamics of warfarin in healthy subjects [Published correction appears in Br J Clin Pharmacol 2004;58:102 Br J Clin Pharmacol 2004;57:592–9.
21 Zhou S, Chan E, Pan SQ, et. al. Pharmacokinetic interactions of drugs with St. John's wort. J Psychopharmacol 2004;18:262–76.
22 Henderson L, Yue QY, Bergquist C, et. al. St John's wort (Hypericum perforatum): drug interactions and clinical outcomes. Br J Clin Pharmacol 2002;54: 349–56.
23 Jiang X, Blair EY, McLachlan AJ. Investigation of the effects of herbal medicines on warfarin response in healthy subjects: a population pharmacokinetic-pharmacodynamic modeling approach. J Clin Pharm 2006;46:1370–8.
24 Kennedy DO, Jackson PA, Haskell CF, Scholey AB. Modulation of cognitive performance following single doses of 120 mg Ginkgobiloba extract administered to healthy young volunteers. Hum Psychopharmacol 2007;22(8):559–66.
25 Robertson SM, Davey RT, Voell J, et. al. Effect of Ginkgo biloba extract on lopinavir, midazolam and fexofenadine pharmacokinetics in healthy subjects. Curr Med Res Opin 2008;24(2):591–9.
26 Jiang X, Williams KM, Liauw WS, et. al. Effect of ginkgo and ginger on the pharmacokinetics and pharmacodynamics of warfarin in healthy subjects. Br J Clin Pharmacol 2005;59:425–32.
27 Mohutsky MA, Anderson GD, Miller JW, et. al. Ginkgo biloba: evaluation of CYP2C9 drug interactions in vitro and in vivo. Am J Ther 2006;13:24–31.
28 Meisel C, Johne A, Roots I. Fatal intracerebral mass bleeding associated with Ginkgo biloba and ibuprofen. Atherosclerosis 2003;167:367.
29 Abebe W. Herbal medication: potential for adverse interactions with analgesic drugs. J Clin Pharm Ther 2002;27:391–401.
30 Bebbington A, Kulkarni R, Roberts P. Ginkgo biloba: persistent bleeding after total hip arthroplasty caused by herbal self-medication. J Arthroplasty 2005;20:125–6.
31 Pierre S, Crosbie L, Duttaroy AK. Inhibitory effect of aqueous extracts of some herbs on human platelet aggregation in vitro. Platelets 2005;16(8):469–7
32 Macan H, Uykimpang R, Alconcel M, et. al. Aged garlic extract may be safe for patients on warfarin therapy. J Nutr 2006;136:793S-795S.
33 Beckert BW, Concannon MJ, Henry SL, et. al. The effect of herbal medicines on platelet function: an in vivo experiment and review of the literature. Plast Reconstr Surg 2007;120(7):2044–50
34 Yuan CS, Wei G, Dey L, et. al. Brief communication: American ginseng reduces warfarin's effect in healthy patients: a randomized, controlled Trial. Ann Intern Med 2004;141(1):23–7.
35 Garrard J, Harms S, Eberly LE, Matiak A. Variations in product choices of frequently purchased herbs: caveat emptor. Arch Intern Med 2003;163:2290–5.
36 Yuan CS, Wei G, Dey L, et. al. Brief communication: American ginseng reduces warfarin's effect in healthy patients: a randomized, controlled trial. Ann Intern Med 2004;141:23–7.
37 Buckley MS, Goff AD, Knapp WE. Fish oil interaction with warfarin. Ann Pharmacother 2004;38:50–2.
38 Desai D, Hasan A, Wesley R, Sunderland E, Pucino F, Csako G. Effects of dietary supplements on aspirin and other antiplatelet agents: an evidence-based approach. Thromb Res 2005;117:87–101.
39 Bender NK, Kraynak MA, Chiquette E, Linn WD, Clark GM, Bussey HI. Effects of marine fish oils on the anticoagulation status of patients receiving chronic warfarin therapy. J Thromb Thrombol 1998;5:257–61.
40 Harris WS. Expert opinion: omega-3 fatty acids and bleeding-cause for concern? Am J Cardiol 2007;99(6A):44C-46C.
41 Celestini A, Pulcinelli FM, Pignatelli P, et. al. Vitamin E potentiates the antiplatelet activity of aspirin in collagen stimulated platelets. Haematologica 2002;87:420–6.

42 Kim JM, White RH. Effect of vitamin E on the anticoagulant response to warfarin. Am J Cardiol 1996;77:545–6.

43 Booth SL, Golly I, Sacheck JM, et. al. Effect of vitamin E supplementation on vitamin K status in adults with normal coagulation status. Am J Clin Nutr 2004;80:143–8.

44 Dereska NH, McLemore EC, Tessier et. al. Short-term, moderate dosage vitamin E supplementation may have no effect on platelet aggregation, coagulation profile, and bleeding time in healthy individuals. J Surg Res 2006;132:121–9.

45 Bagchi D, Sen CK, Bagchi M, Atalay M. Anti-angiogenic, antioxidant, and anti-carcinogenic properties of a novel anthocyanin-rich berry extract formula. Biochemistry (Mosc) 2004;69(1):75–80.

46 Seeram NP, Adams LS, Zhang Y, et. al. Blackberry, black raspberry, blueberry, cranberry, red raspberry, and strawberry extracts inhibit growth and stimulate apoptosis of human cancer cells in vitro. J Agric Food Chem 2006;54(25):9329–39.

47 Bagchi D, Roy S, Patel V, et. al. Safety and whole-body antioxidant potential of a novel anthocyanin-rich formulation of edible berries. Mol Cell Biochem 2006;281(1–2):197–209.

48 Boivin D, Blanchette M, Barrette S, Moghrabi A, Béliveau R. Inhibition of cancer cell proliferation and suppression of TNF-induced activation of NFkappaB by edible berry juice. Anticancer Res 2007;27(2):937–48.

49 Seeram NP. Berry fruits: compositional elements, biochemical activities, and the impact of their intake on human health, performance, and disease. J Agric Food Chem 2008;56(3):627–9.

50 Greenblatt DJ, von Moltke LL, Perloff ES, et. al. Interaction of flurbiprofen with cranberry juice, grape juice, tea, and fluconazole: in vitro and clinical studies. Clin Pharmacol Ther 2006;79:125–33.

51 Li Z, Seeram NP, Carpenter CL, et. al. Cranberry does not affect prothrombin time in male subjects on warfarin. J Am Diet Assoc 2006;106(12):2057–61.

52 Pham DQ, Pham AQ. Interaction potential between cranberry juice and warfarin. Am J Health Syst Pharm 2007;64(5):490–4.

53 Tannergren C, Engman H, Knutson L, et. al. St John's wort decreases the bioavailability of R- and Sverapamil through induction of the first-pass metabolism. Clin Pharmacol Ther 2004;75:298–309.

54 Sugimoto K, Ohmori M, Tsuruoka S, et. al. Different effects of St John's wort on the pharmacokinetics of simvastatin and pravastatin. Clin Pharmacol Ther 2001;70:518–24.

55 Portoles A, Terleira A, Calvo A, et. al. Effects of Hypericum perforatum on ivabradine pharmacokinetics in healthy volunteers: an open-label, pharmacokinetic interaction clinical trial. J Clin Pharm 2006;46:1188–94.

56 Henderson L, Yue QY, Bergquist C, et. al. St John's wort (Hypericum perforatum): drug interactions and clinical outcomes. Br J Clin Pharmacol 2002;54:349–56.

57 Johne A, Brockmoller J, Bauer S, Maurer A, Langheinrich M, Roots I. Pharmacokinetic interaction of digoxin with an herbal extract from St John's wort (Hypericum perforatum). Clin Pharm Ther 1999;66:338–45.

58 Tian R, Koyabu N, Morimoto S, et. al. Functional induction and de-induction of P-glycoprotein by St. John's wort and its ingredients in a human colon adenocarcinoma cell line. Drug Metab Disp 2005;33:547–54

59 McRae S. Elevated serum digoxin levels in a patient taking digoxin and Siberian ginseng. CMAJ 1996;155:293–5.

60 Petchetti L, Frishman WH, Petrillo R, et. al. Nutriceuticals in cardiovascular disease: psyllium. Cardiol Rev 2007;15(3):116–22.

61 Etman M. Effect of a bulk forming laxative on the bioavailablility of carbamazepine in man. Drug Dev Ind Pharm 1995;21:1901–6.

62 Perlman BB. Interaction between lithium salts and ispaghula husk. Lancet 1990;335:416.

63 Walker AF, Marakis G, Simpson E, et. al. Hypotensive effects of hawthorn for patients with diabetes taking prescription drugs: a randomised controlled trial. Br J Gen Pract 2006;56(527):437–43.

64 Sierra M, Garcia JJ, Fernandez N, et. al. Therapeutic effects of psyllium in type 2 diabetic patients. Eur J Clin Nutr 2002;56:830–42.

65 Ziai SA, Larijani B, Akhoondzadeh S, et. al. Psyllium decreased serum glucose and glycosylated hemoglobin significantly in diabetic outpatients. J Ethnopharmacol 2005;102:202–7.

66 Yeh GY, Eisenberg DM, Kaptchuk TJ, et. al. Systematic review of herbs and dietary supplements for glycemic control in diabetes. Diabetes Care 2003;26:1277–94.

67 Kiefer D, Pantuso T. Panax ginseng. Am Fam Physician. 2003;68(8):1539–42.

68 Shimizu K Ozeki M, Tanaka K, et. al. Suppression of glucose absorption by some fraction extracted from gymnema silvestre leaves. J Vet Med Sci. 1997;59:245–262.

69 Inayat-Ur-Rahman, Malik SA, et. al. Serum sialic acid changes in non-insulin-dependant diabetes mellitus (NIDDM) patients following bitter melon(Momordica charantia) and rosiglitazone (Avandia)treatment. Phytomedicine 2009 Apr 9.

70 [No authors listed] Momordica charanti a (bitter melon). Monograph. Altern Med Rev 2007;12(4):360–3.

71 Raju J, Gupta D, Rao AR, et. al. Trigonellafoenum graecum (fenugreek) seed powder improves glucose homeostasis in alloxan diabetic rat tissues by reversing the altered glycolytic, gluconeogenic and lipogenic enzymes. Mol Cell Biochem 2001;224(1–2):45–51.

72 Van den Bout-van den Beukel CJ, Koopmans PP, et. al. Possible drug-metabolism interactions of medicinal herbs with antiretroviral agents. Drug Metab Rev 2006;38(3):477–514.

73 Lee LS, Andrade AS, Flexner C. Interactions between natural health products and antiretroviral drugs: pharmacokinetic and pharmacodynamic effects. Clin Infect Dis 2006;43:1052–9.

74 Gallicano K, Foster B, Choudhri S. Effect of short-term administration of garlic supplements on single-dose ritonavir pharmacokinetics in healthy volunteers. Br J Clin Pharmacol 2003;55:199–202.

75 Mills E, Montori V, Perri D, et. al. Natural health product–HIV drug interactions: a systematic review. Int J STD AIDS 2005;16:181–6.

76 van den Bout-van den Beukel CJ, Koopmans PP, et. al. Possible drug-metabolism interactions of medicinal herbs with antiretroviral agents. Drug Metab Rev 2006;38:477–514.

77 Chauhan AK, Dobhal MP, Joshi BC. A review of medicinal plants showing anticonvulsant activity. Ethnopharmacol 1988;22(1):11–23.

78 Epilepsy Society of Southern New York in the US. Online. Available: www.essny.org/images/Herbalchart.pdf (accessed April 2009).

79 Elferink JGR. Epilepsy and its treatment in the ancient cultures of America. Epilepsia 1999;40: 1041–1046.
80 Kim IJ, Kang JK, Lee SA. Factors contributing to the use of complementary and alternative medicine by people with epilepsy. Epilepsy Behav 2006;8: 620–624.
81 Lai CW, Huang X, Lai YHC, Zhang Z, Liu G, Yang MZ. A survey of public awareness, understanding and attitudes toward epilepsy in Henan province, China. Epilepsia 1990;31:182–7.
82 Dalla Corte CL, Fachinetto R,Colle D, et. al. Potentially adverse interactions between haloperidol and valerian. Food Chem Toxicol 2008;46(7): 2369–75.
83 Grunze H, Langosch J, Schirrmacher K, et. al. Kava pyrones exert effects on neuronal transmission and transmembraneous cation currents similar to established mood stabilizers--a review. Prog Neuropsychopharmacol Biol Psychiatry 2001;25(8):1555–70.
84 Ernst E. St John's Wort supplements endanger the success of organ transplantation. Arch Surg 2002;137(3):316–9.
85 Chiang HM, Fang SH, Wen KC, et. al. Life-threatening interaction between the root extract of Pueraria lobata and methotrexate in rats. Toxicol Appl Pharmacol 2005;209(3):263–8.
86 Kennedy J, Wang CC, Wu CH. Patient Disclosure about Herb and Supplement Use among Adults in the US. Evid Based Complement Alternat Med 2008;5(4):451–6.
87 Gardiner P, Graham RE, Legedza AT, et. al. Factors associated with dietary supplement use among prescription medication users. Arch Intern Med 2006;166:1968–74.

Chapter 38

Adverse reactions to complementary medicines (CMs)

Introduction

The definition of adverse drug reaction is defined as a 'response to a medicine which is noxious and unintended, and which occurs at doses normally used in man'.[1] Overall the risk associated with CMs is generally low considering widespread community use. In Australia, the Therapeutic Goods Administration (TGA) define CMs as 'medicinal products containing herbs, vitamins, minerals, and nutritional supplements, homoeopathic medicines and certain aromatherapy products are referred to as 'complementary medicines'.[2] These are regulated as medicines under the Therapeutics Goods Act 1989i (the Act). CMs also comprise traditional medicines, including traditional Chinese medicines, Ayurvedic medicines and Australian indigenous medicines. See Figure 38.1 for classes of CMs.

According to the TGA, data from adverse events reported to the Australian Drug Reactions Advisory Committee (ADRAC) arising from the use of listed CMs from 2004 to 2008, for example, shows that there were a total of 656 total reports where a CM was the sole suspected possible, probable or certain cause of an adverse patient reaction, with 7 possible death outcomes associated with a CM. During the same period there were 38 337 cases where a medicine (prescription, over-the-counter medication and other products registered on the Australian register of therapeutic goods (ARTG) included registered rather than listed CMs) was the sole suspected possible, probable or certain cause of an adverse patient reaction, and there were 1014 possible death outcomes.[3] In many cases the contribution of the suspected medicine to the death is uncertain, however, based on the information reported it is not possible to entirely exclude the possibility that the suspected medicine contributed to the fatal outcome.

Based on these statistics, the level of reporting for CMs is relatively low compared with pharmaceuticals, considering the widespread usage and the complex diversity of CMs that can be found in Australia, the US and other countries. There may be a number of factors contributing to this, other than having a relatively favourable safety profile (not necessarily efficacy). Other factors include significant under-reporting due to patients failing to communicate adverse events to their medical practitioner and their use of CMs, and medical and allied health practitioners failing to report adverse events to the relevant adverse reporting systems available in each country such as ADRAC in Australia or the FDA in the United States. For example the hepatotoxicity associated with herbal remedies, and naturally occurring plants is extensively under-reported. Hepatotoxicity under-reporting may relate to undetectable subclinical liver disease with mildly abnormal liver chemistry tests thereby endowing many medicinal plants and herbal medicines with a potential for hepatotoxicity with extended use or with overdosing (see Table 38.1).

Knowledge of CM adverse reactions

From the Australian National Prescribing Service (NPS) study, it is clear there is an urgent need for medical practitioners such as General Practitioners to learn more about adverse reactions with CMs.[4] About 40% of general practitioners reported having minimal or no knowledge about black cohosh and *ginkgo biloba*, and less than 40% of the surveyed GPs were aware of some potential side-effects and drug–CM interactions of *ginkgo biloba*, glucosamine and black

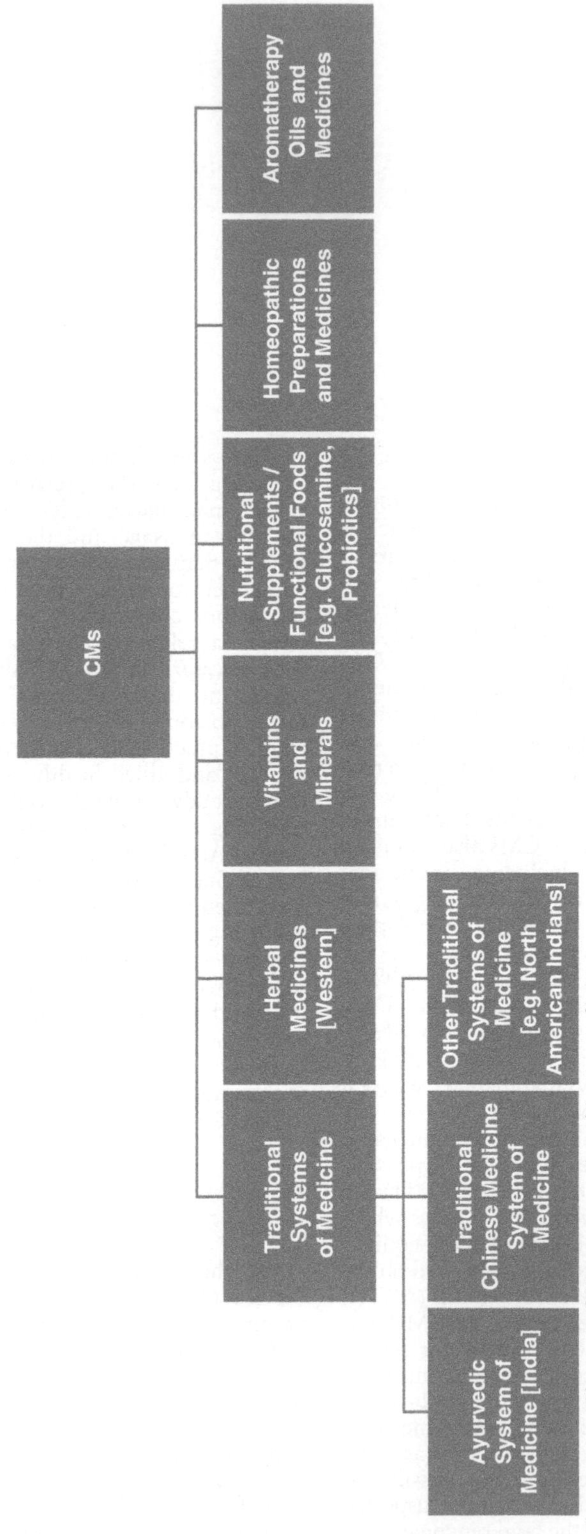

Figure 38.1 Classes of CMs encountered in Australia
(Source: adapted and modified from TGA report http://www.tga.gov.au/DOCS/pdf/cmreport.pdf)

Table 38.1 Hepatotoxicity of medicinal plants and herbal medicines

Potentially hepatotoxic	Unlikely hepatotoxic
Ackee fruit	Aloe vera/*Aloe Barbadensis*
Mediterranean glue thistle/*Atractylis gummifera*	Chamomille/*Anthemis nobilis*
Azadirachta indica	Cranberry/*Vaccinium macrocarpon*
Bajiaolian	
Berberis vulgaris	**Dandelion root/*Taraxacum Officinale***
Black cohosh/*Cimicifuga racemosa*	Feverfew/*Tanacetum parthenium*
Impila/*Callilepsis laureola*	Garlic/*Allium sativum*
Camphor	Ginger/*Zingiber Officinale*
Cascara sagrada	*Gingko Biloba*
Carp gallbladder	Ginseng/*Panax ginseng*
Senna/*Cassia angustifolia*	Goldenseal/*Hydrastis canadensis*
Greater celandine/*Chelidonium majus*	Peppermint/*Mentha piperita*
	St John's Wort/*Hypericum perforatum*
Chinese herbal medicines	Saw Palmetto/*Serenoa repens*
– *Lycopodium serratum/Jin Bu Huan*	
– *Ma-huang Shou-Wu-Pian (Polygonum multiflorum)*	
– *Syo-saiko-to (Xiao-chai-hu-tang)*	
– *Coptis chinensis (Huang lian)*	
– *T'u-san-chi (Compositae)* also a pyrrolizidine alkaloid	
– Green tea extract/*Camellia sinensis*	
Cocaine/*Erythroxylon coca*	
Copaltra	
Cycasin	
Germander/*Teucrium chamaedrys*	
Kava Kava/*Piper methysticum*	
Kombucha mushroom	
Isabgol	
Chapparal; Creosote bush; Greasewood/*Larrea tridentata*	
Lipokinetix	
Hedeoma pulegoides, Mentha pulegium (Pennyroyal)	
Plants/herbs containing pyrrolizidine alkaloids	
– Crotalaria	
– *Heliotropium*	
– Paraquay tea/*Mate*	
– Senecio	
– Comfrey/*Symphytum officinale*	
– Coltsfoot/*Tussilago farfara*	
Sassafras/*Sassafras albidum*	
Skull cap/*Scutellaria lateriflora*	
Shark cartilage	
Felty germander/*Teucrium polium*	
Valerian/*Valeriana officinalis*	
Horse chestnut leaf/*Venencapsan*	
Mistletoe/*Viscum album*	

(Source: adapted and modified from Steadman,[5] Chiturri & Farrell,[6] Ernst,[7] Teschke et. al.,[8] and Schiano[9]) cohosh.[4] Only 38% of GPs were aware that black cohosh has been linked to liver damage despite an ADRAC report published in 2005.[2, 10] This highlights a concern that needs to be addressed through better education about risks associated with CMs and the need to report adverse reports for CMs, especially as there is widespread community use with up to one-quarter of Australians using at least 1 medicinal herb and two-thirds are using some form of CM within the last 12 months of national surveys.[11, 12]

Types of adverse reactions

Idiosyncratic versus non-idiosyncratic reactions

Adverse reactions to any drugs and complementary medicines can be described as *idiosyncratic* reactions involving IgE (type 1 hypersensitivity) such as hepatic reaction or anaphylaxis or allergic reaction, or *non-idiosyncratic* — those that can be expected to occur, interfere with absorption, are dose and duration dependent such as additive effects, overdoses (intentional or unintentional), interactional (e.g. stimulation of cytochrome P450). Potentially any CM can cause an *idiosyncratic* reaction in a sensitive individual at any dosage.

Pharmacodynamic versus pharmacokinetic reactions

Medicine interactions can also be described as pharmacodynamic or pharmacokinetic. Pharmacodynamic reactions are usually complex where medicines can interfere with absorption, metabolism by enzymes such as cytochrome P450 and renal excretion affecting another medicine. Pharmacokinetic interactions involve additive of similar medicines or a cancelling effect.[13]

Common interactions

Most common potential interactions were for pharmaceuticals: aspirin, warfarin, ticlodipine, plus CMs: garlic, gingko, glucosamine, or fish oil potentially resulting in increased risk of bleeding.[14]

Extemporaneous herbs such as Ayurvedic and Traditional Chinese Medicine may be contaminated by heavy metals such as lead, arsenic and mercury, potentially causing metal toxicity[15–18] or contaminated with pharmaceuticals such as steroids or hormones, particularly those imported from overseas countries that have poor regulatory guidelines.[19]

For more detailed information about herb–nutrient–drug interactions, please refer to Chapter 37. A number of papers have explored potential herb drug interactions but adequate research and understanding in this area is still lacking.[20–25]

Reactions to excipients

A reaction can also occur with excipients found in CM products that are not stated on a label. These may include antiadherents (e.g. magnesium stereate), binders (e.g. starches/sugars/cellulose), coatings (e.g. corn protein such as zein), disintegrants (e.g. sodium starch glycolate), fillers/diluents (e.g. vegetable oils, cellulose), flavours (e.g. mint, licorice, vanilla), colours, glidants (e.g. silicon dioxide), lubricants (e.g. vegetable stearin, magnesium stearate), preservatives (e.g. vitamins A, E, sodium citrate), sorbents, or sweeteners (e.g. cough syrup).

Risk factors for adverse reactions

It is important to note that elderly, children, pregnant and lactating women may respond differently to adverse reactions as the physiology and metabolism varies with their weight, age, and many other factors that affect medication dosages.[26] The elderly are particularly prone to adverse reactions as they are more likely to suffer a comorbid disease such as a chronic disease, have some degree of renal and hepatic impairment, low muscle mass, are prone to dehydration especially at times of suffering diarrhoea, and are often taking other medication which puts them at higher risk of herb–drug interactions. Adverse reactions can also be determined by genetic differences which explain why some populations are more prone to reactions. This is known as pharmacogenetics. This phenomenon is recognised with pharmaceuticals but not well recognised with CMs to date.[27]

Table 38.2 summarises likely adverse reactions reported in the literature and to adverse reporting bodies for CMs at the time of writing this chapter.

Table 38.2 Common adverse reaction(s) to CMs

Common name/ scientific name	Administration (e.g. oral or topical)	Type of reaction: idiosyncratic 'I' or non-idiosyncratic 'NIR'	Restrictions or warnings in Australia/ comments
Nutritional supplements			
Vitamins			
Vitamin A	Oral	NIR Toxicity — Hypervitaminosis A — nausea, vomiting, diarrhoea, irritability, drowsiness, dizziness, delirium, coma, raised intracranial pressure, headache (swelling of the optic disc, bulging eyeballs, visual disturbances).	Avoid high doses for prolonged periods of time especially in children. Warning label recommendation in Australia:[28] '1. *The recommended adult daily intake of vitamin A from all sources is 700 μg retinol equivalents for women, and 900 μg retinol equivalents for men.* 2. *WARNING — When taken in excess of 3 000 μg retinol equivalents, vitamin A may cause birth defects.* 3. *If you are pregnant, or considering becoming pregnant, do not take vitamin A supplements without consulting your doctor or pharmacist.'*
Vitamin B3 Niacin Nicotinic acid	Oral	**NIR** Hot flushes (common side-effect), aspirin may also reduce flushing; erythema, sweating. Liver impairment.	Contraindicated: can aggravate gout. Check liver function test. Avoid slow release due to its association with liver toxicity.
Vitamin B6 Pyridoxine Pyridoxal Pyridoxamine	Oral, injection	NIR Neurotoxicity — peripheral neuropathy, burning or electric shock feelings, pins and needles, loss of sensation. Overuse of single vitamin products; avoid use of multiple single-vitamin products (e.g. oral and injectable forms of vitamin B6) or concomitant use of multivitamin products could result in some patients routinely exceeding the upper limit for vitamins associated with severe toxicity. Toxicity in high doses of vitamin B6 includes peripheral neuropathy, such as tingling, burning and numbness of limbs.	Avoid overuse of vitamin B6 (oral or injectable) doses 50mg or above daily.[29, 30] Label warning statement for products containing from 50 to 200mg vitamin B6 (pyridoxine, pyridoxal, pyridoxamine) per recommended daily dose be amended as follows.[30] For single ingredient products: '*WARNING — Stop taking this medication if you experience tingling, burning or numbness and see your healthcare practitioner as soon as possible.'* For multi-ingredient products: '*WARNING — Stop taking this medication if you experience tingling, burning or numbness and see your healthcare practitioner as soon as possible. Contains vitamin B6.'*

(Table 38.2 cont'd)

Vitamin C Ascorbic acid	Oral Intravenous	**NIR** Laxative, gastrointestinal upset in high doses. Common side-effects with high doses: nausea, heartburn, abdominal cramps and diarrhoea. Aggravation of renal impairment especially in patients with renal failure.[31] Intra-renal oxalate crystal formation (oxalosis) in response to high dose vitamin C (oral or intravenous).	*Precautions:* renal impairment, renal calculi, iron overload, haemochromatosis, thalassaemia, leukaemia, gout especially in high doses and prolonged use. Contraindications: can increase iron absorption. Use with caution if glucose-6-phosphate dehydrogenase deficiency.
Vitamin D Cholecalciferol — Vitamin D_3	Oral	**NIR** Sensitivity to vitamin D supplementation. Check serum levels to avoid vitamin D toxicity.	Potentially vitamin D may reduce the effectiveness of Calcium Channel Blockers. If using high doses, care in patients with systemic lupus erythmatosis, hypercalcaemia, sarcoidosis, hyperparathyroidism and patients taking digitalis.
Vitamin E	Oral	**NIR** Side-effects: nausea, vomiting, diarrhoea, sensitivity reactions; avoid high doses >200 IU daily as some research suggests increases all-cause mortality.	Contraindicated: avoid high doses before surgery; pharmaceutical medication such as warfarin especially with vitamin K deficiency, impaired coagulation, hemorrhagic stroke.
Minerals			
Calcium	Oral	**NIR** Hypercalcaemia and kidney stones in those with renal impairment, constipation, GIT upset, metallic taste in mouth.	Contraindicated: avoid if impaired renal function or renal failure. Avoid if patients with hypercalcaemia.
Iodides	Oral Injection	**NIR** Iododerma/acne. Iodine over-consumption can lead to hypo or hyperthyroidism and post-partum thyroiditis. High doses can lead to a brassy taste in mouth, increased salivation, gastric irritations plus skin lesions. Soy can inhibit iodine absorption and T_3 plus T_4 production.	Contraindicated: if thyroid problems exist use with caution.

Iron	Oral Injection	**NIR** Iron toxicity in high doses and prolonged use. Tooth discoloration if liquid (drink with straw). Skin discoloration over injection site. Side-effects: gastrointestinal irritation, abdominal pain, constipation or diarrhoea, nausea, and vomiting. Combine with vitamin C to increase iron absorption.	Contraindicated: haemochromotosis. Ensure that excess iron is not taken; can have adverse outcomes to pregnancy and interfere with absorption of zinc and calcium. Best taken at separate times if calcium and zinc supplementation required.
Gold	Topical Oral	**IR** Pityriasis rosea.	
Colloidal silver Silver	Oral, topical, nasal drops, ophthalmic drops	**NIR** Argyria (silver toxicity) fatigue, irreversible blue skin discoloration, cardiomyopathy, amnesia, incoherent speech, neurologic, cardiac, hepatic, nephrotoxic derangements.	Avoid use of colloidal silver.[33, 34, 35] Topical preparations are available and are prescribed under medical supervision.
Silver sulfadiazine	Topical creams	Silver staining or burn with silver sulfadiazine topically.[32]	
Magnesium	Oral	**NIR** Hypermagnesaemia with high doses and long term use especially if renal impairment. Common side-effects: gastrointestinal irritation, nausea, vomiting, and diarrhoea. The dosage varies from person to person. Although rare, toxic levels can cause low blood pressure, thirst, heart arrhythmia, drowsiness and weakness.	Contraindicated: avoid if renal impairment as reduced renal function may cause high blood levels of magnesium.
Potassium Potassium containing products	Oral	**NIR** Hyperkalemia	Care in patients with renal impairment. Warning statements recommended in Australia:[36] *'Contains (amount of potassium in milligrams) mg of potassium. If you have kidney disease or are taking heart or blood pressure medicines — consult your doctor or pharmacist before use. Keep out of reach of children.'*

(Table 38.2 cont'd)

Selenium	Oral	**NIR** Selenium toxicity.[37, 38] Side-effects: nausea, vomiting, rash, sensitivity reactions, toxicity in high doses; nail changes, irritability, fatigue.	Recommended warning label in Australia:[39] *'This product contains selenium which is toxic in high doses. A daily dose of 150 microgram, for adults, of selenium from dietary supplements should not be exceeded.'* Contraindicated: pregnancy, lactation, children <12 years of age; avoid yeast derived selenium if allergic to yeast.
Zinc	Oral	**NIR** Zinc toxicity Common side-effects: nausea, vomiting, metallic taste in mouth.	Avoid long term use and high dosage as this may cause copper deficiency, impair the immune system and cause anemia. Contraindicated: sideroblastic anemia, above normal blood levels of zinc, severe kidney disease.
Herbal			
Andrographus *Andrographus paniculata*		**IR** Allergic reaction, anaphylaxis, shortness of breath, abdominal discomfort, erythema/rash.[40]	
Aristolochia species	Oral	**IR** Renal failure. Nephrotoxin, carcinogen, renal carcinoma.	No safe level; not permitted in Australia.
Black cohosh *Cimicifuga racemosa*	Oral	**IR** Rare: Hepatotoxicity, hepatitis, liver impairment, fulminant liver failure. Common side-effects include: gastrointestinal upset, headache, dizziness, weight gain, breast discomfort and vaginal spotting or bleeding. Long-term safety data are lacking.	Contraindicated: liver disease. Avoid in children, pregnancy and lactation. Label warnings are required in Australia:[41, 42] *'Warning: Black cohosh may harm the liver in some individuals. Use under the supervision of a healthcare professional.'* Worldwide reports of hepatotoxicity/hepatic failure associated with use of black cohosh although rare.[43, 44, 45, 46]
Cayenne *Capsicum frutescens*	Oral, topical, intranasal	**NIR** Epigastric discomfort; gastritis, gas, bloating, nausea, burning, diarrhoea, and belching; sweating, flushing, lacrimation/irritation of the eyes, sneezing, headaches, dizziness; cough nasal congestion. Topical use can cause dermatitis, burning, stinging, and erythema.	Contraindicated: sensitivity to capsicum; may increase risk of bleeding due to blood thinning effects; avoid concomitant use of herbs and supplements that affect platelet aggregation. Could theoretically increase the risk of bleeding in some people.

Cranberry Cranberry juice *Vaccinium* is a species from the ericaceous plants	Oral	**NIR** Interaction with warfarin.[47]	Contains high levels of oxalate. Avoid in patients with history of nephrolithiasis.
Chaparral (*Larrea tridentate*)	Oral	**IR** Hepatotoxicity Liver impairment.[48]	Label warnings are required in Australia:[49] '*Warning: Chaparral may harm the liver in some people. Use only under the supervision of a healthcare professional*'.
Echinacea *Echinacea purpurea* *Echinacea augustafolia*	Oral	**IR** Urticaria, allergic reaction, rarely anaphylaxis.[50]	Contraindicated: if allergy to *Compositae* family of plants (e.g. chamomile, ragweed). Caution with in asthmatics, if on immunosuppressive medications and long-term use (>8 weeks). Avoid if on immunosuppressive medication.
Elderberry *Sambucus nigra*	Oral	**IR** Allergic reaction, anaphylaxis[51]	
Feverfew *Tanacetum parthenium*	Oral	**NIR** Side-effects: mouth ulcers, allergic reactions, rashes, gastrointestinal irritation, nausea, vomiting, and diarrhoea.	Contraindicated: avoid 2 weeks prior to surgery and concomitant use with blood thinners.
Garlic *Allium sativum*	Oral Topical	**NIR** Interaction with medication such as warfarin.[52] Common side-effects: malodorous breath and body odour; mouth, stomach and gastrointestinal burning or irritation, heartburn, flatulence, nausea, vomiting and diarrhoea. May increase risk of bleeding as garlic can affect platelet function. Some people are allergic to garlic (by ingestion or even topically) and may cause asthma, runny nose, skin irritation and in rare cases severe allergic reactions.	1 study disputed findings of interaction with warfarin.[53] Contraindicated: avoid if allergic to garlic; beware if taking any blood thinning medication such as warfarin; avoid at least 2 weeks prior to any surgery to minimise risk of bleeding; avoid high doses in pregnancy and lactation.

(Table 38.2 cont'd)

Ginger *Zingiber officinale*	Oral	**NIR** Bleeding tendency. Interaction with medication such as warfarin.[54] Common side-effects: nausea, vomiting, heartburn, bloating, stomach irritation. Theoretical risk of bleeding increased with warfarin and antiplatelet drugs.	Avoid use with warfarin. Contraindicated: use with caution if heartburn or gastric ulcers present.
Gingko *Gingko biloba*	Oral	**NIR** Bleeding tendency. Interaction with medication such as warfarin.[14]	Study demonstrates no effect on coagulation.[55] Interaction with warfarin.
Ginseng Panax ginseng Korean ginseng	Oral	**NIR** Interaction with warfarin.[14] Insomnia; even more rarely and with higher doses; breast discomfort, vaginal bleeding, amenorrhea, tachycardia and palpitations.	Contraindicated: avoid stimulants such as excess caffeine and nicotine.
Ginseng American ginseng	Oral	**NIR** May cause gastrointestinal, nervous and hormonal effects, e.g. breast discomfort or vaginal bleeding.	Contraindication: avoid stimulants such as excess caffeine and nicotine.
Greater Celandine *Chelidonum majus*	Oral	**IR** Hepatotoxicity, liver impairment.	Label warnings are required in Australia:[56] '*Warning: Greater Celandine may harm the liver in some people. Use only under the supervision of a healthcare professional.*'
Green tea extract *Camellia sinensis*	Oral	**IR** Hepatitis/liver failure.[57,58,59,60]	In 2003 French and Spanish authorities suspended market authorisation of Exolise, a weight loss product containing green tea extract. Green tea extract should never be taken on an empty stomach. This can increase the risk of liver toxicity. The food supplement Hydroxycut, which contains green tea extract, was removed from sale in New Zealand, Canada and the United States, due to concerns over liver toxicity, seizures, cardiovascular disorders and muscle damage.
Guarana *Paullinia cupana*	Oral	**NIR** Caffeine toxicity, palpitations, tremor, insomnia, agitation.	

Hawthorn berries *Crataegus oxycantha*	Oral	**NIR** May cause fatigue, headache, sweating, arryhthmias, palpitations, dizziness and vertigo.	Contraindicated: pregnancy and lactation; arrhythmias.
Hops *Humulus lupulus*	Oral	**IR, NIR** Side-effects: allergic reactions, drowsiness, dizziness, reduced concentration and alertness following morning. May exacerbate depression.	Contraindicated: young children, pregnancy and lactating mothers. Avoid concomitant use with alcohol, analgesia or hypnotic medication. Depression. Avoid at least 2 weeks before surgery.
Kava Kava *Piper methysticum*	Oral — ethanolic form	**IR** Hepatitis, hepatic impairment, fulminant liver failure.[61, 62]	Contraindicated: pregnancy, lactation, endogenous depression, elderly, those with previous liver problems. Ethanolic form of kava kava linked to hepatotoxic effects is not permitted in Australia. Reports of hepatotoxicity and deaths from liver failure associated with high doses and ethanolic extracts of kava-containing medicines. Following a Therapeutic Goods Administration safety review of kava-containing medicines,[63] there is a limit on the maximum amount of kavalactones (a group of constituents found in Piper methysticum) at 125mg permitted per dosage form (tablet or a capsule), with a maximum daily dose of no more than 250mg of kavalactones.
			Warning labels required in Australia:[64] '*May harm the liver; if symptoms persist seek advice from healthcare practitioner*'. Not for prolonged use. Not recommended for use in pregnancy and lactating women and to stop using the product if they develop adverse liver symptoms.
Licorice *Glychyrriza glabra* *Glychyrriza uralensis*	Oral	**NIR** Hypokalemia, fluid retention, hypertension.	Warning labels recommended in Australia:[65] '*Contains Licorice. Not suitable for people with kidney disease, a history of high blood pressure or during pregnancy*'.
Polygonum *Polygonum multiflorum*	Oral	**IR** Hepatotoxicity, liver impairment	Label warnings are required in Australia:[66] '*Warning: Polygonum multiflorum may harm the liver in some people. Use only under the supervision of a healthcare professional.*'

(Table 38.2 cont'd)

Red clover *Trifolium pratense*	Oral	**NIR** Very mild and rare side-effects: headache, nausea, phytoestrogen activity may stimulate estrogenic receptors causing breast discomfort, heavy menstrual bleeding, vaginal spotting and endometrial hyperplasia (although unlikely). Long-term safety data on individual isoflavones or isoflavone concentrates are not available.	Contraindicated: more evidence is required to determine effect of red clover on patients with existing hormone sensitive cancers such as breast and uterine. Due to its coumarin content, red clover may increase the risk of bleeding. Avoid use 2 weeks prior to surgery.
St John's wort *Hypericum perforatum*	Oral	**NIR** Serotonin syndrome, when used with other anti-depressants. Drug interaction due to stimulation of CYP 450. Common side-effects: very mild and rare such as photosensitivity skin rash, digestion disturbance, dizziness, fatigue, dry mouth.	Avoid high doses, use with other antidepressants (eg SSRIs) or tramadol, medication cleared by the CYP 450 pathway e.g. oral contraceptive pill.[52, 67, 68] Label warnings in place about herb–drug interaction.[69] Recommended warning label in Australia:[70] *'St John's wort affects the way many prescription medicines work, including the oral contraceptive pill. Consult your doctor.'* Contraindicated: pregnancy, lactation, fertility, drug interaction; avoid use with most pharmaceutical medication such as the oral contraceptive pill, other antidepressants, anti-epileptic medication.
Saw Palmetto *Serenoa repens*	Oral	**NIR** Side-effects: abdominal pain, diarrhoea, dyspepsia, nausea, fatigue, headache, decreased libido, erectile dysfunction, gynecomastia and rhinitis.[71]	Contraindicated: pregnancy, lactation, children, fertility, drug interaction; avoid use with pharmaceutical medication such as the anticoagulants (warfarin, aspirin, non-steroidal medication), oral contraceptive pill, androgens, estrogens, immune stimulants.
Senna (*Cassia senna*)	Oral	**NIR** Gastrointestinal discomfort, nausea, abdominal pain. **IR** Rarely hepatic impairment.	Warning on labels in Australia: '*Do not use when abdominal pain, nausea or vomiting is present, if you are pregnant or breast feeding. Seek medical advice before taking this product*'.
Soy phytoestrogen supplements	Oral	**NIR** Side-effects: transient abdominal discomfort; theoretically may stimulate estrogenic receptors causing breast discomfort, heavy menstrual bleeding and endometrial hyperplasia. Soy can inhibit iodine absorption and T_3 plus T_4 production.	Contraindicated: more evidence is required to determine effect of soy on patients with existing hormone sensitive cancers such as breast and uterine.

Turmeric *Curcumin longa*	Oral, Topical	**NIR** Side-effects: gastrointestinal upset e.g. nausea, stomach pains, vomiting, diarrhoea; sensitivity reactions; blood clotting problems; rash when applied topically to skin.	Contraindicated: pregnancy, lactation, children, pharmaceutical medication such as anticoagulant and anti-platelet drugs e.g. aspirin, warfarin, clopidogrel; discontinue turmeric at least 2 weeks before elective surgical procedures.
Valerian *Valerian officinalis*	Oral	**NIR** Side-effects: may cause paradoxical hyperactivity reaction, agitation, restlessness, hyperactivity, insomnia. May cause drowsiness, dizziness, reduced concentration and alertness the following morning. **IR** Liver impairment rare.	Contraindicated: young children, pregnancy and lactating mothers. Avoid concomitant use with alcohol, analgesia or hypnotic medication.
White willow bark *Salix alba*	Oral	**IR** Allergic reaction especially if allergy to salicylates or aspirin; aggravation of asthma.	Contraindicated: avoid allergic or sensitivity to salicylates/ aspirin.
Other CM supplements			
Bee pollen **Royal Jelly**	Oral	**IR** Anaphylaxis, allergic reaction.	Avoid if asthmatic or suffer allergies to bees or its products. Warning labels required in Australia:[72] '*Not to be taken by asthma and allergy sufferers** **Royal jelly may cause severe allergic reactions and in rare cases, fatalities, especially in asthma and allergy sufferers*'.
Co Enzyme Q_{10}	Oral	**NIR** Increased bleeding tendency and INR with warfarin.[73]	Avoid use with warfarin.
Evening Primrose Oil	Oral	**NIR** Propensity to seizures in epileptics. Often well tolerated especially if taken with meals. Very mild and rare side-effects, e.g. gastrointestinal upset; allergic reactions e.g. rash, breathing problems.	Contraindicated: avoid if you suffer epilepsy or seizures.

(Table 38.2 cont'd)

Fish oils Fish oils Krill oil (*Euphausia superba*) Green-lipped muscle extract Omega 3 and essential fatty acids derived from fish oils	Oral	**IR** Allergic reaction if seafood allergy. **NIR** Often well tolerated especially if taken with meals. Very mild and rare side-effects, e.g. gastrointestinal upset; allergic reactions e.g. rash, breathing problems if allergic to seafood; blood thinning effects in very high doses >10gm daily (may need to stop fish oil supplements 2 weeks prior to surgery).	Avoid if seafood allergy. *Warning label required if sourced from seafood.* Drug interactions: caution when taking high doses of fish oils >4 grams per day together with warfarin (your doctor will check your INR test).
Glucosamine May be derived from: Seafood Bovine Vegetables — corn Glucosamine sulfate-potassium chloride complex	Oral Topical	**NIR** Bleeding tendency. Allergic reaction if seafood allergy. Skin reactions including erythematous rash, angioedema, urticaria, rash, pruritis.[74] Dyspnoea, oedema, asthma, anaphylaxis. **NIR** Hyperkalemia especially in patients with renal disease or taking cardiac medication or antihypertensives.	Avoid use with warfarin and in blood disorders, or any disease associated with bleeding e.g. colitis.[75,76,77] *Label warning if derived from seafood.*[78] Recommended warning label if contains potassium in Australia:[79] '*Contains potassium. If you have kidney disease or are taking heart or blood pressure medicines, consult your doctor or pharmacist before use. Keep out of reach of children*'.
Melatonin	Oral	**NIR** Side-effects: drowsiness, dizziness, depressive symptoms, reduced alertness, irritability, headaches; symptoms can be transient.	Contraindicated: young children, pregnant, lactating mothers; epilepsy; taken with alcohol, sedating medication such as benzodiazepines and use with narcotics; depression.
Red Yeast rice extract	Oral	**NIR, IR** Statin side-effects such as muscle aches and pains, fatigue, weakness, falls. Side-effects: abdominal discomfort, heartburn, flatulence and dizziness; liver impairment like cholesterol lowering drugs (statins).	Note contains small quantities of naturally occurring lovastatin. Contraindicated: if hypersensitive to this rice extract; pregnancy and nursing mothers; active liver disease.

SAMe **s-adenosyl methionine**	Oral	**NIR** very mild and rare side-effects: additive effect with other sedating medication and anti-depressants.	Contraindicated: pregnancy, lactation, fertility, bipolar disorder, drug interaction; avoid use with other antidepressants.
Tyrosine	Oral	**NIR** Tyrosine (derived from phenyalanine in food) converts to L-Dopa, then to dopamine and noradrenaline. Consequently it can raise blood pressure.	Contraindicated adrenal disorder, hypertension, when taking antihypertensives.
Essential oils			
Peppermint oil	Oral	**NIR** Side-effects mild and rare: heartburn; stomach upset; peri-anal itch; sensitivity to herb; burning mouth.	Contraindicated: diarrhoea, drug interaction; avoid use with pharmaceutical medication such as anti-ulcer medication.
Eucalyptus oil **Tea tree oil** ***(melaleuca oil)*** **Lavender oil**	Topical Inhalation	**NIR** Skin irritation, rash. Dyspnoea/cough if inhaled; irritation of eyes/nose from fumes.	Contraindications: avoid oral ingestion of oils and always dilute with inactive ingredient. Sample preparation on skin first (patch test) prior to widespread use on the body, especially in babies and young children. Avoid application to eyes or nostrils.

Reporting adverse events

It is imperative that all health practitioners (medical and non-medical) report any *suspected* adverse reactions or interactions to medicines/pharmaceuticals, including CMs, over-the-counter medicines, any traditional or alternative remedies and vaccines, including those suspected of causing death, hospital admission, requiring more treatment and investigations or suspected birth defects if a mother takes a medicine during pregnancy.[80] These reports are analysed by experts using the World Health Organization (WHO) causality assessment algorithm *to determine level of causality of a suspected medicine(s)* (see Who algorithm below). Reporting of adverse reactions provides information that can be gathered for any emerging medicine safety issues and allows further action in each country or internationally to be taken if necessary. Action may include restricting use of the medicine or enforce relevant label warnings and for media alerts to warn the community of concerns.

Reporting systems are in place in many developed countries. These are summarised in Table 38.3.

Table 38.3 International reporting schemes

Country and publications	Mechanism for reporting
Australia Medicines Safety Update (having replaced ADRAC bulletins) in Australian prescriber regularly report common or serious adverse reactions to CMs. To subscribe, go to: www.tga.gov.au/adr/msu/msu1006.htm	Reports of suspected adverse drug reactions are best made by using a prepaid reporting form ('blue card') which is available from the website: http://www.tga.gov.au/adr/bluecard.pdf or from the Adverse Drug Reactions Unit of the Office of Safety Monitoring, phone no: 02-6232-8744. Reports can also be submitted electronically, by going to the TGA website http://www.tga.gov.au and clicking on the 'report problems' tab on the left, by fax: 02-6232-8392, or email: ADR.Reports@tga.gov.au,or by filling in the blue card and posting to ADRAC. Ensure you provide the AUST-L or AUST-R for the CM which is found on the label. This helps the TGA identify the product and its ingredients.
New Zealand Prescriber update bulletin MEDSAFE — New Zealand medicines and medical devices safety authority, a business unit of the ministry of health. Online. Available: www.medsafe.govt.nz Healthcare professionals with any questions on access or availability of the electronic reporting tool should contact BPAC on (03) 477 5418. Prescribers are encouraged to report reactions to the Centre for Adverse Reactions Monitoring (CARM). An electronic version of Prescriber Update is available at: www.medsafe.govt.nz/profs/PUarticles.asp To receive Prescriber Update electronically, register at: www.medsafe.govt.nz/profs.htm Data sheets, consumer medicine information, media releases, medicine classification issues, and adverse reaction forms can be found at: www.medsafe.govt.nz	Report all adverse events occurring with IMMP medicines to: IMMP, NZ Pharmacovigilance Centre, PO Box 913, Dunedin 9054. Use the reporting form provided with each edition of *MIMS New Ethicals* or download it from either the NZ Pharmacovigilance Centre or Medsafe websites: www.otago.ac.nz/carm or www.medsafe.govt.nz/Profs/adverse.htm Further information on IMMP is available at: http://carm.otago.ac.nz/index.asp?link=immp Please report all cases of the following adverse reactions to: CARM, NZ Pharmacovigilance Centre, PO Box 913, Dunedin 9054. Use the reporting form provided with each edition of *MIMS New Ethicals*, or download the form from the CARM or Medsafe web sites: www.otago.ac.nz/carm or www.medsafe.govt.nz/Profs/adverse.htm

Continued

Table 38.3 International reporting schemes—cont'd

Country and publications	Mechanism for reporting
Canada Canada Vigilance Program Phone: 866 234-2345 Fax: 866 678-6789 Online: www.healthcanada.gc.ca/medeffect Health Canada Marketed Health Products Directorate AL 0701C Ottawa ON K1A 0K9 Tel: 613 954-6522 Fax: 613 952-7738	Report an adverse reaction to the Canada Vigilance Program: • by calling toll-free at 1-866-234-2345 • by reporting online at www.healthcanada.gc.ca/medeffect • by completing a form that you can send by: • postage-paid mail or • fax toll-free to 1-866-678-6789 The form and postage-paid label are available at www.healthcanada.gc.ca/medeffect or by calling 1-866-234-2345. The adverse reaction reporting form is also available at the back of the *Compendium of Pharmaceuticals and Specialties* (*CPS*). Reporting Adverse Reactions Canada Vigilance Program Phone: 866 234-2345 Fax: 866 678-6789 Online: www.healthcanada.gc.ca/medeffect
United Kingdom Medicine and Healthcare products Regulatory Agency (UK) www.mhra.gov.uk/mhra/drugsafetyupdate Sign up to receive an email alert when a new issue is published: email registration@mhradrugsafety.org.uk The Medicines and Healthcare Products Regulatory Agency is the government agency which is responsible for ensuring that medicines and medical devices work, and are acceptably safe. The Commission on Human Medicines gives independent advice to ministers about the safety, quality, and efficacy of medicines. The Commission is supported in its work by expert advisory groups that cover various therapeutic areas of medicine.	The Yellow Card Scheme collects information on suspected adverse drug reactions in the UK. See www.yellowcard.gov.uk
United States MedWatch Website is available to the public to voluntarily report a serious adverse event, product quality problem, product use error, or therapeutic inequivalence/failure that they suspect is associated with the use of an FDA-regulated drug, biologic, medical device, dietary supplement or cosmetic. Food and Drug Administration (USA) Contact details: 10903 New Hampshire Ave Silver Spring, MD 20993-0002 or by telephone. The main FDA phone number for general inquiries: 1-888-INFO-FDA (1-888-463-6332) Website: http://www.fda.gov/AboutFDA/ContactFDA/default.htm	Reporting an adverse reaction: Phone 1-800-332-1088 FAX: 1-800-FDA-0178 Electronic reporting: https://www.accessdata.fda.gov/scripts/medwatch/medwatch-online.htm Postage: MedWatch 5600 Fishers Lane Rockville, MD 20852-9787

Country and publications	Mechanism for reporting
Europe/World Health Organization (WHO) Data from the WHO Collaborating Centre for International Drug Monitoring WHO definition of traditional medicine (TM). The Uppsala Monitoring Centre (the UMC) is the fieldname of the WHO Collaborating Centre for International Drug Monitoring, responsible for the management of the WHO Programme for International Drug Monitoring. An independent centre of scientific excellence, the UMC, offers products and services, derived from the WHO database of Adverse Drug Reactions (ADRs) reported from member countries of the WHO program.	**The UPPSALA Monitoring CENTRE (Sweden)** Mail address: Box 1051 SE-751 40 Uppsala Sweden Visiting address only: Bredgränd 7 SE-753 20 Uppsala Sweden Telephone: +46 18 65 60 60 Fax: +46 18 65 60 88 Email: (general enquiries) info@who-umc.org (sales and marketing enquiries) info@umc-products.com (Drug Dictionary enquires) drugdictionary@umc-products.com Internet: www.who-umc.org
Germany **Federal Institute for Drugs and Medical Devices, Bundesinstitut fu¨r Arzneimittel und Medizinprodukte (BfArM)** The BfArM is a federal institute within the portfolio of the Federal Ministry of Health. Website: http://www.bfarm.de/EN/Home/homepage__node.html	Address: Bundesinstitut für Arzneimittel und Medizinprodukte Kurt-Georg-Kiesinger-Allee 3 D-53175 Bonn, Germany Telephone: +49 (0)228 99-307-0 Telefax: +49 (0)228 99-307-5207 Email: poststelle@bfarm.de

World Health Organization causality assessment

Use the following WHO assessment of adverse reports by experts to determine the level of causality of a suspected medicine(s).[81]

Causality Assessment Algorithm

Certain

A clinical event, including laboratory test abnormality, occurring in a plausible time relationship to drug administration, and which cannot be explained by concurrent disease or other drugs or chemicals. The response to withdrawal of the drug (de-challenge) should be clinically plausible. The event must be definitive pharmacologically or phenomenologically, using a satisfactory rechallenge procedure if necessary.

Probable/Likely

A clinical event, including laboratory test abnormality, with a reasonable time sequence to administration of the drug, unlikely to be attributed to concurrent disease or other drugs or chemicals, and which follows a clinically reasonable response on withdrawal (de-challenge). Rechallenge information is not required to fulfil this definition.

Possible

A clinical event, including laboratory test abnormality, with a reasonable time sequence to administration of the drug, but which could also be explained by concurrent disease or other drugs or chemicals. Information on drug withdrawal may be lacking or unclear.

Unlikely

A clinical event, including laboratory test abnormality, with a temporal relationship to drug administration which makes a causal relationship improbable, and in which other drugs, chemicals or underlying disease provide plausible explanations.

Conditional/unclassified

A clinical event, including laboratory test abnormality, reported as an adverse reaction, about which more data are essential for a proper assessment or the additional data are under examination.

Unassessable/unclassifiable

A report suggesting an adverse reaction which cannot be judged because information is insufficient or contradictory, and which cannot be supplemented or verified.

Comments on the Causality Assessment Algorithm

General

While various causality terms are in use, the terms in this algorithm are the ones used most widely among countries participating in the WHO program. Some countries do not use all the terms, and many do not believe that a classification of 'certain' is possible for a single report, while others make no distinction between 'possible' and 'probable.' These definitions have been accepted by countries who do use the terms.

While the terms 'conditional/unclassified' and 'unassessible/unclassifiable' are not causality terms per se, they describe the status of ADR reports and therefore allow for practical communication about ADR issues.

Certain

It is recognised that very few reports will meet the criteria of this stringent definition, but this definition is useful because of the special value of such reports. It is considered that time relationships between drug administration and the onset and course of the adverse event are important in causality analysis. Also important is the consideration of confounding features (i.e. the presence of other disease, drugs or chemicals). But due weight must be placed on the known pharmacological and other characteristics of the drug product being considered. Sometimes the clinical phenomena described will also be sufficiently specific to allow a confident causality assessment in the absence of confounding features and in the presence of appropriate time relationships, for example, penicillin anaphylaxis.

Probable

This definition has less stringent wording than the definition for 'certain' and does not necessitate prior knowledge of drug characteristics or clinical adverse reaction phenomena. As stated, no rechallenge information is needed, but confounding drug administration or underlying disease must be absent.

Possible

This is the definition to be used when the administration of the drug in question is just one of several possible causes of the described clinical event.

Unlikely

This definition is intended to be used when it seems most plausible that the clinical event is attributable to something other than the drug in question.

Reference

1 Safety Monitoring of Medicinal Products. Guidelines for setting up and running a Pharmacovigilance Centre. London: Uppsala Monitoring Centre-WHO Collaborating Centre for International Drug Monitoring. EQUUS; 2002. Online. Available: http://whqlibdoc.who.int/hq/2002/WHO_EDM_QSM_2002.2.pdf (accessed 14 Sept 2009).

2 Australian Government. Department of Health and Ageing. Therapeutic Goods Administration. The regulation of complementary medicines in Australia — an overview. April 2006. Online. Available: www.tga.gov.au/cm/cmreg-aust.htm (accessed 14 April 2009).

3 Statistics provided by the Office of Medicines Safety Monitoring at the Therapeutic Goods Administration, 25 March 2009. Office of Medicines Safety Monitoring adrac@tga.gov.au, Phone: 1800 044 114.

4 Brown J, Morgan T, Adams J, Grunseit A, Toms M, Roufogalis B, Kotsirilos V, Pirotta M and Williamson M. Complementary Medicines Information Use and Needs of Health Professionals: General Practitioners and Pharmacists. National Prescribing Service, Sydney, December 2008.

5 Stedman C. Herbal hepatotoxicity. Semin Liver Dis 2002;22:195.

6 Chitturi S, Farrell GC. Herbal hepatotoxicity: an expanding but poorly defined problem. J Gastroenterol Hepatol 2000;15:1093.

7 Ernst E. Harmless herbs? A review of the recent literature. Am J Med 1998;104:170.

8 Teschke R, Schwarzenböck A, Hennermann KH. Toxic liver disease due to drugs, herbs and dietary supplements: diagnostic approaches. Z Gastroenterol 2007;45(2):195–208.

9 Schiano TD. Hepatotoxicity and complementary and alternative medicines. Clin Liver Dis 2003;7: 453–73.

10 Black cohosh and liver toxicity — an update. Aust Adv Drug Reactions Bull 26(3), Jun 2007 26(3):11.

11 Zhang AL, Story DF, Lin V, Vitetta L, Xue CC. A population survey on the use of 24 common medicinal herbs in Australia. Pharmacoepidemiology and Drug Safety 2008;17:1006–13.

12 Williamson M, Tudball J, Toms M, Garden F, and Grunseit A. Information Use and Needs Of Complementary Medicines Users. National Prescribing Service, Sydney, October 2008. Online. Available: www.nps.org.au/research_and_evaluation/research/current_research/complementary_medicines/cms_users_research#KF (accessed 14 April 2009).

13 Bryant L, Fishman T. Clinically important drug-drug interactions and how to manage them. Journal of Primary Health Care 2009;1(2):150–1.

14 Elmer GW, Lafferty WE, Tyree PT, Lind BK. Potential interactions between complementary/alternative products and conventional medicines in a Medicare population. Ann Pharmacother 2007;41:1617–24.
15 Saper RB, Kales SN, Paquin J, et al. Heavy metal content of ayurvedic herbal medicine products. JAMA 2004;292(23):2868–73.
16 Traditional Indian (Ayurvedic) and Chinese medicines associated with heavy metal poisoning. Australian Adverse Drug Reactions Bulletin 2007;26(1):2.
17 Saper RB, Phillips RS, Sehgal A, et al. Lead, mercury, and arsenic in US- and Indian-manufactured Ayurvedic medicines sold via the internet. JAMA 2008;300:915–23
18 Cooper K, Noller B, Connell D, Yu J, et al. Public Health Risks from Heavy Metals and Metalloids Present in Traditional Chinese Medicines. Journal of Toxicology and Environmental Health, Part A. Current issues 2007;70:1694–9.
19 Adverse reactions to complementary medicines. Australian Adverse Drug Reactions Bulletin 2005;24:2
20 Hu Z, Yang X, Ho PC, et al. Herb-drug interactions: a literature review. Drugs 2005;65:1239–82.
21 Skalli S et al. Drug interactions with herbal medicines. Ther Drug Monit 2007;29:679–86.
22 Horn JR, Hansten PD, Lingtak–Neander CA. Proposal for a new tool to evaluate drug interaction cases. Pharmacotherapy 2007;41:674–80.
23 Bryant L, Fishman T. Clinically important drug–drug interactions and how to manage them. J Prim Health Care 2009;1: Online. Available: www.globalfamilydoctor.com/search/GFDSearch.asp?itemNum=10333 (accessed 14 April 2009)
24 Charrois TL, Hill RL, Vu D, et al. Community identification of natural health product–drug interactions. Ann Pharmacother 2007;41:1124–9.
25 Sood A, Sood R, Brinker FJ, et al. Potential for interactions between dietary supplements and prescription medications. Am J Med 2008;121:207–11.
26 Beggs, S. Adverse drug reactions in children. Paediatrics & Child Health in General Practise. 2009;(5) April;12–13.
27 Howland RH. Pharmacogenetics and pharmacovigilance. Drug Saf. 2009;32(3):265–70.
28 Therapeutic Goods Administration. Online. Available: www.tga.gov.au/docs/html/cmec/cmecdr63.htm(accessed 5 Oct 2009)
29 High-dose vitamin B6 may cause peripheral neuropathy. Australian Adverse Drug Reactions Bulletin 2008;27(4):14–16.
30 Therapeutic Goods Administration. Online. Available: www.tga.gov.au/docs/pdf/cmec/cmecmi66.pdf (accessed 5 Oct 2009).
31 McHugh GJ, Graber ML, Freebairn RC. Fatal vitamin C-associated acute renal failure. Anaesth Intensive Care 2008;36:585–8
32 Fuller FW. The side-effects of silver sulfadiazine. J Burn Care Res. 2009 May–Jun;30(3):464–70.
33 Wan AT, Conyers RA, Coombs CJ, Masterton JP. Determination of silver in blood urine and tissues of volunteers and burn patients. Clin. Chem. 1991; Oct;37(10 Pt 1):1683–7.
34 Therapeutic Goods Administration. Dangers associated with chronic ingestion of colloidal silver. Australian Adverse Drug Reactions Bulletin 2007;26(5):19.
35 White JM, Powell AM, Brady K, Russell-Jones R. Severe generalized argyria secondary to ingestion of colloidal silver protein. Clinical and Experimental Dermatology 2003;28(3): 254–6.
36 Therapeutic Goods Administration. Online. Available: www.tga.gov.au/docs/pdf/cmec/cmecmi60.pdf (accessed 5 Oct 2009).
37 See KA, Lavercombe PS, Dillon J, Ginsberg R. Accidental death from acute selenium poisoning. MJA 2006;185:388–9.
38 Guang-Qi Y, Yi-Ming X. Studies on Juman Dietary Requirements and Safe Range of Dietary Intakes of Selenium in China and Their Application in the Prevention of Related Endemic Diseases. Biomedical and Environmental Sciences 1995;8:187–201.
39 Therapeutic Goods Administration. Online. Available: www.tga.gov.au/docs/html/cmec/cmecdr63.htm (accessed 5 Oct 2009)
40 Farah M, Meyboom R, Ploen M. Acute hypersensitivity reactions to andrographis paniculate containing products, as reported in International Pharmacovigilence. Drug Safety 2008;31:913–14.
41 Agency Search Australia. Online. Available: http://agencysearch.australia.gov.au/search/search.cgi?query=BLACK+COHOSH+WARNING+LABEL&collection=agencies&profile=tga
42 Hepatotoxicity with black cohosh. Australian Adverse Drug Reactions Bulletin 2006;25(2):6.
43 The European Medicines Agency 2008. Online. Available: www.emea.europa.eu/pdfs/human/paediatrics/000006-PIP01-07.pdf (accessed 5 Oct 2009).
44 Whiting PW, Clouston A, Kerlin P. Black cohosh and other herbal remedies associated with acute hepatitis. MJA 2002;177:440–1.
45 Lantos S,Jones RM, Angus PW, Gow PJ. et al. Acute liver failure associated with the use of herbal preparations containing black cohosh. MJA 2003;197:390–1.
46 Chow EC, Teo M, Ring JA, Chen JW. Lessons from practice: liver failure associated with the use of black cohosh for menopausal symptoms. MJA 2008;188:420–2.
47 Suvarna R, Pirmohamed M, Henderson L. Possible interaction between warfarin and cranberry juice. BMJ 2003;327:1454.
48 Kauma H, Koskela R, Mäkisalo H, et al. Toxic acute hepatitis and hepatic fibrosis after consumption of chaparral tablets. Scand J Gastroenterol 2004;39(11):1168–71.
49 Therapeutic Goods Administration. Online. Available: www.tga.gov.au/docs/pdf/cmec/cmecmi50.pdf (accessed 5 Oct 2009).
50 Saunders PR, Smith F, Schusky RW. Echinacea purpurea L. in children: safety, tolerability, compliance, and clinical effectiveness in upper respiratory tract infections. Can J Physiol Pharmacol 2007;85:1195–9.
51 Forster Wadl E, Marchetti M, Scholl I et al. Type 1 allergy to elderberry (Sambucus nigra) is elicited by a 33.2 kDa allergen with significant homology to ribosomal inactivating proteins. Clin Exp Allergy 2003;33:1703–10.
52 Fugh-Berman A. Herb-drug interactions. Lancet 2000;355:134–8.
53 Smith L, Ernst E; Ewings et al. What affects anticoagulation control in patients taking warfarin? British Journal of General Practice 2009;59:590–4.

54 Shalansky S, Lynd L, Richardson K, et al. Risk of warfarin-related bleeding events and supratherapeutic International Normalised Ratios associated with complementary and alternative medicine: a longitudinal analysis. Pharmacotherapy 2007;27:1237–57

55 Jiang X, Williams KM, Liauw WS, et. al. Effect of ginkgo and ginger on the pharmacokinetics and pharmacodynamics of warfarin in healthy subjects. Br J Clin Pharmacol 2005;59(4):425–32

56 Therapeutic Goods Administration. Online. Available: www.tga.gov.au/docs/html/celandine.htm

57 Sarma DN et al. Safety of Green Tea extracts, a systematic review by the US Pharmacopoeia. Drug Safety 2008;31(6):469–84.

58 Molinari et al Acute Liver failure induced by green tea extracts: case report and review of the literature. Liver Transplantation. 2006(12):1892–5.

59 Sarma DN, Barrett ML, Chavez ML, et al. Safety of green tea extracts: a systematic review by the US Pharmacopeia. Drug Saf 2008;31(6):469–84.

60 MEDSAFE New Zealand Government publication. Prescriber Update 2009;30(3):21.

61 Ulbricht C, Basch E, Boon H, et al. Safety review of kava (Piper methysticum) by the Natural Standard Research Collaboration. Expert Opin Drug Saf 2005;4:779–94.

62 Lude S, Torok M, Dieterle S, et al. Hepatocellular toxicity of kava leaf and root extracts. Phytomedicine 2008;15:120–31.

63 Therapeutic Goods Administration. Online. Available: www.tga.gov.au/cm/kavafs0504.htm

64 Therapeutic Goods Administration. Online. Available: www.tga.gov.au/docs/pdf/cmec/cmecmi41.pdf (accessed 5 Oct 2009).

65 Therapeutic Goods Administration. Online. Available: www.tga.gov.au/docs/pdf/cmec/cmecmi71.pdf (accessed 5 Oct 2009).

66 Therapeutic Goods Administration. Online. Available: www.tga.gov.au/docs/pdf/cmec/cmecmi70.pdf (accessed 5 Oct 2009).

67 Adverse reactions to complementary medicines. Australian Adverse Drug Reactions Bull 2005;24(1):2.

68 Voiles KM, Kelly WN. Potential interactions between oral contraceptives and other medication and natural substances. US Pharmacist 2004;29(1).

69 Clauson KA, Santamarina ML, Rutledge JC. Clinically relevant safety issues associated with St John's wort product labels. BMC Complementary and Alternative Medicine 2008 Jul 17;8:42.

70 http://fedcache.funnelback.com/search/cache.cgi?collection=fedgov&doc=http%2Fwww.tga.gov.au%2Fdocs%2Fhtml%2Fcmec%2Fcmecdr50.htm

71 Agbabiaka TB Pittler MH, Wider B, Ernst E. Serenoa repens (saw palmetto). A systematic review of adverse events. Drug Safety 2009;32 (8):637–47.

72 Therapeutic Goods Administration. Online. Available: www.tga.gov.au/docs/html/cmec/cmecdr04.htm(accessed 5 Oct 2009)

73 Shalansky S, Lynd L, Richardson K, et al. Risk of warfarin-related bleeding events and supratherapeutic International Normalised Ratios associated with complementary and alternative medicine: a longitudinal analysis. Pharmacotherapy 2007;27:1237–57.

74 Skin reaction with glucosamine. Australian Adverse Drug Reactions Bulletin 2005;24(6):23.

75 Interaction between glucosamine and warfarin. Australian Adverse Drug Reactions Bull 2008;27(1):3.

76 Yue Q-Y, Stradell J, Myrberg O. Concomitant use of glucosaminepotentiatestheeffectofwarfarin.DrugSafety 2006;29:911.

77 MHRA/CSM. Glucosamine adverse reactions and interactions. Current Problems in Pharmacovigilance. 2006;31:8.

78 Therapeutic Goods Administration. Online. Available: www.tga.gov.au/legis/2008_rasml.htm(accessed 5 Oct 2009)

79 Therapeutic Goods Administration. Online. Available:www.tga.gov.au/docs/pdf/cmec/cmecmi60.pdf (accessed 5 Oct 2009).

80 Therapeutic Goods Administration and Australian Government Department of Health and Ageing. Adverse drug reactions: what to report. Online. Available: www.tga.gov.au/adr/report.htm (accessed 5 Oct 2009).

81 Health Canada. Online. Available: www.hc-sc.gc.ca/dhp-mps/medeff/report-declaration/guide/guide-ldir indust_e.html#a2 9 (accessed 5 Oct 2009).

Appendix 1

Food sources of macronutrients, micronutrients, phytonutrients and chemicals

Dr Antigone Kouris-Blazos

The list below should only be used as a guide because farming, food storage and cooking can significantly alter nutrient levels, and nutrient contents of many fruits and vegetables grown in Australia have not been reanalysed since the 1970s. (Nutrient data from US food composition tables have also been used.)

Foods are listed for each nutrient from highest (best source) to lowest (poorer source).

Abbreviations

ckd = cooked
cnd = canned
conc = concentrate
tbs = tablespoon
tsp = teaspoon

Protein

Fish 100g, ckd (130g raw)	32g
Lamb leg 100g, ckd	30g
Chicken lean no skin 100g, ckd	29g
Beef 100g, ckd (from 130g raw)	27g
Canned salmon/tuna 100g drained	25g
Pork 100g, ckd	23g
Soybeans, ckd ½ cup 100g	16g
Miso ½ cup 140g	16g
Tempeh 1 piece 85g	16g
Amaranth 100g	14g
Lowan Soy flakes 1 cup 70g	13g
Tofu firm raw 100g	12g
Yoghurt, natural, regular 200g	12g
Vegetarian products (e.g. soy burger or lentil patty or 1 slice nutmeat or 2 slices nutolene or 2 soy sausages or 3 felafel patties)	10g
Lentils/chickpeas ½ cup, ckd 100g	9g
Milk cow 200ml	7g
Soy milk 200ml	7g
Cheese 30g	8g
Cottage cheese 2 tbs	8g
All bran cereal ¾ cup	8g
Processed meat 2 slices 50g	8g
Spaghetti/pasta, ckd 1 cup 150g	8g
Split peas ½ cup 100g, ckd	8g
Baked beans ½ cup 150g	7g
Red kidney beans etc 100g, ckd	7g
Linseed 2 tbs 25g	7g
Pumpkin seeds 3 tbs 30g	7g
Sesame seeds 2½ tbs 30g	7g
Sunflower seeds 2½ tbs 30g	7g
Bread wholemeal+grains 1 slice	6.5g
Corn on the cob 1 large 200g	6.5g
Quinoa, ckd ¾ cup (raw 50g)	6g
Egg 1 large (53g)	6g
Nuts 30g (25 almonds or 14 Cashews or 17 walnuts)	6g
Bread wholemeal 1 slice 30g	6g
Special K cereal ¾ cup	6g
Peas ¾ cup 100g	5.5g
Muesli natural ⅓ cup	5g
Ricotta cheese 2 tbs	5g
Rice brown/red/black 1 cup, ckd	5g
Tofu soft 100g	5g
Breakfast cereal flake type 1 cup	3–5g
Weetbix/Vita Brits x 2	4g
Rice, white 1 cup, ckd 150g	4g
Chia seeds 1 tbs 15g	3g
Tahini 1 tbs 20g	3g
Oat milk 1 cup	3g
Bread multigrain/rye 1 slice 30g	3g
Almond milk 200ml	2.6g
Coconut milk 200ml	2.5g
Bread white 1 slice 30g	2.5g
Ryvita crispbread x 2	2g
Ice-cream 1 scoop	2g
Vitawheat dry biscuits x 2	1.5g
Rice milk 1 cup	1g

Essential amino acids

Nine amino acids cannot be made by the body and are called essential amino acids and must come from the diet: **isoleucine, leucine, lysine, methionine, phenylalanine, threonine, tryptophan,** and **valine.** Another amino acid, **histidine,** is considered semi-essential because the body does not always require dietary sources of it.

Animal foods contain all essential amino acids (complete proteins); most **plant foods** are missing one or more amino acids (incomplete proteins) except soy, quinoa, amaranth, chia seeds and spirulina (these have all the amino acids and are thus complete proteins). Lysine is lacking in cereals and methionine is lacking in legumes/nuts.

Leucine

A branched amino acid needed for the maintenance of muscle tissue. It may help preserve muscle stores of glycogen and help prevent muscle protein breakdown during exercise. It promotes growth; hormone synthesis; an important component of haemoglobin. Beneficial for skin, bone and tissue; wound healing.

Good sources: meat, dairy, whey protein.

	g/100g
Whey/soy protein conc	7g
Soy beans raw	2.3g
Lentils raw	2g
Beef, lean, raw	1.8g
Peanuts, raw	1.7g
Fish/crustaceans, raw	1.6g
Chicken, raw	1.5g
Almonds	1.5g
Chickpeas, raw	1.4g
Tahini	1.4g
Flax seed, raw	1.2g
Walnuts	1.2g
Egg, raw	1.0g
Amaranth 100g	0.9g
Milk, sheep	0.6g
Pork, raw	0.4g
Milk, goat	0.3g
Milk, cow	0.3g
Soy milk	0.2g
Asparagus	0.1g
Green beans	0.1g

Isoleucine

A branched amino acid needed for the maintenance of muscle tissue. It may help preserve muscle stores of glycogen and help prevent muscle protein breakdown during exercise. Necessary for the synthesis of haemoglobin, major constituent of red blood cells.

Good sources: meat, dairy, whey protein (4g/100g).

Lysine

Component of muscle protein; needed for growth and to help maintain nitrogen balance in the body; may help absorb and conserve calcium; collagen synthesis in bone cartilage and connective tissues; production of antibodies, hormones and enzymes; may be effective against herpes. Precursor for L-carnitine. Lysine requirements may be greater for athletes and people recovering from injuries, especially burns. Deficiency can cause: tiredness, poor concentration, irritability, blood shot eyes, retarded growth, hair loss, anaemia, and reproductive problems.

Good sources: meat, fish, dairy, eggs, brewers yeast. **Moderate sources:** legumes, nuts/seeds **Poor sources:** wheat/rice/ other cereal grains/corn (except amaranth, quinoa and chia seeds).

	g/100g
Whey protein conc	6.7g
Soy protein conc	5g
Beef/Lamb, ckd	3g
Fish/Seafood	2g
Chicken/Turkey/Pork, ckd	2g
Cheese	2g
Peanuts/almonds	2g
Pumpkin seeds	2g
Egg, whole	1.5g
Legumes, ckd	1.5g
Tofu	1g
Peas green	1g
Amaranth	0.7g
Nuts, other	0.7g
Quinoa, ckd	0.6g

Methionine

Principle supplier of sulfur which prevents disorders of the hair, skin and nails; used to make creatinine; reduces muscle degeneration; lipotropic properties (helps liver process fats) and protects the kidneys; precursor for carnitine; natural chelating agent for heavy metals; regulates formation of ammonia and creates ammonia-free urine which reduces bladder irritation.

Good sources: Meat, fish, dairy, egg, soy. **Moderate sources:** cereal grains (especially amaranth and quinoa). **Poor sources:** legumes and nuts.

	g/100g
Soy/Whey protein conc	1.0g
Soy protein conc	1.0g
Fish/Meat, ckd	1.0g
Cheese, yellow	1.0g
Amaranth	0.2g
Quinoa, ckd	0.2g

Phenylalanine

Beneficial for healthy nervous system. It boosts mood, memory and learning. There are two forms: L-phenylalanine (LPA) and D-phenylalanine (DPA). LPA can be converted to the amino acid L-tyrosine and subsequently to L-dopa, and noradrenaline (a chemical that transmits signals between nerve cells and the brain) and adrenaline. LPA can also be converted (through a separate pathway) to phenylethylamine, a substance that occurs naturally in the brain and appears to elevate mood. It keeps one awake and alert and reduces hunger pains. DPA may be helpful for Parkinson's disease and treatment of chronic pain. A mixture of LPA and DPA has been used as an antidepressant. DPA does not normally occur in foods and so all food sources relate to LPA.

Good sources: red meat, fish, most protein-containing foods.

	g/100g
Soy protein conc	4g
Whey protein conc	2g
Soy beans raw	1.9g
Almonds	1.5g
Lentils raw	1.4g
Chickpeas, raw	1.4g
Tahini	1.4g

Peanuts, raw	1.3g
Flax seed, raw	1.2g
Almonds	1.1g
Chickpeas	1.0g
Egg, raw	1.0g
Flax seed	0.9g
Tahini	0.9g
Beef, lean, raw	0.8g
Crustaceans, raw	0.8g
Chicken, raw	0.7g
Fish	0.7g
Walnuts	0.7g
Milk, sheep	0.6g
Pork, raw	0.4g
Milk, goat	0.3g
Milk, cow	0.3g
Soy milk	0.2g
Asparagus	0.1g
Green beans	0.1g

Threonine

Involved in cardiovascular, liver, central nervous, immune system function (production of antibodies, promotes thymus growth and activity); synthesis of glycine and serine (production of collagen, elastin and muscle tissue); helps build strong bones and tooth enamel; precursor of isoleucine; combines with the amino acids aspartic acid and methionine to help liver break down fats, which reduces accumulation of fat in the liver. Other nutrients are also better absorbed when threonine is present.

Good sources: meat, dairy, eggs.

	g/100g
Soy/Whey protein conc	5g
Soy beans raw	1.6g
Lentils raw	1g
Beef, lean, raw	0.9g
Peanuts, raw	0.9g
Fish/custaceans, raw	0.8g
Chicken, raw	0.8g
Flax seed, raw	0.7g
Tahini	0.7g
Chickpeas, raw	0.7g
Egg, raw	0.7g
Amaranth 100g	0.5g
Milk, sheep	0.3g
Pork, raw	0.2g
Milk, goat	0.16g
Milk, cow	0.14g
Soy milk	0.14g
Asparagus	0.08g
Green beans	0.07g

Tryptophan

Used as a sleep aid due to its ability to increase brain levels of serotonin (a calming neurotransmitter when present in moderate levels) and/or melatonin (a drowsiness-inducing hormone secreted by the pineal gland in response to darkness or low light levels). May assist in treating depression, mood disorders, migraine, obesity and fibromyalgia. Low intake can lead to salt cravings, lower pain threshold, shortness of breath, choking sensation, sleep disorders, appetite disorders/anorexia/bulimia/insatiable hunger, anxiety.

	g/100g
Soy/Whey protein conc	1.0g
Quinoa, ckd1 cup (¹⁄₄cup raw)	0.5g
Flax seed, raw	0.3g
Lentils, raw	0.25g
Turkey, raw	0.25g
Peanuts, raw	0.25g
Chicken, raw	0.23g
Almonds	0.2g
Amaranth 100g	0.18g
Eggs, whole, raw	0.17g
Walnuts, raw	0.17g
Beef, lean, raw	0.14g
Milk, sheep	0.08g
Milk, cow	0.07g
Milk, soy	0.05g
Milk, goat	0.04g
Asparagus	0.03g
Pork, raw	0.02g
Beans green	0.01g

Other sources: salmon, blue fish, mackerel, beetroot, hazelnuts, chocolate, oats, red/brown rice, millet, dried dates, bananas, fish, cottage cheese, sesame/sunflower seeds, hummus, potatoes.

Valine

A branched amino acid needed for the maintenance of muscle tissue. It may help preserve muscle stores of glycogen and help prevent muscle protein breakdown during exercise. Side-effects of high levels of valine in the body include hallucinations.

Good sources: meat, dairy, whey protein.

	g/100g
Soy/Whey protein conc	4.0g
Pork, ckd	2.0g
Cheese	1.5g
Beef/chicken/turkey, ckd	1g
Nuts/seeds	1g

Non-essential amino acids

Eleven amino acids are made by the body: arginine, alanine, asparagine, aspartic acid, cysteine, glutamic acid, glutamine, glycine, proline, serine, and tyrosine. Other amino acids, such as carnitine, are used by the body in ways other than protein-building and are often used therapeutically.

Aspartic acid

Involved in neuroendocrine system and gluconeogenesis; needed during metabolism of other amino acids and biochemicals in the citric acid cycle; involved in synthesis of asparagine, arginine, lysine, methionine, threonine, isoleucine, and several nucleotides; aids in removal of ammonia (ammonia is harmful to the central nervous system); may increase resistance to fatigue and increase endurance; important in the functioning of RNA, DNA; antibody synthesis.

	g/100g
Soy protein conc	10.0g
Whey protein conc	7.0g
Soybeans, raw	4.6g
Pork, ckd	3.0g
Meat, ckd	3.0g
Lentils, raw	3.0g
Peanuts, all types, raw	3.0g
Almonds	2.7g
Chickpeas, raw	2.3g
Fish, salmon, pink, raw	2.0g
Walnuts, English	1.8g
Chicken, thigh, meat only, raw	1.7g
Sesame butter/tahini	1.6g
Egg, whole, raw, fresh	1.3g
Rice, raw	1.0g
Hummus	0.5g
Asparagus	0.5g
Pork, raw	0.4g
Soy milk, fluid	0.4g
Milk, sheep, fluid	0.3g
Snap beans, green, raw	0.3g
Milk, cow, 3% fat	0.2g
Milk, goat, fluid	0.2g

Alanine

Metabolism of glucose, tryptophan and organic acids; important source of energy for muscle tissue, brain and central nervous system; high levels of alanine and low levels of tyrosine and phenylalanine linked to chronic fatigue and glandular fever; removes toxic substances released from breakdown of muscle protein during intensive exercise.

Good sources: meat, dairy, poultry, fish, nuts.

	g/100g
Soy/whey protein conc	3.0g
Pork, ckd	2.0g
Beef, ckd	2.0g
Chicken/turkey/fish, ckd	1.0g
Cheese	1.0g
Nuts	1.0g
Legumes, raw	1.0g

Arginine

Release/synthesis of hormones/enzymes glucagon, insulin, growth hormone, vasopressin, creatinine and other hormones (thus plays a role in glucose tolerance/liver lipid metabolism); promotes wound healing; regeneration of the liver; stimulation of immune function; sperm production/ejaculate (seminal fluid/sperm); precursor to nitric oxide, which the body uses to keep blood vessels dilated (role in lowering blood pressure); component of collagen/skin/connective tissues. Reduces accumulation of ammonia and plasma lactate (by-products of exercise). It may be helpful in congestive heart failure, angina, intermittant claudication, and sexual dysfunction.

Good sources: meat, dairy, poultry, fish, nuts, buckwheat, brown rice, cocoa.

	g/100g
Soy protein conc	6.0g
Peanuts (raw or butter)	3.0g
Nuts/seeds	2.0g
Lentils, raw	2.0g
Peas split, raw	2.0g
Whey protein conc	2.0g
Chicken/turkey/pork, ckd	2.0g
Red meat, ckd	2.0g
Tuna canned drained	1.7g
Beans kidney, raw	1.5g
Salmon, Atlantic farmed	1.2g
Shrimp	1.2g
Beans, green, raw	1.2g
Amaranth	1.0g
Cheese	1.0g
Egg whole raw	0.8g
Tofu, firm (+ nigari)	0.7g
Wheat flour, wholegrain	0.6g
Garlic, raw	0.6g
Pork raw	0.5g
Quinoa, ckd1 cup (1/4 cup raw)	0.4g
Onion, raw	0.1g
Kiwi, raw	0.1g
Milk cow 3% fat	0.08g

Asparagine

Manufactured from aspartic acid; required by the nervous system to maintain equilibrium (aids in balancing state of emotion) and is also required for amino acid transformation from one form to the other in the liver.

Good sources: meat, dairy, poultry, fish.

Cysteine

Required for vitamin B6 utilisation; insulin production; component of protein type abundant in nails, skin and hair (have 10–14% cysteine); healing of burns and wounds; mucolytic; antioxidant and has synergetic effect when taken with other antioxidants such as vitamin E and selenium; increases level of protective amino acid glutathione in the lungs, liver, kidneys and bone marrow; used to make taurine; strengthens the lining of the stomach and intestines, which may help prevent damage caused by aspirin and similar drugs; cysteine is rarely used as a dietary supplement, instead N-acetyl cysteine (NAC), which contains cysteine, is more commonly used.

Good sources: meat, dairy, poultry, fish, soy protein conc (6g/100g), whey protein conc (0.3g/100g).

Glutamine

Glutamine is derived from another amino acid, glutamic acid. The most common excitatory neurotransmitter in the central nervous system; essential for enterocytes, hepatocytes, lymphocytes, macrophages; muscle cells; it is involved in more metabolic processes than any other amino acid. Deficiency may be caused by catabolic stress and gut dysfunction; inadequate levels exacerbate GI disorders; enterocytes use glutamine for fuel and may reduce gut permeability; protective effects on heart muscle in people with heart disease; monosodium glutamate (MSG), the form of glutamic acid that is used as a flavour enhancer, is linked to headache.

Good sources: meat, dairy, poultry, fish/halibut, tomatoes, citrus, brewers yeast, brown rice, broccoli, molasses, liver, organ meats, lentils, potatoes, spinach, lupins, nuts.

	g/100g
Soy protein conc	17.0g
Whey protein conc	11.0g
Lupins, raw	8g
Cheese	6g
Sundried tomatoes	5g
Chicken/turkey/pork, ckd	5g
Red meat, ckd	4g
Fish, ckd	4g
Nuts/seeds/legumes, raw	4g
Wheat/oat products, dry	4g
Rice, raw	1g

Glutathione

A protein made from cysteine, glutamine and glycine; an important intracellular antioxidant that also plays a role in the detoxification and elimination of potential carcinogens and toxins in the liver; studies in animals have found that glutathione synthesis and tissue glutathione levels are significantly lower in aged animals than in younger animals, leading to decreased ability of aged animals to respond to oxidative stress or toxin exposure.

Sources: There is no dietary requirement for glutathione and cannot be absorbed from supplements. Body makes it from scratch, utilising vitamins and common amino acids found in food. Vitamin C, cysteine, (high in soy protein/animal foods), lipoic acid, glutamine, methionine and SAMe can raise levels.

Glycine

Made from serine/threonine, so dietary intake is not essential; protein and nucleic acid synthesis; absorption of calcium; found in prostate fluid; hormone synthesis; needed by immune system; component of skin and is needed for wound healing; retards degeneration of muscles by increasing the supply of extra creatine in the body; acts as neurotransmitter; high levels may cause fatigue.

Sources: meat, dairy, poultry, fish, nuts.

	g/100g
Soy protein conc	3.0g
Pork/chicken/turkey, ckd	3.0g
Red meat, ckd	3.0g
Nuts/seeds	2.0g
Whey protein conc	1.0g

Histidine

Precursor of histamine, released by immune system cells during an allergic reaction; sexual arousal; improves blood flow; needed for growth and for the repair of tissue; red and white blood cell synthesis; removal of heavy metals; production of gastric juices; high intake can cause stress and anxiety.

Sources: meat, poultry, fish.

	g/100g
Soy protein conc	2.0g
Cheese	1.0g
Pork/chicken/turkey	1.0g
Red meat	1.0g
Whey protein conc	1.0g
Lupin	1.0g

Proline

Main amino acid of collagen (15%); collagen in skin contains hydroxy-proline and hydroxylysine, which is formed from proline and lysine, in which ascorbic acid seems to be important in this conversion; needed for bone, skin, and cartilage formation; can be formed from glutamine or the amino acid ornithine; important for the proper functioning of joints and tendons; tissue repair after injury, wound healing; maintains and strengthens heart muscles; important for intracellular signalling.

Good sources: dairy, egg, meat, wheatgerm.

	g/100g
Gelatin	12g
Soy/whey protein conc	4.0g
Cheese	2.0g
Chicken/turkey/pork/beef	1.0g
Cereals/nuts/seeds	1.0g

Serine

Production requires adequate amounts of vitamins B3, B6, and folic acid; constituent of brain proteins thus needed for cognitive function; component of myelin sheath and all cell membranes; aids in synthesis of antibodies; muscle/tissue growth; required for the metabolism of fat; metabolism of nucleic acids in RNA and DNA; creatine synthesis.

Sources: meat, dairy, wheat gluten, peanuts.

	g/100g
Soy protein conc	4.0g
Whey protein conc	3.0g
Soybeans, raw	2.1g
Peanuts, all types, raw	1.3g
Lentils, raw	1.3g
Cheese	1.0g
Egg, whole, raw	1.0g
Chickpeas, raw	1.0g
Chicken/turkey/pork, ckd	1.0g
Nuts/seeds	1.0g
Beef, raw	0.9g
Fish, salmon, pink, raw	0.8g
Milk, sheep, fluid	0.50
Soy milk, fluid	0.20
Milk, goat, fluid	0.20
Milk, cow, 3% fat	0.10
Asparagus	0.10
Green beans	0.10

Tyrosine

Synthesised from the amino acid phenylalanine; deficiency caused by low intake of phenylalanine, prolonged exposure to elevated cortisol/glucocorticoids from endogenous/exogenous sources and elevated oestrogen levels, including oral contraceptive use; precursor of several neuro-transmitters like L-dopa, dopamine, noradrenaline, adrenaline; transmits nerve impulses to the brain and enhances positive mood; abundant in insulin; precursor of thyroxine thus promotes healthy thyroid functioning; adrenal and pituitary gland function; reduces appetite, food addiction, stress, mental fatigue, anxiety.

Sources: meat, fish, wheat germ, tofu, almonds, avocados, bananas, pumpkin seeds, oats, pinto beans, black eyed peas.

	g/100g
Soy protein conc	3.0g
Whey protein conc	2.0g
Cheese	1.0g
Pork/chicken/turkey, ckd	1.0g
Red meat, ckd	1.0g
Fish, ckd	1.0g
Seeds/peanuts	1.0g

L-Carnitine

11–34mg/day synthesised in body from amino acids lysine and methionine and catalysed by SAMe, folate, vitamin C, B6, niacin, and Fe; essential for healthy nervous system function and transport of fats into mitochondria for oxidation and energy production especially in skeletal muscle, heart and spermatozoa; may improve concentration/mood, depression, chronic fatigue, fibromyalgia, diabetic neuropathy and heart disease.

	g/100g
Beef	80mg
Pork	25mg
Fish	6mg
Milk	4mg
Chicken	4mg
Cheese	4mg
Ice-cream	3mg
Avocado	2mg

Taurine

There is no dietary requirement for taurine. Taurine is synthesised from cysteine with the help of iron, molybdenum, B3 and B6; taurine and cysteine are vulnerable to depletion because of physiological demands upon their precursor: methionine. Needed for bile acid conjugation/fat digestion; control of blood cholesterol levels; eye and brain development; stabilises cell membranes/regulates heart beat and prevents brain cell over-activity; aids the movement of potassium, sodium, calcium, magnesium in and out of cells and thus helps generate nerve impulses; may help with anxiety/stress; assists neurotransmitter activity similar to GABA; may be useful for congestive heart failure; improves endothelial function/hypotensive; insulin potentiaition/diabetes modulation. Safe at levels up to 3g/day

Sources: clams, meat, fish, breast milk (and lesser extent cow's milk), seaweed.

Carbohydrate

Following food servings = 15g carbohydrate

Breads/grains/breakfast cereals	
bread roll	½
bread, other, 1 thin slice	30g
breakfast cereal	¾ cup
Burgen wholemeal seed	2 slices
cake, plain thin slice	30g
chocolate, 3–4 pieces	20g
corn thins	4 pieces
crumpet	1 piece
donut	½ donut
English muffin	½
flour	2 tbs
muesli bar	½ bar
muesli/raw oats/all bran	¼ cup
noodles, 2 minute	½ packet
pancake	1 small
pasta, ckd	½ cup
pita bread, 1/2 large	50g
quinoa, ckd	½ cup
rice/noodles, ckd	⅓ cup
sweet biscuits	2 biscuits
sweet muffin, small	½
vitawheat	3
weetbix	1–2
Fruit	
apple/pear	1 small
apricots (fresh/dry)	5 pieces
banana	1 small
figs	3 pieces
fruit juice, ½ cup	100ml
grapes	15
kiwi fruit	2
mandarin	2
mango	½
nectarines/peaches	2 small
orange	1 small
pineapple	2 slices
plums	4
rockmelon, small	¼
sultanas	1 tbs
tinned fruit	½ cup
watermelon	1½ cups
Milk (all types)/yoghurt/custard/icecream	
almond milk	400ml
coconut milk, lite	300ml
coconut milk, regular	700ml
cows milk, regular/lite	300ml
custard	½ cup
fruit yoghurt	100g
ice-cream	1 scoop
natural yoghurt	300g
oat milk	250ml
rice milk	100ml
soy milk, lite	300ml
soy milk, regular	200ml
Legumes	
baked beans	½ cup
lentils/4 bean mix	½ – 1 cup
Vegetables	
beetroot, 1 large	180g
carrots, 2 medium	100g
cherries	15 pieces
corn cob	1 small
corn kernels	⅓ cup
parsnip, 1 medium	150g
peas	1 cup
potato, 1 medium	100g
pumpkin, few pieces	150g
split peas	½ cup
sweet potato, 1 medium	100g

Note: berries, strawberries and nuts are very low in carbohydrates.

Fructose

Apples, clingstone peaches, mango, pears, watermelon, honey, sugar snap peas, tinned fruit in natural juice, fruit juice, dried fruit, tomato juice, wine.

Fructans/galactans

Artichokes, asparagus, beetroot, broccoli, brussel sprouts, cabbage, fennel, garlic, legumes (chickpeas, lentils, red kidney beans, baked beans), okra, onion (white/red/brown/spring/leeks/shallots), peas, custard apple, persimmon, rambutan, watermelon, white peaches, rye, wheat (bread, pasta, couscous, crackers, biscuits), chicory drink (Ecco/Caro), fructooligosaccharides (FOS), inulin.

Sugar polyols

Apples, apricots, avocado, blackberries, cherries, longon, lychee, nashi pears, nectarines, pears, plums, watermelon, cauliflower, mushrooms, snow peas, artificially sweetened gums/mints (containing xylitol, sorbitol, isomalt, mannitol).

Fibre

Recommended 30g/day	**g/serve**
Uncle Toby's Bran Plus ¾ cup	18g
Amaranth 100g	15g
Kelloggs Allbran ¾ cup 50g	14g
Vogels Ultra bran soy lin 45g	14g
Kelloggs Guardian 1 cup 60g	13g
Artichoke globe 200g	11g
Bulgur 1 cup, ckd	8g
Lentils, ckd, ½ cup 100g	8g
Split peas, ckd, ½ cup 100g	8g
Sanitarium Hibran weetbix 2	8g
Lowan Soy flakes 1 cup	8g
Lowan Oat bran and fruit 1 cup	8g
Spaghetti wholemeal, ckd1 cup	8g
Chickpeas, ckd ½ cup 100g	7.5g
Kelloggs Sultana bran 1 cup	7g
Uncle Toby's Healthwise Digestive system 1 cup 45g	6g
Uncle Toby's fibre plus 1 cup 45g	6g
Weight Watchers Fruit & Fibre ½ cup	6g
Bran Wheat 2 tbs 12g	5.5g
Chia seeds 1 tbs 15g	5.5g
Beans dried, ckd, ½ cup	5g
Muesli ½ cup (4 tbs) 45g	5g
Psyllium husk 1 tbs 6g	5g
Parsnip ½ large 100g	5g
Peas ¾ cup 100g	5g
Beetroot 1 med 120g	4.5g
Burgen rye bread 1 slice 40g	4.5g
Orange med 230g	4.5g
Figs dried 2 med 30g	4.5g
Almonds 25–30 30g	4.5g
Bran Oat/Barley/rice 2 tbs 15g	4g
Pear med 150g	4g
Prune juice 150ml	4g
Muesli bars nuts/seeds/fruit 50g	4g
Kelloggs Just right/Sustain 1 cup	4g
Miso ½ cup 140g	4g
Rice black, ckd 1 cup 150g	4g
Burgen wholemeal 1 slice 40g	3.7g
Pistachio nuts dried 30g	3.5g
Sunflowers seed 2 tbs 30g	3.5g
Cauliflower ½ cup100g	3.5g
Corn on the cob small 100g	3.5g
Potatoes 1 med 150g	3.5g
Freedom Foods Cornflakes 1 cup	3.5g

Kelloggs Mini wheats 17 (30g)	3.5g
Kiwi 1 med 100g	3.5g
Figs 2 med 100g	3g
Apple med 150g	3g
Barley pearl, ckd ½ cup	3g
Wheatgerm 20g, 2 tbs	3g
Ryvita 2	3g
Spaghetti, ckd 1 cup 150g	3g
Quinoa, ckd 1 cup 150g	3g
Sweet potato 150g	3g
Capsicum 1 med 140g	3g
Porridge, ckd ¾ cup (40g raw)	2.5g
Rye bread dark 1 slice 30g	2.5g
Pumpernickel 1 slice 25g	2.5g
Rice brown, ckd 1 cup 150g	2.5g
Rice red, ckd 1 cup 150g	2.5g
Banana med 140g	2.5g
Coconut flesh 30g	2.5g
Peanuts 30g	2.5g
Tempeh 1 piece 85g	2g
Bran rice 1 tbs	2g
Wholemeal bread 1 slice 30g	2g
White bread +fibre 1 slice 30g	2g
Rye bread light 1 slice 30g	2g
Strawberries 5 small	2g
Rockmelon 1 cup	2g
Apricots/Plums 2 med	2g
Apricots dried 4 halves 25g	2g
Peach/Nectarine 1 med	2g
Pineapple 1 slice 2cm thick 90g	2g
Sultanas 30g	2g
Blackberries/Raspberries ½ cup	2g
Green beans ½ cup	2g
Carrot ½ cup slices 70g	2g
Tomato 1med 150g	2g
Eggplant 2 slices 60g	2g
Silverbeet/spinach ½ cup	2g
Tahini 1 tbs 20g	2g
Walnuts 15–20 halves 30g	2g
Pepitas 3 tbs 30g	2g
Multigrain bread 1 slice 30g	1.5g
Broccoli tips ½ cup 60g	1.5g
Zucchini 1 small 100g	1.5g
Pumpkin 100g	1.5g
Mango ½ med	1.5g
Bran barley 1 tbs	1.2g
Watermelom 1 cup 150g	1g
Grapes 20 med 120g	1g
Fruit juice	< 1g
Rice white, ckd 1 cup 150g	1g
Linseed 2 tbs 25g	1g
Tofu 100g	1g
Cabbage ½ cup 40g	1g
Snow peas 10 pods 33g	1g
LSA mix 1 tbs	0.5g
White bread 1 slice 30g	0.5g
Lettuce 3 leaves 30g	0.5g
Mushrooms ½ cup	0.5g

Fat

RDI = recommended dietary intake

No RDI; ideal 20–35% energy from fat i.e 40–80g/day	**g/serve**
Fish and chips 1 serve	38g
Coconut milk regular 100ml	29g
Meat pie 190g	26g
Hamburger	25g
Oil all types 1 tbs	20g
Pizza 2 slices meat	18g
Chocolate 40g	16g
Butter 1 tbs	16g
Dairy blend butter 1 tbs	16g
Nuts mixed 30g	15g
Margarine regular 1 tbs	14g
Cheese tasty 30g	10g
Sausage, ckd, regular 50g	10g
Fish oily (salmon/herring) 100g, ckd	10g
Almond milk 200ml 1 cup	9.4g
Cow's milk regular 200ml	9g
Cream 1 tbs unwhipped	8g
Margarine light 1 tbs	8g
Yoghurt natural, regular 200g	8g
Coconut milk lite 100ml	7g
Beef/lamb, lean 120g, ckd	7g
Soy milk regular 200ml	6g
Egg large whole	6g
Seeds mixed 1 tbs	6g
Ice-cream 1 scoop 50g regular	5.5g
Chicken breast no skin 100g, ckd	5g
Fetta cheese goat 30g	5g
Oat milk 200ml	4g
Yoghurt, natural, low fat 200g	3g
Cow's milk lite 200ml	3g
Rice milk 200ml 1 cup	2g
Soy milk lite 200ml	2g
Quinoa, ckd ¾ cup (raw 50g)	2g
Fish white 100g, ckd	2g

Saturated fat

No RDI; ideal <7% energy from saturated fat i.e <15g/day	**g/serve**
Fish and chips 1 serve	35g
Coconut milk regular 100ml	26g
Meat pie 190g	12g
Hamburger	10g
Butter 1 tbs	10g
Palm oil 1 tbs	10g
Chocolate 40g	9g
Dairy blend butter 1 tbs	8g
Lard/Beef fat 1 tbs	8g
Cheese tasty 30g	6.5g
Yoghurt natural, regular 200g	6g
Cow's milk regular 200ml	6g
Cream 1 tbs unwhipped	5g
Sausage, ckd regular 50g	5g
Peanut oil 1 tbs	4g
Rice bran oil 1 tbs	4g
Margarine 1 tbs	4g
Ice-cream 1 scoop 50g regular	3.5g
Fish oily (salmon/herring) 100g, ckd	3g
Beef/lamb, lean 120g, ckd	3g
Fetta cheese goat 30g	3g
Soybean oil 1 tbs	3g
Olive oil 1 tbs	3g
Sesame seed oil 1 tbs	3g
Chicken breast no skin 100g, ckd	2g
Egg large whole	2g
Margarine light 1 tbs	2g
Sunflower/grape seed oil 1 tbs	2g
Tahini paste 1 tbs	2g
Peanut butter 1 tbs	1.6g
Nuts mixed 30g	1g
Fish white 100g, ckd	0.5g
Seeds mixed 1 tbs	0.5g

Cholesterol

No RDI; about 300mg/d has been recommended in the past

Cholesterol is classed as a sterol (a soft waxy substance) and a lipid. Cholesterol is needed for production of hormones, bile acid, cell membranes and vitamin D. The liver makes about 1000mg cholesterol per day from saturated/trans fat, which is almost all the body needs to maintain these vital functions (about 75% of blood cholesterol is made in the liver and about 25% is absorbed through food). When dietary cholesterol increases the body compensates by decreasing its own cholesterol production; this is why changes in dietary cholesterol have little effect on blood cholesterol even when eggs are regularly eaten. Some people make more cholesterol than others because of their genes. Certain conditions (e.g. thyroid) and drugs (e.g. diuretics) can increase cholesterol levels. Cholesterol is transported to and from cells in the blood by special carriers called lipoproteins. High-density lipoprotein or HDL (referred to as good cholesterol) is correlated with a lower risk of heart attack; about 30% of blood cholesterol is transported by HDL away from the arteries and back to the liver. Low-density lipoprotein or LDL (referred to as bad cholesterol) is linked to cardiovascular disease, especially if oxidised. Cholesterol is found in the nervous system, muscle, skin, liver, intestines and heart. Since most cholesterol in the body is made from saturated fat, the need to be overtly concerned about cholesterol in food is being de-emphasised in favour of restricting saturated fat and substituting unsaturated fats. The Heart Foundation does not limit dietary cholesterol in its recommendation and recommends 6 eggs a week for all Australians. Studies have not found a link between the eating of eggs and heart disease risk, even in people with high blood cholesterol. However, some studies have linked egg intake with increased heart disease mortality in people with diabetes.

	mg/serve
Brains 1 set 80g	1500mg
Liver (chicken/beef) 100g, ckd	500mg
Kidney 100g	310mg
Egg, 1	210mg
Crayfish/lobster 100g, ckd	150mg
Duck 90g, ckd	145mg
Sardines 6 med 100g	140mg
Beef/lamb/pork, 120g, ckd	100mg
Chicken 120g, ckd 120g, ckd	100mg
Sausage 50g, ckd	100mg
Fish oily 120g	100mg
Caviar 1 tbs 16g	95mg
Turkey 120g, ckd	70mg
Kangaroo/rabbit 120g, ckd	70mg
Fish white 120g, ckd	70mg
Crab meat 100g, ckd	70mg
Prawns/shrimp ½ cup, ckd 50g	55mg
Oysters, 6 85g	45mg
Chocolate 50g	45mg
Butter 1 tbs	45mg
Mussels 80g	40mg
Cheese 30g	30mg
Milk full cream 1 cup	30mg
Dripping/Lard 1 tbs	20mg
Cream 1 tbs	20mg
Scallops 5 small (30g)	10gg

Omega-9 oleic acid

No RDI; Ideal >10% energy from monounsaturated fat i.e >20g/day

	g/serve
Olive oil 1 tbs	15g
Canola oil 1 tbs	12g
Peanut oil 1 tbs	10g
Peanut butter 1 tbs	8.4g
Palm oil 1 tbs	8g
Canola margarine 1 tbs	6g
Soybean oil 1 tbs	5g
Sunflower oil 1 tbs	5g
Tahini paste 1 tbs	4.7g
Grapeseed oil 1 tbs	4g
Butter 1 tbs	3g

Essential fatty acids

Omega-3 EPA and DHA

RDI: 500mg/day (EPA+DHA); people with heart disease 1000mg/day

Legend:

* Under pressure and may be overfished

** Overfished/significant conservation concern

High mercury levels

	mg/serve
Herring canned 150g*	>1000mg
Pink salmon canned 150g	>1000mg
Red salmon canned 150g	>1000mg
Sardines canned 150g	>1000mg
Mackerel canned 150g	>1000mg
Swordfish# ** 150g	>1000mg
Marlin# 150g	>1000mg
Broadbill# 150g	>1000mg
Spanish mackerel 150g*	500–1000mg
Blue mackerel 150g	500–1000mg
Atlantic salmon 150g (farmed)	500–1000mg
Gemfish* 150g	500–1000mg
Southern Bluefin tuna 150g#**	500–1000mg
Oysters 150g	300–500mg
Squid, arrow 150g	500mg
Mussels 150g	300–500mg
Scallops 150g	200–500mg
Crab, blue swimmer 150g	300–500mg
Baby octopus	300–500mg
Shark# 150g	400–500mg
Australian sardine 150g	400–500mg
Yellow tail kingfish 150g	400–500mg
Australian herring 150g	400–500mg
Sea mullet 150g	400–500mg
Ray# 150g	200–500mg
Catfish# 150g	200–500mg
Flathead 150g	200–500mg
Blue-eye trevalla 150mg*	200–500mg
Smoked cod 150g	300–400mg
Blue Eye Cod 150g	300–400mg
Rainbow trout 150g	300–400mg
Dory 150g*	300–400mg
Jack mackerel 150g	300–400mg
Grey morwong 150g	300–400mg
Blue-spotted goatfish 150g	300–400mg
Small-spotted herring 150g	300–400mg
Australian bass 150g	200–300mg
Blue grenadier 150g	200–500mg
Hoki 150g	300–400mg
Snapper 150g*	200–500mg
Trevally 150g	300–400mg
Flounder 150g	200–500mg
King Dory 150g	300–400mg
Whiting 150g	200–500mg
Wrasse 150g	300–400mg
Blue morwong 150g	300–400mg
Butter fish 150g	300–400mg
Leather jacket 150g	300–400mg
Hussar 150g	300–400mg
Garfish 150g	300–400mg
Dhufish 150g	300–400mg
Mullet 150g	200–500mg
Bream 150g	300–400mg
Mangrove jack 150g	300–400mg
Saddletail 150g	300–400mg
Jackass morwong 150g	300–400mg
Canned tuna * # (if from large tuna) 150g	<200mg
Hake 150g	<200mg
Perch/Orange roughy#** 150g	<200mg
Rockling or Ling ** 150g	<200mg
Barramundi (farmed) 150g	<200mg
Basa (farmed) # 150g	<200mg
Prawns (farmed) 150g	<200mg
Eggs large regular 1	60mg
Turkey 100g	30mg
Lamb 100g (mainly DHA)	25mg
Beef 100g (mainly DHA)	8mg
Chicken/Pork 100g (mainly DHA)	3mg

Omega-3 a-linolenic acid (ALA)

RDI: 1–2g/day or >0.5% energy from linolenic acid

	g/serve
Flaxseed oil 1 tbs	10g
Chia seeds 15g 1 tbs	3g
Flaxseeds 1 tbs	2.2g
Canola oil 1 tbs 20g	2.0g
Walnuts, 30g	1.8g
Bread soy/linseed 2 slices	1.6g
Soybean oil 1 tbs 20g	1.5g
Walnut oil 1 tbs	1.4g
Pumpkin seeds 20g	1.0g
Canola margarine 1 tbs	1.0g
Mustard oil 1 tbs	0.8g
Tofu, firm ½ cup	0.7g
Sunflower margarine 1 tbs	0.5g
Peanut oil 1 tbs 20g	0.4g
Mushroom 75g	0.4g
Rice bran oil 1 tbs	0.2g
Pecans 30g	0.2g
Spinach 75g	0.2g
Lettuce 75g	0.1g
Olive oil 1 tbs	0.1g
Avocado 80g	0.1g
Cheddar cheese 40g slice	0.1g
Sunflower oil/seeds	0g

Omega-6 linoleic acid

RDI: 8–13g/day or 5–10% energy from linoleic acid

	g/serve
Safflower oil 1 tbs	15g
Grape seed oil 1 tbs	13g
Sunflower oil 1 tbs	12g
Walnut oil 1 tbs	11g
Soybean oil 1 tbs	10g
Sunflower seeds 1 tbs	9g
Pine nuts 20g	8g
Walnuts 20g	7g
Corn oil 1 tbs	7g
Peanut oil 1 tbs	7g
Sunflower margarine 1 tbs	6g
Brazil nuts 30g	5.8g
Sesame oil 1 tbs	5.6g
Sesame seeds 20g	5g
Tahini paste 20g	4.7g
Pecans, roasted 20g	4g
Pumpkin seeds 20g	4g
Peanuts 20g	4g
Brazil nuts 20g	4g
Canola oil 1 tbs	4g
Almonds 20g	3g
Pistachios 20g	3g
Canola margarine 1 tbs	2g
Almonds/Hazelnuts 20g	2g
Cashews 20g	2g
Olive oil 1 tbs	1.5g
Avocado 80g	1g
Peanut butter 1 tbs	0.7g

Lipoic acid (thioctic acid)

RDI: nil (intakes 200–400mg/day safe)

Sulfur containing fatty acid and antioxidant synthesised in body, in food it is attached to amino acid lysine; cofactor for several mitochondrial enzymes; chelates heavy metals in body; stimulates glutathione synthesis; enhances insulin signalling and modulating the activity of other cell signalling molecules and transcription factors. May improve insulin mediated glucose utilisation (lowering blood glucose) and treatment of diabetic neuropathy. Deficiency rare but low levels found in diabetes, liver cirrhosis and atherosclerosis.

Source: Spinach, liver/offal, meat, brewers yeast, tomatoes, potatoes, broccoli, peas, brussel sprouts.

Vitamins

RDI = recommended dietary intake
UTI = upper tolerable intake
mcg = micrograms
IU = international units

Vitamin A (retinol)

RDI: 900mcg/RE or 3000IU/day
UTI: 3000mcg or 10000IU/day
Sensitive to light and oxygen, up to 40% loss in cooking; needs zinc to be mobilised from liver stores

Body tissue growth and repair; maintains healthy skin, eyes, body linings of lungs/intestines; involved in production of thyroxine by thyroid and binding of thyroxine (T3) to receptors; reduces susceptibility to infections; protects against air pollutants; counteracts night–blindness and weak eyesight; aids in bone/teeth formation; supports sperm production; may protect against cancer; helps mobilise iron from storage sites so deficiency may exacerbate iron deficiency. Deficiency is rare but certain conditions can cause deficiency (diabetes, Crohn's disease, ulcerative colitis, thyroid conditions).

	mcg/serve
Liver 1 slice 40g	14000mcg
Cod liver oil 1 tbs	3600mcg
Sustagen 250ml	250mcg
Butter/margarine 1 tbs	240mcg
Cheese, cheddar 30g	120mcg
Milo 1 tbs	110mcg
Egg 1	100mcg
Milk full cream 1 cup	80mcg
Swordfish 90g	60mcg
Skim milk 1 cup	5mcg

B Carotene (converts to vitamin A)

1mcg retinol = 2mcg B-carotene
Sensitive to light and oxygen, up to 40% loss in cooking

RDI: converts to vitamin A as needed in digestive tract with help of bile salts/fat, vitamin C, zinc and thyroxine (conversion to vitamin A/retinol may be reduced in thyroid disorders, diabetes and insulin resistance, crohns/coeliac disease, surgical removal of part/all stomach; gall bladder removal, excess alcohol). For chronic disease prevention 5000mcg/day recommended from food.

UTI: non-toxic if from foods (even though large amounts can colour the skin); high levels from supplements may be toxic.

Apart from its role as provitamin A, beta-carotene acts as an antioxidant. Studies suggest a preventive role in cancer, stroke and heart disease when derived from food.

Skin damage by the UV sun rays may be lessened by a diet rich in beta-carotene and other carotenoids. Beta-carotene is just one of hundreds of other carotenoids and probably works best in combination with others.

	mcg/serve
Carrot juice 1 cup	2000mcg
Carrot 1 small 100g	1660mcg
Red palm oil 1 tbs	1400mcg
Spinach, raw, ½ cup	1000mcg
Sweet potato ½ cup 100g	990mcg
Mango, 1 medium	580mcg
Pumpkin, ckd, ½ cup 100g	410mcg
Capsicum (red) ½, 100g	250mcg
Pawpaw, ¼ small, 100g	160mcg
Rockmelon, 1 slice, 100g	130mcg

Persimmon, 100g	130mcg
Tomato, 1 medium, 150g	80mcg
Broccoli, 2–3 clusters, 100g	60mcg
Peas, ckd, ½ cup, 70g	50mcg
Beans, green, ½ cup, 60g	50mcg
Avocado, 100g flesh	50mcg
Peach, 2 medium	50mcg
Plums, 2 medium, 200g	50mcg
Apricots, 2–3 medium, 100g	30mcg
Orange, 1 medium	30mcg
Orange Juice, 250 ml cup	30mcg
Watermelon, 100g flesh	30mcg
Egg yolk, 1	30mcg

Vitamin B1 (Thiamin)

RDI: 1.1mg/day (alcoholics 10–100mg)
UTI: >25mg (non-toxic)
Destroyed by high temp, alcohol, coffee and requires magnesium for conversion to active form.
Every cell in the body needs thiamin to make ATP, especially the heart; essential for normal function of muscles, heart and nervous system; stabilises the appetite; promotes growth and good muscle tone. Deficiency is more common in alcoholics; Crohn's disease; folate deficiency; people on loop diuretics; seafood and herb horsetail can reduce absorption; elderly persons; Beriberi (loss of appetite, fatigue, nerve/muscle degeneration, mental confusion, staggering gait, heart failure, fluid retention); Wernicke–Korsakoff syndrome (double vision, faulty memory, abnormal behaviour). Alcohol interferes with thiamine absorption, storage and conversion into active form. Alcoholics require large doses to combat effects (10–100mg). Australian flour is fortified with thiamin.

	mg/serve
Sustagen, 250ml	0.6mg
Vegemite, ½ tsp, 3g	0.54mg
Milo 1 tbs	0.50mg
Pork, ckd, 120g	0.50mg
Muesli, ½ cup, 60g	0.50mg
Breakfast cereal, 1 cup, 30g	0.47mg
Pasta, wholemeal, ckd, 1 cup	0.36mg
Weetbix, 2 biscuits, 30g	0.28mg
Yoghurt, 200g	0.20mg
Nuts, mixed, ¼ cup, 40g	0.15mg
Peas, green, ckd, ⅓ cup, 55g	0.13mg
Orange, 1 medium	0.13mg
Milk, whole/skim, 1 cup	0.10mg
Lentils, ckd, ⅓ cup, 100g	0.08mg
Meat/Fish, ckd, 120g	0.07mg
Potato, ckd, 1 medium	0.07mg
Bread, w/meal, 1 slice 30g	0.08mg
Chicken, ckd, 120g	0.06mg

Vitamin B2 (Riboflavin)

RDI: 1.7mg/day
UTI: >25mg (non-toxic)
Destroyed by alcohol, light.
Necessary for protein, fat/carbohydrate metabolism; aids in the formation of antibodies and red blood cells; helps maintain good vision, skin, nails and hair; alleviates eye fatigue; may prevent cataracts; may help combat migraines; activates B6 and folate. Deficiency is rare, and causes corneal vascularization, glossitis, cheilosis, seborrheic dermatitis, and impaired wound healing.

	mg/serve
Liver, fried, 1 slice 40g	1.8mg
Vegemite, ½ tsp, 3g	0.66mg
Muesli, ½ cup, 60g	0.55mg
Sustagen 250ml	0.50mg
Breakfast cereal, 1 cup, 35g	0.48mg
Yoghurt, 200g	0.46mg
Milk, whole/skim, 1 cup	0.40mg
Almonds, ¼ cup, 45g	0.38mg
Meat (red), average, ckd, 120g	0.32mg
Milk, evaporated, 100ml	0.3mg
Salmon, pink, cnd, 100g	0.25mg
Egg, ckd, 1 large	0.20mg
Milo 1 tbs	0.20mg
Dark green vegetables ½ cup	0.20mg
Chocolate, 5–6 squares, 30g	0.17mg
Banana, 1 medium	0.15mg
Fish, ckd, fillet, 120g	0.12mg
Pasta, w/meal, ckd, 1 cup	0.12mg
Chicken, ckd, dark meat 90g	0.10mg
Cheese tasty 30g	0.10mg
Wheat germ 2 tbs 20g	0.10m
Bread, w/meal, 2 slices, 60g	0.07mg
Peanuts, 30g	0.03mg

Vitamin B3 (niacin/nicotinic acid/nicotinamide)

RDI: 1.7mg/day
UTI: 35mg for niacin or 900mg for nicotinamide
Relatively stable to heat and light. Little is lost in cooking.
Key role in metabolism of carbohydrates, fat and protein; required for proper function of 50 enzymes;
improves circulation; reduces cholesterol level; helps maintain nervous system; enhances immune system; used to make sex hormones; helps maintain a healthy skin, tongue and digestive system. Deficiency affects the skin, digestive tract and nervous system e.g. pellagra (diarrhoea, dermatitis, dementia); soreness and ulceration of mouth corners. High supplemental dosages (1–4g) used as a drug to lower blood cholesterol, can cause nausea and skin flushing. Nicotinamide may lower blood sugar levels.

Tuna, cnd, ½ cup, 100g	12mg
Fish, ckd, 100g	11mg
Chicken/Turkey, ckd, 100g	8mg
Salmon, canned, ½ cup, 100g	8mg
Liver, fried, 1 slice, 40g	8mg
Sardines, 100g	5mg
Muesli, ½ cup, 60g	5mg
Peanuts, 30g	4mg
Pasta, w/meal, ckd, 1 cup	4mg
Meat (red), ckd, 100g	4mg
Rice, brown, ckd, 1 cup	4mg
Vegemite, ½ tsp, 3g	4mg
Potato, 1 medium	3mg
Soya Beans, ½ cup, 100g	3mg
Fortified Breakfast cereal 1 cup	3mg
Avocado, ½ large, 100g	2mg
Mushrooms, 60g serve	2mg
Baked Beans, ½ cup, 150g	2mg
Lentils, 1 cup, ckd	2mg
Lima beans, 1 cup, ckd	2mg
Egg, boiled, 1 medium	1mg
Bread, w/meal, 1 slice	1mg
Coffee (brewed) 1 cup	0.5mg

Vitamin B5 (Pantothenic acid)

RDI: 5mg/day
UTI: >25mg (non-toxic)
Production of energy in body from macronutrients; manufacture

of red blood cells, antibodies, cholesterol, sex and adrenal hormones and acetylcholine; maintains a healthy digestive tract; helps body use other vitamins (particularly riboflavin) more effectively. Converted to pantethine in body. Pantethine supplements may lower triglycerides and cholesterol.

Deficiency is rare — symptoms include malaise, vomiting, burning feet.

Sources (in a wide variety of foods): liver, meat, fish, brewers yeast, eggs, milk, soy, broccoli, wheat germ, wheat bran, whole grain bread, peanuts, mushrooms, green leafy vegies, peas and green beans, nuts, dried beans.

Vitamin B6 (pyridoxine)

RDI: 1.5mg/day

UTI: 50mg

Better absorbed in small bowel at low pH. Destroyed by alcohol, cooking, processing, contraceptive pill, HRT. Requires magnesium and zinc to be converted to active form (pyridoxal 5 phosphate).

Major role in making proteins, hormones and neurotransmitters; formation of red blood cells and antibodies; reduces muscle spasms/cramps; maintains balance of sodium/phosphorous. Severe deficiency is rare but mild deficiencies are common, especially in the elderly, childern and with use of certain drugs (e.g. OCP, hydralazine, MAO inhibitors). Supplements can reduce morning sickness in pregnancy. Deficiency can cause anaemia, irritability, muscular weakness, insomnia, nervousness, skin eruptions/dermatitis, loss of hair, mouth disorders, water retention, slow learning. Megadoses (>50mg/day) may cause serious nerve damage (numbness in feet or hands, unsteady on feet).

	mg/serve
Oats instant 1pkt	0.74mg
Banana, one medium	0.7mg
Potato, ckd 1med	0.6mg
Chicken, ckd 100g	0.6mg
Chickpeas, ckd ½ cup	0.57mg
Beef liver 100g	0.5mg
Pork 100g	0.5mg
Breakfast cere 1 cup	0.4mg
Turkey, two thin slices	0.4mg
Sunflower seeds, ¼ cup	0.4mg
Watermelon med wedge	0.4mg
Meat, red 100g	0.3mg
Wheat germ, 2 tbs 20g	0.3mg
Pork chop medium	0.3mg
Crab meat ½ cup	0.3mg
Tuna/Sardines/Cod 100g	0.3mg
Artichokes 1 large	0.3mg
Sweet potato 1 med	0.3mg
Wheat bran 2 tbs 12g	0.2mg
Avocado ½	0.2mg
Tomato juice 180ml	0.2mg
Lentils cooked ½ cup	0.18mg
Peanut butter 2 tbs	0.15mg
Brewers yeast 1tsp	0.15mg
Rice brown, ckd ½ cup	0.15mg
Walnuts/hazelnuts 30g	0.15mg
Spinach, ckd ½ cup	0.14mg
Pecans 30g	0.1mg
Potato crisps 50g	0.1mg
Vegemite ½ tsp	0.07mg

Vitamin B12 (Cyanocobalamin)

RDI: 2.4mcg/day

UTI: >1000mcg (non-toxic)

Relatively stable to heat/cooking. Alcohol interferes with absorption.

Maintains healthy nervous system (assists in production of SAMe or S-adenosyl methionine) and improves memory and concentration; production of DNA and RNA; works with folate to regulate the formation of red blood cells and to help iron function properly; needed for calcium absorption; promotes growth in children; reduces heart disease risk by reducing homocysteine levels with the help of folate and vitamin B6; deficiency usually caused by a lack of intrinsic factor, a substance that allows the body to absorb vitamin B12 from the digestive system (symptoms include fatigue, shortness of breath, diarrhoea, pale yellow skin, depression, nervousness, numbness/tingling sensation in the fingers and toes). People with pernicious anaemia do not produce sufficient intrinsic factor and must take high doses of vitamin B12. Some evidence that high doses may reduce kidney function. B12 deficiency is rare in the young, but not unusual in older people because of lower levels of stomach acid needed to release B12 from protein, or due to use of reflux and diabetes medication. Avoiding animal foods increases risk of deficiency as it is not found in plant foods (except sun-exposed mushrooms).

	mcg/serve
Liver 1 slice 40g	30mcg
Sardines 100g	28mcg
Mackerel 100g	19mcg
Oysters 6	16mcg
Tuna/Salmon 100g	4mcg
Beef/Lamb 100g	3mcg
White fish 100g	1.5mcg
Yoghurt 1 cup	1.4mcg
Milk 1 cup	0.9mcg
Fortified soy milk 200ml	0.8mcg
Cottage cheese ½ cup	0.8mcg
Egg 1 med	0.6mcg
Cheese 30g	0.4mcg
Chicken 100g	0.4mcg

Negligible amounts in vegetables, grains, sun-exposed mushrooms, brewers yeast, soy products.

Folate (or folacin/folic/pteroylglutamic acid or vitamin B9)

RDI: 400mcg/day

UTI: 1000mcg from food and supplements

Unstable to heat, light and cooking (especially in water) destroys most of it. Alcohol reduces folate levels in the body.

DNA/RNA synthesis (important during periods of high growth, such as infancy, adolescence and pregnancy); aids in amino acid metabolism and thiamin production; folate works with vitamin B12 and vitamin C in production of red blood cells; helps iron function properly in the body; plays a role in brain function/mental and emotional health; involved in methylation processes. Deficiency is common; animal foods, with the exception of liver, are poor sources of folic acid; plant sources rich in folic acid are frequently not obtained in adequate amounts in the diet. Deficiency more common in pregnant women, elderly, alcoholics and use of certain drugs (eg. methotrexate, H2 blockers, NSAIDS, OCPs). Macrocytic anaemia is an early sign of deficiency. Deficiency in pregnant women increases risk of spina bifida in the growing fetus; risk reduced by supplement (400–600 mcg) daily before/during early months of pregnancy (since defect occurs by sixth week of pregnancy). Deficiency increases risk of cervical cancer and breast cancer but high dose also linked to higher risk of cancer, reduced kidney function and vascular events. Signs of deficiency include loss of appetite, irritability, forgetfulness, mental sluggishness, gingivitis, gastrointestinal disorders, inflammation of the tongue, mouth ulcer, peptic ulcer, poor growth, premature grey hair, elevated homocysteine levels (linked to heart disease). Australian bread is fontified with folate

	mcg/serve
Chicken livers, fried, 100g	500mcg
Cabbage (boiled) 100g	300mcg
Liver, fried, 100g	250mcg
Lentils/dried beans, ckd, ½ cup	180mcg
Spinach, ckd, ½ cup	100mcg
Asparagus 5 spears	100mcg
Artichoke, ckd 1	100mcg
Avocado, ½ medium	100mcg
Cabbage raw 100g	90mcg
Orange Juice, 1 cup	90mcg
Lettuce 1 cup	80mcg
Brussel Sprouts, ½ cup	80mcg
Strawberries 8	80mcg
Kiwi, 1 med	80mcg
Spinach raw 1 cup	60mcg
Oatmeal instant 1pkt	70mcg
Wheat Germ, 2 tbs, 20g	60mcg
Black eye peas, cnd, ½ cup	60mcg
Baked beans 1 cup	60mcg
Capsicum red 1	55mcg
Breakfast cereal fortified	50mcg
Peas, ½ cup	50mcg
Broccoli, ½ cup	50mcg
Corn 1 cob	50mcg
Orange, 1 medium	40mcg
Peanuts, roasted 30g	40mcg
Tomato juice 180ml	35mcg
Wheat bran, 2 tbs	30mcg
Almonds, 30g	30mcg
Bran breakfast cereals, 30g	30mcg
Vegemite/Marmite, ½ tsp, 3g	30mcg
Egg 1	25mcg
Rockmelon ¼ med	25mcg
Bread fortified 1 slice	25mcg
Banana med	20mcg
Shitake mushrooms ½ cup	15mcg

Biotin (vitamin B7 or Vitamin H)

RDI: 30mcg/day
UTI: >2mg/day (non-toxic)
Assists four enzymes with the breakdown of fats, carbohydrates and protein; helps maintain healthy skin, hair, nails and balanced hormonal system. Intestinal bacteria provide most of our biotin requirements. Deficiency can develop from intake of over 12 raw egg whites (contain a protein, avidin, that binds biotin and prevents its absorption; avidin destroyed by cooking). Deficiency symptoms include dermatitis, glossitis, lethargy, muscle pains, nausea. Best sources are listed below.

	mcg/serve
liver 90g	30mcg
egg yolk	20mcg
brewers yeast ½ tsp	5mcg
salmon 90g	5mcg
avocado	4mcg
pork 90g	3mcg
cheese 30g	1mcg
cauliflower 1 cup	1mcg
raspberries 1 cup	0.5mcg

PABA (Para amino benzoic acid)

Metabolism of amino acids; linked to red blood cell formation; linked to hair and skin growth.
Best sources: Brewers yeast, liver, kidneys, wholegrains, mushrooms.

Choline (in food as phosphatidyl choline)

RDI: 500mg/day
UTI: 3500mg/day
Choline is part of a major biochemical process in the body called methylation; used to make acetylcholine for normal muscle function; component of nerve myelin sheath and cell membranes; can be made by intestinal bacteria. Deficiency linked to spina bifida cirrhosis/ fatty liver, memory loss, senile dementia, Alzheimer's disease, multiple sclerosis. Choline/lecithin not shown to lower cholesterol.

	mg/serve
Beef liver 90g	355mg
Lecithin granules 1 tbs	250mg
Egg 1 large	126mg
Chicken/turkey 100g	70mg
Atlantic cod 90g	70mg
Beef cooked 90g	70mg
Broccoli/cauliflower 1 cup ckd	60mg
Shrimp, cnd, 90g	60mg
Salmon 90g, ckd	56mg
Navy beans 1 cup, ckd	50mg
Wheat germ ¼ cup	40mg
Milk 250ml	40mg
Tofu 100g	30mg
Almonds ½cup	25mg
Peanut butter 2 tbs	20mg
Milk chocolate 40g	20mg

Other sources: Oats, brewers yeast 1 tbs.

Inositol

RDI: not essential; suggested intake 100–200mg/day
UTI: not available
Part of cell membranes; plays a role in helping liver process fats; muscle/nerve function. Most dietary inositol is in the form of phytates (inositol hexaphosphate).
Probiotics/good bacteria in bowel help convert phytates in foods to inositol; coffee increases inositol excretion. Deficiency linked to depression. May improve ovulation in women with polycystic ovaries.
Best sources: wheat germ, wheat bran, brown rice, buckwheat, egg, oats, rye, lecithin, brewers yeast, corn, nuts/seeds, liver, dried beans, soy, molasses, oranges, rockmelon, bananas, raisins, probiotics.

Vitamin C (ascorbic acid)

RDI: 45mg/day
UTI: <2000mg/day
Destroyed by boiling food, light, cut food exposed to air, smoking and heat.
Highest concentration of vitamin C in adrenals needed to make cortisol and adrenaline (from

tyrosine); second highest concentration found in brain to make dopamine, serotonin and melatonin (from tryptophan); strengthens walls of body cells/ blood vessels; promotes healthy gums, teeth, bones, joints; promotes formation of collagen/ connective tissue; aids wound healing; stimulates immune system/helps resist infections; aids digestion (especially iron absorption) by activating production of gastrin/stomach acid and secretin/pancreatic enzymes; assists with conversion of lysine to carnitine (which transports fats into muscle mitochondria for oxidation); Deficiency more common in the elderly; smokers; pollution exposure; some medications destroy vitamin C (eg: aspirin, PPIs, OCP). Stress and heavy metal exposure can increase need for vitamin C. Deficiency symptoms: loss of appetite, insomnia, swollen bleeding gums, poor wound healing, easy bruising, aching joints, susceptibility to infection, capillary weakness, nosebleeds, dry/itchy skin, anaemia, fatigue, muscular weakness, impaired digestion, psychological changes.

	mg/serve
Acerola cherries, 1 cup	800mg
Guava, 1 med	180mg
Blackcurrant cordial dil 1 cup	180mg
Capsicum red/yellow, 1 raw	150mg
Kiwi golden, 1 large	130mg
Orange juice 240ml	110mg
Acai juice 240ml	100mg
Capsicum, green, 1 raw	90mg
Kiwi, green, 1 large	70mg
Orange 1 medium	70mg
Cabbage ½ cup	60mg
Broccoli, ckd, ½ cup	60mg
Rockmelon 1 cup	60mg
Papaya 1	50mg
Cauliflower, ckd, ½ cup	50mg
Asparagus	50mg
Mango 1 medium	50mg
Brussel sprouts 4	50mg
Persimmon 1	40mg
Mandarin 1	30mg
Green leafy veg ½ cup	30mg
Peas, black-eye peas ½ cup	30mg
Tomato med	25mg
Strawberries 6	25mg
Raspberries ½ cup	20mg
Potato, ckdmed	20mg
Milo 1 tbs	20mg
Banana med	15mg

Vitamin D3 (calciferol or cholecalciferol or ergosterol)

RDI: 5–15mcg or 200–600IU/day; if sun deprived: 25mcg/1000IU/day
UTI: 80mcg or 3200IU/day (1ug = 40IU)
Is both a vitamin and a hormone
Destroyed by mineral oil.

Made from cholesterol in the skin when exposed to sunshine; converted to active form in liver and kidneys with the help of magnesium; involved in absorption/metabolism of calcium, zinc, magnesium, iron, phosphorus; bone and teeth formation; maintains a stable nervous system; maintains a healthy heart; immune system function and inhibition of auto-immunity; assists cell differentiation and reduces cancer cells; needed for insulin secretion; blood pressure regulation. Deficiency more common in elderly persons (reduced ability to make vitamin D in skin), in the house/office bound, in obese (stored in fat), alcoholics, dark-skinned people, liver and kidney disease, coeliac and Crohn's disease and use of certain drugs (phenytoin, anticonvulsants, steroids, cimetidine, heparin). Symptoms include poor bone growth, rickets (soft bones/enlarged joints), osteomalacia (adult rickets), softening of teeth, muscle twitching/weakness/pain. Low intake linked to osteoporosis, diabetes, hypertension, cancer, autoimmune diseases, heart disease, multiple sclerosis, depression, cognition, fat accumulation, anaemia.

	IU/serve
Cod-liver oil 1 tbs	1300IU
Salmon, cnd, 90g	530IU
Salmon, ckd, 90g	300IU
Sardines, 90g	230IU
Anlene milk, 250ml	200IU
Mackerel, 90g	200IU
Tuna, cnd, 90g	200IU
Soymilk, fortified, 250ml	100IU
Cows Milk, fortified, 250ml	100IU
Orange juice, fortified, 250ml	100IU
Margarine fortified 1 tbs	60IU
Breakfast cereal fortified 1 cup	40IU
Egg 1	20IU
Swiss cheese 30g	12IU

Other sources: Brewers yeast and mushrooms, calf/chicken liver; breast milk has minimal vitamin D.

Vitamin E (alpha tocopherol)

RDI: 10mg or 15IU day
UTI: 300mg or 500IU
Processing, refining and storage can deplete vitamin E. Unstable to heat, light, freezing.

Principal role as an antioxidant; retards cellular aging due to oxidation; prevents oxidation of polyunsaturated fats; helps with red blood cell formation; enhances immunity; may reduce risk of cancer and heart disease but at doses >50IU can increase blood pressure and risk of these diseases; may prevent oxidation of LDL-cholesterol; may reduce arthritis pain; may reduce progression of Alzheimers; protects lungs from air pollutants; may relieve leg cramps, angina, intermittent claudication; may help prevent peripheral neuropathy; may prevent blood clots (has a blood thinning effect) but at doses >50IU can increase risk of bleeding strokes; promotes fertility; reduces/prevents hot flushes in menopause and PMS; may help skin look younger; may promote healing. Deficiency is rare but may be seen in intestinal malabsorption. Symptoms include: haemolytic anaemia and /or elevated bilirubin; neuropathy; dry skin and/or eczema; muscle weakness.

	mg/serve
Wheat germ oil, 1 tbs, 20ml	24mg
Sustagen Sport, powder, 50g	7.7mg
Almonds, dried, 25 nuts, 30g	7mg
Margarine, polyunsat. 30g	7mg
Sweet potato, 1 med. 130g	6mg
Tuna, cnd in oil, 100g	6mg
Almond oil 1 tbs	5mg

Safflower oil, 1 tbs, 20ml	5mg
Sunflower seeds, ¼ cup, 35g	5mg
Cottonseed oil 1 tbs	4.8mg
Acai juice 250ml	4.5mg
Hazelnuts, dried, 30g	4mg
Peanut butter, 1 tbs, 20g	4mg
Rice bran oil, 1 tbs, 20g	4mg
Amaranth breakfast cereal 25g	3mg
Avocado 1medium	2.7mg
Palm oil, 1 tbs, 20ml	2.6mg
Canola oil, 1 tbs, 20ml	2.4mg
Peanuts, dried, 30g	2.4mg
Mango, 1 med	2.3mg
Tuna, cnd, drained of oil, 100g	2mg
Oatmeal, raw, ¼ cup	2mg
Spinach, 3 leaves, 60g	2mg
Corn oil, 1 tbs, 20ml	1.9mg
Olive oil extra virgin, 1 tbs, 20ml	1.7mg
Peanut oil, 1 tbs, 20ml	1.6mg
Wheat germ, 1 tbs, 10g	1.5mg
Pistachios 30g	1.5mg
Navy beans, dry, ½ cup	1.5mg
Parsley sprigs, 2–3, 5g	1.5mg
Soybean oil, 1 tbs, 20ml	1.1mg
Mayonnaise, 1 tbs, 22g	1mg
Egg yolk, 1 large	1mg
Walnuts, dried, 30g	1mg
Asparagus (fresh), 60g	1mg
Broccoli, 100g	1mg
Kiwi, 1 med	1mg
Rice bran 2 tbs 15g	0.7mg

Other forms of vitamin E include beta and gamma tocopherols and tocotrienols which have also been linked to health benefits. Foods high in gamma tocopherol: soybean oil, corn oil, canola oil, peanuts; amaranth and rice bran are high in vitamin E and tocotrienols.

Vitamin K1 (Phylloquinone)

RDI: 70mcg/day
UTI: not available
Can also be made by intestinal bacteria.
Heat stable.

Can be produced in the intestines and this function is improved with the presence of fermented foods high in live cultures. Vitamin K1 (phylloquinone), is found in plants and vitamin K2 (menaquinone) can be synthesised by many bacteria thus is found in cheese/yoghurt; vitamin K3, menadione, is a synthetic form of this vitamin which is man-made; used in the body to control blood clotting/ prevent bleeding; essential for synthesising prothrombin a precursor to the liver protein thrombin that controls the clotting; involved in bone formation and repair and may decrease the incidence or severity of osteoporosis and slow bone loss (helps body transport calcium). Emerging evidence that vitamin K2 can decrease prostate cancer risk. Deficiency is rare but may occur in people with long-term use of antibiotics, chronic diarrhoea, coeliac, crohn's, ulcerative colitis, alcoholics.

	mcg/serve
Amaranth leaves ½ cup, ckd	1200mcg
Chicory, ckd ½ cup	800mcg
Coriander raw ¼ cup	750mcg
Kale 1 cup raw	550mcg
Beef liver 100g	500mcg
Seaweed ½ cup raw	500mcg
Chard, Swiss ½ cup, ckd	500mcg
Green/white tea 250ml	500mcg
Spinach ½ cup, ckd	400mcg
Mint raw ¼ cup	400mcg
Broccoli, ckd 1 cup	250mcg
Chickpeas ½ cup, ckd	250mcg
Parsley raw ¼ cup	240mcg
Endive, ckd, ½ cup	200mcg
Cauliflower, ckd 1 cup	200mcg
Chinese cabbage ½ cup, ckd	200mcg
Mung beans, ckd, ¾ cup	200mcg
Lentils ½ cup ckd	150mcg
Brussel sprouts, ckd 4	120mcg
Soy beans 1 cup, ckd	100mcg
Lettuce raw 1 cup	100mcg
Onions white/spring ⅓ cup	100mcg
Chicken liver 100g	100mcg
Watercress raw 1 cup	85mcg
Okra, ckd1 cup	80mcg
Spinach raw ½ cup	70mcg
Cabbage raw/ckd, 1 cup	60mcg
Peas 1 cup ckd	60mcg
Green apple 1	60mcg
Celery 3 stalks	60mcg
Cucumber 1	60mcg
Green tomato 1 raw	60mcg
Wheat bran cereal 1 cup	40mcg
Avocado 1	40mcg
Green beans ½ cup, ckd	40mcg
Pistachio nuts 30g	40mcg
Coffee 1 cup	30mcg
Asparagus, ckd, 4 spears	30mcg
Kiwi fruit 1	30mcg
Blueberries 1 cup	28mcg
Soy bean oil 1 tbs	26mcg
Mangos 1	25mcg
Oats ½ cup	25mcg
Beans ½ cup, ckd	20mcg
Egg yolk	20mcg
Canola oil 1 tbs	18mcg
Soy milk 1 cup	7mcg
Olive oil	7mcg
Mayonnaise 1 tbs	6mcg

Minerals

Calcium

RDI: 1100mg/day
UTI: 2500mg/day

Absorption of calcium requires adequate stomach acid levels. Calcium plays a vital role in nerve and muscle function; blood clotting; enzyme regulation; insulin secretion; overall bone strength; insomnia; heartbeat; passage of nutrients in and out of cell walls; lowering of cholesterol and blood pressure; prevention of muscle cramps; reducing PMS symptoms; may reduce the incidence of colon cancer. High intakes from supplements may increase risk of prostate cancer and heart attack in older women. To function correctly, calcium must be accompanied by magnesium, phosphorous, vitamins A, C, D, and K. The body can't absorb more than 500mg of calcium at one time and absorption is better in the evening.

	mg/serve
Milk enriched 1 cup	
Anlene	500mg
Physical	400mg
Milk 1 cup cow/sheep/ goat regular/lite	300mg
Soy/Rice milk fortified 1 cup	300mg
Yoghurt 200g tub	300mg
Cheese yellow 40g	300mg
Ricotta cheese ½ cup	300mg
Parmesan cheese 3 tbs	300mg
Sardines/salmon+bones 100g	300mg
Soup stock from bones 1 cup	300mg
Breakfast cereals fortified (e.g. Special K) 1 cup	200mg
Dried figs 5	200mg
Green leafy vegies (e.g. kale, bok choy, spinach, silverbeet,	

Chinese cabbage) 1 cup, ckd 180mg
Milo 1 tbs 160mg
Fetta cheese 40g 150mg
Amaranth 100g 150mg
Prawns 100g 130mg
Chia seeds 15g 120mg
Cottage cheese ½ cup 100mg
Oats ½ cup raw 100mg
Tofu firm (set $CaSO_4$) 60g 100mg
Colombo ice-cream 1 scoop 90mg
Dried beans ½ cup, ckd 80mg
Tahini (sesame paste) 1 tbs 80mg
Philadelphia cheese 3 tbs 80mg
Almonds ¼ cup or 1 tbs paste 70mg
Brocolli 1 cup, ckd 70mg
Ice-cream 1 scoop all types 65mg
Orange 1 50mg
Soy/rice milk regular 1 cup 30mg

Chromium

RDI: 30mcg/day
UTI: 300mcg/day
High sugar diets/diabetes increase chromium losses in urine. Natural chromium levels decline with age.
Part of the low molecular weight chromium binding substance which promotes efficient insulin function; essential for carbohydrate, fat and corticosteriod metabolism; may protect against diabetes; helps regulate appetite. Deficiency is difficult to assess. Some evidence that chromium supplements may help lower blood sugar levels in people with diabetes and prediabetes; may also lower triglycerides and cholesterol.

	mcg/serve
Red wine 150ml	1–13mcg
brocolli ½ cup	11mcg
Turkey ham (processed) 90g	10mcg
Grape juice 1 cup	7mcg
Potatoes 1 cup mashed	3mcg
Garlic dried 1tsp	3mcg
Orange juice 1 cup	2mcg
Beef 100g	2mcg
Bread wholewheat 2 slices	2mcg
Turkey breast 100g	1.8mcg
Apple with peel	1.4mcg
Banana	1.0mcg
Green beans ½ cup	1.0mcg

Other sources: dark chocolate/cocoa, cheese, liver, wheat bran, wheat germ, breakfast cereals brewers yeast (from chromium-rich barley), blackstrap molasses, egg yolk, dried fruit and processed meat.

Iron

RDI: 8mg/day men/women >50yrs 18mg/day women <50yrs
UTI: 45mg/day (100–200mg/day to correct deficiency)
Fibre, phytic acid and other minerals reduce absorption. Absorption of iron requires adequate stomach acid levels.
Needed for 93 enzymes; conversion of lysine to carnitine (which transports fats into muscle mitochondria for oxidation); cofactor in cytochromes for production of energy in mitochondria; cofactor for conversion of tryptophan to serotonin and tyrosine to adrenaline. Major function is to combine with protein and copper to make haemoglobin; increases resistance to stress/disease; formation of muscle myoglobin (supplies oxygen for contraction). Adult men and postmenopausal women lose very little iron except through bleeding. Deficiency can cause fatigue, irritability, pale skin, feels cold, heart palpitations, shortness of breath, constipation, decrease in attention span, anaemia, spoon shaped nails with ridges running lengthwise, finger tingling/numbness. Vitamin A helps mobilise iron from storage sites so deficiency may exacerbate iron deficiency (sometimes seen in hypothyroid and diabetes).

	mg/serve
Chicken liver, ckd, 100g	13mg
Amaranth 100g	7.5g
Liver (beef), grilled, 100g	6.5mg
Sustagen Sports, powder, 60g	6mg
Milo 1 tbs	6mg
Apricots dried 3	5mg
Oysters, 6 med, 60g	5mg
Burgen wholemeal 2 slices	4.8mg
Lentils ½ cup, ckd	4mg
Quinoa, ckd, 1 cup (¼ cup raw)	4mg
Burgen pumpkin seed 2 slices	3.8mg
Molasses 1 tbs	3.5mg
Tofu firm ½ cup	3.4mg
Breakfast cereals e.g. Special K, Oat flakes, Guardian, Just right (All bran is high in iron but phytate/fibre content reduces iron absorption) 1 cup, 30g	3mg
Sustagen Hospital, pder, 60g	3mg
Spinach ½ cup, ckd	3mg
Herring, 100g	3mg
Beef, lean, 100g	3mg
Dried/baked beans, ckd ½ cup	3mg
Prune juice, 1 cup	3mg
Rice red 1 cup, ckd150g	2.5mg
Chia seeds 15g	2.5mg
Lamb, pork, lean, 100g	2.5mg
Turkey, dark meat 100g, ckd	2.3mg
Asparagus, cnd, 5 spears	2mg
Cashews 30g	2mg
Raisins ½ cup	1.5mg
Rice black 1 cup, ckd 150g	1.5mg
Chicken, 100g, ckd	1.3mg
Wheatgerm, 2 tbs, 15g	1.3mg
Pistachios 30g (49 kernels)	1.2mg
Rice brown 1 cup, ckd 150g	1g
Luncheon meats, aver. 50g	1mg
Fish white, ckd, 100g	1mg
Tuna cnd, 100g	1mg
Sardines, 35g	1mg
Egg 1 large	1mg
Soy milk 250ml	1mg
Porridge, ¾ cup	1mg
Broccoli, 100g	1mg
Avocado, ½ medium	1mg
Tomato juice, 1 cup	1mg
Nuts mixed 30g	1mg
Sunflower seeds, 1 tbs	1mg
Pumpkin seeds, 1 tbs	1mg
Pork, 100g, ckd	0.8mg
Potato, 1 medium, 150g	0.8mg
Peanut butter, 1 tbs, 20g	0.5mg
Rice white1 cup, ckd 150g	0.5mg

Magnesium (Mg)

RDI: 300–400mg/day
UTI: 350mg/d (from supplements only)
High sugar diets/alcohol/diabetes/medications increase magnesium losses in urine. Absorption of magnesium requires adequate stomach acid levels, vitamin B6 and vitamin D, selenium.
Needed for the function of 300 enzymes, especially for activation

of most vitamins, like vitamin D, B1 and B6, and metabolism of Ca, K, P, Zn and Na. Major role in glucose/fat metabolism and production of energy/ATP through its help with enzyme activity; where calcium stimulates muscles, magnesium relaxes muscles; helps relax muscle lining of breathing passages and lungs; aids formation of bone/teeth; assists absorption of calcium, potassium, vitamin C; high intake of zinc and vitamin D increases need for Mg; maintains normal heart rhythm, blood pressure, nerve function; helps in glucose metabolism; helps reduce inflammation and C reactive protein; helps mood/ sleep and PMS symptoms due to its involvement in production of hormones and neuro-transmitters. Deficiency found more commonly in some patients with hypertension (and those on diuretic drugs), diabetics, asthmatics, migraine sufferers, patients with arrythmia, osteoporosis, chronic diarrhoea, elderly, dieters, pregnant women, alcohol drinkers and athletes. Symptoms of low intake include muscle cramps, nausea, anorexia, vomiting, diarrhoea, irritability, confusion, tremors, loss of coordination. Magnesium may help migraines, PMT, diabetes, hypertension, heart failure, muscle cramps, constipation, asthma, fatigue.

	mg/serve
Amaranth 100g	260mg
Pumpkin seeds 30g 2 tbs	180mg
Burgen wholemeal 2 slices	140mg
Burgen pumpkin seed 2 slices	140mg
Bran breakfast cereal e.g. All Bran 45g	110mg
Dark chocolate 50g	100mg
Oat Bran ½ cup	100mg
Bread, wholemeal, 4 slices	90mg
Greek coffee 1	90mg
Halibut, ckd, 90g	90mg
Quinoa, ckd 1 cup (¼ cup raw)	90mg
Tofu (hard) fermented 100g	50–90mg
Brown rice 1 cup cooked	86mg
Sustagen Sports, powder, 60g	84mg
Milk Anlene 1 cup	80mg
Spinach cooked ½ cup	80mg
Vegetables, dark green leafy (e.g. swiss chard) ½ cup, ckd	80mg
Porridge, ckd, ¾ cup (40g raw)	70mg
Cashews, 15 nuts, 30g	70mg
Almonds, 15 nuts, 30g	70mg
Soya beans ckd, ½ cup 120g	70mg
Chickpeas ckd, ½ cup	60mg
Chia seeds 15g	60mg
Potato baked with skin 1 med	57mg
Peanuts, shelled, 30 nuts, 30g	50mg
Peanut butter, 2 tbs	50mg
Molasses blackstrap 1 tbs	48mg
Okra ½ cup cooked	47mg
Hazelnuts, 20 nuts	45mg
Walnuts 14 halves	45mg
Pasta wholemeal 1 cup	40mg
Avocado, ½ medium, 150g	40mg
Banana, 1 medium	40mg
Bran, wheat, 1 tbs, 6g	40mg
Beans, haricot, lima, kidney, black eyed peas ½ cup, ckd,	40mg
Baked beans, ½ cup, 150g	40mg
Lentils, ½ cup, ckd	35mg
Wheat germ 2 tbs	35mg
Milo 1 tbs	35mg
Weetbix 2	35mg
Milk cow or soy 1 cup	30mg
Yoghurt 200g	30mg
Salmon/Tuna, cnd, 100g	30mg
Raisins ¼ cup	25mg
Corn ½ cup, ckd	20mg

Zinc (Zn)

RDI: 14mg/day men
8mg/day women
UTI: 40mg/day

Fibre, phytic acid, other minerals and some medications reduce absorption. Increased urinary losses in diabetes.

About 90 enzymes need zinc for activity (e.g. enzymes involved in producing DNA; activation of vitamin B6); zinc is needed to mobilise vitamin A from liver stores; needed for production of thyroxine by thyroid; improves concentration, mood and sleep (zinc helps convert tryptophan to serotonin/melatonin and helps convert B6 to active form pyridoxal phosphate also needed in this reaction); required for digestion (makes stomach acid); needed for blood sugar level regulation (involved in insulin/ glucagon production); necessary for protein synthesis/tissue growth; structure/function of cell membranes; wound healing, healing of gastric ulcers/gut permeability; development of reproductive organs, prostate function, sperm production and male hormone activity; needed for healthy immune system and skin (acne, boils, eczema/dermatitis), required to maintain taste/ smell; maintains body's alkaline balance; aids in digestion/ metabolism of phosphorus and selenium; slows progress of macular degeneration; High doses of zinc (>40mg) can cause nausea, headache, suppression of immune system, lowering of HDL cholesterol, reduced absorption of chromium and copper. Deficiency seen in elderly, dieters, vegetarians, athletes, alcoholics, anorexia, chronic diarrhoea, crohn's disease, diabetics, thyroid conditions and use of certain medications (diuretics, OCP, PPI, ACE inhibitors). Symptoms: retarded growth, poor appetite, loss/change of taste/smell, mental lethargy, slow wound healing, prone to infections, white spots on fingernails, stretch marks, excessive hair loss, reduced sperm count and ejaculatory fluids, reduced sexual libido.

	mg/serve
Oysters, 6 medium, 30g	19mg
Beef steak, grilled, 120g	6mg
Lamb, ckd, 120g	5mg
Scallops, 10 medium, 80g	5mg
Anlene milk 1 cup	4mg
Turkey, roasted 120mg	3 mg
Amaranth seeds 100g	3mg
Burgen wholemeal bread 2 slices	3mg
Burgen pumpkin bread 2 slices	3mg
Sausage, grilled, 2 thick, 130g	3mg
Lobster/crayfish, ½ cup, 80g	3mg
Sustagen Sport, powder, 60g	3mg
Pork, leg, baked, 2 slices, 90g	2.2mg
Cashew nuts, ¼ cup, 40g	2mg
Lentils/chickpeas/beans 1 cup ckd 170g	2mg

All-Bran, ½ cup, 35g	1.8mg
Rice red, 1 cup, ckd, 150g	1.5mg
Pumpkin seeds 20g 1 tbs	1.5mg
Baked beans, ½ cup, 150g	1.2mg
Peanuts, ¼ cup, 40g	1.2mg
Quinoa, ckd 1 cup (¼ cup raw)	1mg
Salmon/tuna, cnd, ½ cup, 100g	1mg
Soy milk, 250ml	1mg
Milk (whole/skim), 1 cup	1mg
Yoghurt, fruit, 200g ctn	1mg
Cheese, cheddar, 30g	1mg
Sunflower seeds, 1 tbs, 16g	1mg
Chia seeds 15g	1mg
Porridge, ckd ¾ cup (40g raw)	0.8mg
Chicken, ckd, 100g fillet	0.8mg
Fish, ckd, 1 fillet, 120g	0.7mg
Peanut butter, 1 tbs	0.7mg
Tahini 1 tbs 15g	0.7mg
Peas, green, ½ cup	0.6mg
Egg, 1 large	0.5mg
Rice, brown, ckd, 1 cup	0.5mg
Sweetcorn, 1 cobette, 85g	0.3mg
Rice white 1 cup, ckd 150g	0.2mg

Potassium

RDI: 2800–4700mg/day

UTI: >10g?

Boiling reduces potassium levels.

The major mineral element in body cells; important role in electrolyte balance, nerve conduction and muscle contraction/heartbeat; energy production; protein synthesis; helps neutralise sodium's tendency to raise blood pressure; may lower risk of death from stroke; preserves proper alkalinity of body fluids; stimulates kidneys to eliminate wastes; promotes healthy skin. Deficiency more common in persons on diuretic drugs and with prolonged vomiting and diarrhoea. Symptoms: muscular weakness, apathy, confusion, abnormal heartbeat, respiratory failure. Toxicity rare in healthy people; over 250mmol (~10g) may cause cardiac arrest; toxicity more likely with kidney, heart or liver disease.

	mg/serve
Avocado, ½ med, 150g	700mg
Lite salt, ½ tsp. 2.5g	660mg
Potato, baked, 120g	660mg
Potato, fried, 120g	660mg
Soyabeans, ckd, 150g	540mg
Prune juice 150ml	500mg
Coconut milk 200ml	500mg
Lima beans ½ cup, ckd	480mg
Meat, average, ckd, 100g	470mg
Potato, boiled, 120g	440mg
Yoghurt, fruit, 200g ctn	440mg
Tomato, raw, 1 medium	430mg
Spinach ½ cup, ckd	420mg
Fish, average, ckd, 100g	400mg
Tomato juice 150ml	400mg
Milk: whole/skim, 1 cup	370mg
Kidney beans /lentils boiled ½ cup,	360mg
Amaranth 100g	360mg
Prunes 50g (5 prunes)	360mg
Orange juice 150ml	350mg
Soy (e.g. So Good), 1 cup	350mg
Banana, 1 med, 150g	350mg
Artichoke, 1 med , ckd	340mg
Baked beans, ½ cup 150g	330mg
Watermelon, med wedge	330mg
Chicken, ckd, 120g	330mg
Kiwi, 1 med	300mg
Molasses blackstrap 1 tbs	300mg
Salmon/tuna, cnd, 100g	300mg
Pumpkin, baked, 100g	300mg
Mango, 1 med	300mg
Dried fruit, average, 30g	270mg
Berries/strawberries 1 cup	250mg
Sunflower seeds 30g	240mg
Peach, 1 med, 120g	230mg
Rockmelon, 1 med wedge	200mg
Nuts, average, 30g	200mg
Brown/wholemeal, 4 slices	200mg
Grapes, 1 cup	170mg
Muesli, average, 45g	170mg
Apple, 150g	150mg
Orange, 1 medium, 130g	150mg
Peas, raw, ¼ cup, 35g	150mg
Cabbage, raw, 50g	130mg
Carrots, raw, 50g	110mg
Vegemite, 1 tsp, 5g	110mg
Porridge ½ cup ckd	100 mg
Weetbix, 2 biscuits	100mg
Chia seeds 15g	100mg
Ice-cream, 1 scoop	100mg
Egg, 1 large	80mg
Spaghetti, ckd, 1cup, 150g	80mg
Rice, boiled, 1 cup, 160g	70mg
Peas, boiled, 35g	50mg

Selenium

RDI: 70mcg/day

UTI: 400mcg/day

Absorption requires adequate stomach acid levels and zinc; reduced absorption due to helicobacter stomach infection, certain medications (proton pump inhibitors).

Promotes more energy in the body by helping thyroid make thyroxine (T4) and helps convert T4 (also found in thyroid medication) to active form (T3); needed for CoQ_{10} production involved in producing energy in mitochondria, especially in heart muscle; protects cell membranes via glutathione peroxidase and prevents free radical generation decreasing risk of cancer/heart disease; preserves tissue elasticity/slows down aging/hardening of tissues through oxidation; treatment/prevention of dandruff; stimulates increased antibody response to infections; helps with alleviating menopausal symptoms; production of healthy sperm; low selenium linked to cancer, heart disease, cholesterol, premature ageing, arthritis, hypothyroid, diabetes, dandruff, psoriasis, depression. Deficiency may be seen in patients with crohn's, ulcerative colitis and taking certain drugs (PP1, H_2 blockers).

	mcg/serve
Brazil nuts 15g (3 nuts)	270mcg
Chicken liver 100g, ckd	80mcg
Tuna, cnd, 90g	65mcg
Couscous, ckd, 1 cup	43mcg
Halibut/herring, ckd 90g	40mcg
Pasta, ckd, 1 cup	37mcg
Pork 90g	35mcg
Shrimp/crab meat 90g	35mcg
Salmon, ckd, 90g	32mcg
Rabbit, ckd, 100g	30mcg
Bagel 1 medium	27mcg
Turkey/chicken 90g	26mcg
Beef, ckd, 90g	20mcg
Wheat germ 2 tbs 20g	15mcg
Egg 1 medium	14mcg
Cottage cheese ½ cup	12mcg
Oatmeal, ckd 1 cup	12mcg
Brown rice ½ cup, ckd	10mcg
Wheat bran 2 tbs 12g	9mcg
Mushrooms ½ cup 60g, ckd	8mcg
Barley pearl ½ cup, ckd	8mcg
Milk 1 cup	5mcg
Walnuts 30g	5mcg
Sunflower seeds ¼ cup	5mcg
Wholegrain bread 1 slice	5mcg
Asparagus 60g 3 spears, ckd	4mcg
Legumes, ckd 100g	4mcg

Peanuts 30g 2mcg
Cabbage red 100g, ckd 2mcg
Garlic 3g 1 clove 0.7mcg
Other sources: brewers yeast.

Sodium

RDI: 460–920 mg/day
UTI: 2300mg (or 1600mg if have hypertension)
1 teaspoon salt = 2000mg sodium
1 teaspoon lite salt = 1000mg sodium
NAS = no added salt

Sodium is essential for nerve and muscle function, to balance the amount of fluid in our tissues and blood and for the production of hydrochloric acid in the stomach.Any extra sodium is excreted by the kidneys. Consuming excess sodium may lead to oedema, increase the risk of osteoporosis (even if calcium intake is adequate), hypertension, Meniere's disease vertigo attacks, premenstrual syndrome and swollen ankles.

Low salt foods <120mg/100g

Sanitarium lite-bix
Weetbix
Weetbix kids
Kelloggs mini-wheats
Kelloggs Just Right
Kelloggs Komplete Muesli
Kelloggs Sustain
Nestle Milo Cereal
Freedom Foods cornflakes
Sunsol Muesli
Uncle Tobys Rolled Oats
Uncle Toby's Oats Temptations
Uncle Toby's Fibre Plus
Uncle Toby's Ots Fruit Bites
Sanitarium Honey Weets
Sanitarium Puffed Wheat
Lowan Healthy Balance
Lowan Oat bran with Fruit
Moores low-salt wholemeal bread
Naturis Organic Salt-free bread
Naturis Wholemeal Buckwheat bread
Naturis Fruit and Nut Loaf
Essene bread
Egyptian bread
Potts VitAmeal bread
Matzos dry biscuits
Trident cheese rice crackers
Ryvita crispbread
Sun Rice Thick Rice Cakes
Freedom Foods corn chips
IGA Way of Life Potato Chips
Freedom foods muesli breakfast bar
Unibic Amaretti almond macaroons
Almond bread biscuits
Arnotts Triple Wafer biscuits
Arnotts Royals Dark chocolate
D'Lush Gluten free biscuits
Select Orange Delights
Naturally Good Gluten Free Peanut
Crunch Cookies
Big Sister Honey and Oat slice
Sara Lee Apple Caramel
Coles Taco shells
Diego's white corn tortillas
Unsalted nuts
Coles Peanut Butter
Scotts Lemon curd
Mayvers Tahini
MeadowLea free margarine
Lemnos Paneer cheese
Pantalica Ricotta cheese
Coles salmon red/pink
Coles fish fillets
King Oscar sardines
Sanitarium Dr Tickell's soup
SPC Bean Cuisine
Heinz NAS baked beans
Woolworth red kidney beans
Heinz toddler food
Edgell stir fry vegies
Farmland NAS asparagus
Golden Circle corn
Coles NAS beetroot
NAS tomatoes
NAS mushrooms
Naked Foods pasta sauce
Fountain tomato paste
Lotus savoury yeast flakes (sprinkle on pasta instead of parmesan)
Mayvers mayonnaise
NAS tomato sauce e.g. Fountain
Beerenberg mint jelly
Maxwell Treats low sodium mustard
Keens hot curry powder
V8 vegetable juice low sodium

Moderate–High salt >120mg/100g

Most breads 400–500mg/100g
Burgen breads 300mg/100g
Muesli bar average 40mg
Breakfast cereals 300–500mg/100g
Kelloggs Coco Pops 1 cup 45g 250mg
Nutrigrain 1 cup 40g 240mg
Rice bubbles 1 cup 215mg
Allbran ¾ cup 200mg
Cornflakes 1 cup 200mg
Special K ¾ cup 160mg
Froot Loops ¾ cup 140mg
Sultana bran 1 cup 130mg
Guardian 1 cup 120mg
Branflakes 2/3 cup 115mg
Uncle Toby's Lite Start 45g 205mg
Vitabrits 2 biscuits 130mg
Weeties 45g 135mg
Weetbix Hi-Bran 1 biscuit 80mg
Most hard yellow cheeses (tasty) 600mg/100g
Most softer yellow cheeses (e.g. Jarslberg) 300–600mg/100g
Processed cheddar >1000mg/100g
Parmesan >1000mg/100g
Most hard white cheeses (fetta) >600mg/100g
Most softer white cheeses (camembert, cream cheese, bocconcini) 300–600mg/100g
Ricotta 120mg/100mg
Cottage cheese 280mg/100g
Butter 1 tbs 20g 145mg
Margarine 1 tbs 20g 160mg
Margarine lite 1 tbs 20g 80mg
Vegemite ½ tsp 100mg
Peanut butter 1 tbs 20g 125mg
Ham leg 1 slice 30g 475mg
Mortadella, Strasburg 30g 250mg
Luncheon meat/chicken 30g 250mg
Canned fish in brine drained (tuna, sardines) 400mg
Smoked fish 100g 1200mg
Packet soups 200ml 800mg
Reduced salt soups 200ml 400mg
Baked beans 100g ¼ cup 350mg
Canned vegetables 100g 100–300mg
Lean cuisine meals 1000mg
Healthy choice meals 650mg
Meat pie average 175g 900mg
Sausage roll large 660mg
Hamburger average 1000mg
Hot dog average 900mg
Doner kebab 400g 1200mg
Fish n chips salted 600mg
Noodles 2 min 70g cup >1500mg
Fried chicken 100g 400mg
Fried rice 1 cup 150g 800mg
Pizza (meat) ¼ medium 1500mg
Sandwich ham/salad 900mg
Hot chips salted 1 cup 300mg
Potato crisps 50g 400–600mg
Corn chips 50g 200mg

Salty biscuits e.g. Jatz	>1000mg/100g
Vitawheat 1	30mg
Sesame wheat biscuits 1	80mg
Salada, 4 squares	160mg
Sweet biscuits average 1	30–60mg
Tomato sauce 1 tbs	200mg
Tomato juice 250ml	730mg
Soy sauce 1 tbs	1500mg
Green olives 4 med	450mg
Black olives 4 med 20g	140mg
Gatorade 600ml	280mg
Powerade 600ml	150mg
Redbull or V drink	250mg

Iodine

RDI: 150mcg/day (>200mcg/day may suppress thyroid function)
UTI: 1100mcg/day
Iodine in foods or supplements is in the inorganic iodide form and is easily absorbed in the stomach and upper small intestine and taken up by the thyroid gland for production of thyroid hormones (inactive T4 converted to active T3 in tissues). T3 'revs up' metabolic rate, heart rate/contractility, blood flow to peripheral tissues; skeletal muscle contraction, glucose production, cholesterol synthesis, lipolysis, thermogenesis. Thyroid gland is important for normal embryonic and post–natal development, speech, hearing, hair, skin, teeth, fertility, gut function (motility/absorption of nutrients), kidney function (glomerular filtration rate, electrolyte balance), heart/blood pressure. Iodine content of food and water depends primarily on the supply of iodine in the soil. All bread in Australia is iodised due to compulsory use of iodised salt. Deficiency or excess linked to enlarged thyroid gland/hypothyroid, dry coarse skin/hair, reduced kidney function/oedema, poor digestion/anaemia/constipation, menstrual irregularities, weight gain, raised diastolic blood pressure/heart rate, insulin resistance/diabetes, depression, memory loss, high LDL cholesterol, inflammation/joint pain. Low vitamin A and zinc contribute to iodine deficiency (needed for uptake of iodine in thyroid) and poor thyroid function. Thyroid disorders can lead to vitamin A deficiency due to reduced ability to convert beta carotene to vitamin A and reduced intestinal absorption of zinc. Iron supplementation improves efficacy of iodine supplementation.

	mcg/serve
Seaweed 10g dried	>4500mcg
Oysters 6	96mcg
Iodised salt pinch (1g)	80mcg
Salmon 120g	72mcg
Sughi, California roll	69mcg
Milo (smart) 1 tbs 20g	32mcg
Milk 200ml	30mcg
Yoghurt 200g	30mcg
Egg 60g	13mcg
Iodised bread 1 slice	12mcg
Shark (flake) 120g	12mcg
Tuna 80g tin	8mcg
Cheese 25g	4mcg

Copper

RDI: 1.5mg/day
UTI: 10mg/day
Involved in the absorption, storage and metabolism of iron (symptoms of deficiency are similar to iron deficiency anaemia); aids in formation of red blood cells; production of ATP; and skin pigment; works with vitamin C to form elastin; proper bone formation/maintenance; thyroid function. Long term high supplemental zinc intake (>50mg/day) may cause copper deficiency. Copper overload occurs in Wilsons disease and potentially from prescribed oestrogen and xeno-estrogens from pesticides/petroleum products/plastics. Overload interferes with Zn, Mg, molybdenum, vitamin C, folic acid, thiamine and vitamin E and can affect brain, liver, hormone and immune function.

	mg/serve
Liver (beef), ckd 30g	4mg
Oysters, ckd 1 med	0.6mg
Clams/crab, ckd 90g	0.6mg
Cashews, 30g	0.6mg
Lentils, ckd1 cup	0.5mg
Sunflower seeds, 30g	0.5mg
Hazelnuts, 30g	0.5mg
Coconut milk 200ml	0.4mg
Mushrooms, raw 1 cup	0.3mg
Almonds/walnuts/pecans 30g	0.3mg
Avocado 100g	0.3mg
Tofu 100g	0.2mg
Salmon 100g	0.2mg
Peanut butter (chunky) 2 tbs	0.2mg
Chocolate (semisweet) 30g	0.2mg
Oats 30g	0.2mg
Buckwheat flour 50g	0.2mg
Raisins 50g	0.15mg
Herring 100g	0.1mg
Shredded wheat cereal 30g	0.1mg
Barley pearl ckd 100g	0.1mg
Eggs 2 medium	0.1mg
Bran wheat 2 tbs	0.1mg
Wheat germ 2 tbs	0.1mg
Tomato puree 50ml	0.1mg
Olives 50g	0.1mg
Prunes 50g	0.1mg
Grapes 100g	0.1mg
Split peas, ckd 100g	0.1mg

Other sources: Tap water that passes through copper pipes, brewers yeast, chestnuts, dandelion greens, Echinacea, fennel, goldenseal, hazelnuts, kelp, lobster, macadamia nuts, molasses, trout, pine nuts, pistachio nuts, sesame seeds, sunflower oil.

Manganese

RDI: 5mg/day
UTI: not available (USA 11mg/day)
Important for the antioxidant enzyme superoxide dismutase manganese is an underrated mineral that can cause severe problems at both low and high intakes. Important for the adrenergic neurotransmitter pathways converting tyrosine to adrenaline: low levels are associated with epilepsy, poor memory, muscle twitching, dizziness, schizophrenia and high levels with aggressiveness, apathy, dementia, hallucinations, speech impairment. Low intake can also cause skin rashes and eczema because it is involved in breakdown of histamine. Also important for glucose regulation (involved in glycolysis and insulin production);thyroid function; production of energy (helps make CoQ10); metabolism of vitamin B1 and E; activation of various enzymes important for proper digestion and utilisation of foods and is a catalyst in the breakdown of

fats and LDL cholesterol. It is necessary for bone production, cartilage repair, joint lubrication and maintains sex hormone production.

	mg/serve
Raisin bran cereal 1 cup	1.9mg
Brown rice 1 cup, ckd160g	1.8mg
Oatmeal 1 pkt	1.7mg
Green tea 1 cup 250ml	0.4–1.6mg
Pecans 30g	1.3mg
Brown rice ½ cup	0.9mg
Spinach ½ cup, ckd	0.8mg
Black tea 1 cup 250ml	0.2–0.7mg
Pineapple fresh/juice ½ cup	0.7mg
Almonds 30g	0.7mg
Wholmeal bread 1 slice	0.6mg
Peanuts 30g	0.5mg
Sweet potato ½ cup mashed	0.5mg
Dried beans 1 cup, ckd	0.4mg

Phosphorus

RDI: 1000mg/day
UTI: 4000mg/day

Cell membranes are composed largely of phospholipids. The inorganic constituents of bone/teeth are primarily a calcium phosphate salt called hydroxyapatite.

Helps in conversion of food to energy (crucial in the production of ATP), vitamin utilisation (especially B vitamins), kidney function, cell growth and heart muscle contraction. Deficiency linked to irregular breathing, fatigue, anxiety, skin sensitivity, changes in body weight.

	mg/serve
Yogurt, plain non-fat,	250mg 385mg
Fish 90g, ckd	250mg
Milk, skim 250ml	247mg
Lentils ½ cup ckd#	180mg
Beef 90g	170mg
Chicken/turkey 90g	160mg
Chia seeds 15g#	160mg
Cheese, mozzarella 30g	130mg
Nuts 30g#	120mg
Egg 1 large, ckd	100mg
Bread, whole wheat 1slice	57mg
Carbonated cola drink 360ml	40mg

#Phosphorus from nuts, seeds, and grains is about 50% less bio available than phosphorus from other sources.

Molybdenum

RDI: 45mcg/day
UTI: 2000mcg/day

Regulates copper–zinc balance; metabolism of iron; conversion of purine to uric acid; important for kidney and nervous system function; formation of tooth enamel; involved in enzyme systems that breakdown environmental toxins and nitrosamines, helps excrete mercury/lead.

Sources: wheat germ, oats, brown rice, cottage cheese, eggs, lentils, green peas, split peas, fish, kidneys, spinach, cauliflower, brewers yeast.

Phytonutrients

Polyphenols

Tyrosol olives, olive oil, grapes.
Oleuropein olives, olive oil, red grapes.
Resveratrol red grape skin, peanuts, blueberries, bilberries, cranberries.

Bioflavanoids

Anthocyanidins

(Cyanidin, delphinidin, malvidin, pelargonidin, peonidin, petunidin) red/blue/purple berries; acai; red/purple grapes; red wine; black/red dried beans, rosehip.

Flavanols (Monomers).

Catechin, Epicatechin, Epigallocatechin Epicatechin gallate, Epigallocatechin gallate (e.g. teas, particularly green/white), rooibos tea, chocolate, grapes, berries, apples.

Flavanols dimers and polymers.

Theaflavins, Thearubigins (e.g. black/oolong); **Proanthocyanidins** (e.g. red wine, red grapes, chocolate, apples, berries/cranberries, olives).

Flavanones **(Hesperidin, Eriodictyol, Naringenin)** (e.g. citrus fruits/juices [oranges, grapefruits, lemons], rosehip).

Flavonols **(Quercetin)** asparagus, apples, blackberries, cranberries, dried beans, buckwheat, broccoli, onions, leeks, garlic, celery, tea, chia seeds, rooibos tea, citrus, rosehip.

Kaempferol kale, swiss chard, endives, raw spinach, chives, dried beans, chia seeds.
Myricetin fennel, blueberries, cranberries, chia seeds, carob.
Isorhamnetin broccoli.
Rutin buckwheat, citus, rosehip.

Flavones

Apigenin, Luteolin (e.g. parsley, thyme, celery, hot peppers, rooibos tea).

Isoflavones (phytoestrogens).

Daidzein, Genistein, Glycitein

Soybeans, soy foods, tofu (30mg/100g); soy linseed bread (114mg/100g); soy milk; legumes (soy beans, tofu, chickpeas), nuts, linseed, sprouted seeds, celery, fennel, green/yellow vegetables, parsley, yams, sweet potato, rice, peas, green beans, cucumber, corn, paw paw, sage, sarsparilla, liquorice.

Lignans (phytoestrogens)

Linseed/flax seeds 30g	85mg
Sesame seeds 30g	11mg
Sesame seed paste 20g	10mg
Kale ½ cup	0.8mg
Broccoli ½ cup	0.6mg
Apricots ½ cup	0.4mg
Cabbage ½ cup	0.3mg
Brussel sprouts ½ cup	0.3mg
Strawberries ½ cup	0.2mg
Tofu 120g	0.2mg
Dark rye bread 1 slice	0.1mg
Flaxseed oil	0mg

Other sources: dried chickpeas, pumpkin seeds, oats, sunflower seeds, berries.

Carotenoids

For chronic disease prevention at least 5000mcg/day recommended from all carotenoids.

Sensitive to light and oxygen, up to 40% loss in cooking.

The relatively low bioavailability of carotenoids from most foods compared to supplements is partly because they are associated with proteins in the plant matrix and they are fat soluble. Therefore, chopping, homogenising, and cooking in oil increase the bioavailability of carotenoids. The bioavailability of lycopene from tomatoes is substantially improved by heating tomatoes in oil.

Alpha carotene

For Retinol equivalents divide by 24

Pumpkin, ckd 1 cup	11748mcg
Carrot juice 1 cup	10247mcg
Carrot, ckd 1 cup	5891mcg
Carrots raw 1 med	2028mcg
Mixed vegies frozen, ckd 1 cup	1762mcg
Squash, ckd 1 cup	1300mcg
Collards, ckd 1 cup	216mcg
Tomatoes raw 1 med	124mcg
Tangerines 1med	85mcg
Peas, ckd 1 cup	85mcg

Beta-cryptoxanthin

Red capsicum raw 1 med	5813mcg
Pumpkin, ckd 1 cup	3553mcg
red capsicum, ckd, 1 cup	2817mcg
papayas raw 1 med	2313mcg
orange juice fresh 250ml	419mcg
Tangerines raw 1 med	342mcg
Carrots, ckd, 1 cup	315mcg
Watermelon, raw 1 wedge	223mcg
Corn frozen, ckd 1 cup	200mcg
Paprika dried 1 tsp	166mcg
Oranges, raw 1 med	152mcg
Nectarines, raw 1 med	133mcg

Lycopene

Tomato puree ½ cup	27200mcg
Tomato soup 1 cup	25615mcg
Vegetable juice 1 cup	23300mcg
Tomato juice 1 cup	22000mcg
Watermelon 1 wedge	13000mcg
Tomato paste 1 tbs	7536mcg
Tomatoes raw 1 cup	4600mcg
Tomato sauce 1 tbs	2550mcg
Pink grapefruit ½	1700mcg
Baked beans, cnd, 1 cup	1300mcg
Red capsicum raw 1 cup	450mcg

Lutein + Zeaxanthin

(quantities not available)
Spinach frozen ckd
Kale frozen, ckd
Turnip greens, ckd
Collards, ckd
Mustard greens, ckd
Dandelion greens, ckd
Green capsicum
Zucchini, ckd
Peas frozen, ckd
Broccoli frozen, ckd
Pumpkin, ckd
Brussel sprouts, ckd
Corn, boiled
Egg yolk
Kiwi fruit
Orange
Mango
Honeydew

Phytosterols

RDI: 2000–3000mg/day

Phytosterols lower LDL-cholesterol by 10% in 3 weeks (little effect on HDL-cholesterol and triglycerides). Found in most plant foods and wood pulp; structurally similar to cholesterol, they can inhibit the intestinal absorption of cholesterol — this displaced cholesterol is then excreted from the body. This action not only interferes with the absorption of cholesterol from food, it has the additional (and probably more important) effect of removing cholesterol from substances made in the liver that are recycled through the digestive tract. Beta-sitosterol in particular may also help manage benign prostatic hyperplasia. They may also play a role autoimmune disease and cancer.

Margarine with added phytosterols 1 tbs	1600mg
Yoghurt with added phytosterols 200g	800mg
Milk with added phytosterols 250ml	800mg
Rice bran oil 1 tbs	160mg
Legumes 100g ½ cup, ckd	130mg
Sesame oil 1 tbs	120mg
Tahini 1 tbs	120mg
Corn oil 1 tbs	100mg
Canola oil 1 tbs	90mg
Pistachios 30g	90mg
Sunflower seeds	90mg
Pumpkin seeds 30g	80mg
Almond 30g	40mg
Peanut butter or peanut/soy oil 1 tbs	40mg
Wheat germ 1 tbs	30mg
Brussel sprouts ½ cup	30mg
Rye bread 2 slices	30mg
Macadamia nuts 30g	30mg
Amaranth 100g	24mg
Olive oil 1 tbs	20mg
Wheat bran 1 tbs	10mg

Other source: Acai berry, soy beans, pumpkin oil.

CoQ_{10} (ubiquinone)

Synthesised in the body from amino acids tyrosine or phenylalanine and vitamin B6.

RDI: not available; suggested intake 30–300mg/day

Plays a critical role in the production of energy (ATP) in mitochondria in every cell of the body, especially the heart. Deficiency is poorly understood, but it may be caused by synthesis problems in the body rather than an insufficiency in the diet. Low blood levels have been reported in people with heart failure, cardiomyopathy, gingivitis, morbid obesity, hypertension, muscular dystrophy, diabetes, AIDS, and in some people on kidney dialysis. People with phenylketonuria (PKU) may be deficient in CoQ_{10} because of dietary restrictions. CoQ_{10} levels are also generally lower in older people. Some evidence suggests that it may help congestive heart failure, hypertension, diabetes, migraines, kidney failure, chronic fatigue syndrome, breast cancer, counteracting side-effects of certain medications.

Meat 90g	2.6mg
Herring marinated 90g	2.3mg
Chicken 90g	1.4mg
Soy bean oil 1 tbs	1.3mg
Canola oil 1 tbs	1.0mg
Trout 90g	0.9mg
Peanuts 30g	0.8mg
Sesame seeds 30g	0.7mg
Pistachio nuts 30g	0.6mg
Broccoli/Cauliflower ½ cup	0.4mg
Orange 1med	0.3mg
Egg 1 med	0.1mg

Prebiotics

Lupin flour, chia seeds, nuts, especially almonds, oats, rye, barley, corn, flaxseed, psyllium, asparagus, garlic, chives, carrots, radishes, tomatoes, artichokes, onions, chickory, greens, legumes, banana, berries, apples, pears.

Alkaline-forming foods

Foods highlighted in **bold type** are the most alkaline-forming foods.

Vegetables
Spinach and other dark green leafy vegetables, chicory, **celery, carrots**, zucchini, cauliflower, potatoes (old), celery, carrots, zucchini, cauliflower, potatoes, eggplant, tomatoes, lettuce, onions, leeks, capsicum (green), mushroom, broccoli, cucumber, asparagus, artichokes, red radish, green beans, cabbage.

Fruits
Raisins, bananas, apricots, kiwi, cherries, pears, pineapple, grapes, peaches, apples (whole/ juice), watermelon, black currants, lemon, oranges (whole/juice), strawberries.

Nuts/seeds
Hazelnuts, almonds, **pumpkin seeds**, sesame seeds, chestnuts.

Other
Beer (draft and stout), cocoa, coffee, mineral water, wine (red/white), tea, honey, marmalade, sugar.

Acid-forming foods
Foods highlighted in **bold type** are the most acid-forming foods.

Nuts/seeds
Walnut. peanuts, pecans, **pistachios, cashews.**

Grains
Brown rice, oats, spaghetti, egg noodles, corn flakes, white rice, rye bread, wheat bread

Legumes
Lentils, peas.

Dairy
Parmesan cheese, processed cheese, hard cheese (all types/ goat/soy), **camembert cheese**, cottage cheese, whole milk, butter, buttermilk, cream, ice-cream, yoghurt.

Meat, fish and eggs
Trout, turkey, chicken, veal, eggs, pork, beef, cod, herring, haddock, **corned beef, sausage, processed meat, salami, bacon**

Other foods
Chocolate, cake.

Amines
Foods highlighted in **bold type** are very high in amines and should be avoided if amine sensitive; non-highlighted foods can be eaten occasionally if amine sensitive. Higher in ripe fruit/ tropical fruit and rich food.

Vegetables/Legumes
Broad bean, broccoli, **choysum** cauliflower, **eggplant, mushrooms, spinach**, tomato, **tomato paste**, sauerkraut, seaweed, humus **baked beans, textured vegetable protein**, rocket, radicchio, **veg soup/juice**

Fruit
Avocado, bananas, citrus, date, fig, grapes, kiwi, lemon, mandarin, **orange juice**, passionfruit, mango, pineapple, plum, raspberry, **currants, berries**, jackfruit, papaya, pawpaw feijoa, **dried fruit.**

Meats, chicken, fish and eggs
Aged meat, improperly stored or spoiled meats/fish/poultry **anchovies**, bacon, **beef liver**, chicken liver, **chicken skin, fish roe, prawns**, mackerel (canned/**dried**), **meat pies, offal, pizza**, pork, sardines (canned/**dried**), **sausages, smoked meat/fish, tuna (canned). surimi**, game meat turkey, salmon (canned), **proccessed meat, chicken nuggets, sausages**

Dairy foods/soy products
Cheese (all, except cottage ricotta, quark, marscapone, cream cheese), **miso**, sour cream, soy sauce, **tempeh**, yoghurt.

Condiments
Bonox, **fish marinades, marmite**, meat extracts, **olives, sauces** (all), **tandoori, stock cubes**, vinegar (all), **pickled vegetables, Fermented products, soysauce, miso, curry, tempeh mustard**

Fats/oils
Coconut oil, copha, **olive oil. Peanut oil, sesame oil, walnut oils**

Nuts
Almond, coconut (dry) macadamia, peanut, pecan, pine nuts, pistachio, sunflower seeds, walnuts, hazelnut, brazil nut, **peanut butter, tahini**, sesame seeds, linseeds, pumpkin seeds, chestnuts

Sweets
Chocolate (milk, white, **dark**, drinking), **jam, maple syrup**

Spreads
Lemon butter, vegemite.

Drinks
Beer (includes non-alcoholic), cider, **chocolate-flavoured drinks, cola drinks, tomato juice**, wine (claret, chianti, fruit wines, port, red/white, sherry), **fruit juice (all), soft drinks, cordial.**

Salicylates
Foods highlighted in **bold type** are very high in salicylates and should be avoided if salicylate sensitive; non-highlighted foods can be eaten occasionally if salicylate sensitive. Higher in unripe fruit and/or tangy fruit. Large reactions to insect bites suggests salicylate intolerance.

Vegetables/legumes
Alfalfa, artichoke, **broad bean, broccoli, capsicum, cauliflower, champignon, chilli**, chicory leaves, corn, cucumber, **eggplant**, endive, **gherkin, mushroom, olive, onion**, pumpkin, rocket, fennel, **seaweed, vegie soup/juice, baked beans, felafel, hummus**, radish, **spinach, tomato**, water chestnut, watercress, zucchini.

Fruit
Apple (Jonathan, granny smith), apricot, **avocado**, berries, **cherry, currant, date**, fig, **grapefruit, grape**, guava, **kiwi, lemon**, lychee, longan, **mandarin**, nectarine, orange, **passionfruit**, peach, **pineapple**, persimmon, rambutan, rhubarb, **plum**, pomegranate, **prune, raisin, dried fruit**, rockmelon, **tangelo, sultana, tomato**, watermelon.

Meats, chicken, fish, eggs

aged meat, chicken liver, chicken skin, **devon,** gravy (meat juice), **meat pies, offal, smoked meat, smoked chicken, salami, sausages, seasoned meats** and **chicken.**

Dairy foods and soy

tasty cheeses, cheeses and **flavoured yoghurt.**

Drinks

Beer, brandy, fruit juices (all), **cider, cola drinks, cordials** and **soft fruit flavoured drinks, coffee,** chamomile, **chai tea liqueur, all herbal teas, port, rum, sherry, tea** (black/green), **tomato juice, wine.**

Herbs, spices, condiments

Spices, herbs (all), gravies, hydrolysed/textured vegetable protein, meat extracts, mustard, **pastes (fish, meat, tomato),** pepper, **sauces (all), stock cubes, tandoori, tomato sauce, vinegar (cider, red** and **white wine), yeast extracts,** pickled vegetables and fermented products.

Cereals/grains/flours

Corn flakes, cornmeal, polenta, breakfast cereals with honey, breakfast cereals with cocoa, breakfast cereals with fruit, nuts and coconut.

Jams/spreads/sugars/sweets

Chewing gum, jellies, maple syrup, fruit flavoured sweets and **ices, honey, jams** (all), **lemon butter, liquorice, mint-flavoured sweets,** molasses, **peppermint,** raw sugar.

Fats/oils

Almond oil, corn oil, peanut oil, **coconut oil, copha, sesame oil, walnut oil,** extra virgin oilve oil

Nuts

Almonds, brazil, **coconut** (dry), hazelnuts, muesli bars, macadamia, peanuts, pecans, pine nuts, pistachio, peanut butter, sesame seeds, sunflower seeds, walnuts.

Phyates (inositol hexaphosphate)

Almonds, walnuts, brazil nuts, hazelnuts, peanut butter, peanuts, raw coconut, raw oats, raw sesame seeds, rye bread, buckwheat, barley, wheat bran, wheat germ, legumes, soy products (especially unfermented textured vegetable protein), cocoa, corn chips.

Oxalates

Foods highlighted in bold type are higher in oxalaten (>99mg/serve).

Bran, wheat germ, barley, rice bran, cornmeal, **almonds, buckwheat, beets (leaves/roots),** carob, chocolate, cocoa, **collards,** gooseberries, apricots (dried), figs, kiwi, apple, **okra,** peanuts, pecans, cashews, **hazelnuts,** pepper, poppy seeds, **tahini, sesame seeds,** turmeric, **purslane,** parsley, **spinach, endive, dandelion greens, rhubarb,** potatoes, sweet potato, carrots, turnips, parsnips, tomato paste, soy milk, **miso,** tofu, textured vegetable protein, white beans (dried), **Swiss chard,** tea (black, green) wholemeal pasta.

Goitrogens

Cruciferous vegetables (broccoli, brussel sprouts, cabbage (all types), cauliflower, mustard greens), bamboo shoots, brazil nuts, canola oil, cassava, Chinese greens, corn, flavanoids (only poly–hydroxyphenolic), garlic, horseradish, kale, lima beans, linseed, millet, mustard oil, onion, peanuts, pine nuts, soy, swede, sweet potato, turnip.

Food additives

Linked to food intolerances and/or allergies.

Food colourings

Tartrazine (102), sunset yellow (110), amaranth (123), erythrosine (127) and annatto extracts (160b) and red colouring E128 in burgers and sausages is linked to cancer (banned in Australia).

Preservatives

Sodium benzoate (e211), sulphur dioxide (220), calcium propionate (282), sodium nitrates (251) and nitrites (250) in processed meat linked to cancer.

Antioxidant

Bha or buylated hydroxyanisole (320).

Flavour enhancers

Monosodium glutamate (MSG) (621) and ribonucleotides (635) artificial sweetener aspartame (951).

References

Choice Magazine 'The Great Dilemma' (article on fish). November 2008.

Colquhoun D, Ferreira-Jardim A, Udell T, et al. Fish, fish oil, n-3 polyunsaturated fatty acids and cardiovascular health. August 2008. Online. Available: www.heartfoundation.org.au (accessed 30 Aug 2008)

Holmes, R P, & Kennedy, M (2000). Estimation of the Oxalate Content of Foods and Daily Oxalate Intake. *Kidney International*, *57*, 1662–1667.

Net Doctor UK. Online. Available: http://www.netdoctor.co.uk/health_advice/facts/vitamins_which.htm (accessed 1 Nov 2008).

Remer T, Manz F. Potential renal acid load of foods and its influence on urine pH. J Am Diet Assoc. 1995; 95:791–797 and www.paleodiet.com

Australian food composition tables:

- website by Dietitian Alan Borushek, www.caloriekin g.com.au (accessed 5 Aug 2008), and Calorie, Fat & Carbohydrate Counter 2009 and 1997
- Online Food Facts, Wahlqvist ML and Briggs D www.healthyeatingclub.org/info/books-phds/books/foodfacts/index.php (accessed 11 Sept 2008)
- Wahlqvist ML (ed.) Food and Nutrition (3rd edn) 2002. Chapter by Wahlqvist ML 'Vitamins and Vitamin like

compounds'. Allen & Unwin Sydney, Australia
- SaltMatters, Menzies Research Institute www.saltmatters.org or Meniere's Australia www.menieres.org.au (accessed 3 Dec 2008)
- website by Professor M Wahlqvist and Dr Antigone Kouris–Blazos www.healthyeatingclub.org (accessed 06-07-08)
- Food Intolerance Network www.fedup.com.au (accessed 5 Jan 2009)
- The low FODMAP diet. Dept Medicine, Eastern Health Clinical School, Monash University, Box Hill, Vic, 2009.

RPAH Elimination Diet Handbook Anne Swain, Valencia Soutter, Robert Loblay: Allergy Unit Royal Prince Alfred Hospital, 2009.

US Food composition tables:
- About.com http://caloriecount.about.com (accessed 18 July 2008)
- Oregon State University Linus Pauling Institute http://www.lpi.oregonstate.edu/
- RealAge Live Life to the Youngest, Dr Oz and Dr Rozien www.realage.com (accessed 30 Sept 2008)
- US National Institutes of Health Office of Dietary Supplements. http://www.ods.od.nih.gov/ (accessed 23 Oct 2008)
- USDA Agricultural Research Service Nutrient Data Laboratory http://www.nal.usda.gov/fnic/foodcomp/search/ (accessed 25 July 2008)

Appendix 2

Drug–nutrient–herb interactions for commonly prescribed medications

Dr Antigone Kouris-Blazos

Disclaimer: This appendix should be used as **a guide only** as most interactions are based on **preliminary data** (especially for herbs). The table may help practitioners better manage their patients by making them more alert to any possible adverse or beneficial effects caused by medications/supplements patients may be taking (or many need to take).

The following drug interaction information is **not** intended to replace information supplied by a doctor, pharmacist or practitioner; neither is it intended to replace package inserts or other printed material that may be available or accompany a particular drug. This appendix reviews known major interactions between pharmaceutical drugs and food, specific nutrients, and herbs. This appendix does not cover interactions between two or more drugs, interactions between alcohol and specific nutrients and interactions between drugs and water (for example, drugs inducing dehydration). Although drug information is extensive, it does not include every drug–nutrient or drug–herb interaction. Therefore, if a drug is not mentioned, there still may be drug–food, drug–nutrient, or drug–herb interactions.

Finally, new adverse or beneficial interactions may be discovered after the publication date. For these reasons, it is **not** sufficient to rely solely on the information presented here. It is always wise for people seeking information about interactions between a prescription drug and food, specific nutrients, or herbs, to talk with their pharmacist, prescribing practitioner, or both. Any trademarks are the property of their respective companies.

As a general rule:

- Some herbal/vitamin/mineral supplements require separation from medications by about 2–4 hours to avoid potential problems with absorption or interactions. See medications in table for more specific advice in relation to this rule.
- Avoid taking psyllium husk, slippery elm, guar gum or other fibre supplements at the same time as medications; separate by a few hours. Slippery elm and marshmallow can coat the lining of the gut forming an inert barrier potentially affecting the absorption of drugs. Limit their use in patients taking medications with a narrow therapeutic range (eg barbiturates, lithium, digoxin, phenytoin, warfarin).
- Cartilage supplements have not been reported to interact with any medications
- Lysine supplements have not been reported to interact with any medications
- Flaxseed/linseed oil may interfere with the absorption of certain medications — separate doses by 2–3 hrs
- milk thistle (*Silybum marianum*) supplements interact with most medications, however, some preparations of milk thistle do not interact (check with manufacturer).
- Aloe skin juice has a laxative effect and can increase potassium excretion; aloe gel juice does not have these effects.

☑ **Possible beneficial interaction (stronger evidence)** Some evidence based on clinical trials, small studies, human case reports. Increased intake of nutrient/herb recommended from food, fortified foods/drinks or supplements improve clinical outcomes by: (a) counteracting nutritional deficiencies caused by drugs (due increased excretion or decreased absorption or altered metabolism of nutrient; (b) complementing drug effects; (c) reducing drug side-effects; (d) reducing drug requirements; (e) alleviating drug withdrawal symptoms; (f) improving patient wellbeing. Commence with low doses and adjust dose under the supervision of a health professional.

☺ **Preliminary/theoretical beneficial interaction (weaker evidence)** Meaningful preliminary evidence from *in vitro* studies, animal studies, human case studies and extrapolation from pharmacology data or traditional use. Increased intake of that nutrient/herb from food, fortified foods/drinks or supplements may help improve action of drug or correct deficiency/adverse effects caused by drug. Commence with low doses and adjust under the supervision of a health professional.

☒ **Possible adverse interaction (stronger evidence)** Some evidence based on clinical trials, small studies, human case reports or traditional use. Nutrient/herb from food, fortified foods/drinks or supplements affects absorption of drug and/or action within body and/or increases the risk of side-effects; separating drug and nutrient/herbal supplement by 2–4 hours can eliminate adverse effects.

☺ **Preliminary/theoretical harmful interaction (weaker evidence)** Meaningful preliminary evidence mainly based on *invitro* studies, animal studies, human case studies and extrapolation from pharmacology data or traditional use. Interactions may not be significant at low doses but the clinician should be alert to the possibility of an adverse interaction.

Figure 1 Interaction evaluation codes

- **High FIBRE foods can reduce effects/absorption of some drugs** e.g cooked barley, cooked bulgur, cooked dried beans, wholemeal pasta, corn chips, corn on cob, fresh broad beans (with pods), fresh coconut, guava, hazelnuts, mango, pepitas (pumpkin seeds), quince, some breads (Burgen), bran breakfast cereals/muesli/soy linseed.
- **High GOITROGEN foods can interfere with iodine utilisation or thyroxine production (but may only be important when iodine intake is low and can be inactivated by cooking) or may interfere with thyroid medication** e.g cruciferous vegetables (broccoli, brussel sprouts, cabbage [all types], cauliflower, mustard greens), bamboo shoots, brazil nuts, canola oil, cassava, chinese greens, corn, flavanoids (only polyhydroxyphenolic), garlic, horseradish, kale, lima beans, linseed, millet, mustard oil, onion, peanuts, pine nuts, soy, swede, sweet potato, turnip.
- **High OXALATE foods can reduce effects/absorption of some drugs** e.g almonds, amaranth, raw beets (leaves/roots), carob powder, cassava root, chocolate, cocoa, collards, gooseberries, leeks, okra, peanut butter, peanuts, pecans, pepper, poppy seeds, purslane, raw parsley, raw spinach, rhubarb, sweet potato, soy products (especially unfermented, textured vegetable protein), swiss chard, tea infusion, wheat germ.
- **High PHYTATE foods can reduce effects/absorption of some drugs** e.g almonds, barley, brazil nuts, cocoa, corn chips, hazelnuts, peanut butter, peanuts, raw coconut, raw oats, raw sesame seeds, rye bread, soy products (especially unfermented, textured vegetable protein), walnuts, wheat bran, wheat germ.
- **High TYRAMINE foods can alter the metabolism of some drugs with the potential to cause serious adverse effects such as hypertensive crises in patients taking monoamine oxidase inhibitors** e.g mature/aged cheeses, aged/cured meats/fish/poultry, improperly stored or spoiled meats/fish/poultry, yoghurt, sour cream, sauerkraut, fava/broad bean pods, beer (including non-alcoholic), avocado, marmite, bananas, pizza, liver, caviar, fermented soy bean products/soy sauce/tofu, wine (red/white).

Figure 2 Food components that can interact with medications (see Table 2 for specific medications)

Table 1 List of abbreviations and symbols

Abbreviation

BSL = blood sugar levels
BTB = breakthrough bleeding
Ca = calcium
CHOL = cholesterol
CoQ_{10} = coenzyme Q_{10}
Cr = chromium
EPO = evening primrose oil
Fe = iron
HPT = hypertension
K = potassium
Mx = medication
Mg = magnesium
Na = sodium
NIDDM = diabetes
TRIG = triglycerides
Zn = zinc
vit = vitamin

Symbol

↑ = increase ↓ =decrease
☑ Possible beneficial interaction
☺ Preliminary/theoretical beneficial interaction
☒ Possible adverse interaction
☹ Preliminary/theoretical harmful interaction

Drug–nutrient–herb interactions

ACARBOSE (amylase inhibitor, NIDDM)

↑ diarrhoea/bloating/wind ↓appetite ↑nausea/vomiting ↓blood CA ↓bloodvit B6, avoid if have inflammatory bowel disease/intestinal obstruction

☑ vit B12

☺ CoQ_{10}, Cr, Mg (>absorbtion of Mx), vit E, aloe vera gel, andrographis, bilberry, bitter melon/karela (*Momordica charantia*), carnitine, cinnamon, fenugreek, garlic, ginger, ginseng, green tea, gymnema, guggul/myrrh, inositol, ipriflavone, lipoic acid, milk thistle (*Silybum marianum*), olive leaf extract, psyllium, turmeric, vanadium (these can ↓BSL and ↓dose of Mx needed)

☒ alcohol, *dong quai*, fenugreek, guar gum, ginkgo, St John's wort

☺ Glucosamine

ACE INHIBITORS (angiotensin-converting enzyme inhibitors, HPT, heart failure, heart attack)

↓ weight ↑constipation/diarrhoea ↑nausea/vomiting ↓appetite ↓taste ↓BSL (and interacts with sulphonylureas to ↓BSL) ↑blood K ↓blood Na ↑anaemia ↑uric acid ↑dry cough ↑skin numbness/tingling (Zn deficiency)

☺ Zn (↓intracellular Zn, drug ↑ deficiency, ↓ taste, ↓appetite, numbness/tingling, supp taken with 2hr gap), Fe (supp can help ↓dry cough but separate doses by at least 2hrs), *coleus forskohlii*, garlic/hawthorn/olive leaf/EPO/fish oil/oats (↑drug effect)

☒ K supplements/high K foods, Mg (drug contains Mg), alcohol, arginine, bitter orange (*Citrus aurantium*), liquorice (deglycyrrhizinated OK)

☺ Black cohosh, don quai, guarana, St John's wort (↓drug levels via ↑metabolism)

ACE INHIBITORS + THIAZIDE DIURETICS

↑ constipation/diarrhea ↓appetite ↑vomit/nausea ↓taste ↑chol ↑trig ↑uric ↑BSL/interacts with sulfonylureas to ↓BSL/impairs glucose tolerance ↓ blood Na ↓ blood Mg ↑ blood K ↑ blood Ca

☑ Mg, Na, Zn, Fe (separate doses by at least 2hrs), EPO/fish oil/oats/olive leaf (↑drug effect)

☺ Garlic/hawthorn/*coleus forskohlii* (↑drug effect)

☒ K, Ca, vit D, alcohol, arginine, bitter orange (*Citrus aurantium*), buckthorn, horsetail, liquorice (deglycyrrhizinated OK), juniper, St John's wort (↑risk sunburn)

☹ Aloe skin, caraway, flaxseed, ginkgo, glycerol, guarana, laxatives, liquorice (deglycyrrhizinated OK), peppermint oil, psyllium, stinging nettle (these can ↑K excretion, limit intake)

ACETAMINOPHEN (Analgesic)

↑ constipation ↑nausea/vomiting ↓appetite ↑risk of stomach/digestion problems (administer with food) prolonged concurrent use with aspirin/salicylates may ↑risk adverse renal effects

☺ Andrographis, CoQ_{10}, garlic, methionine, milk thistle (*Silybum marianum*), N acetyl cysteine, quercetin, schisandra, SAMe, (reduced side-effects)

☒ Vegetarian diets (↓drug absorption), alcohol, vit C (large doses)

☺ Citrate

ACETAZOLAMIDE (diuretic, K depleting, glaucoma)

↓ weight ↑constipation/diarrhea ↓appetite ↑vomit/nausea ↓taste ↑BSL (interacts with anti-diabetic agents to ↓BSL) ↑uric acid ↑chol/trig ↓blood K ↓blood Na

☑ K, Na, Mg, folate

☺ Olive leaf/olive oil (↑drug effect)

☒ Arginine, buckthorn, bitter orange (*Citrus aurantium*), dong quai (↑risk sunburn), horsetail, juniper, salicylates, St John's wort (↑risk sunburn)

☺ Liquorice (deglycyrrhizinated is OK), caraway, flaxseed, glycerol, guarana, peppermint oil, psyllium stinging nettle (can ↑K excretion, limit intake)

ACITRETIN (retinoid, psoriasis, keratolytic)

↓ taste ↑trig ↑chol ↑↓BSL

☒ Vit A, b-carotene, alcohol

ALLOPURINOL (xanthine oxidase inhibitor, antigout)

↑ constipation/diarrhoea ↓taste ↑nausea/vomiting ↓BSL (interacts with sulfonylureas to ↓BSL)

☑ Protein >20g/day, fluid >2L/day

☒ Vit C >500mg, alcohol, salicylates (↓drug effectiveness)

☺ Carnitine, vit D, tryptophan

ALPHA BLOCKERS (HPT, heart failure)

↑ nausea/vomiting ↑constipation/diarrhoea ↑blood uric acid ↑blood Na

☺ Nicotinic acid, hawthorn, *Coleus forskohlii*

☒ Na, alcohol, Black cohosh, bitter orange (*Citrus aurantium*), guarana, liquorice (deglycyrrhizinated OK)

ALTRETAMINE (antitumour)

↑ nausea/vomiting ↓appetite

Multivitamin (low dose), beta-carotene (mouth sores), vit E (applied to mouth sores), chamomile (mouth sores), coriolus versicolor (Japanese mushroom, PSK/polysaccharide krestin ↑immunity, 3g/day, ↑survival time), eleuthero, ginger (nausea), glutamine (↓diarrhoea/mouth sores), melatonin (↓side-effects), milk thistle (*Silybum marianum*), N acetyl cysteine (1800mg/day, nausea), taurine

☹ B6 (↓neurotoxicity but adversely affects response duration), andrographis, astragalus, baical skullcap, echinacea, garlic, ginseng, withania

AMINOGLUTETHIMIDE (Antineopleastic)

↑ weight ↑constipation/diarrhea ↓appetite ↑vomit/nausea ↑blood CA ↓blood Na, interacts with anti-diabetic agents

☹ Andrographis, astragalus, baical skullcap, echinacea, garlic, ginseng, withania

AMINOGLYCOSIDES (antibiotic)

↓ weight ↓appetite ↑nausea/vomiting ↓blood CA

☑ vit B12, Mg/Ca supp with long term therapy (drug ↓ Mg absorption), vit K, probiotics

☺ N-acetylcysteine

☹ Ginkgo

AMINO SALICYLIC ACID (NSAID, contraindicated if sensitive to salicylates, Colitis, Crohns)

↓ weight ↑diarrhoea ↑nausea/vomiting ↓appetite ↓BSL (interacts with sulfonylureas to ↓BSL) ↑headache ↑insomnia ↑hair loss ↑flatulence ↑ rash ↑fatigue/muscle weakness ↓risk of colon cancer

☑ Folate (1mg/d, separate from drug by 2–4hrs), vit C, vit K, Bovine colostrum (<ulcers caused by NSAIDs), fluid, liquorice (deglycyrrhizinated only), psyllium husk, probiotic

☒ Vit E>50IU, K citrate, arginine, feverfew, para amino benzoic acid, policosanol, white willow

☹ Fe (↓drug and Fe effects — separate by 2–4 hrs), chondroitin, don quai, garlic, ginkgo, St John's wort

AMIODARONE (antiarrhythmic, hard on liver/lungs, risk of thyroid disorders, limit sunlight)

↑ weight ↓appetite ↓taste

☺ Vit E (protects lungs from drug side-effects)

☒ Iodine (Mx has ↑ iodine), borage, bitter orange (*Citrus aurantium*), chapparal, coltsfoot, comfrey, don quai (↑risk sunburn), grapefruit, pomegranate, St John's wort (↑risk sunburn)

☹ Mg, astragalus, devil's claw, echinacea, hawthorn (addictive effect)

AMOXICILLIN

↑ diarrhoea ↓appetite ↑nausea/vomiting ↓taste ↑↓blood K ↑blood Na

☑ Vit K, probiotic

☺ Bromelain (↑ antibiotic level)

ANASTROZOLE (antineoplastic, breast cancer, blocks oestrogen)

↑ diarrhoea ↑nausea/vomiting ↓appetite

☹ Andrographis, astragalus, baical skullcap, echinacea, garlic, ginkgo, ginseng, kava kava, St John's wort, withania

ANGIOTENSIN II ANTAGONISTS (HPT)

↑ weight ↑diarrhoea/constipation ↑nausea/vomiting ↑↓appetite ↓taste ↑anaemia ↑chol ↑blood K

☺ Zn (↓intracellular Zn, drug ↑ deficiency, ↓ taste, ↓appetite, numbness/tingling, supp taken with 2hr gap), Fe (supp can help ↓dry cough but separate doses by at least 2hrs), *Coleus forskohlii*, garlic/hawthorn/olive leaf/olive oil/EPO/fish oil/oats (↑drug effect)

☒ K supplements/high K foods, Mg (drug contains Mg, avoid >300mg), alcohol, arginine, bitter orange (*Citrus aurantium*), liquorice (deglycyrrhizinated OK)

☹ Black cohosh, guarana, don quai/St John's wort (>risk sunburn)

ANGIOTENSIN II ANTAGONISTS + THIAZIDE DIURETIC (HPT)

↑ weight ↑constipation/diarrhoea ↑nausea/vomiting ↑↓appetite ↓taste ↑anemia ↑BSL/impairs glucose tolerance (interacts with sulfonylureas to ↓BSL) ↑uric ↑trig ↑chol ↑homocysteine ↑blood Ca ↓blood Na ↓↑blood K ↓blood Mg

☑ B6, B12, folate, Na, K, Mg, all supplements taken with 2hr gap from drug

☺ Nicotinic acid, coleus, hawthorn/garlic/olive leaf/olive oil (↑drug effect) Fe supp (for dry cough), Zn supp (drug ↑ deficiency, ↓ taste, ↓appetite, numbness/tingling), EPO/fish oil/oats (↑drug effects),

☒ Ca supps, vit D supps, alcohol, arginine, bitter orange (*Citrus aurantium*), Black cohosh, Buckthorn, Dong
Quai (↑risk sunburn), liquorice (deglycyrrhizinated OK), horsetail, juniper, St John's wort (↑risk sunburn)

☹ Aloe skin, caraway, dandelion, flaxseed, ginkgo, glycerol, guarana, laxatives, peppermint oil, psyllium, stinging nettle (these can ↑K excretion, limit intake)

ANTACID (GERD, maalox, mylanta, gaviscon, MgOH, Ca carbonate, zoton)

↑ weight/oedema ↑constipation/diarrhoea ↑nausea/vomiting ↓appetite ↓taste ↑thirst ↑blood Mg/aluminium ↓blood K ↑blood Na ↑blood Ca ↑ anaemia (Fe/folate) ↑risk of osteomalacia, avoid taking at mealtimes in the elderly because of binding to nutrients

☑ Fe supp (drug ↓ absorption), Zn supp (drug ↓ absorption), Cr, Cu, vit A, B1, B12, folate supp (drug ↓ absorption), vit D, vit E, vit K (all supplements taken with 2 hr gap from antacid)

☒ Milk/Ca supps, Mg, Phosphorus, vit C/Citrus fruit/Juice/Calcium citrate (↑aluminium absorption, separate doses by at least 2hrs), alcohol, caffeine <400mg/day, guarana, fibre supps/oxalate/phytate (foods to be taken separately, see Fig 2)

ANTIBIOTICS

↓ weight ↑constipation/diarrhoea ↓appetite ↑nausea/vomiting ↓taste ↑↓bloodK ↑bloodNa ↓↑BSL ↓↑uric ↓↑trig ↓↑anaemia ↑risk of IBS ↑candida infections (*vaginal/intestinal*)

☑ B1, B2, B5, B6, Folate(*drug ↓efficacy of supp*), vitC, Probiotic supps (*↓antibiotic induced diarrhoea*)

☹ vit K

☒ Dairy products (*↓drug absorption, separate by 2 hrs*), Minerals/Vitamin supp (*↓absorption of nutrients and antibiotic, separate by > 2hs),* Alcohol, Caffeine, Dandelion root (*↓drug absorption separate by 2 hrs*), Grapefruit, Milk thistle, Para-aminobenzoic acid, Quercetin, Xanthines

☹ Bromelain

ANTICONVULSANTS (epilepsy, depression, mood disorder, migraines)

↑ ↓weight ↑constipation/diarrhoea ↑↓appetite ↑nausea/vomiting ↑megaloblastic anaemia ↓blood Na ↓blood CA ↓bloodfolate ↑chol ↑trig ↑homocysteine ↑risk osteomalacia/osteoporosis ↑insulin ↑BSL/impaired glucose tolerance

☑ Biotin (drug ↓absorption, supp <100ug, separate by >2hrs), B12 supp (drug ↓absorption), Carnitine (↓ transport/uptake, monitor serum levels of free/total carnitine and supplement if low, <2g/day), vit D supp (drug ↑breakdown of vit D, supp or sunlight)

☺ Vit A (avoid during pregnancy), folic acid (drug <absorption, folate supp <drug effect, avoid >400ug supps ↑breakdown of drug/↑seizures), vit E supp (<200IU), vitK supp (drug ↑breakdown of vit K, supplement 20mg/day if drug taken with a steroid or 10mg/day during last trimester of pregnancy, Ca (drug <absorption of Ca and >seizures/osteoporosis), Zn, Cu, carnitine, melatonin

☒ B6 (>50mg may ↓drug levels), alcohol, aspirin, bitter orange (*Citrus aurantium*), borage oil, don quai, ephedra, EPO, glutamine, ginkgo, grapefruit, hops, kava kava, milk thistle (*Silybum marianum*), passionflower, phytoestrogens/ipriflavone, pomegranate, salicylates, St John's wort, valerian, white willow

☹ Niacinamide (↓drug breakdown), milk thistle (*Silybum marianum*) (some preparations don't interact, check with manufacturer), fibre (ispaghula and psyllium husk — separate by 2–3 hrs)

ANTIDEPRESSANTS — see SSRIs, Tricyclic/Tetracyclic

ARIPIRPRAZOLE (Antipsychotic)

↑ weight ↑constipation/diarrhoea ↑thirst ↑nausea/vomiting ↑BSL ↓blood Na

☺ Ginkgo

☒ Alcohol, caffeine, EPO, fatty meal alters drug availability, grapefruit, guarana, St John's wort

☹ Glycine

ASPRIN (Analgesic)

↑ nausea/vomiting ↓appetite ↑risk of stomach/digestion problems ↑GI bleeding ↓blood K ↑anaemia ↓inflammation ↓BSL ↓chol ↑uric acid, avoid in kidney/liver disease, contraindicated in vit K deficiency

☑ B12, folate, vit C, Fe supp (if GI bleeding), Ca, K, Zn, fish oil (<3g EPA + DHA), flaxseed oil (<30g/d), ginger (<10g/d), glucosamine, liquorice deglycyrrhizinated

☺ Colostrum (↓risk of ulcers), Devils' claw, grapeseed extract (additive)

☒ Vit E (>100IU/50mg), alcohol, arginine, bilberry (>160mg/d), caffeine (↑absorption), chamomile, citrate Ca/Mg, garlic (>4g/d), guarana, horse chestnut, lithium, white willow/willow bark (>240md/d)

☹ Andrographis, aloe vera, bitter orange (*Citrus aurantium*) (↑ risk sunburn), cayene (protects stomach from aspirin but high dose can ↑inflammation), chondroitin, coleus, CoQ10, Devil's Claw, don quai (↑risk sunburn), EPO (>1g/d), feverfew, fish oil (>3g EPA + DHA), flaxseed oil *(>30g/d)*, ginger *(>10g/d)*, ginkgo (>100mg/d), ginseng, goji, grapeseed extract, guarana, guggul/myrrh, Kiwi juice (large amounts), krill oil, meadowsweet, pau d'arco (high dose), red clover, red rice yeast extract, policosanol (>10mg/d), saw palmetto, St John's wort (↑risk sunburn), tamarind (↑drug effect), turmeric extracts

AZATHIOPRINE (immunomodifier, rheumatoid arthritis)

↑ nausea/vomiting ↑diarrhoea ↓appetite ↓bloodalbumin ↓uric ↑anaemia ↑steatorrhoea with chronic use

☺ Folate

☹ Alfalfa, andrographis, astragalus, baical skullcap, echinacea, garlic, ginseng, liquorice, withania, Zn

BACLOFEN (Muscle relaxant)

↑ ↓ weight ↑constipation/diarrhoea ↓appetite ↑nausea/vomiting ↓taste ↑BSL (in people with diabetes)

☺ Magnesium, calcium (additive effect)

☒ alcohol, other interactions unknown

BENZODIAZEPINES (tranquilizers)

↑ ↓ weight ↑constipation/diarrhea ↑nausea/vomiting ↑↓appetite ↓taste ↑↓blood K ↑blood Na ↑↓BSL uncertain if ↑chol

☑ Vit A, Biotin, B2, B6, B12, Folic acid (<400ug), vit D, vit K, Ca, Carnitine

☺ Melatonin, periwinkle (*Vinpocetine*). Additive effects: kava kava (piper methysticum), passiflora/passionflower, withania, valerian

☒ Mg to be taken with 2hr gap with Mx, alcohol, bitter orange (*Citrus aurantium*), caffeine, EPO, ephedra, ginseng (>insomnia), grapefruit, green tea, guarana, Lady's slipper (*Cypripedium*), pomegranate, St Johns wort, Yerba mansa (*Anemopsis californica*)

☹ *Calendula officinalis*, catnip (*Nepeta cataria*) chamomile (*additive*) guarana, hops (*Humulus lupulus*) lavender oil, lemon balm (*Melissa officinalis*) pregnenolone, sage, sassafras (*Sassifras officinale*) skullcap (*Scutellaria lateriflora*)

BENZTROPINE (*Cogentin, Parkinson's*) ↓weight ↑constipation ↓appetite ↑nausea/vomit

☺ Niacin, tryptophan

BETA ADRENERGIC BLOCKING AGENTS (HPT, angina, post heart attack, arrythmia)

↑ weight ↑diarrhoea/constipation ↑nausea/vomiting ↑↓appetite ↓taste ↑BSL (especially in the overweight) ↑uric ↑trig ↓HDL chol ↓↑ blood K ↓serum CoQ10

☑ EPO (↑*drug effect*) fish oil/oats (↑drug effects)

☺ Cr, CoQ_{10} supp (↓side-effects) garlic/olive leaf/olive oil (↑drug effects) policosanol, *Coleus forskohlii* (↑drug effect)

☒ K, Ca supps/milk (↓drug absorption, separate from Mx by 2–4 hrs), alcohol, antacids, arginine, bitter orange (*Citrus aurantium*), Black cohosh, grapefruit, hawthorn, liquorice (deglycyrrhizinated is OK), pleurisy root, pomegranate

☹ Vit E (↓drug effect) astragalus, coleus, Devil's claw, guarana, guggul/myrrh (↓drug effect)

BETAHISTINE (*histamine agonist, peripheral vasodilator, ringing in the ears*)

↑ diarrhoea ↑nausea/vomiting; no interactions to date

BIPHOSPHONATES (osteoporosis)

↓ weight ↑constipation/diarrhoea ↓appetite ↑nausea/vomiting ↓taste ↓blood Na ↑↓blood Ca ↓blood Mg ↓blood K ↓blood Phosphate ↑anaemia

☑ Ca/Mg (↓drug absorption but required for optimal drug effects, separate by >2 hrs) phosphate, vit D, Fluid

☒ Antacids (separate by 2–4hrs) high fibre/oxalate/phytate foods/orange juice (to be taken separately, see Fig 2) caffeine, guarana

☹ Fe/Zn supps (↓drug absorption, separate by 2–4 hrs)

BISACODYL (laxative)

↑ nausea ↑constipation/diarrhoea ↓ blood K/Ca

☑ Vit D, vit K, K, Ca, Mg, Na, Fibre

☒ Milk/Ca/Mg not recommended within 1hr of drug

BROMOCRIPTINE (<prolactin, fertility, PMS, antiparkinson)

↑ constipation/diarrhoea ↑nausea/vomit ↓appetite ↓taste

☒ Alcohol

☹ Chasteberry

BUDESONIDE+EFORMOTEROL (inhaled corticosteroid, asthma)

☑ Ca supp

☺ DHEA

CALCITONIN (Ca metabolism)

↑ diarrhoea ↑nausea/vomiting ↓appetite ↑BSL ↓blood Ca ↓bloodphosphate ↑blood Na

☺ Ca supps

☒ Vit D supps

CALCITRIOL//CHOLECALCIFEROL (vit D, bone metabolism)

↓ weight ↑constipation/diarrhoea ↑nausea/vomit ↓appetite ↓taste ↑blood Mg ↑blood Ca ↑blood Phosphate ↑chol

☒ Alcohol, sudden increases in Ca intake due to food or supplements may ↑blood Ca

CALCIUM CHANNEL BLOCKERS (HPT, angina, antiarrhythmic, migraine)

↑ weight ↑constipation/diarrhoea ↑nausea/vomiting ↓↑appetite ↓taste ↑BSL

☑ Carnitine (Mx ↓carnitine transport/uptake), EPO/fish oil/oats (↑drug effect)

☺ Mg/garlic/olive leaf/olive oil/Coleus forskohlii, (↑drug effect)

☒ Ca+vitD supplements (↑blood Ca may ↓drug effects/counter antidysrhythmic effects or HPT effects, avoid high dose), alcohol, arginine, bitter orange (*Citrus aurantium*) Black cohosh, caffeine, grapefruit, guarana, Guggul/myrrh, liquorice (*deglycyrrhizinated is OK*), Peppermint (↑drug effect) pomegranate, pleurisy root, St John's wort (increases metabolism of drug)

☹ Astragalus, citrus bioflavanoids, Devil's claw, ginkgo, Korean Ginseng (↑drug effect), guarana, hawthorn/quercetin (↑drug effect)

CARBAMAZEPINE (anticonvulsant)

↑ ↓weight ↑constipation/diarrhoea ↑↓appetite ↑nausea/vomiting ↑megaloblastic anaemia ↓blood NA ↓blood Ca ↓bloodfolate ↑chol ↑trig ↑homocysteine ↑risk osteomalacia/osteoporosis ↑insulin ↑BSL/impaired glucose tolerance

☑ Biotin (drug ↓absorption, supp <10mg, separate by >2hrs), B12 supp (drug ↓absorption), Carnitine ↓ transport/uptake, monitor serum levels of free/total carnitine and supplement if low, <2g/day), vit D supp/sunlight (drug ↑breakdown of vit D, supp or sunlight)

☺ Folic acid (drug ↓absorption, folate supp ↓drug effect, avoid >400mg daily supps ↑breakdown of drug/↑seizures) vitK supp (drug ↑breakdown of vit K, supplement 20mg/day if drug taken with a steroid or 10mg/day during last trimester of pregnancy, Ca (drug ↓absorption of Ca and ↑seizures/osteoporosis, take supp >2hrs apart)

☒ B6 (>50mg may <drug levels), alcohol, aspirin, bitter orange (*Citrus aurantium*), borage oil, don quai, ephedra, EPO, glutamine, ginkgo, grapefruit, hops, kava kava, milk thistle (*Silybum marianum*), passionflower, phytoestrogens/Ipriflavone, pomegranate, salicylates, St John's wort, valerian, white willow

☹ Niacinamide (<drug breakdown), milk thistle (*Silybum marianum*) (some preparations don't interact, check with manufacturer), Ispaghula & Psyllium husk (separate by 2–3 hrs)

CARBIMAZOLE (hyperthyroid)

↓ weight ↑diarrhoea ↑nausea/vomiting ↑↓appetite ↑BSL/impairs glucose tolerance ↓Chol

☑ Carnitine, lipoic acid, Se (low T3:T4 =impaired Se status), vit A, Iodine, Fe (separate by 4 hrs) goitrogens (see Fig 2)

☒ Amiodarone, Iodine excess >2mg/day (correct Iodine deficiency before correcting Se deficiency), seaweed/kelp, soy flour (↓absorption of drug) Topical disinfectants that contain iodine

CELECOXIB (Cox2 inhibitors, pain relief)

↑ weight ↑constipation/diarrhoea ↑nausea/vomiting ↓↑appetite ↓taste ↓anaemia ↑BSL ↓blood K ↑chol

↑ risk of stomach/digestion problems (administer with food) ↑ risk of CVD/HPT ↓liver finction

☒ Aspirin, NSAIDs, >50mg vit E, >3g EPA/DHA fish oil, arginine, K/Mg/Na citrate, don quai, chondroitin, St John's wort

☹ *Coleus forskohlii*, garlic, ginkgo, ginger, ginseng, grapeseed, policosanol, red clover, white willow

CHOLESTYRAMINE (bile acid seqestrant, hypolipidaemic)

↑ ↓weight ↑constipation/diarrhea ↑nausea/vomiting ↓appetite ↓blood Na ↓blood Ca ↓blood Mg ↓bloodfolate ↓chol, ↑homocysteine ↓absorption of many nutrients/fat soluble vitamins ↑risk of acidosis (<bicarbonate >chloride)

☑ Fat, vit A and b-carotene, carotenoids, vit D, vit E, vit K, B12, folate, Ca, Fe, Cr, Zn, Mg, multivitamin recommended (1hr before or 4–6 hours after Mx), garlic, guggul, oats, psyllium

☹ Policosanol

CISPLATIN (*antineoplastic*)

↓ weight ↑diarrhea ↓appetite ↑nausea/vomiting ↓appetite ↑anaemia↑uric acid ↓blood Na,avoid anti-diabetic agents

☑ Na, K, Mg, Ca, phosphate

☺ Beta-carotene (mouth sores), vit E (↓nerve damage/applied to mouth sores), multivitamin, Se (↓side-effects), Carnitine (↓neuropathy), chamomile (mouth sores), *coriolus versicolor* (Japanese mushroom PSK/polysaccharide krestin ↑immunity 3g/day, ↑survival time), echinacea, eleuthero, glutamine (↓diarrhoea/mouth sores), glutathione (↓nerve damage IV only), lipoic acid, melatonin, milk thistle (Silybum marianum), N acetyl cysteine (1800mg/day ↓nausea), taurine

☹ Vit A, vit C, Black cohosh, garlic, ginseng, ginkgo, kava kava, St John's wort, withania

CLARITHROMYCIN (antibiotic for peptic ulcer)

↑ constipation/diarrhoea ↑nausea/vomiting ↓taste

☑ Fe, B1, B12, vit K, probiotic, saccharomyces

☒ Alcohol, grapefruit, pomegranate

CLOMIPHENE (↑ovulation, ↑FSH)

↑ weight ↑nausea/vomiting ↑chol

☺ N acetyl cysteine (1g/day)

CLONIDINE (HPT)

↑ weight ↑nausea/vomit ↑constipation ↓↑appetite ↑BSL ↓ serum CoQ10

☑ Carnitine (Mx ↓carnitine uptake/transport), EPO/fish oil (↑drug effect)

☺ CoQ_{10}, garlic ↑ drug effect, hawthorn ↑drug effect, olive leaf/olive oil ↑drug effect

☒ Alcohol, bitter orange (*Citrus aurantium*), Black cohosh, liquorice (deglycyrrhizinated liquorice is OK), Yohimbe

☹ *Coleus forskohlii*, guarana

CLOPIDOGREL (Platelet aggregation inhibitor)

↑ nausea ↑constipation/diarrhea ↑chol

☹ Fish oil >3g EPA+DHA/day avoid if patient is bruising easily, capsaicin, chamomile, chondroitin, *Coleus forskohlii*, CoQ_{10}, garlic, grapeseed, ginger, ginkgo (>100mg/d), ginseng, horse chestnut, krill oil, policosanol, red rice yeast extract — see also nutrients/herbs listed under warfarin

CLOZAPINE (antipsychotic)

↑ weight ↑constipation/diarrhoea ↑nausea/vomiting ↑BSL

☺ Vit C, Se, N acetyl cysteine, ginkgo, tryptophan

☒ Alcohol, bitter orange (*Citrus aurantium*) chamomile, EPO, grapefruit, St Johns wort

☹ caffeine — maintain constant intake, guarana, glycine

CODALGIN (Analgesic, paracetamol/codeine)

↑ constipation ↓gastric emptying ↑nausea/vomiting ↓appetite

☑ chondroitin, glucosamine

See also NSAIDs and codeine

CODAPANE — see NSAIDs

CODEINE (narcotic analgesic)

↑ constipation ↓appetite ↓hypoglycaemia

☑ Adhatoda

☒ Alcohol, chronic intake aspirin/paracetamol, chondroitin, glucosamine, kava kava, tannin containing teas (green tea, black tea, uva ursi, black walnuts, red raspberry, oak, witch hazel)

COLCHICINE (antigout)

↓ weight ↑diarrhoea ↑nausea/vomit ↓appetite ↓chol

☑ K, Ca, Na, Fe, B12, vit A, b-carotene

☒ Lactose, low purine diet during acute attack advised — avoid offal, anchovies, crab, fish roe, herring, mackerel, sardines, shrimps, whitebait, port)

☹ Aloe skin, caraway, dandelion, flaxseed, glycerol, liquorice (deglycyrrhizinated is OK), peppermint oil, psyllium (limit intake as these can ↑K excretion)

CONTRACEPTIVE PILL (folate/B6 depleting)

↓ ↑weight ↓↑appetite ↑vomit/nausea ↑blood Ca ↑BSL/↓ glucose tolerance ↑chol ↑trig

☑ B1, B2, B3, B5 pantothenic, B6/B12/folate (drug can cause deficiency) vit C, beta-carotene

☺ Probiotics, chasteberry/vitex (↓premenstrual symptoms)

☒ Bitter orange (*Citrus aurantium*) (↑ risk sunburn) don quai (↑risk sunburn), grapefruit, licorice >100mg/d glycyrrhizin (deglycyrrhizinated is OK) resveratrol, St John's wort (↓drug effects, ↑ risk sunburn, BTB, unplanned pregnancies)

☹ Indole 3 carbinol, milk thistle (*Silybum marianum*) (some preparations do not interact, check with manufacturer), red clover, rosemary

CONTRACEPTIVE PILL (folate/B6 sparing)

↑ ↓weight ↑diarrhoea, uncertain if ↑risk of IBS ↑nausea/vomit ↑↓appetite ↓blood K ↑blood Na ↑blood Ca ↓blood Mg ↓blood Zn ↓bloodB12, ↑bloodFe/↓vit A storage ↑BSL/↓ glucose tolerance ↑trig

☑ B12, Mg, Zn

☺ Fe, vit A, vit C, probiotics, chasteberry/vitex (↓premenstrual symptoms)

☒ Vit C>1g (↑oestrogen levels/↑ risk of toxicity), alcohol, bitter orange (*Citrus aurantium*) caffeine, don quai (>risk sunburn) grapefruit, guarana, liquorice >100mg/d glycyrrhizin (deglycyrrhizinated is OK) resveratrol, St John's wort (↓drug effects, ↑ risk sunburn, BTB, unplanned pregnancies) pommegranate

☹ Folate, vit B6, vit E, indole 3 carbinol, milk thistle (*Silybum marianum*), (some preparations do not interact, check with manufacturer), rosemary

CORTICOSTEROIDS

↑ weight ↑↓appetite ↑vomit/nausea ↑BSL/impaired glucose tolerance ↑chol ↑trig ↓uric ↓blood K ↓blood ↓blood Zn ↓blood Mg ↓blood vit C ↑blood Na ↓vit A storage ↑protein catabolism ↑muscle cramping due to Mg/K/Ca/protein losses ↑bone loss ↑oedema ↑urinary chromium excretion

☑ Protein, B6, B12, folate, vit C, vit D/Ca supp (↓side-effects/bone loss), Cr supp (↓BSL), K supp, Mg supp (↑losses but take 4 hrs from Mx) phosphorus, melatonin

☺ Vit A, vit K, Zn, Se, DHEA, N acetyl cysteine, carnitine, Horny goat weed

☒ Na, alcohol, bitter orange (*Citrus aurantium*) borage, echinacea, ephedra, fenugreek, golden seal, grapefruit, ipriflavone, liquorice (additive effects, deglycyrrhizinated is OK) pomegranate

☹ Aloe laxative, alfalfa, astragalus, asparagus root, buckthorn, butchers broom, caraway, cascara, cleavers, corn silk dandelion, flaxseed, ginseng (additive), glycerol, juniper, Laxatives, liquorice (deglycyrrhizinated is OK) mate, milk thistle (*Silybum marianum*), parsley, peppermint oil, psyllium, senna (limit intake of these, can ↑K excretion)

CYCLOPHOSPHAMIDE (antineoplastic)

↓ weight ↑diarrhea ↓appetite ↑nausea/vomiting ↓appetite ↑anaemia ↑uric acid ↓blood Na

☑ K, Mg

☺ Beta-carotene (mouth sores), vit E (applied to mouth sores), multivitamin, Zn, Se (↓side-effects), carnitine, chamomile (mouth sores), *coriolus versicolor* (Japanese mushroom PSK/polysaccharide krestin ↑immunity3g/day ↑survival time), echinacea, eleuthero, ginger (nausea), glutamine (↓diarrhoea/mouth sores), glutathione (IV only), melatonin, milk thistle (*Silybum marianum*), N acetyl cysteine (1800mg/day nausea), taurine, wheat grass (<side-effects)

☒ Iodine, turmeric

☹ Vit A, vit C, andrographis, astragalus, baical skullcap, garlic, ginseng, ginkgo, kava kava, St John's wort, withania

CYCLOSERINE (Tuberculosis, antibiotic)

☺ B6, B12, folate, vit K, Ca, Mg, probiotcs

☒ Alcohol

CYCLOSPORINE (suppresses immune system/transplants)

↓ weight ↑diarrhea ↓appetite ↑vomit/nausea ↑anaemia ↑BSL ↑uric acid ↑chol/trig ↑blood K ↓blood Mg

☑ Mg supp, Na, vit E

☺ Ginkgo

☒ K, alcohol, baical skullcap, bitter orange (*Citrus aurantium*) *Ephedra,* Grapefruit, Peppermint oil, Pomegranate, Quercetin, Red wine, St John's Wort

☹ Alfalfa, andrographis, astragalus, barberry, bitter orange, echinacea, garlic, ginseng, golden seal, Ipriflavone, liquorice, milk thistle (*Silybum marianum*), Oregon grape, withania, Ca, Zn

DEXTROPROPOXYPHENE (analgesic)

↑ constipation ↑nausea/vomiting ↑dysphagia

☑ Chondroitin, glucosamine

☒ Alcohol

DIGOXIN (dysrhythmias, congestive heart failure)

↓ weight ↑diarrhoea ↓appetite ↑nausea/vomiting ↑confusion ↑fainting ↑palpitations/irregular heart beat ↑visual disturbance ↑↓blood K ↓blood Mg ↓blood Zn

☑ Mg supp (deficiency ↑ digoxin toxicity, supp needs 2 hr gap from Mx), Zn

☒ Ca/vit D supps (may ↑blood CA ↑toxic effects), high fibre foods (to be taken separately to drug, see Fig 2), alcohol, Buckthorn, Digitalis, bitter orange (*Citrus aurantium*) ephedra, guarana, guar gum, ginseng, grapefruit, hawthorn, Laxatives, liquorice (deglycyrrhizinated is OK), milk thistle (*Silybum marianum*), plantain, Pleurisy root, pomegranate, quercetin (↑ drug toxicity), St John's wort (↓ drug effects)

☹ K (can be high or low), aloe skin, caraway, cascara, dandelion, flaxseed, glycerol, horsetail, peppermint oil, pectin, psyllium, sarsaparilla, senna, uzara (limit intake as these can ↑K excretion)

DIPYRIDAMOLE (Anticoagulant)

↑ diarrhoea ↑nausea/vomiting ↓appetite ↑anaemia ↑uric ↑blood K ↓BSL (interacts with diabetes Mx) ↓chol

☑ Vit B12, folate, vit C, Fluids

☺ Fe

☒ Contraindicated if vit K deficient, Nicotinic acid, vit E >50IU, vit K, alcohol, bitter orange (*Citrus aurantium*) fish oil, ginkgo, horse chestnut, policosanol, salicylates, xanthines

☹ Bromelain, caffeine, chamomile, chondroitin, *Coleus forskohlii*, dong quai, EPO, garlic, ginger, grape seed extract, guarana, mesoglycan, papaya enzymes, red clover, reishi, white willow

DISOPYRAMIDE (ventricular arrhythmias)

↑ weight ↑constipation/diarrhoea ↑nausea/vomiting ↓appetite ↓taste ↓blood K ↓BSL ↑Chol/Trig

☒ Alcohol

☹ Mg (high dose), fish oil (high dose), hawthorn

DIURETICS LOOP (HPT, heart failure, oedema)

↑ diarrhoea ↑nausea/vomiting ↓appetite ↓blood K ↓blood Na/Cl ↓blood Mg ↓blood Ca ↓blood Zn ↓ammonium bicarbonate ↓RBCthiamin transketolase (after 4 weeks on drug) ↑BSL ↑uric ↑homocysteine ↑chol ↑trig

☑ Mg/K/Zn supp, Ca, folate, B1 supp (drug ↑excretion, low Mg ↓transketolase activity/B1), B6, vit C

☺ Na (but restricting sodium may enable reduction in medication), olive leaf/olive oil (↓drug effect)

☒ Alcohol, arginine, bitter orange (*Citrus aurantium*), Black cohosh, buckthorn, dong quai (↑risk sunburn) horsetail, juniper, St John's wort (↑risk sunburn)

☹ Aloe skin, caraway, dandelion, flaxseed, guarana, glycerol, liquorice >100mg glycyrrhizin/day for >2 weeks (deglycyrrhizinated is OK), peppermint oil, psyllium, stinging nettle (these can >diuresis and K excretion, limit intake)

DIURETICS THIAZIDE (HPT, heart failure, oedema)

↓ weight ↑constipation/diarrhoea ↑nausea/vomiting ↓appetite ↑blood Ca ↓blood NA/Cl ↓blood K ↓blood Mg ↓blood bicarbonate/phosphate ↓blood Iodine ↑BSL/impaired glucose tolerance (especially in the overweight)/interacts with sulfonylureas to ↑BSL ↑uric ↑trig ↑chol ↑homocysteine ↓serum CoQ10

☑ B6, B12, folate, K/Mg/Zn supp, Iodine

☺ Na (but restricting sodium may enable reduction in medication), CoQ_{10}, olive leaf/olive oil (↑drug effect)

☒ Ca supps/high Ca foods, vit D supps, arginine, bitter orange (*Citrus aurantium*) Black cohosh, buckthorn, dong quai (↑risk sunburn), horsetail, juniper, St John's wort (↑risk sunburn)

☹ Aloe skin, caraway, dandelion, flaxseed, ginkgo, glycerol, guarana, liquorice >100mg glycyrrhizin/day for >2 weeks (deglycyrrhizinated is OK), peppermint oil, psyllium, stinging nettle (these can ↑K excretion, limit intake)

DIURETICS K SPARING (HPT, heart failure, oedema)

↑ constipation/diarrhoea ↑nausea/vomiting ↓appetite ↑anaemia ↑BSL/impaired glucose tolerance/interacts with sulfonylureas to ↑BSL ↑uric ↑trig ↑chol ↑creatinine ↑homocysteine ↑blood Ca ↓blood Na ↓↑blood K ↓blood Mg ↓serum CoQ10

☑ B6, B12, folate, Mg

☺ Na (but restricting sodium may enable reduction in medication) CoQ10, Olive leaf/olive oil (↑drug effect)

☒ Vit D supps, Ca supps/high Ca foods, K supps/high K foods, Mg >300mg/day, aspirin/white willow, arginine bitter orange (*Citrus aurantium*) Black cohosh, guarana

☹ Zn

DOCUSATE (Stool softener)

↓ weight ↑diarrhoea ↑nausea ↓taste ↑BSL ↓blood K

☺ K, Mg

☒ Avoid milk, Ca, Mg within 1hr of drug

DOCUSATE WITH SENNA (Laxative, chronic use causes steatorrhoea)

↓ weight ↑nausea/vomit ↑diarrhoea ↑BSL ↓blood K ↓blood Ca

☑ Fibre, water 2L/day

☺ K, Mg

☒ Na, milk/Ca/Mg not advised within one hour of the drug

☹ Aloe laxative, caraway, dandelion, flaxseed, glycerol, liquorice (deglycyrrhizinated is OK), peppermint oil, psyllium (limit intake as these can ↑K excretion)

DOMPERIDONE (antiemetic, gastroparesis)

↑ constipation/diarrhoea ↑nausea ↑↓appetite ↑thirst ↑breast tissue/cancer
other interactions unknown

DONEPEZIL (Alzheimers disease)

↓ ↑weight ↑constipation/diarrhoea ↑nausea/vomiting ↑↓appetite ↓taste ↑anaemia ↑BSL ↓blood K
other interactions unknown

DONNATAB (Antispasmotic/antiemetic)

↑ constipation ↑vomiting

☒ Alcohol

DOXORUBICIN (antineoplastic)

↓ weight ↑diarrhea ↓appetite ↑nausea/vomiting ↓appetite ↑anaemia ↑uric acid ↓blood Na

☑ K, Mg, CoQ_{10}

☺ Beta-carotene (mouth sores), vit E (applied to mouth sores) Multivitamin, Se (↓side-effects) Carnitine, Chamomile (mouth sores), *Coriolus versicolor* (Japanese mushroom/PSK/polysaccharide krestin ↑immunity, 3g/day ↑survival time), echinacea, eleuthero, ginger (nausea), glutamine (↓diarrhoea/mouth and GI ulcers), glutathione (IV only) melatonin, milk thistle (*Silybum marianum*), N acetyl cysteine (1800mg/day, nausea) taurine, wheat grass (↓side-effects)

☒ Iodine, turmeric

☹ Vit A, vit C, andrographis, astragalus, baical skullcap, garlic, ginseng, ginkgo, kava kava, St John's wort, withania

ERGOTAMINE (caffeine/antimigraine)

↑ nausea ↑diarrhoea ↑vomiting ↑BSL

☑ Ca (supps taken with 2hr gap)

☒ Alcohol, caffeine, cruciferous vegetables (broccoli, cabbage, cauliflower, swede, ↑metabolism of drug), ginkgo, grapefruit, guarana

☹ Bitter orange (*Citrus aurantium*), Ephedra

ERYTHROMYCIN

↑ nausea/vomiting ↑diarrhoea ↓appetite

☑ Vit K, probiotcs

☺ Ca/Mg/folate/B6/B12 with long term therapy, bromelain

☒ Digitalis

EZETIMIBE (↓Cholesterol absorption)

↑ diarrhoea ↑headache ↑myopathy/rhabdomyolysis

☺ CoQ_{10}

FELODIPINE (HPT, congestive heart failure)

↑ nausea ↑constipation

☑ Ca supp, Mg supp, K, EPO/fish oil/oats (↑drug effect)

☺ Garlic/hawthorn/olive leaf (↑drug effect)

☒ Alcohol, arginine, aspirin/white willow, arginine, bitter orange (*Citrus aurantium*), Black cohosh, ephedra, grapefruit/oranges/lime, liquorice (deglycyrrhizinated is OK) pleurisy root, pomegranate, quercetin

☹ Aloe laxative, caraway, dandelion, flaxseed, glycerol, guarana, milk thistle (*Silybum marianum*), psyllium (limit intake as these can ↑K excretion), peppermint oil (>drug effect)

FENOFIBRATE (fibric acid analogue, hypolidaemic)

↓ weight ↑constipation/diarrhoea ↑nausea/vomiting ↑blood thinning with warfarin ↓taste ↑BSL ↑homocysteine ↓blood K

☑ B6, B12, Niacin, folate, Guggul (myrrh), oats

☺ Vit E, Cr, CoQ_{10} (separate doses by 4hrs)

☒ Alcohol, red rice yeast extract

☹ Devil's claw, don quai, red clover, garlic, grapeseed extract, papaya, policosanol — see also herbs listed under warfarin

FLECANIDE (Anti-arrythmia)

↑ constipation/diarrhoea ↑nausea/vomiting ↓appetite ↓taste ↑BSL

☹ Fish oils (high dose), magnesium (high dose) other interactions unknown

FLUDROCORTISONE – see Corticosteroids

FLUOROURACIL (antimetabolite, antitumour)

↓ weight ↑diarrhoea ↑nausea/vomiting ↓appetite ↓taste ↓bloodalbumin

☑ B1, B6 (↓skin problems)

☺ Multivitamin (low dose), Beta-carotene (mouth sores), vit E (applied to mouth sores), Chamomile (mouth sores), *Coriolus versicolor* (Japanese mushroom/PSK/polysaccharide krestin ↑immunity, 3g/day, ↑survival time), echinacea, eleuthero, ginger (nausea), glutamine (↓diarrhoea/mouth and GI ulcers), melatonin (↓side-effects), milk thistle (*Silybum marianum*), N acetyl cysteine (*1800mg/day,nausea*), taurine, wheat grass

FLUTICASONE (inhaled corticosteroid, asthma)

☑ Ca supp

☺ DHEA, other interactions unknown

GABAPENTIN (anticonvulsant, epilepsy)

↑ weight ↑constipation/diarrhoea ↑ ↓appetite ↑nausea/vomiting ↑homocysteine ↑osteomalacia

☑ Biotin, Ca, vitB12, vit D, vitE 100–200IU/day

☺ Vit K or probiotics, folate

☒ Alcohol, EPO (C/Ied in epilepsy), bitter orange (*Citrus aurantium*)

☹ vit A (*high dose avoided during pregnancy*) vitB6 *>80mg/day*

GEFITINIB (antineoplastic)

↑ diarrhoea ↑nausea/vomiting ↑appetite

☹ Andrographis, astragalus, baical skullcap, echinacea, garlic, ginkgo, ginseng, kava kava, St John's wort, withania

GEMFIBROZIL (hypolipidaemic)

↓ weight ↑constipation/diarrhoea ↑nausea/vomiting ↑blood thinning with warfarin ↓taste ↑BSL ↑homocysteine ↓blood K ↓serum CoQ_{10}

☑ B6, B12, Niacin, folate, Guggul (myrrh), oats

☺ Vit E, Cr, CoQ_{10} (separate doses by 4hrs)

☒ Alcohol, Red rice yeast extract

☹ Devil's claw, don quai, red clover, garlic, grapeseed extract, papaya, policosanol — see also herbs listed under warfarin

GONADAL HORMONE (oestrogen, menopause)

↑ weight ↑constipation/diarrhoea, uncertain if ↑risk IBS ↑nausea/vomiting ↑↓appetite ↑BSL/glucose intolerance ↑LDLchol ↑HDL chol ↑trig ↑blood Ca ↑blood K ↑blood Na ↓ blood Mg ↓ blood Zn ↑bloodFe ↑risk of heart attack/strokes/clots/cancer

☑ B12, folate supp, vit D, Ca (additive effects)

☺ B6, Zn supp, Mg supp

☒ Vit A, B-carotene, vit C >1g/day (↑oestrogen levels and risk of toxicity), vit E >50mg, boron, Cu, Fe, alcohol, aspirin, caffeine, grapefruit, guarana, liquorice (↑side-effects, deglycyrrhizinated is OK), NSAIDs, pomegranate, quercetin, resveratrol, St John's wort

☹ Black cohosh, B-sitosterol (additive uncertain if ↑risk cancer), chasteberry, don quai (additive uncertain if ↑risk cancer), fenugreek, ginseng (additive), Hops (additive), Indole-3-carbinol, Ipriflavone (additive uncertain if ↑risk cancer), milk thistle (*Silybum marianum*, some preparations do not interact, check with manufacturer), phytoestrogens (additive uncertain if ↑risk cancer) red clover (↓drug effects or ↑risk cancer), rosemary

HALOPERIDOL (antipsychotic)

↑ ↓ weight ↑constipation ↑nausea/vomiting ↓↑appetite ↑↓BSL (also Interacts with sulfhonylureas to >BSL/may impair control of diabetes) ↑↓blood K ↓blood NA

☑ B2, B12, Quercetin

☺ vit E (↓tardive dyskinesia), ginkgo (↓drug effects ↓side-effects), glycine, milk thistle (*Silybum marianum*), (↓liver damage)

☒ Alcohol, bitter orange (*Citrus aurantium*), ephedra, caffeine (separate by 2hrs) EPO, guarana, pectins/apple juice, tannins/tea

☹ Grapefruit

HEPARIN (anticoagulant)

↑ blood K ↓activation vitD ↑osteopenia

☑ Ca, vit D

☒ Vit E (>400IU), K, alcohol, don quai, bitter orange (*Citrus aurantium*) ephedra, fenugreek, fish oil, garlic, ginkgo, ginger, horse chestnut, krill oil, reishi

☹ Vit C, chondroitin, *Coleus forskohlii*, golden seal, phosphatidyl serine, policosanol, red clover, red rice yeast extract, white willow — see also herbs under warfarin

HISTAMINE RECEPTOR ANTAGONIST (anti-ulcers, GERD)

↓ HCL results in ↓absorption of minerals/vitamins/protein digestion ↑risk anaemia ↑constipation/diarrhoea ↑nausea/vomiting ↓appetite ↑headaches ↑fatigue ↑blood creatine ↑uric acid ↑homocysteine; unlike proton pump inhibitors, H2 receptor antagonists are not linked to bone fractures

☑ Vit B1, B12, folate, vit E, Fe (especially if low haem iron intake), Ca, Zn, Mg, multivitamin (separate doses of all supplements by 2–3hrs from drug), carnitine

☺ Vit D

☒ Alcohol, caffeine/cocoa (drug ↓ clearance), guarana, lipoic acid, salicylates

☹ Antacids/MgOH (separate by 2hrs)

HYDRALAZINE (HPT, vasodilation)

↑ ↓ weight ↑↓appetite ↑nausea/vomiting ↑diarrhoea ↓serum CoQ_{10}

☑ B6 supps (100–200mg corrects drug induced peripheral neuropathy, separate doses by at least 2hrs) EPO/fish oil/oats (↑drug effect)

☺ CoQ_{10}, garlic/hawthorn/olive leaf/olive oil (↑drug effect)

☒ Na, alcohol, arginine, bitter orange (*Citrus aurantium*) ephedra, Black cohosh

☹ Coleus forskohlii, guarana, liquorice (deglycyrrhizinated OK)

HYDROXYCHLOROQUINE (antimalarial, rheumatoid arthritis, lupus)

↓ weight ↑diarrhoea ↑nausea/vomiting ↓appetite

☺ Ca, vit B6, vitD

☹ Mg (or take at different time)

IFOSFAMIDE (antitumour)

↑ constipation/diarrhoea ↑nausea/vomiting ↓appetite

☺ Multivitamin (low dose), beta-carotene (mouth sores), vit E (applied to mouth sores), chamomile (mouth sores), *Coriolus versicolor* (Japanese mushroom, PSK/polysaccharide krestin ↑immunity, 3g/day, ↑survival time), eleuthero, ginger, glutamine (↓diarrhoea/mouth sores), melatonin (↓side-effects), milk thistle (*Silybum marianum*), N acetyl cysteine (*1800mg/day, nausea*), taurine

☒ Fluid

☹ Andrographis, astragalus, baical skullcap, echinacea, garlic, ginseng, withania

IMMUNOSUPPRESSANTS

☹ Alfalfa, andrographis, astragalus, baical skullcap, echinacea, garlic, golden seal, ginseng, liquorice, withania, zinc

INSULIN

↑ weight ↑appetite ↓BSL ↓blood K ↓blood Mg

☺ Mg, Cr, ginseng, fenugreek, bitter melon

☒ Alcohol

INTERFERON ALPHA-2A (*immunomodifier*)

↓ weight ↑constipation/diarrhoea ↑nausea/vomiting ↓appetite ↓taste ↑BSL ↑uric ↓blood CA

☑ Carnitine, fluid

☺ N acetyl cysteine, licorice (*injectable*)

☒ Alcohol, bupleurum, grapefruit, pomegranate

☹ Andrographis, astragalus, baical skullcap, echinacea, garlic, ginseng, withania

INTERFERON ALPHA-2B (immunomodifier)

↓ weight ↑constipation/diarrhoea ↑nausea/vomiting ↓appetite ↓taste ↑BSL ↑anaemia ↑uric (rare) ↑blood Ca ↑bloodphosphate

☑ Carnitine, fluid

☺ N acetyl cysteine, liquorice (injectable)

☒ Alcohol, caffeine, cocoa, bupleurum, grapefruit, guarana, pomegranate

☹ Andrographis, astragalus, baical skullcap, echinacea, garlic, ginseng, withania

INTERFERON BETA-1A (immunomodifier)

↑ ↓weight ↑constipation/diarrhoea ↑nausea/vomiting ↓appetite ↑anaemia

☑ Carnitine, fluid

☹ Andrographis, astragalus, baical skullcap, echinacea, garlic, ginseng, withania

☒ alcohol, bupleurum, grapefruit, pomegranate

☺ N acetyl cysteine, licorice (injectable)

INTERFERON BETA-1B (immunomodifier)

↓ weight ↑diarrhoea ↑nausea/vomiting ↓appetite ↑BSL ↑blood Na

☑ Carnitine, fluid

☹ Andrographis, astragalus, baical skullcap, echinacea, garlic, ginseng, withania

☒ Alcohol, bupleurum, grapefruit, pomegranate

☺ N acetyl cysteine, licorice (injectable)

INTERFERON GAMMA 1-B (immunomodifer)

↓ weight ↑nausea/vomiting ↑diarrhoea ↓appetite ↑BSL ↓blood NA

☑ Carnitine, fluid

☺ N acetyl cysteine, licorice (injectable)

☒ alcohol, bupleurum, grapefruit, pomegranate

☹ Andrographis, astragalus, baical skullcap, echinacea, garlic, ginseng, withania

IRINOTECAN (antineoplastic)

↓ weight ↑diarrhoea/constipation ↑nausea/vomiting ↓appetite ↑anaemia

☹ Andrographis, astragalus, baical skullcap, echinacea, garlic, ginkgo, ginseng, kava kava, St John's wort, withania

ISONIAZID (antituberculotic)

↑ weight ↑constipation/diarrhoea ↑nausea/vomiting ↓blood Na ↑BSL ↑blood K ↓blood Ca ↑bloodphosphataemia ↓bloodvitB6

☑ Vit B3 supp, B6 (100–300mg/d if pre-existing peripheral neuritis or large dose of Mx) B12, folate, vit A/Zn (supplementation earlier elimination of tubercle bacilli from sputum), vitD supp,vitE (drug ↓vitamin absorption), vit K, Ca, Mg, tryptophan, licorice, picrorhiza

☒ Alcohol, amines

ISOSORBIDE (anti-angina)

↑ diarrhoea ↑nausea/vomiting ↓appetite

☑ High fat meal, Mg, K, Zn, Ca (supps with these minerals to be taken with 2hr gap), vit C, N acetyl cysteine

☒ Alcohol, grapefruit, pomegranate, bitter orange (*Citrus aurantium*), ephedra

☹ Aloe skin, caraway, dandelion, flaxseed, glycerol, licorice (*deglycyrrhizinated is OK*), peppermint oil, psyllium (limit intake as these can ↑K excretion)

ISOTRETINOIN (acne)

↓ weight ↓appetite ↑nausea/vomiting ↑blood uric ↑trig ↑chol

☑ Low fat diet

☺ vit E (↓side-effects)

☒ Vit A, B-carotene, alcohol

LACTULOSE (laxative)

↑ diarrhoea ↑nausea/vomiting ↑appetite ↓blood K ↑BSL with extended use

☑ Vit A,D,E,K

☒ Contraindicated if lactose intolerant/disaccharidase deficiency or galactosaemia, grapefruit, pomegranate

LAMOTRIGINE (Anticonvulsants, phenyltriazines, epilepsy, mood disorder, migraines)

↑ diarrhoea ↑nausea/vomiting ↓appetite

☑ Biotin, Ca, Folic acid (<400ug) Carnitine, vit A, B12, B6, vit D, vit K

☺ Carnitine, Melatonin

☒ Alcohol, aspirin, bitter orange (*Citrus aurantium*) borage oil, don quai, ephedra, EPO, Glutamine, ginkgo, grapefruit, hops, ipriflavone, kava kava, milk thistle (*Silybum marianum*), passionflower, phytoestrogens, pomegranate, salicylates, St John's wort, valerian, white willow

☹ Psyllium husk (separate by 2–3 hrs), milk thistle (*Silybum marianum*). (Some preparations don't interact, check with manufacturer)

LATANOPROST — applied to eye to treat glaucoma, nil interactions

LAXATIVES (e.g senna, lactulose, paraffin, psyllium, norgine)

↓ weight ↑diarrhoea/steatorrhea with chronic use ↓blood levels fat soluble vitamins ↑BSL (lactulose) ↓BSL (psyllium) ↓chol (psyllium) ↓blood K/Ca/Na/Mg ↓absorption of medication (separate by 2–4hrs)

☑ B2 (psyllium ↓absorption)

☺ Na, K, Mg, Ca, Fe, vit A, vit D, vit K

☒ Chronic use (longer than 1 week) may cause lazy bowel/dependancy and fatty stools (steatorrhoea), milk/Ca/Mg/medication not recommended within 2hrs of laxative

☹ Aloe skin, caraway, dandelion, flaxseed, ginkgo, glycerol, guarana, laxatives, peppermint oil, psyllium, stinging nettle (these can ↑k excretion, limit intake)

LEFLUNOMIDE (Rheumatoid arthritis)

↓ weight ↑diarrhoea ↓appetite ↑nausea/vomiting ↑anaemia ↑BSL ↓uric ↓blood K ↑chol, contraindicated in severe hypoproteinaemia

☒ Alcohol

☹ Echinacea

other interactions unknown

LEUPRORELIN (Pituitary hormone, antineoplatic, prostate cancer)

↑ ↓weight ↑constipation/diarrhoea ↓appetite ↑nausea/vomiting ↑anaemia ↑BSL ↑uric ↑trig ↑chol ↑blood Ca

☑ K, Mg, Ca

☺ Multivitamin, beta-carotene (mouth sores), vit E (↓nerve damage/applied to mouth sores), carnitine (↓neuropathy), chamomile (mouth sores), *Coriolus versicolor* (Japanese mushroom PSK/polysaccharide krestin ↑ immunity, 3g/day, ↑survival time), echinacea, eleuthero, glutamine (↓diarrhoea/mouth sores), lipoic acid, melatonin, milk thistle (Silybum marianum), N acetyl cysteine (1800mg/day nausea), taurine

☹ Vit A/vit C (high dose), Black cohosh, garlic, ginseng, ginkgo, kava kava, St John's wort, withania

LEVAMISOLE (Immunomodulator, antitumour)

↑ constipation/diarrhoea ↑nausea/vomiting ↓appetite ↓taste

☑ Mg, K

☺ Multivitamin, beta-carotene (mouth sores)

☒ Alcohol, aspirin, St John's wort

☹ Folate (↓side-effects but can ↓drug effect, deficiency ↑methotrexate toxicity — should not take folate if methotrexate tx for cancer) vit C, vit E (applied to mouth sores), Se (↓side-effects), chamomile (mouth sores) echinacea, eleuthero, ginger (nausea), glutamine (←diarrhoea/mouth sores), glutathione (IV only), melatonin, milk thistle (*Silybum marianum*), N acetyl cysteine (1800mg/day nausea), taurine

LEVODOPA (anti-Parkinson's disease)

↑ ↓weight ↑constipation/diarrhoea ↓appetite ↑nausea/vomiting ↑taste ↓blood K

☑ Folate, vit C (↓side-effects)

☺ SAMe

☒ Amino acid/protein supps, high protein intake (keep high protein foods to evening meal, restrict high biological protein intake to 0.5g/kg/day to stabilise drug effects), B6 supp >5mg or B6 rich food can ↓drug effect (banana, brewers yeast, brown rice, lentils, eggs, oats, peanuts, potatoes, soy flour, spinach, tuna, turkey, walnuts, vegemite, wheat bran/germ), Fe/Ca/Mg/Zn supps (chelate drug separate by 2 hrs), kava kava, phenylalanine, policosanol, tryptophan, tyrosine

☹ Ginkgo (↑'off' periods in Parkinson's disease patients)

LITHIUM (manic depression)

↑ ↓weight ↑diarrhoea ↓appetite ↑nausea/vomiting ↑taste ↑BSL (interacts with sulfonylureas to >BSL) ↓blood K ↓blood NA ↑blood Mg ↑blood Ca ↑bloodphopshate

☑ Na consistant intake (avoid low/highNa) Cu, Inositol, fish oil, folate

☺ Tryptophan

☒ Iodine supps (↑ risk of hypothyroidism) alcohol, bitter orange (*Citrus aurantium*) ephedra, buchu, caffeine/cocoa (may ↓ lithium levels), celery seed, cleavers, corn silk, couchgrass, dandelion, ginseng, guarana, goldenrod, horsetail, juniper, parsley, psyllium, rosemary

LUMIRACOXIB (Cox2 inhibitors, pain relief)

↓ liver finction

☒ Aspirin, arginine, NSAIDs, vit E (>50mg), fish oil (>3g EPA+DHA) chondroitin, citrate (K/Mg/Na) don quai, St John's wort

☹ Coleus forskohlii, garlic, ginkgo, ginger, ginseng, grapeseed, policosanol, white willow, red clover

MAO INHIBITORS (MonoAmineOxidase inhibitor, antipsychotic)

↑ ↓weight ↑constipation ↑nausea/vomiting ↑↓appetite ↓BSL and interacts with sulfonylureas to <BSL ↑blood Na

☑ B6 supps, ginkgo

☒ Alcohol, anise, aspartame, bitter orange (*Citrus aurantium*) caffeine, EPO, ephedra, ginseng, green tea, guarana, hawthorn, parsley, passionflower, phenylalanine, pleurisy root, St John's wort, SAMe, tryptophan, tyramine (avoid during treatment and 14 days after discontinuation, see Fig 2), tyrosine, verbena

MEDROXYPROGESTERONE (gonadal hormone)

↑ weight ↑nausea ↑↓appetite ↓glucose tolerance ↑BSL in people with diabetes ↑chol ↑trig ↑anaemia ↑blood K ↑blood Na ↑blood Ca

☺ Ca (additive effects), vit D

☒ Licorice (↑side-effects, deglycyrrhizinated is OK), vitex (chasteberry)

☹ Vit A, folate, Mg, Zn

MEMANTINE (dementia)

↑ weight ↑constipation/diarrhoea ↑nausea/vomiting ↓↑appetite ↑anaemia ↑BSL ↑uric ↑ blood Na ↓ blood K

☒ Significant changes in diet may alter urinary pH and alter renal clearance of drug

METFORMIN (biguanide, NIDDM)

↓ weight or stable ↑constipation/diarrhea ↓appetite ↑nausea/vomiting ↓taste ↓chol ↓trig ↑homocysteine ↓ CoQ_{10}

☑ Vit B12 (drug ↑malabsorption), folate (drug ↑malabsorption) Ca (may ↓metformin induced B12 malabsorption)

☺ Vit E, Mg,Cr, CoQ_{10}, aloe vera gel, andrographis, bilberry, bitter melon/Karela (*Momordica charantia*), carnitine, cinnamon, damiana, fenugreek, garlic, ginger, ginseng, goat's rue, green tea, gymnema, guggul/myrrh, inositol, ipriflavone, lipoic acid, milk thistle (*Silybum marianum*), olive leaf extract, psyllium, turmeric, vanadium (these can ↓BSL and ↓dose of Mx may be needed)

☒ Citrates (Mg/Ca/K), alcohol, bitter orange (*Citrus aurantium*) (↑ risk sunburn), Don quai (>risk of sunburn) ephedra, guar gum, ginkgo

☹ Niacin (>BSL), DHEA, feverfew, gotu kola, licorice

METHADONE (Opioid analgesic)

↑ constipation ↑nausea/vomiting ↓appetite

☑ Chondroitin, Glucosamine

☒ Alcohol, kava kava, St John's wort

☺ Melatonin, periwinkle (*Vinpocetine*). Additive effects: chamomile, passiflora/passionflower, valerian

METHOTREXATE (antimetabolite, antitumour, immunosuppressant, psoriasis,rheumatoid arthritis)

↓ weight (↓fat absorption) ↑diarrhoea ↓appetite ↑nausea/vomiting ↓taste ↑anaemia ↑uric ↑homocysteine

☑ Ca, B6, B12

☺ Multivitamin (low dose), Se (↓side-effects), beta-carotene (mouth sores), vit E (applied to mouth sores), chamomile (mouth sores), *Coriolus versicolor* (Japanese mushroom, PSK/polysaccharide krestin ↑immunity 3g/day ↑ survival time), eleuthero, ginger (nausea), glutamine (↓diarrhoea/mouth and GI ulcers),glutathione (IV only), melatonin, milk thistle (*Silybum marianum*), N acetyl cysteine (1800mg/day, nausea), taurine

☒ Alcohol, aspirin, borage, citrates e.g Mg/K/Na, don quai, ipriflavone, para-aminobenzoic acid, St John's wort, white willow, vit A/retinoids

☹ Zn, vit C, folate (↓side-effects but can ↓drug effect, deficiency ↑methotrexate toxicity — should not take folate if methotrexate tx for cancer), alfalfa, andrographis, astragalus, echinacea, ginseng, licorice, lipoic acid

METHYLDOPA (HPT)

↑ constipation/diarrhoea ↑nausea/vomiting ↑uric ↑blood K ↑blood Na ↓serum CoQ_{10}

☑ B12 supp, folate, EPO/fish oil/oats (↑drug effects)

☺ CoQ_{10}, garlic/hawthorn/olive leaf/olive oil (↑drug effects)

☒ Protein/amino acid drinks/supps (↓drug absorption), K, Na, Fe (↓drug absorption, separate by 2–4hrs), alcohol, arginine, black cohosh, guarana, licorice (deglycyrrhizinated licorice is OK)

METHYLPHENIDATE (CNS stimulant with actions similar to amphetamines)

↓ weight ↑nausea/vomiting ↓appetite

☑ Fluid

☒ Alcohol, bitter orange (*Citrus aurantium*), ephedra, caffeine, guarana

☺ Melatonin, periwinkle (*Vinpocetine*). Additive effects: kava kava (*Piper methysticum*), chamomile, passiflora/passionflower, withania, valerian

METOCLOPRAMIDE (dopamine receptor antagonist, antiemetic, GERD)

☺ Willow

☒ Alcohol, caffeine, guarana, N acetyl cysteine, lactose

METRONIDAZOLE (antibacterial)

↑ constipation/diarrhoea ↓appetite ↑nausea/vomiting ↓taste

☑ Vit K, Probiotics

☺ Milk thistle (*Silybum marianum*)

☒ Alcohol, vinegar

☹ Flavanoids/diosmin

MEXILETINE (anti-arrhythmia)

↑ nausea/vomiting ↓taste

☒ Caffeine, high dose fish oils, high dose magnesium, hawthorn

MINOXIDIL (HPT, hair loss)

↑ weight (may be due to fluid retention) ↑nausea/vomiting ↑BSL in people with diabetes ↑blood Na

☑ Fish oil/EPO/oats (↑drug effects),

☺ garlic/hawthorn/olive leaf/olive oil (↑drug effect)

☒ Na, alcohol, arginine, bitter orange (*Citrus aurantium*), Black cohosh, ephedra, liquorice (deglycyrrhizinated liquorice is OK)

☹ Guarana

MISOPROSTOL (prostaglandin E1 analogue, ulcer prevention if on NSAIDs, ulcer treatment)

↑ diarrhoea ↑nausea/vomiting

☑ Fe, Ca, B1, vitE (separate doses by 4hrs)

☹ MgOH (↑ diarrhoea)

MORPHINE (narcotic analgesic) ↑constipation ↑nausea/vomiting ↓appetite ↓taste

☑ Chondroitin, fluid, glucosamine

☺ Withania (reduced morphene tolerance so may be used in opiate withdrawal under supervision)

☒ Alcohol, kava kava

☹ Tyrosine

NEOMYCIN (aminoglycoside antibiotic)

↑ diarrhoea ↑nausea/vomiting ↓appetite

☑ Fats, Na, K, Ca, Fe, Mg, vit A, B carotene, folate, B6, B12, vit D, vit K, probiotics, mutlivitamin (if drug taken for more than a few days)

NICORANDIL (synthetic nicotine derivative, antiangina, potassium channel opener)

↑ constipation/diarrhoea ↑vomit/nausea ↓appetite ↑risk of ulcers at multiple sites

☒ Caffeine, guarana, nicotinamide, nicotinic acid other interactions unknown

NICOTINIC ACID (hypolipidaemic)

↑ diarrhoea ↑nausea/vomiting ↑uric acid ↑homocysteine ↑BSL/impairs glucose tolerance

☑ Folate, B6, B12

NITROGLYCERIN (glyceryl trinitrate, transiderm nitro, angina)

↑ nausea/vomiting

☑ Vit C (↓drug tolerance)

☺ Folate (↓drug tolerance, ↓nitric oxide synthase dysfunction), vit E/arginine/N-acetyl cysteine (↓nitrate tolerance)

☒ Alcohol, bitter orange (*Citrus aurantium*), Ephedra, guarana

NO-DOZ (caffeine, stimulant)

↑ diarrhoea ↑nausea/vomiting ↑BSL in people with diabetes ↓blood K ↑homocysteine

☑ B12, folate, B6, B12

☺ Ca/Fe supps (2hr gap with drug), cruciferous vegetables (↑ caffeine metabolism)

☒ Caffeine, bitter orange (*Citrus aurantium*), ephedra, guarana

NORGINE (Laxative)

↓ weight ↑diarrhoea ↑nausea ↓appetite ↓lowblood K ↓lowblood Na ↓lowblood Ca, chronic use may cause lazy bowel/dependancy

☹ Aloe skin, Caraway, Dandelion, Flaxseed, Glycerol, liquorice (deglycyrrhizinated is OK), peppermint oil, psyllium (limit intake as these can ↑K excretion)

NSAIDs (Ibuprofen/Naproxen/Diclofenac/Piroxicam)

↓ ↑weight ↑constipation/diarrhoea ↑nausea/vomiting ↓↑appetite ↑anaemia ↓↑BSL ↑blood K ↑GI disturbance/ulcer ↑ risk of CVD/HPT (Naproxen safest if patient has CVD) ↑bleeding problems (aspirin has ↑ blood thinning effect than Ibuprofen), avoid in kidney/liver disease ↓melatonin

☑ Folate supp, Devil's claw/fish oils/ginger/glucosamine (additive)

☺ Vit E (additive), celery seed extract (↓side-effects), chamomile (↓side-effects), chondroitin (additive), colostrum (↓side-effects), glutamine (↓side-effects), green lipped mussel (additive), licorice deglycyrrhizinated, SAMe (additive), slippery elm, stinging nettle (additive), tryptophan, willow bark

☒ Zn (↓absorption, separate by 2–4hrs), alcohol, arginine, feverfew, garlic, grapefruit, lithium, pomegranate, reishi, salicylates/aspirin

☹ Bitter orange (*Citrus aurantium*) (↑ risk sunburn), Citrate, don quai (↑ risk sunburn), ginkgo, krill oil, policosanol, red rice yeast extract, St John's wort (↑risk sunburn)

OCTREOTIDE (pituitary hormone)

↑ constipation/diarrhoea ↑nausea/vomiting ↓appetite ↓↑BSL ↑malabsorption of fat soluble vitamins

☑ Vit A, B carotene, vit E, vit D, vit E, vit K

OLANZAPINE (atypical antipsychotic)

↑ weight ↑constipation ↑appetite ↑BSL

☺ Ginkgo

☒ Alcohol, bitter orange (*Citrus aurantium*), ephedra, grapefruit, pomegranate, St John's wort

☹ Glycine

ORLISTAT (anorectic, reduced fat absorption by 30%)

↑ nausea/vomiting ↓↑appetite ↓taste ↓BSL ↓blood K, may interact with warfarin (↓ vitamin K status)

☑ Multivitamins recommended and to be taken 2hrs before/after drug, vit A, beta-carotene, vit D, vit E (↓vitamin absorption, separate doses by at least 4hrs), vit K, probiotic, psyllium

☒ Fat (>67g/day)

OXYBUTYNIN (antispasmodic)

↑ constipation ↑nausea/vomiting ↑dysphagia

☒ Alcohol

OXYCODONE (analgesic narcotic)

↑ diarrhoea/constipation ↑↓appetite ↑nausea/vomiting ↓taste ↓blood Na

☑ Chondroitin, glucosamine

☒ Alcohol

OXPENTIFYLLINE (sedative)

↑ ↓ weight ↑constipation ↑nausea/vomiting ↓appetite ↓taste ↑↓BSL

☒ Caffeine, cocoa, bitter orange (*Citrus aurantium*), guarana

☹ Baical skullcap, chamomile, ginseng, golden seal, gotu kola, guarana, hops, kava kava (*Piper methysticum*), lavender oil, passionflower, sage, St John's wort, valerian

PANCRELIPASE (pancreatic enzymes) ↓weight ↑constipation/diarrhea ↑fibrosing colonpathy ↑vomit/nausea ↑uric acid

☒ High pH foods/drugs separate by 1 hr (e.g. milk, proton pump inhibitors)

PANTOPRAZOLE — see proton pump inhibitors

PARACETAMOL

↑ constipation ↑nausea/vomiting ↓appetite

☺ Andrographis/garlic/quercetin/milk thistle (*Silybum marianum*), SAMe/Schisandra (hepatoprotective)

☹ Vegetarian diets ↓absorption, alcohol, salicylates

PARACHOC (Paraffin, laxative)

↓ weight ↑diarrhoea ↑nausea ↓appetite ↓lowblood K administer at bedtime to minimise loss of vitamins

☑ Supplement fat soluble vitamins (vit A, D, E, K), Ca, K, vit K

PENICILLAMINE (chelating agent, Wilsons disease, antirheumatic)

↑ diarrhoea ↑nausea/vomiting ↓appetite ↓low blood Zn

☑ B6 (25–50mg/day to ↓drug induced peripheral neuropathy), Na, Fe/Zn supp (separate by 2hrs)

☒ Cu (contraindicated in Wilsons disease), Ca, Mg, K

☹ Guar gum (separate by 2hrs)

PHENOBARBITONE (barbiturates, anticonvulsant, anxiety, insomnia, seizures, migraines)

↑ ↓weight ↑constipation/diarrhoea ↑↓appetite ↑nausea/vomiting ↓blood Ca ↑homocysteine ↑risk of osteomalacia ↓BSL if on sulfonylureas

☑ Ca, Mg, Biotin supp (separated from drug by 2hrs), vit A, B6 (<10mg/day), Folic acid (<400ug), vit D (↑ inactivation 25–oH vit D), vit E supp (100–200IU/day), vit K supp (if drug taken with a steroid or if pregnant 10mg/day last trimester), carnitine

☒ Alcohol, bitter orange (*Citrus aurantium*), ephedra, kava kava, withania, valerian, EPO (in epilepsy)

☹ Vit B12 (drug can increase blood levels of B12), celery supp/juice, don quai, glutamine, hops, passionflower, St John's wort

PHENTERMINE (non-amphetamine anorectic)

↓ weight ↑constipation/diarrhoea ↑nausea/vomiting ↓appetite ↓taste ↓↑BSL (can alter insulin/sulfonylurea effects in people with diabetes)

☒ Alcohol, caffeine, guarana
other interactions unknown

PHENYTOIN (anticonvulsant)

↑ weight ↑constipation ↓↑appetite ↑nausea/vomiting ↓blood albumin ↑insulin ↑BSL/impaired glucose tolerance

☑ Biotin (drug ↓absorption, supp <10mg, separate by >2hrs), B12 supp (drug ↓absorption), carnitine (drug ↓ transport/uptake//↑side-effects, monitor serum levels of free/total carnitine and supplement if low, <2g/day), vit D supp/sunlight (drug ↑breakdown of vit D)

☺ Folic acid (drug ↑absorption, folate supp ↑drug effect; suggest 400mcg daily; avoid > 1mg daily as ↓drug bioavailability>↑seizures), B6 supp (<80mg, drug ↓ B6, supp can ↓ drug levels), vit K supp (drug ↑breakdown of vit K, supplement 20mg/day if drug taken with a steroid or 10mg/day during last trimester of pregnancy), Ca (drug <absorption of Ca and >seizures/osteoporosis, Ca supp ↓absorption, separate by 2–4hrs), carnitine, melatonin

☒ Alcohol, aspirin, bitter orange (*Citrus aurantium*), borage oil, don quai, ephedra, EPO, glutamine, ginkgo, grapefruit, hops, kava kava, milk thistle (*Silybum marianum*), passionflower, phytoestrogens/ipriflavone, pomegranate, salicylates, St John's wort, valerian, white willow, ispaghula and psyllium husk (separate by 2–3 hrs)

☹ Vit B12 (drug can increase blood levels of B12)

PHENINDIONE (anticoagulant)

↑ diarrhoea ↑vomiting

☒ Vit B complex, Nicotinic acid, vit E (>400IU), vit K, alcohol, fish oil, bitter orange (*Citrus aurantium*), ephedra, salicylates, theophylline (cocoa), xanthines — see also herbs under warfarin

PHENOTHIAZINES (antipsychotic)

↓ ↑weight ↑constipation ↑nausea/vomiting ↑↓appetite ↑↓BSL (interacts with sulfonylureas to >BSL/may impair control of diabetes) ↓blood Na ↓blood Ca ↑chol

☑ B2 increased requirement

☺ B6, vit E, CoQ_{10}, DHEA, fish oil, glycine, milk thistle (*Silybum marianum*)

☒ alcohol, antacids, bacopa, bitter orange (*Citrus aurantium*), caffeine, don quai (↑risk sun burn), EPO, ephedra, ginkgo, ginseng, guarana, grapefruit, hops, kava kava, inositol/lecithin supps, lithium, melatonin, passionflower, pectin/apple juice, phenylalanine, pomegranate, SAMe, St John's wort (↑risk sun burn), tannins/tea, tryptophan, tyrosine, valerian, yohimbe

PICOSULPHATE (osmotic laxative, bowel cleansing)

↑ diarrhoea ↓blood K ↑blood Mg, avoid using for >24 hours, avoid using in elderly, crohns/colitis, toxic megacolon, intestinal obstruction and in kidney disease, ↓absorption of medications

PIOGLITAZONE (NIDDM)

↑ weight ↓BSL ↑risk of heart attack

☑ Vit B12 (drug >malabsorption)

☺ Biotin, niacinamide, CoQ_{10}, Cr, Mg (>absorbtion of Mx), vit E, aloe vera gel, andrographis, bilberry, bitter melon/karela (*Momordica charantia*), carnitine, cinnamon, fenugreek, garlic, ginger, ginseng, green tea, goat's rue, gymnema, guggul/myrrh, inositol, ipriflavone, lipoic acid, milk thistle (*Silybum marianum*), olive leaf extract, psyllium, turmeric, vanadium (these can ↓BSL and ↓dose of Mx may be needed)

☒ Bitter orange (*Citrus aurantium*) (↑ risk sunburn), citrates, niacin, alcohol, don quai (>risk of sunburn), guar gum, St John's wort (>risk of sunburn)

☹ Ginkgo

PIZOTIFEN (Serotonin antagonist, migraines)

↑ weight ↑constipation ↑nausea ↑appetite

☒ Alcohol, St John's wort
other interactions unknown

PRIMIDONE (anticonvulsant, see also phenobarbitone)

↑ ↓weight ↑↓appetite ↑nausea/vomiting ↓blood Ca ↑megaloblastic anaemia

☑ Ca, Mg, biotin supp (separated from drug by 2hrs), vit A, B6 (<10mg/day), folic acid (<400ug), vit D
(↑ inactivation 25–oH vit D), vit E supp (100–200IU/day), vit K supp (if drug taken with a steroid or if pregnant 10mg/day last trimester), carnitine

☒ Nicotinamide (↑ blood levels of drug), alcohol, bitter orange (*Citrus aurantium*), ephedra, kava kava, withania, valerian, EPO

☹ Don quai, ginkgo, glutamine, hops, passionflower, St John's wort

PROBENECID (antigout)

↑ nausea/vomiting ↓appetite ↑anaemia

☑ K, Mg, Ca, B2, pantothenic acid, carnitine

☒ Salicylates

PROPYLTHIOURACIL (antithyroid, thionamide)

↓ weight ↑diarrhoea ↑nausea/vomiting ↑↓appetite ↑BSL/impairs glucose tolerance ↓Chol

☑ Carnitine, Lipoic acid, Se (low T3:T4 =impaired Se status), vit A, Iodine, Fe (separate by 4 hrs)

☺ Goitrogens (see Fig 2)

☒ Amiodarone, Iodine excess >2mg/day (correct Iodine deficiency before correcting Se deficiency), Seaweed/Kelp, Soy flour (↓absorption of drug), topical disinfectants that contain iodine

PROTON PUMP INHIBITORS (GERD/reflux oesophagitis)

↓ HCL may ↓absorption of minerals/vitamins/protein digestion ↑risk anaemia ↓weight ↑constipation/diarrhoea ↑nausea/vomiting ↓taste ↓BSL ↓blood Na ↓blood K ↑bacterial overgrowth in small intestine due to low acidity, contraindicated if fructose intolerant/sucrase-isomaltase insufficiency, contraindicated for use in elderly or in osteoporosis due to ↑risk of bone fracture (HCL needed to absorb Ca)

☑ Multivitamin supp (drug ↓absorption) (separate by 2–4hrs), B1, B12/folate, vit C, vit E, Fe (especially if low haem iron intake), Ca, Zn, Mg, (separate doses of all supps by 2-3 hrs from drug), acid foods/cranberry (↑absorption B12, minerals), garlic (↓ growth of H Pylori)

☺ Vit D, Indole 3 carbinol, b-carotene, probiotics

☒ Alcohol, caffeine, guarana, lipoic acid, MgOH, salicylates, St John's wort

PSYLLIUM (laxative)

↑ diarrhoea/steatorrhoea with chronic use ↓appetite ↑nausea/vomiting ↓BSL ↓chol

☑ B2 (psyllium ↓ absorption)

☺ K, Mg, Ca, Fe, Na, vit A (psyllium can ↓ absorption)

QUETIAPINE (atypical antipsychotic)

↑ weight ↑BSL ↑chol ↑headache/dizzy ↑stomach upset ↓blood pressure, ↓thyroid ↑chol ↑trig

☺ Ginkgo

☒ Alcohol, caffeine, MgOH, Lipoic acid, St John's wort

☹ Glycine

QUINIDINE (anti-arrhythmic)

↑ diarrhoea ↑nausea/vomiting ↓appetite

☑ Carnitine, Mg and K supps if taking K depleting diuretics, B-carotene (↓sun sensitivity)

☒ Na and sodium bicarbonate, bitter orange (*Citrus aurantium*) ephedra, guarana, grapefruit, Citrus juices, pomegranate

☹ Aloe laxative, caraway, dandelion, flaxseed, glycerol, licorice (deglycyrrhizinated is OK), peppermint oil, psyllium (limit intake as these can ↑K excretion)

QUININE (leg cramps, antimalaria)

↑ diarrhea ↑nausea/vomiting ↓BSL ↑blood insulin

☑ Riboflavin (effective in killing malaria and ↑activity of quinine), carnitine

☒ Grapefruit, pomegranate

QUINOLONE ANTIBIOTICS

↑ constipation/diarrhoea ↑nausea/vomiting ↓appetite ↓taste ↑halitosis ↓↑BSL

☑ B1, B5, vit K, Probiotics

☒ Multivitamin (2 hr gap), Fe/Zn/Mg/Ca (↓ drug absorption, separate by at least 2 hrs), caffeine, dandelion root (↓drug absorption, separate by at least 2 hrs), guarana, quercetin (↓drug effect)

RALOXIFENE (Oestrogen receptor modulator, osteoporosis)

↑ weight ↑nausea/vomiting ↓chol ↓trig ↓fibrinogen

☑ Phytoestrogens, Ca, vit D

☺ Ginkgo, ginseng (mild estrogenic properties)

REBOXETINE (antidepressant, selective noradrenaline reuptake inhibitor [SNRI])

interactions unknown

REPAGLINIDE (NIDDM)

↑ constipation/diarrhoea ↑nausea/vomiting ↓BSL

☺ CoQ_{10}, Cr, Mg (>absorbtion of Mx), vit E, aloe vera gel, andrographis, bilberry, bitter melon/karela (*Momordica charantia*), carnitine, cinnamon, fenugreek, garlic, ginger, ginseng, green tea, gymnema, goat's rue, guggul/myrrh, inositol, ipriflavone, lipoic acid, milk thistle (*Silybum marianum*), olive leaf extract, psyllium, turmeric, vanadium (these can ↓BSL and ↓dose of Mx needed)

☒ Vit B3,alcohol, salicylates, bitter orange (*Citrus aurantium*) (↑ risk sunburn)) dong quai (↑risk sunburn) ephedra, guar gum, ginkgo, St John's wort(↑risk sunburn)

☹ Feverfew, gotu kola, liquorice

RILUZOLE (glutamate antagonist, movement disorders)

↑ ↓weight ↑constipation/diarrhoea ↑nausea/vomiting ↓↑appetite ↑anaemia ↓blood Na absorption

☒ Caffeine, guarana, high fat meals after drug other interactions unknown

RISPERIDONE (atypical antipsychotic)

↑ weight ↑constipation ↑appetite ↑nausea/vomiting ↓blood Na ↓BSL (interacts with sulfonylureas)

☺ B6, vit E, ginkgo, licorice (deglycyrrhizinated is OK), white peony

☒ Alcohol, bitter orange (*citrus aurantium*), caffeine, ephedra, guarana, lithium, St John's wort

☹ Glycine

SAQUINAVIR (protease inhibitor, antiviral, HIV)

↓ ↑weight/↑trunkal fat ↑constipation/diarrhoea ↑nausea/vomiting ↓appetite ↓taste ↑anaemia ↑↓BSL/affects diabetes control ↑↓blood Na ↓↑blood K ↑↓blood Ca ↓blood phosphate ↑trig

☺ Milk thistle (*Silybum marianum*)

☒ Vit C, garlic, grapefruit, pomegranate, St John's wort

SELEGILINE (movement disorders/ Parkinson's disease)

↓ weight ↑constipation/diarrhoea ↑nausea/ vomiting ↓appetite ↓taste ↓↑BSL

☑ Ginkgo

☒ Alcohol, aspartame, bitter orange (*Citrus aurantium*), caffeine, ephedra, ginseng, green tea, guarana, St John's wort, SAMe, tryptophan, tyramine foods (if drug dose >10mg, see Fig 2), tyrosine

SENNA LAXATIVE

↓ weight ↑nausea/vomit ↑diarrhoea ↑BSL ↓blood K ↓blood Ca

☒ Chronic use may cause lazy bowel/dependancy and fatty stools (steatorrhoea), milk, Ca or Mg supplements, not recommended within 1 hr of drug

☹ Aloe skin, caraway, dandelion, flaxseed, glycerol, licorice (deglycyrrhizinated is OK), peppermint oil, psyllium (limit intake as these can ↑K excretion)

SILDENAFIL (erectile dysfunction)

↑ diarrhoea ↑nausea/vomiting ↑anaemia ↑↓BSL ↓uric ↓blood Na

☒ Arginine, grapefruit, nitrites (preserved meat, cheese, spinach, beets, radish, eggplant, celery, lettuce, collards, turnip greens), pomegranate

SIMETHICONE (antacid)

↑ anaemia

☑ Ca, Fe, Cu, B1, folate

SIROLIMUS (immunosuppressant)

↑ diarrhoea ↑anaemia ↑trig ↑chol ↓blood K

☒ Fat (alters drug availability), grapefruit, pomegranate

☹ Andrographis, astragalus, baical skullcap, echinacea, garlic, ginseng, withania

SODIUM BICARBONATE (antacid)

↑ weight/oedema ↑nausea ↓appetite ↓blood K ↑blood Na ↑anaemia/folate

☑ Folate

☒ Fe supps 1 hr before or 2 hrs after drug, milk/Ca supplements may cause alkali syndrome

SODIUM CITROTARTATE (urinary alkaliniser)

↑ blood Na ↑anaemia/folate

☑ B1, folate

☒ Fe supps 1 hr before or 2 hrs after drug, milk/Ca supplements may cause alkali syndrome

SODIUM VALPROATE (anticonvulsant)

↑ weight ↑diarrhoea ↑appetite ↓taste ↑nausea/ vomiting ↑megaloblastic anaemia ↓blood Ca ↓bloodfolate ↑homocysteine ↑risk osteomalacia/ osteoporosis ↑insulin ↑BSL/impaired glucose tolerance

☑ Biotin (drug ↓absorption, supp <10mg, separate by >2hrs), carnitine supp (drug ↓ transport/uptake/↑side-effects, monitor serum levels of free/total carnitine, supplement if low, <2g/day), vit D supp/sunlight (drug ↑breakdown vit D)

☺ Folic acid (drug ↓ absorption, folate supp ↓ drug effect, avoid >400ug supps ↑breakdown of drug/↑seizures), B6 supp (<80mg, drug ↓ B6, supp can ↓ drug levels), B12, vit E (<200IU), Se, Ca, Zn, Cu, melatonin

☒ Vit A (↑risk of birth defects), alcohol, aspirin, bitter orange (*Citrus aurantium*), borage oil, don quai, ephedra, EPO, glutamine, ginkgo, grapefruit, hops, kava kava, milk thistle (*Silybum marianum*), passionflower, phytoestrogens/ipriflavone, pomegranate, salicylates, St John's wort, valerian, white willow, ispaghula and psyllium husk (separate by 2–3 hrs)

SSRIs (antidepressant)

↑↓ weight ↑constipation/diarrhoea ↑↓appetite ↑risk of anorexia in elderly ↑nausea/vomiting ↓taste ↑↓BSL ↑chol/trig ↓blood Na ↓blood K ↑anaemia ↑risk of intestinal bleeding ↑ risk of developing IBS

☑ Folate/B3/B6/B12/Zn, (↑ drug effect/prefer low dose/avoid sudden changes in dose levels/ termination), vit C, Na, Leucine

☺ DHEA, fish oil, ginkgo, (<sexual dysfunction), Cr

☒ Alcohol, bitter orange (*Citrus aurantium*), ephedra, ginseng, grapefruit, hops, inositol, lecithin supps, kava kava (*Piper methysticum*), milk thistle (*Silybum marianum*), passionflower, pomegranate, pregnenolone, SAMe, St John's wort, tryptophan, tyrosine, valerian

☹ Aloe skin, caraway, dandelion, flaxseed, glycerol, melatonin, licorice (deglycyrrhizinated is OK), peppermint oil, psyllium (limit intake as these can ↑K excretion)

STATINS (HMGCO reductase inhibitors, chol)

↓ appetite ↑diarrhoea/constipation ↑nausea/ vomiting ↓↑BSL↓LDL chol ↓Trig ↑HDL cholesterol (rosuvastatin only) ↓serum CoQ_{10} ↑myopathy ↑liver and kidney problems ↑insomnia/nightmares (Simvastatin) ↓serum vit A

☑ Cr/Fish oil/Garlic/Guggul/myrrh/Krill oil/Oats/ Phytosterols/Psyllium husk (additive effects), CoQ_{10} (especially if there is muscle pain)

☺ Niacin (additive effects but sustained release form may be unsafe), Zn, Peppermint oil

☒ Chinese skull cap, grapefruit, pomegranate, red rice yeast extract, St John's wort (↓drug effects)

☹ Vit A, Mg antacids/MgOH, vit E (>100IU), vit C (>100mg), gotu kola, milk thistle (*Silybum marianum*), (some preparations do not interact, check with manufacturer), policosanol, green tea supplements

SULFONYLUREAS (NIDDM)

↑ weight ↑constipation/diarrhea ↑↓appetite ↑vomit/nausea ↓iodine uptake by thyroid (↑weight) ↓blood Na ↓ CoQ_{10} ↑anaemia (B12/folate)

☑ vit B12, Folic, Na, Ca, Iodine

☺ CoQ_{10}, Cr, Mg (>absorbtion of Mx), vit E, Aloe vera gel, andrographis, bilberry, bitter melon/karela (*Momordica charantia*), carnitine, cinnamon, fenugreek, garlic, ginger, ginseng, goat's rue, green tea, gymnema, guggul/myrrh, inositol, ipriflavone, lipoic acid, milk thistle (*Silybum marianum*), olive leaf extract, psyllium, turmeric, vanadium (these can ↓BSL and ↓dose of Mx needed)

☒ B3 at high doses >BSL, alcohol, bitter orange (*Citrus aurantium*) (↑ risk sunburn), don quai (↑risk of sunburn), ephedra, guar gum, ginkgo, St John's wort (↑risk of sunburn)

☹ Feverfew, gotu kola, licorice

SUMATRIPTAN (anti-migraine)

↑ vomit/nausea

☑ Vit B2, CoQ_{10}, feverfew

☒ Alcohol, tryptophan

SYMBICORT (budesonide+eformoterol) (inhaled corticosteroid, asthma)

☑ Ca supp

☺ DHEA other interactions unknown

TADALAFIL (erectile dysfunction)

↑ diarrhoea ↑nausea/vomiting ↑anaemia ↑↓BSL ↓uric ↓blood Na

☒ arginine, grapefruit, nitrites (preserved meat, cheese, spinach, beets, radish, eggplant, celery, lettuce, collards, turnip greens), pomegranate

TAMOXIFEN (antioestrogen drug to treat breast cancer)

↓ weight ↓appetite ↑nausea/vomit ↑blood Ca ↓chol

☺ Ca/Mg supp (2hr gap with drug), gamma linolenic acid (3g/day), melatonin, soy isoflavones (low dose can ↓ actions of drug but high dose can ↑action of drug), tocotrienols/red palm fruit

☹ Citrus bioflavanoids supps, citrus peel

TAMSULOSIN (bladder function disorders, benign prostatic hyperplasia)

↑ weight ↑constipation/diarrhoea ↑nausea/vomiting ↑BSL

Interactions unknown

TEMOZOLOMIDE (antineoplastic)

↓ weight ↑constipation/diarhoea ↑nausea/vomiting ↓appetite ↓taste ↑anaemia

☹ Andrographis, astragalus, baical skullcap, echinacea, garlic, ginkgo, ginseng, kava kava, St John's wort, withania

TERAZOSIN (bladder function disorders)

↑ weight ↑constipation/diarrhoea↑vomit/nausea ↓chol ↓albumin ↓bloodprotein

☒ Alcohol, licorice (deglycyrrhizinated licorice is OK), other interactions unknown

TERBUTALINE (bronchodilator)

↑ diarrhoea ↑nausea/vomiting ↓taste ↓blood K ↑BSL in people with diabetes

☒ Caffeine, cocoa, guarana

other interactions unknown

TESTOSTERONE

↑ appetite ↑nausea ↑oily stools ↑interacts with anti-diabetic drugs

☺ Beta-carotene, vit A

☹ Zn, DHEA (check levels and dosage)

TETRABENAZINE

☒ St Johns Wort, SAMe

TETRACYCLINE antibiotics

↓ diarrhoea ↓appetite ↑nausea/vomiting ↓blood Na ↓BSL ↑risk of IBS ↑candida infections (vaginal/intestinal)

☑ Folate, B2, nicotinamide, B6, B12 vit C, vit K (supps with long term use), probiotics

☺ Bromelain (↑ levels of antibiotic)

☒ Bitter orange (*Citrus aurantium*) (↑ risk sunburn), ephedra, don quai/St John's wort (↑ risk sunburn)

☹ Ca/Milk/Fe/Mg/Zn/B12 (↓drug absorption, separate doses by 4hrs), Citrates, Golden seal

THEOPHYLLINE (bronchodilator)

↑ diarrhoea ↑nausea/vomiting ↓appetite ↓taste ↑BSL

☑ Vit B6 (drug may cause deficiency), B12, Mg, K

☒ Caffeine/tea/coffee, cayenne, chamomile, charcoal-broiled foods (↑clearance), cocoa, high protein diets/drinks (↓asthma control), grapefruit, guarana, ipriflavone, pomegranate, tannin-containing herbs (green tea, black tea, uva ursi, black walnut, red raspberry, oak, and witch hazel)

☹ Cruciferous vegetables, milk thistle (*Silybum marianum*), soy, St John's wort

THYROXINE

↓ ↑weight ↑diarrhoea ↑nausea/vomiting ↓↑appetite ↑BSL/glucose intolerance ↓chol, low stomach acidity ↓absorption of drug ↑Ca excretion, may reduce levels of antibodies in Hashimoto's thyroiditis, take 1 hour before food or 2 hours after food

☺ Iodine, (<150ug/day, check urinary iodine levels first), Fe, zinc, selenium, vitamin A, B2, B3, B6, vit C are needed for T4 and T3 production; correcting deficiency of any of these nutrients, especially iodine, may result in improved thyroid frunction requiring reduced dose of thyroxine; vit A and Iodine deficiency should be corrected before Se deficiency (T4:T3 should be 3:1, if higher may be due to impaired Se status); Tyrosine (additive effects, precursor to thyroxine), withania (additive effects), vit A/fish oil (helps T3 bind to receptors), CoQ_{10} (may affect T4/T3 levels — monitor)

☒ High fibre meal/Soy/Mg/Ca/Zn/Fe/Cr supps (↓drug absorption, separate doses by 2–4hrs), Kelp/seaweed and Iodine >150ug/day can also be goitrogenic, potassium iodide, bungleweed, isoflavones (genistein/daidzein, <T3/T4 production), lemonbalm, SAMe

☹ Carnitine (blocks thyroid hormone at cellular level), celery supps (↓ drug effect), goitrogenic foods reduce utilisation of iodine by the thyroid and may only be important if iodine intake is low (e.g broccoli, cauliflower, cabbage, garlic, horseradish, onion, linseed, rapeseed, lima beans, soy, peanuts, swede, sweet potato, millet — see Fig 2), lipoic acid (↓ conversion T4 to T3)

TICLOPIDINE (anticoagulant)

↑ diarrhoea ↑nausea/vomiting ↓appetite ↓blood Na ↑trig ↑chol

☒ >400IU vit E, fish oil, krill oil, alcohol, bitter orange (*Citrus aurantium*), *Coleus forskohlii*, fenugreek, garlic, ginkgo, salicylates

TIOTROPIUM BROMIDE (anticholinergic, COPD); interactions unknown

TRAMADOL (analgesic)

↑ constipation/diarrhoea ↑nausea/vomiting ↑↓appetite

☑ Chondroitin, glucosamine

☒ Tryptophan, St John's wort, SAMe

TRICYCLIC ANTIDEPRESSANT

↑ weight ↑constipation/diarrhoea ↑nausea/vomiting ↑↓appetite ↓taste ↑↓BSL ↑blood uric ↓blood Na ↓blood K ↑chol ↑muscle pain/tremor/headache ↑fatigue ↑secretion melatonin

☑ B1, B2 (deficiency common), B3, B5, B6, B12, andrographis, ginkgo

☺ CoQ_{10}

☒ Alcohol, bitter orange (*Citrus aurantium*), caffeine, carbonated drinks, chamomile, ephedra, fibre dense foods/supplements <drug effect, ginseng, grape juice, guarana, grapefruit, pomegranate, hops, inositol/lecithin supps, kava kava, melatonin, milk thistle (*Silybum marianum*), passionflower, pregnenolone, St John's wort, SAMe, tryptophan, tyrosine, valerian, yohimbe

☹ Tea — separate by 2 hrs

TRIMETHOPRIM Antibiotic

↑ nausea/vomiting ↑anaemia ↑blood K ↓BSL (interacts with sulfonylureas) ↑candida infections(vaginal/intestinal)

☺ Ca, Mg, folate, B6, B12, (if antibiotic taken for more than 2 weeks), vit K, probiotics

☒ Bitter orange (*Citrus aurantium*) (↑ risk sunburn), para-amino benzoic acid, white willow, Don quai/St John's wort (↑risk sunburn)

VALACYCLOVIR (antiviral, cold sores/herpes/shingles)

↑ constipation/diarrhoea ↑nausea/vomiting ↓appetite

☺ Echinacea, zinc, lysine

WARFARIN

INR ideal 2–3.5 (>3.5 ↑risk bleeding <2 ↑risk thrombosis) ↑diarrhoea ↑nausea/vomiting

☒ Vit K (avoid major changes to diet, keep vit K intake 65–80ug/d, high intake of vitamin K rich foods, even for single day, will alter plasma coagulation for several days afterward,variation in vit K should not exceed 250–500ug/d) vit A (>RDI), vit C (>1000mg), vit D (>RDI), Fe, Mg, Zn (>RDI), alcohol, alfalfa supps, andrographis, aspirin/salicylates, beef liver, bilberry (high doses), bitter orange (*Citrus aurantium*), caffeine, canola oil, carnitine, cinnamon supp, dandelion, danshen salvia miltorrhiza, Devils claw, dong quai, egg yolk, ephedra, EPO, fish oil (>12g/day), flaxseed oil, garlic (>4g/day), ginger (>10g/day), korean ginseng, korean glucosamine, grapefruit, green leafy vegetables (lettuce, spinach, endive, kale), broccoli/cabbage/green peas/green beans (avoid large serves), green tea extract, guarana, horse chestnut, licorice (deglycyrrhizinated is OK), meat tenderiser, milk thistle (*Silybum marianum*), papain/papaya, pau d'arco (high doses), pistachios, pomegranate, policosanol (>10mg/d), quinine, reishi, royal jelly, rosemary, soy oil, spring onions, St John's wort (<warfarin effect), white willow

☹ Low carbohydrate diet high protein diets, charbroiled foods, vit E (>1000IU), agrimony, anise, avocado, barley grass, Black cohosh, borage oil, bromelain, celery seed, chamomile tea, chondroitin, clove, *Coleus forskohlii*, CoQ_{10}, cranberry (>1 cup), fenugreek, feverfew, fish oil (12g/d), ginkgo (>10Mg/d), Siberian ginseng, goji berry, grapefruit seed extract, green lipped mussel, grape seed extract, green tea (>2 litres/day), guar gum, guggul/myrrh, horsechestnut, horseradish, inositol, ipriflavone/isoflavones, Kiwi juice (large amounts), krill oil, mango, meadowsweet, mesoglycan, oligomeric proanthocyanidins, onions raw/fried/boiled (>60g/day), passionflower, phosphatidyl serine, phytoestrogens, psyllium (separate by at least 1hr), red clover, red rice yeast extract, sea weed, soy protein (↓drug effectiveness), turmeric extracts, wheat grass

ZALCITABINE (antiviral, AIDS)

↓ weight ↑constipation ↑nausea/vomiting ↓appetite ↓taste ↓↑BSL ↑uric ↑↓blood Na ↓blood Ca ↓blood Mg

☒ Alcohol, St John's wort

☹ CoQ_{10}

ZOLMITRIPTAN (antimigraine)

↑ constipation ↑nausea ↑↓appetite

☑ B2, CoQ_{10}, feverfew

☒ Alcohol, tryptophan

ZOLPIDEM (sedative)

↑ constipation/diarrhoea ↓appetite ↑nausea/vomiting

☒ Alcohol

☹ Baical skullcap, chamomile, ginseng, golden seal, gotu kola, guarana, hops, kava kava (piper methysticum), lavender oil, passionflower, sage, SAMe, St John's wort, tryptophan, valerian

ZOPICLONE (sedative)

↑ constipation/diarrhoea ↑↓appetite ↑nausea/vomiting ↓taste

☒ Alcohol

☹ baical skullcap, chamomile, ginseng, golden seal, gotu kola, guarana, hops, kava kava, lavender oil, passionflower, sage, St John's wort, valerian

ZUCLOPENTHIXOL (antipsychotic)

↑ constipation/diarrhoea ↑nausea/vomiting ↓appetite ↓taste ↑BSL

☒ Alcohol, bitter orange (citrus aurantium), ephedra other interactions unknown

References

Blackmores Complementary Medicine Interaction Chart. Online. Available: www.blackmores.com.au (accessed 1 June 2008).

Braun and Cohen Herbs & Natural Supplements: An Evidence-Based Guide (2006). (2nd edn). Sydney: Elsevier.

EBSCO Publishing Health Library — Drug Nutrient Herb Interactions. Online. Available: http://www.bidmc.harvard.edu/YourHealth/HolisticHealth/DrugInteractions.aspx (accessed 1 June 2008). The EBSCO Publishing Health Library site is free, referenced/peer reviewed/continually updated; hosted on university websites (e.g Harvard University http://healthlibrary.epnet.com/GetContent.aspx?token=1edc3d6e-4fec-4b20-baca-795e48830daa (accessed 1 June 2008).

Fugh-Berman, A (2000). Herb-drug interactions. *The Lancet*, *355*, 134–138.

Hamilton Smith, C, & Bidlack, W R (1984). Dietary concerns associated with the use of medications. *J Am Diet Assoc*, *84*(8), 901–914.

Rx list the Internet drug index www.rxlist.com acceessed 2/2/2009.

HEALTH NOTES — Drug Nutrient Herb Interactions. Online, free referenced/peer reviewed/continually updated; hosted on pharmacy websites. Available: http://www.pccnaturalmarkets.com/health/2411003/(accessed 1 June 2008).

Heimburger, D C (2006). *Ard Jamy. Handbook of Clinical Nutrition* (4th edn). USA: Elsevier.

Holbrook, A M, et al. (2005). Systematic overview of warfarin and its drug and food interactions. *Arch Intern Med* (165), 1095–1106.

Journal of Complementary Medicine, January/February 2004; March/April 2006.

Skalli, S, Zaid, A, & Soulaymani, R (2007). Drug Interactions with herbal medicines. *Ther Drug Monit*, 6(29), 679–686.

Stargrove, M B, Treasure, J, & McKee, D L (2008). *Herb, Nutrient and Drug Interactions*. USA: Elsevier.

Wahlqvist, M L (1997). *Nutrition and health problems related to substance abuse and medications. Food and Nutrition*. Sydney: Allen and Unwin.

Yvonne Coleman (Dietitian). (1998). *Drug Nutrient Interactions:The Manual*. Vic: Nutrition Consultants Australia.

Index

Page numbers followed by 'f' denote figures; those followed by 't' denote tables